MEDICAL SCIENCES

Dedication

We would like to dedicate this book to all medical students, past and future, and to all future doctors. You have to know the science in order to understand the practice of medicine.

Jeannette Naish

Denise Syndercombe Court

Senior Content Strategist: Pauline Graham
Senior Content Development Specialist: Ailsa Laing
Project Manager: Sukanthi Sukumar
Designer: Christian Bilbow
Illustration Manager: Jennifer Rose
Illustrator: Robert Britton, Antbits

MEDICAL SCIENCES

Second Edition

EDITED BY

Jeannette Naish

MBBS MSc FRCGP

Clinical Senior Lecturer, Wolfson Institute of Preventive Medicine,
Barts and The London School of Medicine and Dentistry, London, UK

AND

Denise Syndercombe Court

CBiol MSB CSci FIBMS DMedT MFSoc PhD

Honorary Research Fellow, Queen Mary University of London;
Reader in Forensic Genetics, King's College London, London, UK

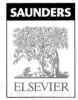

SAUNDERS

ELSEVIER

Edinburgh London New York Oxford Philadelphia St Louis Sydney Toronto 2015

First edition 2009
Second edition 2015

ISBN   9780702051388

British Library Cataloguing in Publication Data
A catalogue record for this book is available from the British Library

Library of Congress Cataloging in Publication Data
A catalog record for this book is available from the Library of Congress

Notices
Knowledge and best practice in this field are constantly changing. As new research and
experience broaden our understanding, changes in research methods, professional practices, or
medical treatment may become necessary.
Practitioners and researchers must always rely on their own experience and knowledge in
evaluating and using any information, methods, compounds, or experiments described herein. In
using such information or methods they should be mindful of their own safety and the safety
of others, including parties for whom they have a professional responsibility.
With respect to any drug or pharmaceutical products identified, readers are advised to check the
most current information provided (i) on procedures featured or (ii) by the manufacturer of each
product to be administered, to verify the recommended dose or formula, the method and duration
of administration, and contraindications. It is the responsibility of practitioners, relying on their own
experience and knowledge of their patients, to make diagnoses, to determine dosages and the best
treatment for each individual patient, and to take all appropriate safety precautions.
To the fullest extent of the law, neither the Publisher nor the authors, contributors, or editors,
assume any liability for any injury and/or damage to persons or property as a matter of products
liability, negligence or otherwise, or from any use or operation of any methods, products, instructions, or
ideas contained in the material herein.

 your source for books,
journals and multimedia
in the health sciences
www.elsevierhealth.com

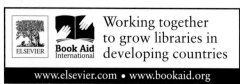

The
Publisher's
policy is to use
**paper manufactured
from sustainable forests**

Printed in China

Contents

Contributors   vii

Preface   ix

Acknowledgements   xi

1   Introduction and homeostasis   **1**
Jeannette Naish

2   Biochemistry and cell biology   **15**
Marek H. Dominiczak

3   Energy metabolism   **57**
Mark Holness, Mary Sugden and Jeannette Naish

4   Pharmacology   **101**
Walter Wieczorek and Jeannette Naish

5   Human genetics   **155**
Denise Syndercombe Court and David P. Kelsell

6   Pathology and immunology   **211**
Denise Syndercombe Court, Paola Domizio and Armine M. Sefton

7   Epidemiology: science for the art of medicine   **277**
Jeannette Naish and Denise Syndercombe Court

8   The nervous system   **337**
Brian Pentland

9   Bone, muscle, skin and connective tissue   **403**
Lesley Robson and Denise Syndercombe Court

10   Endocrinology   **451**
Joy Hinson and Peter Raven

11   The cardiovascular system   **493**
Andrew Archbold and Jeannette Naish

12   Haematology   **567**
Drew Provan, Adrian C. Newland and Denise Syndercombe Court

13   The respiratory system   **613**
Gavin Donaldson

14   The renal system   **655**
Girish Namagondlu and Alistair Chesser

15   The alimentary system   **699**
John Wilkinson

16   Diet and nutrition   **749**
Amrutha Ramu, Penny Neild and Jeannette Naish

Index   785

Contributors

Andrew Archbold MD FRCP
Consultant Cardiologist, Barts Health NHS Trust,
London Chest Hospital, London, UK

Alistair Chesser MB BChir FRCP PhD
Consultant Nephrologist, Barts Health NHS Trust, The
Royal London Hospital, Whitechapel, London, UK

Marek H. Dominiczak dr hab med FRCPath
FRCP (Glas)
Honorary Professor of Clinical Biochemistry and
Medical Humanities, University of Glasgow; Consultant
Biochemist, NHS Greater Glasgow and Clyde,
Department of Biochemistry, Gartnavel General
Hospital, Glasgow, UK

Paola Domizio BSc MBBS FRCPath
Professor of Pathology Education, Institute of Cell and
Molecular Science, Barts and the London School of
Medicine and Dentistry, Queen Mary University of London;
Department of Cellular Pathology, Barts Health NHS Trust,
The Royal London Hospital, Whitechapel, London, UK

Gavin Donaldson BSc PhD
Reader in Respiratory Medicine, National Heart and
Lung Institute, Faculty of Medicine, Imperial College
London, London, UK

Joy Hinson BSc PhD DSc FHEA
Professor of Endocrine Science, Dean for
Postgraduate Studies, Barts and the London School
of Medicine and Dentistry, Queen Mary University of
London, UK

Mark Holness BSc PhD
Reader in Diabetes and Metabolism, Institute of Cell
and Molecular Science, Barts and The London School
of Medicine and Dentistry, Queen Mary University of
London, UK

David P. Kelsell BSc PhD
Professor of Human Molecular Genetics, Blizard
Institute, Barts and The London School of Medicine and
Dentistry, Queen Mary University of London, UK

Jeannette Naish MBBS MSc FRCGP
Clinical Senior Lecturer, Wolfson Institute of
Preventive Medicine, Barts and The
London School of Medicine and Dentistry,
London, UK

Girish Namagondlu MBBS, MRCP
Consultant Nephrologist, Barts Health NHS Trust, Royal
London Hospital, Whitechapel, London, UK

Penny Neild MD FRCP
Consultant Gastroenterologist and Honorary Senior
Lecturer, St George's Hospital, St. George's University
of London, London, UK

Adrian C. Newland BA MB BCh MA FRCP(UK)
FRCPath
Professor of Haematology, Institute of Cell and
Molecular Science, Barts and the London School
of Medicine and Dentistry, Queen Mary University of
London, London, UK; Department of Haematology,
Royal London Hospital, Whitechapel, London, UK

Brian Pentland BSc MB ChB FRCP(Ed) FRCSLT
Consultant Neurologist (retired), Astley Ainslie Hospital,
Edinburgh; Head of Rehabilitation Studies (retired),
University of Edinburgh; Professor (Honorary), Queen
Margaret University, Edinburgh, UK

Drew Provan BSc MB ChB MD FRCP FRCPath
Reader in Autoimmune Haematology, Institute of Cell
and Molecular Science, Barts and the London School
of Medicine and Dentistry, Queen Mary University of
London; Department of Haematology, Royal London
Hospital, London, UK

Amrutha Ramu MBBS BSc MRCP MRCPGastro MSc
Senior Clinical Fellow in Nutrition and Intestinal Failure,
Salford Royal Hospital, Salford, UK

Peter Raven BSc PhD MBBS MRCP MRCPsych FHEA
Faculty Tutor, Faculty of Medical Sciences, UCL;
Honorary Consultant Psychiatrist, Camden and
Islington Mental Health Trust, London, UK

Lesley Robson BSc PhD
Senior Lecturer, Institute of Cell and Molecular Science,
Barts and the London School of Medicine and Dentistry,
Queen Mary University of London, UK

Armine M. Sefton MBBS MSc MD FRCP FRCPath
FHEA
Professor of Clinical Microbiology, Centre of
Immunology and Infectious Disease, Blizard Institute,
Barts and The London School of Medicine and
Dentistry, Queen Mary University of London, UK

Mary Sugden MA DPhil (Oxon) DSc (Lond)
Professor of Cellular Biochemistry, Institute of Cell
and Molecular Science, Barts and the London School
of Medicine and Dentistry, Queen Mary University of
London, UK

Denise Syndercombe Court CBiol MSB CSci FIBMS
DMedT MFSoc PhD
Honorary Research Fellow, Queen Mary University of
London; Reader in Forensic Genetics, King's College
London, London, UK

Walter Wieczorek MIBiol PhD
Senior Lecturer, Institute of Dentistry, Barts and The
London School of Medicine and Dentistry, Queen Mary
University of London, UK

John Wilkinson BSc (Hons) PhD
Academic Manager (Retired), School of Life Sciences,
University of Hertfordshire, Hatfield, UK

Preface

We were extremely pleased to be invited to compile a second edition of *Medical Sciences*. In the first edition, we tried to be scientifically comprehensive, but limit the amount of core information to focus on the facts that are relevant and important to clinical medicine. As this was the first time anyone had attempted to integrate information from the diverse branches of medical science in a book based on all the systems of the human body in health, and link it to clinical phenomena, we were most anxious to receive feedback both from students and faculty. While the students who kindly reviewed the first edition were extremely polite and complimentary, we believed that – while we achieved most of our aim – there were areas which could be improved. Some of the reviews by faculty members from different institutions confirmed this.

Medical science has marched on in the past 5 years and this edition has been substantially updated, particularly in genetics. Some chapters have been completely re-written. Once again, we have tried to avoid chemical formulae and physical equations that medical students are unlikely to use as future practitioners, while providing an understanding of the scientific processes that these relate to.

Some chapters include more clinical content than others, as clinical and information boxes. This is because those systems relate to more common, and therefore important, clinical conditions. The student, however, must never forget that uncommon and rare conditions do exist that affect the patient just as much, and are therefore equally important.

It was never an easy task to get the right balance between the basic and clinical sciences. Any feedback will be very much valued, and we sincerely hope that you will enjoy reading this book and find it useful throughout your studies.

Jeannette Naish
Denise Syndercombe Court
London

Acknowledgements

We thank all the contributors to this second edition of *Medical Sciences*. We would especially like to thank our new contributors, as we recognise that joining an established writing team is often as difficult as to undertake an entirely new commission.

We welcome Elsevier's decision to commission this second edition, giving us the opportunity to improve on the previous content. As Editors we have been well supported through this project. A very special thank you goes to Ailsa Laing, Senior Content Development Specialist, who saved our sanity with saintly patience and ensured delivery with gracious firmness. Pauline Graham, Senior Content Strategist, was instrumental in the commissioning of this second edition. We thank her wholeheartedly for handling this project with clarity, and for being so very supportive. The whole production team have been wonderfully efficient and thorough, especially Sukanthi Sukumar, Project Manager in production. We will be eternally grateful.

To the students and faculty members who reviewed *Medial Sciences I*, we extend our grateful thanks. Your feedback was invaluable, and we hope that *Medical Sciences II* will be all the better for it.

Not least, we owe a vote of thanks to the original contributors to *Medical Sciences I*, without whom we would not be here today:

Alison Chambers BSc PhD
Alan Longstaff BSc PhD BSc FRAS
Jeremy Powell-Tuck MD FRCP
Patricia Revest BSc PhD
Malcolm Segal BSc PhD MPS
Nigel Yeatman MBBS BSc MRCP DCH DRCOG

1

Introduction and homeostasis

Jeannette Naish

Chapter 2 Biochemistry and cell biology 1

Chapter 3 Energy metabolism 1

Chapter 4 Pharmacology 1

Chapter 5 Human genetics 2

Chapter 6 Pathology and immunology 2

Chapter 7 Epidemiology 2

Systems of the body 2

Chapter 16 Diet and nutrition 3

Homeostasis 3

Homeostatic regulation mechanisms 3

Water and electrolytes: homeostatic control of body fluids 7

Acid–base balance: homeostatic control of hydrogen ions 10

Disease ensues when normal physiological mechanisms and processes are disrupted. These processes take place in the basic unit of living organisms, the cell. It is therefore essential that all clinicians understand normal cellular and molecular mechanisms and processes in order to understand disease. The chapters address specific mechanisms related to particular areas of human function and systems of the body.

The basic science concepts that attempt to explain disease processes cannot be undervalued. The best diagnostic and most effective therapeutic decisions made by clinicians need to be underpinned by sound scientific principles. The inclusion of all the relevant basic sciences in one book will, hopefully, be useful.

CHAPTER 2 BIOCHEMISTRY AND CELL BIOLOGY

This chapter gives an overview of the principles of mechanisms that enable the body to work as a biochemical system. The functional unit of the human organism is the cell (see Fig. 2.32). All cells are surrounded by a **cell membrane**, also known as the **plasma membrane**. Other cell components are contained in the **cytoplasm** in which the cellular elements (organelles), including the nucleus, are suspended in the **cytosol** (**intracellular fluid** or **cytoplasmic matrix**).

Cells are suspended in fluid composed of water and a variety of biologically active molecules. Movement of these molecules into and out of cells, involving both active and passive transport, triggers the physiological mechanisms that enable the cells to perform their normal physiological functions. Examples include protein synthesis, regulation of cell function (signalling), cell movement, metabolism (glucose and respiration), cell division and death (apoptosis), skeletal and cardiac muscle contraction, the transmission of signals along nerve fibres, the digestion and absorption of nutrients in the alimentary system, the synthesis and secretion of hormones by the endocrine system, transport of oxygen and carbon dioxide by blood, the exchange of respiratory gases and the important functions performed by the renal system. These cells perform different functions and therefore possess different properties, as described in detail in the chapters on the systems of the body.

Understanding cell and molecular biology – the similarities and differences between cell types, their components and functions – is essential to understanding the clinical sciences because disease results from the disruption of normal mechanisms. These principles underpin the development of disease, therapeutics and, in particular, the understanding of cancers and their treatment.

CHAPTER 3 ENERGY METABOLISM

This chapter discusses the cellular mechanisms that enable human beings to produce the energy needed for survival, maintenance of body temperature and physical work. Most biological processes are driven by energy in the form of adenosine triphosphate (ATP), produced through metabolism of the food that we eat. The main metabolic fuels are carbohydrate, protein and fat. The most important source of energy is glucose, but the body has intricate and dynamic adaptive mechanisms for using alternative fuels under particular physiological conditions. Metabolism occurs in cells, and is tightly regulated by the actions of enzymes, gene expression and transcription in response to changing demands on the need for energy, and the action of hormones, which may take place rapidly or gradually. Energy metabolism is essential for life, and disturbances can lead to important diseases, such as diabetes mellitus.

CHAPTER 4 PHARMACOLOGY

Chapter 4 describes how drugs work (pharmacodynamics) and how they are absorbed, distributed around the body (pharmacokinetics), metabolised and then eliminated. Knowledge of cell and molecular biology underpins the understanding of pharmacology and therapeutics.

The pharmacokinetics and pharmacodynamics of synthetic drugs depend on their individual properties. Specific classes of drugs share common properties, but there are variations between individual drugs. It is vital to remember that how a drug performs in the laboratory (in vitro) is not necessarily how it performs in the body (in vivo), which is relevant to the safety and effectiveness of drugs. Generally, pharmacokinetics follows the principles of cell biology. Pharmacodynamics, on the other hand, looks at how drugs work by targeting cellular processes to either enhance or inhibit the process. Examples include the targeting of enzymes, transport processes and receptors on cell surfaces. Here, understanding of the autonomic nervous system is essential because most drugs are designed to target elements of this system.

CHAPTER 5 HUMAN GENETICS

The understanding of human genetics dates back to Charles Darwin's (1809–1882) *On the Origin of Species* (1859), later further explained by Gregor Mendel's (1822–1884) principles of inheritance and mutations. The most exciting modern development in genetics was the Human Genome Project, which mapped the complete set of genetic codes stored as DNA sequences in the whole 23 chromosomes of the human cell nucleus. This project started in 1990, and was originally sponsored by the USA government, directed through the Office of Biological and Environmental Research in the US National Institutes of Health and the National Human Genome Research Institute. Most of the publically sponsored sequencing was performed in universities from the USA, the UK, Japan, France, Germany and Spain – the Human Genome Sequencing Consortium.

The Human Genome Project published the working draft of the human genome in 2000; the complete genome was published in 2003. A parallel project, privately sponsored by the Celera Corporation – Celera Genomics – was started in 1998 using some of the data already obtained by the Human Genome Project. This competition speeded up the work of mapping the human genome, which has now become an essential component of medicine.

The 'genome' of individual human beings has unique characteristics. Even identical twins have small differences. Together with understanding molecular and cellular biology, medical genomics will extend our understanding of disease processes and aid the development of preventive measures, diagnosis, prognosis and therapeutic strategies. The proposal to sequence the genome of all bacteria, for example, will revolutionise the management of infectious diseases. It behoves all budding physicians to really study modern genetics and to follow the ongoing research.

CHAPTER 6 PATHOLOGY AND IMMUNOLOGY

Pathology and immunology are essential for understanding disease processes and to enable the clinician to formulate sensible diagnostic and therapeutic decisions. Infectious diseases and the body's response to them – immunology – are discussed. Disorders of the immune system, including autoimmunity and hypersensitivity are also discussed. In these conditions, it is thought that there is a defect in the genetic regulation of the immune response. The inflammatory response underpins the body's defence mechanisms and needs to be fully understood.

Immunology is followed by the pathology of neoplasia – cancers — which cause about 25% of all deaths in the UK. The pathology of common degenerative diseases is discussed in the chapters on systems of the body. Once again, molecular and cellular biology and medical genomics form the basis for understanding these processes.

CHAPTER 7 EPIDEMIOLOGY

Chapter 7 is about the epidemiological principles that underpin the discovery of patterns of diseases and their occurrence in populations, and how the effectiveness of therapeutic intervention is evaluated. It is, perhaps, unusual to consider this as a basic science. However, epidemiology and the epidemiological approach underpin the art of clinical medicine. Observational studies form the cornerstone of clinical medicine.

For example, how do we know how to diagnose disease from patients' descriptions of symptoms? How disease presents and progresses clinically is based on repeated, multiple observations by many doctors and the sharing of their observations. For example, whooping cough starts like a common cold, then the cough develops and continues for up to 100 days. The cough is characteristic in being spasmodic and prolonged, often ending in a sharp intake of breath – the 'whoop'.

In the example of John Snow and the Broad Street Pump, Snow found the association between the water from the Broad Street Pump, in London, and the cholera epidemic. The actual cause of cholera, the organism *Vibrio cholerae*, was not discovered until later by Filippo Pacini, an Italian anatomist, and not widely known until published by Robert Koch some 30 years later. Until the comma-shaped bacterium was identified, treatment and prevention could not be formulated. Careful and systematic observation thus formed the basis for further research into the cause of this disease.

Moreover, how do we select therapeutic interventions, whether pharmacological or surgical? How do we know that this intervention is effective, or more effective than another one? Here, the methodology for experimental studies, e.g. randomised controlled trials, and the statistical concepts that underpin the proof for the likelihood of a positive effect need to be understood. The mathematics might be daunting, but understanding the principles is essential. These principles also apply to diagnostic and screening tests.

SYSTEMS OF THE BODY

The next eight chapters are on all the systems of the body, and discuss the cellular makeup of different organs, their functions, normal metabolic processes in health and the biological basis for disturbance leading to disease. Understanding these processes forms the rationale for diagnostic and therapeutic decisions. Despite their separation, the systems interconnect so that the body functions as a whole, so it might be more helpful to think about the cellular mechanisms that ensure normal physiological function. These basic mechanisms are common to all living organisms, including *Homo sapiens*.

As mentioned before, the basic unit of the human organism is the cell, and normal biological functioning is determined by molecular and cellular processes and controlled by human genomics. The cells in each system vary according to their physiological function. For example, hepatic (liver) and muscle cells both store glycogen, but the primary function of the liver is to release glucose converted from glycogen into the whole circulation when there is a shortage of glucose, whereas muscle cells (myocytes) primarily need to break down the stored glycogen for generating ATP for muscle contraction. Skeletal muscle thus lacks the enzyme (glucose-6-phosphatase, G6Pase) for breaking down glycogen to glucose through glycogenolysis for export into the circulation.

Another example, where the influence of genomics is more obvious, is sickle cell disease (SCD). This is a condition where there is a mutation in the haemoglobin gene (β-globin gene), leading to the red cells assuming a sickle shape and becoming rigid. Sickle cells confer a resistance to malaria infection, and the mutation arose historically among populations in tropical and subtropical regions where malaria is endemic. The disadvantage is that under conditions of reduced oxygenation, infection, cold or dehydration, the sickle haemoglobin elongates and cannot flow smoothly through small blood vessels, sticks to the vessel lining, leading to occlusion of the vessels and causing sickle cell crises, which may be life-threatening. Understanding of molecular and cell biology and human genomics for the cells in each system is therefore necessary for understanding disease processes.

CHAPTER 16 DIET AND NUTRITION

This chapter is about the nutritional needs for humans to stay alive, and more importantly, the principles for assessing these needs in health and disease. What makes a human being eat or not eat is also addressed, with implications for dietary control of conditions, such as obesity, and some therapeutic diets for chronic conditions, such as inflammatory bowel disease. The association between diet and disease is also discussed. Nutritional support during severe illness, artificial nutrition and associated complications are discussed.

Artificial nutrition includes enteral feeding, i.e. putting feeding liquid directly into the stomach or small intestine, and parenteral nutrition, which is intravenous feeding. The makeup of the feeding fluid will depend on the nutritional needs of the patient. These principles are important, especially during the foundation years. Inclusion of nutrition as a basic science in this book is perhaps also unusual, but clinicians need to know about these principles for sustaining life.

HOMEOSTASIS

To maintain the normal physiological processes for sustaining life, all living organism and cells have to maintain a stable internal environment in response to changes in external conditions. Physiologists have called this function **homeostasis**,

from the Greek *homeo* meaning same or unchanging, and *stasis* meaning standing still. It is a complex system of processes that adjusts an attribute (such as pH or temperature) within the organism or cell back to the constant level needed for physiological functioning, whenever the attribute changes for whatever reason. This attribute is labelled a **variable**, something that is changeable.

Homeostatic systems are multiple, dynamic mechanisms that are **regulated** (or controlled) for making the adjustments necessary for a stable internal environment, unlike simple dynamic equilibrium or steady states that are not regulated. Many examples of human homeostasis are discussed throughout the book. Disease ensues when homeostatic mechanisms break down, and the body exhibits **symptoms** (what the patient experiences) and **signs** (what the clinician finds on clinical examination).

Many physiological parameters such as the balance of blood glucose (Chapter 3), water and electrolytes (sodium, potassium, calcium and so on) and body temperature are examples of precise control by homeostatic mechanisms. Of the homeostatic mechanisms that control body fluids, **fluid balance** (the control of fluid volumes) and **acid–base balance** (the control of acidity [H⁺ ions]) are important to understand.

HOMEOSTATIC REGULATION MECHANISMS

Homeostatic control mechanisms have three (sometimes more) interdependent components for the variable being regulated:

- A receptor that detects, monitors and responds to changes (sometimes wide variation) in a variable in the external environment; known as the **sensor**.
- The sensor sends information to a **control centre** that sets the physiological range for the variable, and determines the necessary response for bringing the variable back to the set point. In humans, the control centre is usually in the brain, and many examples are discussed in Chapter 8.
- The control centre sends signals to the tissues and organs, known as the **effector**, that have to effect, i.e. make the adjustment, to changes in the relevant variable to bring it back to its set point.

A simplistic analogy would be ambient temperature control in air conditioning systems, where the thermostat is the sensor responding to changes in environmental temperature, set at a comfortable level. It also acts as the control system that switches heating or cooling systems on and off. The effector would be the heating and cooling systems with their own, separate mechanisms.

Once the control centre receives the stimulus that a variable has changed from the set point, it sends signals to effectors to correct the change by:

- Negative feedback to depress the change if the variable level has increased beyond the narrow, set range. This is the commonest mechanism.
- Positive feedback to effect an increase or acceleration in the output variable that has already been triggered. The result is to push the level beyond the physiological range.
- Feedforward control to either depress or enhance the level of a variable before the change is needed, i.e. anticipatory.

Negative feedback

Negative feedback mechanisms can either increase or reduce the activity of tissues or organs back to normal, set levels, and the system is sometimes called a negative feedback loop (Fig. 1.1). Numerous examples of negative feedback exist in metabolic processes in all physiological systems.

Homeostatic control of glucose metabolism

An example of a negative feedback system is the homeostatic control of blood glucose. Among the tissues of the body, red blood cells and the brain (under normal conditions) can only use glucose to generate the energy needed to drive metabolic processes. Glucose is essential to ensure an adequate supply of energy for the vital functions performed by these and other tissues. Blood glucose concentration (measured as fasting blood glucose) is therefore tightly maintained within a narrow range (3.5–8.0 mmol/L) normally. Here, the sensor is specialised pancreatic cells that receive blood from the portal circulation. The control is the autonomic nervous system, and the effector is the α (secreting glucagon) and β (secreting insulin) pancreatic cells in the islets of Langerhans. A simplified version for glucose homeostasis would be something like that shown in Figure 1.2.

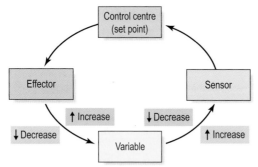

Fig. 1.1 **Negative feedback loop.** An increase in the variable produces an effector response to decrease it and vice versa.

- When blood glucose concentration is abnormally low (hypoglycemia), as in prolonged fasting, glucagon is released from the pancreas to trigger alternative metabolic pathways to bring the glucose level up. Glycogenolysis, the process in which glucose stored in the form of glycogen is broken down to glucose, and when glycogen stores are depleted, gluconeogenesis, in which other metabolic fuels such as fat and protein are converted to glucose, and alternative fuels, such as fatty acids and ketone bodies, are used for generating energy.
- When blood glucose concentration is too high (hyperglycaemia), e.g. following a high carbohydrate meal or the ingestion of excessive amounts of alcohol, the secretion of the hormone insulin rises to increase the take-up of glucose into cells, thus lowering blood glucose concentration to normal. These processes are described in detail in Chapters 3 and 16.

Thermoregulation

Another example of a physiological homeostatic negative feedback system, addressed elsewhere in Chapter 8, is the control of body temperature: **thermoregulation**. Ambient environmental temperature can vary widely (−50°C to +50°C), but human body temperature needs to be set at about 37°C (range 36°–38°C) for normal physiological functioning. For example, some mechanisms in glucose metabolism require energy, and if body temperature falls below a certain level, there will not be enough energy to drive the process. Figure 1.3 shows the mechanisms for controlling body temperature by negative feedback.

Body temperatures outside the normal range are defined as:

- Hyperthermia when core temperature rises above 40°C
- Hypothermia when core temperature falls below 35°C.

Prolonged and significant elevation (as in hyperthermia) or depression (as in hypothermia) in core body temperature (see below) can have fatal consequences.

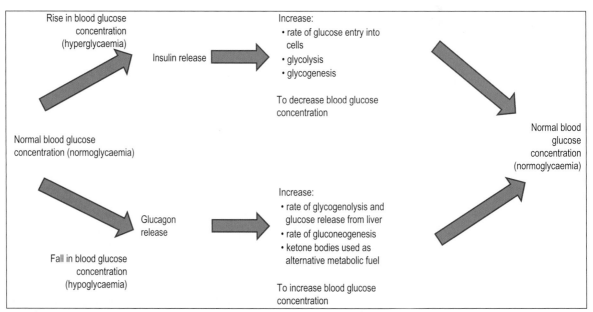

Fig. 1.2 **Simplified scheme for glucose homeostasis.** Increased blood glucose concentration leads to increased insulin secretion to lower blood glucose concentration back to normal, and a reduction in blood glucose concentration leads to the release of glucagon to raise blood glucose concentration to normal.

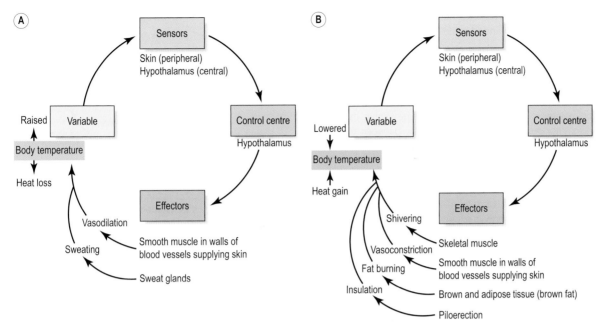

Fig. 1.3 **Control of body temperature by negative feedback.** (A) Responses to an increase in body temperature; (B) responses to a decrease in body temperature.

Human body temperature (Clinical box 1.1)

As mentioned above, human body temperature is set at about 37°C. This can be measured through different anatomical orifices, such as oral, rectal, vaginal, external auditory meatus. These are measurements of peripheral temperature, and will vary between healthy subjects depending on where the measurement is taken. The **core** temperature (or core body temperature) is the temperature needed for normal physiological functions in deep organs such as the liver or brain, and is different from peripheral temperatures. Core temperatures have to be measured by inserting a deep probe, which is not always possible, so that rectal or vaginal temperatures are taken as an accurate reflection of core temperature.

Body temperature also varies according to the time of day, known as the **circadian rhythm**, an endogenous biological process driven by light and darkness in the external environment. Rhythmical physiological and behavioural patterns can be adjusted to follow the oscillations in circadian rhythm, a phenomenon known as *entrainment*. Sleep and wakefulness is an example (see Ch. 8). Core temperatures are higher in the evenings and lower in the morning, with the lowest temperature during the second half of sleep, about 2 hours before waking.

Behavioural and environmental factors can affect body temperature when homeostatic mechanisms will be called into play. For example, eating, drinking and exercise can raise body temperature; jet lag and shift work upset circadian rhythm and thus the pattern of body temperature. Ambient temperatures will affect body temperature.

Using the negative feedback loop:

- The main **sensor** of temperature is the skin.
- The body temperature **control centre** is the hypothalamus (see Ch. 8 for details).
- The effectors for adjusting to core temperature change will be the skin and muscles.

Heat loss mechanisms

The skin is responsive to peripheral temperature, where capillary blood can be heated or cooled. When carried to the

hypothalamus, the temperature of this blood is measured as core temperature. The hypothalamus then sends signals to the effector organs (see Figure 1.3).

Heat loss through the skin occurs when blood flow through the skin increases by vasodilation, and the skin becomes reddened and 'hot'. Heat is then lost through radiation to the atmosphere. Sweat glands in the skin also promote heat loss. Increased sweating increases water evaporation from the surface of the body, and lowers temperature through the latent heat of evaporation. This mechanism is less effective in humid atmospheres. Also, excessive loss of water through sweating can lead to dehydration. For example, the combined effects of lack of drinking water and the hot, dry atmosphere in deserts are well documented and could be fatal.

Heat gain mechanisms

Falls in core temperature trigger heat gain mechanisms. Physiological adjustments include:

- In the skin, arteriolar vasoconstriction, leading to pallor and even cyanosis, reduces blood flow to prevent heat loss.
- Sweating almost ceases so that there is minimal heat lost through water evaporation.
- Body hair becomes erect through the action of erector pili muscles in the skin, piloerection, which traps warm air between the hairs that also acts as insulation.
- Increased muscular activity to cause shivering to generate heat.
- Direct conversion of fat stores to heat energy by mitochondria to raise the temperature in cells (see also Ch. 3). Brown fat stores in infants are a form of fat specialised for conversion to heat energy; they are also abundant in hibernating animals.

Behavioural mechanisms can also operate; e.g. exercise to generate heat, putting on more clothing to conserve body heat and reduce heat loss, turning up the air conditioning thermostat. In furry animals, piloerection is equivalent to putting on clothes. The erect hairs trap air, which provides insulation, and the warmed air helps to conserve body heat.

Thermoneutral zones

In humans and other warm blooded animals, the **thermoneutral zone (TNZ)** is the range of body temperatures in which the organism only needs to use a minimum amount of energy for maintaining normal body temperature. Within the TNZ, vasomotor responses control blood flow between the core and periphery to adjust for the amount of heat loss or gain from the body surface. Organisms use different mechanisms for adjusting body temperature within the TNZ; for example by changing posture or going into the shade to avoid heat, and into the sun for warmth. In humans, the TNZ is about 27°C at rest, and energy is expended at temperatures above and below this for maintaining body temperature.

Positive feedback (Clinical box 1.2)

Once triggered, some homeostatic mechanisms need to continue. This continuation is known as **positive feedback**. Unlike negative feedback, positive feedback has no set point, so the process can continue indefinitely if unchecked. As the process proceeds, small deviations from the original variable become amplified, and the process becomes a cascade.

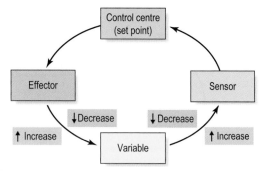

Fig. 1.4 Positive feedback loop. An increase in the variable produces an effector response to increase it, and vice versa, until the loop is terminated.

The 'brake' is usually the desired physiological outcome that ends the feedforward cascade, so normally, this is a self-limiting mechanism. Figure 1.4 shows diagrammatically a positive feedback loop. Uncontrolled feedforward leads to disease.

Feedforward (Information box 1.1)

Feedforward mechanisms trigger the change in a variable before the change is needed; it anticipates the need for the change and accelerates the change.

Clinical box 1.1   **Fever**

The set point for temperature control is not always fixed. In infection, toxins released from bacteria and chemicals produced by cells of the immune system change the set point upwards (see Ch. 6). The normal mechanisms to generate heat, such as shivering, are triggered leading to an increase in body temperature, known as fever or **pyrexia**. The cause for this fever is thought to be a mechanism to help kill off bacteria. The higher rate of metabolism will also produce a faster rate of healing and more rapid induction of defence mechanisms. If the temperature becomes too high, however, the proteins inside the cells may be damaged.

Clinical box 1.2   **Some examples of positive feedback**

- The coagulation cascade is described in Chapter 12. A positive feedback loop is triggered by tissue damage after injury, which triggers the coagulation cascade to stop bleeding. Coagulation (blood clotting) which arrests the bleeding then terminates the cascade.
- In the menstrual cycle (see Ch. 10), the rise in oestrogen levels during the follicular phase reaches a spike that triggers ovulation, after which event oestrogen levels fall, terminating the follicular phase.
- During childbirth, the rhythmic uterine contractions for expelling the foetus are activated by the hormone oxytocin secreted by the pituitary gland (triggered by the hypothalamus). The pressure of the foetal head on the lower uterine segment continues to stimulate oxytocin release until the baby is delivered, when oxytocin secretion stops.
- In genetics, the production of gene transcription factors is accelerated by feedforward loops (see Ch. 5). The process is normally self-limiting, as the loop terminates when the target gene is achieved.
- In cancer genetics (see Ch. 5), the proliferation of mutated cancer cells occurs through feedforward mechanisms, which are unchecked.
- In neural signalling, long-term potentiation (LTP) to strengthen synapses is achieved through feedforward mechanisms (see Ch. 8).

Information box 1.1   **Some examples of feedforward control**

Many examples of physiological feedforward control exist, some of which are:
- Salivation and increased stomach secretion in anticipation of food being eaten, discussed in Chapter 15, Alimentary system.
- In response to eating, a fast phase of insulin secretion by the β cells of the pancreas is triggered even before blood glucose levels rise in the portal circulation in anticipation of the requirement for insulin for glucose metabolism. When blood glucose levels rise, a negative feedback mechanism takes over for glucose homeostasis. This is discussed in Chapter 3, Energy metabolism, and Chapter 10, Endocrinology: endocrine control of energy metabolism.
- When blood glucose is plentiful, as in the fed state (Ch. 3), muscle and fat cells express a glucose transporter, GLUT4, which is regulated by insulin, in anticipation of the need to transport glucose into the cells for storage.
- In gene regulation, the sequence of events that activate transcription factor genes may be seen as feedforward control, where cell differentiation is controlled by a network of factors each activating the next in sequence. This is discussed in Chapter 5, Human genetics: genes and development.
- In haematology (Ch. 12), the development of mature blood cells from stem cells follows a haemopoietic cell lineage, which is a feedforward mechanism.
- In the motor system, fast movements are controlled by feedforward mechanisms that anticipate what is required, based on learned, pre-existing motor programs, e.g. playing the piano (Chapter 8, motor control and pathways; see also Information box 8.10). Feedforward failure, where feedforward commands to alternating agonist/antagonist muscles cannot be properly timed, can lead to tremor, speech impairment and other rapidly alternating movements. Negative feedback, based on muscle stretch, is too slow. Training (practice) can accelerate feedforward.
- During exercise, a neurological feedforward mechanism can be triggered, where blood lactate levels rise in anticipation of the increased need for glucose. Lactate is a precursor for glucose in gluconeogenesis.

WATER AND ELECTROLYTES: HOMEOSTATIC CONTROL OF BODY FLUIDS

The functional unit of the human organism is the cell; the human body is made up of some 10 trillion cells (10^{12}). The structure of the human cell is discussed in Chapter 2 (Biochemistry and cell biology). Each cell contains fluid, which is a solution of electrolytes and a variety of biochemical compounds, and in which organelles, including the nucleus, are suspended (see Fig. 2.32). Separated by the cell wall are extracellular fluid compartments. The cells and extracellular compartments of different organs have different components that perform biological processes that determine their functions. Depending on the requirements for these biological processes, the fluids, electrolytes and biochemical compounds are constantly being transferred from one compartment to another. The precise mechanisms for maintaining this balance are not yet fully understood, so laboratory measurements of serum electrolytes can only be a rough guide to the state of the internal environment.

The ensuing chapters describe the makeup of the various human organs, their composition and functions. In particular, Chapter 4 discusses drug distribution through the body, the mechanisms concerned with transferring fluids, electrolytes and chemical compounds into and out of cells; and Chapter 16 discusses the requirements for water and electrolytes, the balance of these substances in health, and the processes that could disrupt normal function.

Fluid compartments

Total body water in a healthy 70 kg adult male is between 40 and 45 litres. The amount of total body water relates inversely to body fat (adipose tissue), where a higher proportion of fat leads to a lower proportion of water.

Basically, there are two compartments of fluid in the human body (Fig. 1.5): an **intracellular compartment (ICF)** that is fluid within all the cells, which is the larger of the two, and the **extracellular compartment (ECF)** that surrounds the cells. The intracellular compartment occupies about two-thirds of total body water (40% body weight).

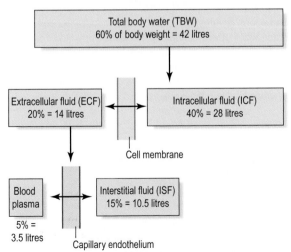

***Fig. 1.5* Distribution of body fluid in compartments.** Approximate values in an adult weighing 70 kg, showing percentage of total body water.

The extracellular compartment is further divided into:

- **Interstitial fluid** (ISF) between the cells. The larger of the extracellular fluid compartments, this occupies two-thirds of the ECF.
- **Intravascular fluid** (IVF), which is mainly **plasma**, is contained in blood vessels, comprising about 25% of ECF. All blood constituents, such as red and white blood cells, platelets, plasma proteins, various nutrients and electrolytes, are carried in plasma. Plasma makes up about 60% of blood volume (see Ch. 12). The lymphatic system contains the remainder of ECF.

Each compartment has a different ionic composition (see Ch. 2, Table 2.4). In health, the distribution and constitution of the fluid compartments are homeostatically controlled to enable normal physiological function. Homeostatic imbalance leads to disease (Information box 1.2).

A third space, where small amounts of fluid are collected – interstitial fluid – includes extracellular fluids in particular regions, which is further discussed in the chapters on systems of the body. Examples include the cerebrospinal fluid, which bathes the brain, the fluid inside the eye (Ch. 8), fluid in joints (Ch. 9) and fluid secreted into the intestines (Ch. 15).

Information box 1.2   Some clinical effects of homeostatic failure in fluid compartments: intravascular volume

Dehydration occurs when there is insufficient fluid (water) in all the compartments; some effects are described in Clinical box 1.6. Water overload leads to fluid accumulation in the tissues, particularly in the interstitial compartment, as described in Clinical box 1.7.

Homeostatic disturbance also occurs when there are abnormalities in the intravascular compartment, principally in blood plasma, known as **intravascular volume status**:

- Fluid depletion in plasma is known as **hypovolaemia**. This may be related to overall fluid depletion through severe diarrhoea and vomiting, or from renal or other extrarenal causes. Depending on whether the fluid loss is primarily water or solutes, hypovolaemia may be isonatraemic, hyponatraemic or hypernatraemic, related to plasma sodium (Na^+) levels (see later). Plasma concentrations of Na^+, K^+, urea and proteins will rise, as will the volume of red cells – **packed cell volume** (PCV), also known as the haematocrit (see Ch. 12). The raised haematocrit (and to a lesser extent plasma protein concentration) increases blood viscosity so that blood flow through the vessels is much slower. Red cells and other blood constituents, such as platelets, tend to aggregate and stick together, increasing the risk of intravascular coagulation. The increased plasma protein concentration, particularly of some proteins such as fibrinogen and immunoglobulins, also increases red cell aggregation. When chronic, increased blood viscosity is associated with the development of atheroma and coronary heart and peripheral vascular diseases. When there is acute and severe fluid or blood loss, as in dehydration or haemorrhage, hypovolaemic shock may occur. The heart is no longer effective as a pump to supply essential organs with blood, and multiple organ failure occurs. This is a medical emergency as the consequences could be fatal.
- **Hypervolaemia** occurs when there is fluid overload, usually associated with increased body sodium. The excess sodium causes an increase in extracellular fluid volume, which in turn leads to the entry of water into the intravascular compartment. The increase in sodium is related to homeostatic failure in sodium handling, as in congestive heart (CHF), renal or hepatic failure. Other causes include excessive sodium intake, intravenous infusions of saline or blood and some drugs.

The body fluid compartments are separated by **semi-permeable barriers**.

- The intracellular compartment is separated from the extracellular compartments by the cell membranes that allow water to move in and out of cells but restrict the movement of the main extracellular ion, sodium, so that water can move freely between the compartments but sodium cannot move into cells except in disease conditions.
- In the extracellular compartment, interstitial fluid is separated from blood plasma by the endothelium in blood vessels (see Ch. 11, Cardiovascular system). In health, the movement of blood cells and proteins between the interstitial and intravascular compartments is restricted. Water and ions can move freely between the two compartments.

Movement of fluids between compartments

In health, fluids constantly move between the different compartments of the human body. The driving forces consist of:

- Pressure generated by the pumping of the heart; **hydrostatic pressure** in the circulation refers to the pressure exerted by the volume of blood in a blood vessel (see Ch. 11). Capillary hydrostatic pressure drives fluid out of the capillary bed (also known as filtration). It is highest at the arteriolar end and lowest at the venule end of the capillary bed. Interstitial hydrostatic pressure, determined by interstitial fluid volume and tissue compliance, opposes capillary hydrostatic pressure.
- **Osmotic pressure**, exerted by substances in solution, prevents the flow of water across a semi-permeable membrane, i.e. the cell membrane. Osmosis is the passage of a solvent through a semi-permeable membrane from a solution of higher concentration of solute to one of a lower concentration, and occurs when two solutions of different concentration are separated by a membrane which will selectively allow some solutes to move across. Thus, water osmotically moves from more dilute to more concentrated solutions, and osmotic pressure is pressure exerted by the solutes that must be applied to the solution from outside to end osmosis (Fig. 1.6).

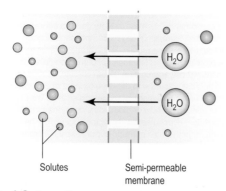

Solutes   Semi-permeable membrane

Fig. 1.6 Osmotic movement of water across a membrane. The membrane is semi-permeable. It is permeable to water, but not all solutes. Osmotic pressure is the pressure exerted by the solutes that cannot move across the membrane to oppose the movement of water across the membrane.

Disturbance of either the efficiency of the heart as a pump or the composition of body fluids as a consequence of disease would lead to manifestations of disease as symptoms and signs. These mechanisms are discussed in almost all the chapters on systems of the body, particularly in Chapters 11 (Cardiovascular system), 13 (Respiratory system), 14 (Renal system) and 15 (Alimentary system).

Properties of forces that drive fluid movement between compartments

The movement of water between compartments is driven by characteristics of the body fluids in the different compartments. These are complicated mechanisms, and perhaps best understood by considering the osmolarity and tonicity of the solutions.

Osmolarity

Osmolarity is a measure of the osmotic pressure exerted by a solution across a perfect semi-permeable membrane which allows free passage of water and completely prevents movement of solute. Osmolarity depends on the number of particles in solution, but not the nature of the particles. If two solutions contain the same number of particles they are **iso-osmotic (isosmotic)** with each other. If one solution has a greater osmolarity than another solution, it is **hyperosmotic** compared to the weaker solution. If one solution has a lower osmolarity than another solution then it is **hypo-osmotic (hyposmotic)** compared to the stronger solution.

Tonicity (Clinical box 1.3)

Tonicity is a measure of the osmotic pressure that a substance exerts across a semi-permeable membrane compared to blood plasma (as opposed to water for osmolarity), and is almost the same as osmolarity for substances that are impermeable to cell membranes. Tonicity depends on the number of particles in solution, but also on the nature of the solute. If a cell is suspended in a solution that exerts no osmotic pressure, the solution is **isotonic**, where there is no movement of water across the cell membrane. A solution containing more osmotically active particles than the cell is **hypertonic**, will draw water out of the cell, which shrinks. A solution with fewer particles is **hypotonic**, causing water to move into the cell, which swells and eventually bursts.

Effect of solutes on body fluids

Some ions (solutes) in solution can penetrate the cell membrane while others cannot, so the three body fluid compartments contain different solutes. For example, cell membranes are impermeable to sodium (Na^+), but permeable to potassium (K^+) so Na^+ cannot move into cells by simple diffusion, whereas K^+ can diffuse out.

Clinical box 1.3   **The effect of tonicity in disease**

Uraemia, abnormally high levels of plasma urea, occurs in renal failure (see Ch. 14). Cell membranes are permeable to urea, so high levels in the extracellular compartment allow urea to enter the cell. The concentration of urea becomes higher in the intracellular compartment. Urea molecules are osmotically active, so the intracellular fluid becomes hypertonic. Water is drawn into the cell, which swells and then bursts, resulting in cell death. This can occur in any cell, but may be lethal in the brain.

Within cells, the intracellular ions are K^+ (together with phosphate and some large anions, e.g. proteins). Outside the cells, extracellular ions are mainly Na^+. These ions are moved in and out of cells by Na^+ and K^+ transporters, discussed in all the chapters about the systems of the body, and particularly in Chapter 4 (Pharmacology), where the action of drugs depends on their movement in and out of cells.

In the extracellular compartment, the solutes in interstitial fluid differ from those in intravascular fluid. While the ionic content of interstitial fluid and blood are the same, proteins in blood are barred from the interstitial compartment by vascular endothelium. The higher hydrostatic pressure in blood tends to push water out, but the proteins exert a **colloid osmotic pressure** that opposes the blood hydrostatic pressure so that excess fluid does not enter the ISF, and blood volume is maintained at a constant level.

Homeostatic control of fluid balance

The physiological processes that maintain life depend on the constant movement of fluids and solutes in and out of cells, and between extracellular compartments. Fluids are also lost as urine and sweat and through respiration. In health, fluids in the different body compartments have the same osmolarity (and tonicity). In disease, when there are changes in either the water or solute content in the fluids, there will be a net movement of fluid between the compartments. The fluid and solutes lost have to be replaced by fluid intake and vice versa, so that the volume and composition of body fluids in each compartment are maintained in status quo. This is achieved through hormonal mechanisms. Human behaviour, such as drinking fluids in response to fluid loss, also helps to maintain fluid balance.

Hormonal control of fluid balance (Clinical box 1.4)

The renal system has a major role in the control of balancing fluid intake to fluid loss, discussed in Chapter 14 (Renal system). The kidney forms urine in a process that filters fluid, retaining essential nutrients (e.g. protein and glucose) but excreting waste products of metabolism (e.g. urea), and some electrolytes (e.g. Na^+) are lost. These are complex processes that require hydrostatic pressure to drive filtration, and changes in osmolarity (or tonicity) in the different parts of the renal system for recovering water, small molecules, sugars, amino acids and electrolytes from the primary filtrate. The control of mechanisms that balance fluid intake to fluid loss is an osmoreceptive complex in the hypothalamus that secrets vasopressin (antidiuretic hormone, ADH) (see also Chapter 8, Nervous system). Vasopressin is the hormone that regulates urine volume; it is released from the posterior pituitary gland in response to small changes in osmotic pressure. Failure of any part of these mechanisms would lead to failure in fluid balance.

Behavioural control of fluid balance (Clinical box 1.5)

In health, loss of body fluid is replaced through drinking. The daily amount lost varies, in part, on environment and physical activity. For example, fluid loss increases with sweating in hot climates (see above, heat loss mechanisms), and during exercise (Clinical box 1.6). The excretion of urea and salt (Na^+) is affected by dietary intake; a high protein, high salt diet would lead to increased urea and Na^+ excretion accompanied by increased urine output, whereas a low protein, low salt diet has the opposite effect (Clinical box 1.7). This effect is utilised

| Clinical box 1.4 | Some examples of renal causes for homeostatic failure in fluid balance |

Disorders in the control of fluid balance related to renal mechanisms may be central, as in failure of control by the brain, or peripheral, as in kidney disease. Chapter 14 discusses these in detail.

Failure of central control:
- Under secretion or lack of vasopressin, due to hypothalamic or posterior pituitary damage. There are a variety of causes, discussed in Chapter 14, including tumours, trauma (head injury) and surgical damage among others. This results in the daily excretion of a high volume of dilute urine (**polyuria**), accompanied by excessive drinking of water (**polydipsia**), which is characteristic of a condition known as diabetes insipidus. There is also a condition in which the receptors in renal tubules become unresponsive to vasopressin.
- Over secretion of vasopressin, known as the syndrome of inappropriate ADH secretion, may be caused by low fluid intake or ectopic tumours and others. This can also occur post-operatively.

Failure due to kidney disease:
This is more common than the failure of central control.
- Impairment to filtration due to abnormal hydrostatic pressure may be caused by failure of the heart as a pump, or abnormality of the blood vessel supplying the renal apparatus. Examples include heart failure, hypertension (high blood pressure), damage to renal vasculature from whatever cause, particularly atheroma/arteriosclerosis and related conditions such as diabetes mellitus.
- Disease of the renal apparatus responsible for producing urine which could lead to disturbance in renal handing of either water, molecules (e.g. protein, glucose) or electrolytes (e.g. Na^+). This explains, in part, the appearance of glucose and protein in the urine in conditions such as diabetes mellitus. Significant conditions include acute or chronic renal failure from whatever cause.

in some therapeutic diets, discussed in Chapter 16 (Diet and nutrition). Thirst is the sensation that drives the behaviour of drinking water.

Thirst

Chapters 14 (Renal system) and 8 (Nervous system) describe the osmoreceptors in the hypothalamus. These also cause the sensation of thirst in response to stimulation by an increase in plasma osmolarity, and less so by a fall in plasma volume. The behavioural response to thirst is drinking. The presence of fluid in the mouth and pharynx abolishes thirst before the restoration of normal osmolarity and plasma volume.

| Clinical box 1.5 | Some behavioural effects leading to disturbance of fluid balance |

Excessive drinking (**polydipsia**) may be driven by thirst or be psychogenic. Polydipsia leads to a dilution of extracellular fluid, decreasing the osmolarity. The hypothalamus responds to the reduced osmotic pressure with decreased vasopressin secretion, leading to the passing of high volumes of dilute urine – polyuria. In extreme cases, water intoxication may occur, when the Na^+ concentration in extracellular fluid falls to the extent that water enters the cells, causing them to swell. In the brain, this can lead to coma and convulsion, and may be lethal. Water overload may also occur through parenteral nutrition (Ch. 16, Diet and nutrition).
- Polydipsia may be caused by thirst as the side effect of some drugs, e.g. phenothiazines, diuretics, anti-diabetic agents. It is also a symptom associated with diabetes mellitus (see Ch. 3, Energy metabolism).
- Psychogenic polydipsia is associated with some mental illnesses, such as schizophrenia or some form of intellectual disability, but may also be psychological, as in a panic attack. This could lead to an inaccurate diagnosis of diabetes insipidus.

Urine overproduction, excessive loss of body fluids or inadequate fluid intake leads to **dehydration**. Dehydration occurs when the input of water is less than water loss. Physiologically, it also involves the loss of electrolytes, mainly Na^+.

- If electrolyte loss is the main problem, then it is known as hyponatraemic or hypotonic dehydration.
- If water is the primary loss, body fluids become hypertonic, i.e. hypernatremic or hypertonic dehydration.
- If water and Na^+ loss is balanced, then dehydration is isonatraemic or isotonic.

These issues are important when considering fluid replacement therapy (Ch. 16, Diet and nutrition). Water moves from the intravascular to the extravascular compartment in hypotonic dehydration, which in turn affects intracellular osmolarity and, particularly if brain cells are affected, may lead to seizures. In hypertonic dehydration, the reverse occurs, and may result in osmotic cerebral oedema if rehydration is too rapid.

To compensate for the reduced plasma volume, the heart and respiratory rates increase, leading to hypotension (low blood pressure). Further complications of hypotension include reduced renal perfusion (low hydrostatic pressure), which can cause renal failure. Body temperature rises due to the shutdown of heat loss mechanisms that involve water loss.

- Symptoms of mild dehydration include dry mouth and thirst, and signs include decreased skin turgor (stays puckered if pinched gently) and low urine output. Infants may have a sunken anterior fontanelle.
- Moderate to severe dehydration leads to anuria (reduced or no urine output). Symptoms of lethargy, delirium, seizures and orthostatic hypotension (fainting) may also occur. Death may ensue with increasing severity.

Dehydration may be caused by excessive fluid loss or inadequate intake:

Excess loss of fluids:
- Increased urine output, as in diabetes mellitus (Ch. 3, Energy metabolism) and diabetes insipidus.
- Loss of other body fluids as in severe vomiting and diarrhoea due to gastrointestinal disease (Ch. 15, Alimentary system) or infection, such as cholera, and following surgical bowel resection (e.g. colostomy).
- Loss of plasma as in haemorrhage or burns and following some surgical procedures.

Inadequate fluid intake occurs:
- In malnutrition and fasting (Ch. 16).
- In the elderly as behavioural consequence, and in infants due to inadequate feeding.

Underproduction of urine leads to water overload, resulting in the accumulation of water in the tissues – **oedema**. Oedema may be a symptom or a sign, and is clinically important. Patients may complain of facial puffiness or shoes feeling 'tight'. Clinical examination may demonstrate 'pitting' (a dent in the skin on gentle pressure that persists after pressure is released) over the ankles, shins or sacrum. There are many causes for oedema, including:

- Failure of renal mechanisms or due to abnormalities in hydrostatic pressure as the consequence of heart failure (see Ch. 11, Cardiovascular system)
- Failure of renal clearance of water and electrolytes (Ch. 14, Renal system), or
- Failure of the lungs to clear CO_2 (Ch. 13, Respiratory system).

It is important to distinguish which physiological mechanisms are disordered, to properly formulate the diagnostic and therapeutic decisions. Oedema is commonly treated with diuretics (Ch. 4, Pharmacology).

ACID–BASE BALANCE: HOMEOSTATIC CONTROL OF HYDROGEN IONS (Clinical box 1.8)

Acid–base balance is the regulation of hydrogen ion (H^+) concentration in body fluids. The concentration of free H^+, i.e. not bound to other molecules such as proteins, determines the acidity of body fluids. This is measured as the partial pressure of free H^+ in solution in body fluids (pH). The partial pressure of a gas in solution is the pressure that the gas would exert if it were the sole occupant of that volume of fluid. Thus, the total pressure of a mixture of gases in solution is the sum of the partial pressures of each gas.

The pH of body fluids determines the rate of activity of the thousands of enzymes that control physiological processes. Enzymes are biological molecules that catalyse (accelerate) chemical reactions in cells at a rate sufficient to sustain life. Enzymes in general are discussed in detail in Chapter 2 (Biochemistry and cell biology) and also in almost all the systems. The various mechanisms for maintaining acid–base balance are discussed in detail under various headings in Chapters 3 (Energy metabolism), 12 (Haematology), 13 (Respiratory system) and 14 (Renal system). Disturbances of acid–base balance can lead to life-threatening conditions.

Partial pressure of hydrogen ions

The pH of a neutral solution such as water is 7. Increased H^+ concentration lowers the pH, rendering the solution acid, whereas reduced H^+ concentration raises the pH, making the solution alkaline. In health, the H^+ concentration in body fluids is regulated within a narrow physiological range (see below). Homeostatic failure, as the result of disease, leads to deviation of pH outside the physiological range and gives rise to specific signs and symptoms. These mechanisms are discussed in detail in Chapters 13 (Respiratory system) and 14 (Renal system). Extreme deviations outside of this range are incompatible with life.

Cellular glucose metabolism is a two-stage process in which glucose is finally broken down to water (H_2O) and carbon dioxide (CO_2) (see Ch. 3). Put simply, glycolysis first breaks glucose down to pyruvate, which is then oxidised in mitochondria to CO_2 and H_2O. The second stage requires oxygen. If there is inadequate oxygen, either due to tissue oxygen lack or a metabolic abnormality, the pyruvate is converted to lactate, which is released into the blood stream, but may accumulate over time.

Lactic acidosis occurs when there is an accumulation of lactic acid, and blood and tissue pH is very low (acidosis). This can occur during conditions of extreme low blood pressure as in cardiogenic or septic shock, when there is a reflex vasoconstriction to abdominal organs, skin and other peripheral structures, leading to lack of oxygen. The acidosis compromises cardiac function, causing further vasoconstriction, oxygen lack and lactic acid production. This is potentially lethal if not corrected.

Some other causes of lactic acidosis include extreme, severe exercise, poisoning (e.g. ethylene glycol or anti-freeze), decreased lactate metabolism by the liver, and some drugs (such as the accumulation of metformin in diabetics with chronic renal disease).

Physiological range of pH

The normal pH of blood is about 7.4. Arterial blood is slightly less acidic at pH 7.45 than venous blood (pH 7.35). **Acidosis** occurs when blood pH falls below 7.35 and **alkalosis** is present at pH over 7.45. Death would ensue if blood pH falls below 6.8 or rises above 8 for a significant period.

Some physiological processes work best at pH values that are different from blood pH. Table 1.1 shows the pH values for some fluids. For example, muscle activity produces lactic acid, bringing the pH in myocytes to between 6.8 and 7, and sometimes below 6.4 (see Ch. 9).

Effect of pH on physiological processes

Many intracellular chemical reactions need to perform within a narrow range of pH, known as the **optimal pH**, at which they occur more quickly. Generally, optimal pH is similar to blood pH. However, depending on the normal pH of the compartment in which the reaction takes place, optimal pH can vary.

Chapter 8 (Nervous system) discusses the effects of changes in pH on the brain and peripheral nerves. A reduction in pH (acidosis) causes a reduction in excitability, especially in the brain, which can lead to confusion and, in extreme cases, coma and death. Conversely, an increase in pH (alkalosis) will produce unwanted nervous activity in the peripheral and central nervous systems. Nerves become hypersensitive and transmit signals in the absence of normal stimuli, producing symptoms such as numbness and tingling, caused by overactivity of sensory nerves. Overactivity in the nerves that excite the muscles can cause muscle spasms, which, in severe cases, can lead to paralysis of the muscles required for breathing. Excessive nervous activity in the brain may lead to convulsions.

Chapter 13 (Respiratory system) discusses the mechanisms for the respiratory control of blood pH, and the effects of pH changes on respiration – known as respiratory acidosis or alkalosis. Chapter 14 (Renal system) discusses the renal control of acid–base balance, and the effects of homeostatic imbalance – known as metabolic acidosis or alkalosis.

Sources of acid and alkali

Acids are by-products of metabolism. Carbon dioxide (CO_2), essential for the adjustment of pH, is a by-product of energy metabolism. Metabolism of dietary fats and proteins produce acid, and exercising muscles release lactic acid. Chapters 3 (Energy metabolism) and 16 (Diet and nutrition) discuss the breakdown of ingested food to provide energy for metabolic processes. Chapter 15 (Alimentary system) outlines the absorption and digestion of food, water and minerals. Chapter 14 (Renal system) describes how the kidneys produce acid.

Alkalis (bases) are not by-products of metabolic processes, but ingested in food (vegetables). The excess meat (protein and fat) in Western diets may lead to an increased production of acid. In health, this excess acid is dealt with by homeostatic mechanisms to maintain acid–base balance:

- Chemical buffers act to limit the free H^+ concentration of body fluids in the short term.
- Renal and respiratory homeostatic mechanisms increase the excretion of CO_2 and H^+.

Buffer systems

A **buffer system** limits changes in free hydrogen ions [H^+] in body fluids. The H^+ (acid) combines with weak acids (bases) in free solution, thus limiting any large changes in [H^+]. These systems consist of buffer pairs, which, at normal pH ranges found in the body, are only partially dissociated so both acid and base are present. If hydrogen ions are added to the system, they can bind to the base to prevent a fall in pH. If hydrogen ions are removed, then more acid dissociates to form H^+ so that the pH is unchanged. The amount of change that can be prevented depends on the amount of the buffer pair present. Three main buffer systems maintain a relatively constant pH in body fluids:

- Bicarbonate/carbon dioxide
- Proteins, particularly haemoglobin
- Phosphate.

The amount of H^+ that each buffer system is able to buffer is known as the **buffer capacity** (Table 1.2). Changes in pH are seen when the buffer capacity is exceeded.

Blood contains all the three buffer systems. In interstitial fluid, buffering is done by the bicarbonate and phosphate systems because there is very little protein in the ISF. The intracellular compartments also use all three systems, being rich in protein and phosphate, although the bicarbonate concentration is lower than in extracellular fluid (see Ch. 2, Table 2.4).

Bicarbonate/carbon dioxide

In blood, the bicarbonate/carbon dioxide buffer system performs an important role in acid–base balance. It is the main buffering system in extracellular fluids. It buffers H^+ from mechanisms that do not involve either bicarbonate ($H_2CO_3^-$)

Table 1.1	pH values for some fluids
Solution	**pH**
Hydrochloric acid (0.1 moles/L)	1.0
Gastric juice	1.0–2.5
Lemon juice	2.1
Tomato juice	4.1
Urine (average)	6.0
Saliva	6.8
Milk	6.9
Pure water (25°C)	7.0
Blood (average)	7.4
Sea water	7.9–8.3
Ammonia (NH_3, 0.1 moles/L)	11.1

Table 1.2	Buffer capacity of the main buffer systems in the blood	
Buffer system	**Capacity (mmoles H^+/L)**	
Bicarbonate/carbon dioxide	18	
Protein	1.7	
Haemoglobin	8	
Phosphate	0.3	
Total	28	

or CO_2, e.g. falls in H^+ in response to lactate production in exercise, or the use of fat as fuel substrate in diabetes. These processes are discussed in Chapter 3 (Energy metabolism).

In aqueous solutions, CO_2 forms carbonic acid (H_2CO_3), which dissociates into H^+ (acid) and HCO_3^- (base):

$$CO_2 + H_2O \rightleftharpoons H_2CO_3 \rightleftharpoons H^+ + HCO_3^-$$

The rate at which acids dissociate is known as the dissociation constant (K), referred to as the pK. A buffer is most effective when its pK is close to the desired pH.

Protein buffers

The acidic and basic protein side chains accept or donate H^+ to limit changes in pH. Chapter 2 (Biochemistry and cell biology) discusses the structure of proteins. The carboxyl and amino groups found at the ends of each protein chain also accept H^+. Proteins, e.g. albumin, in plasma buffer significant amounts of H^+.

Haemoglobin buffer system

Haemoglobin, a protein in red cells, is discussed in detail in Chapter 12 (Haematology). Its main function is oxygen transport in the circulation. Carbon dioxide, a waste product of metabolism, has a complex transport system, but haemoglobin also has a role in CO_2 transport. When CO_2 from tissues is taken up by haemoglobin, it is converted by the enzyme carbonic anhydrase in red cells to carbonic acid ($H_2CO_3^-$) which takes part in the bicarbonate/carbon dioxide buffer system. Haemoglobin also absorbs H^+ when H^+ combines with deoxyhaemoglobin (formed by the release of O_2 from oxyhaemoglobin), which has a higher affinity for H^+ ions. The movement of HCO_3^- into plasma is counterbalanced by the chloride shift of chloride ions (Cl^-) into red cells (Fig. 1.7).

Bicarbonate diffuses back into the plasma to be transported by the venous circulation to the lungs, where haemoglobin takes up oxygen to form oxyhaemoglobin. Oxyhaemoglobin has a low affinity for CO_2, which is released and exhaled.

About 10% of CO_2 in haemoglobin is carried as **carbamino haemoglobin**, where the combination of CO_2 with the haemoglobin molecule results in the release of further H^+ ions in addition to those generated from carbonic acid. Not all the H^+ ions are taken up by haemoglobin, so venous blood is slightly more acid than arterial blood (see Ch. 12).

Chapter 13 (Respiratory system) discusses disturbances in acid–base balance when the lung function is compromised: metabolic acidosis and alkalosis.

Phosphate buffer system

The phosphate buffer system is intracellular. It consists of dihydrogen phosphate, an acid, which dissociates to hydrogen phosphate and H^+.

$$H_2PO_4^- \rightleftharpoons HPO_4^{2-} + H^+$$

Phosphate buffering is an important mechanism for H^+ ion excretion by the kidneys. This is discussed in detail in Chapter 14 (Renal system). Whilst buffering systems control H^+ concentration, the excess H^+ ions have to be excreted. This is a renal function, where phosphate and ammonia are excreted and act as buffers for the H^+ secreted into the urine.

Control of acid–base balance

The control of acid-base homeostasis is performed by the lungs and the kidneys.

Respiratory control of pH (Clinical box 1.9)

The respiratory control of pH is dependent on the bicarbonate/carbon dioxide buffer system, which has the highest capacity of all the buffering systems. Chapter 13 (Respiratory system) discusses the mechanisms in detail.

In essence, the removal of CO_2 by the lungs restricts the amount of circulating free H^+ ions and thus the pH. If the pH falls, i.e. acidosis occurs, respiration increases either in the rate or depth of breathing to remove more CO_2. The removal of CO_2 allows the pH to rise. Conversely, if the pH rises (alkalosis), a compensatory decrease in respiration takes place, CO_2 is retained and pH falls. Breathing is therefore partly controlled by blood pH. Chronic lung diseases, with or without impairment of the respiratory centre, could lead to **respiratory acidosis** or **alkalosis** (Clinical box 1.9).

Clinical box 1.9   **Disturbance of acid–base balance related to lung ventilation: respiratory acidosis or alkalosis**

Gas exchange in the lung relies on two mechanisms:
- The bellows, consisting of respiratory muscles, and the chest wall, that pump the gases in and out of the lungs; and
- The lung structures, i.e. the airways, alveoli and blood vessels, responsible for gas exchange.

If either or both are damaged, then the take up of oxygen and the removal of carbon dioxide will be affected. The CO_2 content in blood is the main determinant of acidity (pH) in respiratory acidosis or alkalosis.

Respiratory acidosis is caused by CO_2 retention, when the ability of the lungs to remove CO_2 is reduced. Failure of any part of the gas exchange mechanisms could do this. Some examples include:
- Disease of the airways: chronic obstructive pulmonary disease (COPD), asthma, bronchial tumours
- Lung disease: emphysema
- Impairment of bellows: neuromuscular disease, chest wall and/or spinal deformities, interstitial fibrosis, disease of central respiratory control mechanisms (depression of respiratory centre, narcotics overdose, cardiopulmonary arrest).

Respiratory alkalosis is caused by abnormal, excessive removal of CO_2 through hyperventilation, which may be caused by anxiety or hysteria, brain injury or stroke, excessive mechanical ventilation and overdose of some drugs.

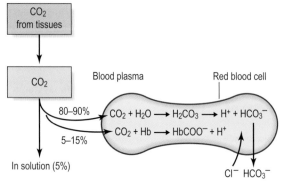

Fig. 1.7 Carriage of carbon dioxide in blood. Most of the CO_2 is converted to bicarbonate (HCO_3^-). The remainder is either in solution or combined with haemoglobin.

Renal control of pH *(Clinical box 1.10)*

The kidneys contribute to acid-base homeostasis by excreting H^+ and HCO_3^- in the urine. These are complex mechanisms, discussed in detail in Chapter 14 (Renal system). The renal secretion of H^+ and reabsorption of bicarbonate are the functions that control blood pH.

Renal H⁺ excretion

Carbon dioxide diffuses into the kidney tubule cells, where carbonic anhydrase converts CO_2 and H_2O to H_2CO_3. H_2CO_3 dissociates to H^+ and HCO_3^-; HCO_3^- is transported to blood, and H^+ is excreted in urine (Fig. 1.8). Nearly all the H^+ found in urine is secreted by the kidneys. To prevent H^+ diffusing back into the tubules, urine is kept at a pH of not less than 4.5.

Renal bicarbonate reabsorption

Bicarbonate is indirectly reabsorbed from the renal tubules because the cells lining the renal tubules are impermeable to HCO_3^-. The HCO_3^- in tubules reacts with secreted H^+ to form H_2CO_3 (Fig. 1.9). On the surface of the tubule cells,

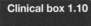

Clinical box 1.10	**Disturbance of acid–base balance related to renal mechanisms: metabolic acidosis and alkalosis**

Disturbance in acid–base balance from renal causes, known as metabolic acidosis or alkalosis, primarily affects the bicarbonate component of a system (see also Ch. 14).

Some causes of metabolic acidosis include:

- Over-production of acid, as in lactic acidosis (see Clinical box 1.8)
- Chronic renal failure when renal H^+ excretion is reduced
- Diabetic ketoacidosis, where alternative metabolic fuels other than glucose are used
- Bicarbonate loss from gastrointestinal disease
- Some drugs.

Some causes of metabolic alkalosis, although uncommon, include:

- Excessive acid loss, as in severe, prolonged vomiting of acid gastric contents
- Renal disease
- Some drugs, such as diuretics.

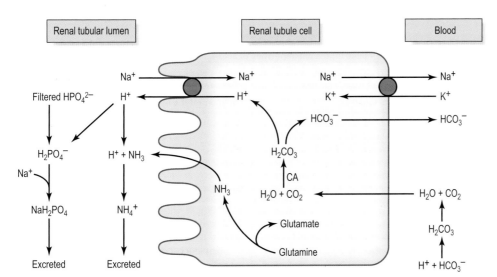

Fig. 1.8 **Renal excretion of hydrogen ions.** H^+ combines with phosphate or ammonia before being excreted. H^+ combines with phosphate (HPO_4^{2-}) and sodium ions (Na^+) to form NaH_2PO_4, which is excreted. If there is insufficient phosphate available, ammonia (NH_3), synthesised from glutamine in the tubule cells, is secreted into the urine where it combines with the H^+.

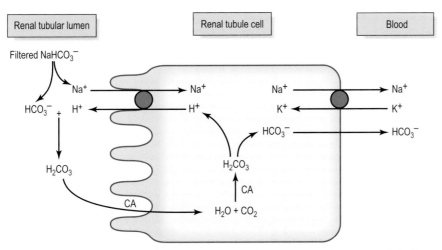

Fig. 1.9 **Renal reabsorption of bicarbonate.** One molecule of HCO_3^- is transferred from the tubular lumen to blood. CA carbonic anhydrase.

Clinical box 1.11   **An example of acid–base disturbance**

Table 1.3 was constructed using data from patients with different respiratory and metabolic acid–base disorders. This shows the range of changes in H^+, HCO_3^- and pH (Fig. 1.10) and is used to identify the type of acid–base disorder. Serial measurements for individual patients in graphic form are used to monitor the progress and effectiveness of treatment.

The arterial blood gases of an elderly man with emphysema showed the following:

- pH = 7.30
- pCO_2 = 50 mmHg
- Standard $[HCO_3^-]$ = 32 mM

As the pH is below 7.35, the patient therefore has acidosis. The pCO_2 is more than 45 mmHg, showing that the primary cause of the acidosis is respiratory. The standard $[HCO_3^-]$ is greater than 28 mM so he therefore has respiratory acidosis with renal compensation.

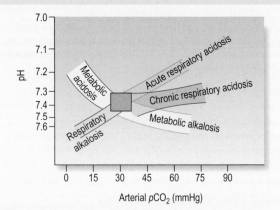

Fig. 1.10 **Acid–base graphs showing H^+ and pCO_2 ranges for acid–base disturbance.** Normal range = red shaded area.

Table 1.3   **Investigation of acid–base disturbance**

1. Measure arterial pH (normal range 7.35–7.45)

pH < 7.35: **Acidosis**	pH > 7.45: **Alkalosis**

2. Measure arterial pCO_2 and $[HCO_3^-]$ (standard bicarbonate). Normal values pCO_2 35–15 mmHg (4.8–6.1 kPa), $[HCO_3^-]$ 22–28 mM. The following shows the values for the different types of acid–base disturbance

pCO_2 > 45 mmHg (6.1 kPa): **Respiratory acidosis**	$[HCO_3^-]$ < 22 mM: **Metabolic acidosis**	pCO_2 < 35 mmHg (4.8 kPa): **Respiratory alkalosis**	$[HCO_3^-]$ > 28 mM: **Metabolic alkalosis**
3. Interpret the two measurements together		**3. Interpret the two measurements together**	
$[HCO_3^-]$ > 28 mM: Respiratory acidosis with renal compensation	pCO_2 < 35 mmHg (4.8 kPa): Metabolic acidosis with respiratory compensation	$[HCO_3^-]$ < 22 mM: Respiratory alkalosis with renal compensation	pCO_2 > 45 mmHg (6.1 kPa: Metabolic acidosis with respiratory compensation

carbonic anhydrase converts H_2CO_3 to H_2O and CO_2. The CO_2 diffuses freely into the tubule cells where intracellular carbonic anhydrase catalyses the reverse reaction to produce H_2CO_3. This then dissociates into HCO_3^- and H^+. The H^+ is secreted into the urine and the HCO_3^- diffuses into the blood. The net result is the transfer of one molecule of HCO_3^- from the urine to the blood.

When a mechanism fails, for example in respiratory acidosis, a compensatory renal mechanism may operate to retain bicarbonate, and $[H^+]$ could return to normal. In respiratory alkalosis, when CO_2 levels are persistently low, a compensatory metabolic acidosis may occur, although the response is usually slight (Clinical box 1.11 and Table 1.3).

Respiratory compensation of metabolic acidosis also occurs, when respiration increases to 'blow off' CO_2 and allows $[H^+]$ to rise in a respiratory alkalosis. There is usually a delay in this respiratory compensatory mechanism. Similarly, respiratory compensation for metabolic alkalosis, although slight, can occur.

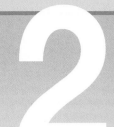

Biochemistry and cell biology

Marek H. Dominiczak

PRINCIPLES OF MOLECULAR INTERACTIONS   **16**
Atoms   16
Ions   16
Acids and bases   16
Chemical bonds   16
Organic compounds   17
Chemical reactions   18
The energy cycle in biology   18

CHEMICAL COMPOSITION OF THE HUMAN BODY   **20**
Chemical elements that form the human body   20
Water content and the main fluid compartments   20
Organic biomolecules   20

CARBOHYDRATES   **21**
Monosaccharides, disaccharides and polysaccharides   21
Complex carbohydrates   23

Lipids   **23**
Fatty acids   23
Cholesterol and other steroids   24
Complex lipids   26

Purines and pyrimidines   **26**

Nucleic acids   **28**
Deoxyribonucleic acid   28
Ribonucleic acids   31

Amino acids   **32**

Proteins   **33**
Structure of proteins   34
Protein synthesis and processing   36

Functions of proteins   39
Structural proteins   39
Catalytic proteins: enzymes   40

THE CELL   **43**
Cytoplasm   44
Cytoskeleton   44
Nucleus   45
Endoplasmic reticulum   45
Golgi apparatus (Golgi complex)   45
Mitochondria   45
Lysosomes   45
Proteasomes   46
Peroxisomes   46
Cell junctions   46
Cell adhesion and recognition   46
Signal transduction in cells   46
Receptors   47

Membrane transport   **48**
Passive diffusion   48
Carrier mediated transport   48
Coordinated action of transporters   50
Endocytosis   50
Exocytosis   51
Transcytosis   51
Receptor-mediated endocytosis   51
Transport of substances in the blood   51

Organs and tissues   **51**
Epithelial tissues   51
Connective tissue   53
Muscle   54
Nervous tissue   55
Integrated learning: the systemic approach   56

This chapter describes basic principles of chemistry and cell biology that underpin a large part of medical knowledge. Cell biology tells us about the structure and functions of the cell and its organelles, while biochemistry translates much of it into the language of molecules, their interactions and metabolic pathways.

We know increasingly more about pathways of cellular metabolism and, particularly, about their regulation by intracellular signalling systems and gene expression. The very aim of most medical therapies is to control these pathways when the normal regulatory mechanisms fail. Therefore, understanding these basics is not just intellectual indulgence: it provides one with tools to understand better the effects of disease and of therapeutic interventions.

We will start by considering fundamentals of the atomic structure, chemical bonds and chemical reactions, putting particular emphasis on the energy flow in biological systems.

We will then consider the chemical composition of the human body and discuss the most important classes of compounds: carbohydrates, fats, proteins and the nucleic acids. We will also discuss more complex molecules that are synthesised by combining the main classes of molecules.

In the third part of the chapter we will consider the cell and its organelles. We will highlight the function of cell membranes and associated structures which enable cells to communicate, transport nutrients and interact with other cells, forming tissues and organs.

PRINCIPLES OF MOLECULAR INTERACTIONS

ATOMS

Chemical reactions are exchanges of protons and electrons, and formation of a range of chemical bonds between atoms and molecules. They are associated with energy transfer – some require energy to proceed, and others release it during the process.

All atoms have a nucleus surrounded by an outer shell(s) of electrons. The nucleus contains **protons** and **neutrons**. The number of protons is the **atomic number** of an element and the total of protons and neutrons the **atomic mass**. The atomic mass of an element varies between **isotopes** (the hydrogen atom has just a single proton as a nucleus). See also Information box 2.1. Each of the electron shells contains a defined number of electrons in their orbitals:

- The first (innermost) shell has a maximum of 2 electrons
- The second shell has a maximum of 8 electrons
- Third shell: up to 18 electrons
- Fourth shell: up to 32 electrons.

A fully occupied shell makes an atom chemically inert (examples are the noble gases such as helium and neon). Atoms that have incompletely filled outer shells can react, until the shells are fully occupied. Finally, atoms that possess an unpaired electron that is not shared with other atoms are known as free radicals, and are highly reactive.

IONS

Normally there is a balance between the positive charge of the protons and the negative charge of the electrons, the atom being electrically neutral. However, when an atom loses or gains electrons, it becomes electrically charged: such an atom is called an ion. Charge can also be associated with groups of atoms.

- Anions are negatively charged ions and result from the gain of electrons.
- Cations are positively charged ions and result from the loss of electrons.

Electrical charge and electrical potential play a fundamental role in cellular functions such as membrane transport and in transfer of nerve impulses. Therefore ionic composition and ionic balance are key elements of human biochemistry. Formation of ionic bonds between atoms is one of the main mechanisms of chemical reactions.

ACIDS AND BASES

The concept of acid and base is also related to the balance between protons and electrons in atoms and chemical groups. It is particularly important in considering body buffers and the acid–base balance (see Ch. 1 and Information box 2.2). There are two closely related definitions of an acid.

According to the **Brönsted-Lowry** definition, an acid is a molecule that can donate protons, and a base is a molecule that accepts protons. Note that each acid molecule in a sense 'contains' a base (it is known as the conjugate base). Thus, when an acid loses a proton, the remaining species (now negatively charged) is its conjugate base:

$$HA \rightleftharpoons H^+ + A^-$$

Conversely, a base that accepts the proton becomes an acid.

According to the **Lewis** definition, an acid is a molecule that can accept electrons and a base is an electron donor. Note that a transfer of electrons from an acid to a base results in the formation of a covalent bond.

In this context it is worth remembering the definition of an **acid anhydride**: a substance formed by elimination of a water molecule during the reaction of two molecules of acid.

CHEMICAL BONDS

Chemical bonds determine how molecules join together. Atoms can form chemical bonds with other atoms of the same or different kind (Fig. 2.1). Bonds differ in their strength and stability, and are also a crucial determinant of the spatial conformation of molecules. The bonds most relevant to biomolecules are:

- Ionic bonds
- Covalent bonds
- Hydrogen bonds.

Ionic bonds

Ionic bonds are formed when ions are attracted to each other by their opposite electrical charge. An electron(s) from one atom moves closer to the nucleus of another. Importantly, such molecules dissociate into their component ions in an

---

Information box 2.1 **The carbon atom**

Carbon is the element contained in all organic molecules. The carbon atom is assigned an atomic number of 6 because it has 6 protons. However, it can have 6, 7 or 8 neutrons, forming different isotopes with different atomic masses. Carbon isotopes show no differences in chemical reactivity (Table 2.1).

Table 2.1 **Atomic mass of carbon isotopes**

	Number of protons	Number of neutrons	Atomic mass
Carbon 12	6	6	12
Carbon 13	6	7	13
Carbon 14	6	8	14

Information box 2.2 **Strength of acids**

Acids and bases have different 'strengths'. The strength of an acid is the ease with which it donates proton or accepts electrons. Strong acids dissociate completely, whereas weak acids dissociate to a limited extent. This tendency is described by the acid's unique dissociation constant (K_a), which is a ratio between its undissociated and dissociated forms:

$$K_a = [H^+] + [A^-] / [HA]$$

The derivative of the dissociation constant is its negative logarithm, the pK. The lower the pK_a, the more active is a molecule as a proton donor (a stronger acid).

Conversely, increasing pK_a means an increase in the basicity (alkalinity) of the conjugate base. Examples of strong acids are inorganic acids such as hydrochloric or sulphuric acid. The weak acids are carbonic acid (an important blood buffer) and the carboxylic acids. **The acidity or alkalinity of a solution also relates to the concentration of hydrogen ions (H^+) measured as its negative logarithm, the pH.** The neutral pH of pure water is close to 7.0. Solutions with pH less than 7.0 are acidic and solutions with pH greater than 7.0 are alkaline. The normal range of human blood pH is 7.35–7.45. The maintenance of stable pH of the body fluids is necessary for survival (see Ch. 1).

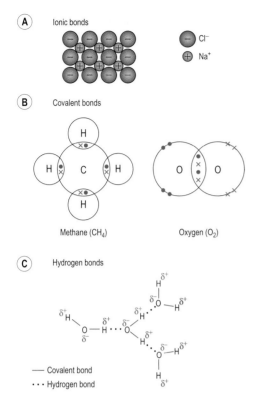

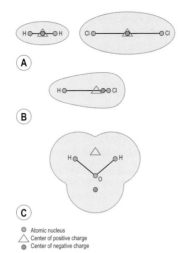

Fig. 2.1 **Different types of chemical bond.** In (C) δ$^+$ and δ$^-$ are partial positive and partial negative charges, respectively.

Fig. 2.2 **Polar and non-polar covalent bonds.** (A) Covalent bonds formed between atoms of the same kind are usually non-polar and the shared electrons are equidistant from both atomic nuclei. (B) A polar covalent bond may form between atoms of different elements, where the electrons are closer to the nucleus of one element than the other. Such a molecule acquires a partial electric charge. (C) Water is a dipolar molecule. Oxygen has a higher electronegativity than hydrogen and results in a charged molecule. Dipole-dipole interactions are the basis of attraction between many molecules known as hydrogen 'bonding' (see Fig 2.1C).

aqueous solution. For instance, **sodium chloride** (table salt) is formed when sodium (Na) and chlorine (Cl) atoms attract each other. In aqueous solution, Na loses an electron, becoming a cation, Na$^+$, while Cl acquires the electron, forming an anion, Cl$^-$. A strong ionic bond forms sodium chloride, NaCl. When the water is removed, salt crystals consisting of Na$^+$ and Cl$^-$ held together by ionic bonds are formed (Fig. 2.1A).

Covalent bonds

The covalent bond is fundamentally important in organic chemistry and biochemistry. The principle behind its formation is **electron sharing**. A pair of electrons is shared between two atoms making both atomic shells complete. This may occur between atoms of the same or different elements. Examples include oxygen (O$_2$), where two oxygen atoms form a double bond (O=O), hydrogen atoms sharing electrons with a single bond (H–H), and when carbon and hydrogen atoms share electrons to form methane (CH$_4$) (Fig. 2.1B).

Polar covalent bonds

A covalent bond is electrically neutral when the electrons remain equidistant from the two atoms that share them. However, when the nuclei of two bound atoms differ in their positive charge, the distance may become unequal, creating partial electric charges across the covalent bond. Such a bond becomes a **polar covalent bond** (Fig. 2.2) and the resulting molecule becomes a **dipole**. The water (H$_2$O) molecule is an example of a dipole. The strongly negative oxygen atom attracts electrons away from the two hydrogen atoms, which become positive. Because of this, they keep at a distance from each other. The water dipole can form hydrogen bonds with non-water molecules: this is the principle behind solubilisation of substances by water. The hydrogen ions can also associate

with other water molecules. This results in **water dissociation** into the hydronium ion (H$_3$O$^+$) and the hydroxide ion (OH$^-$):

$$H_2O + H_2O \rightleftharpoons H_3O^+ + OH^-$$

We normally simplify this in our notation and show water dissociation as:

$$H_2O \rightleftharpoons H^+ + OH^-$$

Hydrogen bonds

The hydrogen atom has a single proton as nucleus, and only one electron shell occupied by a single electron. When this electron is lost, the cation (H$^+$) forms. Such a cation can attract the negative pole of a dipolar molecule to form a hydrogen bond (Fig. 2.1C). These bonds are weaker than covalent and ionic bonds, and are easily disrupted by pH and temperature changes. They are important in stabilising the spatial structures of proteins and nucleic acids. Many large molecules contain numerous hydrogen bonds.

Non-polar molecular interactions

Non-polar molecules are water-insoluble (**hydrophobic**). Such molecules tend to aggregate in polar solvents; this is known as **hydrophobic interaction**. An example is the behaviour of lipid molecules in the plasma membrane. Another type of weak interaction, the **Van der Waals force**, makes molecules align in an energetically optimal conformation. These forces are effective at a relatively long range (up to 50nm) and are easily reversible. They, for example, contribute to the binding of substrates to enzyme molecules, and the binding of antibodies to antigens.

ORGANIC COMPOUNDS

An organic compound is a compound containing carbon atoms linked by covalent bonds. This definition usually excludes some small molecules such as carbon dioxide. Organic compounds may also contain oxygen, nitrogen and sulphur.

Table 2.2	Common functional groups and classes of compounds	
Group	**Formula**	**Class**
Hydroxyl	R-OH	Alcohols
Aldehyde	R-COH	Aldehydes
Ketone	R-COR′	Ketones
Carboxy	R-COOH	Carboxylic acids
Ester	R-COO-R′	Esters
Amino	R-NH$_2$	Amines
Imino	R-NH	Imines
Sulphydryl	R-SH	Thiols

The carbon atoms commonly bond with each other and with hydrogen, forming **hydrocarbon chains**. The hydrogen atoms in hydrocarbons may be replaced by other atoms or functional groups. Also, carbon atoms can share more than one electron with another atom, forming double or triple covalent bonds. Table 2.2 shows examples of the chemical groups that occur in different classes of organic compounds.

The carbon atoms may share four electrons with other atoms, including carbon atoms (Fig. 2.1B). For example, in methane (CH$_4$) the carbon atom links covalently with four hydrogen atoms. Importantly the carbon can form long chains (e.g. some fatty acids), which can also branch, or form rings (e.g. the steroids), containing either carbon only or carbon linked to other atoms such as nitrogen.

Spatial arrangement of organic molecules

A carbon atom within an organic molecule that shares its four available electrons with four different atoms (or groups) is known as the **chiral centre**. The chiral compound cannot be superimposed on its mirror image. Such a molecule can exist as variants which, while having the same formula, have different spatial orientations (they are **stereoisomers**). Stereoisomers are identified by the way they rotate the plane of polarised light. Those that rotate the compound anticlockwise (to the left) are l-isomers and those that rotate it clockwise (to the right) are the d-isomers. (These should not be confused with L- and D- forms which relate compounds to the l- and d-isomers of glyceraldehyde.)

Another type of isomerism is *cis-trans* isomerism, which relates to the arrangement that exists across the carbon–carbon double bonds. The *cis* configuration is when the two linked atoms reside on the same side of the double bond, and *trans* when they reside on the opposite sides. *Cis-trans* isomerism is particularly important in lipid chemistry.

CHEMICAL REACTIONS

The basic types of chemical reactions are:

- **Synthesis,** when a larger molecule is formed from smaller substrates
- **Lysis,** when a molecule is broken down into smaller compounds
- **Exchange reactions** where atoms, or groups of atoms, are exchanged between molecules (e.g. transamination reactions, where the amino group is transferred between molecules).

Electrophiles and nucleophiles

During a chemical reaction, atomic structures of reacting molecules are modified by transfer of electrons (or protons). The excess electrons from one atom may 'invade' the orbitals of another, forming new shared orbitals. The relevant terminology is as follows:

- **Nucleophiles** are negatively charged atoms that are electron-rich. They have a tendency to lose pairs of electrons.
- **Electrophiles** are positively charged atoms that are electron-poor. They accept electrons.
- A **nucleophilic attack** is a situation where the electrons from a nucleophile move into an electrophilic atom. Nucleophilic attack, for instance, underpins very common reactions of hydrolysis.

Oxidation–reduction (redox) reactions

Oxidation–reduction (redox) reactions are paired reactions in which electrons pass from one molecule to another. In the process, the energy trapped in the chemical bonds in the molecule being oxidised is transferred to the molecule being reduced.

Oxidation is a net *loss* of electrons with an *increase* in oxidation state by a molecule (the complete oxidation state is when an atom is maximally charged after all its electrons have participatd in ionic bonds).

Reduction is a net *gain* of electrons (or protons – hydrogen ions) with a *decrease* in oxidation state by a molecule.

Redox reactions are common and are fundamental for cellular energy transfer in biology. They underpin electron transfer from the reactants to coenzymes such as nicotinamide adenine dinucleotide (NAD) or nicotinamide adenine dinucleotide phosphate (NADP) and the operation of the mitochondrial electron transfer chain (ETC), the main cellular generator of adenosine triphosphate (ATP).

THE ENERGY CYCLE IN BIOLOGY

Energy required by living organisms is trapped in foodstuffs by plant photosynthesis, which consumes carbon dioxide and generates oxygen. Organic molecules thus produced then become metabolic fuel for animals. Their absorption and digestion by living organisms provide energy necessary for their survival. This energy is released in a highly controlled, stepwise manner during biological oxidations, resulting finally in the production of carbon dioxide and water. The released energy is used for the building up of sophisticated biological structures. It is used to support cellular transport, neural transmission and mobility as well as growth, reproduction, defence and repair.

Potential energy of chemical bonds

The formation of a chemical bond requires energy input and some potential energy accumulates in the formed bond (Table 2.3). This energy can be recovered when the bond is broken. An analogy is putting a bucket of water on a high shelf (inputting energy) and recovering the energy when the water is poured down to drive a wheel. The biologically important bonds that have a particularly high potential energy are the phosphoanhydride bonds formed between phosphate groups in molecules such as ATP.

Another mechanism of energy trapping is building up an ion gradient across a biological membrane. Energy input is

Table 2.3	Potential energy of some chemical bonds in biological systems	
Type of bond	**Energy (kJ/mol)**	
Ionic	12.6–29.3	
Covalent (single)	210–160	
Covalent (double)	500–710	
Covalent (triple)	815	
Hydrogen	4.2–8.4	
Van der Waals interactions	4.2	

required to create such a gradient; it is released when the ions 'return' across the barrier.

Energy flow in chemical reactions

The content of free energy (G) changes during chemical reactions. We describe the energetics of reactions in relative terms, indicating free energy change (G), which is negative when the energy content decreases, or positive when it increases. If a reaction releases energy it is **exergonic**, and when it requires energy input to proceed it is **endergonic**. The products of exergonic reactions have a lower potential energy than their substrates, and the products of endergonic reactions have higher potential energy.

Reactions where products have less potential energy than the substrates tend to occur spontaneously, whereas those where the potential energy of substrates increases require energy input. The key concept in biochemistry is that the energetically favourable reactions are used to drive the unfavourable ones. Let's imagine two reactions:

1. A+B > X and (endergonic reaction)
2. X+Y > Z (exergonic reaction).

Reaction 1 is energetically unfavourable. It occurs only very slowly yielding small amounts of the product X, according to its equilibrium. Reaction 2, on the other hand, proceeds spontaneously. Since its substrate is X, it depletes it, shifting the equilibrium of reaction 1 and 'forcing' it to proceed. This is a common pattern in various metabolic pathways. Note that the hydrolysis of ATP has highly negative G. Thus ATP can drive otherwise energetically unfavourable reactions.

Activation energy

Activation energy is the minimum energy needed to initiate a chemical reaction. This can be increased by increasing the temperature and/or the concentration of the reactants. A catalyst added to a chemical reaction lowers the activation energy and increases the rate of reaction, while itself remaining unchanged. The proteins called enzymes are biological catalysts. They make reactions proceed under the mild conditions of physiological temperature and pH.

Metabolic energy generation

The cellular energy flow depends on biological oxidations. The overall oxidation reaction in living organisms is the multistep conversion of organic compounds, in the presence of oxygen, to carbon dioxide and water. This is analogous to a combustion reaction but the difference is that in biology this 'combustion' proceeds by minute, carefully controlled, stages and under physiological conditions. The substrates for oxidation are highly reduced compounds, mainly carbohydrates and fats, known as

metabolic fuels (Information box 2.3). The process yields energy, a substantial part of which is chemically trapped for subsequent use. There are three major stages in this process:

1. **Ingestion of nutrients** and the liberation of the molecules of metabolic fuels (such as glucose and fatty acids) from more complex compounds. This is essentially the function of digestive processes in the gut. The fuels are then absorbed into the system.
2. **Metabolic conversions of the fuel molecules**: the oxidation of nutrient molecules. At this stage, the electrons (and protons) are transferred to 'mobile' intracellular coenzymes such as nicotinamide adenine dinucleotide (NAD) and nicotinamide adenine dinucleotide phosphate (NADP), forming the reduced NADH and NADPH, respectively. The NADH carries the electrons, accompanied by protons, to the mitochondria and transfers them to the ETC. (The NADPH is used in biosynthetic reactions.)
3. In the ETC, electrons and protons enter the sequence of further oxidations involving ferric iron complexes, cytochromes and other electron carrier molecules. The final recipient of electrons is the oxygen atom and a molecule of water is formed.

As the electrons proceed through the ETC, the 'remaining behind' protons are pumped out forming a gradient across the inner mitochondrial membrane (as said above, such a gradient acquires potential energy). These protons then return to the mitochondrial matrix through a membrane channel, which is part of the enzyme ATP synthase; the energy released by the returning protons is trapped in high energy bonds by converting ADP to ATP. The process is known as oxidative phosphorylation and the ATP formed becomes the 'energy bank' for the cell.

Anabolic and catabolic pathways

Metabolic pathways are chains of chemical reactions, classed according to their purpose. The **anabolic pathways** use energy in order to build up large molecules, and are usually associated with reductions; the **catabolic pathways**, on the other hand, break down large reduced precursor molecules. This is associated with oxidations.

Apart from NAD and NADH a number of other **coenzymes** are involved in the transfer of chemical groups between molecules (see below).

Information box 2.3	Metabolic fuels

Metabolic fuels are highly reduced compounds that can be oxidised in the body to release energy. The main metabolic fuels are carbohydrates and fats. Among the carbohydrates, the most important fuel is glucose. Its caloric value is 16.7 kJ (4 kcal) per gram. Importantly, under normal circumstances it is the only fuel used by the brain. Red blood cells also rely completely on glucose for energy. Muscle preferentially uses glucose at the start of exercise, switching subsequently to the use of fatty acids. A limited amount of glucose, sufficient for approximately 12 hours, is stored in the body in the form of glycogen.

Fatty acids, which yield 37.7 kJ (9 kcal) per gram, are the most efficient metabolic fuel. The amount of fat stored in the adipose tissue of a lean average human is sufficient for survival for more than 2 months without food.

Proteins can be converted to fuel (glucose) when glucose supply is insufficient. Their caloric value is also 16.7 kJ (4 kcal) per gram. The pathway of conversion of non-carbohydrate compounds to glucose is known as gluconeogenesis. The primary substrates for gluconeogenesis are the amino acid alanine and also glycerol and lactate.

CHEMICAL COMPOSITION OF THE HUMAN BODY

CHEMICAL ELEMENTS THAT FORM THE HUMAN BODY

The body contains mostly organic compounds, excluding the skeleton, which for a substantial part has an inorganic, mineral structure. Carbon, oxygen, hydrogen and nitrogen make up 88.5% of the dry body mass. The most abundant mineral is calcium (4%), followed by phosphorus 2.5%, potassium, sulphur, sodium, chlorine and magnesium (0.1%). Other elements are present in much lesser amounts: iron, for instance, constitutes only 0.01%. The elements that are present in less than 0.01% are known as the trace elements (e.g. manganese constituting 0.001%, or iodine 0.00005%, of the body mass). In spite of their minute amounts, many of them are needed as prosthetic groups or cofactors of enzymes.

WATER CONTENT AND THE MAIN FLUID COMPARTMENTS

Water makes up about 60% of lean body mass (see Chs 1 and 16). A 70 kg adult male has about 42 L total body water in two main compartments. Two-thirds of it is in the **intracellular fluid** (ICF) and one-third is in the **extracellular fluid** (ECF). ECF is further compartmentalised into the interstitial fluid, blood plasma and transcellular fluids, such as lymph and cerebrospinal fluid (CSF). The ionic compositions of ICF and ECF differ (Table 2.4). The transfer of water, ions and metabolites across cell membranes is fundamental to body functions. The main cations are sodium and potassium. Sodium and potassium ions are differentially distributed across the plasma membrane, with higher concentrations of sodium in the ECF (outside the cell) and higher concentrations of potassium inside. ICF also has a higher concentration of proteins and phosphates than ECF.

The ICF–ECF **ion gradient** is fundamental for cellular transport and **impulse transmission,** including **nerve impulses**. The differential distribution of sodium and potassium ions across the cell membrane creates an electrical potential known as the **resting membrane potential**. In most cells it is of the order of −60 mV, inside being negative (see Ch. 8). Changes in the electrical potential underlie the electrical signals generated by excitable cells (Clinical box 2.1; see also Information box 2.4).

Table 2.4 Composition of the extracellular and intracellular fluids

Ion	Approximate extracellular concentration (mmol/L)	Approximate intracellular concentration (mmol/L)
Na$^+$	140	12
K$^+$	4	140
Cl$^-$	110	4
Bicarbonate, HCO$_3^-$	25	12
Phosphates	2	13
Protein anions	9	138
Ca^{2+}	2.4	<0.0002
Mg^{2+}	1.0	0.8

Clinical box 2.1 Cardiac muscle is very sensitive to changes in K$^+$ concentration

Changes in the extracellular K$^+$ concentration alter the resting membrane potential of cardiac myocytes, which can change their excitability. Normal extracellular potassium concentration is 3.5–5.0 mmol/L but if levels fall below this then the myocytes will become hyperpolarised and cardiac excitation is reduced. If the K$^+$ concentration rises above 5.5 mmol/L, cardiac excitation increases. This carries the potential risk of arrhythmias and cardiac arrest (see Ch. 11).

Information box 2.4 Laboratory tests used in the assessment of water and electrolyte balance

The water and electrolyte balance of a patient is assessed by maintaining a record of intake and output of fluids known as the fluid chart (the record includes the amount drunk, the volume of intravenous solutions given, the urine volume and the volumes of fluids obtained during surgical drainage etc.).

This is complemented by measurements of ionic balance of the plasma. The set of common measurements, called in hospital jargon 'urea and electrolytes', includes measurements of sodium and potassium as the main cations, and chloride and bicarbonate as the main anions. The measurements of plasma urea and creatinine are normally included because they reflect kidney function – the most important determinant of the ionic balance.

Normally, the sum of sodium and potassium is greater than the sum of bicarbonate and chloride. The difference, which is normally around 10 mmol/L, is known as the anion gap (AG):

$$AG = (Na^+ + K^+) - (Cl^- + HCO_3^-)$$

The ions that contribute to the anion gap are all the anions that are not routinely measured, such as lactate or ketones. The gap can increase substantially when these anions accumulate as a result of pathological process (e.g. ketones in poorly controlled diabetes), and thus is of diagnostic significance for the physician.

Calcium ions (Ca^{2+}) are essential for muscle contraction (see Ch. 9), neurotransmission and most secretory processes.

ORGANIC BIOMOLECULES

The three main classes of organic biomolecules are carbohydrates, fats and proteins.

They exist in the body in their 'pure' forms but many important molecules combine them into molecules such as glycoproteins, glycolipids, nucleotides and nucleic acids. Amino acids, the components from which proteins are assembled, and lipid molecules such as cholesterol, also serve as precursors of a wide range of biologically important molecules including hormones and neurotransmitters (Table 2.5).

From the **energy flow point of view**, carbohydrates and fats are the main body 'fuels'. Proteins can be transformed into fuel when the supply of carbohydrates is poor.

From the **structural point of view** proteins form the main framework of tissues and organs, with lipids making a major contribution to the structure of cell membranes, and minerals to the skeleton.

Table 2.5	Macromolecules	
Macromolecules	**Monomers**	**Major functions**
Protein	Amino acids	Structural material, biological catalysts
Carbohydrates	Sugars	Energy source, cell surface markers
Nucleic acids	Nucleotides	Genetic information (DNA and RNA)
Lipids		Energy storage (triacylglycerols), cell membranes

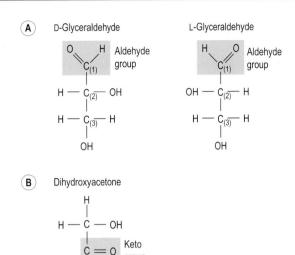

Fig. 2.3 **The trioses.** (A) Aldoses (showing stereoisomerism). (B) A ketose.

From the **functional point of view** proteins in the form of enzymes, transducer (signalling) molecules and antibodies provide the major part of body functions. They are synthesised, maintained and regulated according to the genetic information contained in the DNA, which itself is a molecule containing amino-acid derived structures (the purine and pyrimidine bases), carbohydrates and phosphate.

CARBOHYDRATES

Carbohydrates form about 2% of the body mass. They consist of carbon, oxygen and hydrogen, with a ratio of hydrogen to oxygen of about 2:1 (same as in water), hence the name 'hydrated carbon'. Carbohydrates have the general formula $(CH_2O)_n$ where n is the number of carbon atoms. They may exist as single molecules (simple sugars, **monosaccharides**), or their polymers (**polysaccharides**), which may contain thousands of units.

MONOSACCHARIDES, DISACCHARIDES AND POLYSACCHARIDES

Monosaccharides

The body obtains monosaccharides directly from the diet **or** by digestion of more complex carbohydrates. They can also be synthesised in the body from non-carbohydrate sources, and therefore their external supply is not required for survival. The simplest of the monosaccharides are the three-carbon sugars (trioses). Those that contain an aldehyde group are known as **aldoses**, and those with a ketone group are called **ketoses** (Fig. 2.3).

Like other types of organic molecules, the carbohydrates exhibit **isomerism**. In glyceraldehyde, a triose, the central carbon atom is chiral, and therefore it can exist as two (D- and L-) stereoisomers. All sugars larger than trioses have chiral groups and are divided into D- and L-series, according to which isomer of glyceraldehyde they originate, dextrorotatory (d/D) or laevorotatory (l/L), depending on the arrangement of atoms around the asymmetrical carbon furthest from C1. Virtually all sugars found in biological systems are D-isomers.

The five-carbon sugars (pentoses)

Two important pentoses are **ribose** and **deoxyribose**. They are components of the nucleic acids RNA and DNA, respectively.

The six-carbon sugars (hexoses)

The most important hexose is glucose, $C_6H_{12}O_6$, the central molecule in human energy metabolism. In aqueous solution, it can exist in four different forms (Fig. 2.4) forming both straight chain (less than 1% of all glucose molecules) and ring structures. Further, α- or β-glucose anomers differ by the arrangement of the hydrogen atoms and hydroxyl (–OH) groups on C1.

Other common hexoses are **mannose, galactose** and **fructose** (Fig. 2.5). Mannose and galactose are aldoses, and fructose is a ketose. Mannose and galactose only differ from glucose in the configuration of one of the carbons (mannose around C2 and galactose around C4) and are called **epimers**.

Amino sugars and sugar-derived acids

Monosaccharide molecules can be modified by other chemical groups. The introduction of an amino group on C2 of glucose and galactose yields the amino sugars **glucosamine** and **galactosamine**, respectively. The amino sugars, as well as sugars containing carboxyl groups (glucuronic and sialic acids), or sulphate, are components of the proteoglycans, key substances present in the extracellular matrix (ECM).

Disaccharides

Disaccharides are formed from two either identical or different monosaccharide units linked together by **glycosidic bonds**. These bonds link C1 of one sugar and the hydroxyl group of another. They are either α or β linkages, depending on the orientation around C1 (Table 2.6). Sucrose, the ordinary sugar, is a disaccharide made up of α-glucose and β-fructose linked by an α1→2 linkage. Two other dietary disaccharides are **maltose,** a dimer of glucose molecules, and **lactose** (milk sugar), made from glucose and galactose.

Polysaccharides

Polysaccharides are important storage compounds. **Starches,** which are polymers of glucose, serve as storage carbohydrates in plants. The simplest, **amylose,** has long linear glucose chains linked by α1→4 bonds. **Amylopectin,**

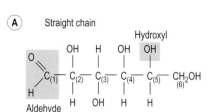

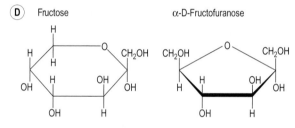

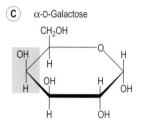

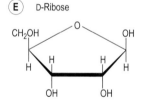

Fig. 2.4 Different forms of glucose. Each of these molecules has an identical chemical composition. A reaction between the hydroxyl group on C5 and the aldehyde on C1 produces the pyranose ring structure (B, C). If the hydroxyl group is on C4 then the furanose ring is produced (D).

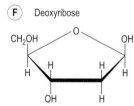

Fig. 2.5 Common monosaccharides. In (B) and (C) the part of the molecule which differs from glucose is highlighted.

which makes up about 80% of the starch in foods, has 1→4 linked glucose chains, which also contain 1→6 bonds, producing a branched molecule. The starches found in grains such as wheat, rice and potatoes are the major source of dietary carbohydrates. Amylases secreted by the pancreas and the salivary glands digest them releasing glucose, maltose and isomaltose.

Cellulose is the principal component of plant cell walls and is the most common organic compound on the planet. It is an unbranched glucose polymer linked by β1→4 bonds. Humans have no enzymes capable of hydrolysing these bonds. Cellulose and other non-metabolised polysaccharides form **dietary fibre**.

In humans, the carbohydrate storage molecule is **glycogen**. It is a large glucose, similar to amylopectin but with a more extensive branched structure. The high level of glycogen branching means that the molecule has a large number of free ends. This facilitates its rapid degradation to glucose. Glycogen stores glucose in a highly concentrated form, without the osmotic problems (attraction of large amounts of water, and thus increased volume) associated with a large number of separate glucose molecules. The size of glycogen stores is modest in humans, with approximately 75 g present in the liver and 250 g in skeletal muscle. It can supply glucose for 12–18 hours, after which time glucose needs to be synthesised from non-carbohydrate sources through **gluconeogenesis**.

Table 2.6 Principal disaccharides

Disaccharide	Carbon-1 sugar	Other sugar	Linkage	Digesting enzyme
Sucrose	α-Glucose	β-Fructose	1→2	Sucrase-isomaltase
Lactose	β-Galactose	β-Glucose	1→4	Lactase
Maltose	α-Glucose	β-Glucose	1→4	Maltase
Isomaltose	α-Glucose	β-Glucose	1→6	Sucrase-isomaltase

Table 2.7 Major glycosaminoglycans (GAGs)

GAG	Main source
Hyaluronic acid	Joints, ECF
Chondroitin sulphate	Cartilage
Keratan sulphate	Cornea
Dermatan sulphate	Skin
Heparan sulphate	Basement membranes
Heparin	Mast cells

Clinical box 2.2 Atherosclerosis

There is a link between raised plasma cholesterol (mostly in the form of low-density lipoprotein (LDL-cholesterol); see Ch. 16), and increased risk of coronary events such as angina or heart attacks. It is beneficial to reduce plasma cholesterol levels particularly in persons who already suffer from heart disease. Diets rich in polyunsaturated fats reduce serum cholesterol to some extent. Drugs that inhibit cholesterol synthesis by competitively inhibiting the regulatory enzyme 3-hydroxy-3-methylglutaryl-CoA reductase (HMG-CoA reductase), the statins are commonly used for cardiovascular disease prevention.

COMPLEX CARBOHYDRATES

Complex carbohydrates are carbohydrates that are covalently linked to proteins or lipids.

Glycoproteins contain carbohydrate chains bound to serine and threonine residues of proteins. Their carbohydrate content is 10–15%. The carbohydrates involved are most commonly mannose, galactose, fucose, xylose, the amino sugars such as N-acetylglucosamine and N-acetylgalactosamine, and glucuronic and sialic acids. The carbohydrate chains are relatively short, 10–15 molecules, and most often look like two- or three-pronged forks. They form highly variable structures important for cell and immune recognition including a variety of membrane receptors. Glycoproteins and glycolipids (see below) present on the surface of red cells constitute **blood group antigens**, the most important being the **ABO blood group system**.

Formation of a bond between the hydroxyl group of the amino acid side chain and the C-1 of N-acetylgalactosamine is known as **O-glycosylation** and the linkage between the amide group of the amino acid asparagine and the C-1 of N-acetylglucosamine is **N-glycosylation**.

Complex carbohydrates linked to proteins, known as proteoglycans, are key components of the ECM. They typically contain 95% carbohydrate. The carbohydrates are attached to a polypeptide chain, forming long, linear chains. The molecules are known as glycosaminoglycans (GAGs) or **mucopolysaccharides** (Table 2.7). Many GAGs are negatively charged and thus attract cations and large amounts of water, forming a gel-like substance. This imparts a degree of flexibility to the tissue, and acts as a shock absorber.

LIPIDS (Clinical box 2.2)

The lipids make up about 20% of body mass in adults of normal weight, more in women. They play a number of essential roles:

- They are key components of cell membranes.
- They are the major form of energy storage.
- They play important roles in cell signalling.

FATTY ACIDS

Fatty acids are hydrocarbon chains (Fig. 2.6A, B), with a carboxy group at one end (the α-carbon) and a methyl group (CH_3) at the other (the ω-carbon):

- **Saturated** fatty acids have all the carbon atoms in the chain linked by single bonds.
- **Monounsaturated fatty acids** possess a single double bond in the hydrocarbon chain.
- **Polyunsaturated** fatty acids have more than one double bond.

Most of the double bonds in biological molecules are in the *cis* configuration, which puts a kink in their hydrocarbon chains. Many of the fatty acids found in cells have 16, 18 or 20 carbon atoms and up to three double bonds. The most common fatty acid is the C18 **palmitic acid** (see Information box 2.5). The C20 **arachidonic acid** is one of the fatty acids incorporated into membrane phospholipids. It can be released from the membrane by the action of the enzyme phospholipase A_2 (PLA_2) on phosphatidylcholine, one of the membrane phospholipids. **Eicosapentaenoic** acid is the precursor of some prostaglandins. One of the double bonds in this acid is placed three carbons from the ω-carbon (such fatty acids are known as the ω-3 fatty acids). The ω-3 fatty acids are found in fish and originate from accumulated algae. Although thought to confer cardiac benefits, a recent meta-analysis has not found any evidence to support this.

Triacylglycerols

Glycerol is a C3 sugar alcohol, formed by the reduction of the aldehyde group of a triose to the hydroxyl group (Fig. 2.6C).

The **triacylglycerols** (also called triglycerides) are the storage form of lipids. They are esters of glycerol and fatty acids formed by dehydration reactions between the carboxyl group (COOH) of a fatty acid at each of the three hydroxyl (OH) groups of the glycerol molecule (Fig. 2.6D). Triacylglycerols are stored in the adipose tissue mainly as subcutaneous fat, and also as visceral fat, which surrounds the abdominal organs.

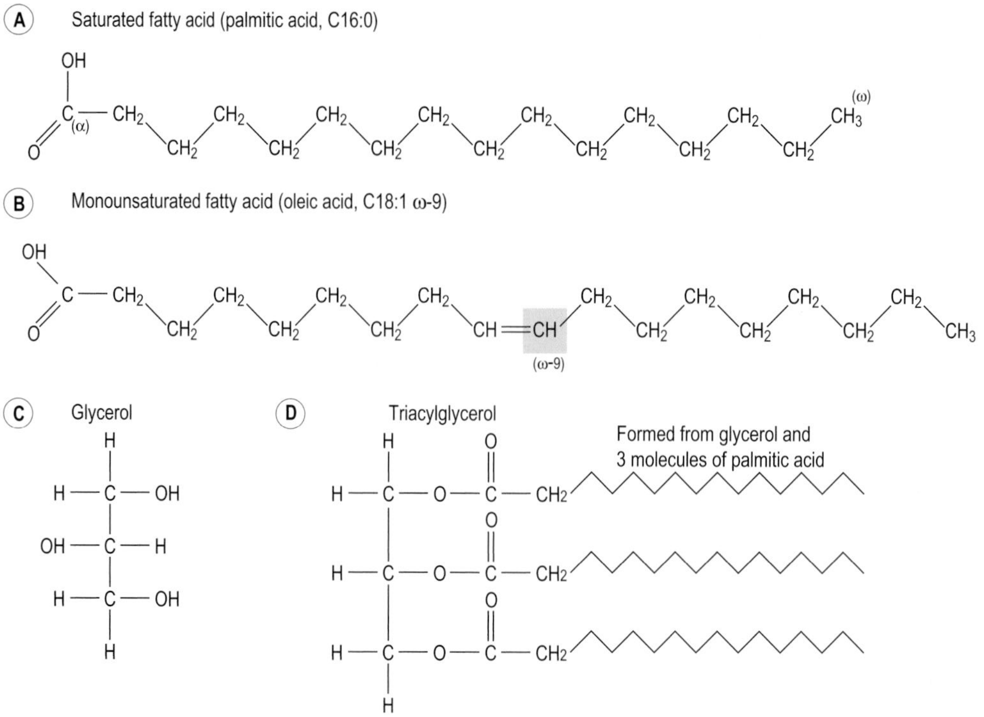

Fig. 2.6 **Triacylglycerols and their components.**

Information box 2.5	**Fatty acids can be named in several ways**

Fatty acids can be described according to the number of carbon atoms in the chain and the number and position of the double bond/s.

A shorthand notation that is widely used gives the number of carbon atoms, the number of double bonds and the position of the first double bond, counting from the ω-carbon. For example, the saturated fatty acid found in palm oil is called palmitic acid. The formula for palmitic acid is $CH_3(CH_2)_{14}COOH$, its chemical name is *n*-hexadecanoic acid and the shorthand notation is C16:0, indicating that it has 16 carbon atoms and no double bonds.

For arachidonic acid, its chemical name is *cis*-5,8,11,14-eicosatetraenoic acid, and the shorthand notation is C20:4 ω-6. The positions of all of the double bonds are noted as C20:4 all *cis*-$\Delta^5,\Delta^8,\Delta^{11},\Delta^{14}$ (see Fig. 2.7).

Dietary fats

Triacylglycerols are the main components of both solid and liquid dietary fats. The fatty acids which make up the triacylglycerol molecules determine the physical properties of the fat. Triacylglycerols composed of short-chain fatty acids, or unsaturated fatty acids, are liquid at room temperature. Examples of these are olive oil (containing oleic acid) and sunflower oil (which contains polyunsaturated fatty acids). Triacylglycerols that contain more saturated fats and longer fatty acid chains (for example, butter) yield fats solid at room temperature.

Essential fatty acids

Most of the fatty acids used in the body are supplied in the diet. Saturated fatty acids can be synthesised from carbohydrates (see Ch. 3). The saturated fatty acids can be converted to unsaturated fatty acids. However, **linoleic acid** and **linolenic acid** are **essential fatty acids**. They cannot be manufactured in the body, because none of the human enzymes can insert double bonds beyond C-10 in a fatty acid molecule.

Eicosanoids

Eicosanoids are derived from C20 fatty acids with between 3 and 5 double bonds. **Arachidonic acid,** synthesised from the linoleic acid, is the precursor of a large number of eicosanoids. The different groups of eicosanoids are prostaglandins, thromboxanes and leukotrienes. They are locally acting hormones with a very short half-life. They are important in the response to inflammation, and in the control of vascular smooth muscle contraction (Information box 2.6).

CHOLESTEROL AND OTHER STEROIDS

The **Cholesterol** molecule has a four-ring structure known as the sterol ring (Fig. 2.8). There is a hydroxyl group attached to ring number 1, and it can interact with water. Cholesterol is the major sterol in animals, while plants produce related sterols such as sitosterol and campesterol. Cholesterol is an essential structural component of the cell membranes. It decreases the fluidity of cell membranes. It is also an important precursor of a range of biologically important substances: bile salts, vitamin D and steroid hormones.

Most cells are capable of synthesising cholesterol. It can also be absorbed from the diet. It is distributed to tissues by lipid-transporting particles known as the lipoproteins.

Cells have a complex system, which precisely regulates their cholesterol supply, balancing the rate of synthesis against the external provision. The key regulatory points are the enzyme **HMG-CoA** reductive (regulating cholesterol synthesis) and the **LDL** receptor (regulating cholesterol uptake). The dysregulation of cholesterol balance leads to its high concentrations in plasma and contributes to the formation of atherosclerotic plaques.

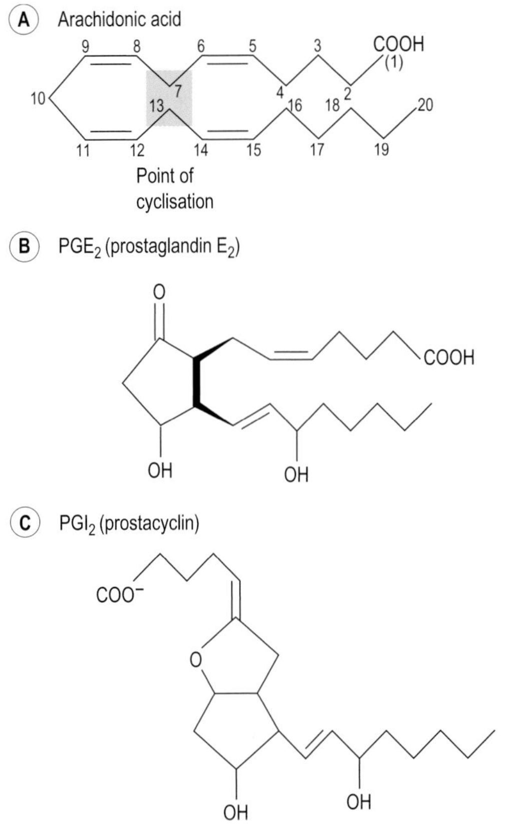

(A) Arachidonic acid

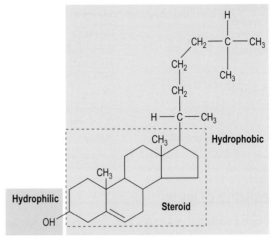

Point of cyclisation

(B) PGE$_2$ (prostaglandin E$_2$)

(C) PGI$_2$ (prostacyclin)

Fig. 2.7 **Arachidonic acid.** All *cis* 5,8,11,14-eicosatetraenoic acid (or alternatively C20:4 ω-6 Δ^5,Δ^8,Δ^{11},Δ^{14}) and two of the many eicosanoids derived from it, prostaglandin E$_2$ (PGE$_2$) and prostacyclin (PGI$_2$).

Information box 2.6	**Prostanoids facilitate blood flow through vessels and aspirin acts by inhibiting the synthesis of prostaglandin**

Prostacyclin released from the blood vessel wall acts as a vasodilator, thus encouraging blood flow. It inhibits the aggregation of blood platelets which leads to clot formation.

In contrast to prostacyclin, thromboxane A$_2$ acts as a vasoconstrictor, thus reducing blood loss through the leaking vessel wall, and stimulates platelets to aggregate, plugging the hole in the vessel.

The enzyme which acts on arachidonic acid in the first step of the production of the prostanoids is cyclo-oxygenase (COX). Aspirin (acetylsalicylic acid) belongs to a group of drugs called non-steroidal anti-inflammatory drugs (NSAIDs) which inhibit COX and reduce inflammation and pain. Aspirin is also used in cardiovascular prevention, to inhibit blood clotting.

Bile acids

Bile acids are essential for the absorption and digestion of fats in the intestine. They are synthesised in the liver from cholesterol, and are secreted as conjugates with the amino acids taurine or glycine. They are stored in the gallbladder and are secreted into the duodenum. They act as detergents in the gut, emulsifying dietary fats to aid their absorption (see Ch. 15). The secreted bile acids (primary bile acids) are further modified by the intestinal bacteria (forming the secondary bile acids). Bile acids are conserved by the body through reabsorption in the large intestine. This secretion-reabsorption cycle is known as the enterohepatic circulation of the bile acids.

Fig. 2.8 **Structure of cholesterol.** The figure inside the dashed blue lines is the basic steroid structure.

Vitamin D

Vitamin D is essential for calcium absorption and bone metabolism. Its precursor (cholecalciferol) is synthesised from 7-dehydrocholesterol in the skin under the influence of ultraviolet light. It requires two hydroxylations to yield the active forms of vitamin D. The first one, in the liver yields 25-hydroxycalciferol, and the second one, in the kidney, generates the active form, 1,25-dihydroxycholecalciferol. Vitamin D facilitates absorption of calcium in the intestine, its reabsorption in the kidney, and stimulates bone resorption. Analogously to steroid hormones, vitamin D acts through binding to an intracellular receptor (see Ch. 16).

Steroid hormones

Steroid hormones are all derived from cholesterol (Information box 2.8), after its conversion to another key metabolite, pregnenolone. The subsequent reactions lead to the synthesis of glucocorticoids such as cortisol, mineralocorticoids such as aldosterone, and oestrogens and androgens, including progesterone, the hormone that is important in maintaining pregnancy (Table 2.8) (see also Ch. 10).

Because steroids are lipid soluble, they cross plasma membranes and bind to cytoplasmic receptors – which, after activation by their ligands, become transcription factors and influence gene expression. They are usually carried in the plasma bound to binding proteins such as the cortisol binding globulin (CBG) (Table 2.9).

Table 2.8	**Key steroid hormones**	
Group	**Example**	**Major actions**
Glucocorticoids	Cortisol	Carbohydrate and lipid metabolism, proteolysis
Mineralocorticoids	Aldosterone	Sodium and potassium homeostasis, blood pressure control
Progestogens	Progesterone	Pregnancy and ovarian cycles
Androgens	Testosterone	Male sexual development and characteristics
Oestrogens	Oestradiol	Female sexual development and characteristics

Table 2.9	Selected transport proteins in plasma
Protein	**Ligand**
Albumin	Metal cations, free fatty acids, steroids, bilirubin, haem, therapeutic drugs
Transferrin	Iron
Thyroid-binding globulin	Thyroxine (T_4), Tri-iodothyronine (T_3)
Cortisol-binding globulin	Cortisol
Sex-hormone-binding globulin	Androgens and oestrogens

COMPLEX LIPIDS

Complex lipids are molecules that have lipid and non-lipid (particularly carbohydrate) components. The lipid component is hydrophobic and the non-lipid component is often hydrophilic. Therefore, they are **amphipathic** (both hydrophilic and hydrophobic) molecules that can orient themselves at lipid/water interfaces. They are important components of cell membranes. Their hydrophilic part faces the 'outside' of the membrane and the hydrophobic part orients towards the membrane core. Complex lipids also play a major role as components of the extracellular matrix (ECM).

Phospholipids

The complex lipids include **glycerophospholipids** and **sphingolipids**. They are formed from phosphatidic acid and from diacylglycerol. Phosphatidic acid is essentially a triglyceride molecule with one fatty acid residue substituted by phosphate. Diacylglycerol is a triglyceride where one fatty acid residue is substituted by a hydroxyl group.

Linking choline to the phosphate group of the phosphatidic acid produces lecithin, an important cell membrane phospholipid. Instead of choline, serine, ethanolamine and inositol can also be linked. The structure of phosphatidylserine is shown in Figure 2.9A.

Many of the phospholipid head groups are negatively charged, and thus the overall surface charge of the membrane is negative.

Sphingolipids

Sphingolipids have a structure similar to phospholipids, but instead of glycerol contain the alcohol **sphingosine** (an alcohol formed from palmitic acid and serine) (Fig. 2.9B). A molecule consisting of sphingosine with a linked fatty acid, (acylsphingosine) is known as a ceramide. When ceramide is linked to a choline, it forms sphingomyelin. When it binds a sugar it forms a cerebroside, and when it binds sialic acid it forms a ganglioside.

Sphingomyelin, cerebrosides and gangliosides are components of nerve tissue and the brain. Glycoproteins and sphingolipids also contribute to the structure of blood group substances.

Defects in the degradation of cerebrosides and gangliosides result in several rare clinical disorders known as the lysosomal storage diseases.

PURINES AND PYRIMIDINES

Purines and pyrimidines contain nitrogen in their carbon rings. They also have amino groups that are basic (thus the alternative name 'nitrogenous bases'). They are components of nucleotides and nucleic acids (Fig. 2.10). Purines are two-ring structures. The major purines are adenine and guanine. Pyrimidines consist of a single ring. The major pyrimidines are cytosine, thymine and uracil.

Nucleosides are molecules in which a sugar phosphate (**ribose** or **deoxyribose**) is linked to a purine or a pyrimidine

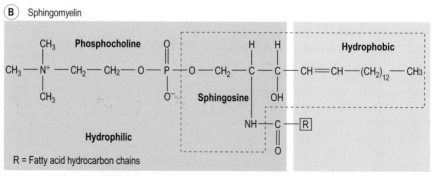

Fig. 2.9 **The structure of phosphatidylserine and sphingomyelin.**

(A) Purines

NH₂ Adenine (A)

Guanine (G)

(B) Pyrimidines

Cytosine

Thymine

Uracil

Fig. 2.10 Structure of purine and pyrimidine bases.

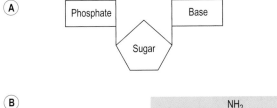

(A)

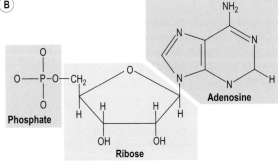

(B)

Fig. 2.11 Nucleotide structure. (A) Components of a nucleotide. (B) Structure of ribo-adenosine monophosphate (rAMP), usually referred to more simply as adenosine monophosphate.

(Fig. 2.11). **Nucleotides** are phosphorylated nucleosides (Table 2.10). There could be one, two or three phosphates attached to C5 of the sugar; each via phosphoanhydride bonds, forming nucleotide mono-, bi- or tri-phosphates. Nucleotides are the modules that form nucleic acids. In

addition, the free nucleotides play important roles in energy transfer and cell signalling.

Purines are components of nucleotide coenzymes such as ATP and GTP (Fig. 2.12 and Information box 2.7). The cyclic nucleotides derived from them, also containing purines, are cyclic adenine monophosphate (**cAMP**) and cyclic guanosine monophosphate (**cGMP**). Both are involved in signal transduction (Table 2.10). Other key coenzymes, **NAD**, the **NADP**, the flavin adenine dinucleotide (**FAD**) and **coenzyme A**, are all derived from the adenine nucleotide (Clinical box 2.3).

Synthesis and degradation of nucleotides

The purines can be synthesised de novo from 5-phosphoribosyl pyrophosphate (PRPP), a derivative of ribose supplied by the pentose phosphate pathway, a pathway which branches off from the glycolysis. They are synthesised in reactions involving the amino acids glutamine, aspartate and glycine, CO_2 and the coenzyme tetrahydrofolate, which transfers single carbon residues between molecules. The result is the nucleotide inosine monophosphate (IMP), the precursor of the purines (See also Information box 2.7).

The precursor of pyrimidines is a 1-carbon molecule, carbamoyl phosphate. The pyrimidine synthesis pathway involves the amino acids glutamine and aspartate, and also the bicarbonate anion. The pathway yields uridine monophosphate (UMP) from which other pyrimidines are synthesised.

Table 2.10	Nucleosides and nucleotides (nucleoside phosphates)				
Base	Nucleoside	Nucleoside monophosphates	Nucleoside diphosphates	Nucleoside triphosphates	Cyclic nucleotides
Adenine	Adenosine	AMP	ADP	ATP	cAMP
Guanine	Guanosine	GMP	GDP	GTP	cGMP
Cytosine	Cytidine	CMP	CDP	CTP	
Uracil	Uridine	UMP	UDP	UTP	
Thymine	Thymidine	TMP	TDP	TTP	

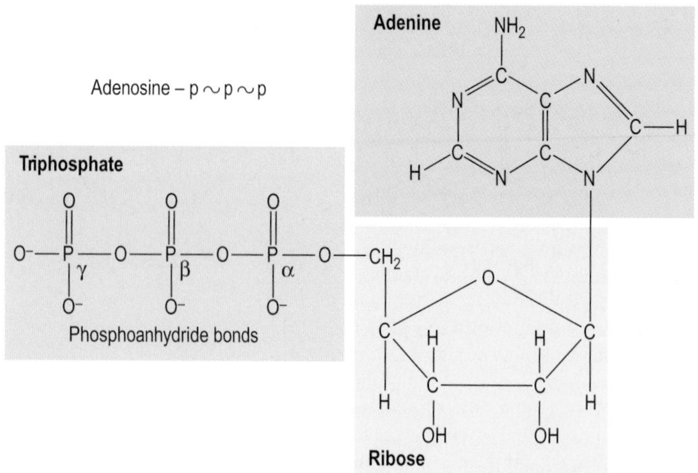

Adenosine – p ～ p ～ p

Adenine

Triphosphate

Phosphoanhydride bonds

Ribose

Fig. 2.12 **Structure of adenosine triphosphate (ATP).** The symbol ~ denotes high-energy bonds.

Information box 2.7 **Adenosine triphosphate (ATP)**

The most important of the nucleoside phosphates is adenosine triphosphate or ATP (Fig. 2.17). ATP is a highly mobile cellular energy store. It also participates in many metabolic regulatory loops, controlling the activity of key enzymes.

The phosphoanhydride bonds between the second (β) and third (γ) phosphate groups of the ATP release energy on hydrolysis, yielding about 7.3 kcal/mol each. These bonds are usually depicted by ~, indicating that they are high-energy bonds.

Most of the ATP in the cell is formed during oxidative phosphorylation in the mitochondrial electron transfer chain (ETC). A reaction that results in ATP synthesis by the transfer of a phosphate group from another phosphorylated compound outside the ETC is known as substrate-level phosphorylation.

Clinical box 2.3 **Excess purines can cause disease**

In humans, excess purines are broken down to uric acid. If large amounts of uric acid are produced and not removed by the kidneys, uric acid crystals are deposited in joints and soft tissues, resulting in gout. One treatment of gout blocks the enzyme xanthine oxidase, which catalyses the last steps in the production of uric acid. The intermediate breakdown products are more water soluble than uric acid and can be excreted.

Deficiencies in one of the enzymes involved in the recycling pathways leads to increased purine synthesis and a concomitant increase in uric acid, leading to a condition known as Lesch–Nyhan syndrome. One of the features of Lesch–Nyhan syndrome is gout. Patients may also go on to develop arthritis and severe mental disorders.

Information box 2.8 **Anti-cancer drugs may act by inhibiting nucleotide synthesis**

One of the ways of treating cancer is by blocking the rapid proliferation of the cancer cells. Many of the side-effects of anti-cancer drugs can be accounted for by their effect on cells that are normally rapidly dividing, such as hair and intestinal cells.

A commonly used anti-cancer drug, methotrexate, acts by inhibiting an enzyme involved in the production of thymidine nucleotides. Methotrexate is an analogue of dihydrofolate, which acts as a competitive inhibitor of the enzyme dihydrofolate reductase. Other cytotoxic agents act by inhibiting other points in the production of nucleic acids.

Ribonucleotides are reduced to deoxyribonucleotides by nucleotide reductase, producing purine and pyrimidine nucleotides that make up the DNA. Folic acid (a B vitamin) is required for the synthesis of the deoxyribonucleotides TMP (a thymidine nucleotide) from deoxyuridine monophosphate (dUMP) (see also Information box 2.7).

Purines are degraded to uric acid, and pyrimidines to a Krebs cycle metabolite, succinyl-CoA.

Nucleotide recycling: the salvage pathways

De novo synthesis of nucleotides requires a large amount of energy. There are, however, the so-called salvage pathways which recycle the purines and pyrimidines before they are completely degraded, and re-incorporate them into nucleotides.

NUCLEIC ACIDS

Deoxyribonucleic acid (DNA) and the **ribonucleic acids** (RNAs) contain and transmit genetic information in all biological organisms. They ensure structural and functional continuity of an organism through generations. Both DNA and RNA are polymers of nucleotides. DNA forms very long chains, while RNAs are of very variable size. Both DNA and RNA are made from only four different nucleotides each.

DEOXYRIBONUCLEIC ACID

DNA is found in all cells capable of dividing. Most of the DNA within a cell is found in the nucleus. A small amount is present in the mitochondria. In the prokaryotic cells (bacteria) and some viruses (DNA viruses) DNA is present in the cytoplasm.

DNA is a polymer of deoxyribonucleotides, and forms a double-stranded molecule, with a characteristic double-helical structure. There are four nucleotide 'modules' in the DNA and RNA: two are purine and two pyrimidine nucleotides. The purines, adenine (designated A) and guanine (G), are found in both DNA and RNA. With regard to pyrimidines,

DNA contains cytosine (C) and thymine (T), and RNA contains cytosine (C) and uracil (U) (Fig. 2.10).

The primary structure of the nucleic acids

The primary structure of the nucleic acids is their sequence of nucleotides (Information box 2.9). In the nucleic acid chains nucleoside phosphates are linked by phosphodiester bonds between the sugar and phosphate groups (Fig. 2.13). The hydroxyl group at C-3 of the sugar links with the phosphate on the C-5 on the next nucleotide. The bases are attached to the C-1 of each sugar.

When nucleotides are being attached to the nucleic acid during its synthesis, the substrates are nucleotide triphosphates, and a pyrophosphate (PPi) is released during the reaction. The nucleotide chain grows in the 5'→3' direction.

Secondary structure of DNA

The secondary structure of DNA is the spatial arrangement of the nucleotide chains. The two strands of the DNA molecule are held together by hydrogen bonds. Its secondary structure is dependent on the **pairing** between the bases that project from the sides of the sugar–phosphate backbone of each of the two strands.

The pairs of nitrogenous bases, each consisting of a purine and a pyrimidine, are linked by hydrogen bonds. The bases can only form specific pairs (AT and GC) (Fig. 2.14). The AT pairs form two hydrogen bonds, and the GC pairs have three hydrogen bonds. The two types of pairs are the same width, therefore the double strands are held at the same distance apart throughout their length. The two complementary strands of the DNA molecule run in opposite directions from one another (they are anti-parallel). One is the 3'→5' chain and the other the 5'→3' chain.

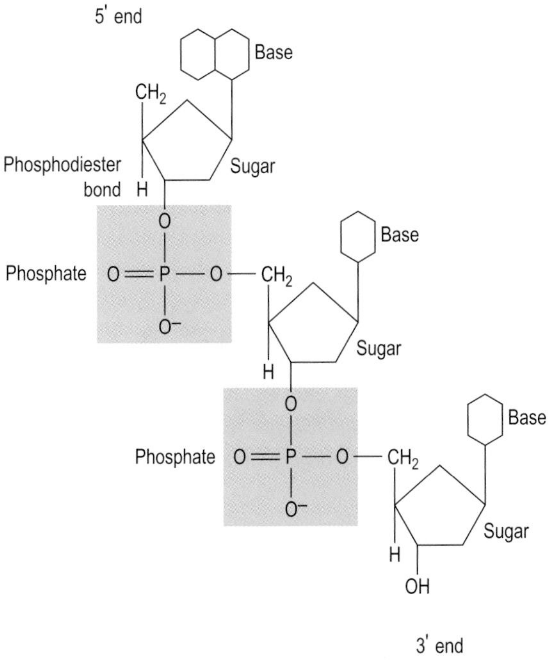

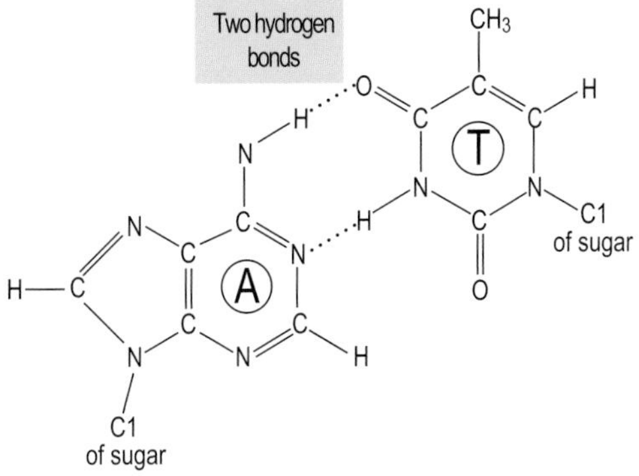

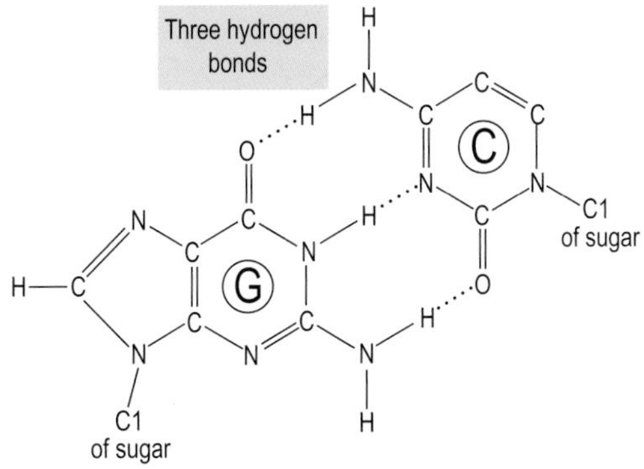

Fig. 2.14 Base pairing between adenine and thymine (or uracil) (A-T; or U) and guanine and cytosine (G-C).

The base pairs have a planar structure, and therefore can be 'stacked' one on top of another in the core of the DNA molecule. In addition to the hydrogen bonds between the bases, hydrophobic interactions occur 'vertically' between the stacked base pairs. The negatively charged phosphate groups and the sugar backbone remain on the outside.

The double helix

The DNA molecule forms a right-handed helix with 10 base pairs (bp) and 3.4 nm distance for each turn. Since there are no 'vertical' hydrogen bonds between nucleotides, the DNA molecule is not rigid. There are two grooves with different widths, the major and the minor groove, formed along the outside of the molecule. Most DNA exists in this form, called the B form (Fig. 2.15).

Fig. 2.13 The strand of nucleotides in a nucleic acid.

Information box 2.9	Deletion of a single base from DNA will frame shift the protein

If a single nucleotide is removed from a gene, the entire subsequent triplet sequence of the genetic code will change (this is known as a frameshift mutation). If the deletion is near the end of the coding sequence, then the protein may be nearly normal, but if it is close to the beginning then changes can be major. Normal haemoglobin is composed of two polypeptide chains, α- and β-globin, folded to hold the haem molecule. β-Thalassaemia is an inherited anaemia characterised by a point mutation in the β-globin chain. The resulting frame shift produces a protein that is unstable. The globin chains in red cells can precipitate causing haemolysis, and a severe anaemia in those individuals who have inherited the abnormality from both parents.

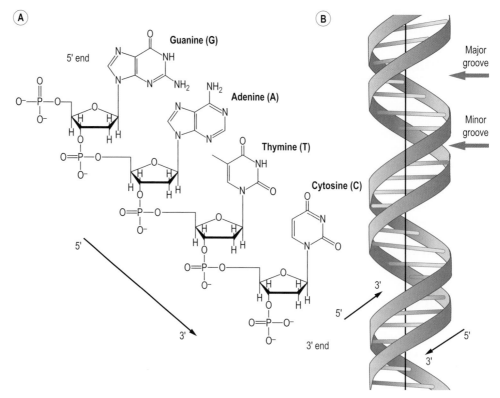

Fig. 2.15 **The structure of DNA.** (A) The details of nucleotide sequence in a fragment of the DNA strand. (B) The double helix showing the major and the minor grooves. Reproduced with permission from Dominiczak MH 2012 Flash cards in biochemistry. London, Elsevier.

Complementarity of the DNA strands

The two strands of DNA are **complementary**. This means that a particular sequence on one strand is reflected by a specific sequence on the other. For example, the sequence TGCT in one strand would be reflected by the sequence ACGA in the other. Complementarity is fundamental for the generation of identical copies of DNA during its replication.

Tertiary structure of DNA: chromatin and the nucleosomes

The largest human DNA molecules are nearly 10 cm long when fully extended, and have $2–3 \times 10^8$ nucleotide pairs. This large molecule must be packed into the cell nucleus and must uncoil easily when its segments are about to be copied.

In the nucleus, DNA is combined with protein, forming **chromatin**. Chromatin consists of a series of structures called **nucleosomes** (Fig. 2.16). Each nucleosome contains a core of proteins called histones, around which loops of DNA are wrapped, with a piece of linker DNA between each nucleosome (Fig. 2.16A). The nucleosome 'string' is then folded again, forming a supercoiled structure (Fig. 2.16B,C). Such multiple folding reduces the length of the DNA molecule about 8000-fold.

The genetic material in eukaryotes is organised into the chromosomes, each of which contains a single DNA molecule. There are 23 pairs of chromosomes in human cells, each characterised by a specific size and shape. When cells are about to divide, the chromatin concentrates still further (Fig. 2.16D), and the chromosomes become visible under a light microscope.

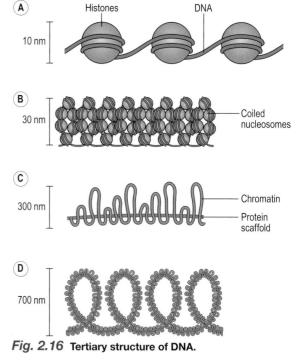

Fig. 2.16 **Tertiary structure of DNA.**

Mitochondrial DNA

The mitochondria contain their own mitochondrial DNA (mtDNA) as well as the machinery to make proteins. mtDNA is present in the mitochondrial matrix and codes for some of the molecules needed by the mitochondrion, including its own rRNA and tRNA. The mtDNA is a circular molecule similar to bacterial DNA. This is used as evidence that mitochondria originated as free-living bacteria, before forming a symbiotic relationship with what later became eukaryotic cells.

DNA replication

DNA replication ensures the continuity of genetic material through generations. The DNA molecule is copied during the interphase, which precedes cell division (Ch. 5). During replication the DNA unwinds, and a new complementary strand is synthesised against each of the two parent strands. Thus each new DNA molecule contains one new and one old strand: the replication is **semi-conservative**.

The double-stranded DNA is unwound by the action of a number of enzymes, including helicases, which separate the strands at a location called the **origin of replication**. In eukaryotes there are many such replication sites. The separation is maintained by proteins that bind to the separate strands (Fig. 2.17). The two DNA strands are called sense and antisense.

The replication process is 'primed' by the binding of the priming RNA polymerase called primase. The new antisense strand is then synthesised by **DNA polymerase III**; the RNA primer is subsequently removed. Replication can proceed in both directions away from the primer.

The DNA polymerase travels along the leading strand in the 3′ to 5′ direction, adding new nucleotides to the 3′ end of the new strand. The other strand, known as the lagging strand, is replicated in fragments known as Okazaki fragments. At the end of the process the fragments are joined together by DNA ligase.

DNA proofing and repair

DNA polymerase III also controls the accuracy of replication by checking that the bases on the original strand and the new strand are complementary. If they are not, then the incorrect nucleotide is excised and replaced (Clinical box 2.4). The error rate in replication is very low. It is estimated that the error rate before proofreading is about 1 in 10 000, but with the replacement of wrong nucleotides this falls to 1 in 10^8–10^{12}. However, it does not eliminate all errors.

There are two other major mechanisms of continuous repair of the DNA. They have been studied extensively in bacteria. The repair process is initiated by **DNA glycosylases,** enzymes that remove nitrogenous bases but leave the

sugar-phosphate chain intact. Larger segments are repaired by removal of the damaged section by **DNA helicase**, and its replacement by DNA polymerase. The new fragment is attached to the DNA strand by **DNA ligase**.

Damage to DNA

The DNA of a cell is subjected to damage by high-energy radiation, the reactive oxygen species (the free radicals), and many mutagenic chemicals. These processes have been estimated to produce up to 60 000 base modifications per day. Many of the modifications produce no discernible effect, possibly because they occur in non-essential regions of DNA or do not change the activity of the gene product. Some, however, are detrimental to the cell. Mutations in somatic cells can lead to cancers, with the uncontrolled proliferation of cells. Mutations in gametes can lead to inherited metabolic errors.

RIBONUCLEIC ACIDS

RNA is found in all cells (except red blood cells), including prokaryotes and some viruses. Several types of RNA are present in eukaryotic cells. These are:

- **Messenger RNA** (mRNA) serves as a template for protein synthesis and is synthesised during transcription. It is a copy of the transcribed gene. It subsequently moves from the nucleus to the cytoplasm, where it binds protein-synthesising ribosomes.
- **Transfer RNAs** (tRNAs) are a range of relatively small molecules which bind specific amino acids in the cytoplasm and move them to the ribosome for protein synthesis. About 50 different tRNA molecules are produced in animal cells, each between 70 and 90 nucleotides long.
- **Ribosomal RNA** (rRNA) together with proteins contributes to the structure of the ribosome.
- **Small nuclear RNAs** (snRNAs) are involved in mRNA processing.
- **Micro RNAs** (**miRNAs**) including small interfering RNA (siRNA) participate in the regulation of gene expression.

Secondary structure of RNA

RNA molecules are single-stranded and have variable coiling patterns. Parts of the molecule can form loops or hairpins between complementary regions of its single strand. The tRNAs have a cloverleaf shape with four stem-loops, each of which forms a short double helix (Fig. 2.18).

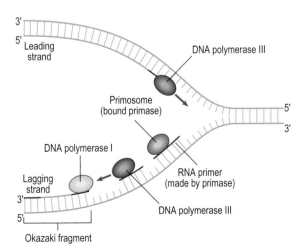

Fig. 2.17 **DNA replication.**

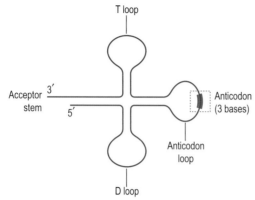

T loop

Acceptor stem 3′
5′

Anticodon (3 bases)

Anticodon loop

D loop

Fig. 2.18 **General structure of tRNA.**

AMINO ACIDS

Amino acids are the structural units of proteins. They contain short hydrocarbon chains of variable length, oxygen atoms and nitrogen. Apart from being incorporated into proteins, amino acids are precursors of nucleosides, neurotransmitters and haem, among many other molecules (see Ch. 3). They can also be converted into carbohydrates through gluconeogenesis, and therefore are a potential energy source.

In contrast to carbohydrates and fats, amino acids are not stored in the body. The amino acid 'reserve' is the muscle mass. Thus, when the fuel supply is short, muscle proteins are used up to synthesise glucose. This is why starvation – or chronic disease – is associated with muscle wasting.

Note that amino acids are designated by a set of three-letter abbreviations and a set of single-letter abbreviations. In humans, 20 amino acids are used in protein synthesis (Table 2.11). Of these, 8 (9 in infants) are known as **essential amino acids**, because they must be supplied by the diet (see Ch. 16).

Table 2.11	Amino acids found in human proteins		
Classification	**Amino acid**	**Abbreviations**	
	Glycine	Gly	G
	Alanine	Ala	A
	Valine	Val	V
	Leucine	Leu	L
	Isoleucine	Ile	I
	Proline	Pro	P
Non-polar aromatic	Phenylalanine	Phe	F
	Tyrosine	Tyr	Y
	Tryptophan	Trp	W
Polar uncharged	Serine	Ser	S
	Threonine	Thr	T
	Asparagine	Asn	N
	Glutamine	Gln	Q
Polar negatively charged	Glutamic acid	Glu	E
	Aspartic acid	Asp	D
Polar positively charged	Lysine	Lys	K
	Arginine	Arg	R
	Histidine	His	H
Sulphur-containing	Cysteine	Cys	C
	Methionine	Met	M

Structure of the amino acids

The structure of an amino acid includes a chiral carbon atom (the α-carbon), attached to four different chemical groups (Fig. 2.19): the hydrogen atom (–H), the amino group (–NH$_2$), the carboxyl group (–COOH) and a side chain (–R). The chirality means that amino acids (except glycine) can exist as two stereoisomers (enantiomers) named D and L. With very few exceptions, only the L-amino acids are incorporated into proteins. D-Amino acids are present in bacterial walls. The side chains of the amino acids vary in length and chemical complexity, and determine the characteristics of these molecules.

Dissociation of amino acids

Amino acids are dipolar ions (zwitterions): they carry a positive charge at one end and a negative charge at the other end of the molecule. The carboxyl group ionises at the physiological pH forming an anion (COO$^-$) and the amino group becomes a cation (NH$_3^+$) (Fig. 2.19). In addition, there might be different charged groups in the side chains. Amino acids that have polar side chains form hydrogen bonds with water and thus tend to locate on the 'outside' of protein molecules. In contrast, the non-polar, hydrophobic, amino acids locate in the core of protein molecules where they are not exposed to water.

Classification of amino acids

Amino acid side chains vary from a single hydrogen atom (in glycine) to the relatively complex cyclic side chains of tryptophan and the branched molecules of lysine and valine (Fig. 2.20). Amino acids are classified into the following groups:

- **Non-polar aliphatic**: amino acids with linear hydrocarbon side chains.
- **Non-polar aromatic**: amino acids with side chains containing ring structure.
- **Polar neutral**: amino acids with side chains containing polar hydroxyl or amide groups. The hydroxyl groups of serine, threonine and tyrosine on the surface of proteins may undergo phosphorylation.
- **Polar negatively charged**: amino acids with side chains containing carboxyl groups that are negatively charged at pH 7.

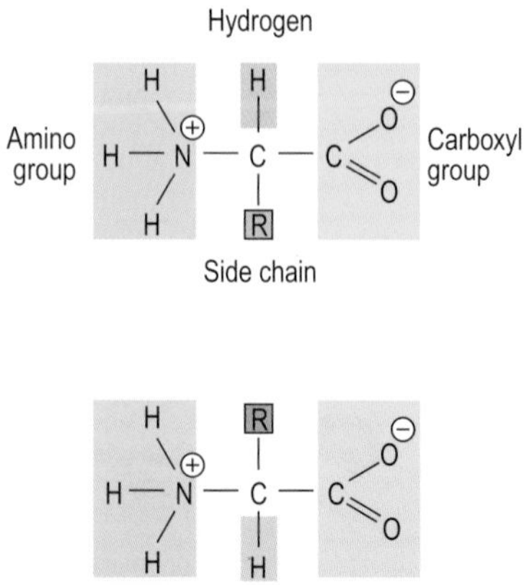

Hydrogen

Amino group

Carboxyl group

Side chain

Fig. 2.19 **Two stereoisomers of an amino acid with ionised NH$_3^+$ and COO$^-$ groups.** The two molecules are mirror images of each other and cannot be superimposed.

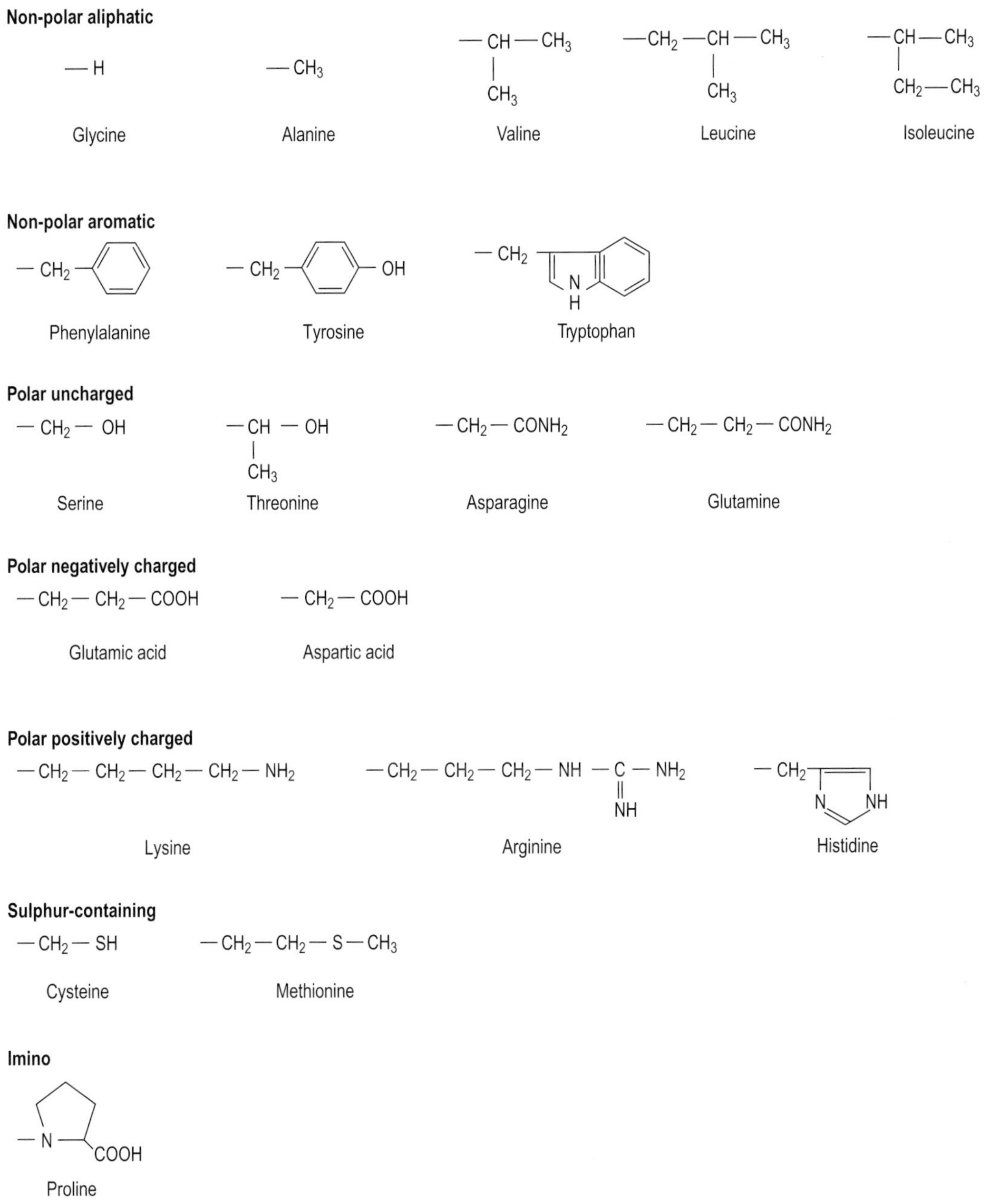

Non-polar aliphatic

—H	—CH$_3$	—CH—CH$_3$
		     |
		    CH$_3$
			—CH$_2$—CH—CH$_3$
			         |
			        CH$_3$
				—CH—CH$_3$
				    |
				   CH$_2$—CH$_3$

Glycine	Alanine	Valine	Leucine	Isoleucine

Non-polar aromatic

Phenylalanine — Tyrosine — Tryptophan

Polar uncharged

—CH$_2$—OH   —CH—OH (CH$_3$)   —CH$_2$—CONH$_2$ —CH$_2$—CH$_2$—CONH$_2$

Serine   Threonine   Asparagine   Glutamine

Polar negatively charged

—CH$_2$—CH$_2$—COOH   —CH$_2$—COOH

Glutamic acid   Aspartic acid

Polar positively charged

—CH$_2$—CH$_2$—CH$_2$—CH$_2$—NH$_2$ —CH$_2$—CH$_2$—CH$_2$—NH—C—NH$_2$ (‖NH)   —CH$_2$— (imidazole)

Lysine   Arginine   Histidine

Sulphur-containing

—CH$_2$—SH   —CH$_2$—CH$_2$—S—CH$_3$

Cysteine   Methionine

Imino

Proline

Fig. 2.20 **The side chains of the common amino acids.**

- **Polar positively charged**: amino acids with side chains containing amino group that is positively charged at pH 7.
- **Sulphur-containing**: amino acids with sulphydryl (–SH) groups in the side chain. These amino acids are able to form disulphide bridges between two sulphydryl groups and thus link different parts of a protein molecule.
- **A note on proline**. Proline is not actually an amino acid but an amino acid with an –NH group instead of the amino (–NH$_2$) group. This has structural consequences for proline-containing proteins.

Clinical box 2.5	Errors in amino acid metabolism

When the metabolic pathway of an amino acid is disrupted, its precursors may accumulate in the blood, or appear in the urine (normally, most amino acids are absorbed in the kidney proximal tubules). In clinical practice, measurements of serum and urine levels have diagnostic significance particularly in the detection of conditions known as the inborn errors of metabolism.

For example, in phenylketonuria (PKU), where there is a deficiency in the enzyme phenylalanine hydroxylase (or two other enzymes in the same pathway), the intermediate metabolites phenylacetate, phenylacetylglutamine and phenylpyruvate accumulate. Untreated PKU leads to brain damage (see Chs 3 and 5).

PROTEINS

Proteins are polymers of amino acids. Each protein has a unique number and sequence of amino acids, which has been assembled according to the information encoded in the DNA. Molecules with shorter amino acid chains are known as **peptides** (dipeptides, tripeptides etc., or poly-peptides). Those with a chain longer than 50 amino acids are **proteins** (Clinical box 2.5).

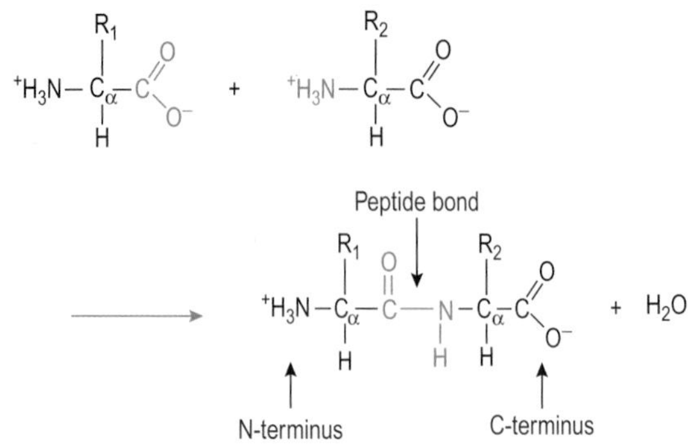

Fig. 2.21 The peptide bond.

The peptide bond

The amino acids are linked by **peptide bonds**. Such a bond is formed when the amino group ($-NH_3^+$) of one amino acid covalently bonds with the carboxyl group ($-COO^-$) of another (Fig. 2.21).

In a polypeptide chain, the amino acid with a free amino group at one end is known as the N-terminal amino acid, and this is by convention the start of a peptide chain. The amino acid with the free carboxyl group is the C-terminal amino acid, and forms the end of a chain.

STRUCTURE OF PROTEINS

There are four levels of protein structure:

1. **Primary structure**: the sequence of amino acids in the peptide chain.
2. **Secondary structure**: the spatial arrangement of the primary structure determined by hydrogen bonding.
3. **Tertiary structure**: further folding of the polypeptide chain stabilised by a wide range of bonds and interactions between the side chains of amino acids.
4. **Quaternary structure**: the arrangement of protein subunits in multimeric proteins.

Primary structure

The primary structure of a protein is its sequence of amino acids. Incidentally, it also determines the secondary and tertiary structures of the molecule: for instance, an amino acid chain with a large number of hydrophobic residues will have completely different properties from one with many polar side chains. Some amino acids introduce specific structural features to a protein: the presence of proline leads to kinks in the protein chain, and glycine, because it has only a single hydrogen as the side chain, contributes to the formation of tight loops in the structure.

Secondary structure

Secondary structure is the folding pattern of the polypeptide chain. It is stabilised by the hydrogen bonds. The common types of secondary structure are the **α-helix** and **β-sheet** (Fig. 2.22). An important structural motif is the **U-turn**, which allows protein chains to change direction.

The α-helix is formed when the polypeptide chain twists into a 'spring' with the carbonyl group of each peptide bond hydrogen-bonded to the hydrogen of the amide group four residues down the chain (Fig. 2.22A). Such coiling turns clockwise and

has a pitch of 3.6 residues per turn. All the amino acid side chains face outwards (See also Information box 2.10).

The β-sheet is a structure where hydrogen bonds form between peptide chains that lie alongside each other (Fig. 2.22B). It has a pleated appearance, with the side chains protruding above and below its plane. Some proteins are formed from multiple layers of β-sheets.

The U-turn consists of three to four amino acid residues, commonly glycine and proline, which form a short loop. This makes the tertiary structure more compact.

Tertiary structure

Tertiary structure specifies the spatial arrangement of the secondary structure. It is determined by multiple interactions between the amino acid side chains and may include:

- **Hydrogen bonds** between side chains that have partial positive (δ^+) and negative (δ^-) charges, e.g. between serine and asparagine side chains.
- **Ionic bonds** between oppositely charged side chains, e.g. between lysine and glutamic acid.
- **Hydrophobic interactions** in regions where there are large numbers of non-polar, aliphatic and aromatic side chains.
- **Disulphide bonds,** between cysteine residues (Information box 2.11).

Some proteins require other protein molecules, known as **molecular chaperones,** to facilitate their folding.

Protein denaturation

The secondary and tertiary structures of proteins can be disrupted by heating, pH changes, by high concentrations of substances such as urea, or by reducing agents which break the disulphide bonds. The process is called **denaturation** and it destroys the protein's biological activity. Some proteins recover their activity when the denaturing agent is removed: this illustrates that the secondary and tertiary structures are to a significant extent determined by the amino acid sequence.

Quaternary structure

Many proteins consist not of a single chain but of several **subunits** held together by non-covalent bonds. Spatial arrangement of such subunits is the **quaternary** structure of a protein. An example of this is immunoglobulin G (IgG), the antibody molecule. Its Y-shaped structure consists of four protein subunits, two heavy and two light chains, joined by disulphide bridges and hydrogen bonds (see Ch. 6).

Cooperativity between protein subunits

The subunits of multimeric proteins interact with each other: this is known as **cooperativity**. It is particularly important when a protein binds other molecules. In a protein that exhibits cooperativity, when one subunit binds a molecule, there is a change in the quaternary structure which affects its affinity for subsequent molecules. For example, haemoglobin binds four oxygen molecules. The binding of the first molecule to a four-subunit deoxygenated form of haemoglobin (deoxyhaemoglobin) causes a conformational change in

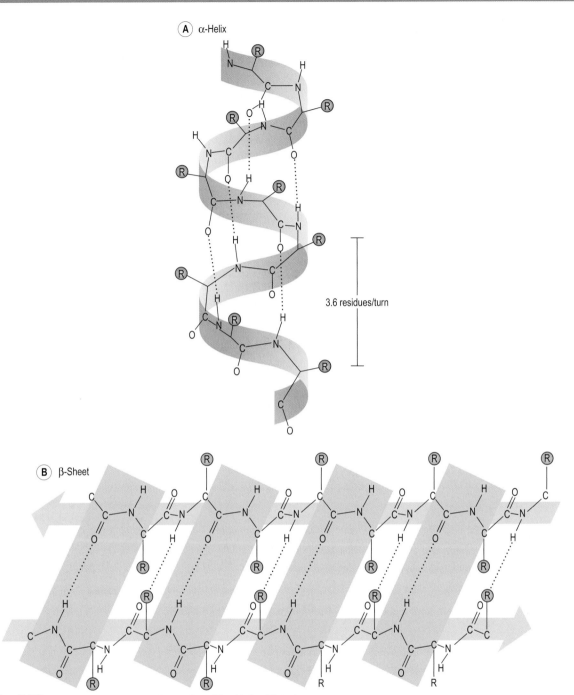

Fig. 2.22 Secondary structure of proteins. (A) α-Helix; (B) β-sheet.

Information box 2.10	Hair is made up of many α-helices

Hair is made up largely of a protein called keratin. Single hairs are made up of hundreds of microfibrils embedded in a protein matrix. Each microfibril is formed from a number of α-helices that are wound around each other in a superhelix. Hairs can be stretched by elongating the α-helices, which breaks the hydrogen bonds in the helices. When the hair is released it reverts to its previous length because the covalent disulphide bonds between cysteine residues in the α-helix and the protein matrix remain intact. Hair can be permanently curled or straightened by applying chemicals which first break these disulphide bonds and then re-form them in the new conformation.

Information box 2.11	Disulphide bond

Disulphide bonds between cysteine residues in polypeptides affect the folding and the stability of protein structure. Disruption of these bonds, caused for instance by mutations, would lead to loss of protein function.

Fibrillin is a glycoprotein needed for the manufacture of elastic fibres in the connective tissue. It is rich in cysteine residues. Homocysteine, a homologue of cysteine, can disrupt the disulphide bond. In homocystinuria, the high level of circulating homocysteine disrupts disulphide bonds in the fibrillin that supports the lens. This may lead to lens dislocation. In another rare connective tissue disorder, the Marfan syndrome, fibrillin mutation may lead to loose and overextending joints.

the other subunits. It increases their affinity for oxygen, making the second oxygen molecule bind more readily. This, in turn, increases the affinity of the remaining binding sites. The reverse also occurs: if one oxygen molecule dissociates, the other molecules are lost more easily (see Ch. 13).

PROTEIN SYNTHESIS AND PROCESSING

The amino acid sequence of a protein is encoded in the DNA. The principles of this encoding are the genetic **code** (see Ch. 5 and Clinical box 2.6). In essence, DNA uses three nucleotide sets (triplets) to code for an amino acid. The triplets are known as **codons** (Table 2.12) which the mRNA transcript translates on the ribosome. For example, GUU, GUC, GUA and GUG all code for valine. Three of the codons are stop codons (UAA, UAG and UGA) and signal the end of a polypeptide chain. The start codon initiates protein synthesis and in eukaryotes coders for methionine, and is usually AUG.

Protein synthesis includes three major steps: the transcribing of the DNA code into the much shorter and more 'mobile' mRNA molecule (**transcription**) (Fig. 2.23), the transfer of the mRNA from the nucleus to the cytoplasm and the assembly of a ribosome around it, and translation of the sequence of the mRNA bases into the sequence of the amino acids in the new polypeptide chain (**translation**).

Subsequently, the synthesised proteins are often further modified before they reach their mature form. This is known as **post-translational modification**.

Ribosomes

Ribosomes are globular structures consisting of rRNA and proteins. They are assembled in the nucleus. They translocate to the cytoplasm through nuclear pores, and either remain free in the cytosol, or become attached to the rough endoplasmic reticulum (ER) (see below). Each ribosome has a large and a small subunit: they join together when the ribosome attaches to mRNA in preparation for protein synthesis (Fig. 2.24).

Transcription

Transcription is accomplished in the nucleus by RNA polymerases. The template is the sense strand of the DNA. Thus, the newly synthesised mRNA has the antisense sequence (it becomes a 'photographic negative' of the sense strand). Therefore, when it binds complementary tRNAs on the ribosome, the codons on the tRNA are in the same as the sequence of the DNA sense strand (Table 2.13).

Post-transcriptional modification of mRNA: splicing

Transcription proceeds until the RNA polymerase encounters the stop codon. However, genes include regions that code for amino acids (coding sequences or **exons**) as well as

Table 2.12	The mRNA genetic code (in DNA thymine (T) replaces uracil (U))				
1st position	**2nd position**				**3rd position**
	U	**C**	**A**	**G**	
G	Val	Ala	Asp	Gly	U
	Val	Ala	Asp	Gly	C
	Val	Ala	Glu	Gly	A
	Val	Ala	Glu	Gly	G
A	Ile	Thr	Asn	Ser	U
	Ile	Thr	Asn	Ser	C
	Ile	Thr	Lys	Arg	A
	Met (start)	Thr	Lys	Arg	G
C	Leu	Pro	His	Arg	U
	Leu	Pro	His	Arg	C
	Leu	Pro	Gln	Arg	A
	Leu	Pro	Gln	Arg	G
U	Phe	Ser	Tyr	Cys	U
	Phe	Ser	Tyr	Cys	C
	Leu	Ser	Stop	Stop	A
	Leu	Ser	Stop	Trp	G

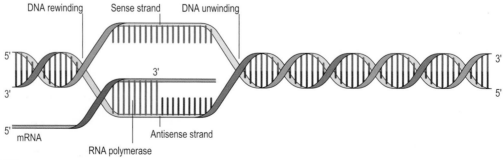

Fig. 2.23 **Transcription.**

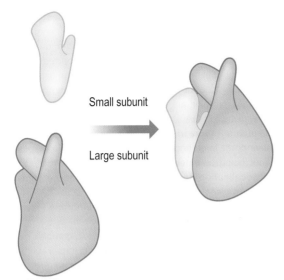

Fig. 2.24 Structure of the ribosome.

Table 2.13	Complementary DNA and mRNA sequences	
Sequence	**Direction**	**Codons or amino acids**
DNA coding strand (sense)	5' → 3'	ATG AGA CTA TTC AGC TAA
Complementary DNA (antisense)	3' → 5'	TAC TCT GAT AAG TCG ATT
mRNA	5' → 3'	AUG AGA CUA UUC AGC UAA
Amino acids	N → C	Met (start) Arg Leu Phe Ser

Spaces are shown between the codons for clarity.

non-coding regions (**introns**). The primary transcript needs to be edited before its transfer to the cytoplasm. Such editing is known as post-transcriptional modification of the mRNA. During the editing the introns are excised and the exons are joined together. This is known as **splicing**. Importantly, different exons of a gene may be joined in different combinations: this is known as **alternative splicing** and increases the number of proteins that can be produced from one gene (see also Ch. 5).

Translation

Translation includes three stages: initiation, elongation and termination of the new peptide chain. Before it takes place, the substrate amino acids are bound to their specific tRNA molecules, producing aminoacyl-tRNAs. The reaction is catalysed by the aminoacyl-tRNA synthetase.

The **initiation** stage starts with the binding of the small ribosome subunit to the mRNA. In bacteria, this is followed by the binding of the first amino acid-tRNA complex, which carries a methionine. This Met-tRNA is released when the peptide chain synthesis is completed. Then the large subunit binds to the small one, completing the ribosome which now possesses three tRNA binding sites which span the two subunits (Fig. 2.25). They are known as the P (peptidyl) site, the A (aminoacyl) site and the E (exit) site (Fig. 2.26).

Elongation of the polypeptide chain

The growing polypeptide chain is attached to the P-site. The tRNA, carrying an amino acid to be added, binds to the A-site. A peptide bond is formed between the new amino

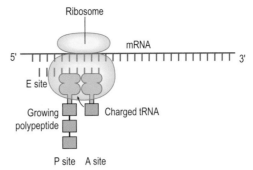

Fig. 2.25 Translation of mRNA.

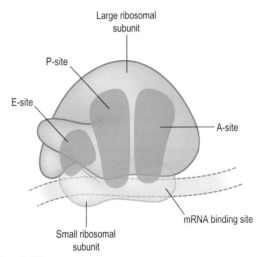

Fig. 2.26 Ribosomal tRNA binding sites. The P-site is occupied by peptidyl-tRNA (the growing polypeptide chain). The A-site is occupied by aminoacyl-tRNA (tRNA carrying new the amino acid to be inserted into the polypeptide chain). The E-site holds the tRNA derived from the P-site, after the polypeptide chain has attached to the new aminoacyl-tRNA.

acid and the last amino acid in the peptide chain. As a result, the peptide chain transfers from the P-site to the A-site. At this stage the ribosome moves along the mRNA, so that the peptide chain now occupies the P-site, and the A-site becomes vacant to accept a new aminoacyl-tRNA. The peptide chain grows from the N-terminal towards the C-terminal end. **Termination** of synthesis occurs when the A-site encounters a stop codon. At this stage, the protein known as the releasing factor frees the polypeptide chain from the ribosome. The ribosome subsequently dissociates into subunits.

Several ribosomes can bind to one mRNA simultaneously. Such 'sets' are known as **polyribosomes** (Fig. 2.27). Ribosomes attached to the ER give the characteristic appearance to the rough ER.

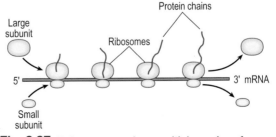

Fig. 2.27 Polysomes produce multiple copies of a protein from a single mRNA.

Post-translational modification of proteins

Almost all proteins are further modified after their synthesis is completed. Some of the post-translational modifications are permanent while others are reversible.

Acetylation involves the addition of an acetyl (CH_3CO) group to the N-terminal end. It protects proteins against degradation. **Glycosylation** is important in the formation of glycoproteins and **proteoglycans**. **Phosphorylation** is a common modification, which reversibly modifies the activity of many enzymes and intracellular signal transducing proteins. Enzymes called **kinases** add phosphate groups to the hydroxyl groups of serine, threonine and tyrosine. **Phosphatases** remove these groups.

Proteolytic cleavage is another form of post-translational modification. Several proteins are synthesised in a precursor form and are subsequently split to yield mature proteins. An example is insulin, which actually undergoes a two-stage proteolysis. First, a single peptide chain, preproinsulin, is split to yield proinsulin, which is then cleaved again just before the secretion stage to yield insulin and the connecting peptide (C-peptide). Several pancreatic enzymes are also synthesised as inactive proenzymes (zymogens), and are activated by partial digestion in the duodenum.

Cellular protein targeting

The large number of proteins that need to be synthesised at any given time requires a complex machinery to sort and target them to different organelles, or mark them for secretion (Fig. 2.28).

Proteins that are synthesised within the cytosol are either destined to remain there or are targeted for the nucleus, mitochondria or peroxisomes. Proteins synthesised in the rough ER are destined for insertion into membranes, lysosomes or for secretion.

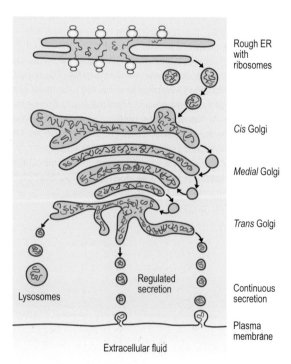

Fig. 2.28 **Protein processing in the rough endoplasmic reticulum (ER) and the Golgi apparatus.**

Proteins synthesised in the cytosol but destined for the mitochondria possess N-terminal signal sequences that determine their transport into the mitochondria. They are unfolded by molecular chaperones, transported through the mitochondrial membranes, and then refolded using other chaperones inside the mitochondria. A limited number of mitochondrial proteins are synthesised on mitochondrial ribosomes, using mtDNA.

Proteins for use in the nucleus are transported through nuclear pores large enough for the protein to be transported without being unfolded. Fragments of proteins, called **nuclear localisation sequences**, interact with these pores to facilitate uptake.

Proteins destined for secretion or membrane insertion possess the N-terminal signal sequence which, as the protein is being synthesised, binds to an RNA–protein complex called a **signal recognition particle** (SRP). This halts further synthesis until the ribosome reaches the ER. At this point the SRP is released and synthesis resumes. The newly synthesised peptide is passed into the lumen of the ER through a special pore.

Protein processing in the endoplasmic reticulum

In the ER further protein modifications such as N-linked and O-linked glycosylation or proteolytic cleavage takes place. Also, excess protein subunits are eliminated and misfolded proteins are retained.

Clinical box 2.6 **Genetic code mutation**

Sickle cell disease
Gene mutations may distort protein synthesis and result in the manufacture of functionally impaired, or inactive, proteins.

Sickle cell disease is caused by a single point mutation in the genetic code that changes a single codon to specify valine instead of the normal glutamine during protein synthesis. This leads to a structural abnormality in the haemoglobin molecule and results in the production of sickle haemoglobin (HbS). Under reduced oxygenation, red cells containing HbS become elongated and sickle shaped. They aggregate and adhere to the vascular endothelium. This leads to vascular occlusion, and haemolytic anaemia.

Clinical box 2.7 **Clinical conditions associated with disordered protein structure**

Normal protein function depends on the correct primary structure, followed by correct folding. An abnormal amino acid sequence resulting from gene mutation can lead to abnormal folding; this in turn may give rise to clinical disorders. An example of this is collagen, where substitution of amino acids in the chain prevents the correct coiling of the chains. **Osteogenesis imperfecta** results from the replacement of glycine in the collagen chain. The **Ehlers–Danlos syndrome**, with its characteristic joint hypermobility, fragility of blood vessels, easy bruising and loose skin, also results from a defect in collagen synthesis.

Prions are misfolded proteins that can invade cells and cause misfolding and aggregation of host proteins. **Creutzfeldt–Jakob disease** (CJD) is a prion disease in which the infecting prion (prion protein – scrapie; PrPCS) induces the misfolding of the normal protein (prion protein – cellular; PrPC).

Alzheimer disease is associated with amyloid plaques composed of the protein amyloid beta (Aβ) which has a protein fold similar to those in prion diseases. Other diseases associated with protein misfolding include Parkinson disease and amyotrophic lateral sclerosis.

Protein processing in the Golgi apparatus

In the Golgi apparatus, proteins that are destined for secretion – after being transferred from the ER – are separated according to whether or not they are to be continuously secreted, or stored before secretion in response to a stimulus (Fig. 2.28) (see Ch. 8).

Protein secretion

Protein secretion is by extrusion of vesicles that contain the synthesised product. They are released into the extracellular space by exocytosis (see below). Release may be continuous, or the secretory vesicles may be stored. Continuous (constitutive) secretion is, for instance, the mode of secretion of immunoglobulins by the plasma cells. The regulated secretion responds to a particular stimulus, which often involves a rise in intracellular calcium concentration, which releases the stored secretory granules. In many neurons one can identify different populations of vesicles in nerve terminals, which contain different substances and are released in response to different stimuli (see Ch. 8).

FUNCTIONS OF PROTEINS

Proteins are responsible for much of the body's structure and functions (Clinical box 2.7). Their most important roles are described below.

Structural proteins form large structures such as muscle and collagen fibres and also are essential for the cytoskeleton of individual cells, providing a framework that maintains cell shape, and internal structure (see Ch. 9).

Catalytic proteins: the entire metabolism relies on biological catalysts, enzymes, which facilitate and – under the influence of other factors – regulate the great majority of chemical reactions that occur in the organism.

Signalling proteins. Transfer of signals that regulate cell functions relies on the **signalling cassettes**, sets comprising molecules that contain the metabolic information (e.g. hormones or cytokines), their cellular receptors, and the downstream signal transducing proteins that change the activity of genes or enzymes.

Many hormones and all cytokines are peptides or proteins. They carry biological signals either locally or over a distance, via plasma. Receptors are proteins located either in the cell membrane, or intracellularly, that bind these molecules and relay the signals to the cell interior, through the series of proteins that make up intracellular signal-amplifying cascades. Some intracellular receptors bind to DNA and regulate gene expression: such molecules are known as transcription factors (Fig. 2.29).

Proteins that interact with DNA. Protein-nucleic acid interactions are essential for cell biochemistry. Proteins help DNA packing in the nucleus, stabilise it in its coiled or uncoiled state, form a significant part of ribosomes' structure, and extensively assist in DNA replication and protein synthesis. As mentioned above, many proteins act as transcription factors, binding to gene promoters and modifying gene expression.

Proteins that transport substances in plasma. The universal transporter is the albumin. In addition to albumin, many specific binding proteins are present in plasma (see below).

Proteins that transport molecules across biological membranes. The membrane embedded proteins that transport

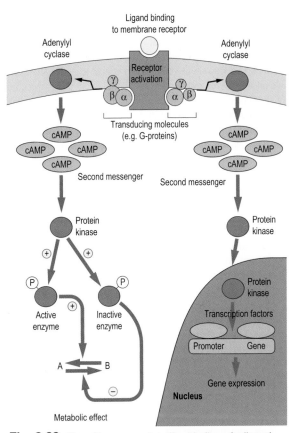

Fig. 2.29 Signalling cascades. The binding of a ligand to a membrane receptor leads to receptor activation, and the activation of sets of transducing molecules. They in turn activate an enzyme (for instance the adenylyl cyclase) which generates a second messenger (cAMP). The second messenger activates protein kinases which initiate phosphorylation cascades that result either in change in the rate or direction of individual reactions, or change in gene transcription. Reproduced with permission from Dominiczak MH 2012 Medical biochemistry flash cards, London, Elsevier.

substances across the cell membrane, the mitochondrial membrane or other intracellular structures are fundamental for the functioning of a cell (see below).

Proteins that participate in immunity. The immunoglobulins are the principal tool of the acquired immunity, and a wide range of other proteins (such as the components of complement) participate in the innate immunity, which includes response to inflammation. (see Ch.6)

STRUCTURAL PROTEINS

Structural proteins form the scaffolding (cytoskeleton) of every cell (see Ch. 9). They also make up the muscles, bones, skin and connective tissues. The three major groups of structural proteins are collagens, cytoskeletal proteins and muscle proteins.

Collagens and proteins present in the extracellular matrix

The **collagens** are the most abundant type of fibrous protein. They make up about 25% of the total protein of the body and are the major component of the **extracellular matrix** (ECM). At least 20 different types of collagen have been described to date.

Collagen is made up of three polypeptide chains, each of which can be up to 3000 amino acids in length. Each chain forms a left-handed helix that is tighter than the standard α-helix, with just three amino acids per turn. This 'tightness' is achieved because every third amino acid in the collagen chain is a glycine, which, with its single hydrogen, can fit into the core of the molecule. The other amino acids are very often proline and its hydroxylated derivative, hydroxyproline. The three collagen helices are wound round each other into a right-handed triple superhelix stabilised by hydrogen bonding. The commonest type of collagen (type I) forms fibrils, with its molecules packed side by side. Other collagens form sheets which produce large flexible networks. Type IV collagen is a component of the basement membrane, which underlies the epithelial cells.

Elastin is a flexible globular protein, associated with collagen. It is found mostly in ligaments and blood vessel walls, and also in the skin, tendons and connective tissues. Many elastin molecules are cross-linked between lysine residues. When a tissue is stretched, the globular proteins extend, and when the tension is released they shorten, reverting to their globular form.

Two glycoproteins, **laminin and fibronectin**, are important components of the basement membranes, These molecules can simultaneously bind to proteins on the cell surface and to those in the ECM.

Muscle

The main contractile proteins in muscle cells (myocytes) are **actin** and **myosin**. They form the filaments of skeletal muscle, which interact to produce muscle contraction. Other proteins which participate in muscle contraction are tropomyosin and the troponins (see Ch. 9 for details).

Cytoskeletal proteins

Cytoskeleton consists of several types of filaments. All cells contain **cytoskeletal proteins** (Table 2.14). The types of filaments are described in more detail in the table.

Immunoglobulins

The immune system is capable a range of 'standard' responses known as innate immunity, and highly flexible, specific responses called adaptive immunity (see Ch. 6). Adaptive immunity relies on the production of **immunoglobulins** or **antibodies,** which bind to the invading organism or **antigen**, enabling the latter to be removed and destroyed.

Transport (binding) proteins

Many proteins are transported in the plasma. **Albumin** makes up 50% of the plasma proteins and is present at a concentration

Table 2.14	Cytoskeletal proteins	
Filament types	**Main protein constituent**	**Major role**
Microfilaments	Actin	Cell movement
		Form core of microvilli
Intermediate filaments (IFs)	Keratins*	Mechanical strength
Microtubules	Tubulins	Chromosome separation
		Intracellular transport

*The proteins making up IFs vary between cell types.

of 35–45 g/L. It is the main protein that maintains the oncotic pressure of the plasma. This balances the outward-directed hydrostatic pressure in the blood vessels ensuring the correct distribution of fluid between the vascular and interstitial compartments (see Ch. 11). Low albumin concentration is a common cause of generalised oedema (Ch. 1 and Clinical box 2.8). Albumin is also a non-specific transport protein capable of binding many substances, including therapeutic drugs. It has a negative charge at physiological pH, which means that it can bind cations such as copper and iron. Many hydrophobic molecules such as, for instance, fatty acids can also be transported bound to albumin (see Ch. 3). There are other binding proteins in plasma that transport specific substances (Table 2.9).

CATALYTIC PROTEINS: ENZYMES

Almost all the biochemical reactions that take place in the body require the presence of protein catalysts, **enzymes**. Enzymes lower the activation energy of the reaction so that it can proceed under physiological temperature, pH and pressure. They speed up the reaction rate 10^6–10^{12}-fold.

The active site of each enzyme has a structure that allows the substrate to fit into it exactly, like a **lock and key**. Some enzymes are strictly specific in their substrates, only catalysing the reaction involving a single substrate, whereas others may accept a range of related substrates.

Enzymes are classified into six classes, depending on the type of catalysed reaction (Table 2.15). Most enzymes also have a 'common' name.

Enzyme kinetics

The basic enzymatic reaction proceeds as follows:

$$E + S \rightarrow ES \rightarrow E + P$$

where E is the enzyme, S is the substrate and P is the product.

The rate of the enzyme-catalysed reaction is affected by **temperature, pH** and **substrate concentration**. For many enzymes the optimal pH is close to pH 7. However, there are some that work in pretty extreme environments: for instance, pepsin has an optimal pH of about 2, which is the pH of the gastric juice (see Ch. 15).

Another major factor which determines the rate of enzymatic reactions is the concentration of the substrate [S]. As [S] increases, the rate of the reaction increases: the increase is linear until it reaches a plateau, where further increase in [S] does not produce any increase in the **reaction rate**. This occurs because at low [S] the rate of reaction is limited by the number of substrate molecules available to bind to the active site, and as the number of molecules increases further, the enzyme becomes saturated, i.e. all the binding sites are

Table 2.15   Classes of enzymes (see also Clinical box 2.9)

Class	Type	Action	Examples of common names
I	Oxidoreductases	Oxidation–reduction reactions	Dehydrogenase, oxidase, peroxidase, reductase
II	Transferases	Transfer of amino, carboxyl, acyl, carbonyl, methyl, phosphate and other groups between molecules	Transaminase, transcarboxylase
III	Hydrolases	Cleavage of bonds coupled with inserting water	Esterase, peptidase, amylase, phosphatase, pepsin, trypsin
IV	Lyases	Cleavage of carbon-carbon, carbon-sulphur and carbon-nitrogen (but not peptide) bonds	Decarboxylase, aldolase
V	Isomerases	Rearrangement of bonds	Epimerase, mutase
VI	Ligases	Formation of bonds between carbon and oxygen, sulphur, nitrogen	Synthetase, carboxylase

Clinical box 2.9   Enzymes as biomarkers

Each tissue has a particular enzyme complement. Physical or functional damage to cells caused by disease, trauma, or side effects of therapeutic drugs, may release enzymes into the blood. Thus elevated activities of certain enzymes in plasma are used as biomarkers.

The **liver** profile includes two aminotransferases: alanine aminotransferase (ALT) and aspartate aminotransferase (AST) which are present in hepatocytes, and alkaline phosphatase and gamma-glutamyl transpeptidase (GGT) which are present in bile canaliculi and are markers of biliary obstruction. These enzymes are usually measured in conjunction with measurements of serum bilirubin and albumin – the tests being known as 'liver function tests'.

Alkaline phosphatase is also used as a marker of **bone disease** (different isoenzymes of the alkaline phosphatase are present in liver and bone).

Creatine kinase (CK) is a marker of **muscle damage**. Another isoenzyme is more common in heart muscle was for a long time used as an early marker of myocardial infarction. This has now been superseded by measurements of cardiac troponins.

which the rate is half V_{max}. The K_m reflects the **affinity** of the enzyme **for its substrate**. A low K_m indicates a high affinity. It means that only a low concentration of substrate is required to saturate the enzyme. The two constants, V_{max} and K_m, characterise each enzyme–substrate pair. The Michaelis–Menten curve can be mathematically rearranged into **Lineweaver–Burk** and **Eadie–Hofstee** plots (Fig. 2.31).

Importantly, the same mathematical models can be used to describe **membrane transport**, **receptor-ligand binding** (see Ch. 3) and **drug interactions** with a variety of targets.

The Michaelis–Menten equation applies only to a reaction with a single substrate. Reactions that involve multiple substrates can have curves of different shapes. In particular, reactions characterised by cooperative interactions between substrate molecules yield sigmoidal curves.

An enzyme catalysing the same reaction can exist in different tissues in different forms, called **isoenzymes**. Isoenzymes differ in substrate affinities and patterns of inhibition.

constantly occupied by substrate. The rate of the reaction is the maximum reaction velocity (designated $\boldsymbol{V_{max}}$) (Fig. 2.30).

If the initial rate of the reaction *(v)* at different [S] is plotted, the resulting curve is described by the **Michaelis–Menten equation:**

$$v = (V_{max} + [S]) / (K_m + [S])$$

The maximum reaction rate (V_{max}) can be estimated from the plateau of the curve in Figure 2.30 where the rate of reaction is plotted against concentration. The other constant of the Michaelis constant ($\boldsymbol{K_m}$) is the substrate concentration at

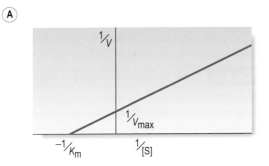

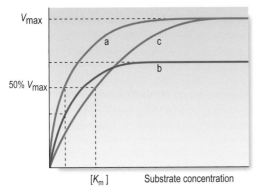

Fig. 2.30 **Michaelis–Menten curves.** Curves a and c have the same V_{max}, whereas curves a and b have the same K_m.

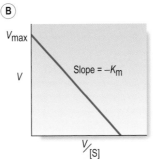

Fig. 2.31 **(A) Lineweaver–Burk plot:** *x*-intercept = $-1/K_m$, *y*-intercept = $1/V_{max}$. **(B) Eadie–Hofstee plot:** *y*-intercept = V_{max}, slope = $-K_m$.

Enzyme inhibition

Enzyme inhibition is a fundamental regulatory mechanism in the cell. Many therapeutic drugs work through enzyme inhibition. There are two types of reversible inhibition: competitive and non-competitive inhibition (see also Ch. 4)

Competitive inhibition occurs when an inhibitor binds reversibly to the active site of the enzyme. At low substrate concentrations the enzyme activity is inhibited, but as [S] rises the inhibitor is displaced from the active site and the enzyme activity returns towards normal. The presence of the inhibitor, however, causes an increase in the K_m for the substrate (more substrate is required to saturate the enzyme). V_{max} remains unchanged (see Clinical box 2.10).

Non-competitive inhibition occurs when the inhibitor binds to a site other than the active site of the enzyme, and by doing so reduces the reaction rate. Since the binding of the substrate is unaltered, the K_m remains unchanged. However, the V_{max} decreases. Several chemotherapeutic drugs act in this way.

Regulation of enzyme activity

Enzyme activity can be controlled in several ways:

- **Feedback loops**. The feedback inhibition is inhibition by the product of a given reaction, or a pathway. This is a very common regulatory mechanism.

- **Feed forward activation**. This is a relatively rare regulatory mechanism where a product of reaction activates a downstream enzyme, increasing substrate flow through a pathway.
- **Allosteric regulation**. An allosteric regulator binds to a site other than the enzyme's active site. It changes the enzyme's activity through changes in the tertiary or quarternary structure.
- **Phosphorylation–dephosphorylation sequence**. Many enzymes and proteins in the signalling pathways can be reversibly altered by phosphorylation. It is a common mechanism of signal transduction. For many enzymes phosphorylation/dephosphorylation acts as an on/off switch. Phosphorylation requires an enzyme called kinase. Dephosphorylation is performed by phosphatases.
- **Proteolysis**. Enzymes can be irreversibly activated or inactivated by proteolytic enzymes.
- **Changes in gene expression**. The amount of an enzyme can be altered through increased or decreased gene transcription and the consequent change in enzyme synthesis. Gene expression is controlled by a wide range of metabolic signals and is mediated by proteins known as transcription factors.

Enzyme cofactors

Cofactors are non-protein substances required for an enzymatic reaction to proceed. Cofactors are easily removable from the enzyme and are often metal ions such as copper or magnesium. Organic cofactors are known as **coenzymes**. Vitamins often act as coenzymes. Coenzymes are frequently involved in oxidation–reduction reactions, acting as electron donors or acceptors such as nicotinamide adenine dinucleotide (NAD) and flavin adenine dinucleotide (FAD) (Table 2.16).

Finally, a **prosthetic group** of an enzyme is a non-protein group that is an integral part of the enzyme molecule.

Clinical box 2.10	Competitive inhibition of alcohol dehydrogenase can be used to treat methanol poisoning

Methanol is poisonous to humans and can cause blindness. The metabolism of both methanol and ethanol involves the enzyme alcohol dehydrogenase. Part of the treatment of methanol poisoning is the administration of ethanol in order to block methanol metabolism, as it is the breakdown products of methanol that are toxic. Ethanol has a higher affinity (lower K_m) for the active site of alcohol dehydrogenase than methanol and therefore blocks its binding to the enzyme. It can then be removed from the blood by dialysis.

Table 2.16 Some coenzymes involved in metabolism

Coenzyme	Group transferred	Oxidised	Reduced
Nicotinamide adenine dinucleotide (NAD)	2H	NAD^+	$NADH + H^+$
Nicotinamide adenine dinucleotide phosphate (NADP)	2H	$NADP^+$	$NADPH + H^+$
Flavin adenine dinucleotide (FAD)	2H	FAD^+	$FADH_2$
Coenzyme A (CoA)	Acyl groups	CoA	Acetyl-CoA

THE CELL

Cells are the fundamental structural units of an organism. They are enclosed by the plasma membrane. Eukaryotic cells (with a few exceptions) possess a nucleus and cytoplasm which contains different subcellular organelles (Fig. 2.32). The details of structure vary widely in different cell types (Information box 2.12). Cells perform a wide range of specialised functions.

There are also significant differences between animal and plant cells with regard to their organelles and cell membranes. The subcellular organelles are distinctive structures within the cytoplasm. They enable cells to compartmentalise biochemical processes, and maintain different conditions (such as low pH) in the local cell areas.

Many organelles are enclosed by single or double membranes, but there are also structures which are non-membranous such as the ribosomes. Glycogen or lipids can be stored in the cytoplasm in the form of granules or droplets. In multicellular organisms they are units that make tissues.

Cell can be structurally polarised. This means that different functions are performed in different areas of the cell. A good example is the enterocytes, the epithelial cells lining the lumen of the intestine (Fig. 2.33). They have an apical surface which remains in contact with the lumen and may have one of a number of membrane specialisations such as cilia or microvilli (see below). The other pole of the cell, the basolateral surface, is in contact with the basement membrane.

Cell membranes

All cells, both prokaryotic and eukaryotic, are surrounded by the **cell membrane**. It maintains the integrity of the cell and is fundamental for its survival. The plasma membrane also regulates the movement of molecules in and out of the cell. The membrane is hydrophobic but it contains proteins that

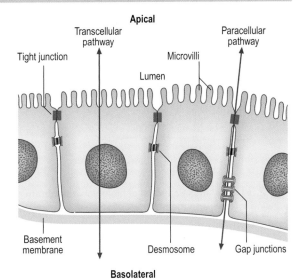

Fig. 2.33 **A sheet of epithelial cells.**

allow the movement of hydrophilic molecules across (see below). The outside of the plasma membrane also contains glycoproteins, which participate in cell-to-cell interactions and cell recognition. Plants and bacteria in addition possess cell walls, which surround the plasma membrane (Ch. 6).

The structure of plasma membranes was proposed by Singer and Nicholson in 1972 and is known as the **fluid mosaic model** (Fig. 2.34). All cell membranes, including the plasma membrane, consist in part of a **bilayer** of phospholipids, sphingolipids and cholesterol.

Phospholipids and sphingolipids are **amphipathic** molecules. In an aqueous environment phospholipids aggregate so that their acyl tails form the hydrophobic core of the membrane. The phospholipid bilayer is remarkably dynamic. Individual phospholipid molecules are free to migrate within their side of

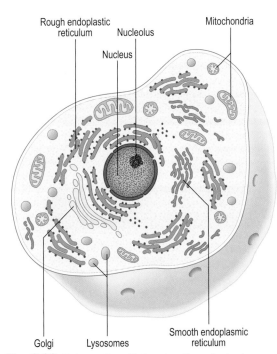

Fig. 2.32 **Eukaryotic cell showing the principal organelles.** Not all organelles are present in all cells.

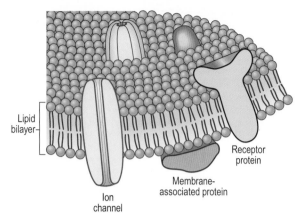

Lipid
bilayer

Receptor
protein

Membrane-
associated protein

Ion
channel

Fig. 2.34 **Fluid mosaic model of biological membranes, showing integral and membrane-associated proteins.**

the bilayer. However, transfer of a phospholipid between the sides of the bilayer (flipping) is rare. Some membranes, particularly in the endoplasmic reticulum and in erythrocytes, contain **flippases**, which can move phospholipids from one side of the bilayer to the other. Overall, a phospholipid bilayer allows the passage of small molecules, such as water, oxygen and carbon dioxide, and anything that is fat soluble, but excludes almost all polar molecules and charged solutes.

The cholesterol molecule also has hydrophobic and hydrophilic regions, and the presence of cholesterol reduces the fluidity of the membrane. It inserts itself between the phospholipids with its hydrophilic hydroxyl group facing outwards, and it reduces the movement of phospholipid molecules.

Proteins in cell membranes

The amount of protein varies greatly between different membranes. The erythrocyte plasma membrane is about half lipid and half protein with about 8% carbohydrate. In contrast, the myelin membrane, which surrounds nerve cell axons and acts as an insulator, is almost 80% lipid. On the other hand, the inner mitochondrial membrane, which contains many embedded enzymes, is over 75% protein.

The cell membrane proteins include enzymes, transporters, transmembrane channels, receptors, molecules associated with cell adhesion and recognition, and proteins that link the cytoskeleton and the ECM.

The **integral membrane proteins** can only be removed by disrupting the membrane structure. Many of these proteins span the bilayer and have hydrophobic amino acid residues in their transmembrane section, while the parts inside and outside the cell are hydrophilic and may also carry charged groups. The charged groups present on the extracellular side are often glycosylated residues.

Peripheral membrane proteins, in contrast, may be removed without disrupting the membrane. They may be associated with the cytoskeleton or may be attached to the ECM. Many are involved in signal transduction across the membrane.

CYTOPLASM

Cytoplasm is a viscous, aqueous solution criss-crossed by the cytoskeleton fibres. It fills the space between the plasma membrane and the nucleus and forms a suspending medium for other subcellular organelles.

CYTOSKELETON

All cells have an internal skeleton (**cytoskeleton**) consisting of protein fibres (Table 2.14) made up of microfilaments, microtubules and intermediate filaments.

Microfilaments are double strands of actin about 7 nm thick (Fig. 2.35A) which form a mesh below the plasma membrane. Its components are linked to proteins embedded in the membrane. These in turn may connect with molecules present in the ECM. This enables a cell to fix its shape with respect to the external environment and, if necessary, even move around.

Actin filaments provide support for the cell membranes. They also form a core of membrane projections such as **microvilli**, present in cells that are required to absorb substances from the extracellular medium, such as those found in the intestine and kidney. There may be up to 3000 microvilli per cell, forming what is known as the brush border. They are small (<1 μm) cell membrane projections and may increase the surface area for absorption up to 30-fold. They are attached to a network of filaments running under the surface of the cell.

Microtubules participate in the intracellular movement of organelles. They are made up of two globular proteins, α- and β-tubulin polymerised into a protofilament. Thirteen protofilaments are arranged to form a tube called a singlet (Fig. 2.35C) which can be enlarged to a doublet or triplet.

Centrosomes are formed from microtubules and locate near the nucleus. The microtubules are embedded in it at one end, and radiate from there towards the plasma membrane.

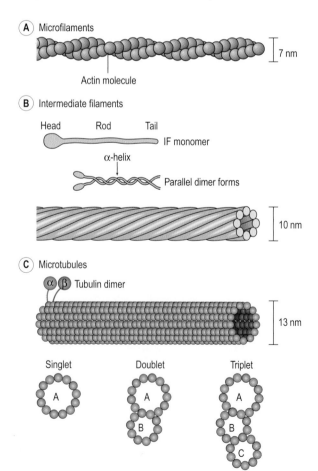

Ⓐ Microfilaments

7 nm

Actin molecule

Ⓑ Intermediate filaments

Head   Rod   Tail

IF monomer

α-helix

Parallel dimer forms

10 nm

Ⓒ Microtubules

α β Tubulin dimer

13 nm

Singlet   Doublet   Triplet

Fig. 2.35 **Structure of cytoskeletal elements.** IF, intermediate filament.

The microtubules are used as tracks along which organelles can be moved. The centrosome contains two **centrioles** that direct the movement of the chromosomes during cell division.

An example of the function of microtubules is transport of substances in the neurons. There, the proteins required by the synapse are manufactured in the cell body and transported along the microtubules. This is known as fast **axonal transport**. It occurs in both directions along the same microtubule: the **anterograde transport** carries new material from the cell body to the synapse and is carried out by **kinesins**. **Retrograde transport** carries materials back to the cell body for destruction in the lysosomes and is carried out by the motor proteins, **dyneins**.

A number of proteins known as **microtubule-associated proteins** are attached to microtubules. They crosslink microtubules in the cytoplasm, or bind to the intermediate filaments. One of such proteins found in nerve cells is called **tau**. Its accumulation and cross-linking can lead to the formation of the so-called neurofibrillary tangles found in the brains of many people with Alzheimer disease.

Cilia and flagella are mobile projections of the plasma membrane composed of microtubules. They are anchored to the basal body just underneath the membrane. They are moved by dyneins, using energy derived from ATP. Cilia are up to 10 μm long, and move fluids or particles across the cell surface. For instance, cells that line larger airways have cilia that move mucus and small particles out of the lungs. Flagella are much longer: the only human cells that have flagella are sperm.

Intermediate filaments are made from a variety of proteins. They form α-helical dimers which twist around one another (Fig. 2.35B). They form the most stable element of the cytoskeleton and provide support to the nucleus and the plasma membrane.

NUCLEUS

Most eukaryotic cells possess a nucleus. Some cells have more than one nucleus, whereas mammalian red blood cells lose their nucleus as they mature (see Ch. 12). The nucleus is the only organelle that can be seen under the light microscope without staining.

The nucleus is surrounded by a double layer of membrane, the **nuclear envelope**. The inner membrane is smooth, whereas the outer membrane may be continuous with the endoplasmic reticulum. The nuclear envelope is studded with pores about 9 nm in diameter, through which proteins and RNA can pass.

The nucleus contains chromatin, which is not normally visible as an organised structure. Inside the nucleus are one or more dark-staining spherical areas called **nucleoli**. They are the place of assembly of the ribosomes and contain large amounts of RNA and proteins. Surrounding the chromatin and the nucleoli is a gel-like substance called the **nucleoplasm**.

ENDOPLASMIC RETICULUM

The endoplasmic reticulum (ER) is a network of interconnected tubules and sacs extending from the nucleus into the cytoplasm (Information box 2.13). There are two types of ER within the cell. The **rough ER** membranes are covered with dense granules which are **ribosomes**. Not surprisingly, the rough ER is extensive in cells that have high levels of protein synthesis. The smooth ER is continuous with rough ER but is granule-free. It contains enzymes that synthesise membrane phospholipids, cholesterol and steroid hormones.

In the hepatocytes, the rough ER is involved in the synthesis of plasma proteins, such as albumin. Enzymes present in the smooth ER are involved in the detoxification of a wide range of non-polar molecules, including drugs, which they transform into polar metabolites that are subsequently excreted by the kidney (see Ch.14). In these cells, the smooth ER is also associated with glycogen granules.

GOLGI APPARATUS (GOLGI COMPLEX)

The Golgi apparatus consists of stacks of flattened containers (they are described as miniature cisterns or sacs) located in the cytosol, in the space extending concentrically from the endoplasmic reticulum surrounding the nucleus towards the cell membrane (Fig. 2.28). The segments close to the nucleus are known as the cis-Golgi, the segments located in the intermediate distance are median Golgi, and the parts closest to the cell membrane are the trans-Golgi. The system remains in contact with cytoskeletal filaments.

The two important functions of the Golgi apparatus are modification of proteins and lipids, primarily by attachment of carbohydrates (glycosylation), and their sorting and distribution to other organelles within the cell, or packaging for subsequent secretion from the cell.

The proteins which are to be processed are transferred to the Golgi apparatus from the endoplasmic reticulum within the membranous vesicles. Complex carbohydrates (e.g. glycosaminoglycans) are synthesised within the Golgi. Once this is completed, new vesicles bud off from the trans-Golgi and fuse with the cell membrane or other organelles. Vesicles containing substances subject to regulated secretion (secretion in response to a stimulus, see above) are transported towards the membrane along the cytoskeletal filaments.

MITOCHONDRIA

Mitochondria are generally sausage-shaped and about 1 μm wide and 7 μm long. They are enclosed by a double layer of membrane separated by the intermembrane space. The outer membrane is permeable to small molecules, due to the presence of **porin**, a pore-forming protein. The inner membrane contains many embedded proteins that are involved in oxidative phosphorylation. This membrane has multiple folds (**cristae**) projecting inwards. The interior of the mitochondrion is called the **matrix**.

Mitochondria contain the enzymes of the electron transport chain and several other major pathways such as the Krebs cycle and the pathway of the beta-oxidation of fatty acids. Mitochondria generate most of the cellular ATP through oxidative phosphorylation. They are particularly plentiful in cells, which consume large amounts of energy.

In plants, the organelle equivalent to the mitochondrion is the **chloroplast**, which generates organic substances using solar energy, water and CO_2 by photosynthesis, and produces oxygen as a 'waste product'.

LYSOSOMES

Lysosomes are spherical or oval organelles measuring up to 400 nm in diameter. The important function of the lysosomal membrane is that it compartmentalises intracellular degradative enzymes. The lysosomes contain **acid hydrolases** that can digest most biological molecules. The pH inside is around 4.8 and is optimal for their activity. Also, such pH denatures many proteins and this facilitates their degradation. If many lysosomes are ruptured, the cell self-digests. This is known as **autolysis** and occurs physiologically, for instance during the breakdown of the uterine lining during menstruation.

Vesicles from the Golgi apparatus and other membrane-bound structures fuse with lysosomes, delivering their contents for degradation. These include phagosomes containing bacteria and viruses retrieved from the extracellular space by endocytosis and phagocytosis. The lysosome also destroys aged cell organelles, which are first engulfed by the ER, forming vesicles and subsequently are passed to the lysosomes.

PROTEASOMES

Proteasomes are specialised structures that degrade cytosolic proteins. They are protein complexes arranged in four rings around a central core. Proteins destined for destruction are first tagged with multiple copies of a protein called **ubiquitin**. This directs them into the core of the proteasome where they are degraded. Only proteins tagged with ubiquitin are able to enter the proteasomes.

PEROXISOMES

Peroxisomes resemble the lysosomes and are particularly abundant in the hepatocytes. They contain enzymes such as **oxidases** and **catalases**. The oxidases oxidise substrates such as fatty acids, using molecular oxygen as a substrate, and generating hydrogen peroxide (H_2O_2). Other oxidases are involved in the biosynthesis of cholesterol and other membrane components. H_2O_2 is also produced by some cells of the immune system in order to kill bacteria. Catalase uses H_2O_2 to oxidise other potentially toxic compounds, or breaks it down to water.

CELL JUNCTIONS

Cells adhere to each other forming tissues, organs and sheets, which anatomically separate different body compartments. This adhesion is through the interactions of cell adhesion molecules described below. There are several types of junctions between cells, and between cells and the ECM (Fig. 2.33):

- **Tight junctions**, which prevent movement of substances between cells
- **Adhering junctions**, which maintain cellular positions
- **Gap junctions,** which allow movement of substances between cells.

Tight junctions

Tight junctions form a belt around the cell attached to the neighbouring cells. Each is formed from a complex of proteins that connect two membranes tightly together. Tight junctions also separate different parts of the surface of polarised cells. This allows each region of membrane to perform its distinct functions. Tight junctions also prevent the passage of molecules between cells forming a sheet.

Adhering junctions

Adhering junctions are bound to cytoskeletal elements, lying just below the plasma membrane. They connect to elements of neighbouring cells, or, through integrins, to the ECM.

Gap junctions

The gap junctions are formed from integral membrane proteins called **connexins**. A pore in the membrane, a **connexon,** is formed from six connexin molecules, and is aligned with the connexon in the opposing cell, forming a channel, which allows free passage of water, ions and small molecules. Electrical coupling of cells via gap junctions allows the dissemination of excitation signals (this is particularly important in smooth muscle and cardiac cells).

CELL ADHESION AND RECOGNITION

In multicellular organisms, a cell interacts both with the surrounding cells and with the components of the extracellular space. During development, where cells are forming into tissues, there are considerable movements of cells from place to place. In the adult, to divide and grow in a controlled manner, cells need to sense their surroundings. The sensors are the cell adhesion molecules. The cell–cell adhesion in, for instance, muscle cells and in the skin is permanent. On the other hand, the interactions between circulating white blood cells and the endothelial cells are transitory.

There are four types of adhesion molecules that allow cells to make connections between each other and the ECM. The **cadherins** and the **selectins** are calcium-dependent, and the **integrins** and the cell adhesion molecules are calcium-independent. They are all transmembrane proteins with intracellular and extracellular domains.

There are more than 80 **cadherins**. Their intracellular domain interacts with actin via other proteins called catenins, and the extracellular section consists of a dimer with four calcium-binding sites. The dimer binds to the cadherin on the neighbouring cell. The removal of calcium reduces cell adhesiveness (this is exploited during preparation of tissue extracts for cell culture).

Selectins bind to the glycoproteins, especially on the surface of leucocytes, and this, for instance, helps to target sites of inflammation. When the endothelial cell is stimulated by inflammatory factors, the selectins are inserted into the cell membrane and interact with circulating leucocytes, facilitating leucocyte movement across the endothelial layer.

The **integrins** mediate interactions between the cell and the ECM. They bind to laminin and fibronectin in the ECM. Inside the cell, they bind to cytoskeletal proteins.

Intercellular adhesion molecules (ICAM) and **vascular adhesion molecules** (VCAM) mediate interactions between the vascular endothelial cells and leucocytes. These molecules have a structure similar to immunoglobulin G.

SIGNAL TRANSDUCTION IN CELLS

Cells communicate through signals that may be chemical, electrical or mechanical. The signal transfer molecules are hormones, cytokines, growth factors and neurotransmitters. They bind to receptors present on the cell surface (or intracellularly, see below). The membrane receptors then initiate what is called the intracellular signal cascade: a further transfer and amplification of the signal. This process may involve a molecule known as the second messenger and a chain of events which usually involves a series of protein phosphorylations and dephosphorylations (Fig. 2. 29).

Some signal transfer molecules do not require membrane receptors: they cross cell membranes and bind to (and thus activate) intracellular receptors that become transcription factors. They transfer to the nucleus and bind to the response elements on DNA. This alters gene expression and thus protein synthesis in the cell.

Hormones

A hormone is a substance secreted in very small amounts by a group of cells (the endocrine gland) and is then transported to its target cells, on which it exerts a regulatory action. Hormones differ in the distance over which they exert their actions and the wider definition includes endocrine, paracrine and autocrine hormones. The endocrine hormones are transported in the blood and can reach the entire organism. The paracrine hormones act on a close group of cells. Finally, an autocrine hormone affects the cells by which it has been produced (Fig. 2.36).

The paracrine and autocrine hormones are called **cytokines**. They affect cell growth and differentiation, and the inflammatory and immune responses. **Growth factors,** substances that promote growth of cells in culture, or the growth of an organism, are also cytokines. Another group of cytokines are the interferons, which act against viruses and cancer cells.

Neurotransmitters

Neurotransmitters are released from nerve endings. They are small molecules, such as acetylcholine, epinephrine (adrenaline) or norepinephrine (noradrenaline). Nerves may also secrete peptide neurotransmitters, such as the natural painkiller β-endorphin. The neural responses are faster than the hormonal responses.

RECEPTORS

Hormones, cytokines and neurotransmitters produce an effect on target cells by interacting with their **receptors**. The receptors are proteins that specifically bind one molecule or a closely related group of molecules (the **receptor's ligands**) and transmit the signal contained in the ligand molecule to the cell interior (See Information box 2.14).

Cell surface (membrane) receptors

Membrane receptors are proteins embedded in the cell membrane, with the binding site located on the cell surface. Binding of a **ligand** causes a conformational change in the receptor, often associated with its self-phosphorylation. The receptor possesses tyrosine kinase activity and phosphorylates itself when the ligand binds. It often also phosphorylates a number of other molecules to initiate different signal cascades.

Signal transduction cascades

Signal transduction cascades are series of reactions which disseminate and amplify intracellular signals generated by hormones and neurotransmitters. Many of the molecules that transduce the signal are enzymes and thus each turn over a large number of molecules. This explains the amplification – the fact that hormones present in minute concentrations precipitate major metabolic changes which can be, for instance, activation of multiple enzymes and change of direction of major metabolic pathways, or change in the expression pattern of genes that influence growth and differentiation.

The sequence of events is initiated by the binding of a molecule (a ligand) to its receptor, followed by the receptor activation. The activated receptor in turn activates transduction molecules, which stimulate synthesis of a second messenger, a key molecule that will activate or inhibit key intracellular enzymes (usually kinases). Actually, the key kinases often initiate chains of kinase-catalysed phosphorylations, which eventually affect the regulatory enzymes in cellular pathways. Kinases such as protein kinase A, protein kinase B (also known as Akt) or protein kinase C play a particularly important role in signalling cascades.

Endocrine

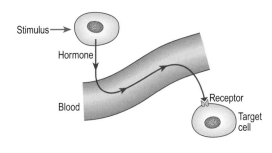

Paracrine

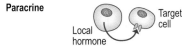

Autocrine

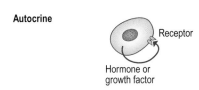

Neural signalling

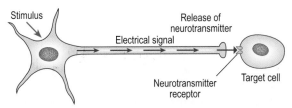

Fig. 2.36 **Different types of cell signalling.**

| Information box 2.14 | High levels of plasma cholesterol can be caused by a defect in LDL receptors |

A genetic disorder known as familial hypercholesterolaemia leads to a raised concentration of cholesterol in the blood. This defect occurs in about 1 in 500 of the normal population and is also associated with a family history of early heart disease and lipid deposition in the tendons known as xanthoma. It also carries a substantially increased risk of premature heart disease, particularly in the homozygotes.

There are a number of genetic mutations responsible for the disease, but the common theme is a reduction in the removal of LDL particles from plasma via the LDL receptors. In some cases the receptor numbers are reduced. In others, the receptor itself is defective.

There are a large number of transducing molecules that link membrane receptors to second messengers (see below). Perhaps the best known are the guanine nucleotide binding proteins (G-proteins). They are composed of subunits (designated, for instance, Gα, Gβ and Gγ). A ligand which binds to a receptor stimulates the Gα subunit to bind GTP and to dissociate from other subunits; the remaining subunits can now bind other activating molecules and in turn activate other proteins in the cytosol. Different G-proteins either activate or inhibit other proteins (enzymes). Some G-proteins such as Ras and Raf are themselves serine/threonine protein kinases. Other involved molecules are GTPases such as Rho protein, or guanine nucleotide exchange factors (SOS1). The G-proteins stimulate the enzyme adenylate cyclase, which produces cyclic AMP (cAMP) from ATP.

cAMP is the key intracellular second messenger. In this concept, the hormones are regarded as the first messengers and the second messengers are key signal transduction molecules that initiate new signalling cascades. cAMP, for instance, links downstream to protein kinase A (PKA) and mediates, among others, the action of hormones such as glucagon and epinephrine.

G-proteins also activate (through the control of calcium channels) the enzyme phospholipase C which cleaves a phospholipid, phosphatidylinositol 4,5-bisphosphate (PIP_2), generating two lipid second messengers, inositol 1,4,5-trisphosphate (IP_3) and diacylglycerol (DAG). IP_3 also activates calcium channels in the ER.

An example of a complex set of signalling pathways is the action of insulin. Insulin signalling involves membrane receptor autophosphorylation and concomitant phosphorylation of the proteins belonging to the insulin receptor substrate (IRS) family. IRS proteins, in turn, have domains that allow binding of several proteins that, through different pathways, link to protein kinase C and, in parallel, to the Ras/mitogen activated protein kinase (MAPK) growth-stimulating pathway. Another path involves phosphoinositide-3-kinase (PI3K) (which generates phosphatidylinositol phosphates) and protein kinase B/Akt which stimulates glycogen synthesis as well as protein synthesis and transcription factors involved in programmed cell death (apoptosis). A third pathway, also involving PI3K, Akt and another series of transducing proteins, affects the membrane recruitment of the glucose transporter GLUT4 (see below). Still other pathways affect lipid metabolism and gluconeogenesis.

Intracellular receptors

Hydrophobic signalling molecules, such as the steroid hormones (e.g. cortisol, testosterone or oestrogens), cross the cell membrane and bind to receptors that are present in the cytoplasm. After binding of the hormone, the activated hormone-receptor complex transfers to the nucleus, where it binds to response elements in the DNA, affecting gene expression (it acts as a transcription factor). Some receptors/transcription factors need two different ligand molecules for activation: this refines their regulatory potential.

MEMBRANE TRANSPORT

Membrane transport is a fundamental biological function that sustains life. The movement of molecules across biological membranes depends on their size and lipid solubility.

Hydrophobic molecules move into cells by simple diffusion through the lipid phase, but hydrophilic substances which cannot cross the membrane bilayer require **transport systems** for this.

PASSIVE DIFFUSION

Passive diffusion is the diffusion of a substance down its concentration gradient (from a high concentration to a low concentration). This is the mode of transport of small molecules such as water, oxygen, carbon dioxide and fat-soluble molecules (Fig. 2.37).

CARRIER MEDIATED TRANSPORT

Carrier mediated transport requires the presence of special proteins (transporters) within the membrane. They bind the molecule to be transported on one side of the membrane and move it to the other side. Carrier mediated transport is the mode of transport of molecules that are either polar or charged and therefore unable to spontaneously diffuse through cell membranes. The transporters are specific and saturable. The binding characteristics of a transported molecule can be described using the Michaelis–Menten equation.

There are three types of carrier-mediated transport:

- Facilitated diffusion
- Active transport
- Secondary active transport.

Facilitated diffusion

Facilitated diffusion is transport of a molecule by a membrane transporter down its concentration gradient. The transporters involved are also called **permeases**. They span the entire thickness of the membrane. Transporters that bind a single substrate are called **uniporters**. Maximal rates of transport mediated by permeases are in the order of 10^2–10^4 molecules per second. An example of facilitated diffusion is the transport of glucose in the erythrocytes. The glucose transporter

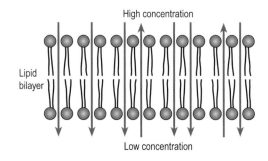

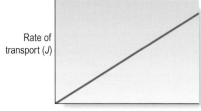

Fig. 2.37 **Passive diffusion.** The graph shows the relationship between rate and concentration difference.

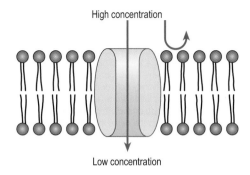

High concentration

Low concentration

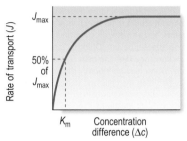

Fig. 2.38 Facilitated transport via an ion channel.
The graph shows the relationship between rate and concentration difference.

involved is known as GLUT1 and is one of a number of such transporters (GLUT1–GLUT5).

Ion channels

Facilitated diffusion also involves the movement of ions (Fig. 2.38). Charged ions can cross plasma membranes via protein pores called ion channels (see Ch. 4). They are selective for specific ions, e.g. sodium, potassium or calcium. About 40 different types of ion channels have been identified so far. Some channels open in response to chemical signals, either directly (**ligand-gated ion channels**) or indirectly (**receptor-operated channels**). Others are opened by changes in the electrical potential (**voltage-gated channels**). Ion channels allow a faster rate of transfer of the transporters: 10^7–10^8 ions per second.

Active transport

Active transport is carrier-mediated transport that requires energy input and moves molecules against their concentration gradient. The enzymes involved in active transport are known as ATPases. They use ATP and are critical for cell function.

Na⁺/K⁺-ATPase

The most important of the ATPases is **Na⁺/K⁺-ATPase**, a cation pump located in the plasma membrane (Fig. 2.39). It pumps intracellular Na⁺ out of the cell in exchange for K⁺, which it moves from the extracellular space into the cytoplasm (See also Information box 2.15).

Other ATPases

Apart from Na⁺/K⁺-ATPase, several other ATPase exist in a cell. H⁺/K⁺-ATPase locates in the membranes surrounding the lysosomes. It transports H⁺ into the lysosome, decreasing the intra-lysosomal pH. The Ca²⁺-ATPases are active in removing ionised calcium from the cytoplasm, either by pumping it into organelles or across the plasma membrane. In the mitochondria, an ATPase known as ATP synthase runs

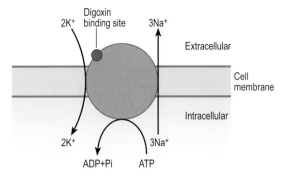

Fig. 2.39 Na⁺/K⁺-ATPase. Pi, phosphate.

Information box 2.15 **Na⁺/K⁺-ATPase**

Na⁺/K⁺-ATPase consists of four protein subunits ($\alpha2\beta2$), all of which span the cell membrane. Na⁺/K⁺-ATPase removes three Na⁺ ions from the cell in each cycle, in exchange for two K⁺ ions (Fig. 2.39). The sequence of events is as follows:
1. The ATPase binds ATP.
2. The ATPase binds three Na⁺ ions.
3. ATP phosphorylates the α-subunits. This induces conformational changes and three Na⁺ ions are released into the extracellular fluid.
4. Two K⁺ ions bind from the extracellular fluid.
5. The α-subunits are dephosphorylated. The ATPase reverts to its previous conformation and two K⁺ ions are released into the cell.

Information box 2.16 **Two transport processes are involved in the action of digoxin on the heart**

Na⁺/K⁺-ATPase can be inhibited by a number of compounds extracted from the foxglove (*Digitalis purpurea*), called cardiac glycosides, the most important of which is digoxin. Digoxin binds to a site on the external face of the ATPase and inhibits it. The consequence is an increased force of contraction of the heart, which can be exploited in the treatment of heart failure.

This is due to an increase in the intracellular concentration of calcium. Usually calcium is removed from the cardiac muscle by the action of a secondary active antiporter, the Na⁺/Ca²⁺ exchange pump, which exchanges extracellular sodium for intracellular calcium. When the Na⁺/K⁺-ATPase is inhibited, the intracellular sodium concentration rises and the exchange is inhibited due to the reduction in the sodium gradient, which powers the transport. Calcium builds up inside the cell and inactivates the protein troponin, which normally inhibits the actin – myosin interaction, thus facilitating cardiac muscle contraction.

'in reverse', using the energy of the H⁺ gradient to synthesise ATP from ADP. Virtually all cells have cation pumps in their plasma membranes. It is estimated that as much as 30% of all ATP generated in the cell is used to power these pumps.

Secondary active transport

Na⁺/K⁺-ATPase maintains a Na⁺ concentration gradient across the cell membrane (high extracellular and low intracellular Na⁺ concentration). Such a gradient accumulates energy (see above). Many membrane transporters other than ATPase exploit this by allowing Na⁺ ions to diffuse back to the cell. This releases energy, which is then used to pump other substances out of the cell against their concentration gradients. This method of transport is known as **secondary active transport**. An example is the transport of many amino acids into cells which occurs by coupling the amino acid uptake to the diffusion of Na⁺.

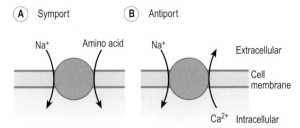

(A) Symport   (B) Antiport

Fig. 2.40 **Secondary active transport.**

Two types of transporters are engaged in secondary active transport (Fig. 2.40). Transporters that transport sodium and the accompanying ion in the same direction (as described above) are **symports**. Those that transport the accompanying ion in the direction opposite to the Na^+ are **antiports**. For example, a Na^+/Ca^{2+} antiport is present in heart muscle (see Information box 2.16 and Ch. 4).

COORDINATED ACTION OF TRANSPORTERS

The movement of substances through cells usually requires the coordinated activity of different transport systems. An example is the transport of glucose from the intestine into the blood (Fig. 2.41). The transported glucose crosses both the apical and basolateral membrane of enterocytes lining the intestinal lumen. This involves the concerted action of three different transport systems. The transport of glucose across the luminal brush border is by secondary active transport via a sodium-dependent symport called sodium/glucose linked transport-1 (SGLT1). The SGLT uses the energy stored in the sodium ion gradient created by the Na^+/K^+-ATPase situated on the basolateral membrane. The transport of glucose from the enterocyte into the extracellular space involves the GLUT2 transporter also located in the basolateral membrane (See also Clinical box 2.11).

ENDOCYTOSIS

Endocytosis involves the enclosure of transported substances by the plasma membrane, which is then pinched off inside the cell (Fig. 2.42). It is the mode of transport of large molecules that cannot be moved into the cell by protein transporters. There are three major categories of endocytosis: phagocytosis, pinocytosis and receptor-mediated endocytosis.

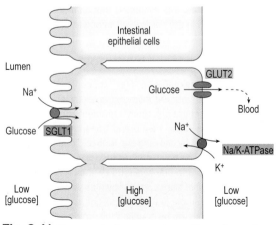

Fig. 2.41 **Transport of sugars across the enterocytes.**

Clinical box 2.11	Oral rehydration therapy relies on the action of transporters

Diarrhoea causes (sometimes massive) loss of water and salts from the intestine. A key part of the treatment involves rehydration of the patient. It was observed during a cholera epidemic that when severely dehydrated patients were treated with sodium chloride solution alone, the response was poorer than when a combination of sodium chloride and glucose was administered. This led to the development of the oral rehydration solution (ORS), which is now recommended by the WHO. Its use has saved millions of children worldwide, and its development has been hailed as one of the most important medical achievements in the twentieth century.

ORS is a powder, which contains a mixture of glucose, potassium salt and sodium chloride, to be dissolved in water for oral ingestion. When it reaches the intestine, the SGLT transporter is activated, and sodium, glucose and amino acids are transported across the epithelium. Chloride ions are drawn through the tight junctions between the cells by the positively charged sodium ions. Water is subsequently drawn through the paracellular pathway between the cells and hence into the blood (see also Ch. 16).

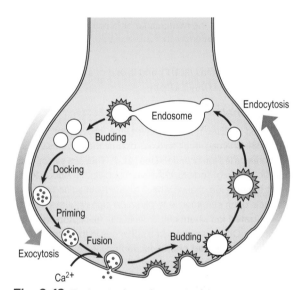

Fig. 2.42 **Endocytosis and exocytosis.**

Phagocytosis involves the uptake of large particles into vesicles called **phagosomes**. It is mainly carried out by macrophages and neutrophils, cells belonging to the immune system. It forms a part of the body's defence against pathogens. Recognition of bacteria, or other particles, by the phagocyte (see Ch.6) triggers a rearrangement of their actin cytoskeleton so that the plasma membrane is extended around the particle, forming an intracellular phagosome. Once the particle is engulfed, the phagosome is moved to the lysosomes for digestion. Anything that cannot be degraded remains in the lysosome as a residual body. In long-term smokers, for example, lung tissue is blackened by the accumulation of macrophages in the septa of the alveoli that contain black particles derived from inhaled smoke.

Pinocytosis is carried out by small vesicles that take up external fluid and solutes. Cells can also ingest large amounts of fluid and solutes by macro-pinocytosis, where an extension of the plasma membrane spreads around an area of extracellular fluid. Cells in the thyroid gland use this method to take up thyroglobulin.

EXOCYTOSIS

Exocytosis is the inverse of endocytosis. It involves the fusion of intracellular vesicles with the plasma membrane, and the release of their contents into the extracellular fluid. Exocytosis is the mechanism by which receptors are returned to the cell surface and also the mechanism of secretion of hormones and neurotransmitters (see Ch. 8).

TRANSCYTOSIS

Some substances are moved across cells by transcytosis. This is a combination of endocytosis and exocytosis. It takes place, for instance, in the intestinal epithelium. The transported molecules are moved by receptor-mediated endocytosis into endosomes, which travel across the cell and fuse with the opposite plasma membrane, releasing the transported species. The membrane of the vesicle containing the receptors is then endocytosed, and exocytosed on the other side, completing the cycle. An example of transcytosis is the movement of immunoglobulins derived from the mother's milk across the intestine of the newborn.

RECEPTOR-MEDIATED ENDOCYTOSIS

Receptor-mediated endocytosis is a mechanism for concentrating and internalising proteins. The substrate first binds to cell surface receptors, which are clustered in the area of membrane that is coated with a lattice of a protein called **clathrin**. The binding causes the membrane to fold inward, forming a coated pit. The edges of the pit fuse together and a clathrin-coated intracellular vesicle is formed. The clathrin then dissociates from the vesicle, which fuses with another endosome with a low internal pH, and this makes the ligand-receptor complex dissociate. The membrane is then returned to the cell surface, and the ligand is either delivered to lysosomes, or transported into the cytoplasm (Information box 2.17).

TRANSPORT OF SUBSTANCES IN THE BLOOD

The membrane transport processes described above move substances over very short distances. The fastest mode of transport over longer distances is transport in the blood. The flow of blood allows the movement of large quantities of nutrients, signalling molecules, gases and waste products. For instance, in humans, blood transports oxygen from the lungs to the furthest blood vessels in the limbs in about 30 seconds (see Ch. 11).

ORGANS AND TISSUES

Almost all the cells in the body show some specialisation, and most are organised into tissues and organs. Tissues are collections of cells adapted to perform a specific function. Organs are structures where more than one tissue contributes to a functional unit.

The embryo contains non-specialised (pluripotent) stem cells that differentiate into all specialised cell types. At the very early stage of embryo development, by 16 days, three layers of cells develop. They are called, from the surface inwards, **ectoderm, mesoderm** and **endoderm**. All cell types form from these three germ cell layers. Some, such as epithelial cells, form from all three germ cell layers. Others are derived from a single layer. For example, the nervous tissue is derived from ectoderm, muscle and connective tissue mainly from mesoderm, and most mucosal membranes from endoderm.

In the adult only some cell types, such as epithelial and blood-forming cells, remain highly mitotic. Others, such as nervous tissue, rarely divide. Some new cells are produced by division of mature differentiated cells, but many are derived from relatively undifferentiated stem cells. Stem cells have now been observed in different tissues. The possibility of using stem cells from easily accessible sources, such as the blood, to produce replacement cells in organs such as the brain, where local stem cells are rarer, has a great therapeutic potential (see Information box 2.18).

There are four primary tissue types in the body:

- Epithelial tissues
- Connective tissues (including blood)
- Muscle
- Nervous tissues.

EPITHELIAL TISSUES

Epithelial tissues are sheets of cells which cover body surfaces and form secretory glands. They perform a variety of functions, which include secretion, absorption, protection and transport. Epithelial tissues exhibit polarity. They are joined by intercellular junctions. The basement membrane provides mechanical support and attachment for the cells. Many epithelial cells have specialisations of their apical surfaces, such as **microvilli** and **cilia**.

Information box 2.17	Low-density lipoproteins (LDL) and transferrin are taken into cells by receptor-mediated endocytosis

The LDL particles are spherical, measure about 20 nm in diameter, and are composed of a single phospholipid and cholesterol-containing layer surrounding a core consisting of hydrophobic cholesterol esters. A protein, known as apolipoprotein B, is embedded in the phospholipid monolayer. Apolipoprotein B binds to the LDL receptors, 'fixing' the particle to the cell surface. Subsequently the LDL-receptor complex is ingested in a clathrin-coated vesicle. The receptor is recycled to the cell surface and LDL is degraded inside the cell.

The uptake of transferrin loaded with iron also occurs through receptor mediated endocytosis but with a slightly different sequence of events. Transferrin is an iron-binding protein present in plasma. Transferrin with the bound iron binds to transferrin receptors, and the complex is endocytosed in clathrin-coated vesicles. Subsequently the iron dissociates from the transferrin. When the receptors are returned to the plasma membrane, the iron-free **transferrin** is released to the plasma.

Information box 2.18	Neural stem cells

During the development of the nervous system, cells in the neural tube become **multipotent stem cells** that can divide into all the different cells of the brain. Stem cells in other tissues, for example **haematopoietic stem cells** in the bone marrow, can produce all the blood cells. While the blood stem cells remain active throughout life, until recently it was thought that stem cells were not present in the nervous system after the initial phase of brain development. Neural stem cells have now been isolated from both foetal and adult brains. They normally do not divide in adults, but current research is aimed to identify conditions under which these cells can be stimulated.

Epithelial tissues, which form linings, may form a simple epithelium made up of either a single layer of cells, or from several layers (stratified epithelium). The cells may have different shapes: cuboidal, flattened (squamous), columnar or transitional (where the cells vary in shape across the different layers) (Fig. 2.43).

Glandular epithelial cells store and secrete substances such as enzymes or hormones. The simplest types of glandular epithelium are the goblet cells, which secrete mucus into the intestinal lumen. Epithelial cells can be organised into glands. The **exocrine glands** secrete either to the outside of

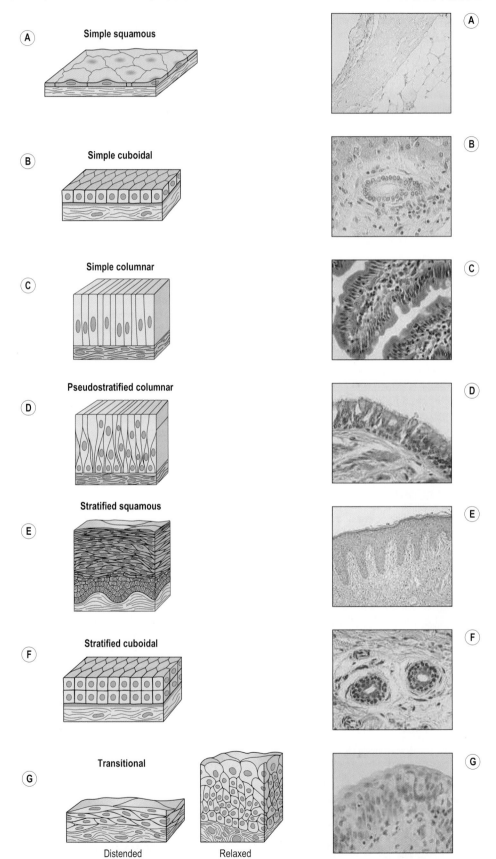

(A) Simple squamous

(B) Simple cuboidal

(C) Simple columnar

(D) Pseudostratified columnar

(E) Stratified squamous

(F) Stratified cuboidal

(G) Transitional

Distended   Relaxed

Fig. 2.43 Epithelial cell types.

the body or into luminal spaces via an excretory duct, and **endocrine glands,** which are ductless and secrete directly into the bloodstream.

CONNECTIVE TISSUE

There are four types of connective tissue (see also Ch. 9):

- Fibrocollagenous tissues
- Cartilage, teeth and bone
- Adipose tissue
- Blood.

Fibrocollagenous tissues

Fibrocollagenous tissues can be in turn divided into three main types (Fig. 2.44):

- **Loose connective tissue**, with abundant ground substance, some collagen and elastic fibres, and many different cells.
- **Dense connective tissue**, which has little ground substance, abundant collagen and few cells. It provides mechanical support and tensile strength.

Cells that are found in the connective tissue include **fibroblasts**, which are spindle-shaped with an oval nucleus. They have a well-developed ER and a Golgi apparatus, which reflects their role in the secretion of ECM components. They produce proteoglycans of the ECM as well as the precursors of the collagens and the elastins. Fibroblasts are active in wound healing. Fibrocollagenous tissue also contains small numbers of **fat cells** (adipocytes), **stem cells** and a variety of cells belonging to the **immune system** such as macrophages, mast cells and plasma cells (see Ch. 6). It also contains **blood vessels**.

Extracellular matrix

The ECM contains **ground substance**, made up of three main elements: the **glycosaminoglycans** (**GAGs**), structural proteins such as **laminin** and **fibronectin,** and either **collagen** or **elastin** fibres.

Cartilage, teeth and bone

Cartilage is less dense than bone. It is solid but flexible and resists compression, while allowing diffusion of water through its matrix. It lacks blood vessels, so all metabolites are exchanged by diffusion. The ground substance of cartilage has a large amount of glycosaminoglycans bound to a lattice of **type II collagen**. Growing cartilage contains **chondroblasts**, metabolically active cells, which secrete proteins and contain energy reserves in the form of lipids and glycogen. Adult cartilage contains the much less active mature **chondrocytes**. The three types of cartilage reflect the varying proportion and types of fibres:

- **Hyaline cartilage** contains type II collagen only, forms most of the embryonic skeleton, and in the adult forms the sternal parts of the ribs and also the cartilage found in the nose, trachea and larynx. It also covers the ends of the long bones where it can absorb compressional stresses.
- **Elastic cartilage** has more elastic fibres than hyaline cartilage. It supports the pinna of the external part of the ear and forms the epiglottis.

(A)

Loose or areolar connective tissue
Submucosa of large intestine

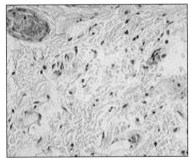

(B)

Dense connective tissues
Dermis of the skin

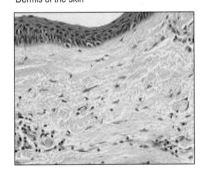

(C)

Tendon

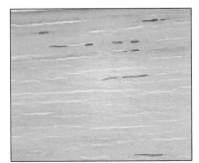

(D)

Reticular tissue
Liver

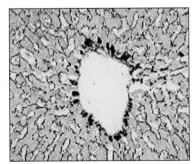

Fig. 2.44 **Types of fibrocollagenous tissue.**

Clinical box 2.12 Osteoporosis is caused by increased reabsorption of bone

Post-menopausal women are deficient in sex steroid hormones, oestrogens, and the consequence is a reduction in bone density due to an increase in the numbers of osteoclasts leading to an increase in bone reabsorption. This makes the bones fragile and more likely to fracture.

- **Fibrocartilage** has less matrix than hyaline cartilage and contains type I collagen. It is more compressible than hyaline cartilage and is found in areas where there are high pressures, such as the intervertebral discs and the knee joints.

Teeth are made up of three layers. The external surface, or crown, of the tooth is covered by **enamel,** the hardest substance in the body. It is principally made up of calcium phosphate. The middle layer consists of a mineralised matrix, called **dentine**, which is similar to bone although cell-free. Inside the dentine is the **pulp cavity**, which contains the cells producing the dentine, the odontoblasts, as well as the nerves and blood vessels supplying the tooth. These enter the tooth through the **root canal**, a narrow channel at the root of the tooth. The part of the tooth embedded in the jawbone is covered by a thin layer of a calcified tissue called **cementum**, which serves both to anchor the tooth and protect it.

Bone is similar to cartilage, except that its ECM contains more collagen fibres and its matrix is mineralised. This produces a very rigid tissue that forms the skeleton. Bone is initially formed by the bone-forming cells, **osteoblasts**, which produce matrix called **osteoid**; this is followed by the deposition of crystals of **calcium hydroxyapatite** around the osteoblasts, which become **osteocytes**. Mature bone is continually being remodelled due to the activity of osteoblasts and the bone-resorbing cells, **osteoclasts** (see Ch. 9 and Clinical box 2.12).

Fat (adipose) tissue

Adipocytes are specialised mesenchymal cells, and contain large amounts of triacylglycerols. Fat serves as an energy store and performs an insulating function. Adipose tissue forms the subcutaneous fat and the visceral fat surrounding major organs in the abdominal cavity. Fat can also be deposited in other places, such as liver and muscle. The excess tissue deposition of fat underlies, for instance, the condition called fatty liver (liver steatosis).

It is now recognised that the adipose tissue is an active endocrine organ. It secretes cytokines specific to the adipose tissue (adipokines) such as leptin or adiponectin, and also pro-inflammatory cytokines such as interleukin-6 and tumour necrosis factor-α (TNF-α). Leptin regulates the adipose tissue mass, decreasing food intake by acting in the central nervous system (see Chs 8 and 16). It stimulates fatty acid oxidation and decreases triglyceride deposition. Adiponectin stimulates glucose oxidation and fatty acid metabolism. Low levels are associated with resistance to insulin and the development of hepatic steatosis. The size and number of adipocytes increase in obesity.

Blood

Blood is a connective tissue because it is derived from the mesoderm. It consists of red blood cells, white blood cells and platelets suspended in the aqueous matrix, the plasma. Different elements of blood carry nutrients and waste products and

Clinical box 2.13 Tests performed on plasma or serum

Anticoagulants and preservatives are used when blood is sampled for laboratory analyses.
Centrifugation of an unclotted blood sample yields plasma and the red blood cells. Centrifugation of blood which had been allowed to clot yields serum (which is plasma devoid of fibrinogen).

Laboratory tests can be performed on plasma or serum. To obtain plasma the blood is taken into sample tubes that contain anticoagulant. The most commonly used anticoagulant is EDTA. Heparin is used for some tests. When glucose is to be measured, a sample tube containing sodium fluoride is used to inhibit red cell glycolysis.

contribute to immunity by transporting white blood cells and antibodies. The coagulation system, which includes platelets and plasma coagulation factors, controls bleeding (see Ch. 12). Plasma contains the soluble protein **fibrinogen**, which is converted into insoluble fibrin during blood clotting (forming serum if the blood is allowed to clot in vitro) (See also Clinical box 2.13).

MUSCLE

Muscle is made up of **contractile cells** (**myocytes**) (Fig. 2.45). There are three types of muscle: skeletal muscle, smooth muscle and cardiac muscle. Another classification separates muscle into:

- **Voluntary**, which remains under conscious control, such as the muscles that move elements of the skeleton
- **Involuntary**, controlled by the autonomic nervous system.

(A)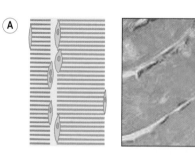

(B)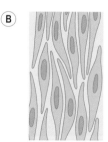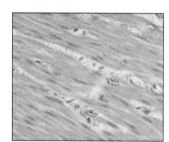

(C)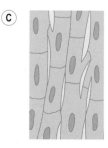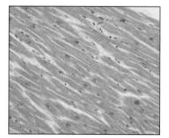

Fig. 2.45 **Muscle types.** (A) Skeletal muscle; (B) smooth muscle; (C) cardiac muscle.

Table 2.17	Comparison of the different types of muscle		
	Skeletal	**Smooth**	**Cardiac**
Morphology	Multinucleated, long, thin	Single nucleus, spindle-shaped	Single or double nuclei, cylindrical, branched, prominent intercalated discs
Appearance	Striated appearance due to overlapping bands of actin and myosin	No obvious striations	Striated appearance, but less organised than skeletal muscle
Unit of excitation	Groups of fibres called motor units	Linked by gap junctions	Linked by gap junctions
Contraction	Discontinuous	Usually continuous (resting tone), often rhythmic (wavelike)	Continuous, rhythmic
Regenerative ability	Limited regeneration	Can regenerate	No regeneration

Skeletal muscle is voluntary, and smooth muscle is involuntary (Table 2.17).

Skeletal muscle is made up of long, multinucleated cells, forming muscle **fibres** from the fusion of many single cells during development (see Ch. 9). The myocytes have a distinct banded appearance due to the arrangement of the myosin and actin filaments into repeating units called **sarcomeres**. The **myofilaments,** which make up the sarcomeres, are arranged in cylindrical **myofibrils,** which are themselves grouped together to form muscle fibres.

Muscle fibres are studded with muscle precursor cells called **satellite cells**. These quiescent cells resume proliferation when the muscle is either damaged or stressed. This activity is particularly obvious in weight lifters and body builders, who can remodel their muscles by increasingly stressing them.

Smooth muscles are made up of elongated spindle-shaped cells. The cells usually have a single nucleus and are much shorter than skeletal muscle cells. They are often joined together in sheets, and are electrically coupled through gap junctions. This enables the cells to contract in a coordinated manner. Their contraction is controlled by the autonomic nervous system, hormones and local factors such as stretching. Smooth muscle cells retain their ability to divide, and **hypertrophy** in response to increased stress.

Cardiac muscle is in some ways intermediate in type between skeletal and smooth muscle. It contains myofibrils, although the muscle cells are much shorter than in skeletal muscle. Cardiac muscle fibres are branched. They have large numbers of **gap junctions**, allowing electrical communication between cells, and **adhering junctions**, which bind the cells together to form an electrically and mechanically interconnected network. Due to their high energy requirement they have large numbers of mitochondria and a rich blood supply (see Ch. 11 and Clinical box 2.14).

NERVOUS TISSUE

The nervous tissue of the body is divided into the **central nervous system** (**CNS**), which consists of the brain and spinal cord, and the **peripheral nervous system** (**PNS**), which consists of all remaining nervous tissue.

Both the central and peripheral nervous systems are principally made up of two types of cells: **neurons** and **glia** (see Ch. 8). Minor types of cells present in the brain are the **ependymal cells** (epithelial cells, which line the brain ventricles) and **choroid epithelial cells** (cells involved in the secretion of the cerebrospinal fluid which bathes the brain).

Neurons are the cells of the brain that receive signals, process them and transmit the appropriate response either to another neuron or to an effector such as a secretory cell or a myocyte (Fig. 2.46). Neurons in general have a very high metabolic rate, which means that they require a continuous supply of oxygen and glucose. Energy-deprived neurons die rapidly.

During development, the epithelial cells lining the neural tube give rise to **neuroblasts**. They divide mitotically to produce amitotic neurons, which then migrate to their final positions in the brain. This occurs during foetal development and

Clinical box 2.14	Nitric oxide relieves the pain of angina pectoris

The pain of angina pectoris is due to the heart muscle not receiving enough oxygen delivered in the blood. In 1867 the pharmacologist Lauder Brunton observed that amyl nitrite inhalation relieved the pain of angina, but the mechanism of this effect was unknown. Amyl nitrite has since been superseded by nitroglycerin (glyceryl trinitrate), which is degraded in plasma, releasing nitric oxide. This acts to relax vasculars smooth muscle cells, thus increasing the diameter of the vessels and the blood flow. This increases the oxygen supply, reducing the pain.

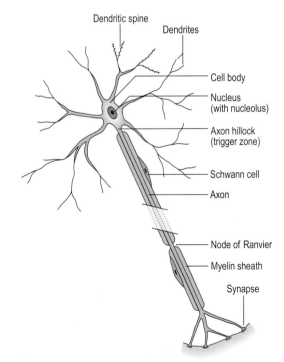

Dendritic spine

Dendrites

Cell body

Nucleus
(with nucleolus)

Axon hillock
(trigger zone)

Schwann cell

Axon

Node of Ranvier

Myelin sheath

Synapse

Fig. 2.46 **A typical multi-polar neuron.**

is completed in early childhood. The mature brain does not contain neurons which can divide (however, see Information box 2.18). Therefore, neurons that have died cannot usually be replaced. This is why brain tumours derived from neurons are very rare and occur almost exclusively as **neuroblastomas** in children.

The **glial cells** make up about half the brain mass and outnumber neurons about 10-fold. Their functions include structural and metabolic support, electrical insulation of the axons and immune functions. The glial cells include astrocytes, microglia and oligodendrocytes and Schwann cells.

INTEGRATED LEARNING: THE SYSTEMIC APPROACH

Organs and tissues are functionally integrated. Different organs and tissues together contribute to a particular set of organism's functions. The systemic approach integrates the aspects of anatomy, physiology, pathology and treatment. It has also been a basis for the emergence of medical specialties, and remains the most commonly used framework for learning medicine. The functions of the organism can be divided into the following systems:

- Cardiovascular system
- Respiratory system
- Gastrointestinal system
- Kidney and the urinary tract
- Endocrine system
- Reproductive system
- Blood and the immune system
- Nervous system
- Musculoskeletal system
- Skin.

The systemic approach has been adopted in the subsequent sections of this book.

3

Energy metabolism

Mark Holness, Mary Sugden and Jeannette Naish

Introduction to metabolism	**57**
Energy is released by catabolism and consumed by anabolism	57
Tricarboxylic acid cycle	59
Electron transport chain and oxidative phosphorylation	59
Regulation of fuel metabolism	61
Further considerations in fuel metabolism	62
Carbohydrate metabolism	**63**
Regulation of blood glucose (glycaemia)	63
Sources of blood glucose	63
Four key pathways maintain and utilise blood glucose	64
Glucose transport	64
Glycolysis – the anaerobic catabolism of glucose	65
Oxidative glucose metabolism – aerobic glycolysis	71
Glycogen – The storage form of glucose	72
Synthesis of glycogen	72
Glycogenolysis – the breakdown of glycogen	75
Regulation of glycogenolysis	75

Mechanism of glucagon regulation of glycogenolysis – hormone signalling	76
Sympathetic stimulation	76
Regulation of hepatic glycogen phosphorylase	77
Gluconeogenesis – glucose synthesis	78
Amino acid metabolism	**83**
Metabolic classes of amino acids	83
Absorption of amino acids	83
Nitrogen in amino acid metabolism	84
Amino acids in gluconeogenesis	87
Essential amino acids	87
Amino acids and signalling molecules	88
Lipid metabolism	**88**
Sources of fatty acids	88
Storage of lipids	90
Fatty acids	90
Triacylglycerols (triglycerides)	91
Lipoproteins	91
Fatty acid oxidation	93
Lipogenesis – fatty acid synthesis	96
Fine-tuning of fatty acid synthesis, oxidation and ketogenesis	99
Regulation of fat metabolism	100

INTRODUCTION TO METABOLISM

The human organism needs a constant supply of energy:

- For survival (e.g. for the chemical reactions that take place in the processes of transport and storage, and in the biosynthesis of new molecules for tissue repair)
- To maintain body temperature
- To perform work (see Ch. 16).

Fuel for producing energy is taken in as food, which is processed through digestion and absorption (see Ch. 15) into circulating blood and energy is produced from the breakdown – **catabolism** – of metabolic fuels. Glucose and lipids (fatty acids) are the main energy substrates (metabolic fuels), with amino acids being used during fasting, illness and injury.

ENERGY IS RELEASED BY CATABOLISM AND CONSUMED BY ANABOLISM

The metabolic fuels – carbohydrates, lipids and proteins – are ultimately metabolised to yield energy, carbon dioxide (CO_2) and water (H_2O) and, in the case of amino acids derived from proteins, urea. The two types of metabolic pathway in fuel metabolism are:

- **Catabolism**, when biochemical reactions break down molecules of fuel substrate to release energy
- **Anabolism**, when chemical reactions consume energy in the synthesis of new molecules.

Energy is stored in **adenosine triphosphate** (**ATP**), to be released and used in energy-requiring reactions.

Energy is used to synthesise:

- Glycogen (the storage form of glucose)
- Lipids for storage (e.g. as triacylglycerol)
- Proteins for tissue regeneration and cell growth (Fig. 3.1).

Carbohydrates, lipids and amino acids are metabolised in separate pathways, but there are intricate adaptive processes for integrating fuel metabolism (Information box 3.1). The metabolic pathways rely on energy supplied by the breakdown of large molecules (fuels), often stored in the body as carbohydrates or fats, but ultimately derived from ingested nutrients.

ATP is an **energy-coupling agent** and not a fuel. It consists of a purine base (adenine), and a five carbon sugar (ribose), which together form **adenosine**. A phosphoester bond binds the initial phosphate group to the sugar and a further two phosphate groups are attached by anhydride linkages (bonds that form between two phosphate groups (Fig. 3.2). The anhydride bonds are 'high energy' unstable bonds that readily release the attached phosphate, with little energy loss, in a reaction coupled with another reaction, and the terminal phosphate (Pi) is transferred by hydrolysis from ATP to another compound, leaving adenosine diphosphate (ADP) and releasing energy to drive metabolic processes. This process is called **phosphorylation**.

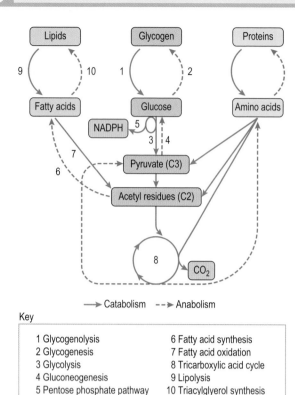

Key

1 Glycogenolysis	6 Fatty acid synthesis
2 Glycogenesis	7 Fatty acid oxidation
3 Glycolysis	8 Tricarboxylic acid cycle
4 Gluconeogenesis	9 Lipolysis
5 Pentose phosphate pathway	10 Triacylglyerol synthesis (esterification)

Fig. 3.1 **General layout of fuel metabolism.**

Information box 3.1	Metabolic pathways are dynamic, inter-related networks

- Some of the products of metabolic pathway intermediary metabolites are activators or inhibitors of enzymes in the pathway, or in the pathway of another substrate
- Catabolic and anabolic pathways are at least partially reversible in response to the availability of fuel substrates and to the changing energy requirements of the body
- The pathways intersect; for example, variation in the plasma concentration of glucose can activate or inhibit pathways in lipid metabolism, and vice versa
- Metabolic intermediates from one substrate can enter the pathway of another; for example, intermediates from glucose breakdown serve as substrates for amino acid and fatty acid synthesis.

Other molecules are also involved in metabolism, transferring other groups between molecules and are referred to as **coenzymes** (Table 3.1). These include:

- Nicotinamide adenine dinucleotide (**NAD**)
- Nicotinamide adenine dinucleotide phosphate (**NADP**)
- Flavin adenine dinucleotide (**FAD**).

These are all involved in the transfer of two hydrogen groups between, for example, the oxidised form NAD$^+$ to its reduced form, NADH+H$^+$.

Another important coenzyme is coenzyme A (**CoA**) which transfers acyl groups from the oxidised form CoA to its reduced form, **acetyl-CoA**.

Acetyl-CoA is the common end-product of the metabolism of carbohydrates, fatty acids and amino acids. These acetyl residues are further oxidised in a common pathway, the **tricarboxylic acid cycle** (**TCA cycle**), also known as the citric acid cycle or Krebs' cycle (see Fig. 3.3), providing free energy for the synthesis of ATP by the **electron transfer chain** in a process known as **oxidative phosphorylation**.

Table 3.1	Some coenzymes involved in metabolism		
Coenzyme	**Group transferred**	**Oxidised**	**Reduced**
Nicotinamide adenine dinucleotide (NAD)	2H	NAD$^+$	NADH+H$^+$
Nicotinamide adenine dinucleotide phosphate (NADP)	2H	NADP$^+$	NADPH+H$^+$
Flavin adenine dinucleotide (FAD)	2H	FAD$^+$	FADH+H$^+$
Coenzyme A (CoA)	Acyl groups (CH$_3$(CH$_2$)$_n$CO), e.g. the acetyl group (CH$_3$CO, where $n=0$)	CoA	Acetyl-CoA

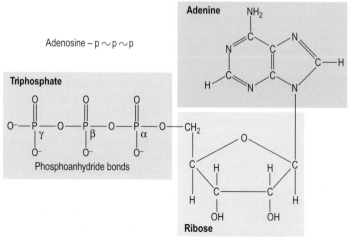

Fig. 3.2 **Structure of adenosine triphosphate (ATP).** The symbol ~ denotes the so-called high energy bonds.

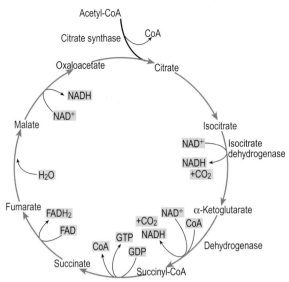

Fig. 3.3 **The TCA cycle.**

TRICARBOXYLIC ACID CYCLE

The **tricarboxylic acid (TCA) cycle** is the metabolic 'engine' in the mitochondria, where acetyl-CoA is oxidised to produce CO_2 and reduced nucleotides (conversion of NAD^+ to NADH and of $NADP^+$ to NADPH; Fig. 3.3). All of the enzymes involved in the TCA cycle lie within the mitochondrion. The molecule acetyl-CoA cannot cross the inner mitochondrial membrane and so its utilisation within the cycle is separated from its use in the cytoplasm, where it is involved in fatty acid synthesis.

The cycle begins when any of the three major metabolic precursors (pyruvate from carbohydrates, fatty acids from lipids or amino acids from proteins) produce acetyl-CoA.

- Pyruvate needs to be actively transported by a carrier protein into the inner mitochondria where it is decarboxylated through **pyruvate dehydrogenase** to acetyl-CoA. Pyruvate can also be converted to **oxaloacetate** through the action of **pyruvate carboxylase** (also synthesised within the TCA cycle).
- Fatty acids are broken down into two carbon chains by β-oxidation (at the beta position in the fatty acid chain), producing one $FADH_2$ and one NADH molecule. The oxidised fatty acids attach to CoA and are transported through the membrane in special channels.
- Amino acids are transported by various carriers. Glucagonic amino acids (see later) can be metabolised into pyruvate or other TCA cycle intermediates; ketogenic amino acids can only be metabolised into acetyl-CoA, acetoacetate or acetoacetyl-CoA.
- All of these processes result in the production of acetyl-CoA which primes the start of the cycle by combining with oxaloacetate to form **citrate**, through the first enzyme in the cycle, **citrate synthase**, with the release of CoA.

A series of eight enzyme reactions transform citrate into other molecules, finally regenerating oxaloacetate to start the cycle again. Early in the cycle are two oxidative decarboxyl-ation reactions in which NAD^+ is reduced to form NADH and CO_2 is released, leading to the formation of succinyl-CoA, which has a high energy thioester bond. The subsequent hydrolysis of this bond conserves the energy by forming GTP from GDP and Pi. A further enzyme, a flavoprotein, involved

in the oxidation of the next molecule in the sequence, enables the reduction of FAD (flavin adenine nucleotide) to $FADH_2$. The final enzyme oxidises malate to form oxaloacetate, again involving the reduction of NAD^+ to form NADH.

Therefore, for every acetyl-CoA molecule that enters the cycle several coenzymes are produced that are subsequently used for energy production through oxidative phosphorylation. The TCA cycle yields:

- Three NADH molecules
- One $FADH_2$ molecule
- One GTP molecule.

Intermediates in the cycle may also be used as substrates in other pathways:

- Citrate may be used in fatty acid synthesis
- Succinyl-CoA may be used to synthesise haem
- Oxaloactate can be converted into aspartate and used:
  - to manufacture amino acids and nucleic acids
  - within the urea cycle (see later)
  - to synthesise glucose (gluconeogenesis).

Control of the TCA cycle

Three enzymes are key regulators: **citrate synthase**, whose activity is sensitive to the availability of oxaloacetate, and the two dehydrogenase enzymes (**isocitrate dehydrogenase** and **α-ketoglutarate dehydrogenase**) which depend on the availability of NAD^+; this molecule in the mitochondria provides the link between work, in which ATP is consumed, and fuel consumption.

ELECTRON TRANSPORT CHAIN AND OXIDATIVE PHOSPHORYLATION

Oxidative phosphorylation is the process through which electrons are transferred from fuels through a series of coenzymes (NAD^+, FAD and FMN – flavin mononucleotide), with conservation of the energy released through oxidation by forming ATP, rather than simply wasting it in the form of heat. ATP may then be used for work in the body: molecule biosynthesis, molecule transport and physical activity. For example, the high energy phosphate anhydride bonds in ATP can be used to drive unfavourable reactions; the breakdown of ATP releases sufficient free energy to synthesise glucose-6-phosphate from glucose as the first step in glycolysis (see later).

Electron transport chain

This involves a series of reactions in which the final fuel metabolites are transformed into an energy source through a series of reactions located on the inner membrane of the mitochondrion. Reduced coenzymes, produced in the TCA cycle, enable electron transfer to complexes which release free energy as the electrons move down a gradient of redox potentials, each more electronegative than its predecessor, finally transferring to oxygen, which is reduced as it combines with hydrogen to form water. The free energy released from the electron transfer enables the movement of protons from the inner mitochondrial membrane to the space between this and the outer mitochondrial membrane.

Figure 3.4 illustrates the electron transport processes taking place within the mitochondrion.

- Fuel oxidation and involvement of the TCA cycle release CO_2 and reduced coenzymes (NADH and $FADH_2$).

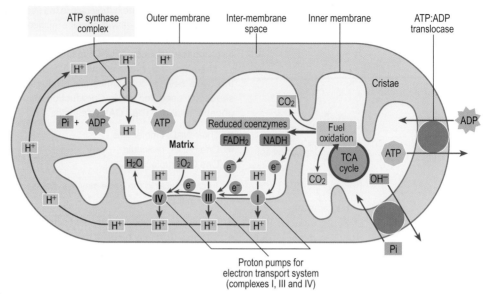

Fig. 3.4 **Energy transfer in the mitochondrion.** Adapted with permission from Baynes J, Dominiczak M 2005 Medical biochemistry, 2nd edn. Elsevier Mosby, Edinburgh.

- On the inner membrane are a series of large protein complexes, complex I through to complex IV, which also function as proton pumps.
- The release of an electron pair from NADH can combine with complex I, a flavoprotein containing FMN and provides the energy to pump sufficient protons through into the intermembrane space to eventually form 1 mole of ATP. These electrons are subsequently transported through two more complexes (III and IV), each pumping protons out of the inner mitochondrial space.
  - Each electron pair from NADH therefore enables the production of 3 moles of ADP, once they have been transported through each of the proton pump complexes.
- NADH produced in the cytoplasm of cells during carbohydrate metabolism cannot pass through the inner mitochondrial membrane. Instead the electrons are moved through a redox shuttle.
  - The glycerol-3-phosphate shuttle involves an enzyme that reduces FAD to $FADH_2$.
- Electrons from $FADH_2$ can only combine with complex II, which is composed of three flavoproteins. Both pathways merge at a small hydrophilic molecule, ubiquinone, which accepts electrons and transfers them to complex III and then IV.
  - Each electron pair from $FADH_2$ enables the production of 2 moles of ADP, because the proton pumping ability of complex I is bypassed.
- Complex III is an enzyme complex that involves a haem protein, cytochrome c, to shuttle electrons between this complex and complex IV through a three-dimensional change in the protein.
  - Transport of two electrons to cytochrome c allows the pumping of sufficient protons to produce 1 mole of ATP, as part of the ATP generating chain that starts at complex I and II.
- Complex IV, or cytochrome c oxidase, conducts electrons through other cytochromes, finally reducing oxygen to water.
  - Again this process pumps sufficient protons to produce an additional mole of ATP per electron pair transported.

Some electrons may directly leak to oxygen and form superoxide free radicals. These are highly reactive molecules that contribute to oxidative stresses associated with ageing and some diseases (see Ch. 16).

Oxidative phosphorylation

The efflux of protons across the inner mitochondrial membrane creates an electrochemical gradient as the outside space becomes more acidic and more positively charged as H^+ protons accumulate. The chemiosmotic theory describes the process in which electron transport is linked to the production of energy through oxidative phosphorylation.

- The electrochemical gradient drives protons back into the inner space through a fifth complex, ATP synthase, which acts as an ion channel (the F_0 component) and drives the synthesis of ATP from ADP and inorganic phosphate within the inner mitochondrial space. This reaction is catalysed by the F_1 component of the ATP synthase enzyme and the protons force a rotational change to one of the subunits of this complex, actively releasing ATP on its conversion.
- ATP is, therefore, mostly made in the mitochondrion, but it needs to be transported to the cytoplasm to be utilised in reactions requiring energy.

Coupling of the electron transport chain and oxidative phosphorylation

The electron transport chain and oxidative phosphorylation are tightly coupled. This can be shown in vitro by measuring oxygen utilisation (a measure of the end-point of the electron transport chain) while controlling ATP synthesis. If ADP is not available, then oxygen utilisation stops. When ADP is included, oxygen use increases until it is all converted to ATP. Various poisons and toxins can affect this process at the different points within the electron transport chain (see below).

Uncoupled phosphorylation occurs when other substances enable protons to move back into the inner mitochondrial space, bypassing ATP synthase. This leads to stimulation of respiration as the body rapidly oxidises more fuel in order to restore the proton gradient. Because ATP is not formed, the oxidative energy is released as heat. Although exposure to some synthetic uncouplers (such as 2,4-dinitrophenol (DNP)) can be lethal in high doses, they may also be useful therapeutically. There are also natural mechanisms where uncoupling can be protective. For example, neonates do not shiver when they get cold, possibly because their nervous system is not sufficiently developed to coordinate the muscular activity required. However, within specialised adipose tissue (brown fat), which contains large numbers of mitochondria, a naturally occurring protein, thermogenin, uncouples the process under certain conditions to allow heat to be generated instead of ATP.

Electron transport chain inhibition

Various toxic substances can inhibit different parts of the electron transport chain, preventing or reducing ATP synthesis and oxygen uptake:

- Complex 1 can be inhibited by an insecticide, rotenone. Electron transport, although reduced, is not stopped because $FADH_2$ can still enter the chain through Complex II. Normally excess ADP will stimulate ATP synthesis, which rotenone inhibits. Subsequent addition of succinate into the system returns the levels to normal as ATP synthesis is allowed to continue.
- Antimycin-A from *Streptomyces* bacteria binds to cytochrome C reductase, blocking the transfer of electrons to ubiquinol, part of Complex III, and therefore inhibiting ATP production. Succinate does not help here but ascorbic acid reduces cytochrome C and will restore respiration.
- Both cyanide and carbon monoxide inhibit Complex IV. This is the final electron transfer step and its action cannot be bypassed leading to a lack of reduction of components earlier in the transport chain and the failure of the proton pump. Dependent on the exposure, death can occur rapidly. Methylene blue treatment alleviates this by accepting electrons from Complex III so that proton pumping can continue while cyanide is converted to a harmless ion, or oxygen administration overcomes the effect of carbon monoxide buildup.
- Oligomycin is another *Streptomyces* product which blocks ATP synthase, leading to a build-up of protons outside the mitochondrial inner membrane. DNP can assist here by dissipating the proton gradient through uncoupling stimulating oxygen uptake and re-established the proton gradient.
- Other plant toxins can also inhibit ATP:ADP translocase. Again, protons build up and electron transport stops but uncouplers can also assist here.

Energy output

The metabolism of one mole of glucose through glycolysis, although it begins with consumption of two moles of ATP, with the subsequent involvement of the TCA and electron transport chain, produces a net output of about 38 moles of ATP, although this varies a bit as the ratio of ATP production and proton pumping fluctuates. Table 3.2 summarises the output.

Table 3.2	Summary of ATP generated during the complete oxidation of glucose	
Stage	**Net change in coenzymes (per mole glucose entering glycolysis)**	**ATP equivalents***
Glycolysis	2 ATP	2
	2 NADH	6
Link reaction	2 NADH	6
TCA cycle	2 GTP	2
	6 NADH	18
	2 FADH	4
		Total 38

*During aerobic metabolism 1 NAD = 3 ATP and 1 FAD = 2 ATP.

A comparative calculation for the 16-carbon fatty acid, palmitic acid, gives a total of 129 moles of ATP per mole. This increases by 17 moles of ATP for each subsequent 2-carbon increase in fatty acid length. So stearic acid (C18) metabolism yields 146 moles of ATP per mole, which shows why fats provide so much more energy than carbohydrates.

REGULATION OF FUEL METABOLISM

Generally, metabolism takes place in cells, both within the cytoplasm and in cellular organelles. The processes of human metabolism are tightly regulated to maintain internal functionality, but have to be flexible at the same time to respond to changes in the external environment of the cells.

The overall rate of reaction in a complex metabolic pathway is limited by its slowest step: the 'rate-limiting' (also known as flux-generating) step. The key enzyme in the 'rate-limiting' step regulates the metabolic pathway; however, there can be more than one step in a pathway that is involved in regulating flux. Methods for controlling metabolism include:

- Binding of small molecules (**allosteric effectors**) to sites on an enzyme, other than the catalytic site, to increase or inhibit its affinity for substrates, thereby affecting the rate of reaction
- Reversible activation/deactivation of enzymes by covalent modification
- Regulation of gene expression and transcription (and thus ultimately enzyme protein concentration) in response to changing metabolic demands (see Ch. 5)
- Hormone action inhibiting or activating particular enzymes.

Binding of allosteric effectors to an enzyme to alter its affinity for substrate

The binding of allosteric effectors to a site on an enzyme that is separate from the substrate binding site can alter the enzyme affinity for the substrate. Binding of different molecules can fluctuate rapidly. For example, when the demand for energy is low, e.g. while resting after a meal, cellular ATP and NADH accumulate to allosterically inhibit isocitrate dehydrogenase (a major regulatory enzyme in the TCA cycle), whereas when energy demand is high, e.g. during exercise, ADP and NAD^+ accumulate to allosterically stimulate isocitrate dehydrogenase.

Reversible activation and deactivation by covalent modification

This process involves the binding of groups (most commonly phosphate, but also acetyl groups) that alters the structure of a protein to affect its function. Phosphorylation (by protein kinases) or dephosphorylation (by protein phosphatases) is a commonly used mechanism in the regulation of enzyme activity.

- **Kinase activity** involves transfer of a phosphate group, normally from ATP, to an amino acid, binding covalently with a free hydroxyl group, predominantly on serine, threonine and tyrosine residues. There are a large number of different kinases. Phosphorylation results in functional changes to proteins by changing the activity of an enzyme, or enabling binding to activators or inhibitors; phosphorylation can also influence the cellular location of the molecule. Because of the profound affect that protein kinases have on a cell they are themselves highly regulated and turned on or off by phosphorylation, sometimes by the kinase itself (autophosphorylation). Different kinases can form dimers which interact, enabling a highly varied response to extracellular signals.
- **Phosphatase activity** leads to dephosphorylation, removing a phosphate ion to leave a free hydroxyl group, reversing the action of kinases. Alkaline phosphatase is a commonly found phosphatase.

Regulation of gene expression and transcription in response to changing metabolic demands

Changes in metabolic demands can alter gene expression and transcription. For example, iron is necessary to produce haemoglobin for oxygen transport and is stored as ferritin. When iron concentrations are low, a repressor protein binds to ferritin mRNA so that no more ferritin is made. When iron is plentiful, iron binds to the repressor protein, so altering its shape, which releases the mRNA, again allowing ferritin to be produced and excess iron stored in a safe form (see Ch. 12). There are many other examples in carbohydrate and vitamin metabolism.

Action of hormones

Hormones (see Ch. 10) inhibit or activate essential enzymes in response to the body's internal environment (e.g. arising from a high-fat or a weight-reducing diet, or in response to stress and disease). This regulation may take effect rapidly, over days or gradually over weeks.

The hormones insulin, glucagon, epinephrine (adrenaline), tri-iodothyronine, cortisol and growth hormone are involved in the regulation of metabolic fuels – carbohydrates, lipids and proteins – and can exert short-term and/or long-term effects on the direction and rates of fluxes in metabolic pathways.

Both the catabolic and anabolic pathways of fuel metabolism have to be partially reversible to adapt to environmental changes because we alternately eat food (feed) and fast between meals. The fasting state can begin just a few hours from the last meal. The processes of fuel metabolism are reversible within this feed–fast cycle.

Information box 3.2 **Maintenance of normal blood glucose concentration is the starting point in regulating fuel metabolism**

Maintenance of a normal blood glucose concentration within a narrow range of 3.5–8.0 mmol/L is essential for life, and abnormal variation in this level triggers alternative metabolic pathways:

- Hypoglycaemia occurs when plasma glucose falls below 2.1 mmol/L, which can lead to acute neurological complications because glucose is an essential requirement for brain function in the short term. Although hypoglycaemia may occasionally occur in healthy people after fasting, exercise or alcohol consumption, it is most commonly seen as a complication of the treatment of diabetes mellitus by insulin.
- Consistently elevated fasting blood glucose concentrations above 7 mmol/L (hyperglycaemia) are a consequence of failed regulation of glucose metabolism by insulin, as in untreated diabetes mellitus, and can lead to both acute complications, due to increased production of ketone bodies (ketones, diabetic ketoacidosis), and long-term potentially life-threatening complications of micro- and macrovascular disease (i.e. hypertension, coronary artery disease, diabetic glomerulosclerosis leading to renal failure, neuropathy, and retinopathy that can lead to blindness).

When nutrients are plentiful

When nutrients are plentiful (the fed or absorptive state), the active pathways are:

- Fuel breakdown and storage of excess metabolic fuel through glycogen and lipid synthesis
- Protein synthesis for regenerating tissues (anabolism).

Glucose uptake into cells, the storage of carbohydrates and lipids, and protein synthesis are promoted by **insulin**, an anabolic hormone. For example, insulin stimulates lipoprotein lipase to break down dietary triacylglycerols to glycerol and fatty acids. Fatty acids are then transported into adipose tissue for storage (Information box 3.2).

Metabolic adaptation to changes in energy requirement

During the fasting state, the direction of the metabolic pathways is reversed:

- Stored fuels are broken down (catabolism) – glycogen, lipids, proteins – to produce energy
- Biosynthesis is slowed.

The complex interactions between the biochemical pathways also have to adapt to changes in energy requirements, as in increased physical activity – the difference between a 100 m sprint versus a marathon – and some extreme changes from changing diets, fasting and starvation (see Ch. 16).

The action of insulin to suppress endogenous glucose production is opposed by glucagon, growth hormone, epinephrine and cortisol, which promote endogenous glucose production. (Clinical box 3.1)

FURTHER CONSIDERATIONS IN FUEL METABOLISM

The processes by which different tissues metabolise different energy substrates, store and transport fuel are integrated and adapted for varying functions (Information box 3.3).

Clinical box 3.1 **Diabetes mellitus – a disorder of fuel metabolism**

Importance of diabetes mellitus
- A common condition in which the normal pathways for fuel metabolism are disrupted by defective insulin secretion and/or action.
- Characterised by persistently high concentrations of blood glucose (hyperglycaemia) leading to life-threatening complications and long-term organ damage.
- Although no 'diabetic gene' has been identified, the patterns of family history and a higher incidence in some racial groups suggest genetic susceptibility, particularly for type 1 diabetes (see below).

  There are **two main types** of diabetes mellitus:
- Type 1 diabetes – onset predominantly in children and young adults, but can occur at any time in adult life. The condition is associated with high morbidity (end-stage renal disease and retinopathy) and premature death.
- Type 2 diabetes – usually of late onset, but is increasingly being seen in younger people, adolescents and even children:
  - Complex interactions between genetic and environmental factors seem to influence the development of this disease; however, 90% of individuals that develop the disease are also obese and cardiovascular co-morbidity also increases the risk.
  - Type 2 diabetes is a major public health issue. In East London, UK, for example, about 1 in 10 people are at high risk (>20%); the number of people diagnosed is expected to double to 80 000 by 2020. Socio-economic deprivation increases the risk and this is exacerbated by being of non-Caucasian origin. This is particularly prominent in the people of South Asian ancestry, doubling the risk.

  Other forms of diabetes mellitus include:
- Gestational diabetes (during pregnancy) occurs in fewer than 10% of pregnancies with incidence much higher in higher risk non-Caucasian populations and is a risk factor for continuing metabolic problems later.
- Maturity-onset diabetes of the young (MODY) is a rare genetic disease of dominant inheritance in which there is a defect in insulin secretion. Mutations in the glucokinase gene in the milder type 2 disease, or in the hepatocyte nuclear factor 1α gene, leading to the more serious type 3 disease are the most common.

Information box 3.3 **Advantages and disadvantages of glycolysis**

Advantages
- Ability to provide ATP without using oxygen for red blood cells (RBCs) and when a tissue loses its oxygen supply
- Provides many intermediates, which interlink with the metabolic pathways of proteins and fats (see Fig. 3.3).

Disadvantages
- A relatively inefficient pathway for producing energy – the first part uses energy (two molecules of ATP for each molecule of glucose), though it continues with the release of four molecules of ATP – therefore it recovers only about 5% (two molecules) of the 36–38 ATP molecules that can be produced by the complete oxidative metabolism of glucose, which occurs in any cell containing mitochondria, provided that there is a sufficient supply of oxygen.

Different tissues metabolise different energy substrates

Red blood cells, the main carrier and transporter of oxygen (O_2), do not have mitochondria and rely on metabolising glucose through anaerobic glycolysis. This process does not consume O_2, thus maximising red cell capacity for carrying and delivering O_2.

Under normal circumstances, the brain uses only glucose as metabolic fuel, but under prolonged starvation conditions it can use ketone bodies which are produced in the liver from the breakdown of fats.

How fuel is stored and transported between tissues

Liver and skeletal muscle are both involved in the storage of glucose as glycogen, but:

- The liver is able to release glucose into the bloodstream to prevent hypoglycaemia
- In contrast, muscle cannot release glucose into the circulation because it lacks glucose-6-phosphatase (see below).

The glucose phosphate produced by muscle glycogenolysis is used within the muscle to produce energy for contraction.

CARBOHYDRATE METABOLISM

Carbohydrates are present in high concentration in plants, making up most of the dry tissue weight. For the body to make use of the many ingested carbohydrates, they must first be broken down by digestive enzymes into monomer sugars (e.g. glucose, fructose) and disaccharides (e.g. maltose, lactose). Disaccharide sugars can be converted to glucose, the major carbohydrate fuel for all tissues.

Even more importantly, some tissues (including the brain and RBCs, see above) have an obligatory requirement for glucose as a metabolic fuel. Blood glucose concentration (glycaemia) is governed by the balance between:

- Glucose absorption from the intestine
- Glucose production by the liver and kidneys
- Glucose uptake and metabolism by all tissues of the body.

REGULATION OF BLOOD GLUCOSE (GLYCAEMIA)

Glucose is the only metabolic fuel used by red cells, and under normal fed conditions glucose is the only fuel that brain can use. Glucose is also the preferred fuel for skeletal muscle during short bursts of exercise. A continuous supply of glucose is therefore needed to ensure that there is an adequate energy supply for the vital functions performed by these and other tissues. Fuel metabolism is highly regulated to ensure adequate energy for cellular function.

SOURCES OF BLOOD GLUCOSE

Metabolic fuels are stored for use in times of fuel shortage.

- Carbohydrates are stored as glycogen, the liver being the main glycogen source for maintaining blood glucose concentrations. However, liver glycogen stores will be depleted after a 16-hour fast.
- Dietary lipid that is surplus to requirement is stored in adipose tissue adipocytes (fat cells) as triglyceride. Triglycerides are esters formed from glycerol with three fatty acid molecules, and its glycerol moiety can be converted to glucose via gluconeogenesis (see below) to generate energy. The fatty acid moiety of triglyceride cannot be converted to glucose.

- Protein from muscle breakdown can also be converted to glucose via gluconeogenesis in the liver.
- Carbohydrates can also be converted to fats for storage.

FOUR KEY PATHWAYS MAINTAIN AND UTILISE BLOOD GLUCOSE

Maintenance of blood glucose levels and glucose utilisation are governed by four key interacting metabolic processes (Fig. 3.5):

- **Glycolysis** – the process by which glucose is broken down to form pyruvate and energy in the form of ATP
- **Glycogenesis** – the process by which glucose is converted to glycogen for storage
- **Glycogenolysis** – the process by which glycogen is broken down
- **Gluconeogenesis** – the process by which glucose can be produced when glycogen stores are depleted.

GLUCOSE TRANSPORT

Before glucose can be metabolised, it must be transported into the cell. Molecules such as sugars cannot move through membranes by simple diffusion. Instead this is achieved via special transmembrane proteins by facilitated diffusion. **Glucose transporters (GLUTs)** are specific for glucose or, in certain cases, fructose, and facilitate the movement of glucose down a concentration gradient which does not require energy.

Originally, five members of the GLUT family were identified, GLUT1–5, which have been well characterised. However, a further eight have been identified through cloning of the human genome. GLUT1–4 are primarily glucose transporters with distinct tissue distribution and kinetic characteristics (Table 3.3). GLUT5 is a fructose transporter.

GLUT1

GLUT1 molecules (found in most cells) do not require the stimulus of insulin and transport glucose under most conditions, including fasting (blood glucose concentration ≤5 mmol/L). They also work with GLUT3 (which does not have to be activated by insulin) to allow glucose to cross the blood–brain

Table 3.3	Tissue location of glucose transporters	
Transport protein	**Tissue location**	**Characteristics**
GLUT1	Most, including red cells	Low K_m*
GLUT2	Liver and pancreatic β cells	High K_m
GLUT3	Mainly brain	
GLUT4	Liver, muscle and adipose tissue	Insulin sensitive
GLUT5	Mainly intestinal tissue, kidney and spermatozoa	Fructose transporter

*K_m is a property of enzymes, defined as the concentration of the substrate that allows 50% of the *maximal* rate of enzyme reaction at normal body temperature and pH.

barrier, enter neurons and the placenta. GLUT1 deficiency syndrome impairs glucose transport into brain. GLUT 1 is also overexpressed in cancers.

GLUT2

GLUT2 only transports glucose into cells when blood glucose concentration is high, such as after a high carbohydrate meal, allowing glucose entry. It can act as a metabolic trigger to coordinate insulin secretion with high blood glucose concentration.

- In the rodent endocrine pancreas: GLUT2 mediates the uptake of glucose into pancreatic β cells. The increase in intracellular glucose metabolism stimulates the β cell to secrete insulin. GLUT2 thus acts as a 'glucose sensor' in the β cells.
- In the liver: GLUT2 activity facilitates glucose transport into hepatocytes from the blood for glycogenesis (temporary glucose storage), and from the liver into the blood after glycogenolysis (see Fig. 3.5).

GLUT3

GLUT3 has a higher affinity for glucose than the other glucose transporters and its high expression in neuronal tissues is useful for glucose transport under conditions where glucose levels are about five times that of blood glucose.

GLUT4

GLUT4 is present in intracellular vesicles in insulin-sensitive tissues (liver, muscle, fat). When blood glucose concentration is high (e.g. fed state), insulin is released from the pancreatic β cells and binds to insulin receptors in the cell membrane, activating the insulin signal pathway. In response to insulin stimulation, GLUT4 translocates from intracellular vesicles to the cell membrane, allowing glucose transport into the cell. This process is reversed when the blood glucose concentration falls, with a concomitant fall in insulin concentration. GLUT4 is recycled back to intracellular vesicles so that it can no longer transport glucose into the cell. **Insulin resistance**, a state in which cells respond poorly to insulin stimulation, is associated with deficits in glucose transport. Exercise, like insulin stimulation, increases GLUT4 translocation in skeletal muscle and so is beneficial to help remove excess glucose from the blood in insulin resistance.

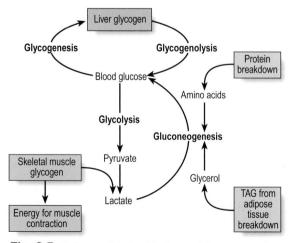

Fig. 3.5 Pathways involved in the maintenance and utilisation of blood glucose. TAG, triacylglycerol.

GLYCOLYSIS – THE ANAEROBIC CATABOLISM OF GLUCOSE

Glycolysis is the first step in the production of energy from glucose. It is a metabolic pathway that breaks down (catabolises) glucose to lactate without using oxygen (anaerobic). Insulin stimulates glycolysis in skeletal muscle and adipose tissue.

Glycolysis is also the main final pathway for the metabolism of other important dietary components, including fructose (found in sugar, sucrose) and galactose (found in milk, lactose). It also produces several intermediate metabolites that are the starting points for the synthesis of amino acids, proteins, lipids, DNA, RNA and nucleotides (Fig. 3.6). In a sedentary man, the brain consumes approx. 60% of blood glucose. Other tissues requiring glucose are, e.g., tissues of the eye, RBCs, kidney medulla, proliferating cells and skin epithelium.

Importance of the anaerobic nature of glycolysis

The crucial biomedical significance of glycolysis is its ability to provide ATP in the absence of oxygen (anaerobic metabolism) or in cells that lack mitochondria. For example:

For red blood cells

Mature RBCs have no mitochondria, and so cannot carry out oxidative metabolism, or oxidise fats for energy purposes (see later). RBCs rely entirely on glucose as fuel, but do not consume oxygen during metabolism, thus fulfilling their primary role of oxygen transport and delivery.

When a tissue's oxygen supply is cut off

When the oxygen supply to a tissue is cut off (**anoxia**), ATP levels can still be maintained by glycolysis for a short period of time. The capacity for glycolysis is particularly important in the brain, in skeletal muscle during exercise, in ischaemic heart muscle, and during birth. The brain is most sensitive to oxygen lack – irreversible damage may occur after only 3 minutes of anoxia. During hypoxic events (anaemia, poor tissue perfusion, low atmospheric O_2), adaptations occur that aim to:

- Limit ATP use by switching off non-essential cellular functions (often involving activation of **AMPK** – AMP activated protein kinase)
- Improve the efficiency of anaerobic ATP production
- Limit oxidative stress, providing protection against ischaemia.

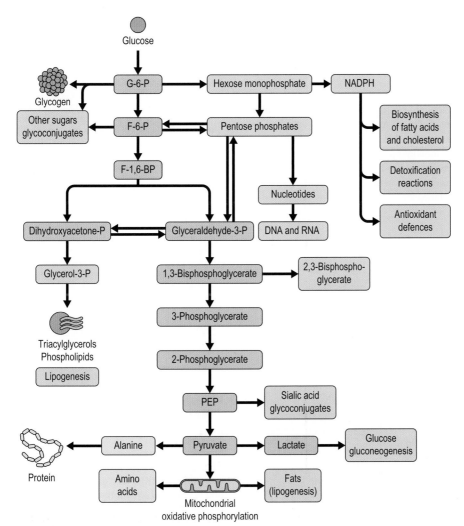

Fig. 3.6 Glycolysis and associated metabolic pathways. F, fructose; G, glucose; P, phosphate; PEP, phosphoenolpyruvate. Adapted with permission from Baynes J, Dominiczak M 2005 Medical biochemistry, 2nd edn. Elsevier Mosby, Edinburgh.

Metabolic adaptations to hypoxia can be mediated via changes in gene expression, predominantly involving the transcription factor **hypoxia-inducible factor 1** (HIF1). In normoxia, the HIF1α subunit is degraded. However, when oxygen is limited, HIF1 is stabilised and binds to **hypoxia response elements** (HREs) in the promoter regions of metabolic genes. These include glycolytic enzymes. Glycolysis is upregulated as a result.

Energy-using reactions in glycolysis – glucose phosphorylation

Glycolysis proceeds through the formation of a series of phosphorylated intermediate metabolites, which are eventually metabolised to pyruvate and lactate with the production of ATP. In the first part of the pathway, two molecules of ATP are used up per molecule of glucose metabolised (Fig. 3.7), but this deficit is more than made up in the remainder of the pathway.

Glycolysis is initiated by the formation of the phosphorylated intermediate **glucose-6-phosphate** (**G6P**) from glucose. Glucose phosphorylation to G6P is catalysed in an irreversible process by **hexokinase** at normal blood glucose concentrations and by glucokinase in liver and pancreatic β cells at higher blood glucose concentrations (e.g. after a meal).

- Synthesis of G6P is energy dependent, using one molecule of ATP as a phosphate donor, per molecule of G6P. This is the **first energy requiring step**. However, ATP expenditure at this stage is a long-term investment because it enables the production of ATP later as G6P is broken down.

Phosphate esters are charged and water soluble, rather than lipid soluble, so do not readily penetrate lipid-rich cell membranes (see also Chs 1, 2 and 4). Because there are no transport systems for sugar phosphates in the plasma membranes of mammalian cells, the phosphorylated product, G6P, is trapped within cells, and glucose is thus committed to intracellular metabolism.

Hexokinase

The enzyme **hexokinase** (**HK**) is found in most tissues, including red blood cells and muscle. It has a low K_m (0.1 mM) for its substrate, glucose, relative to blood glucose concentration (approximately 5 mM). At low K_m levels, enzymes have a high affinity for their substrate and so HK is normally saturated with both ATP and glucose. By phosphorylating all the glucose that enters the cell (because of the low K_m), HK maintains a large glucose concentration gradient between the blood and the intracellular environment, ensuring a continued intracellular supply of glucose, even at low blood glucose concentrations.

HK is inhibited, allosterically, by its product G6P (i.e. feedback control, Information box 3.4). This is an important regulatory feature because it prevents HK from sequestering all the inorganic phosphate (Pi) of the cell in the form of phosphorylated glucose, which would make Pi unavailable for other biochemical reactions (Fig. 3.8). As well as acting on glucose, HK can also catalyse the phosphorylation of other hexoses (e.g. fructose), but at a much slower rate. Inhibition of HK will suppress glucose uptake because the intracellular glucose concentration will rise. In addition, since HK is inhibited allosterically by its product, G6P, a failure to dispose of G6P within the cell will cause HK inhibition.

Information box 3.4	Glucokinase affects insulin release into the systemic circulation

There is evidence to suggest that glucokinase (GK) participates in the mechanism by which the pancreatic β cell monitors an increase in blood glucose concentration and delivers an appropriate quantity of insulin into the systemic circulation:
- Genetic mutations of GK can inactivate the enzyme, leading to diabetes, or activate it to cause hypoglycaemia.
- Mutations in the GK gene are associated with one form of maturity-onset diabetes of the young (MODY).
- In sustained hyperglycaemia, and when there are high levels of insulin (e.g. in people with insulin resistance leading to increased risk of type 2 diabetes), GK gene expression is enhanced, leading to increases in GK enzyme protein and activity that takes place over several hours. In this way the liver also contributes to the lowering of blood glucose levels.
- In hypoglycaemia (as a result of starvation or as a complication of the treatment of diabetes mellitus), GK gene and protein expression is decreased. This change influences hepatic glucose handling, with a sustained switch to increase net glucose output, and impairs blood glucose 'buffering'. Insulin release by the pancreas is also impaired.

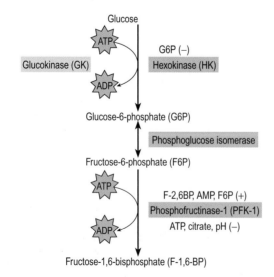

+ Allosteric activator
− Allosteric inhibitor

Fig. 3.7 Energy-utilising steps in glycolysis.

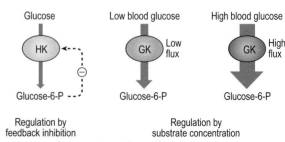

Fig. 3.8 **Regulation of glucokinase (GK) and hexokinase (HK).** Hexokinase has a low K_m for glucose and is inhibited allosterically by its product, glucose-6-phosphate. In contrast, glucokinase has a higher K_m for glucose and is not inhibited by glucose-6-phosphate. Glucokinase phosphorylates glucose only when blood glucose levels are high.

Glucokinase

Glucokinase (**GK**) is an isoenzyme of HK with strikingly different kinetic properties from other hexokinases. It is specific for glucose and found only in liver parenchymal cells and pancreatic β cells where GK assumes a more primary role than HK. In contrast to HK:

- GK has a much higher K_m for glucose than HK, and operates optimally at blood glucose concentrations above 5 mM
- GK is not inhibited by G6P, so neither the liver nor the pancreatic β cell is subject to any feedback inhibition as the result of G6P accumulation
- GK activity in liver cells (not the pancreas) is inhibited by a GK regulating protein (GKRP) that competes with glucose for binding to GK.

This means that, when glucose concentrations are high, GK is the only enzyme responding to increases in glucose concentration. Its high concentration in the liver provides for the synthesis of glycogen, the storage form of glucose. Because the K_m of GK for glucose (approximately 10 mM) is considerably greater than normal blood glucose concentrations (approximately 5 mM), any increase in glucose concentration leads to a proportional increase in the rate of glucose phosphorylation by GK and vice versa (see Fig. 3.8). This is called **substrate concentration regulation**. Therefore:

- GK is the rate-limiting enzyme for glucose uptake into liver cells. The liver uses glucose at a significant rate only when blood glucose levels are greatly elevated. Mice with liver-specific knockout of GK have a mild hyperglycaemia and cannot synthesise liver glycogen.
- In the pancreatic β cell, glucose utilisation and oxidation closely track the release of insulin as glucose concentrations increase. GK in the pancreatic β cell has been termed the glucose sensor (glucostat) for insulin secretion (Information box 3.4).

One of the intermediate metabolites of glycolysis is G6P and at this point the pentose phosphate pathway branches off

Pentose is a sugar containing five carbons. The **pentose phosphate pathway** (or **hexose monophosphate shunt**) is present in all cells, but is only active in a few specialised cells, e.g. cells synthesising fatty acids and rapidly dividing cells. The pentose phosphate pathway branches from glycolysis at the G6P stage (see Fig. 3.6). The pathway is sited in the cytosol. It is the main pathway for the formation of pentose phosphates, necessary for the synthesis of DNA, RNA and nucleotides. It is also important as a generator of **reduced nicotinamide adenine dinucleotide phosphate** (**NADPH**) in the cytosol.

G6P enters into an irreversible redox stage (a reduction-oxidation (redox) reaction that transfers a pair of electrons through G6P oxidation and concomitant reduction of NADP) to synthesise NADPH and pentose phosphates (see Fig. 3.6). There is also a reversible interconversion stage where excess pentose phosphates are recycled back into glycolysis.

Red cells have no nuclei and so have little need for DNA and RNA synthesis, and G6P is re-routed back into the next stage of glycolysis. About 90% of red cell glucose is metabolised to pyruvate, but the rest is diverted through the pentose phosphate shunt to provide NADPH, which is particularly important to red cells (Clinical box 3.2). NADPH is also needed

---

> **Clinical box 3.2** **G6PD deficiency is a cause of haemolytic anaemia**
>
> G6PD deficiency is a common X-linked genetic defect that results in an inability to synthesise NADPH. NADPH is used to maintain reduced glutathione, which protects the cell from the toxic effects of oxidation (i.e. provides antioxidant protection). Red cells are particularly vulnerable to G6PD deficiency because they have no nucleus and so cannot make proteins for repair. As a result of oxidation, haemoglobin is oxidised to methaemoglobin and cannot deliver O_2 to the tissues; the red cell membrane becomes rigid and breaks up.
>
> Acute, life-threatening intravascular haemolysis may be precipitated in G6PD deficiency by:
> - Drugs (e.g. aspirin, some antimalarials and antibiotics) undergo redox reactions in red cells to produce oxidants (e.g. superoxide, hydrogen peroxide) that set off a toxic chain reaction, which disrupts the cells (see Ch. 16).
> - Ingestion of fava (broad) beans – these contain high levels of oxidants and result in haemolytic anaemia in some deficiency variants.
> - Infections and inflammatory processes are associated with increased oxidative substance production. For example, phagocytes kill bacteria by exposure to the strong oxidant, hypochlorous acid (HOCl) produced within the cell from hydrogen peroxide catalysed by myeloperoxidase.
>
> The prevalence of G6PD deficiency is highest in certain African, Mediterranean, Middle Eastern and South East Asian populations. It offers protection against malaria which probably explains the high gene frequency in these populations.

in the redox reactions used for the biosynthesis of fatty acids, steroid hormones, cholesterol and bile acids. The first part of the conversion of G6P into NADPH is dependent on oxidation by the enzyme **glucose-6-phosphate dehydrogenase** (**G6PD**).

Phosphofructokinase-1 (PFK-1)

The second stage in glycolysis is the conversion of G6P into **fructose 6-phosphate** (**F6P**) by the enzyme **phosphoglucose isomerase** (see Fig. 3.7). This process is freely reversible and not subject to regulation. The product, F6P, may then be phosphorylated at a specific carbon, C-1, by another enzyme termed **phosphofructokinase-1** (**PFK-1**) to yield the product **fructose-1,6-bisphosphate** (**F-1,6-BP**).

This is the **second-energy requiring stage** of glycolysis, consuming one molecule of ATP for each molecule of F-1,6-BP produced.

PFK-1 catalyses a reaction that is biochemically reversible, but physiologically irreversible. Like HK, PFK-1 is a key regulatory enzyme in glycolysis that accepts a phosphate group from ATP to form a more phosphorylated product. PFK-1 has the dominant role in the regulation of the overall rate at which glycolysis operates. By controlling the flux of F6P through glycolysis, PFK-1 indirectly controls the level of G6P and therefore the activity of HK.

PFK-1 activity is highly sensitive to the energy status of the cell

ATP serves as both a substrate and an allosteric regulator of PFK-1. As an allosteric regulator, ATP can bind at a second site within the enzyme structure that is quite distinct from the substrate site (involved in the enzyme reaction) and inhibit PFK-1. PFK-1 is inhibited by high intracellular levels of ATP. Adenosine monophosphate (AMP) and adenosine diphosphate (ADP) relieve the inhibition of PFK-1 by ATP. Therefore, the rate of glycolysis depends on the ratio of (AMP + ADP) to ATP (Information box 3.5).

Life or death can depend on intense muscle activity and there must be a large supply of energy available at all times

One mechanism for providing this energy is to increase production through glycolysis, and glycolysis is therefore amplified:

- During exercise (when ATP is used for muscle contraction)
- During hypoxia and in anaerobic muscle (which limits ATP production by oxidative ATP-generating electron transport pathways within mitochondria).
  Mechanism for increasing ATP production through glycolysis
- In muscle, ATP is used up during bursts of activity, with the accumulation of ADP.
- ADP is then converted to AMP + ATP by adenylate kinase (also referred to as myokinase).
- As a result, when ATP is used up there is a large increase in AMP concentration. (This is because the sum of ATP + ADP + AMP remains nearly constant and the intracellular ATP concentration is much greater than that of AMP at equilibrium (approximately 50 times); relatively small fractional changes in ATP concentration therefore lead to relatively large fractional changes in the concentration of AMP.)
- AMP, the positive allosteric effector of PFK-1, acts as a metabolic amplifier – PFK-1 is therefore activated, increasing glycolysis.

Regulation of PFK-1

PFK-1 is pivotal in regulating the rate and direction of glycolysis, being highly sensitive to the energy requirements of the cell. The enzyme is regulated by several mechanisms (see Fig. 3.7). In muscle there is an involvement of a specific protein kinase (AMPK). PFK is also allosterically regulated.

Regulation by energy status and allosteric effectors

In muscle, a change in AMP concentration coordinates glycolytic flux with glucose uptake via glycolysis. This involves the activation of a specific regulatory enzyme, a protein kinase (PK). In general, PKs enable phosphorylation of specific amino acid residues in enzymes and proteins. This often results in altered catalytic activity in enzymes.

One particular PK, **AMP-activated protein kinase (AMPK)**, is sensitive to cellular energy status because its activity is acutely increased when AMP (and ADP) levels rise. Activation of AMPK by AMP is achieved directly by an allosteric mechanism, as well as by phosphorylation induced by other kinases that phosphorylate AMPK itself. This constitutes a phosphorylation cascade, which regulates the rate of glycolysis.

Activation of AMPK, like insulin, leads to recruitment of GLUT4 protein to the plasma membrane of skeletal muscle cells. This allows increased glucose entry into the cell for ATP production, and is of particular importance for fast-twitch skeletal muscle during anaerobic exercise.

Fructose-2,6-bisphosphate

PFK-1 has a second potent allosteric effector, F-2,6-BP, which is not an intermediate of glycolysis, but a key regulator. F-2,6-BP activates PFK-1 and counters the inhibition by ATP of PFK-1.

F-2,6-BP is formed by phosphorylation of F6P through the regulatory enzyme **phosphofructokinase-2 (PFK-2)**, which is also responsible for F-2,6-BP breakdown to F6P. PFK-2 is therefore a bifunctional enzyme that also has F-2,6-bisphosphatase (F-2,6-BPase) activity, exhibiting kinase activity when dephosphorylated and phosphatase activity when phosphorylated.

In the liver

In the liver, PFK-2 is under the allosteric control of F6P. High concentrations of F6P (due to an abundance of glucose) stimulate the kinase activity and inhibit the phosphatase activity, thereby stimulating glycolysis. This is an important mechanism for determining whether the predominant direction of hepatic glucose flux is towards glycolysis or towards glycogen synthesis.

During starvation, the hormone glucagon is released (by pancreatic α cells) in response to low blood glucose concentration. The hepatic priority then becomes glucose synthesis (gluconeogenesis) for export to extrahepatic tissues. Consumption of the newly synthesised glucose by hepatic glycolysis would be wasteful. Under the influence of glucagon, PFK-2 exhibits F-2,6-BPase activity, bringing about a fall in cellular F-2,6-BP levels, simultaneously:

- Inhibiting glycolysis (PFK-1)
- Reducing the inhibition on gluconeogenesis.

In muscle

Muscle contains a different form of the bifunctional enzyme PFK-2, both in its amino acid sequence and its response to phosphorylation by protein kinases. Muscle PFK-2 is an isoenzyme, catalysing the same reaction, but it has different regulatory properties. Unlike the liver, striated muscle has no glucagon receptors. Instead, as part of the 'flight-or-fight' mechanism, a rise in the catecholamine stress hormone epinephrine stimulates glycolysis in the heart muscle. This is part of a mechanism to meet the increased demand for ATP caused by an epinephrine-induced increase in workload (e.g. increased cardiac output).

Citrate and pH

PFK-1 is inhibited by citrate (from the TCA cycle) and hydrogen ions (low pH) (see Fig. 3.7).

In oxidative tissues such as the heart during increased exercise, a rise in cytosolic citrate concentration signals the availability of fuels that are alternatives to glucose, namely fatty acids and ketone bodies.

Crossover analysis (Information box 3.6) has demonstrated that inhibition of PFK-1 by citrate is important in suppressing cardiac glycolysis when the heart is oxidising lipid during starvation. This decreases glucose utilisation and

Crossover analysis is used in experiments to determine the likely regulatory enzymes in a metabolic pathway

For a hypothetical pathway with the intermediates A, B, C, D (A → B → C → D), the crossover theorem proposes that in the conversion of C to D:

- If a regulatory enzyme is inhibited the amount of substrate C will build up and the concentration of D will decrease. This is described as a crossover in the metabolic profile between C and D. (In the absence of an inhibitor the substrate C will decrease in concentration as D production increases under control of the enzyme.)
- Inhibiting a non-regulatory enzyme will cause little change in the intermediates concerned, unless the enzyme is completely inhibited.
- When steady-state concentrations of intermediates in the presence or absence of an inhibitor are compared, the intermediates before the site of inhibition (i.e. C) accumulate in response to the inhibitor, whereas the intermediates after the site (i.e. D) are depleted.

conserves glucose for tissues that contain few mitochondria (where anaerobic glycolysis predominates) such as RBC and the central nervous system.

Hydrogen ions shut off glycolysis through inhibition of PFK-1. Unless lactic acid and the H⁺ ions formed by glycolysis are transported out of the cell, the intracellular pH will drop, decreasing PFK-1 activity so that further lactic acid production by glycolysis is stopped. This helps to prevent intracellular pH falling to a level where the cell is rendered non-viable. An accumulation of lactate and the reduced pH in muscle results in the severe muscle cramp experienced by athletes during prolonged exercise.

Energy-producing stage of glycolysis – production of pyruvate and lactate

In the energy-producing stage of glycolysis, four molecules of ATP are produced.

Once F-1,6-BP is formed, the molecule is split into two 3-carbon phosphorylated intermediates (triose phosphates: dihydroxyacetone phosphate (DHAP) and glyceraldehyde 3-phosphate). These two compounds are interconvertible, but only glyceraldehyde 3-phosphate enters the later stages of glycolysis (Fig. 3.9). DHAP enters a pathway for fatty acid synthesis (see later). Each triose phosphate can provide one phosphate, which is subsequently transferred to ATP.

Two additional phosphate molecules are recruited in the next stage (one for each triose phosphate) as glyceraldehyde 3-phosphate traps soluble phosphate in the form of an acyl phosphate. This reaction is catalysed by glyceraldehyde 3-phosphate dehydrogenase (G3PDH) to form 1,3-bisphosphate glycerate (1,3-BPG), with the simultaneous reduction of NAD⁺ to NADH.

Reactions yielding ATP

During the next stage of glycolysis, ATP is produced by substrate-level phosphorylation in which a 'high-energy' phosphate intermediate of the pathway (a pathway substrate) transfers its phosphate to ADP to form ATP. The two reactions that yield ATP and pyruvate are catalysed by the enzymes phosphoglycerate kinase and pyruvate kinase, which together yield 2 moles of ATP per mole of triose phosphate, a total of **4 moles of ATP per mole of glucose**. The energy-producing stage of glycolysis also generates reduced nicotinamide adenine dinucleotide (NADH) from the coenzyme NAD⁺ in the reaction catalysed by G3PDH.

After adjustment for the ATP invested in the phosphorylations catalysed by the HK and PFK-1 reactions, the conversion of glucose to pyruvate yields a **net gain of two molecules of ATP, together with two molecules of NADH**. Pyruvate can potentially enter oxidative phosphorylation, the process by which energy is released in the form of ATP as pyruvate is broken down into CO_2 and water.

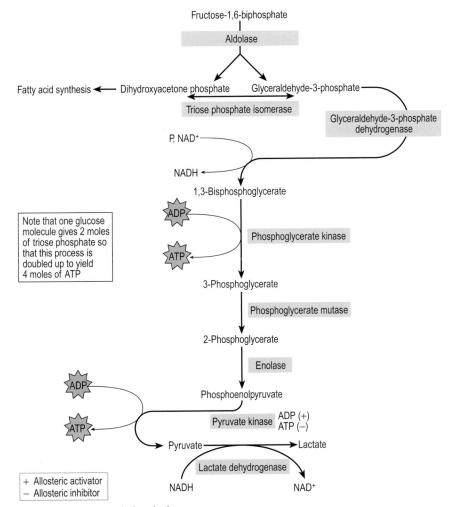

Fig. 3.9 **Energy-producing stage of glycolysis.**

Pyruvate kinase

Pyruvate kinase not only catalyses substrate-level phosphorylation yielding ATP (Clinical box 3.3), but it is also another regulatory enzyme of glycolysis, though its action is in direct contrast to the ATP-consuming reactions catalysed by the other regulatory enzymes, HK and PFK-1.

Kinetic studies have revealed three classes of pyruvate kinase isoenzymes, with qualitative differences in regulatory properties. For example, the pyruvate kinase isoenzyme found in liver is activated by the product of the PFK-1 reaction, F-1,6-BP, and shows allosteric inhibition by ATP. This links the regulation of pyruvate kinase with that of PFK-1. When glucose is abundant, conditions favour increased flux through PFK-1, and the level of F-1,6-BP increases. The rise in F-1,6-BP concentration acts as a feed-forward activator of pyruvate kinase.

Liver pyruvate kinase, like glucokinase, is induced by higher steady-state concentrations of glucose and insulin. This increase in enzyme concentration is a major reason why the liver of a well-fed person has a greater capacity for utilising carbohydrate than in a fasting person.

Fate of pyruvate

Pyruvate is metabolised in different ways, depending on the availability of glucose, as in the fed state or fasted state (Fig. 3.10).

In mitochondria-containing cells

Fed state

In the fed state, pyruvate is diverted into the more energy efficient metabolic pathway, the TCA cycle. The enzyme **pyruvate dehydrogenase complex** (**PDC**) converts pyruvate to CO_2 and acetyl-CoA. Acetyl-CoA can then:

- Enter the TCA cycle for complete oxidation – this generates far more ATP than glycolysis alone
- Be converted to citrate (in the TCA cycle), and then be transported to the cytosol to enter fatty acid synthesis, where the first step is the conversion of acetyl-CoA to malonyl-CoA.

PDC activity can either determine or reflect fuel preference (carbohydrate versus lipid), and therefore occupies a pivotal position in fuel homeostasis. Importantly, the initial decarboxylation of pyruvate catalysed by PDC begins a process that

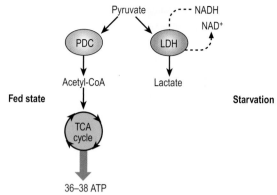

Fig. 3.10 Fate of pyruvate in the fed and fasted states. **Fed state**. When PDC is active, pyruvate can be converted to acetyl-CoA via PDC. Acetyl-CoA can enter the TCA cycle for complete oxidation. This generates far more ATP than glycolysis alone. Acetyl-CoA can also be converted to citrate (in the TCA cycle), and then can be transported to the cytosol to enter fatty acid synthesis. **Starvation**. When PDC is inactive, pyruvate is converted to lactate, which is released into the circulation. This also regenerates NAD^+. LDH, lactate dehydrogenase; PDC, pyruvate dehydrogenase complex; TCA, tricarboxylic acid.

is physiologically irreversible, committing glucose-derived pyruvate to acetyl-CoA production (see Fig. 3.10).

Fasted state

In the fasted state, PDC is inactive, and, in liver and kidney, pyruvate is directed towards gluconeogenesis. Pyruvate is converted to:

- Oxaloacetate by pyruvate carboxylase (the water soluble vitamin biotin acts as coenzyme, see Ch. 16).
- Alanine by alanine aminotransferase (ALT).

In cells that lack mitochondria, when oxygen is limited, and in starvation

In cells that lack mitochondria (e.g. RBCs) or tissues that contain relatively few mitochondria (e.g. cornea, lens, retina, kidney medulla and white muscle) pyruvate is converted by **lactate dehydrogenase** (**LDH**) to **lactate** as the principal end-product. Conversion to lactate in other tissues also predominates when oxygen is limited or the activity of PDC is low. Glycolytic ATP production is therefore important for brief high intensity exercise, ageing (loss of mitochondria), and in the disease state atherosclerosis (loss of oxygen supply to muscle).

Lactate production becomes important under conditions where dietary glucose is scarce (e.g. starvation) and glucose must be conserved for 'glucose-dependent' tissues. It is also important because lactate production from pyruvate regenerates NAD^+ so that glycolysis can continue.

Lactate dehydrogenase

Pyruvate can be converted to lactate via LDH. In this process, NAD^+ is regenerated from NADH. LDH catalyses a near-equilibrium reaction, and is not regulatory for glycolysis.

The regeneration of NAD^+ by LDH is crucial under anaerobic conditions and in cells lacking mitochondria, because NAD^+ is an essential cofactor for glycolysis. Lactate is moved out of the cell by facilitated diffusion. A family of membrane bound proteins, **monocarboxylate transport proteins** (**MCT1–4**), has been identified that transport lactate into and out of cells. The MCT

Clinical box 3.4 **Enzyme defects that cause lactic acidosis**

Lactic acidosis occurs when there is excessive accumulation of lactic acid in the bloodstream. It can be a metabolic emergency. The clinical features are those of metabolic acidosis. Tissue oxygen deprivation stimulates respiration, giving rise to 'air hunger' – Kussmaul respiration. Treatment should be aimed at the primary cause. Lactic acidosis can be caused by:
- Severe exercise – the condition is self-limiting
- Defective tissue perfusion when cells are deprived of oxygen and undergo anaerobic glycolysis (type A lactic acidosis)
- Decreased enzyme activity for degrading lactic acid (type B lactic acidosis).

Type A lactic acidosis
- Clinically much more common than type B lactic acidosis
- Occurs in shock – i.e. general circulatory insufficiency of any cause leading to poor tissue perfusion or reduced blood oxygenation

Type B lactic acidosis
This is less common, and occurs in the absence (at least obviously) of circulatory failure, and may be caused by:
- Decreased pyruvate dehydrogenase activity in diabetes, sometimes after diabetic ketoacidosis
- Reduced lactic acid metabolism by the liver
- Drug-induced (e.g. biguanide accumulation in people with diabetes with chronic renal failure, some treatments for malaria)
- In association with inborn errors of metabolism (G6PD deficiency for example)

family proteins (produced by solute carrier (SLC) gene *SLC16A*) also transport other simple monocarboxylates such as pyruvate and ketone bodies across the plasma membrane. Released lactate is transported to the liver and converted back to glucose for re-use (Cori cycle, see later). Lactate release is vital for some cells under normal conditions, including white muscle fibres, and rapidly proliferating cells (e.g. activated lymphocytes and cancer cells), and for all cells under hypoxic conditions. MCT4 is the major MCT form found in white (glycolytic) muscle. Fast-twitch muscle fibres produce lactate, which is transported outwards by MCT4. Lactate is then taken up by the slow-twitch muscle fibres, which express another MCT form, MCT1, for oxidation. The MCT system is a pH dependent antiport.

When NAD^+ is regenerated from NADH, lactate and H^+ ions accumulate in the cell, leading to a fall in pH. This creates the pH gradient that activates the MCT system, and lactate diffuses out of the cell to enter the blood. Excessive accumulation of lactate leads to lactic acidosis (Clinical box 3.4). This can be caused by physiological lactate production, when there is inadequate tissue oxygen supply (as in intense exercise), or if there is defective pyruvate clearance or increased pyruvate production.

Under fasting conditions, even cells capable of oxidative metabolism produce lactate because PDC is inactivated (see above). In the fed state when PDC is active, cells (e.g. muscle cells) can take up circulating lactate derived from other tissues (e.g. the red blood cell) for conversion to pyruvate via the reversible LDH reaction and entry into the TCA cycle for energy (ATP) production.

OXIDATIVE GLUCOSE METABOLISM – AEROBIC GLYCOLYSIS

The conversion of glucose to CO_2 and water takes place in two stages: the anaerobic conversion of glucose to pyruvate, followed by the complete oxidation of pyruvate to CO_2 and water in two stages:

- In the TCA cycle, reduced coenzymes, such as NADH, are produced within the inner membrane of mitochondria
- NADH is then oxidised to NAD^+ in the electron transport system, coupled with the reduction of oxygen.

The ATP yield from glucose degradation is massively increased when pyruvate is oxidised completely through this process.

Glycolysis produces two molecules of ATP for each molecule of glucose, whereas the **complete oxidative metabolism of glucose can yield up to 36–38 molecules of ATP**.

Acetyl-CoA is the molecule at the starting point of the TCA cycle and is a metabolite that is also common to the breakdown of lipid and proteins. Entry of acetyl-CoA derived from carbohydrates is under the control of the the pyruvate dehydrogenase complex (PDC). When PDC is active, pyruvate is converted to acetyl-CoA. When PDC is inactive, pyruvate is generally converted to lactate, which is released into the circulation (see above).

Pyruvate dehydrogenase complex

The PDC is a tightly organised arrangement of polypeptides and cofactors working sequentially in the multienzyme complex catalysing a multi-step reaction in which pyruvate is converted to acetyl-CoA (Clinical box 3.5). The intermediate substrates and products remain bound to the complex, increasing overall efficiency. In this process, carbon is lost in the form of CO_2, and NAD^+ is reduced to NADH. This is **oxidative decarboxylation**.

Unlike the key controlling glycolytic enzymes HK, PFK-1 and pyruvate kinase, which are located in the cytosol, PDC is located in the mitochondria. Pyruvate produced by glycolysis must first be transported by a specific pyruvate transporter into the mitochondria for entry into the TCA cycle.

Regulation of PDC activity

Regulation of PDC activity (Fig. 3.11) is an important component of glucose homeostasis. Active PDC facilitates the entry of glucose carbon into the TCA cycle when fuel is abundant. When there is a lack of glucose (e.g. during prolonged starvation) suppression of PDC activity is crucial to glucose conservation.

Clinical box 3.5 **Defective pyruvate dehydrogenase complex activity**

PDC activity requires coenzymes from the B vitamin family, notably thiamine (B$_1$), but also riboflavin (B$_2$), pantothenic acid and nicotinamide (B$_3$). Dietary (beriberi) and alcohol-related thiamine deficiency leads to defective coenzyme synthesis so that PDC activity is impaired, and pyruvate entry into the TCA cycle is reduced (see Ch. 16).

PDC deficiency
PDC converts pyruvate to acetyl-CoA, needed for the production of citrate, which is essential for the TCA cycle. In PDC deficiency (PDCD), mitochondrial oxidation of pyruvate in the TCA cycle cannot proceed, so pyruvate is converted to lactate with consequent high blood pyruvate and lactate concentrations, with or without overt lactic acidosis. Total PDCD is incompatible with life.

The extremely rare Leigh disease is associated with an X-linked genetic PDC defect. Prenatal PDCD may lead to congenital brain malformations, Symptoms present early in infancy, including hypotonia, developmental delay, seizures and early death. Treatment is aimed to stimulate PDC activity with thiamine supplementation and to provide alternative metabolic fuels to glucose, e.g. low carbohydrate, ketogenic diet.

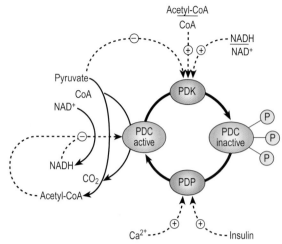

***Fig. 3.11* Mechanisms regulating pyruvate dehydrogenase complex (PDC) activity.** PDK, pyruvate dehydrogenase kinase; PDP, pyruvate dehydrogenase phosphatase.

Acetyl-CoA and NADH are competitive inhibitors. These are also generated by fat oxidation.

PDC is also inactivated through phosphorylation by pyruvate dehydrogenase kinases (termed PDKs or PDHKs). These are structurally related proteins of which four isoforms have been identified: PDK1–4. Most tissues contain at least two and often three isoforms. Changes in tissue PDK isoform expression occur in response to:

- Starvation
- Variations in dietary composition
- Hormonal status: e.g. insulin increases PDC activity in adipose tissue.

The common products of glucose and fatty acid metabolism, acetyl-CoA and NADH, inhibit PDC activity. They also both activate PDK, which in turn inactivates PDC.

Intermediates of glucose and fatty acid metabolism have opposing effects on PDC and PDK:

- PDK is suppressed by pyruvate, generated via glycolysis or from circulating lactate
- High mitochondrial acetyl-CoA/CoA and NADH/NAD$^+$ concentration ratios (which are generated when rates of fatty acid β-oxidation are increased) activate PDK.

PDC is re-activated by pyruvate dehydrogenase phosphatases (PDPs), of which two isoenzymes exist. One of these is activated by Ca^{2+}. Ca^{2+} activation of PDP increases PDC activity, leading to increased ATP generation from pyruvate. Cytoplasmic Ca^{2+} concentrations increase when there is increased demand for ATP (e.g. in muscle during exercise).

GLYCOGEN – THE STORAGE FORM OF GLUCOSE

Glycogen, a branched polysaccharide, is the principal storage form of glucose in mammalian cells. The two quantitatively major tissue sites of glycogen storage are the liver and skeletal muscle. When carbohydrate is supplied in excess of tissue requirements, it is used for the synthesis of storage molecules:

- **Glycogen**, the storage form of glucose. Liver glycogen is readily mobilised, and provides a defence against a declining blood glucose concentration.

- **Triacylglycerol** (TAG; also known as triglyceride), the storage form of fatty acids.

When the supply of metabolic fuels is restricted, tissue energy demands are met by the mobilisation of stored (endogenous) fuels. Metabolic stores can either:

- Provide substrates directly – glucose from glycogen (glycogenolysis), fatty acids from TAG, or
- Provide precursors such as lactate and glycerol for glucose synthesis via gluconeogenesis.

In the liver

In the liver, glycogen is mainly present as a glucose reservoir for other tissues, and the amount of glycogen stored in the liver changes constantly with changes in nutritional status. Liver glycogen degradation generates glucose directly to maintain blood glucose concentrations between meals. Thus, during the post-absorptive state – between meals – glucose is produced directly from hepatic glycogenolysis. Hepatic glycogen is essentially depleted after overnight starvation because total hepatic glycogen stores (typically 50–100 g) are only sufficient to maintain blood glucose over a 12-hour fast.

In skeletal muscle

Skeletal muscle glycogen can be rapidly mobilised and utilised for ATP production via anaerobic glycolysis (in the absence of oxygen). In skeletal muscle, glycogen cannot be broken down to glucose through glycogenolysis directly because it lacks the enzyme glucose-6-phosphatase (G6Pase). Glucose cannot therefore be supplied to the circulation by skeletal muscle.

Information box 3.7	Liver and muscle glycogen have different functions

- Hepatic glycogen is primarily directed towards glucose release to counteract a dangerously low blood glucose concentration (hypoglycaemia).
- Muscle glycogen breakdown is primarily directed towards the provision of ATP for muscle contraction.

SYNTHESIS OF GLYCOGEN

The general mechanism of glycogen synthesis is the same in all tissues. The first step is the conversion of G6P into glucose-1-phosphate (G1P) by the enzyme phosphoglucomutase. To be converted into glycogen, G1P has to be converted into a form that can be acted on by the next enzyme in the sequence, **glycogen synthase (GS)**. Glycogen can only be synthesised if a small branched oligosaccharide primer is present. This is synthesised by a protein glycogenin by self-glycosylation. Glycogenin forms a complex with glycogen synthase (GS), which extends the oligosaccharide chain using the sugar nucleotide, uridine diphosphate (UDP)-glucose as the substrate adding glucose residues by α1→4 glycosidic linkages. The combination of G1P with uridine triphosphate (UTP) forms UDP-glucose, in an activation process catalysed by the enzyme UDP-glucose pyrophosphorylase. Apart from glycogen synthesis, UDP-glucose also takes part in the synthesis of other sugars, glycoproteins and glycolipids. Therefore it is the next enzyme in the pathway, GS, and not UDP-glucose pyrophosphorylase, which is regulatory for glycogen synthesis (Fig. 3.12) (see below).

Glycogenin, the glycogen primer

As noted previously, a primer is required for glycogen synthesis when cells are totally depleted of glycogen: the protein called **glycogenin**. Glycogenin can attach glucose molecules to its own amino acid residues, a process called self-glucosylation.

- The 'C-1' of glucose is autocatalytically attached by glycogenin to one of its own tyrosine residues, using UDP-glucose to donate the glucose residue (UDP-glucose is a glucosyl donor). This forms the core glycogen sequence.
- Glycogenin then autocatalytically extends the 'glucan' chain by up to six or seven glucose residues to form the 'primed' glycogen. The glucose residues are joined together by α1→4 links (Fig. 3.11).

Glycogen synthase (GS)

The 'primed' glycogen is further elongated by GS, a member of the class of enzymes known as glycosyl transferases.

- GS elongates the primed glycogen by adding glucose molecules via α1→4 linkage
- Glycogen branching enzyme transfers some of the α1→4-links to a α1→6 branch when the α1→4 chain reaches 6–8 glucose residues, so that the glycogen molecule becomes tree-like (see Fig. 3.12).

Glycogen limits its own synthesis by end-product inhibition so that its accumulation in liver and muscle does not become excessive.

Structure of glycogen

A mature glycogen particle has a structure resembling the head of a cauliflower (see Fig. 3.12), with branches that form a left-handed helix with 6.5 glucose residues per turn.

About half of the glycogen mass is attributable to the external branches, which provide ready access to the glucose residues for the enzymes involved in their release from the glycogen polymer. The internal branches carry side chains separated by about four glucose units.

The cauliflower-like structure of glycogen accounts for the spherical shape of beta-particles (30 nm diameter, up to 60 000 glucose units), which are present in most cells. In the liver, about 20–40 beta-particles are associated into larger complexes known as alpha rosettes, which are visible under the electron microscope.

Control of glycogen synthesis

Glycogen synthesis occurs during and immediately following meals. In response to a rising blood glucose concentration, insulin is secreted from the β-cells of the pancreatic islets, lowering blood glucose concentration by promoting:

- cell glucose uptake
- cellular glucose metabolism
- glycogen synthesis.

Insulin and glucagon are the main hormones concerned with controlling blood glucose concentration. Glucose stimulates the secretion of insulin and inhibits the secretion of glucagon. Insulin reverses the action of glucagon on enzyme phosphorylation, inhibiting glycogen phosphorylase, the enzyme catalysing glycogen breakdown, and activating GS, so initiating the metabolic processes that transform glucose to glycogen in liver and muscle.

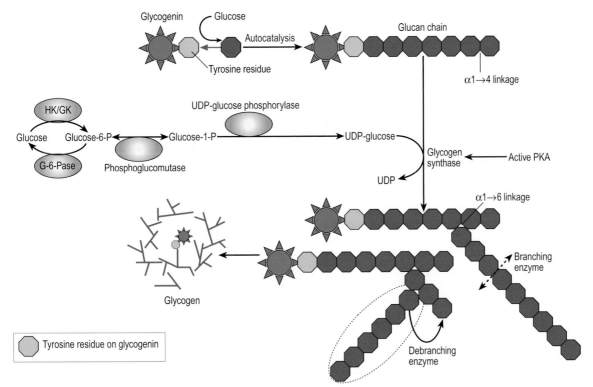

Fig. 3.12 **Glycogen synthesis and its regulation.** GK, glucokinase; G6Pase, glucose-6-phosphatase; HK, hexokinase; UDP, uridine diphosphate.

Glucose that is not stored in the liver proceeds to the peripheral circulation where it is taken up by:

- skeletal muscle (for glycogen synthesis)
- adipose tissue (to provide glycerol 3-phosphate for fatty acid esterification to form triglyceride and fatty acid synthesis de novo).

Allosteric activation of glycogen synthesis

Because glucose can enter liver cells without insulin, the liver is responsive to the direct stimulus of a post-prandial rising blood glucose concentration, initiating glycogen synthesis before insulin concentration rises. This occurs by:

- Direct allosteric inhibition of glycogen phosphorylase by glucose, inhibiting glycogen breakdown (see Fig. 3.12)
- Secondary stimulation of a protein phosphatase activity (dephosphorylation of glycogen phosphorylase; see below).

Covalent mechanisms regulating glycogen synthesis

Glycogen synthase (**GS**) is the key regulatory enzyme for glycogen synthesis. Acute regulation of GS activity operates through covalent mechanisms achieved in part by a reversible phosphorylation (see Fig. 3.12).

- GS is activated by dephosphorylation, a reaction catalysed by protein phosphatases.
- GS is inactivated by phosphorylation, a reaction catalysed by protein kinases.

Glycogenolysis is catalysed by glycogen phosphorylase, which breaks the $\alpha1\rightarrow4$ links in glycogen. Glycogen phosphorylase is activated by phosphorylation (to promote glycogenolysis) and inactivated by dephosphorylation. By using common kinases and phosphatases, GS can be activated when glycogen phosphorylase is inactivated, and vice versa.

There is a strong linear correlation between the activity of the activated form of GS-a (glycogen synthase a) and the rate of glycogen synthesis in liver. This positive correlation is also observed in fast-twitch skeletal muscle, where glycolysis from glycogen is a vital source of ATP for contraction.

Glycogen synthesis in the liver

The cell membranes of hepatocytes contain the glucose transporter GLUT2. Glucose is freely transported into the cells even when glucose is delivered at high concentration in the portal blood during the absorption of a carbohydrate-rich meal. Because the transport capacity of GLUT2 is not rate-limiting for hepatic glucose uptake, the liver functions as a blood glucose sensor.

The hepatocytes are rich in GK, which converts glucose into G6P. Unlike HK, GK is not inhibited by G6P, so the concentration of G6P increases rapidly in the liver cells following a carbohydrate-rich meal, leading to GS activation by dephosphorylation. If liver glycogen concentrations are not at maximum, G6P is channeled into the glycogen synthesis pathway; as hepatic glycogen becomes replenished, excess G6P enters glycolysis.

Direct versus indirect pathway of hepatic glycogen synthesis

After a meal, ingested glucose is converted first into liver glycogen, stimulated by the secretion of insulin, which:

- Inhibits glycogen phosphorylase
- Activates GS.

After fasting, however, when blood glucose falls and liver glycogen becomes the immediate source of glucose, liver glycogen can be replenished from the product of glycolysis – lactate – which is converted into G6P via gluconeogenesis.

Thus the liver has both direct (via glucokinase) and indirect (via gluconeogenesis) pathways for glycogen replenishment.

Glycogen synthesis in skeletal muscle

Skeletal muscle is a major tissue site for glucose disposal when insulin levels are elevated (e.g. after a carbohydrate-rich meal).

Glycogen synthesis represents the primary pathway for the non-oxidative disposal of glucose in normal healthy human subjects, and skeletal muscle glycogen synthesis is a major pathway of overall glucose metabolism (Information box 3.8). Impaired glycogen synthesis in skeletal muscle, due to defective insulin action or insulin resistance, is a major intracellular metabolic defect in type 2 diabetes mellitus (Clinical box 3.6).

Information box 3.8 **Non-invasive techniques for studying the rate of glycogen synthesis**

Glycogen concentrations can be measured accurately with a time resolution of several minutes using carbon-13 nuclear magnetic resonance spectra of human muscle glycogen. Used in combination with indirect calorimetry, the rate of muscle glycogen synthesis during insulin stimulation can then be related to whole body glucose disposal.

Clinical box 3.6 **Insulin resistance in type 2 diabetes mellitus**

Diabetes mellitus is the result of disordered metabolism secondary to defects in the production and/or effectiveness of the hormone insulin, secreted by pancreatic β-cells.

In type 2 diabetes, resistance to insulin action is the major problem, but insulin secretion becomes impaired. Some β-cells are still active initially, but there is a suboptimal insulin response to glucose stimulation. Treatment would therefore be to stimulate the remaining β-cells to secrete more insulin, or to improve insulin sensitivity.

Insulin resistance results from inefficient glucose utilisation by target cells

Patients with type 2 diabetes often have hyperglycaemia despite the presence of plasma insulin, even at inappropriately high concentrations. The cause of this hyperglycaemia is uncertain, but has been postulated as the result of inefficient glucose utilisation by insulin target cells (insulin resistance), which may be due to:

- Defective insulin-receptor binding due to down-regulation of insulin receptors
- Gene mutation causing abnormality in insulin-receptor binding
- Defective key enzymes, such as glycogen synthase or pyruvate dehydrogenase
- Increased pyruvate dehydrogenase kinase (PDK) isoform expression in muscle leading to inactivation of muscle pyruvate dehydrogenase complex (PDC)
- Possible genetically determined post receptor defect, i.e. defective signal transduction
- Defects in signalling pathway, due to defects in the insulin receptors (e.g. absence of tyrosine kinase) or in the post receptor cascade
- Defects in insulin-induced glucose transport, such as defective translocation of GLUT4 to cell membrane.

Energy metabolism in muscles

Skeletal muscles generally comprise two types of muscle fibre:
- Fast-twitch fibres in white muscle (as in chicken breast meat) are relatively low in mitochondria, blood flow (hence 'white') and fat, but rich in glycogen. These muscles contain a large number of fast-twitch fibres, which perform rhythmic contractions using glycogen stores and anaerobic glycolysis for short bursts of additional energy, since glycogen stores only last a short period of time.
- Slow-twitch fibres in dark muscle (as in red meat) are well perfused, have a high fat content and are rich in mitochondria. These muscles use aerobic (oxidative) metabolism of fatty acids for the energy required for prolonged, strenuous exercise.
- Cardiac muscle contracts continuously. It is has a rich blood supply and mitochondria, and relies mainly on oxidative fatty acid metabolism for ATP synthesis, similar to slow-twitch muscles.

Short-distance versus long-distance running
- Athletes specialising in short-distance running (e.g. 100 or 200 m sprinting) primarily use anaerobic metabolism for energy.
- Energy for long-distance running (e.g. 5000 m or marathon) is mainly obtained by aerobic metabolism.

Hitting the wall
Long-distance athletes sometimes 'hit the wall' when their glycogen stores are depleted. The popular high-carbohydrate diet before a race is intended to build up glycogen stores.

The pathway for glycogen synthesis from glucose in skeletal muscle differs from that in liver. Muscle contains the glucose transporter GLUT4 (recruited to the cell surface following insulin stimulation) and the glucose phosphorylating enzyme, HK. HK has a low K_m for glucose and is inhibited by G6P. Hence, efficient use of glucose by muscle for glycogen synthesis requires the continuous removal of G6P (unlike in the liver, which uses GK).

Intracellular glycogen content exerts a regulatory effect on glucose uptake in fast-twitch muscle (needed for short bursts of energy; Clinical box 3.7). However, in the period after prolonged and heavy physical activity, glycogen re-synthesis is of high priority and both glucose transport and glycogen synthesis are increased to replenish the depleted glycogen stores.

GLYCOGENOLYSIS – THE BREAKDOWN OF GLYCOGEN

Glycogenolysis is the process by which glycogen is broken down to glucose for use in energy metabolism. This is achieved not by simple hydrolysis, but by phosphorylation. Because of the branching nature of the glycogen molecule, separate enzymes are needed.

Glycogenolysis in liver

Liver glycogen is broken down to provide a rapid source of blood glucose as a short-term buffer to a fall in blood glucose concentration, and is particularly important between meals. The degradation of glycogen requires the concerted action of two enzymes:

- **Glycogen phosphorylase**, which breaks down the long chains of glucose molecules
- **Debranching enzyme**, which lops off the branches.

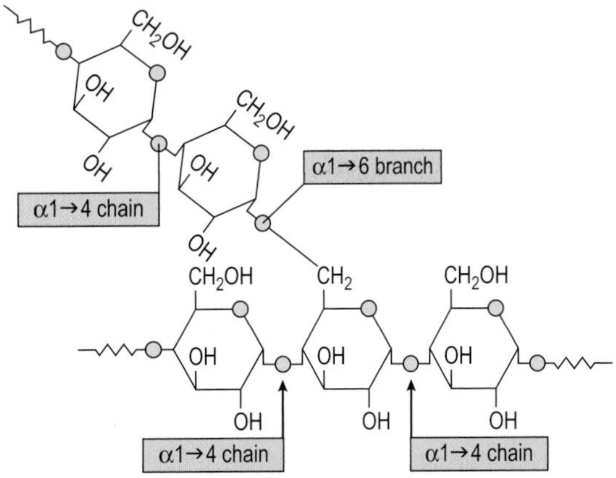

Fig. 3.13 **Pathways for hepatic glycogenolysis.**

The pathway of glycogenolysis begins with the removal of the terminal glucose residue of the abundant external $\alpha1\rightarrow4$ linked chains of glucose residues by glycogen phosphorylase, releasing G1P (see Fig. 3.13). G1P is converted into G6P by the enzyme phosphoglucomutase. G6P is then hydrolysed to glucose by G6Pase. Glucose is transported out of the cell by GLUT2 into the bloodstream.

Glycogenolysis in muscle

Unlike liver, skeletal muscle does not express the enzyme glucose 6-phosphatase (G6Pase) and therefore cannot convert G6P to glucose. This action keeps glucose within the cell (is glucose sparing) Instead, muscle G6P enters glycolysis to produce energy for muscle contraction (see Fig. 3.5). Although more of the body's glycogen is stored in muscle than in the liver, muscle cannot release glucose into the bloodstream. However, lactate generated from skeletal muscle glycogen can be transported by the blood to the liver and used as a precursor for the synthesis of glucose (gluconeogenesis).

REGULATION OF GLYCOGENOLYSIS

Regulation of glycogenolysis is achieved by:

- Hormones, mainly glucagon, epinephrine (sympathetic control), cortisol and to some extent human growth hormone (GH).
- Intracellular enzymes to catalyse the breakdown of glycogen.

Glycogen phosphorylase 'nibbles' at the external glucose residues until all external chains of the glycogen molecule have been shortened to four glucose units. At a branch point, debranching enzyme then removes a short segment of glucose residue by a glucose transferring activity (transglycosylase) and transfers the stub to the end of an adjacent chain. The remaining glucose molecule at the stub of the branch point is then liberated by the exo-α-glucosidase activity of the same debranching enzyme, which is bifunctional. The newly formed $\alpha1\rightarrow4$-linked glucose residues become available for phosphorylase to proceed with degradation until another branch point is reached.

Because the production of glucose from glycogen serves different purposes in the liver and skeletal muscle, the presence of hormone receptors and enzymes in their cells is specific to their needs.

Regulation of hepatic glycogenolysis

A range of metabolic pathways have to be activated to mobilise glucose stores. Glycogenolysis in the liver is activated in response to falling blood glucose levels in the fasting state and in preparation for an increased demand for glucose, for example in response to:

- Physiological stress, as in increased or prolonged exercise
- Pathological stress, as in severe shock from blood loss
- Psychological stress as in fear and preparation for 'flight or fight'.

Hormone regulation of hepatic glycogenolysis

Hepatic glycogenolysis during fasting or moderate exercise is increased by the hormone **glucagon**, secreted by pancreatic α-cells in response to low blood glucose. Glucagon has the major function of activating glycogenolysis to maintain normoglycaemia. It has a half-life in the plasma of only a few minutes so the plasma concentration of glucagon fluctuates constantly in response to the body's need for glucose.

In severe acute stress and severe hypoglycaemia, epinephrine works in tandem with glucagon to amplify hepatic glycogenolysis. This may in part explain the symptoms of tachycardia, sweating and shaking in hypoglycaemia and fear. Glucagon and epinephrine (via β-adrenergic receptors) activate glycogenolysis through a mechanism resulting from binding to their target cell surface receptors. The resultant increase in cAMP activates glycogen phosphorylase (and inactivates glycogen synthase) by a kinase cascade. Epinephrine has a second glycogenolytic pathway, via α-adrenergic receptors (see below).

In chronic stress (or in response to prolonged exposure to cold), plasma cortisol levels rise in response to the need for glucose, and stimulate glycogen synthesis. **Cortisol** is a glucocorticoid that has a major role in glucose homeostasis. Like glucagon, the action of cortisol leads to increases in blood glucose concentration, but has a much slower effect. It acts through gene expression to stimulate the transcription of mRNA to synthesise enzymes that increase glycogenesis and gluconeogenesis. Cortisol is secreted by the adrenal glands, controlled by the hypothalamic-pituitary axis. Secretion varies according to circadian rhythm (see Ch. 10).

MECHANISM OF GLUCAGON REGULATION OF GLYCOGENOLYSIS – HORMONE SIGNALLING

Glucagon binds to a liver cell plasma membrane receptor, setting off a cascade of reactions to release glucose into the bloodstream. The glucagon receptor is coupled to the **G protein**, adenylate cyclase-cAMP second messenger system (see above, Ch. 4 and Fig. 4.14). The binding of glucagon to its receptor protein causes dissociation of a subunit from the G protein complex in the cell membrane.

G proteins are so named because they bind guanosine nucleotides and consist of three subunits – α, β and γ. In its resting state, guanosine diphosphate (GDP) is bound to G protein. Binding of glucagon to its plasma membrane receptor in the liver starts a cascade involving the G proteins as follows (Fig. 3.14):

- GTP loses one P to become GDP and the α-subunit dissociates from the other two subunits

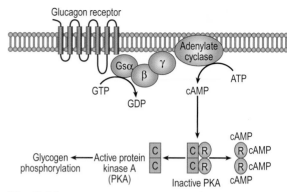

Fig. 3.14 Signalling pathway from glucagon to cAMP-dependent protein kinase A. PKA, cyclic AMP-dependent protein kinase A; GDP, guanosine diphosphate; GTT, guanosine triphosphate; C, catalytic; R, regulatory (inhibitory).

- Adenylate cyclase is activated by the stimulatory Gα-subunit, catalysing the conversion of ATP to cAMP and pyrophosphate
- cAMP binds to protein kinase A (PKA), a tetrameric enzyme with two pairs of subunits, releasing its inhibitory R-subunits, thus activating PKA
- PKA phosphorylates a series of enzymes (phosphorylase kinase and glycogen phosphorylase), which break down glycogen to form G1P, thus initiating glycogenolysis.

The activation of PKA by cAMP is instantaneous, thus providing very dynamic control of glycogenolysis.

SYMPATHETIC STIMULATION

Epinephrine (adrenaline) is an important neurotransmitter acting through the sympathetic nervous system. Acute stress, regardless of its cause, activates glycogenolysis through the action of epinephrine, which is released from the adrenal medulla as part of a 'flight or fight' response or during prolonged exercise.

In both liver and skeletal muscle, binding of epinephrine to β-adrenergic membrane receptors, like glucagon, leads to a cAMP-mediated increase in glycogenolysis. The action of epinephrine can also be mediated via α-adrenergic receptors in a different process involving the phospholipase C-Ca²⁺ (PLC-Ca²⁺) second-messenger system (see Ch. 4 and Fig. 4.16) as follows:

1. Binding to the α-receptor produces a conformational change in the G protein, which activates membrane-bound PLC
2. PLC splits a membrane phospholipid producing two second messengers: diacylglycerol (DAG, also known as diglyceride) and inositol trisphosphate (IP_3)
3. DAG activates PKC, initiating protein phosphorylation
4. IP_3 promotes entry of Ca^{2+} into the cytosol where it binds to the cytoplasmic protein, calmodulin
5. Ca^{2+}-calmodulin activates phosphorylase kinase, initiating phosphorylation to produce glucose via glycogenolysis.

Enzyme regulation of hepatic glycogenolysis

The rate-limiting step in glycogenolysis is catalysed by the enzyme glycogen phosphorylase. In the late 1930s, Carl and Gerti Cori discovered that there were two forms of the enzyme: a and b (Fig. 3.15):

- **Phosphorylase b** is the inactive form and is activated to phosphorylase a through phosphorylation. This reaction is regulated by a specific enzyme, phosphorylase kinase.

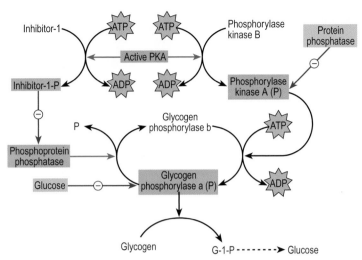

Fig. 3.15 **Regulation of hepatic glycogen phosphorylation.** Activated enzymes are shown in red and inhibitors are shown in blue.

- **Phosphorylase a** is the active form and is inactivated through reconversion to phosphorylase b by dephosphorylation. Dephosphorylation is catalysed by a phosphate-releasing protein (phosphatase enzyme).

There are three mammalian glycogen phosphorylases, designated muscle, brain and liver isoenzymes according to the tissue in which they are preferentially expressed.

REGULATION OF HEPATIC GLYCOGEN PHOSPHORYLASE

Activation of PKA sets off a series of phosphorylation reactions. In the liver, glycogen phosphorylase is very tightly controlled by phosphorylation (Fig. 3.15), as expected from an enzyme responding to extracellular signals involved in the maintenance of normoglycaemia, rather than responding to altered hepatic energy requirement. In addition, phosphorylase a acts as a glucose receptor in the liver. When blood glucose concentration is high, direct binding of glucose to phosphorylase a inactivates the enzyme by allosteric inhibition, which arrests glycogenolysis, a unique feature of the regulation of hepatic glycogenolysis.

Regulation of phosphorylase kinase by covalent modification – phosphorylation
Phosphorylase kinase is itself regulated by a phosphorylation-dephosphorylation mechanism:

- Dephosphorylation inactivates phosphorylase kinase, and is catalysed by a protein phosphatase that removes phosphate groups
- PKA catalyses the phosphorylation of hepatic phosphorylase kinase and activates it
- PKA also phosphorylates glycogen-associated protein phosphatase 1 (PP1G), which inhibits the phosphoprotein phosphatases that would otherwise decrease the response to glucagon by reversing the phosphorylation of:
  - phosphorylase kinase
  - glycogen phosphorylase
  - glycogen synthase (see Fig. 3.12).

Amplification of the signalling cascade
Cyclic AMP regulates the activity of PKA, which is a key signalling enzyme in the interconversion of glycogen and glucose

through the phosphorylation of phosphorylase kinase and glycogen synthase in the liver. PKA is very sensitive to small changes in cAMP concentration.

The activation of glycogen phosphorylase involves the phosphorylation and activation of many molecules of phosphorylase kinase by PKA (an example of a regulatory cascade).

Ca²⁺ as a second messenger
A subunit of phosphorylase kinase is functionally identical to the Ca²⁺-binding protein calmodulin (see Ch. 4). It acts as a Ca²⁺ receptor when there is an influx of Ca²⁺, activating phosphorylase kinase, and produces a conformational change.

Regulation of muscle and brain glycogenolysis

In contrast to liver, glycogenolysis in skeletal muscle is activated in response to increased energy requirement. Muscle cells lack glucagon receptors. Muscle glycogenolysis is activated by epinephrine via muscle β-adrenergic receptors acting via cAMP, mostly during 'flight or fight', but also during prolonged exercise.

Muscle glycogenolysis is also activated during short bursts of activity by two other mechanisms:

- In response to neural stimulation, Ca²⁺ enters the myocyte to activate unphosphorylated phosphorylase kinase, which contains calmodulin as a subunit, by forming a Ca²⁺-calmodulin complex, rapidly activating glycogenolysis. Muscle phosphorylase kinase activity is thus coordinated with muscle contraction and associated with muscle calcium influx.
- Allosteric activation of phosphorylase by AMP: ATP is depleted during bursts of muscle contraction, leading to an accumulation of ADP. The enzyme myokinase (adenylate kinase) catalyses a reaction that converts part of the excess ADP to ATP and AMP:

  $$2ADP \rightarrow ATP + AMP$$

The rapid rise in AMP concentration activates phosphorylase and the rate of glycogenolysis increases. Muscle and brain isoenzymes are allosterically:

- Activated by AMP, irrespective of whether they are phosphorylated or dephosphorylated
- Inhibited by G6P.

Genetic defects in glycogenolysis

Disorders of glycogen metabolism occur when there are defects in the enzymes that enable glycogenolysis. These rare conditions, known as glycogen storage diseases (Clinical box 3.8), are inherited. All are autosomal recessive, presenting in childhood. The genes concerned may be expressed in either liver or muscle.

GLUCONEOGENESIS – GLUCOSE SYNTHESIS

- Liver glycogenolysis is important for maintenance of blood glucose in the short term only. During progressive starvation, hepatic glycogenolysis in the short term and gluconeogenesis in the longer term compensates for the lack of glucose. When liver glycogen is depleted, tissues that require glucose are dependent on glucose synthesis from non-carbohydrate precursors, the process of **gluconeogenesis**. Thus gluconeogenesis becomes increasingly important after hepatic glycogen is depleted.
- These changes occur within 24 hours of fasting, depending on:
  - how well fed the individual was before the fast
  - how much hepatic glycogen was present
  - the amount of physical activity occurring during the fast.

Glycogenolysis cannot replace all the glucose oxidised by tissues in the post-absorptive period. Some new ('neo') glucose must be synthesised even at the expense of muscle protein breakdown. Gluconeogenesis is crucial for survival because of the continual fuel requirements of tissues that use only glucose as their primary energy substrate (e.g. brain in the short term, RBCs, kidney medulla, lens). For example, brain dysfunction occurs in hypoglycaemia; if severe, coma, death or (rarely) permanent brain damage may ensue. Therefore, even when fat may be supplying most of the energy requirements, a basal requirement for glucose has to be met. Furthermore, gluconeogenesis removes its products of metabolism from the blood (e.g. lactate). Lactate is generated in large quantities by glycolysis in RBCs and in anaerobically exercising muscle. Elevated lactate concentrations are characteristic of impaired gluconeogenesis (Clinical box 3.9).

Precursors of gluconeogenesis

Gluconeogenesis occurs mainly in the liver and kidneys, requiring a source of carbon for the backbone of the glucose molecule and a source of energy.

Energy for gluconeogenesis is provided by fatty acids released from fat cells (adipocytes). Fatty acid oxidation not only generates the ATP required to fuel gluconeogenesis, but also generates acetyl-CoA and NADH. Acetyl-CoA activates a key gluconeogenic enzyme, pyruvate carboxylase. Acetyl-CoA and NADH generated by fatty acid oxidation also inhibits the pyruvate dehydrogenase complex (PDC), which decarboxylates pyruvate to yield acetyl-CoA. This conserves pyruvate and prevents the loss of carbon as CO_2 (via PDC and the tricarboxylic acid cycle). Thus PDC inhibition directs available pyruvate towards glucose formation (via pyruvate carboxylase) and away from acetyl-CoA formation and degradation (oxidation).

Major carbon sources are (see Fig. 3.16):

- Lactate from anaerobic glycolysis and exercising muscles
- Gluconeogenic amino acids, including alanine and glutamine from protein breakdown
- Glycerol from triglyceride breakdown in adipocytes.

Gluconeogenesis from lactate

Whilst sharing the reversible enzymes of glycolysis, three irreversible kinase reactions in glycolysis must be overcome to produce glucose from lactate via gluconeogenesis. Thus gluconeogenesis from lactate is the reversal of glycolysis with three irreversible steps. Reversing the glycolysis pathway, the irreversible steps are:

- Last step in the generation of pyruvate, catalysed by pyruvate kinase (see Fig. 3.9)
- Conversion of F6P to F-1,6-BP, catalysed by PFK-1 (see Fig. 3.7)
- First step in the conversion of glucose to G6P, catalysed by GK (see Fig. 3.7).

These reactions are all non-equilibrium, and therefore physiologically irreversible. The liver and kidney use four additional enzymes that bypass these reactions:

- Pyruvate carboxylase and phosphoenolpyruvate carboxykinase (PEPCK) bypass pyruvate kinase.
- GK and PFK are bypassed by phosphatase enzymes, G6Pase (glucose 6-phosphatase) and F-1,6-BPase (fructose 1,6-bisphosphatase). F-1,6-BPase bypasses PFK-1 and G6Pase bypasses glucokinase. In liver, G6Pase also allows the direct generation of glucose from G6P generated via glycogenolysis.

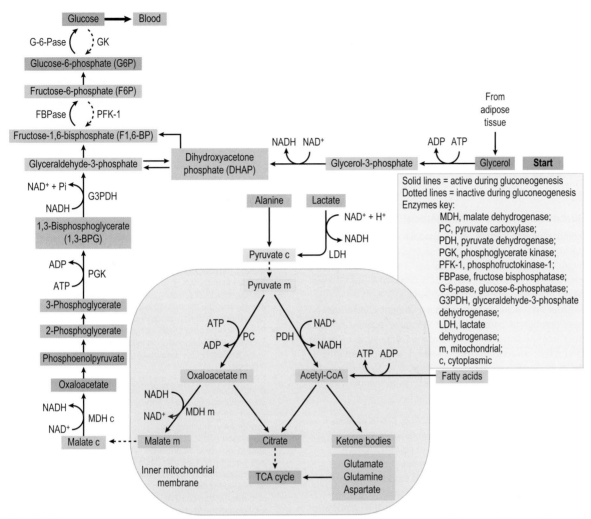

Fig. 3.16 Gluconeogenic pathway. Gluconeogenesis requires carbons to form the glucose skeleton and energy. The carbons are derived from lactose, alanine and glycerol. Energy is provided by the metabolism of fatty acids released by adipose tissue. Adapted with permission from Baynes J, Dominiczak M 2005 Medical biochemistry, 2nd edn. Elsevier Mosby, Edinburgh.

The pathway for gluconeogenesis from lactate involves both mitochondrial and cytosolic enzymes, and substrates have to be shuttled between the two intracellular areas.

Lactate is converted to pyruvate by LDH in the cytosol. NADH is generated from NAD+ in this reaction, and this co-enzyme is required for a subsequent step in the pathway (see Fig. 3.16). Reversal of the PK reaction is achieved by pyruvate carboxylase, malate dehydrogenase and PEPCK. This requires the investment of two ATP equivalents. Thus, a net expenditure of 4 moles of ATP is required per mole of glucose produced from pyruvate.

1. Pyruvate enters the mitochondrion where it is converted into oxaloacetate by intramitochondrial pyruvate carboxylase. Oxaloacetate is reduced to malate by mitochondrial malate dehydrogenase for export from the mitochondrion (see below, Malate shuttle, Fig. 3.28). Within the cytosol, malate is then reoxidised to oxaloacetate by cytosolic malate dehydrogenase. Cytosolic oxaloacetate is converted to phosphoenolpyruvate (PEP) by the key gluconeogenic enzyme PEPCK.

   The high mitochondrial NADH/NAD+ ratio generated from a brisk rate of β-oxidation of fatty acid facilitates the reduction reaction (see below, Lipid metabolism).

2. Gluconeogenesis proceeds in the reversal of glycolytic reactions to the next irreversible step, where F-1,6-BP has to be reconverted to F6P. PFK-1 is bypassed by a hydrolysis reaction catalysed by FBPase, without the production of ATP.

3. In the penultimate step, equivalent to the second step in glycolysis, phosphoglucose isomerase is freely reversible and functions in both glycolytic and gluconeogenic pathways. Finally, the irreversible GK is bypassed by the hydrolysis of G6P to glucose by G6Pase, again without the production of ATP. In the liver, the free glucose generated by G6Pase is then released into the blood by facilitated diffusion via GLUT2.

Gluconeogenesis from protein

The carbon atoms of gluconeogenic amino acids released by protein breakdown can be converted into glucose. The main amino acids used in gluconeogenesis are alanine and gluta-mine, from muscle protein hydrolysis, but all amino acids that yield pyruvate, oxaloacetate, ketoglutarate or succinyl-CoA (glucagonic amino acids) can be used. Thus, if catabolism of an amino acid can yield either net pyruvate or net oxaloac-etate formation, then net glucose synthesis can occur from that amino acid.

Protein breakdown is facilitated by low insulin levels when glucose is scarce.

The liver extracts alanine from blood, removes its amino nitrogen by transamination (see Fig. 3.20 below) to re-form pyruvate, and converts this via the gluconeogenic pathway to glucose, which is returned to the blood (as for gluconeogenesis from lactate; see above). Some of the glutamine released from muscle is used for energy by the gastrointestinal tract. The rest is converted to glucose in the renal cortex.

The carbon skeletons of amino acids can also be converted via TCA cycle intermediates to oxaloacetate, and malate is then released into the cytosol (see above, Gluconeogenesis from lactate, and Fig. 3.20 below).

Gluconeogenesis from glycerol

During nutrient scarcity, when glucose is in short supply, triacylglycerols (TAGs from adipose tissue) are broken down (hydrolysed) via lipolysis (see below). The products of adipose tissue lipolysis are fatty acids and free glycerol. Glycerol mainly enters hepatic gluconeogenesis.

Most fatty acids in humans have straight chains with an even number of carbon atoms. Because acetyl-CoA and other intermediates of even-numbered fatty acid oxidation cannot be converted to oxaloacetate or any other intermediate of gluconeogenesis, it is impossible to synthesise glucose from such fatty acids. An exception to this general rule applies to:

- Fatty acids with methyl branches, e.g. phytanic acid, a breakdown product of chlorophyll
- Fatty acids with an odd number of carbon atoms – metabolism of these fatty acids yields the 3-carbon compound propionyl-CoA, which is a good, if minor, precursor for gluconeogenesis in humans
- Propionyl-CoA, which is also produced in the catabolism of the branched-chain amino acids valine and isoleucine, and in the conversion of cholesterol into bile acids.

Free glycerol liberated via activated lipolysis cannot be reutilised by adipose tissue to re-form TAG; it therefore passes into the blood and can then be converted back to glucose by the liver and kidney. The release of glycerol from the adipocyte is facilitated by a transport protein, one of the family of the **aquaporin membrane proteins** (**AQPs**). Of the AQPs, which transport glycerol as well as water, AQP7 (AQPap/7 in man) is expressed at high levels in adipose tissue.

In times of nutrient excess, blood glucose entering glycolysis is the source of glycerol 3-phosphate, which is esterified in the synthesis of adipose tissue TAG. Glucose/glycerol cycling can therefore contribute to glucose homeostasis in starvation.

Glycerol enters gluconeogenesis at the level of the triose phosphates, with phosphorylation by glycerol kinase to form glycerol 3-phosphate. This is converted by glycerol 3-phosphate dehydrogenase to dihydroxyacetone phosphate (DHAP) for entry into the gluconeogenic pathway (see Fig. 3.16).

Peroxisome proliferator-activated receptors in energy homeostasis

From the foregoing, it seems clear that metabolism of the main metabolic fuels, glucose and fatty acids, follow dynamic, inter-related pathways in order to maintain energy balance. It has been shown that the associated chronic

***

Clinical box 3.10 | **Peroxisome proliferator-activated receptors**

There is evidence to suggest that the hyperlipidaemia, central obesity, insulin resistance, atherosclerosis and hypertension associations comprising the metabolic syndrome (syndrome X) are linked to an interplay of genetic propensity, nutrition and environmental factors (see Ch. 16). In this context, recent research has focused on a family of nuclear receptors, the peroxisome proliferator-activated receptors (PPARs), which may have a major role in glucose and fatty acid metabolism in relation to energy balance in humans. The discovery that PPAR activity can be modulated by certain drugs has prompted an increase in research effort into such drugs.

PPARs are transcription factors activated by the binding of specific ligands, usually hormones, to them. Three isoforms, PPARα, PPARβ (also known as δ) and PPARγ, have been identified. More research is needed, but available data so far suggest that PPARγ promotes insulin sensitivity and lipid storage.

- PPARα is most abundant in liver cells and is also present in skeletal muscle, kidney and heart. It is actively involved in fatty acid catabolism in the peroxisomes, mitochondria and microsomes during fasting, when fatty acid oxidation and ketogenesis are strongly stimulated. PPARα also stimulates cellular uptake of fatty acids and lipoprotein synthesis.
- PPARα agonists are therefore hypolipidaemic. Fibrates, synthetic PPARα agonists, have been used for lipid lowering in the prevention and treatment of cardiovascular disease, for example.
- PPARγ is more active in the fed state, when glucose and chylomicrons in the circulation are abundant. It is lipogenic, stimulating the uptake of fatty acids and glucose and their conversion to TAG for storage in adipose tissue, and has hypoglycaemic properties.
- Decreased PPARγ expression in experimental animals may lead to increased leptin levels, which decreases food intake and weight gain (see also Ch. 16).
  - Thiazolidinediones (TZDs) are synthetic PPARγ agonists developed for the treatment of insulin resistance and type 2 diabetes. Increased PPARγ levels, however, can theoretically suppress leptin secretion, which could lead to weight gain.
- PPARβ is less well researched, but may be associated with colon cancer.
- PPARs have also been identified as anti-inflammatory transcription factors, so that they could be potential targets for the development of drugs in the treatment of the metabolic syndrome.

***

conditions hyperlipidaemia, insulin resistance, hypertension, obesity, atherosclerosis and coronary heart disease (which make up the metabolic syndrome, also known as syndrome X, and can lead to type 2 diabetes) are the result of the interplay between changes in gene expression, nutrition and lifestyle. There is evidence to suggest that a family of nuclear receptors, the **peroxisome proliferator-activated receptors** (**PPARs**), have a major role in the control of glucose and fatty acid metabolism in energy homeostasis (Clinical box 3.10).

Energy for gluconeogenesis

As noted above, gluconeogenesis is an energy-requiring process. In the liver, oxidation of the fatty acids concomitantly generated by adipose tissue lipolysis provides most of the ATP required for gluconeogenesis. Metabolic conditions under which the liver is required to synthesise glucose favours the increased availability of fatty acids in the blood. Therefore prolonged fasting, malnutrition or starvation, whether voluntary or involuntary, are all characterised by loss of both adipose stores and muscle mass. Ketone bodies, the water-soluble products of fatty acids via hepatic ketogenesis, are an alternative source of energy during starvation but are not used by the liver itself.

Cori and glucose–alanine cycles

The **Cori cycle** refers to the inter-organ carbon recycling that takes place during hepatic gluconeogenesis from lactate. Lactate is formed continuously by tissues that lack mitochondria or are anoxic. In addition, during prolonged fasting, skeletal muscle switches from the use of glucose to the use of lipid fuels as the primary oxidative fuel, and then it too releases lactate.

Alanine is a plentiful, simple amino acid. The **glucose–alanine cycle** moves carbon between tissues, like the Cori cycle, but also cycles nitrogen:

- Under conditions where muscle protein is being broken down (e.g. starvation), a proportion of available pyruvate is converted to alanine.
    - Glutamate + pyruvate ↔ α-ketoglutarate + alanine
- Alanine, released from muscle into the blood, is converted in the liver to pyruvate, with removal of the amino group by **transamination** (see Fig. 3.20 below) to form urea for urinary excretion.

This prevents a build-up in muscle of nitrogen in the form of ammonium ions, which are toxic. Pyruvate can then enter gluconeogenesis and glucose can be returned to muscle for use in its various pathways.

Both the Cori and glucose–alanine cycles depend on gluconeogenesis in the liver, followed by glucose output and delivery to extrahepatic tissues. They can only operate between liver and tissues that can release either lactate (Cori cycle) or alanine (alanine cycle) as the end-products of glucose metabolism.

The Cori and glucose–alanine cycles are important because they ensure continued provision of substrate for gluconeogenesis. It should be emphasised that the Cori cycle does not provide carbon for net synthesis of glucose. Glucose formed from lactate merely recycles the carbon to the glucose to replace that which was converted to lactate by extrahepatic tissues.

Gluconeogenesis from sugars

Humans consume considerable quantities of fructose as one of the component sugars of the disaccharide sucrose (table sugar), which is composed of glucose and fructose. In the liver:

- Fructose is phosphorylated by an ATP-linked kinase, fructose kinase, to yield fructose-1-phosphate
- A specific aldolase, fructose-1-phosphate aldolase, then cleaves fructose-1-phosphate to yield one molecule of DHAP and one of glyceraldehyde
- Glyceraldehyde is reduced to glycerol for entry into gluconeogenesis via glycerol kinase
- Two molecules of DHAP can either be converted:
    - into glucose via the gluconeogenic pathway, or
    - into pyruvate or lactate by glycolysis.

Gluconeogenesis also uses galactose as a precursor (Clinical box 3.11). Lactose (milk sugar) is a disaccharide composed of glucose and galactose. Galactose can be enzymically converted to glucose by galactose kinase, and is an important source of glucose in the human diet, particularly for infants.

Clinical box 3.11 **Some inborn errors of sugar metabolism**

Defects of fructose metabolism

Fructose is normally metabolised in the liver via glycolysis. Defects in fructose metabolism occur when essential enzymes in the metabolic pathway are deficient; such defects are inherited autosomal recessive conditions.

- Fructose kinase deficiency leads to unconverted fructose being excreted in the urine – fructosuria, which is a benign condition, but carries a risk of early cataract formation, owing to high blood fructose concentrations.
- In fructose intolerance, caused by fructose-1-phosphate aldolase deficiency, glycogenolysis and gluconeogenesis are decreased. This leads to hypoglycaemia; hepatomegaly and renal tubular damage may be associated features. This can be managed with a fructose- and sucrose-free diet. People with the genetic deficiency learn to avoid the discomfort caused by eating sweet food; children are very resistant to eating fruit and will not eat sweets. One advantage is that the incidence of dental caries is significantly reduced.
- In F-1,6-BPase deficiency, failure of gluconeogenesis gives rise to hypoglycaemia, ketosis and lactic acidosis. This condition can cause death in infancy. About 50% present during the first few days of life with severe metabolic derangement. Early intervention with frequent carbohydrate feeds is the treatment of choice.

Galactosaemia

Galactosaemia, the accumulation of galactose in the blood, is an inherited, autosomal recessive condition in which there is deficiency in the enzymes that convert galactose to glucose. There are two main types of enzyme deficiency, namely:

- Galactokinase deficiency: this enzyme catalyses the first step in the conversion of galactose to glucose, when galactose-1-phosphate (Gal-1-P) is formed. Galactokinase deficiency leads to an accumulation of galactose in the blood, but causes less severe tissue damage.
- Galactose-1-phosphate uridyl transferase deficiency: this mediates the conversion of galactose-1-phosphate (Gal-1-P) to G6P, a necessary step for the interconversion of galactose and glucose. Gal-1-P uridyl transferase deficiency leads to an accumulation of galactose and Gal-1-P in the blood.
    Galactokinase deficiency mainly causes cataracts. The transferase deficiency is much more severe. Feeding breast or cow's milk to infants with galactosaemia leads to vomiting and diarrhoea, failure to thrive, liver damage, cataracts and developmental delay. A galactose-free diet, as in formula milk containing sucrose instead of galactose, ameliorates the condition, but the child may still have poor growth, impaired speech and intellectual development, especially if diagnosis is delayed.

Regulation of gluconeogenesis

The pathways of hepatic glycolysis and gluconeogenesis are tightly controlled and counter-regulated by enzymes under the control of insulin and glucagon. This is to ensure that the glucose from gluconeogenesis is not used up by hepatic glycolysis but released into the bloodstream for glycaemic control. Glycogenolysis and gluconeogenic flux are suppressed by insulin and increased by glucagon, epinephrine and other insulin counter-regulatory hormones.

A lowering of blood glucose concentration lowers insulin secretion, but increases glucagon secretion. Thus, the insulin:glucagon ratio in the blood:

- Decreases with falling blood glucose, stimulating gluconeogenesis
- Increases with rising blood glucose, and the shift in the insulin:glucagon balance in diabetes leads to unopposed lipolysis (Clinical box 3.12).

Clinical box 3.12   Metabolic defects in diabetes mellitus

The principal hormone defect in diabetes mellitus is a lack of insulin secretion from the pancreatic β-cells in type 1 diabetes, and insulin resistance and inadequate insulin secretion to combat hyperglycaemia in type 2 diabetes. Glucagon levels are inappropriately elevated for the increase in blood glucose. Knowledge of the defects in fuel metabolism due to insulin deficiency and the relative excess of glucagon is important for understanding the clinical features of diabetes mellitus.

Type 1 diabetes
- Results from the destruction of pancreatic β-cells due to the production of autoantibodies to β-cells, possibly related to an autoimmune reaction triggered by viral infection.
- No insulin, or only a trace amount, is secreted.
- Often diagnosed in childhood, but can be at any age. Latent autoimmune diabetes of adults (LADA) may be unrecognised and can develop in people with type 2 diabetes.
- Patients are dependent on exogenous insulin for survival.

Type 2 diabetes
- Insulin secretion is abnormal, but some β-cells are still active, with an inadequate response to glucose stimulation, relative to the degree of insulin resistance, which seems to be the primary defect.
- Normally diagnosed in middle age, but can occur in the young, even children.
- About half of the people with type 2 diabetes are unaware that they have the condition.

Clinical features of diabetes mellitus
The clinical features of type 1 and type 2 diabetes are similar, but with important differences. Some patients with type 2 diabetes may have no symptoms so that they are undiagnosed until they present with complications or are identified by incidental urine testing or blood glucose measurement. This is why some countries, such as the UK, recommend screening for type 2 diabetes so that patients can be identified before complications occur. The main clinical feature is a persistently elevated blood glucose concentration, hyperglycaemia. Increased glycogenolysis and gluconeogenesis are the major causes of hyperglycaemia.

Thirst and polyuria
Insulin deficiency leads to the inability of insulin-responsive tissues (e.g. muscle and adipose tissue) to take up glucose because transport into cells is impaired. Glycolysis and lipogenesis are thus inhibited; blood glucose concentration rises (hyperglycaemia). In addition, owing to inadequate insulin secretion by pancreatic β-cells, the insulin:glucagon ratio decreases, driving gluconeogenesis and further increasing blood glucose concentration.

Hyperglycaemia in type 1 and many cases of type 2 diabetes causes the symptoms of:
- Excessive urination (polyuria) resulting from an osmotic diuresis caused by high blood glucose levels in blood and urine
- Thirst (polydipsia) due to loss of fluid.

Glucose tolerance curve in diabetes
In healthy subjects, blood glucose concentration rises sharply after a meal but falls to normal levels after 2 hours. In people with diabetes, this return to normal does not occur. Owing to insulin deficiency, glucose entry into cells is impaired, so that glycolysis cannot take place to maintain cellular energy. Hepatic glycogenolysis, lipolysis and gluconeogenesis are stimulated to generate increased levels of endogenous glucose. Together with impaired glucose transport, increasing amounts of glucose remain in the blood, leading to sustained hyperglycaemia after meals, characterised by the diabetic glucose tolerance curve. In the long term (after years), fasting hyperglycaemia occurs.

Metabolic ketoacidosis and ketonuria
The shift in the insulin:glucagon balance leads to unopposed lipolysis and fatty acid oxidation in the liver. This leads to the accumulation of excess acetyl-CoA, which stimulates the ketogenic pathway in the liver. When insulin secretion becomes inadequate to maintain anti-lipolysis in the fat stores, or under acute metabolic stress, the rising levels of ketone bodies (e.g. β-hydroxybutyrate and acetoacetate) lower blood pH and cause life-threatening ketoacidosis. Ketonuria develops if renal function remains normal. Ketoacidosis is more common in type 1 diabetes, either at presentation or when insulin is omitted. Although less common in type 2 diabetes, metabolic acidosis can develop during stress, e.g. myocardial infarction.

Microvascular and macrovascular disease
Increased fat breakdown results in raised plasma lipoprotein concentration, either low-density lipoproteins (LDLs) or very-low-density lipoproteins (VLDLs), which eventually leads to atheroma formation and subsequent arterial narrowing. In diabetes with poor glycaemic control, the resultant ischaemic organ damage leads to the long-term vascular complications of diabetes, depending on the size and site of the arteries affected:
- Macrovascular disease (larger arteries) gives rise to peripheral vascular disease and a high risk of coronary arterial disease. Renal artery stenosis may lead to hypertension.
- Microvascular disease (arterioles, capillaries): damage to the glomerular basement membrane leads to renal damage and results in hypertension. In diabetic retinopathy, microaneurysms and haemorrhages lead to leaking blood vessels and new vessel formation; macula oedema and degeneration, and ischaemia can lead to visual impairment and eventual blindness. Restricted blood supply to peripheral nerves may be a factor in peripheral neuropathy.

Clinical features resulting from glycated protein
Glucose entry into some tissues is independent of insulin (e.g. red blood cells, lens). For some other tissues (e.g. liver, renal, peripheral nerves and brain), glucose entry can be insulin independent or dependent. The persistent, very high intracellular glucose level leads to non-enzymic attachment of glucose to proteins (protein glycation, the Maillard reaction). Protein structures become altered to form advanced glycation end-products (AGE). Typical sites of glycated protein are in:
- Lens, leading to opacities, the formation of cataracts and impaired vision
- Renal glomeruli, leading to albuminuria, glomerulosclerosis and eventually renal failure
- Vessels supplying peripheral nerves, a further contribution to peripheral neuropathy.

The glycated protein in haemoglobin is the basis for the measurement of glycosylated haemoglobin (HbA_{1c}), which gives a guide to glycaemic control over the previous 6 weeks in both type 1 and type 2 diabetes.

The glycolysis/gluconeogenesis pathways are antagonistic, so if they operated simultaneously at the same rate, there would be no net production of glucose for export from the liver. This situation would create a 'futile cycle' so called because the expended ATP is 'wasted'. However, normally one pathway prevails over the other.

Gluconeogenesis is excessive in poorly-controlled diabetes mellitus because of an increased supply of gluconeogenic precursors (glycerol, amino acids) and fatty acids to the liver, and an increased glucagon/insulin ratio.

Regulation of gluconeogenesis can occur both by short-term effects on enzyme activities and at the gene level, influencing the concentration of enzyme proteins. Gluconeogenesis is stimulated by increasing gene expression of G6Pase and PEPCK. A rise in glucagon leads to activation of transcriptional activators (e.g. PGC-1α, which activates PPARα) allowing increased gene expression. cAMP also activates a transcription factor FoxO (allowing its nuclear localisation) to increase G6Pase expression, whereas insulin inactivates FoxO.

AMINO ACID METABOLISM

In contrast to carbohydrates and fats, amino acids are not stored in designated sites in the human body. Although protein is not a major metabolic fuel under normal conditions, amino acids have key roles in human metabolism.

- Amino acids are a source of metabolic energy – in starvation, muscle protein can be broken down to keto acids for gluconeogenesis to maintain blood glucose concentration
- The carbon skeletons of amino acids are the building blocks for the biosynthesis of all proteins and other important biomolecules (e.g. nucleotides) essential for cell growth, and haem
- The carbon skeletons of amino acids are precursors of neurotransmitters, hormones and other important biomolecules (e.g. thyroxine, epinephrine, 5-hydroxytryptamine and melanin)
- Some amino acids are metabolised to form precursors of lipids and ketone bodies (see below, Lipogenesis)
- The carbon atoms of some amino acids may be used to produce energy via oxidative metabolism in the later stages of glycolysis and in the TCA cycle.

METABOLIC CLASSES OF AMINO ACIDS
(Clinical box 3.13)

Twenty amino acids are needed for human protein synthesis (Fig. 3.17):

- Non-essential amino acids can be endogenously synthesised, using the carbon skeletons from metabolism
- Essential amino acids cannot be endogenously synthesised. There are 10 of these amino acids, which have to be present in the diet (see Chs 2 and 16).

Another way of classifying amino acids depends on their ability to be converted to glucose or lipids. Because the body does not have protein stores, amino acid metabolism is dynamic. The carbon skeletons of amino acids are used in central metabolic pathways for energy production in oxidative metabolism. Any excess (and amino acids during starvation) is converted in one of two ways:

- Gluconeogenic amino acids are converted by gluconeogenesis to glucose, which may be released into the blood or stored as glycogen:
  - **Alanine**, cysteine, glycine, serine and threonine degrade to form pyruvate
  - Asparagine and aspartate degrade to form oxaloacetate
  - **Glutamine**, glutamate, histidine and proline degrade to form α-ketoglutarate
  - Isoleucine, methionine and valine degrade to form succinyl-CoA
- Ketogenic amino acids are oxidised to acetyl-CoA or acetoacetate, and then converted to precursors of ketone bodies and lipids (see below, Lipogenesis):
  - Leucine and lysine are exclusively ketogenic
  - Isoleucine, phenylalanine, tryptophan, tryosine and threonine can be ketogenic or glucogenic.

ABSORPTION OF AMINO ACIDS

After a meal, dietary protein is hydrolysed to:

- Peptides (containing two or three amino acid residues)
- Free amino acids.

The peptides are transported into intestinal epithelial cells (enterocytes) by specific membrane transporters and then rapidly hydrolysed to free amino acids within the cells (see Ch. 15). The uptake of free amino acids from the gut is analogous to the uptake of glucose. It is worth noting that di- and tri-peptides are more rapidly absorbed than the amino acids themselves.

An SLC protein (SLC15A1), also known as PepT1, localised in the brush border membrane of intestinal epithelium facilitates di- and tri-peptide transport into the enterocytes along with H^+ ions where they are then hydrolysed further into amino acids.

Clinical box 3.13   **Inborn errors of amino acid metabolism**

Inborn errors of amino acid metabolism can be due to:
- Enzyme defects in the urea cycle
- Deficiencies in the enzymes involved in the metabolism of the carbon skeletons of various amino acids
- Inherited autosomal recessive disorders (most are this).

Phenylketonuria (PKU)
- Deficiency of phenylalanine hydroxylase, an enzyme required for tyrosine synthesis
- Untreated individuals excrete phenylpyruvate and phenylacetate in the urine, and develop brain damage, mental retardation and epilepsy
- The rate of incidence of around 1 in 20000 births in the UK and USA is one of the reasons for screening infants soon after birth
- Dietary control by restricting phenylalanine, and giving tyrosine supplementation, is successful, but there is generally some limitation of intellectual development.

Alkaptonuria (also known as black urine disease)
- Deficiency of **homogentisic acid oxidase**. Homogentisic acid is an intermediate metabolite in the breakdown of phenylalanine and tyrosine
- Very rare condition, occurring in about 1:1000000 births
- Homogentisic acid accumulates and is excreted in the urine, which turns a black-brown colour on standing.

- Deposition of the pigment in cartilage and other tissues causes distinctive (sometimes visible) brown discoloration (ochronosis), and tissue damage leading to arthritis.

Maple syrup urine disease
- Rare condition (1 in 300000 births in the USA)
- Related to metabolism of branched-chain amino acids, leucine, valine and isoleucine
- After transamination, the resulting keto acid is normally decarboxylated with a **keto acid decarboxylase**. A defect in this enzyme results in an accumulation of keto acids, giving a characteristic 'maple syrup' smell to the urine.
- Clinically, the infant suffers fits, neonatal acidosis and severe brain damage, leading to early death. There is no effective treatment.

Albinism
Albinism is a benign condition.
- Deficiency of tyrosinase, an enzyme catalysing the hydroxylation of tyrosine to dihydroxyphenylalanine (DOPA), a precursor of the skin pigment melanin
- Results in amelanosis: a lack of colour in the skin, hair and irises (pinkish), and a risk of damage by sunlight
- Although DOPA is an intermediate in the synthesis of neurotransmitters, there are no neurological defects.

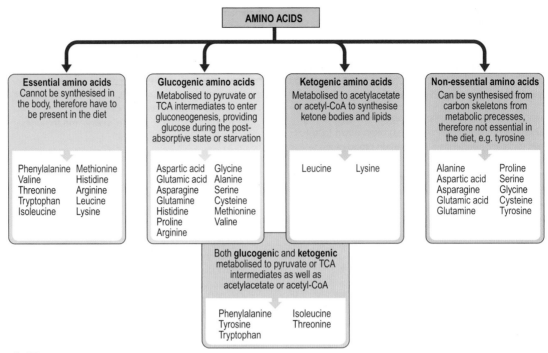

Fig. 3.17 **Metabolic classes of amino acids.**

Not all amino acids are released from the enterocytes into the portal vein blood.

- Dietary glutamine, derived from glutamic acid, is the major fuel of the intestine and is oxidised by enterocytes in preference to glucose to provide the energy needed for the intestinal absorption of digestion products
- Dietary aspartate and glutamate are also used in enterocyte metabolism.

As aspartate, glutamate and glutamine metabolism produce alanine, much more alanine appears in the portal vein blood after feeding than was originally present in the ingested protein. Thus, intestinally absorbed glucose is spared for the rest of the body and the alanine produced can be converted to glucose (see above, Gluconeogenesis).

NITROGEN IN AMINO ACID METABOLISM

The nitrogen component, the α-amino group of amino acids, has to be removed before the carbon skeleton can be metabolised. This is achieved by:

- Transamination (Fig. 3.18) – the transfer of the amino group to a corresponding α-keto acid acceptor, or
- Deamination, the oxidative removal of the amino group to give oxo acids, releasing ammonia (NH_3).

Transamination

Transamination is a reversible reaction catalysed by enzymes known as **aminotransferases (transaminases)** (Clinical boxes 3.14 and 3.15).

The process of transamination merely removes nitrogen in the form of an amino group from the amino acid donor to a suitable corresponding α-oxo acid acceptor. Conversely, amino groups can be added to the appropriate carbon skeleton to synthesise non-essential amino acids.

This takes place through the transamination of the α-keto acid corresponding to that amino acid.

Aminotransferases are specific for particular amino acids, but most of them will transfer amino groups:

- Most commonly to 2-oxoglutarate (α-ketoglutarate) to form glutamate
- To a lesser extent to oxaloacetate to give aspartate.

In some skeletal muscle, pyruvate can act as an amino acceptor to form alanine, which is transported to the liver where it may either be used for protein synthesis or undergo transamination in the opposite direction to release NH_3 that enters the urea cycle. The liberated pyruvate then participates in gluconeogenesis (glucose–alanine cycle, see above).

Glutamine is synthesised from malate from the TCA cycle, when malate accepts amino nitrogen from skeletal muscle breakdown. Alanine and glutamine thus transport amino groups from the tissues to the liver.

Amino acid release by skeletal muscle in the post-absorptive state

In the post-absorptive state, two amino acids – alanine and glutamine – are released from skeletal muscle in large amounts (over 50% of the amino acid outflow). This does not reflect their relative concentration in muscle protein; rather, that other amino acid residues present in muscle protein are metabolised to give intermediates, pyruvate and 2-oxoglutarate, which accept amino groups to yield alanine and glutamine, respectively (see Fig. 3.20).

Branched-chain amino acids are a major source of nitrogen for the production of alanine and glutamine in muscle. They are oxidised within the muscles for energy, and the nitrogen is removed and trapped for disposal by the conversion of pyruvate to alanine. The alanine is released into the blood via amino acid membrane transporters.

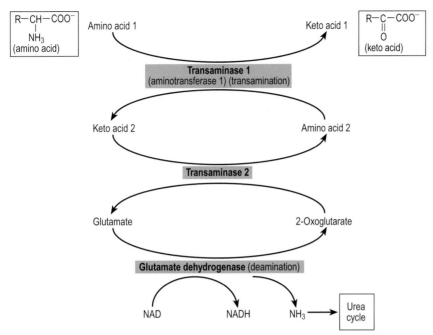

Fig. 3.18 **Conversion of surplus amino groups to ammonia (NH₃).**

Plasma transaminase levels rise when there is liver cell damage, allowing the enzymes to leak into the blood.

- Aspartate aminotransferase (AST) is a mitochondrial enzyme
- Alanine transaminase (ALT) is a cytosolic enzyme.

These enzymes are used as clinical markers of liver cell damage. Their serum levels are raised in various forms of cellular liver disease.

AST is also present in heart and skeletal muscle, kidney and brain cells, so high levels in blood plasma may also be seen in muscle damage, e.g. myocardial infarction or rhabdomyolysis (muscle injury).

Transamination needs an essential cofactor, pyridoxal phosphate, derived from vitamin B_6 (pyridoxine). Dietary vitamin B_6 deficiency is rare, but some drugs interact with pyridoxal phosphate to cause vitamin B_6 deficiency. Certain antituberculosis drugs (e.g. isoniazid) are examples:

- Vitamin B_6 deficiency characteristically causes peripheral neuropathy; there may also be anaemia and dermatitis
- When vitamin B_6 deficiency causes any serious problems for amino acid metabolism, vitamin B_6 supplementation reverses the unwanted effects.

Branched-chain α-keto acids produced from the branched-chain amino acids by transamination are partially released into the blood. These are taken up by the liver, which synthesises:

- Glucose from the keto acid of valine
- Ketone bodies from the keto acid of leucine
- Both glucose and ketone bodies from the keto acid of isoleucine.

Deamination

The α-amino group is finally removed from an amino acid molecule through deamination, although to a lesser extent than occurs with transamination. Deamination is the oxidative removal of the amino group from the amino acid molecule by amino acid oxidases. This activity results in the release of keto acids and NH_3. Glutamate (from hydrolysis of glutamine), the commonest intermediate in nitrogen removal, is oxidatively deaminated by glutamate dehydrogenase to form 2-oxoglutarate and ammonia (NH_3) (see Fig. 3.18). The NH_3 enters the urea cycle in the liver.

Glutamine in acid–base homeostasis

Maintaining blood pH at a constant 7.4 is a coordinated activity by the liver, kidneys and lungs (see Ch. 14). One of the mechanisms for acid–base homeostasis uses the products of amino acid breakdown. In an alternative pathway to the ones in liver and skeletal muscle, glutamine is hydrolysed by glutaminase to glutamate and ammonium ion (NH_4^+) in the proximal renal tubules (Information box 3.9)

Glutamate is subsequently oxidised to 2-oxaloglutarate and more NH_4^+ is generated. NH_4^+ in these two steps is positively charged and water soluble. Some NH_4^+ is secreted into the tubular lumen, the rest is diverted to the liver, where one molecule of NH_4^+ and one of bicarbonate (HCO_3^-) combine to form carbamoyl phosphate, which starts off the urea cycle (see below and Fig. 3.19).

In many forms of acidosis, glutaminase is upregulated so that more NH_4^+ appears. This excess NH_4^+ is diverted from the liver where it would normally be converted to urea. Urine has a minimum pH of 4.5 to be compatible with life. It is more acid than blood (pH 7.4), so a pH gradient is established between urine and blood. At the minimum urine pH of 4.5, the pH gradient is markedly increased, so increasing the NH_4^+ gradient between urine and blood. Urinary NH_4^+ excretion increases. In diabetic ketoacidosis, for example, urinary NH_4^+ excretion can increase from 50 mmol/24 h to 200–500 mmol/24 h (up to 10-fold).

This urinary excretion of NH_4^+ deprives the liver of the opportunity to consume HCO_3^- in urea synthesis. Thus, the HCO_3^- derived from the peripheral oxidation of amino acid skeletons (see above) remains unconsumed, and tends to counteract the metabolic acidosis.

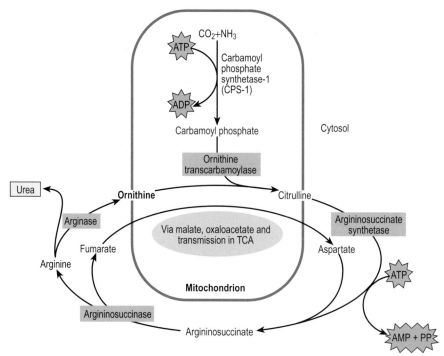

Fig. 3.19 **The urea cycle.**

The HCO_3^- consumed in the liver in this way deals with the major quantity of HCO_3^- derived from oxidation of amino acid carbon skeletons, thus regulating acid–base status.

Ammonia

The waste product of the deamination process is NH_3, which is associated with toxicity (Clinical box 3.16). NH_3 is usually rapidly converted to urea via the urea cycle.

Urea cycle (Clinical box 3.16)

Urea synthesis takes place in the liver, involving both mitochondrial and cytosolic reactions. A key compound in the urea cycle (Fig. 3.19) is ornithine, which is derived from the dietary and endogenously derived amino acid arginine. Arginine is split by the enzyme arginase to yield ornithine and urea.

Clinical box 3.16 | **Urea cycle defects**

A number of enzyme defects in the urea cycle have been identified. Apart from ornithine transcarbamoylase deficiency, which has an X-linked dominant inheritance, they are autosomal recessive.

Carbamoyl phosphate synthetase (CPS-1) deficiency
- The most severe form of urea cycle defect (UCD)
- Symptoms (vomiting, poor feeding, convulsions, ataxia, coma) are due to the high levels of NH_3 (hyperammonaemia), and begin immediately after birth when the foetal and maternal circulations are separated
- Invariably fatal within a few days if undiagnosed and untreated.

Deficiency in other enzymes of the urea cycle
- Ornithine transcarbamylase, argininosuccinate synthetase, argininosuccinase, arginase
- Give rise to varying degrees of hyperammonaemia.

Treatment of urea cycle defects
- Restriction of dietary protein
- Removal of NH_3 (e.g. antibiotics to eliminate NH_3-producing intestinal bacteria, drugs such as benzoate and phenylacetate to promote the excretion of NH_3 nitrogen in faeces).
- Replacement of missing urea cycle intermediates by intravenous infusion.

The urea cycle generates new urea molecules from recycled ornithine. Urea is excreted; all other intermediates in the urea cycle are recycled.

- Carbamoyl phosphate is synthesised from NH_3, CO_2 and ATP in the hepatic mitochondria, catalysed by carbamoyl phosphate synthetase 1 (CPS-1)
- Cytosolic ornithine is transported to the mitochondrion where it condenses with carbamoyl phosphate to form citrulline, catalysed by ornithine transcarbamoylase
- Citrulline diffuses into the cytosol where it condenses with aspartate to form argininosuccinate, catalysed by argininosuccinate synthetase and requiring ATP
- Argininosuccinate is split into arginine and fumarate by argininosuccinase
- Arginine is split by arginase to give urea, regenerating ornithine, which re-enters the urea cycle
- Aspartate, re-used for condensation with citrulline, is regenerated from fumarate.

The urea diffuses into the blood to be transported to the kidneys for excretion in urine. Note that ornithine and citrulline are amino acids that are not part of the set of 20 amino acids used for protein synthesis.

The urea cycle intersects with the TCA cycle at the point where fumarate branches off in the conversion of argininosuccinate to arginine. Some fumarate is converted to malate by the enzyme fumarase, then to oxaloacetate through the action of malate dehydrogenase. Oxaloacetate is then transaminated to aspartate by AST (see Fig. 3.19).

Regulation of the urea cycle

In the short term, the urea cycle is rate limited by the allosteric activator for mitochondrial CPS-1 (carbomyl phosphate synthetase 1), *N*-acetylglutamate. The function of the urea cycle is to:

- remove surplus nitrogen
- to consume bicarbonate generated in peripheral tissues (see above).

The urea cycle is controlled through regulation of the activity of its various enzymes through gene expression. For example, glucagon and glucocorticoids interact with various receptors to form complexes that interact with the promoter region of the CPS-1 gene (Clinical box 3.16). The enzyme CPS-1 concentration:

- Rises on high-protein diets and during starvation when proteins are degraded to provide carbon skeletons for energy, thereby increasing the amount of surplus nitrogen to be excreted
- Declines with more normal, balanced diets.

Nitrogen balance

The continuous turnover of amino acids, proteins and nucleic acids in healthy human beings underpins the concept of nitrogen balance, in which dietary intake and excretion of nitrogen are approximately equal (see Ch. 16).

- Positive nitrogen balance takes place when the body receives more nitrogen than it excretes, as in healing wounds, growth and pregnancy
- Negative nitrogen balance occurs in protein malnutrition, severe exercise or starvation, when muscle protein is degraded to carbon skeletons for gluconeogenesis, so that more nitrogen is lost than is taken in.

AMINO ACIDS IN GLUCONEOGENESIS

Figure 3.20 sets out the flux of key amino acids in gluconeogenesis. Nearly all the carbons can be converted to intermediates for entry into:

- Glucogenesis or ketogenesis
- The TCA cycle
- Lipogenesis.

Information box 3.10 **Fate of amino acids in the liver**

In the well-fed state
- Carbon skeletons of excess amino acids are eventually used for ATP production
- Glucogenic amino acids are converted to glucose, which may be stored as glycogen
- Ketogenic amino acids are converted to lipids and transported to adipose tissue, ultimately to be stored as fat (see below).

In the fasting state
- Incoming amino acids are used for glucose production.

There are complex inter-relationships between amino acid, glucose and lipid metabolism. Most amino acid nitrogen ends up in the liver (see Information box 3.10), having either been generated there or reached there from muscle or from intestinal cells, and is converted to urea for excretion by the kidneys in urine.

ESSENTIAL AMINO ACIDS (See also Clinical box 3.17)

Some individual amino acids must be conserved for protein synthesis because, apart from collagen, all 20 of those that form proteins must be present together for protein synthesis. This applies particularly to the essential amino acids, which cannot be synthesised fast enough for requirements in the body and must be obtained from food (see Fig. 3.17 and Ch. 16).

The hepatic extraction of the branched-chain amino acids that cannot be synthesised by humans is less than the extraction of the other amino acids. Furthermore, although used for hepatic protein synthesis, these essential amino acids are not degraded to any great extent by the liver, and so they are found in higher concentrations in peripheral blood

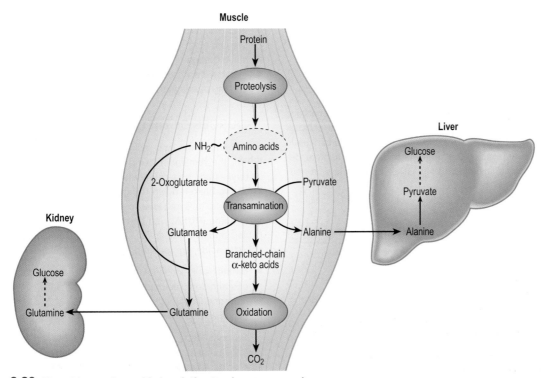

Fig. 3.20 **Flux of key amino acids in relation to gluconeogenesis.**

Although the mechanism is not well understood, NH_3 in the blood diffuses into cells and crosses the blood–brain barrier and is associated with encephalopathy (a brain disorder). Even low concentrations are neurotoxic. The uptake of NH_3 by the brain causes glutamate to be converted to glutamine, resulting in glutamate deficiency.

Glutamate is an important excitatory neurotransmitter and the encephalopathy is associated with glutamate deficiency. Decreased levels of γ-aminobutyric acid (GABA), which is synthesised from glutamate, also result. GABA is an important inhibitory neurotransmitter (see Chs 4 and 8).

Enzyme defects in infants leading to excessive accumulation of NH_3 result in life-threatening cerebral oedema requiring haemodialysis.

than other amino acids. Whereas they typically constitute about 15–20% of dietary protein, valine, leucine and isoleucine represent at least 70% of the total amino acids entering the general circulation after a meal.

Valine, leucine and isoleucine are, therefore, taken up by skeletal muscle to a greater extent than the other amino acids, accounting for 60–80% of the total amino acid uptake by muscle. Branched-chain amino acids that are not used for protein synthesis can be oxidised in the muscles to provide energy.

The use of the branched-chain amino acids preferentially by muscle underlies their inclusion in parenteral feeding solutions for patients in situations of negative nitrogen balance (e.g. stress, trauma, burns), where there is excessive protein breakdown (see Ch. 16).

AMINO ACIDS AND SIGNALLING MOLECULES

Certain derivatives of amino acids are precursors for neurotransmitters and hormones. Some amino acids, notably glutamate and glycine, act directly as neurotransmitters. Others undergo metabolism to form neurotransmitters or hormones.

Amino acids as neurotransmitters
(Clinical boxes 3.17 **and** 3.18)

Glutamate is an excitatory transmitter in the central nervous system (CNS), transported into neurons and glial cells. γ-Aminobutyric acid (GABA), the major inhibitory transmitter in the brain, is synthesised from glutamate by glutamate decarboxylase (Clinical box 3.18). Glycine also acts as a neurotransmitter in the spinal cord.

The Chinese restaurant syndrome, also known as Kwok's Quease, is a syndrome that occurs in some individuals after a meal. Only a very few individuals are susceptible. Symptoms include:
- Sudden onset of temporary headache, sweating and nausea after a meal in a Chinese restaurant.
- Attributed to the high content of monosodium glutamate (MSG) used in Chinese cuisine, and may be due to the action of glutamate or its derivative, GABA, on the CNS.
- No permanent damage has been demonstrated, although it can trigger bronchospasm in people with severe asthma.

Amino acids as precursors of neurotransmitters and hormones

The hormones epinephrine and norepinephrine (adrenaline and noradrenaline) are derived from the amino acid tyrosine. Their mode of action is described in Chapter 4.

- **Dopamine** is an intermediate metabolite in the synthesis of epinephrine and norepinephrine, and is also a neurotransmitter. It acts on the basal ganglia to control voluntary movement, and its deficiency is associated with the tremor and difficulties in the initiation and control of movement in Parkinson disease.
- **Tyrosine** is also a precursor of thyroid hormones (see Ch. 10).
- **Serotonin** (5-hydroxytryptamine) is derived from the amino acid tryptophan and affects mood (see Ch. 8).

LIPID METABOLISM (Clinical box 3.19)

Apart from cells that contain few mitochondria, such as red cells and neural cells, which can use only glucose as metabolic fuel, lipids are the major and immediate source of energy in liver, muscle, kidney and other tissues. The term 'lipids' includes triacylglycerols (TAGs; also known as triglycerides), phospholipids and glycolipids.

TAG is constructed from fatty acids and glycerol (a 3-carbon sugar alcohol) by a process of 'esterification'. Non-esterified fats are known as 'free' fatty acids (FFA) and are the major fuel for metabolism. They are an immediate source of energy, and their importance as metabolic fuels arises because their oxidation yields much more ATP than the oxidation of either carbohydrate or protein (see below).

Lipids also contribute to the construction of cell membranes and intracellular membranes. Therefore, in addition to their functions as energy substrate, lipids are important for:

- maintenance of the integrity of lung alveoli (surfactant, see Ch. 13)
- solubilisation of non-polar substances in body fluids
- metabolic and cellular regulation (e.g. steroid hormones and the prostaglandins).

SOURCES OF FATTY ACIDS

In humans, most fatty acids are supplied as dietary TAG (90%), the remainder being made up of cholesterol, cholesteryl esters, non-esterified fatty acids and phospholipids. TAGs are broken down to fatty acids via lipolysis. Humans are unable to synthesise or desaturate **polyunsaturated fatty acids** (PUFA) with particular complex structures (e.g. linoleic and linolenic acids). These PUFAs, known as essential fatty acids, are required for specific functions, including:

- synthesis of eicosanoids (biologically active derivatives of arachidonic acid, found in cell membranes, with hormone-like functions)
- acting as second messengers (diacylglycerol).

Essential fatty acids such as n-3PUFA and n-6PUFA, must be present in the diet or synthesised from other dietary fatty acids. They can be obtained from dietary plant or fish oils (see Ch. 16).

Clinical box 3.19   Disorders of lipoprotein metabolism – dyslipidaemias

Disturbances of lipoprotein metabolism result in abnormalities in plasma lipoprotein concentrations, known as dyslipidaemias. Dyslipidaemias are associated with defects in either the fuel transport or overflow pathways, and in most cases will increase the risk for cardiovascular disease and atheroma. Clinical clues include family history of heart disease or acute pancreatitis, and physical signs in severe cases include xanthomata, lipaemia retinalis (specific for high VLDL) and retinal vein thrombosis. Available treatments include dietary control of fat intake, lipid-lowering diets, increased dietary fruit and vegetable content, exercise and lipid-lowering drugs (see Ch. 16).

Primary dyslipidaemia may be classified according to genetic/functional defects of lipoprotein metabolism.

Disorders of chylomicron and VLDL metabolism

Mechanisms for disordered chylomicron and VLDL metabolism are poorly understood.

- Polygenic hypertriglyceridaemia is a polygenic disorder possibly associated with a moderately elevated plasma VLDL concentration, with LPL or apoC deficiency, and is rare.
- Lipoprotein lipase (LPL) deficiency and apoC-II deficiency are rare conditions characterised clinically by high TAG levels and plasma chylomicrons persisting in the fasting state. The TAG in chylomicrons cannot be metabolised because either the LPL enzyme is absent, impairing TAG hydrolysis, or LPL cannot be activated owing to the absence of apoC-II.

Disorders of LDL metabolism – hypercholesterolaemia

- Heterozygous familial hypercholesterolaemia is the commonest disorder of LDL metabolism, more common is some racial groups (e.g. South Africans, Finns). It is an autosomal dominant, monogenic disorder, where there is defective gene coding for apoB/E receptor. Impaired apoB/E receptor production affects both fuel transport and overflow pathways, giving impaired LDL clearance.
- Homozygous familial hypercholesterolaemia is extremely rare, characterised by the absence of hepatic apoB/E receptors. Plasma LDL concentration is greatly elevated, and patients die in late childhood or adolescence from ischaemic heart disease. Possible treatments are LDL apheresis to remove LDL from the circulation or liver transplant. Research into gene therapy is ongoing.

- Mutations in apoB-100 is a single gene disorder, affecting LDL binding to hepatic clearance receptors, and results in hypercholesterolaemia. The condition clinically resembles heterozygous familial hypercholesterolaemia, but is less common.
- Polygenic hypercholesterolaemia is the most common type of hypercholesterolaemia that is not one of the monogenetic disorders. The nature of this condition is not well understood.
- Familial dysbetalipidaemia is a rare condition characterised by mutation of apoE gene to apoE isoforms (E2) that have a low affinity for apoB/E receptor, resulting in lipoprotein remnants not being taken into hepatocytes, with consequent cholesterol and TAG accumulation in blood.

Combined hyperlipidaemia–hypercholesterolaemia and hypertriglyceridaemia

Familial combined hyperlipidaemia is the commonest dyslipidaemia in which there is both hypercholesterolaemia and hypertriglyceridaemia, thought to be associated with an overproduction of apoB-100, leading to VLDL overproduction and consequent LDL overload. The high plasma concentration of LDL suppresses HDL synthesis. Both fuel transport and overflow pathways are overloaded. The inheritance is autosomal dominant.

Secondary hyperlipidaemia

Hyperlipidaemia can be associated with diabetes, hypothyroidism and liver disease (particularly alcohol related). Treatment of the underlying condition is essential.

In type 2 diabetes and metabolic syndrome, excess VLDL synthesis overloads the fuel transport pathway with increased remnant concentration which is accompanied by lowered HDL concentration. LDL concentration may be normal as the overload pathway is not compromised.

Disorders of HDL metabolism – Tangier disease

The role of HDL in cholesterol transport was elucidated from the study of the extremely rare dyslipidaemia, Tangier disease. Patients have almost no circulating HDL, with extrahepatic deposition of cholesteryl esters leading to corneal opacities and an orange discoloration of the tonsils, spleen and intestinal mucosa. Mutation in the CERP (also known as *ABC1*) gene prevents cellular cholesterol ester efflux. Plasma TAG and cholesterol concentrations are normal.

Dietary fatty acids

Dietary fats are digested by pancreatic enzymes (lipases) in the intestine to form free fatty acids, monoacylglycerols and glycerol, which are absorbed into the enterocytes. The enterocyte re-esterifies the free fatty acids and monoacylglycerols to synthesise TAG. **Chylomicrons** are then assembled from the TAG, together with cholesterol, apolipoproteins and phospholipids (see later).

Endogenously synthesised fatty acids

Humans can synthesise fatty acids from intermediates derived from the breakdown of sugars (glucose, fructose), some amino acids and other fatty acids. In general, the de novo synthesis pathway is primarily used under conditions of excess carbohydrate intake. Carbohydrate is converted to fatty acids in the liver and stored as TAG in adipose tissue.

- Fatty acids used for hepatic TAG synthesis are released (see storage of lipids, below).
- In adipose tissue, lipoprotein-derived fatty acids are used almost exclusively for TAG synthesis (for storage). These are predominantly derived from dietary TAGs in circulating chylomicrons (Fig. 3.21).
- The liver is the major site of fatty acid synthesis.

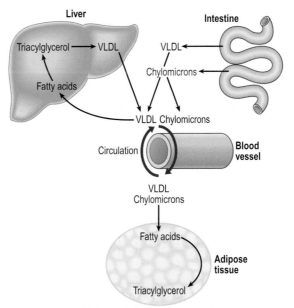

Fig. 3.21 **Lipid homeostasis in the fed state.** VLDL, very-low-density lipoprotein.

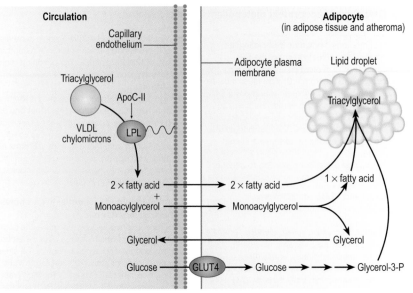

Fig. 3.22 **Pathway of triacylglycerol uptake and storage by adipose tissue.** LPL, lipoprotein lipase; VLDL, very-low-density lipoprotein; ApoC-II, apolipoprotein CII.

STORAGE OF LIPIDS

Fat metabolism is controlled primarily by the rate of stored TAG breakdown (**lipolysis**) although there is also local generation of fatty acids from circulating lipoproteins by the enzyme **lipoprotein lipase** (**LPL**) (Fig. 3.22).

The fatty acids used for adipose tissue TAG synthesis are derived from TAG contained in chylomicrons and very-low-density lipoproteins (VLDLs; see below), acted upon by LPL. Adipose tissue LPL is found attached to the basement membrane glycoproteins of capillary endothelial cells.

- LPL hydrolyses fatty acids from the 1 and/or 3 position of triacylglycerols and diacylglycerols present in VLDLs and chylomicrons.
- Apolipoprotein C-II must be present within the lipid particles to activate LPL. A deficiency in apolipoprotein C-II leads to increased plasma TAG levels (see below).
- Adipocyte LPL generates fatty acids locally for direct uptake and use by the adipocyte, without entering the general circulation.
- A rise in plasma insulin stimulates adipocyte LPL to release fatty acids from chylomicrons and VLDLs.

FATTY ACIDS

Lipids contain a mixture of fatty acids of different chain length, degree of saturation and branching. In contrast to carbohydrates, which are converted to water-soluble glucose, lipid fuels have to be transported by processes that are specific for varying chain lengths. In humans, lipids are catabolised only through oxidative processes, which take place primarily in the mitochondria and peroxisomes (see below).

Non-esterified (or free) fatty acids (FFA) may be:

- derived from dietary fats
- endogenously synthesised de novo when there is energy excess (see below).

FFAs are not water soluble. Their soap-like detergent effect would dissolve lipid cellular and intracellular membranes. This is avoided as fatty acids are transported:

- bound to albumin, in the blood

- esterified as TAG for transport between tissues and organs, and for storage
- in lipoproteins (TAGs are highly hydrophobic, i.e. insoluble in water; see below).

Protein-bound fatty acids

In plasma, fatty acids are bound to albumin for delivery to tissues. Each albumin molecule can bind up to eight fatty acid molecules and carry them to cells for metabolism. The molecular mechanism of fatty acid uptake into cells is controversial, but may be achieved via diffusion across the plasma membrane according to concentration differences and/or via **fatty acid transport proteins** (**FATP**).

Two major classes of FATPs have been described: CD36 (GP-IV, membrane glycoprotein IV) and FATPs 1–6.

- Mice lacking CD36 exhibit decreased FA uptake in muscle (cardiac and skeletal) and adipose tissue
- FATP1 knockout mice are resistant to lipid-induced insulin resistance in muscle since uptake of fatty acids into muscle (and excess accumulation of lipid in muscle, which causes insulin resistance) is impaired.

Long-chain fatty acids (<C12) are bound to **fatty acid binding proteins** (**FABPs**) to diffuse down a concentration gradient into cells, in proportion to their concentrations inside and outside the cells. To maintain the concentration gradient, fatty acids within cells are sequestered by tissue-specific FABPs (also known as lipid-binding proteins, LBPs). The presence of fatty acid binding proteins within the cell facilitates cellular fatty acid uptake by reducing intracellular FFA concentration. FATP4 may be localised to the endoplasmic reticulum as well as the plasma membrane where it also catalyses the esterification of fatty acids with CoA and so drives transport of fatty acids by altering the concentration difference. FA transport/binding proteins are regulated by FA-activated transcription factors (PPARs, LXR (liver X receptor), SREBP-1 (sterol regulatory element-binding protein 1)). In the small intestine, protein-bound short- and medium-chain fatty acids (<C10) diffuse into cells directly and subsequently into the hepatic portal circulation (see Ch. 15).

TRIACYLGLYCEROLS (TRIGLYCERIDES)

There are limited stores of glucose in the body. In times of need alternative metabolic fuels are produced to ensure the continuous provision of glucose for certain tissues. Storage of fatty acids in the form of TAG, with subsequent breakdown in times of energy need, is more efficient and quantitatively more important for energy production than the storage of glycogen. Plasma TAGs constitute the major transport form of fat.

Triacylglycerols are formed by the esterification of one molecule of glycerol with three molecules of fatty acids: the carboxylic acid terminals of fatty acid condense with the hydroxyl terminal of glycerol (see Fig. 2.6).

In both liver and adipose tissue, TAGs are produced by a pathway that involves the 3-carbon molecule **glycerol 3-phosphate (gl-3-P)**. The gl-3-P is of different origin in the two tissues:

- In liver, glycerol provides the gl-3-P, catalysed by glycerol kinase
- Adipose tissue lacks glycerol kinase, so glucose is the source of gl-3-P via glycolysis.

When there is plenty of glucose, insulin is secreted and stimulates glucose uptake by the adipocyte via GLUT4. The immediate precursor of gl-3-P in adipose tissue is **dihydroxyacetone phosphate (DHAP)** (see Fig. 3.6). Fatty acid storage as TAG in adipose tissue can take place only when glycolysis is activated in the fed state.

Regulation of triacylglycerol breakdown

Triacylglycerols deliver fatty acids from adipose tissue stores to peripheral cells for catabolism. **Lipolysis** (degradation of TAG) releases three fatty acids and one glycerol. Fatty acids are transported via blood (bound to albumin) to oxidative tissues (e.g. muscle) for entry into β-oxidation and ATP production. In liver, fatty acids can also be utilised for **ketone body production (ketogenesis)**. The hydrolysis of stored TAG in adipocytes is tightly regulated by the enzyme **hormone-sensitive lipase**, so-called because it is sensitive to a range of hormones (Fig. 3.23).

Lipolysis is:

- Activated by glucagon and epinephrine (β receptor), which increase cAMP levels
- Inhibited by insulin, which lowers cAMP levels.

Lipid droplets (adiposomes) in adipocytes consist of a neutral lipid core containing TAGs and cholesteryl esters, surrounded by a single layer of phospholipids. Several proteins are anchored in the phospholipid layer which constitutes a family of structurally related proteins (PAT proteins) which are classified according to their stability. Perilipins are the most abundant proteins on the surface of lipid droplets. There are three isoforms, A, B and C, A being predominant. Uniquely of the PAT proteins, perilipin can be phosphorylated. β-Adrenergic agents cause the phosphorylation of perilipin A at specific serine residues by cAMP-dependent protein kinase (protein kinase A, PKA). Phosphorylated perilipin targets **hormone-sensitive lipase (HSL)** on the surface of the lipid droplet, enabling lipolysis of the contents. Perilipin is an important regulator of lipid storage and perilipin null mice are more likely to develop insulin resistance.

Research has also shown that hormone-stimulated lipolyis is impaired, but not eliminated, in HSL knockout mice, which accumulate cellular diacylglycerol (DAG) with reduced release of glycerol. This observation led to the discovery of a second lipase, **adipose triglyceride lipase (ATGL)**, which has strong TAG hydrolase activity and may therefore generate DAG, known to be the preferred substrate for HSL. HSL then removes the remaining two fatty acids from TAG, stepwise. ATGL expression is sensitive to nutritional status but, unlike that of HSL, ATGL activity is not acutely regulated by cAMP.

The liberated fatty acids and glycerol are then released to circulating blood.

LIPOPROTEINS

Lipoproteins are molecular combinations of lipids and protein components called **apolipoproteins**. Lipoproteins are classified according to density. Apolipoproteins emulsify the lipoprotein particle to make it more stable in aqueous solution for carriage in plasma, and interact with cellular receptors that determine how and where lipoprotein particles are metabolised. Each lipoprotein particle has a specific set of apolipoproteins (see later).

Lipoprotein particles are constructed by hepatocytes and enterocytes from (Fig. 3.24):

- TAG
- Cholesterol
- Apolipoproteins
- Phospholipids.

The hydrophobic TAG and cholesteryl esters make up the 'core' of lipoprotein particles, with apolipoprotein strands, cholesterol molecules and phospholipids in the outer shells. Hepatocytes assemble VLDLs and high-density lipoproteins (HDLs). HDLs are also derived from

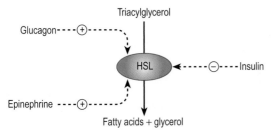

Fig. 3.23 Hormonal regulation of hormone-sensitive lipase (HSL) activity.

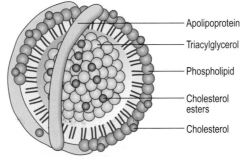

***Fig. 3.24* Generalised structure of lipoproteins.** The external monolayer contains phospholipids, cholesterol and apolipoproteins. Cholesterol esters and triacylglycerols are located in the particle core.

the gut. These are distinguished by the difference in their size, density, lipid composition and apolipoprotein content (Clinical box 3.20).

Apolipoproteins

Apolipoproteins are protein strands embedded in the surface of lipoproteins (Fig. 3.24). They activate and inhibit enzymes in lipoprotein metabolism, and are ligands for the cellular apoB/E (LDL) receptors and scavenger receptors. ApoB/E receptors and scavenger receptors are responsible for LDL clearance (see below).

The important apolipoproteins are:

- **ApoA** (A-I and A-II) present in HDLs. Binding of apoA-I to cellular receptors mediates the efflux of cholesterol from peripheral cells, and the influx of cholesterol into hepatocytes (see below).
- **ApoB**: apoB-100 recognises apoB/E receptors and facilitates cellular uptake of LDL. ApoB-100 is derived from liver and forms part of low-density lipoprotein (LDL). ApoB-48 is derived from the gut and is found in chylomicrons.
- **ApoC** is made in the liver and is a peripheral activator of lipoprotein lipase (LPL). It is transferred between lipoproteins.
- **ApoE** stabilises VLDL (and possibly intermediate-density lipoprotein (IDL) and remnant particles) for cellular uptake, and is a ligand for the apoB/E receptor.
- **Apo(a)** links with apoB-100 to oxidise LDL, giving Lp(a) lipoprotein particles.

On large particles, e.g. VLDLs, the apolipoproteins are stretched. As the particles shrink with increasing density, apoB and apoE change conformation so that they can no longer bind to apoB/E receptors. However, apoE adapts to a shape that allows binding to apoE receptors for uptake into hepatocytes. As lipoprotein particles travel around in the circulation, apoC-II on chylomicrons and VLDLs allow TAG to be removed by LPL in the capillary endothelium.

Apolipoproteins are important because they control lipoprotein metabolism. Apolipoprotein and LDL receptor genes have been identified, sequenced and mapped to chromosomes. Apolipoprotein disorders are known to lead to rare defects of lipid metabolism and particular apolipoproteins have also been linked with various neurodegenerative conditions, such as Alzheimer disease.

Lipoprotein classes and functions

Lipoproteins vary in size and density, the denser being smaller. A high TAG content makes the lipoprotein particle less dense, and therefore larger in size. Intestinal, adipose and skeletal muscle lipoprotein lipase (LPL) and hepatic triacylglycerol lipase (HTGL), present in capillary endothelial cells, remove TAG from TAG-rich lipoproteins. Progressive removal of TAG increases the protein:lipid ratio and thus the density of the particle remnants.

Chylomicrons

The least dense and largest lipoproteins are **chylomicrons**, which are globules assembled by enterocytes following lipid digestion and composed principally of TAG, apoB-48, apoA-I and apoA-II, a smaller amount of cholesterol and cholesteryl esters. In the bloodstream, apoC-II and apoE are acquired from HDLs (see below). They transport products from dietary fat digestion to peripheral tissues (see Ch. 15). Progressive removal of TAGs by LPL leads to the formation of remnant particles, which are taken up and catabolised by the liver.

Very-low-density lipoprotein

VLDL is synthesised continuously in the liver. It is the main source of TAGs exported from liver to muscle and adipose tissues:

- TAG forms about 50% of the particle
- Contain apoB-100 as an essential component
- ApoC-II and apoE are incorporated by transfer from high-density lipoprotein (HDL).

Intermediate-density lipoprotein

IDL is a particle remnant derived from VLDL by the removal of TAG by LPL in extrahepatic tissues with loss of apolipoprotein. IDLs are precursors of LDLs. Some IDL particles are taken up by hepatocytes, when TAG is removed by HTGL:

- TAG content in the particle remnant is decreased, with a proportional rise in cholesterol
- Contains apoB-100 and apoE
- Loses apoC-II.

Low-density lipoprotein

LDL is also a particle remnant, resulting from further removal of TAG in liver and peripheral tissues when the molecule:

- Is depleted of almost all of its TAG, and mainly consists of cholesterol
- Contains a single apoB-100 molecule and some apoE.

LDL is the main cholesterol carrier, delivering cholesterol to liver and peripheral tissues.

High-density lipoprotein

HDL particles are synthesised in both the liver and intestines. They carry cholesterol from adipose tissue directly to liver – **reverse cholesterol transport** – and to tissues that synthesise steroid hormones (e.g. adrenal glands, ovaries and testes). HDL also takes part in the metabolism of other lipoproteins by exchanging apolipoproteins, cholesteryl ester, TAG and phospholipids.

- HDL is rich in cholesteryl esters
- Only about 5% of the particle is TAG
- It contains apoA (A-I and A-II) and also apoC and apoE.

Lipoprotein receptors

Activation of membrane-bound lipoprotein receptors in hepatic and peripheral cells enables cholesterol entry. The main receptor is the **apoB/E** (also known as LDL) **receptor**, present on cell surfaces. ApoB/E receptors bind either apoB-100 or apoE, but not apoB-48 (cellular uptake of chylomicron remnants is mediated by apoE and apoB/E related receptors). Gene expression of apoB/E receptor is regulated by intracellular cholesterol concentration.

Binding of LDL to apoB/E receptors stimulates endocytosis. LDL is taken into hepatic (about 80% of total LDL) and peripheral cells, then broken down to cholesterol by lysosomes, destroying the LDL particle. The receptor is recycled back to the cell membrane.

Scavenger receptors

Scavenger receptors are membrane-bound receptors on phagocytic cells, e.g. macrophages. Unlike the apoB/E receptor, scavenger receptors do not bind intact LDLs, but rather the oxidised form – Lp(a) particles. The scavenger receptors (scavenger receptor type A) on macrophages are not regulated by raised intracellular cholesterol concentration, so they can be overloaded by the ligand – oxidised LDL – which can disrupt the macrophage, leading to atherogenesis (see Chs 11 and 16). Scavenger receptor type BI takes part in cholesterol removal in HDL metabolism (see below).

Elevated Lp(a) concentration is associated with increased risk of atherogenesis.

Lipoprotein metabolism

Lipoprotein metabolism involves a series of processes:

1. Assembly of chylomicrons in enterocytes from TAGs, cholesterol, phospholipids and apolipoproteins.
2. Endogenous synthesis of VLDL in the liver from apoB-100, apoE, TAGs, cholesterol esters and phospholipids, but predominantly TAGs.
3. Fatty acids: LPL and HTGL catalyse the cleavage (by hydrolysis) of TAGs and fatty acids from chylomicrons and VLDLs to form remnant particles. IDLs, LDLs and HDLs (VLDL–IDL–LDL–HDL cascade) are delivered to peripheral cells for energy metabolism. LPL and HTGL are activated by apoC-II binding.
4. Cellular uptake of remnant particles through activation of membrane receptors by apoB/E binding.
5. The cell surface of an LDL particle has a single apoB-100 and some apoE.
6. Removal of cholesterol from cells by HDL particles – reverse cholesterol transport – for delivery to liver for VLDL synthesis or conversion to bile salts for excretion in bile.

Reverse cholesterol transport

HDLs are lipid-poor particles formed in the liver and intestine. Newly formed (nascent) HDL particles resemble flat, bi-layered discs, and mainly contain phospholipid and apoA-I. As they travel around the circulation, nascent HDL particles remove cholesterol from cells, mediated by the action of **cholesterol efflux regulatory protein** (**CERP**, also known as ATP-binding cassette transporter A-I; ABC1). CERP is activated by apoA-I, facilitating the movement of cholesterol out of cells to apoA-I.

ApoA-I also activates the enzyme **lecithin-cholesterol acyl transferase** (**LCAT**), which catalyses the synthesis of cholesteryl esters. The cholesteryl esters move deeper into the HDL particle to give it a more spherical shape (see Fig. 3.24). As HDL moves through the circulation, some cholesteryl esters are exchanged for TAGs from TAG-rich lipoproteins, and the HDL particle becomes larger as the space between the bilayer fills.

In reverse cholesterol transport, HDL transports cholesterol away from peripheral cells, delivering cholesterol directly to the liver and tissues that synthesise steroids. In the liver, binding of apoA-I to scavenger receptor type BI mediates the removal of cholesterol into the hepatocytes for excretion as bile salts and sterols. HDL is then released in the disc form to enter a new cycle of cholesterol transport.

ApoA-I is thus essential for both the efflux of peripheral cellular cholesterol into HDL, and the uptake of cholesterol from HDL into hepatocytes and steroid synthetic cells. Defects of apoA-I are associated with defective cholesterol excretion, and consequently hypercholesterolaemia.

Lipoprotein fuel transport and overflow pathways

The lipoprotein fuel transport pathway includes the VLDL–IDL–LDL–HDL cascade, cellular uptake of lipoprotein remnant particles and reverse cholesterol transport. Fatty acids, mainly in the form of TAGs, are transported to adipose tissue for storage and to peripheral tissues for energy metabolism.

TAG is depleted from lipoprotein remnants in the fuel transport pathway to generate LDL, which can no longer deliver TAG. The metabolic pathway of LDL is therefore unrelated to the supply of fuel, and may be considered an 'overflow pathway'.

FATTY ACID OXIDATION

The catabolism of fatty acids is entirely oxidative and requires both mitochondrial and cytosolic phases, intermediary metabolites being shuttled between the cytosol and mitochondrion. Fatty acids are delivered to cytosol bound to fatty acid binding proteins (see above), and have to be 'activated' to their fatty acyl-CoA derivatives in the cytosol before they can enter the mitochondrion for β-oxidation (see below).

Fatty acid activation and transport into mitochondria

Fatty acid activation is catalysed by the enzyme **acyl-CoA synthetase** (also known as acyl-CoA thiokinase), sited in the outer mitochondrial membrane (see Fig. 3.25). Two ATP molecules are used as the energy source.

- The acyl-CoA derivatives of short- and medium-chain fatty acids enter the mitochondrion directly by simple diffusion across the mitochondrial membranes.
- Very-long-chain fatty acids (C22–24) have to be shortened to long-chain fatty acids, and branched-chain fatty acids are oxidised in the **peroxisomes**, before being shuttled to the mitochondrion.

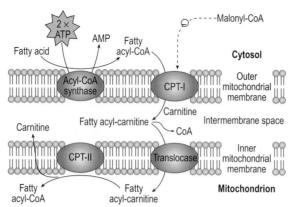

Fig. 3.25 Carnitine shuttle. The fatty acyl-CoA formed from short- and medium-chain fatty acids diffuses across the mitochondrial membranes into the mitochondrion. Fatty acyl-CoA from long-chain fatty acids has to be transported via the carnitine shuttle. CPT, carnitine palmitoyltransferase.

- Long chain-fatty acids are converted to their acyl-CoA derivatives in the cytosol. Long-chain fatty acyl-CoA derivatives cannot cross the outer mitochondrial membrane by simple diffusion, and have to be transported across via the carnitine shuttle (Fig. 3.25).

  Peroxisomes are cellular organelles that selectively import their content from the cytosol, like mitochondria, but differ in that they only have a single membrane and don't contain DNA or ribosomes. They therefore rely on importing all of their proteins for their function.

Carnitine shuttle

The carnitine shuttle is an **antiport** transport mechanism.

1. The large and polar long-chain fatty acyl-CoA molecule is transferred to the small carnitine molecule by carnitine **palmitoyltransferase-I** (**CPT-I**), located in the outer mitochondrial membrane.
2. Long-chain fatty acylcarnitine is formed, releasing CoA. An acyl-carnitine carrier (a translocase) in the inner mitochondrial membrane then carries fatty acyl-carnitine into the mitochondrion. CPT-1 transports a range of long-chain acyl-CoAs.
3. On entry into the mitochondrion, a second transferase, **carnitine palmitoyltransferase-II** (**CPT-II**), regenerates the long-chain acyl-CoA and releases free carnitine, which diffuses out back through the inner mitochondrial membrane.
4. The entry of acyl-carnitine into the mitochondrion is obligatorily linked to the exit of carnitine from the mitochondrion (an antiport mechanism) for the shuttle to continue.

Carnitine shuttle in the regulation of fatty acid oxidation

The carnitine shuttle is an important site in the regulation of mitochondrial long-chain fatty acid oxidation. In the liver, inhibition of mitochondrial CPT-I by malonyl-CoA (see below) prevents the mitochondrial catabolism of newly-synthesised fatty acids. Malonyl-CoA is formed predominantly when glucose is abundant and therefore, in the fed state, malonyl-CoA inhibits CPT-I suppressing mitochondrial long-chain fatty acid oxidation. Because long-chain fatty acids remain

in the cytosol, their esterification to form TAG is favoured. Ultimately, this liver TAG will be exported as VLDL. In liver, total CPT-I activity increases following prolonged fasting and in uncontrolled diabetes mellitus.

Regulation of CPT-I in muscle, which is not a major site of fatty acid synthesis from glucose, is an important aspect of metabolic fuel selection (Clinical box 3.21).

β-Oxidation of fatty acids in mitochondria

Fatty acids are catabolised via β-oxidation in the mitochondrial matrix. Most tissues containing mitochondria oxidise fatty acids, but the brain cannot.

The β-oxidation of fatty acyl-CoA takes place by the removal of two carbon atoms at a time from the fatty acyl-CoA molecule at the β-carbon position to form a ketone (C=O). The chain reaction finally releases:

- Acetyl-CoA
- Reduced nucleotides flavin adenine dinucleotide ($FADH_2$) and nicotinamide adenine dinucleotide (NADH). $FADH_2$ and NADH donate electrons to the electron transport chain. The reduced nucleotides are used directly for synthesis of ATP by oxidative phosphorylation.
- Acetyl-CoA is oxidised either:
  - in muscle, in the TCA cycle to CO_2 and water, releasing free CoA
  - in liver, predominantly for ketone body formation.

The net ATP yield for the complete oxidation of such a fatty acid is far higher that the yield from glucose catabolism. The caloric value of palmitate is 37.6 kJ/g (9 kcal) compared with that of glucose, 16.4 kJ/g (4 kcal).

Oxidation of acetyl-CoA in the TCA cycle

The oxidation of acetyl-CoA in the TCA cycle begins with the condensation of acetyl-CoA with **oxaloacetate** (**OAA**) to form citric acid with the release of free CoA. This reaction is catalysed and regulated by **citrate synthase**.

Another key enzyme in the TCA cycle is **isocitrate dehydrogenase**, which catalyses one of the subsequent oxidative reactions when NAD^+ is reduced to NADH, releasing CO_2.

Inhibition of the β-oxidation spiral by excess CoA

Under fasting and starvation conditions, the balance of metabolic processes in the TCA cycle is shifted to favour of gluconeogenesis. One of these shifts occurs through changes in OAA-malate equilibrium (see below, Malate shuttle, Fig. 3.28). Under physiological conditions, OAA is converted to malate in the mitochondrion in a ratio of 1:1. In starvation, the OAA-malate equilibrium shifts towards malate. Malate then leaves the mitochondrion and is consumed in gluconeogenesis. As a result, less OAA is available to take part in the citrate synthase reaction within the TCA, so less acetyl-CoA can be oxidised to free CoA. Excess acetyl-CoA then accumulates.

Free CoA is essential to the initiation and continuation of β-oxidation. When there is a deficiency in free CoA, an alternative pathway, the ketogenic pathway in the liver, is activated for the breakdown of acetyl-CoA to liberate free CoA.

Ketogenesis in the liver

Ketone bodies (acetoacetate and 3-hydroxybutyrate) are produced in the liver from acetyl-CoA generated by oxidation of fatty acids. This is termed **ketogenesis**. Thus, ketogenesis is a hepatic pathway for the metabolism of acetyl-CoA. The free CoA needed for the initiation and continuation of the β-oxidation spiral is generated in this process, which also results in the release of ketone bodies.

Ketone bodies are the water-soluble lipid derivatives:

- Acetoacetate
- β-Hydroxybutyrate
- Acetone, a metabolic waste product formed by the non-enzymic decomposition of acetoacetate.

Under physiological conditions, only the liver is able to synthesise and export ketone bodies, the entire process taking place in the mitochondrial matrix. There is excessive ketogenesis in uncontrolled type 1 diabetes because of a lack of insulin, which increases delivery of the precursors, fatty acids, from the adipocyte to the liver.

Oxidation of acetyl-CoA in the ketogenic pathway

In the ketogenic pathway (Fig. 3.26), acetyl-CoA is converted to acetoacetate in the mitochondrion via the hydroxymethylglutaryl-CoA (HMG-CoA) pathway. Acetoacetate can decompose to acetone, or be converted to β-hydroxybutyrate enzymatically. Free CoA is liberated in this pathway for initiating and continuing the β-oxidation spiral.

There are three stages in the conversion of acetyl-CoA into ketone bodies:

1. Condensation of two molecules of acetyl-CoA to form acetoacetyl-CoA; releasing one CoA molecule.
2. Catalysis by mitochondrial HMG-CoA synthase (Information box 3.11), releasing a second CoA molecule.

Information box 3.11	Mitochondrial HMG-CoA synthase versus cytosolic HMG-CoA synthase

- Mitochondrial HMG-CoA synthase is involved in the ketogenic pathway.
- Cytosolic HMG-CoA synthase is involved in cholesterol synthesis. This enzyme is inhibited by the statins used in the treatment of hyperlipidaemia.
- Their modes of regulation are quite different.

Acetoacetate and β-hydroxybutyrate are inter-convertible by the mitochondrial enzyme, β-hydroxybutyrate dehydrogenase. Their relative concentrations therefore reflect the mitochondrial redox state, with β-hydroxybutyrate predominating when the $NADH/NAD^+$ ratio is high due to brisk rates of β-oxidation. Thus, considerably more β-hydroxybutyrate than acetoacetate is released from the liver.

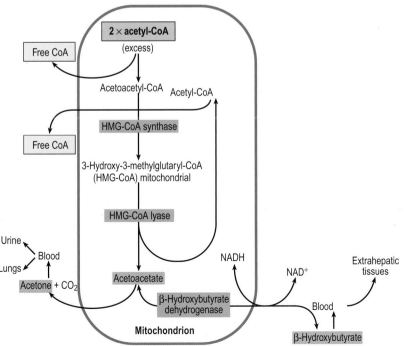

Fig. 3.26 **Mitochondrial ketogenic pathway.** Ketone bodies are in purple; enzymes are in red. HMG-CoA, hydroxymethylglutaryl-CoA.

3. Catalysis by HMG-CoA lyase. Together the synthase and lyase enzymes catalyse the conversion of acetoacetyl-CoA to acetoacetate.

HMG-CoA synthase is regulatory for ketogenesis in prolonged starvation and its gene expression is increased by the lipid-regulated transcription factor PPARα. HMG-CoA synthase is also acutely regulated by protein acetylation/deacetylation (which is analogous to protein phosphorylation/dephosphorylation). Deacetylation by a NAD⁺ dependent **mitochondrial sirtuin enzyme, SIRT3**, activates the enzyme.

Role of ketone bodies in fuel homeostasis

As well as enhancing hepatic ATP production by providing free CoA for continued β-oxidation, the formation of ketone bodies by the liver is vital to whole-body fuel homeostasis during starvation and uncontrolled diabetes.

In brief, fatty acids are converted, through hepatic ketogenesis, to water-soluble products, the ketone bodies, which, unlike fatty acids, can readily be transported in aqueous solution in the blood. Moreover, ketone bodies can be used for energy production by the brain during starvation (see below), whereas long-chain fatty acids are unable to cross the blood–brain barrier.

Ketone body utilisation

During starvation, the brain adapts to use ketone bodies, which fuel more than 50% of its energy requirements. Ketone bodies are also important energy substrates for heart and oxidative skeletal muscle. Although the liver is able to synthesise ketone bodies, it is deficient in the key enzyme needed for their metabolism. Thus, for further metabolism, ketone bodies are exported from the liver and taken up in extrahepatic tissues. In tissues other than the liver, ketone bodies appear to be used in proportion to their plasma concentration. They are, therefore, an efficient source of energy during starvation and in other conditions in which they are produced in large quantities (Clinical box 3.22).

LIPOGENESIS – FATTY ACID SYNTHESIS

Whereas the degradation of fat, β-oxidation, occurs in the mitochondria, fatty acid synthesis occurs in the cytosol. Generally, **palmitic acid** (palmitate), a simple straight-chain saturated fatty acid containing 16 carbon atoms, is synthesised first; many other fatty acids are made by chain elongation and/or desaturation of palmitic acid. Not all fatty acids can be endogenously synthesised. The carbon atoms in the palmitate chain originate only from acetyl-CoA (see below). Insulin has a major role in promoting lipogenesis.

Fatty acid synthesis takes place in two stages (Fig. 3.27). Both stages use acetyl-CoA as the carbon source, and require multienzyme complexes. The acetyl-CoA units are derived from mitochondrial oxidative glycolysis via the pyruvate dehydrogenase pathway, then transported into the cytosol via the malate shuttle (see below).

- Stage 1: acetyl-CoA is converted to malonyl-CoA by **acetyl-CoA carboxylase (ACC)**
- Stage 2: fatty acid chain elongation, catalysed by **fatty acid synthase (FAS)** to form palmitate.

Stage 1: ACC – the committed step of lipogenesis

In stage 1, acetyl-CoA is converted, or 'activated', by the action of ACC to form malonyl-CoA. This reaction commits acetyl-CoA to fatty acid synthesis. The ACC enzyme is synthesised in an inactive single unit (protomer) form. The synthesis of ACC, like many enzymes that carry CO_2, requires the water soluble B vitamin **biotin** as cofactor (see Ch. 16). The protomer is activated to its polymeric form by citrate (or isocitrate). The ACC reaction takes place in two stages:

- Carboxylation (transfer of CO_2) of biotin, requiring energy in the form of ATP
- Transfer of the carboxyl group to acetyl-CoA to produce malonyl-CoA, releasing the biotin–carboxyl complex.

Clinical box 3.22 **Ketone bodies accumulate in starvation, uncontrolled type 1 diabetes mellitus and with serious loss of control in type 2 diabetes**

- The ketone body level in the blood rises to 2–3 mM after a few days of starvation, increasing to 7–8 mM or more after prolonged starvation.
- Certain pathological conditions, notably diabetic ketoacidosis, are characterised by excessive accumulation of ketone bodies in the blood with acidosis, even if blood glucose levels are not much increased.

Diabetic ketoacidosis
- Blood ketone body levels can increase to up to 15–20 mM in uncontrolled type 1 diabetes mellitus.
- Blood pH falls because the ketone bodies are acid, giving rise to metabolic acidosis.
- In diabetic coma due to ketoacidosis, the β-hydroxybutyrate:acetoacetate ratio can rise to as high as 3 (from excessive adipose-tissue lipolysis, hepatic fatty acid oxidation and ketogenesis). Because a rapid 'dip stick' test for ketonuria detects only acetoacetate, the increased excretion of ketone bodies (ketonuria) may go unrecognised.
- Acetone, from acetoacetate decomposition, is expired by the lungs, producing a characteristic fruity (pear) odour on the patient's breath.
  During short-term starvation (overnight fast, or up to 3 days), ketone bodies are important in providing a fuel for

muscle, kidney and intestine. As the period of starvation is extended, the brain also converts to the use of ketone bodies for more than 50% of its energy. This metabolic switch allows considerable glucose conservation, reducing the demand for degraded muscle protein, which provides precursors for gluconeogenesis.
  Ketone bodies are converted to CoA derivatives for oxidation as follows:
1. β-Hydroxybutyrate is first oxidised to acetoacetate by NAD⁺ in a reaction catalysed by β-hydroxybutyrate dehydrogenase. This is a direct reversal of hepatic synthesis (see Fig. 3.23).
2. Activation of acetoacetate – its conversion to acetoacetyl-CoA – occurs by the transfer of CoA from succinyl-CoA, catalysed by the enzyme β-oxoacid CoA-transferase, which is absent in the liver.
3. Acetoacetyl-CoA is then split to acetyl-CoA by the reversal of the thiolase reaction, the direction of which depends on the concentration ratio of its substrates and products.
4. The major source of succinyl-CoA for the β-oxoacid CoA-transferase is the TCA cycle.
  The increased production of succinate at the expense of succinyl-CoA allows increased production of oxaloacetate (via the TCA cycle), which facilitates the entry of more acetyl-CoA into the TCA cycle.

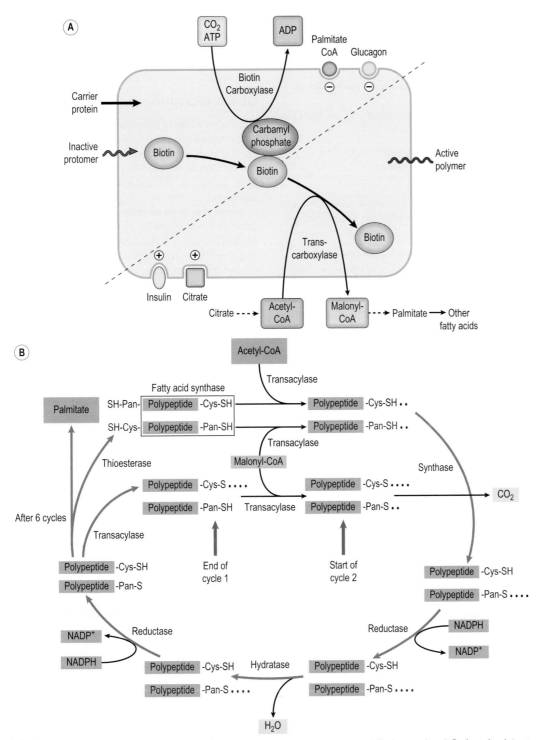

Fig. 3.27 **(A) The acetyl-CoA carboxylase (ACC) complex.** ACC converts acetyl-CoA to malonyl-CoA and exists as a small complex (protomer) in its inactive state, forming a polymer when activated. The diagram illustrates the molecule in its inactive and active states. Fatty acid synthesis is regulated by the activity of ACC in two ways: (1) allosteric binding of citrate (promotes ACC) or palmitate CoA (inhibits ACC) at one site; and (2) hormonal binding by insulin (promotes ACC by dephosphorylating the enzyme) or glucagon (inhibits ACC by phosphorylating the enzyme) at a second binding site. **(B) The fatty acid synthase (FAS) enzyme.** FAS is composed of two identical polypeptides, placed head to tail. They each contain a carrier protein and a series of seven enzymes that catalyse the addition of four carbon units (•) at each end of the enzyme in the first step, then adding two additional carbon units in a cyclical set of reactions. Carbon units are added to both the cysteine (Cys) and pantetheine (Pan) ends of the enzyme and the growing fatty acid chain is transferred from one to the other between the two polypeptides. The diagram shows only the processes taking place on one end of the polypeptide pair. After six cycles there are 16 carbon units attached to the pantetheine-carrier part of the enzyme. At this point the enzyme complex is saturated and thioesterase cleaves off the 16-carbon fatty acid chain (palmitate) and FAS re-enters the cycle at the top of the diagram. ATP, adenosine triphosphate; ADP, adenosine diphosphate; Cys, cysteine; Pan, pantetheine; S, sulphur group; H, hydrogen; •, carbon unit; NADP, nicotinamide adenine dinucleotide phosphate (NADP$^+$ oxidised, NADPH reduced).

Regulation of ACC activity

In the short term, ACC activity is tightly controlled by two independent mechanisms.

Acetyl-CoA contains an allosteric site for the binding of citrate or palmitoyl-CoA

Citrate is a TCA cycle intermediate, which, on exit from the mitochondrion, acts both as:

- the immediate source of the cytosolic acetyl-CoA, required for the ACC reaction, and as
- a feed-forward activator of the ACC protomer.

When energy supply is high, storage of energy through lipogenesis is promoted by increased insulin secretion to prevent overproduction of fatty acids.

- Insulin acts indirectly to increase the availability of citrate through its promotion of glucose uptake, aerobic glycolysis and the TCA cycle
- Palmitoyl-CoA, a product of stage 2 of lipogenesis, acts as an allosteric inhibitor of the ACC protomer, acting at the same site as citrate.

ACC control by hormone-dependent covalent modification

Independent of the citrate/palmitoyl-CoA mechanism, ACC is also controlled by hormone-dependent covalent modification, a phosphorylation-dephosphorylation mechanism. The phosphorylated ACC enzyme is less active than the dephosphorylated one. Under low-energy conditions, the AMP-dependent protein kinase (AMPK) is activated by glucagon or epinephrine to phosphorylate ACC. When cellular energy level is high (metabolic pathway moves towards fatty acid synthesis for storage), dephosphorylation is activated by a protein phosphatase stimulated by insulin.

The rate of ACC synthesis is highly regulated

Long-term regulation of ACC synthesis is exerted mainly at the level of changes in gene expression, induced by specific transcription factors.

Experimental data suggest that more ACC enzyme is produced by animals on high-carbohydrate or fat-free diets, whereas starvation and high-fat/low-carbohydrate diets decrease enzyme synthesis. A high insulin level therefore acutely increases ACC gene expression.

Stage 2: fatty acid synthase (FAS)

The second stage of fatty acid synthesis (Fig. 3.27B) is catalysed by FAS. Starting with acetyl-CoA as the carbon source, fatty acids are synthesised by the addition of two-carbon units, one at a time, to the activated carboxyl end of a growing chain, ending with an even number of carbon atoms.

FAS is a complex enzyme system in the cytoplasm containing seven enzymes and an **acyl-carrier protein (ACP)**. Acetyl-CoA and malonyl-CoA are transferred to ACP, initiating the fatty acid synthesis cycle. All the reactions in the cycle are catalysed by fatty acid synthase. As the fatty acid chain grows, the carbon moiety is moved to a second site in ACP, freeing the original binding site, allowing the cycle to continue. The cycle is repeated six times until there is a saturated 16-carbon complex on the carrier protein, a palmitate molecule.

Thioesterase splits palmitate from the carrier protein to release the FAS molecule to restart synthesis.

Chain elongation

With the exception of the essential PUFAs, palmitate is the basis for synthesising other long-chain fatty acids. Chain elongation occurs by the addition of two-carbon units derived from malonyl-CoA by another enzyme complex, **fatty acid elongase**, located on the endoplasmic reticulum (mitochondrial membrane).

Short- and medium-chain fatty acids can also be elongated in mitochondria in a process that is the reversal of β-oxidation, using acetyl-CoA as the carbon source. Very-long-chain fatty acids (C22–24) are produced in the brain, which contains additional elongation systems. Elongation of stearoyl-CoA (C18) in the brain increases rapidly during myelination to generate the fatty acids required for the synthesis of brain-specific lipid (sphingolipids).

Fatty acid elongation is greatly reduced during starvation, secondary to decreasing insulin secretion.

Desaturation

Chain elongation produces saturated fatty acids only. Desaturation takes place in the endoplasmic reticulum, catalysed by mixed function oxidases: **desaturases**. Oxygen and energy in the form of NADH are needed. The enzymes produce double bonds in the fatty acid chain.

An initial step in the formation of unsaturated fatty acids from palmitate (C16), or stearate (C18), is the introduction of a double bond between C-9 and C-10 atoms to produce palmitoleic or oleic acid, respectively. The desaturase system in humans cannot introduce double bonds between C-9 and the terminal methyl ω carbon atom. This is despite fatty acids with double bonds in this inaccessible region being necessary precursors of eicosanoids.

Regulation of fatty acid synthase and rate of lipogenesis

The regulation of FAS occurs primarily by long-term effects of changes in nutritional status on its rate of synthesis and degradation. Increased insulin secretion in the fed state stimulates ACC and FAS synthesis, starvation leads to decreased synthesis. FAS levels are:

- High in individuals eating a high-carbohydrate/low-fat diet, promoting lipogenesis.
- Low after starvation, or in individuals eating a high-fat/low-carbohydrate diet, inhibiting lipogenesis. The effect of consuming a high-fat diet to depress insulin secretion and inhibit lipogenesis is partly the basis for the 'Atkins diet'.

In the short term, substrate flux (the presence of phosphorylated sugars) causes allosteric activation of FAS.

Malate shuttle – production of acetyl-CoA for lipogenesis

Acetyl-CoA, the carbon source for lipogenesis, is produced from pyruvate, via glycolysis. Pyruvate is transported into the

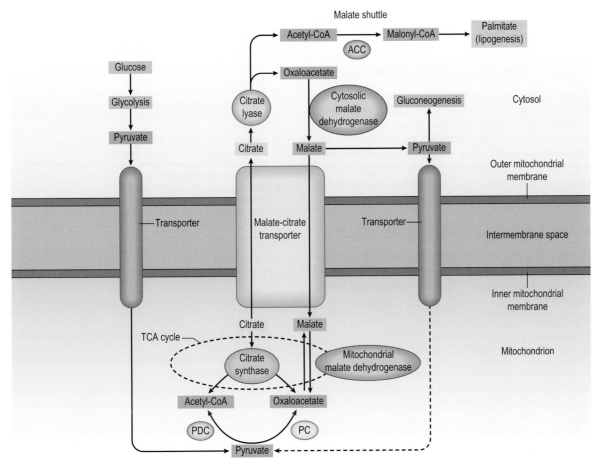

Fig. 3.28 **The malate shuttle.** Acetyl-CoA and oxaloacetate do not easily cross the mitochondrial membrane and are transported between the mitochondrion and cytosol via the malate-citrate antiporter. The malate shuttle is a method of transporting electrons (and reducing equivalents) from the cytosol to the mitochondrion. PDC, pyruvate dehydrogenase complex; PC, pyruvate carboxylase; ACC, acetyl-CoA carboxylase.

mitochondrion to undergo oxidative decarboxylation (losing CO_2) to form acetyl-CoA via the PDC (see Fig. 3.10) and oxaloacetate by **pyruvate carboxylase** (**PC**). PDC and PC are located in the mitochondrial matrix, whereas ACC and FAS are found in the cytosol. Acetyl-CoA does not readily traverse the mitochondrial membrane, and needs to be transported. This is achieved by the **malate shuttle**.

The malate shuttle is a complex antiport system. Acetyl-CoA combines with oxaloacetate in the TCA cycle to form citrate, catalysed by citrate synthase. Citrate is then translocated to the cytosol via the malate-citrate antiporter. At the same time, a molecule of malate is transferred to the mitochondrion (Fig. 3.28).

In the cytosol, citrate undergoes cleavage by citrate lyase to form acetyl-CoA and oxaloacetate. The action of ACC then converts acetyl-CoA to malonyl-CoA to enter lipogenesis.

Like acetyl-CoA, oxaloacetate does not readily cross the mitochondrial membrane. To re-enter the mitochondrion, oxaloacetate is converted to malate by cytosolic malate dehydrogenase. Malate is then transported back into the mitochondrion, via the malate-citrate antiporter, to be reconverted to oxaloacetate by mitochondrial malate dehydrogenase.

In starvation, malate is converted to pyruvate to enter gluconeogenesis.

FINE-TUNING OF FATTY ACID SYNTHESIS, OXIDATION AND KETOGENESIS

In the liver, inhibition of mitochondrial CPT-I by malonyl-CoA, the product of ACC reaction, prevents the catabolism of newly synthesised fatty acids, favouring their esterification to TAG, which is subsequently exported as VLDL.

With carbohydrate feeding (high insulin/low glucagon), the liver is actively engaged in fatty acid synthesis. Tissue malonyl-CoA content is high, and the capacity for mitochondrial long-chain fatty acid oxidation (and consequently ketogenesis) is depressed. Conversely, in starvation and uncontrolled diabetes mellitus, malonyl-CoA levels fall. Hepatic fatty acid synthesis is attenuated, and fatty acids reaching the liver from adipose tissue are efficiently oxidised.

The transition between normal and ketotic states is accompanied by marked shifts in the sensitivity of CPT-I to inhibition by malonyl-CoA. As a result, the liver continues to oxidise fat immediately on re-feeding after starvation, enabling gluconeogenesis to continue, and thereby allows glycogen formation via the indirect pathway.

The suppressive effect of malonyl-CoA on CPT-I is not restricted to liver. Regulation of CPT-I in muscle, not a major site of fatty acid synthesis, appears to be an important aspect of metabolic fuel selection in muscle. Muscle malonyl-CoA concentrations fall with starvation, and also acutely in response to exercise, both conditions being associated with increased β-oxidation (when fatty acids become a major source of metabolic energy, ATP).

REGULATION OF FAT METABOLISM

Fat metabolism is controlled by the coordinated action of insulin, glucagon, epinephrine, cortisol and human growth hormone, and interacts with the regulation of carbohydrate metabolism. Insulin stimulates and regulates fatty acid synthesis and storage, promoting glucose uptake in both liver and adipose tissue. The rate of fat catabolism is controlled by the rate of TAG hydrolysis in adipose tissue, activated by rising concentrations of glucagon.

In the fasting (post-absorptive) state

As blood glucose concentration falls, glucagon activates hepatic gluconeogenesis, coordinating the release of amino acids and TAG hydrolysis. This results in increasing plasma concentrations of:

- Fatty acids
- Glycerol
- Ketone bodies.

Epinephrine secretion, in response to physiological or psychological stress, has a similar effect. Cortisol has a more long-term effect (over weeks) and may cause insulin resistance (see Clinical box 3.23).

Clinical box 3.23   **Cushing syndrome**

Increased cortisol secretion in Cushing syndrome has a major long-term influence on fat metabolism by:

- Increasing gluconeogenesis
- Inhibiting glucose uptake and metabolism in peripheral tissues (insulin resistance)
- Stimulating glycogen synthesis and lipolysis.
  High plasma cortisol concentrations result in:
- Hyperglycemia, which may lead to diabetes mellitus
- Muscle wasting
- Redistribution of adipose tissue from glucagon-sensitive depots to areas such the face, upper back and abdomen, giving the typical appearance of central obesity (apple versus pear shape, see Ch. 16)
- Osteoporosis.

The characteristic moon face and 'dowager's hump' in Cushing syndrome is the result of facial fat deposition and thoracic spinal vertebral collapse from osteoporosis leading to kyphosis.

Although Cushing syndrome can be the result of advanced adrenal or pituitary disease, it occurs more commonly because of long-term administration of therapeutic steroids.

In the fed (absorptive) state

When there is excess energy intake, especially excess dietary carbohydrate, the pathways for de novo fatty acid synthesis (lipogenesis) are activated by insulin. The carbohydrate is converted to fatty acids in the liver, then stored as TAG in adipose tissue.

4 Pharmacology

Walter Wieczorek and Jeannette Naish

Introduction	**101**
Digoxin – an example in clinical pharmacology	102
PHARMACOKINETICS	**103**
Absorption – transfer of drugs across cell membranes	**103**
Passive diffusion through lipid membranes	103
Carrier-mediated transport	104
Endocytosis and exocytosis	106
Diffusion through aqueous and intercellular pores	106
Drug distribution	**106**
Blood flow	106
Capillary permeability and gap junctions	106
Accumulation of drug in fat and redistribution in other tissues	107
Binding of drugs to proteins	107
Distribution of drugs in the body	108
Drug metabolism	**109**
Phase I metabolic reactions (pre-conjugation reactions)	110
Phase II metabolic reactions (conjugation reactions)	112
Factors affecting drug metabolism	112
Conversion of inactive pro-drug to active metabolite	113
Excretion of drugs and metabolites	**113**
Renal system	113
Hepatobiliary excretion and enterohepatic circulation	116
Routes of drug administration	**116**
Oral administration	116
Parenteral administration	118
Other forms of injection	118
The mathematics of pharmacokinetics	**119**
First-order kinetics	119
Zero-order (non-linear or saturation) kinetics	120

Steady state and multiple dosing	121
PHARMACODYNAMICS	**123**
Drug targets	**123**
Enzymes	123
Carrier proteins (transporters)	124
Ion channels	124
Receptors	125
Receptor classification	126
The safety and effectiveness of drugs	**132**
Graded dose–response curves	132
Classification of drugs according to performance	133
Quantal dose–response curves	135
Factors that affect the performance of drugs	135
Tolerance, desensitisation, tachyphylaxis	137
THE AUTONOMIC NERVOUS SYSTEM	**138**
Neurotransmitters	**138**
Functions of the autonomic nervous system	**138**
Overview of the autonomic nervous system	**139**
The parasympathetic system	139
The sympathetic system	139
The reflex arc	139
Anatomy of the autonomic nervous system	**140**
The parasympathetic system	140
The sympathetic system	140
Neurotransmitters and receptors of the autonomic nervous system	**140**
Parasympathetic (cholinergic) system	141
Sympathetic (adrenergic) system	144
General anaesthetics	151

INTRODUCTION

Pharmacology studies the effects of chemical substances on the function of living organisms. Initially, tissue and animal experiments enabled observation of the qualitative effects and measurement of quantitative effects of these chemicals. Therapeutic uses were discovered for human beings, and later, drugs were developed and even designed to exert specific effects. More recently, advances in the study of cell and molecular biology have moved the theoretical basis of pharmacology rapidly forward. Newer concepts have replaced the historical theories, and biotechnology now underpins the development of drugs.

The typing and cloning of the human genome has given further, exciting prospects for therapeutic development. The genetic makeup of individuals determines their response to drugs, and genetic variation is complex. Pharmacogenetics is an evolving subject, and although still theoretical, the future of pharmacogenomics could be far reaching.

There are, of course, therapies other than drug therapy. Surgical procedures and other forms of medicines are alternative approaches to ill health. These are beyond the scope of this chapter.

The components of pharmacology discussed in the following sections include:

- Pharmacokinetics – how drugs are taken into the body, distributed, metabolised and eliminated.

- Pharmacodynamics – the effects that drugs have on the functions of human organs, and the mechanisms through which these effects occur.
- The autonomic nervous system (ANS) – this controls nearly all the major human organs. Most clinically important groups of drugs act on this system.
- Some drugs work selectively on physiological processes. Others have a more diffuse action. Disturbance in absorption, distribution, metabolism and elimination can potentiate or inhibit the action of drugs resulting in a variation in the speed of onset, duration of action, drug interactions, toxic and other unwanted side effects. It is therefore important that these processes are understood when prescribing drugs.

DIGOXIN – AN EXAMPLE IN CLINICAL PHARMACOLOGY

Digoxin is therapeutically the most important member of the family of cardiac glycosides, which are extracts from the foxglove plant *(Digitalis purpurea)*. The general principles described here will be discussed in greater detail in later sections. Digoxin is an example of how a commonly prescribed and important drug works in the context of pharmacology.

Clinically, digoxin is used for its effects on the heart, which may be direct and indirect.

- Digoxin increases the force of contraction of cardiac muscle by a direct action on the myocytes, improving pumping efficiency in heart failure – **positive inotropic effect**.
- Indirect activity mediated through increased parasympathetic vagal stimulation reduces the rate of contraction of cardiac muscle, e.g. slows ventricular rate in atrial fibrillation – **negative chronotropic effect**.

Pharmacodynamics – how digoxin works

The positive inotropic effect of digoxin on heart muscle is probably caused by:

- Inhibition of the Na^+/K^+ pump in the membrane of the cardiac myocyte
- Intracellular Na^+ increases, while Ca^{2+} diffusion out of the cell via the separate Na^+/Ca^{2+} exchange transporter slows down
- The retained intracellular Ca^{2+} ions are stored, increasing the amount of Ca^{2+} available for subsequent release for muscle contraction
- The increased release of Ca^{2+} increases the action potential of the muscle and thus the force of contraction.

The negative chronotropic action of digoxin is due to central nervous system (CNS) effects that increase parasympathetic vagal activity (see later, ANS), potentiating the action of acetylcholine (ACh) to:

- Decrease the rate of firing at the sino-atrial (S-A) node to slow the heart rate

- Block conduction via the atrio-ventricular (A-V) node, increasing the intervals between ventricular contractions, allowing more time for ventricular filling in diastole, thus improving pumping efficiency.

Pharmacokinetics – how the body handles digoxin

Orally administered digoxin is well absorbed from the gastrointestinal tract and excreted by the kidneys, unchanged. The drug stays in the body for a long time, the half-life being about 1.5 days.

Unwanted effects

The unwanted effects of digoxin are related to the non-specific nature of some of its actions.

- Excessive accumulation of intracellular Ca^{2+} produces ectopic discharges at the A-V node, giving rise to tachycardia and ventricular ectopics. The clinical sign is known as coupled beats or **pulsus bigeminy**. Each normal pulse is followed by an ectopic beat. Fatal ventricular tachycardia may ensue.
- Excessive vagal activity at the S-A node can lead to atrial bradycardia and A-V block. Progressive A-V block leads to bradycardia and potentially fatal complete heart block. Paradoxically, excessive parasympathetic activity in atria will result in tachycardia due to a more rapid repolarisation phase of the atrial action potential.
- Excessive parasympathetic activity on the gastrointestinal tract causes nausea, vomiting, anorexia and diarrhoea.
- CNS effects include tiredness, vertigo, confusion and yellow vision. The precise mechanism for yellow vision is not known, but attributed to inhibition of the Na^+/K^+ pump in retinal cones.
- The steroid-like chemical structure of digoxin can lead to gynaecomastia.

Factors that contribute to digoxin toxicity

- Hypokalaemia – co-administration with K^+ losing diuretics leads to hypokalaemia, which potentiates the action of digoxin, causing toxic effects.
- Renal function impairment – common in elderly patients – slows down excretion, prolonging the half-life of digoxin as digoxin is eliminated unchanged. The drug accumulates with rising plasma concentrations, which could reach toxic levels.
- The toxic dose is only slightly higher than the therapeutic dose (very narrow therapeutic window).
- Drugs that displace digoxin from tissue (protein binding) sites increase plasma concentration with an increased risk of toxicity (e.g. verapamil, a Ca^{2+} channel blocking drug also used in the treatment of cardiac arrhythmias).
- Hypoxia – potentiates digoxin-induced cardiac arrhythmias.

PHARMACOKINETICS

Clinicians need to understand how the human body deals with drugs, the aim of drug therapy being to rapidly deliver and maintain therapeutic levels. Pharmacokinetics is a study of the interactions that determine the speed of onset, intensity and duration of drug action, which, following release from its formulation (see below), is the product of four simultaneous processes (Fig. 4.1):

- Absorption, into the body and into cells
- Distribution, around the different compartments of the body
- Metabolism, when the drug is broken down and inactivated, or sometimes transformed into an active form
- Elimination or excretion from the body

To produce a pharmacological response, a drug needs to achieve an adequate concentration at the site of action. The two fundamental processes that determine the concentration of a drug in any given part of the body are:

- **Absorption**, the process of transfer of a drug from its site of administration into the systemic circulation, and into tissues where the drug exerts its therapeutic effect. Both necessitate the transfer of a drug across cell membranes.
- **Distribution** of drug molecules from the site of administration to either their site of action or to storage depots.

ABSORPTION – TRANSFER OF DRUGS ACROSS CELL MEMBRANES

Absorption is important for all routes of drug administration except intravenous injection. The degree of absorption depends on the route chosen and the physico-chemical properties of the drug. Cell membranes form barriers between intracellular and extracellular aqueous compartments in the body. A drug must cross at least one cell membrane to be absorbed, reach its site of action and eventually be eliminated.

The ways that drugs, nutrients and other substances (solutes) in aqueous solution cross a membrane barrier are by:

- Passive diffusion through cell membranes
- Carrier-mediated transport
- Endocytosis and exocytosis
- Diffusion through aqueous pores and intracellular pores.

PASSIVE DIFFUSION THROUGH LIPID MEMBRANES

The majority of drugs pass through cell membranes by passive diffusion of molecules down a concentration gradient, a process which does not involve energy expenditure (see Ch. 2) and is not saturable. As cell membranes are composed of a double layer of phospholipid molecules, the drug has to be lipid soluble to diffuse across them. The rate of diffusion across the membrane depends on:

- The lipid solubility of the drug
- The area over which absorption occurs
- The concentration gradient across the membrane.

Molecular size has little effect on diffusion because most drugs have a molecular mass of below 1000 daltons.

Lipid solubility

The human body largely consists of water, which forms the major part of extracellular and intracellular fluids (see Ch. 2). A drug must be water soluble to be distributed throughout the body. However, cell membranes that separate the extracellular from the intracellular compartments are mostly composed of lipids. The ability of a drug to enter or exit cells will depend on its lipid solubility. Some drugs are sufficiently lipid soluble to permeate the lipid membrane. Drugs that are not lipid soluble need to be transported across the cell membrane (Information box 4.1).

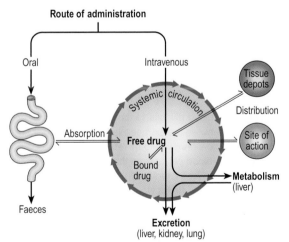

Fig. 4.1 The relationship between absorption, distribution, metabolism and excretion of a drug. The route of administration determines the degree of absorption, and thus the dose required for sufficient drug to enter plasma in the systemic circulation. The drug leaves the plasma to be distributed to its site of action and to storage sites (fat deposits). Finally, the majority of drugs are metabolised before excretion.

Information box 4.1	The relative ease with which drugs permeate cell membranes

The lipid solubility of a drug determines whether it can permeate cell membranes through passive diffusion.
- Aminoglycoside antibiotics are sufficiently lipid soluble for the whole molecule to permeate cell membranes.
- Thiopental, a general anaesthetic, is highly lipid soluble and can rapidly permeate cell membranes in the CNS and therefore has a rapid onset of action, making it useful as a general anaesthetic.
- Phenobarbital, of the same family of barbiturates as thiopental, used for its sedative and anti-epileptic action, is much less lipid soluble. Phenobarbital enters the CNS much more slowly, and is used in more long-term treatment.

Ionised and non-ionised forms of a drug

Most drug molecules exist in solution as a mixture of ionised and non-ionised forms. The ionised form carries an electrical charge, has very low lipid solubility and cannot easily permeate lipid membranes. Most ionised drugs are weak organic acids. The non-ionised form of a drug molecule carries no net electrical charge, so less ionised drugs are weak organic bases. The non-ionised fraction of a drug is highly lipid soluble and easily diffuses across cell membranes.

The proportion of the drug that is non-ionised determines its lipid solubility. Since only this fraction is capable of passive diffusion across cell membranes, the amount of administered drug that reaches the interior of cells depends on the proportion that is non-ionised.

Degree of ionisation of a drug

The degree of ionisation of a drug will depend upon its **hydrogen ion dissociation constant** (pK_a) and the pH of the medium in which it is dissolved. pK_a can be defined as the pH at which 50% of the drug is ionised and 50% non-ionised. The pK_a values for different drugs vary widely (Table 4.1).

The pH of the medium in which the drug is dissolved affects the degree of ionisation (see Ch. 2, Information box 2.2). There is significant variation in the pH of different aqueous environments in the body (see Table 4.1). For example, the very acid gastric juices have a pH that varies between about 1.0 and 3.0, whereas plasma is normally maintained at a constant pH of 7.4.

Figure 4.2 shows the difference in the degree of ionisation between an acidic (A) and a basic (B) drug in the acid medium of the stomach and the basic medium of the plasma.

Passive diffusion across cell membranes

If the pH on either side of a cell membrane is different, the degree of ionisation of a drug on either side of the membrane will also be different (Fig. 4.2).

- Only the non-ionised form of the drug permeates lipid membranes readily.
- The pH in an aqueous compartment and the pK_a of the drug determine how much of the drug is ionised (or remains non-ionised).

- The difference in pH on either side of the cell membrane gives unequal concentration of non-ionised drug on each side – known as **pH partitioning of drug molecules**. This is more pronounced where the pH difference is large, e.g. pH difference between gastric juices and plasma (see Fig. 4.2).
- The unequal non-ionised drug concentration on each side of the cell membrane gives rise to a concentration gradient. The non-ionised, lipid soluble form of the drug will passively diffuse down the concentration gradient across the cell membrane.
- The rate of diffusion will be proportional to the concentration difference of the non-ionised form of drug on either side of the membrane (see Ch. 2 and Fig. 2.37).
- The distribution of the non-ionised form of the drug on each side of a cell membrane will reach equilibrium. This is known as the **steady state** distribution. Equilibrium is rarely achieved in vivo because the blood circulation and gastric motility constantly remove the drug. Also, the ionised form of the drug has some degree of permeability and can cross the lipid membrane down its concentration gradient.

Ion trapping

The effect of pH partitioning results in the accumulation of weak acids in compartments with relatively high pH (basic), and weak bases accumulate in compartments with a relatively low pH (acidic). This is the concept of **ion trapping**. Applying this principle, the degree of drug ionisation on one or other side of a cell membrane can be changed by increasing or decreasing intra- or extracellular pH, altering the concentration gradient of the non-ionised (lipid soluble) fraction of drug across the membrane, to increase or decrease the rate of passive diffusion into or out of the cell (see Clinical box 4.1 for clinical application).

Effects of acidosis or alkalosis on absorption and distribution

The effects of metabolic or respiratory acidosis or alkalosis on drug absorption and distribution are of importance when treating patients with conditions such as respiratory failure and diabetic ketoacidosis. Restoration of acid–base balance in these patients is essential for avoiding ineffective drug treatment, adverse effects, overdose and toxicity.

Changes in plasma pH due to acidosis or alkalosis can have a significant effect on the pH partitioning or 'ion trapping' of drugs:

- In acidosis, blood pH falls so that the pH difference, or gradient, between the extracellular and intracellular fluids rises. An acidic drug would be retained in the cells.
- In alkalosis, blood pH rises so that, indirectly, the difference between interstitial pH and intracellular pH decreases. Acidic drugs would tend to accumulate in the extracellular fluid.

CARRIER-MEDIATED TRANSPORT

Drugs that are ionised in plasma and will not diffuse into the cells require specialist transmembrane proteins, **transporters**, to carry them across cell membranes. The ionised drug molecules combine with the protein on one side of the membrane, the transporter then changes its conformation and releases the drug on the other side. Drugs have been

Table 4.1	Variation in pK_a of drugs and pH of body fluids		
Variation in pK_a of drugs		**Variation in pH of body fluids**	
	Normal pK_a		**Normal pH**
Acidic drugs			
Aspirin	3.5	Gastric juices	1.0–3.0
Thiopental	7.6	Intestinal fluids	4.8–8.0
Ethosuximide	9.5	Blood	7.4
Basic drugs			
		Cerebrospinal fluid	7.2
Diazepam	3.3	Urine	6.0–7.4
Codeine	7.9		
Amphetamine	9.8		

pK_a, hydrogen ion dissociation constant.

Gastric juices pH 2.4   Plasma pH 7.4

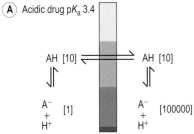

(A) Acidic drug pK_a 3.4

AH [10] ⇌ ⟶ AH [10]

A⁻ [1]   A⁻ [100000]
+   +
H⁺   H⁺

Ratio across membrane 1:9091

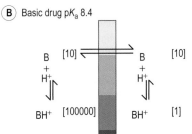

(B) Basic drug pK_a 8.4

B [10] ⇌ ⟶ B [10]
+   +
H⁺   H⁺

BH⁺ [100000]   BH⁺ [1]

Ratio across membrane 9091:1

AH – an acidic drug is less ionised in an acid medium, so that a large proportion of the drug is the lipid soluble, non-ionised form in the stomach (pH 2.4). The non-ionised form crosses the cell membrane by passive diffusion into the plasma.

AH – the acidic drug in the more alkaline medium in the plasm (pH 7.4) is more ionised. The ionised form cannot diffuse back in the opposite direction.

At equilibrium, the concentration of non-ionised drug will be the same on both sides of the membrane, but the total concentration on the plasma side will be 9091 times higher.

BH – a basic drug is more ionised in the acid medium (pH 2.4) of the stomach so that very little of the non-ionised form of the drug can be absorbed by passive diffusion into plasma.

BH – in plasma, the basic drug is less ionised in the more alkaline medium. A high concentration of the non-ionised drug potentially could diffuse out of the plasma into the stomach.

In gastric juices at pH 2.4, the degree of ionisation for an acidic drug (pK_a 3.4) is: 10
 • for every 10 non-ionised molecules there is 1 ionised molecule (ratio 10:1)

The same drug in plasma (pH 7.4), the degree of ionisation is: 10 000
 • for every 10 non-ionised molecules there are 100 000 ionised molecules.

The reverse happens for a basic drug.

Fig. 4.2 **Effect of pH partitioning on passive diffusion across the gastric cell membrane.**

developed to facilitate or inhibit transporter activity (see Clinical box 4.2 for examples).

Cells have two major classes of transmembrane proteins:

- Transporters (carrier proteins)
- Ion channel proteins.

Transporters (carrier proteins)

A given transporter is selective for a small group of related substrate molecules, which compete for the transporter. Protein transporters can be the sites of drug action, when the drug is similar to the substrate and competitively binds to the transporter. The process saturates when the number of drug molecules exceeds the number of transporter molecules. The drug then 'blocks' the action of the substrate (e.g. Na⁺, K⁺, neurotransmitter) on the cell.

Clinical box 4.1 **Therapeutic application of ion trapping: treatment of overdose**

Most drugs are excreted through the kidneys. If the pH gradient across the glomerular basement membrane can be increased, renal excretion is increased. This can be achieved by making the urine either more acid or more alkaline:
- Urinary acidification increases tubular excretion of weak bases and decreases excretion of weak acids
- Urinary alkalinisation accelerates the excretion of weak acids and slows down the excretion of weak bases.
  Therefore, in:
- **Aspirin overdose**: renal excretion of aspirin (weak acid) can be increased if urinary pH is increased (made more alkaline, i.e. basic) by the administration of sodium bicarbonate or a carbonic anhydrase inhibitor such as acetazolamide. Aspirin concentration in the more alkaline renal tubule could be increased fourfold.
- **Amphetamine overdose**: amphetamine is a weak base, so an acceleration in tubular excretion can be achieved by lowering urinary pH (making more acidic) by the administration of ammonium chloride.

Clinical box 4.2 **Drugs acting on protein transporters**

- Probenecid competes for the transporter associated with the reabsorption of uric acid from the lumen of the nephron (facilitated diffusion). The resulting increase in uric acid excretion is exploited in the treatment of gout, a painful joint disease caused by deposition of uric acid in joints.
- Probenecid also competes for the transporter that is involved in the renal excretion of penicillin; competition reduces penicillin excretion, which helps to maintain plasma concentration.
- Digoxin inhibits the Na⁺/K⁺ pump in the membrane of cardiac myocytes so that Na⁺ is retained in the cell. A related Na⁺/Ca²⁺ symporter slows down in response to Na⁺ retention. Intracellular Ca²⁺ increases, is stored, then released for muscle contraction.
- Omeprazole, a proton pump inhibitor of the benzimidazole group, irreversibly inhibits the H⁺/K⁺-ATPase pump (proton pump) in the last step in the pathway for acid secretion in the stomach. Omeprazole is prescribed for conditions in which excessive acid secretion causes gastritis, peptic ulceration and symptoms of gastro-oesophageal reflux (GORD).
- Amitriptyline and other tricyclic drugs used in the treatment of depression compete with norepinephrine (noradrenaline)/serotonin neuronal uptake transporters to produce their effects (see also The autonomic nervous system, below).

There are three classes of transporters (see Ch. 2):

- Uniporters
- Symporters
- Antiporters.

Uniporters are proteins of a specific size which allow specific compounds to be carried across the cell membrane, by **facilitated diffusion** down a concentration gradient, which does *not* require the expenditure of metabolic or electrochemical energy. **Ion channels** and glucose transporters are an example of uniporters where specific ions are allowed through. These are particularly important to the action of drugs (see below).

Symporters and antiporters are secondary active transporters, or **pumps**, requiring energy expenditure. Active transport can carry substances *against* a concentration gradient. Two substances are transported together across the cell membrane in the same direction by **symporters**, and in opposite directions (exchanged) by **antiporters**. For example, Na$^+$/K$^+$-ATPase is an antiporter ion pump, which removes 3 ions of Na$^+$ from the cytoplasm of the cell in exchange for 2 ions of K$^+$ using ATP as energy.

P-glycoproteins (PGPs) are antiporter transport proteins that use ATP to 'pump' noxious substances from cells. Recent research has shown that drugs may be expelled from cells in the same way. If this occurs in the gut lumen then bioavailability of an orally administered drug is reduced, and PGPs effectively 'block' absorption. Some cancer cells overproduce PGPs, driving out anti-cancer drugs, effectively causing 'resistance'.

Ion channel proteins

Ion channel proteins are large proteins forming water-filled pores that span the lipid bilayer of cell membranes. These pores, or channels, allow ions of appropriate size and charge, that otherwise cannot permeate cell membranes, to be transferred across. The flux, or flow, of ions can be into or out of the cell.

All ion channel proteins allow solutes to cross membranes by facilitated diffusion without energy expenditure. The channel, or pore structure, is either open or closed and the conformational change is called gating.

- With uncharged solutes, facilitated diffusion takes place down a concentration gradient without the expenditure of energy.
- If the solute carries a net charge then both its concentration gradient and the membrane potential influence the transport process. The concentration gradient and the membrane potential combine to produce the net driving force known as the **electrochemical gradient**.

ENDOCYTOSIS AND EXOCYTOSIS

Very large molecules (macromolecules), such as proteins, cannot be transported across the cell membrane by transporters, and have to be taken into or out of the cells through the processes of endocytosis and exocytosis. These are the most complex method of transport across a biological membrane (see Ch. 2). Drugs can facilitate or inhibit these processes.

- **Endocytosis**: a substance gains entry into a cell by first being captured into an invagination of the cell wall, which is then pinched off as a vesicle. The drug thus enters the cell without having to cross the cell membrane (e.g. botulinum toxin).
- **Exocytosis**: membrane-coated vesicles fuse with the plasma membrane to release their contents into the extracellular compartment, e.g. neuronal synapse (see Ch. 2). Examples are the vesicles associated with the storage of neurotransmitters (norepinephrine, acetylcholine) and with pancreatic enzymes (see later).

DIFFUSION THROUGH AQUEOUS AND INTERCELLULAR PORES

Most biological membranes are relatively permeable to water that passes across the cell membrane via **aqueous pores**, either by diffusion or by bulk flow that results from osmotic differences across the membrane, carrying extremely small, water-soluble molecules with a mass of less than 100 daltons with it (e.g. lithium, urea, ethanol).

Gap junctions

Junctions between cells (intercellular pores) may allow the transfer of free, not protein bound, drug molecules in solution, a process known as **filtration**. These junctions are known as **gap junctions**. Other junctions prevent the transfer of molecules, and are known as **tight junctions**.

The ability of drugs to penetrate the endothelial membrane varies from one tissue to another. Gap junctions in vascular endothelium allow bulk transfer of drug molecules free in solution but not those bound to plasma proteins. In contrast, in the blood–brain barrier and the placenta, the capillary membranes are tightly joined together with only a few tight junctions, so that drugs can only pass through the membrane either by passive diffusion (lipid soluble molecules) or carrier-mediated transport. In the liver, the capillary endothelium is porous, allowing for free passage of large molecules.

DRUG DISTRIBUTION

Depending on pH, ionisation and lipid solubility, drugs can be moved for short distances by diffusion and membrane transport. Rapid transport over long distances around the body has to be done in the bloodstream, partly in solution as **free** (unbound) drug and partly **bound** to blood components (plasma proteins, blood cells). The bound and unbound forms are in **equilibrium**, and *only* the unbound drug is available for passive diffusion from the bloodstream to tissue sites where the pharmacological effects occur.

Drug distribution is the process by which a drug is transferred from the bloodstream (plasma) to tissues (interstitial fluid and cells). The rate and degree of drug distribution throughout the body depends on:

- Blood flow
- Capillary permeability
- Protein binding (affinity of the drug for various constituents of cells)
- Accumulation in and redistribution to other sites.

BLOOD FLOW

The rate at which a drug reaches different organs and tissues depends on the blood flow to those regions. Equilibration of free drug between plasma and tissue is rapidly achieved in well-perfused tissues, for example the liver, kidneys, brain and skeletal muscle. Equilibrium in poorly perfused tissues, such as fat (adipose tissue), takes much longer.

CAPILLARY PERMEABILITY AND GAP JUNCTIONS

The ability of drugs to leave plasma and enter the interstitial fluid is determined by their physico-chemical properties (e.g. lipid solubility and ionisation) and via intercellular pores, the **gap junctions**, in the vascular endothelium. Gap junctions can be 4–10 nm in diameter, i.e. wide enough to allow the passage of ionised water-soluble drugs, even those as large as albumin, into the interstitial fluid. The capillaries in the liver are extremely permeable, with gap junctions that allow the passage of large protein molecules, whereas the vascular epithelium to the brain is the opposite, so that only drugs that are highly lipid soluble or have a selective transporter can enter the CNS.

Drug distribution to special organs

Central nervous system

Many drugs cannot gain access to the brain because of the **blood–brain barrier**. By virtue of tight junctions, much reduced number of aqueous pores in the cell membrane, the blood–brain barrier only allows drugs that are lipid soluble (e.g. thiopental, a general anaesthetic) or have a selective transporter protein (e.g. L-dopa for Parkinsonism) to enter the CNS. However, inflammation of the capillary epithelial layer, for example in meningitis, may increase the permeability of the blood–brain barrier and allow charged or polar drugs to attain therapeutic concentrations; this is exploited in the use of penicillin in the treatment of meningitis.

Foetus

Lipid soluble drugs given to the pregnant mother can cross the placental barrier to the foetus by passive diffusion. Some drugs need active transport. Large, highly ionised molecules (e.g. heparin) do not cross the placental barrier easily. Compared with well-perfused organs such as liver and lungs, the placental circulation is slow, equilibrates slowly with maternal blood, and relies on maternal elimination for drug excretion. Although foetal plasma concentration of the drug will be much lower than in maternal blood, the foetus could still be affected:

- Serious foetal abnormalities can develop if the foetus is exposed during the first trimester, when the brain and major organs are developing. Thalidomide (α-phthalimido-glutarimide), marketed as Distaval and used to relieve symptoms of nausea in early pregnancy, caused an epidemic of severe birth defects.
- Toxic effects during the second and third trimesters are similar to those in the mother, but are exaggerated: tetracyclines can affect developing teeth and bones, warfarin can damage foetal brain.
- Drugs of addiction such as heroin or cocaine have a profound effect on the foetus, as can alcohol and nicotine (cigarette smoking).
- Drugs given just before delivery, e.g. analgesics and tranquillisers, can cause respiratory impairment in the newborn.

ACCUMULATION OF DRUG IN FAT AND REDISTRIBUTION IN OTHER TISSUES

When a drug is administered directly into the bloodstream, as in intravenous injection, the drug will rapidly reach well-perfused tissues, such as brain, liver and lungs, to reach equilibrium at high tissue concentrations. The drug will also be transported to, and enter, poorly perfused tissues, but

---

| Information box 4.2 | Termination of the action of thiopental |

Thiopental, a highly lipid-soluble general anaesthetic, achieves equilibrium and a therapeutically effective concentration in the CNS in a matter of seconds. In muscle, which has a lower blood flow, it takes about 30 minutes to achieve equilibrium, and in adipose tissue it takes 4–8 hours. Thus, when the concentration of thiopental in the brain has reached equilibrium and may be declining due to redistribution, tissue concentration in muscle and adipose tissue is still rising. Thiopental will diffuse out of the brain to be redistributed to adipose tissue, lowering the concentration in the brain. The general anaesthetic effect of thiopental is terminated by redistribution of the drug into adipose tissue and not through metabolism.

---

at a slower rate, lowering the plasma concentration. If the concentration gradient between plasma and well-perfused tissue reverses, the drug will diffuse back into plasma for redistribution to poorly perfused tissues, terminating the action of the drug in well-perfused tissue (see Information box 4.2).

Fat, or adipose tissue, is poorly perfused. A few, highly soluble drugs can accumulate in body fat. Of importance to long-term administration are drugs such as benzodiazepine and some insecticides (e.g. DDT). The accumulation of long-acting benzodiazepine (e.g. diazepam) and their subsequent release can give cumulative effects. Other drugs such as the general anaesthetic, thiopentone, can have their action terminated by accumulation in adipose tissue.

BINDING OF DRUGS TO PROTEINS

At therapeutic plasma concentrations, many drugs bind extensively to plasma and intracellular proteins. This limits the amount of drug available for distribution outside the bloodstream. The protein-bound drug molecules cannot permeate cell membranes, be metabolised, excreted or produce their effect.

- Drug–protein complex has no pharmacological effect
- Protein binding lowers the plasma free drug concentration
- Protein binding reduces the amount of drug available for acting on receptors.

The major plasma proteins that bind drugs are **albumin**, **γ-globulin lipoproteins** and **α₁-acidic glycoprotein**. There are also binding sites on intracellular proteins. The ionic binding between drug and protein is competitive and readily reversible so that the protein acts as a reservoir for the drug. As the drug is eliminated, the ratio between bound and unbound drug is maintained by more drug dissociating from the proteins.

The degree of protein binding depends upon the drug and varies from almost 100% (warfarin, diazepam) to less than 30% (digoxin) (Table 4.2). This difference is of clinical importance because of its effect on the duration of action of the drug after administration. As the intracellular concentration of free drug falls, the drug will dissociate from its protein-binding site, sustaining drug concentration. If the proportion of bound drug is high, then a higher concentration of free drug will be maintained for longer, so that dosing intervals have to be adjusted to avoid overdose.

Table 4.2	Examples of drugs that bind to plasma albumin		
Drug (chemical class)	% of drug bound	% of occupied binding sites on proteins	
Warfarin (acid)	99.5	<1	
Diazepam (base)	99	<1	
Digitoxin (neutral)	90–97	<1	
Propranolol (base)*	90–96	<1	
Phenytoin (acid)	90–94	<1	
Amitriptyline (base)*	82–96	<1	
Sodium valproate (acid)	80–90	50–60	
Imipramine (base)	80–95	<1	
Lidocaine (base)*	45–80	<1	
Salicylate (acid)	50–90	50	
Phenobarbital (acid)	50–60	<1	
Digoxin (neutral)	20	<1	
Lithium (ion)	0	<1	

*Also bind to α_1-acid glycoprotein. The majority of drugs occupy less than 1% of the binding sites available to them. Drugs that occupy 50% or more of binding sites may induce displacement of other drugs.

Competitive protein binding

Competition for binding sites can take place between drugs and between drugs and endogenous ligands. A drug with a high affinity for protein-binding sites (e.g. aspirin) can saturate its binding sites at therapeutic concentrations. This will displace a less highly bound drug (e.g. warfarin) from its binding site, increasing the concentration of free drug (see Clinical box 4.3). If drug A is 98% bound then only 2% of this drug is available to give its therapeutic effect. If the binding is reduced to 96% through displacement by a second drug, the plasma concentration of drug A is doubled.

The importance of competitive interactions may sometimes be overstated because the number of binding sites occupied by any one of the majority of drugs is only a small fraction of the total available for binding that molecule (i.e. the binding sites are not saturated).

Hypoproteinaemia

If the number of protein-binding sites in plasma are reduced, for example due to hypoalbuminaemia, drugs that are normally present in a predominantly bound form will be present in the free form at an elevated concentration, so that their therapeutic effect will be increased and drug dosages need to be adjusted to avoid adverse effects.

Clinical box 4.3	Aspirin potentiates the action of warfarin

Aspirin (salicylate), a non-steroidal anti-inflammatory drug, is highly protein bound, where up to 90% of the drug is bound, and occupies over 50% of the protein-binding sites. If warfarin is administered at the same time, the aspirin molecules will displace warfarin molecules so that less warfarin is protein bound, making more free warfarin available to exert its anticoagulant effect, thus 'potentiating' the effect of a given dose of warfarin. Spontaneous bruising, haematoma and prolonged bleeding after minor trauma will occur.

Information box 4.3	Consequences of drug sequestration

The antimalarial drug chloroquine only needs to be taken once per week: because of its binding to DNA, drug concentration in liver and white blood cells is several thousand times higher than its concentration in plasma. The sequestered drug in the liver and white cells is slowly released into the circulation as plasma concentration falls due to metabolism and excretion, prolonging the action and duration of chloroquine in the body.
- **'Bone seekers'** such as fluoride and strontium-90 may be deposited with bone salts in an insoluble form, making them difficult to remove. Fluoride deposition in teeth benefits mineralisation and prevents dental caries. Strontium-90, however, is harmful and can cause leukaemia.
- **Calcium chelators**, such as tetracyclines, are deposited with bone salts in an insoluble form, making them difficult to remove. Deposition in developing teeth causes discoloration. Tetracyclines should not be prescribed for pregnant women or young children.

Hypoalbuminaemia can occur as a consequence of liver disease, nephrotic syndrome, malnutrition, burns and renal failure, when less albumin is available to bind drugs. This is particularly important in elderly people, when dosages may have to be reduced to avoid overdose.

Sequestration of drugs in tissues

In addition to protein binding, a drug may bind to and accumulate within tissues, prolonging its duration in the body. This is because the stored (sequestered) drug is in equilibrium with drug in plasma, so as the drug is eliminated from the body, sequestered drug moves into plasma from the storage tissue (see Information box 4.3). However, the binding between the drug and the tissue element may be so stable that the drug may not be readily available for release.

DISTRIBUTION OF DRUGS IN THE BODY

Distribution is the pharmacokinetic stage in which a drug in the plasma is transferred to tissues to exert its therapeutic action. Once a drug enters the body, it can be distributed between four major aqueous compartments (Fig. 4.3), separated by barriers composed of cell membranes:

- Plasma
- Interstitial
- Intracellular
- Transcellular.

Total body water, as a percentage of body weight, varies from approximately 50% to 75%, depending on age and sex. Women tend to have lower body water due to increased body fat.

Drug molecules also exist in free and protein-bound forms. Therefore, in each aqueous compartment, drug molecules may be:

- Free in aqueous solution or bound to protein
- In ionised and non-ionised form in equilibrium.

The degree of ionisation of free drug depends on whether the drug is a weak acid or weak base (pK_a value) and on the pH of the aqueous compartment.

Typical volumes of fluid compartments
in a 70 kg man

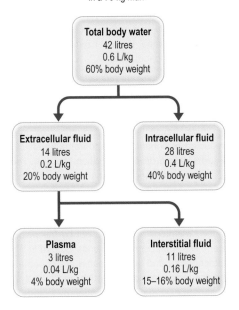

Fig. 4.3 **The approximate distribution of body fluids in a 30-year-old man weighing 70 kg.** (Expressed as total volume (L), volume per kg body weight (L/kg) and percentage of body weight.)

Body water is distributed between three major compartments:

- **Extracellular fluid** (20% of body weight) composed of:
  – blood plasma (4–5% of body weight)
  – interstitial fluid (16% of body weight)
  – lymph (1%).
- **Intracellular fluid** (30–40% of body weight), the total amount of fluid in all the cells of the body.
- **Transcellular fluid** which includes synovial, cerebrospinal, peritoneal, pleural and intraocular fluids. These constitute approximately 2.5% of the total body weight.

Extent of drug distribution into aqueous compartments

Free drug is distributed between the four major aqueous compartments of the body, but most drugs are not exclusively associated with any one. The majority of drugs are:

- Distributed into a number of aqueous compartments
- Bound to cellular components, such as protein
- Dissolved into lipid stores.

The **pattern**, or extent of drug distribution into the compartments depends on:

- Permeability across cell membranes
- Protein binding within compartments
- pH partitioning
- Accumulation in adipose tissue.

The estimated amount of drug that is distributed from plasma to other aqueous compartments is important, because the pharmacological effects of drugs are exerted in the interstitial, intracellular and transcellular compartments.

- Some drugs remain in the plasma because their molecules are too big to cross capillary membranes into tissues (e.g. heparin)
- Highly protein-bound drugs tend to remain in the plasma.

The amount of drug needed to reach a plasma concentration that enables adequate distribution to effector tissues depends on the extent of distribution from plasma. This will determine the therapeutic **dosage** that needs to be administered.

The concept of an apparent volume of distribution is an estimate of the extent of drug distribution from plasma to effector tissues.

Apparent volume of distribution

While it is possible to measure drug concentration in total body water in animal experiments, only plasma concentration is measurable in humans, as tissue biopsies merely to measure drug concentration would be impossible. The **apparent volume of distribution** measures the concentration of free and protein-bound drug remaining in the plasma after distribution is completed, and is used to predict distribution of the drug in the various compartments of the body.

The apparent volume of distribution of a drug is a calculated volume of fluid containing the total amount of drug in the body at the same concentration as plasma concentration, expressed as the ratio of the total dose of drug to plasma concentration and reflecting the amount of drug left in the plasma after distribution. It does *not* indicate where and how much drug has been taken up by effector tissues.

Apparent volume of distribution does have pharmacological importance. It:

- Gives an estimate of total drug in the body in relation to plasma concentration, and the concept is useful for monitoring progress when treating drug toxicity and overdose
- Is related to drug clearance from the body (see later), and indicates the overall rate of drug elimination and thus the drug half-life (see below)
- Can predict tissue drug concentration from the above two estimates.

DRUG METABOLISM

Drug metabolism is the process by which the body produces a change to the chemical structure of a drug molecule by enzyme activity to produce a new chemical with different pharmacological properties. Metabolic processes determine how long a drug is active in the body, drug interactions and toxicity.

The outcomes of drug metabolism may be:

- To produce metabolites with less biological activity
- To produce **active metabolites** that may be more potent and persist longer than the parent compound
- To convert an **inactive pro-drug** to the active form
- To produce toxic metabolites
- To produce inactive metabolites that are water soluble for excretion (by conjugation, see below)

The liver is the major organ for drug metabolism. After absorption from the gastrointestinal tract, orally administered drugs pass through the liver via the portal vein before distribution to other organs. The liver may extensively metabolise and inactivate some drugs. This is the concept of first pass metabolism (see later), which can make a difference to how much of the administered drug reaches the target tissues.

Metabolic reactions for drugs are classified as:

- **Phase I reactions**, or pre-conjugation consisting of oxidation, reduction and hydrolysis reactions followed by
- **Phase II reactions**, consisting mainly of conjugation but also including acetylation reactions.

These reactions are not always sequential. The enzymes involved in both phases have low substrate specificities and can metabolise a wide range of drugs. They are associated with the following cell constituents:

- Smooth endoplasmic reticulum (where the enzymes are called microsomal enzymes)
- Cytoplasm
- Mitochondria.

PHASE I METABOLIC REACTIONS (PRE-CONJUGATION REACTIONS)

Phase I reactions – oxidation, reduction, hydrolysis – mainly take place in the liver and are mediated by **microsomal enzymes**. The collective term, the **mixed function oxidase (MFO) system**, is used to describe the hepatic microsomal enzymes involved in phase I reactions.

Oxidation

Oxidation is the most important of the phase I reactions, mainly catalysed by microsomal enzymes.

Microsomal oxidation reactions

There are two types of microsomal oxidation reaction:

- One in which an oxygen molecule is added to the substrate
- One in which the primary oxidation leads to a loss of the oxygen atom in a small fragment of the original molecule – e.g. **deamination** and **dealkylation**.

Microsomal oxidation reactions require:

- Molecular oxygen
- NADPH (nicotinamide adenosine dinucleotide phosphate (reduced form))
- NADPH-cytochrome c reductase
- The haemoprotein cytochrome P450 mono-oxygenase enzymes that bind both the drug and O_2 molecules.

Cytochrome P450 system

Cytochrome P450 is the most important enzyme system in the diverse group of enzymes that catalyse oxidation in humans. They are so named because cytochrome P450 reacts with carbon monoxide to produce a pink (P) complex with an absorption peak at 450 nm.

The cytochrome P450 system is a superfamily of related but distinct microsomal liver enzymes, subject to genetic variation (see below). Although drug metabolism by cytochrome P450 takes place mainly in the liver, the enzyme also occurs elsewhere in the body, for example in the small intestine. These enzymes also take part in the biosynthesis of endogenous substances such as arachidonic acid, steroids, prostaglandins, cholesterol and thromboxane (made by platelets causing vasoconstriction and platelet adhesion).

For human beings, cytochrome P450 enzymes are named as CYP in capitals (human), subsequent number (the isoform family), subsequent letter (the subfamily), and final number (the individual gene product in the subfamily). Table 4.3 lists examples of cytochrome P450 isoenzymes. These enzymes differ from each other because of:

- Difference in amino acid sequence
- Specificity for the drugs that they metabolise
- The drugs that can inhibit or induce them.

Some drugs cause enzyme induction or inhibition, thereby reducing or enhancing the therapeutic effect of another, co-administered drug (Information box 4.4). These effects are discussed further in relation to enzyme induction and inhibition.

Non-microsomal oxidative reactions

Not all phase I reactions are carried out by the cytochrome P450 system. Non-microsomal enzymes located in the cytoplasm, mitochondria and in the plasma are capable of oxidation and the less common reduction and hydrolysis (see below). Important examples for drug therapy include:

- The soluble liver cytoplasmic enzyme, **alcohol dehydrogenase**, metabolises alcohol to acetaldehyde, which is further metabolised by aldehyde dehydrogenase to acetic acid (in addition to CYP2E1).
- **Xanthine oxidase** – also located in liver cytoplasm is important in the metabolism of purines to produce uric acid. Excessive accumulation of uric acid in joints leads to gout.

Information box 4.4 **Examples of enzyme induction and inhibition**

- Some anticonvulsants (e.g. phenytoin) and rifampicin induce cytochrome P450 enzymes, which increase the rate of metabolism and thus reduce the therapeutic effect of warfarin if administered at the same time. Patients on anticoagulant therapy being prescribed rifampicin or phenytoin will need a higher dose of warfarin.
- Cytochrome P450 enzyme induction by rifampicin (and phenytoin) also increases the metabolism of oestrogens so that the efficacy of the combined oral contraceptive pill is reduced. Breakthrough bleeding or contraceptive failure may occur. Patients prescribed rifampicin (or anticonvulsants) need to be warned about this effect and advised to use alternative contraception.
- Components of grapefruit juice inhibit CYP3A4, slowing down the metabolism of substrates that use the same enzyme, such as simvastatin and atorvastatin, leading to elevated blood levels. The effect on calcium channel blockers, used for the treatment of angina, leads to elevated plasma levels with potentially disastrous consequences, such as hypotension and asystole.
- Grapefruit juice also enhances the effects of some antihistamines such as terfenadine, by inhibiting the action of CYP3A4 in the gut, reducing the breakdown of the drug and increasing bioavailability. Hay fever sufferers taking terfenadine should be cautioned about drinking grapefruit juice because they might become excessively drowsy, risking accidents when driving a car or operating machinery.
- Grapefruit juice is associated with a reduction in blood level of some drugs. This has been attributed to an interaction with p-glycoproteins in the gut, which pumps the drug out of the cells into the lumen, thus reducing absorption. Further research is needed to explain this phenomenon.

Table 4.3 Examples of drugs and their interaction with the isoenzymes of cytochrome P450*

Isoenzyme	Substrate	Inducer	Inhibitor
CYP1A2	Paracetamol	Barbiturates	Cimetidine
	Amitriptyline		Erythromycin
	Clozapine	Nicotine	Grapefruit juice
	Diazepam		Diltiazem
	Methadone	Polycyclic aromatic hydrocarbons found in cigarette smoke and in the charred parts of charcoal-grilled meats	
	Caffeine		
	Calcium channel antagonists		
	Antihistamines		
	Tamoxifen		
CYP2B6	Tamoxifen	Phenobarbital	Orphenadrine
	Cyclophosphamide	Phenytoin	
CYP2C8	Diazepam	Phenobarbital	Omeprazole
	Diclofenac	Primidone	
	Tolbutamide		
CYP2C9	Amitriptyline	Carbamazepine	Amiodarone
	Diclofenac	Rifampicin	Cimetidine
	Indometacin		Fluvoxamine
	Phenytoin		
	Warfarin		
CYP2C19	Omeprazole	Barbiturates	Fluoxetine
	Phenytoin		Tolbutamide
	Valproic acid		
CYP3A4†	Amiodarone	Carbamazepine	Cimetidine
	Tamoxifen	Glucocorticoids	Diltiazem
	Paracetamol	Phenytoin	Omeprazole
	Diazepam	Rifampicin	Quinidine
	Dexamethasone		
	Imipramine		
	Oestrogens		
CYP2E1	Paracetamol	Ethanol	Disulfiram
	Enflurane	Isoniazid	Ritonavir
	Ethanol		
	Isoniazid		

*Drugs given in italics are substrates for a number of the isoenzymes.
†Involved in the metabolism of 50% of all drugs.

- **Allopurinol** – metabolised by xanthine oxidase, but also a competitive inhibitor of xanthine oxidase. This characteristic is exploited in the use of allopurinol in the treatment of gout to reduce uric acid production.
- **Tyrosine hydroxylase** and **tryptophan hydroxylase** are important neuronal cytoplasmic enzymes (see The autonomic nervous system, below). Tyrosine hydroxylase oxidises the amino acid tyrosine to levodopa in the sequence of reactions during the synthesis of the neurotransmitter norepinephrine (see later). Tryptophan hydroxylase catalyses the oxidation of tryptophan in the synthesis of 5-hydroxytryptamine (5-HT, serotonin).
- Mitochondrial **monoamine oxidase** (MAO) is important in the metabolism of catecholamines, some sympathomimetic amines and 5-HT. Dietary 5-HT is completely metabolised by MAO in the intestines and liver (first pass metabolism, see below). MAO also metabolises 5-HT in the neuron (see The autonomic nervous system).

Reduction

Reduction is much less common, or important, than oxidation in drug metabolism, and can be performed by body tissues or intestinal flora. The enzymes catalysing reduction include both cytochrome P450 and cytochrome P450 reductase.

Hydrolysis – hydroxylation

Hydrolysis reactions involve the addition of a water (H_2O) molecule to the drug, and the process splits the drug. The reaction takes place in plasma, not mitochondria. This can occur spontaneously because of unstable groups in the drug molecule, or be catalysed by enzymes capable of hydrolysing amide and ester bonds in many drugs (Information box 4.5). Intestinal flora can also hydrolyse drug molecules, when metabolites are excreted in the bile or faeces.

A number of non-specific esterases and amidases are present in the endoplasmic reticulum of cells of the liver, intestine and kidneys, and in blood and other tissues. The

- Cholinesterase, which is found in plasma as well as in the cytoplasm of cholinergic neurons, is important in the termination of action of acetylcholine and a wide variety of drugs
- Pethidine (US meperidine), an opiate analgesic, is de-esterified by a membrane bound microsomal esterase to meperidinic acid
- Procaine, a local anaesthetic, is metabolised by both plasma pseudocholinesterase and a liver microsomal esterase
- Suxamethonium, a neuromuscular blocker, is predominantly hydrolysed by plasma pseudocholinesterase.

alcohol and amine groups exposed following the hydrolysis of esters and amides are suitable for conjugation (phase II metabolism, see below), inactivating the drug and making it water soluble for excretion.

PHASE II METABOLIC REACTIONS (CONJUGATION REACTIONS)

Phase II reactions, known as **conjugation**, involve the synthesis of a covalent bond between a highly polar, normal substance in the body (endogenous) with a phase I metabolite or sometimes with the parent drug. Energy is needed for synthesising the bond. The conjugate is a less lipid-soluble, more water-soluble compound that is readily excreted in urine and/or bile and nearly always pharmacologically inactive. There are, however, exceptions, e.g. morphine 6-glucuronide has greater analgesic potency than the parent compound morphine.

Conjugation by glucuronidation

The most important phase II reaction is **glucuronidation**, when a molecule of glucuronic acid is transferred to the drug molecule. This is catalysed by microsomal uridine diphosphate (UDP)-glucuronyltransferase.

Other conjugation reactions

Other phase II reactions are catalysed by enzymes in the cytoplasm:

- **Sulphate conjugation,** catalysed by sulfotransferase
- **Methylation,** catalysed by transmethylase and
- **Acetylation,** catalysed by *N*-acetyltransferase.

Acetylation, in contrast to other forms of conjugation, sometimes produces metabolites that are less water soluble than the original substance. For example, the acetyl metabolites of some of the earlier sulphonamides (a class of antibacterial agents) produced crystalluria because they were precipitated in the renal tubules.

Drug detoxification

Conjugation with **glutathione** represents a major detoxification pathway for a number of drugs. Glutathione conjugates are cleaved to give cysteine derivatives, which in turn are acetylated to produce mercapturic acids. Many of the substrates for the enzyme glutathione-*S*-transferase are reactive metabolites, and depletion of the endogenous hepatic stores of glutathione can result in hepatotoxicity (Information box 4.6).

Although conjugation is a major detoxification pathway for many drugs, some reactions produce metabolites that are more toxic than the parent drug.

Paracetamol (US acetaminophen) undergoes conjugation with sulphate or glucuronide. However, in a phase I reaction, it is also metabolised by the P450 mixed function oxidase to produce a reactive metabolite (*N*-acetyl-*p*-benzoquinone imine). This reactive metabolite then interacts with glutathione to produce mercapturic acid. In paracetamol overdoses, glutathione eventually becomes depleted. The reactive metabolite accumulates and interacts with cellular proteins causing hepatotoxicity and nephrotoxicity, resulting in cell death in the liver and kidneys.

FACTORS AFFECTING DRUG METABOLISM

The ability of an individual to metabolise a drug can be influenced by a variety of factors including genetic factors, age, sex and disease. Exposure to a drug or environmental chemicals causing induction or inhibition of the enzymes associated with metabolism will also affect the way that patients metabolise drugs. These factors have an impact on the therapeutic effect of the drug and potential drug interactions that can give rise to adverse side effects, overdose and toxicity.

Genetic factors

When known, differences in the expression of metabolic enzymes in different groups of people need to be taken into account when prescribing. There is genetic variation in the ability of unrelated individuals to metabolise drugs. Most of the metabolic enzymes are under polygenic control. For some enzymes, however, there is polymorphism at a single gene. Although there is a 'normal' (Gaussian) distribution of enzyme activity in the general population, some people are 'fast' and some 'slow' metabolisers.

The earliest example to be identified of polymorphism at a single gene is the fast and slow acetylation of isoniazid (antituberculous drug). **Slow acetylator** status is an autosomal recessive trait that shows a race-dependent distribution. It is found in about 60% of Europeans but in only 5% of the Japanese population. Clinically, slow acetylators are more likely to develop peripheral neuropathies with isoniazid. Procainamide (used in cardiac arrhythmia) and hydralazine (antihypertensive) show a similar pattern of 'slow' metabolism. Slow metabolisers will show a high concentration of the parent drug with lower concentrations of metabolites.

Environmental contaminants and drugs

The activity of drug metabolising enzymes can be induced (increased) or inhibited (decreased) by chemicals contained in environmental contaminants and drugs.

- Organochlorine insecticides (e.g. DDT)
- Organophosphate pesticides (e.g. sheep dip)
- Polycyclic aromatic hydrocarbons (contained in cigarette smoke and the charred parts of char-grilled [broiled] meat)
- Alcohol in chronic alcohol consumption.

Enzyme induction

Repeated exposure of the liver to certain lipid-soluble substances can cause an increase in microsomal enzyme activity by increasing the de novo synthesis of cytochrome P450 enzymes – **enzyme induction**. Examples of inducers of specific cytochrome P450 enzymes are given in Table 4.3.

Induction can be non-specific: for example, phenobarbital and rifampicin are non-selective inducers that act on a number of cytochrome P450 families (CYP1, 2 and 3). In contrast, chronic ethanol consumption induces a specific isoenzyme, CYP2E1. Enzyme induction has clinically important effects (Clinical box 4.4).

Induction by broad-spectrum inducers of cytochrome P450, such as phenobarbital, leads to:

- Hepatic hypertrophy, proliferation of smooth endoplasmic reticulum
- Increased protein and phospholipid synthesis
- Increased synthesis of cytochrome P450 isoenzymes and NADPH cytochrome P450 reductase.

The induction occurs over a period of time (weeks) and is slowly reversible after the cessation of the drug. The mechanism of induction is not fully understood.

Enzyme inhibition

Enzyme inhibition slows down the metabolism of a drug so that it persists for longer periods in the body. Most cytochrome P450 enzymes that metabolise drugs are not very specific. A single enzyme is usually capable of metabolising several different drugs, and two or more enzymes with overlapping substrate specificities can contribute to the metabolism of a single compound. As a result, two or more drugs may *compete* for the active site of a single cytochrome P450 enzyme, interfering with the normal metabolism of a co-administered drug or endogenous compound. For example, imidazole-containing drugs, such as cimetidine (a histamine (H$_2$) receptor antagonist), bind competitively to a number of cytochrome P450 enzymes, reducing the metabolism of endogenous steroids and co-administered drugs such as warfarin, phenytoin, quinidine. Plasma levels of these drugs will be elevated, and may contribute to adverse reactions or toxicity.

Enzyme inhibition by metabolites

Metabolites of cytochrome P450 can form a complex with the enzyme that inactivates the enzyme. This process is reversible. Another form of enzyme inhibition, known as 'suicide' inhibition, is irreversible. A reactive metabolite of cytochrome P450 binds to the enzyme and destroys it. Furthermore, a drug may be an inhibitor of a specific cytochrome P450 enzyme without necessarily being a substrate for that enzyme. For example, quinidine is a potent inhibitor of CYP2D6 but is metabolised by CYP3A4.

CONVERSION OF INACTIVE PRO-DRUG TO ACTIVE METABOLITE

Some drugs are inactive pro-drugs, only becoming therapeutically active after metabolism (Clinical box 4.5). The inactive pro-drug is sometimes designed to bypass problems with drug administration (see later).

EXCRETION OF DRUGS AND METABOLITES

Water-soluble drugs may be excreted unchanged, whereas metabolic inactivation makes drugs more soluble for excretion. The main routes of excretion for drugs and their metabolites are via:

- The renal system
- The hepatic/biliary system
- The lungs: this route is important in the excretion of gaseous anaesthetics; the lungs also have a role in the biotransformation of prostaglandins (see Ch. 13).

Losses of drugs via sweat and milk play only a small part in the overall excretion of drugs. However, excretion in milk is important because of the potential exposure of the breastfed infant.

RENAL SYSTEM

Although the renal system is fully discussed in Chapter 14, renal functions concerned with drug excretion will be discussed here. Figure 4.4 is a schematic representation of

---

Clinical box 4.4   **Clinical importance of enzyme induction**

Induction of a specific cytochrome P450 will increase the metabolism of its substrate drugs; this will reduce the amount of drug that is available to give a therapeutic effect.

This is an important consideration in prescribing drugs that induce liver metabolic enzymes: dosages of other medication, e.g. oral contraceptives and antibiotics, may need adjustment. Alternative methods for contraception will be needed.

Examples

Rifampicin, phenobarbital and many anticonvulsant drugs used in the treatment of epilepsy increase the rate of metabolism of a wide range of drugs (e.g. phenytoin, warfarin, oral contraceptives). Their own rate of drug metabolism also increases, thereby reducing their therapeutic effectiveness.

The measurement of serum levels of hepatic enzymes is used as an indicator of liver disease. An elevated serum γ-glutamyl transpeptidase (γ-GT, a hydrolysing enzyme) could be an early sign of either alcohol- or drug-related liver enzyme induction.

Clinical box 4.5   **Examples of pro-drugs designed for bypassing problems with drug administration**

- Olsalazine, a member of the sulfasalazine family of drugs used to treat inflammatory bowel disease, is a pro-drug. Olsalazine is inactive until metabolised by colonic bacteria in the distal colon, the desired site of action.
- Azathioprine, an immunosuppressant drug, is inactive until metabolised to mercaptopurine. It is well absorbed in the gastrointestinal tract, so oral administration would not damage the intestinal mucosa.
- Enalapril, an angiotensin-converting enzyme (ACE) inhibitor used in the treatment of hypertension, has to be hydrolysed to enalaprilat to become active.
- Cortisone and prednisone are inactive pro-drugs that have to be converted to hydrocortisone and prednisolone respectively, in vivo, to be become active drugs.
- Cyclophosphamide, a cytotoxic agent, only becomes active after metabolism in the liver. Therefore, cyclophosphamide can be orally administered as the pro-drug that should not damage the intestinal mucosa.

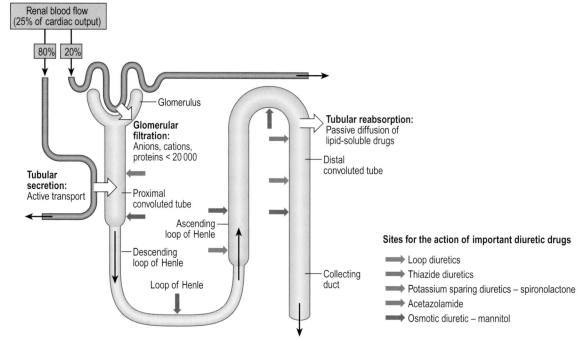

Fig. 4.4 **Renal excretion systems.**

the renal tubular system, where renal excretion mainly takes place. The processes are:

- Glomerular filtration
- Tubular secretion
- Tubular reabsorption.

Glomerular filtration

Drugs and metabolites are excreted via renal glomeruli by filtration. The kidneys are highly perfused organs and receive about 25% of cardiac output of which 20% is filtered (180 L/day) to produce the initial urine. Glomerular capillaries allow the filtration of molecules with a molecular weight of below 20000, irrespective of whether they are anions or cations, ionised or non-ionised. Plasma proteins, which have a molecular weight of 68000 or more, and protein-bound drugs are not normally filtered. Therefore protein binding of drugs significantly affects their elimination via glomerular filtration.

Tubular secretion

Tubular secretion takes place in the proximal renal tubules, where the 80% of the renal blood flow that is not filtered by the glomerulus passes through to the peritubular capillaries of the proximal convoluted tubule. Here the tubule removes a wide variety of substances from plasma into the lumen of the tubule through **active transport** *against* a concentration gradient – tubular secretion. In the proximal tubule there are two non-specific carrier-mediated transport processes:

- A cation transporter for weak bases (e.g. quinine, morphine)
- An anion transporter for weak acids (e.g. penicillin, furosemide).

These two processes are rapid and saturable. In contrast to glomerular filtration, protein binding of the drug has no effect on drug clearance via tubular secretion. The affinity

of drugs for the transporter is greater than that of the drug for plasma protein and results in maximum drug clearance. Substances that are transported by the same transporter compete with each other, resulting in drug interactions (Clinical box 4.6)

Tubular reabsorption

Tubular reabsorption of drugs takes place in the distal convoluted tubules of the kidney. There are specific transporters in the nephron for the reabsorption of essential constituents of tubular filtrate (e.g. amino acids, glucose, vitamins, water), but only very rarely are drugs reabsorbed in this way. The majority of drugs that are reabsorbed are lipid soluble and pass through the distal convoluted tubule membranes by passive diffusion.

The urine is concentrated during its passage to the distal convoluted tubule as water is reabsorbed. This increases the tubule to plasma concentration gradient for drugs that have been filtered or secreted into the lumen. While polar and ionised molecules (water soluble) remain in the urine, only the non-ionised (lipid-soluble) fraction of a weak acid or base contributes to the concentration gradient. As the degree of ionisation of a drug depends upon the pH of the urine and pK_a of the drug, altering the pH of urine can promote drug excretion (see Clinical box 4.1).

| Clinical box 4.6 | Competition for transporters: clinical examples |

- **Exploitation in drug development**: probenecid was developed to compete with penicillin for its transporter, reducing the secretion and prolonging action of penicillin when it was scarce and expensive
- **Causing interactions**: e.g. low doses of salicylates or probenecid compete with uric acid for active secretion into renal tubules. This can lead to hyperuricaemia and gout
- **Influencing dose**: high doses of probenecid compete with uric acid to prevent its active reabsorption and is used in the treatment of gout.

Diuretic drugs

Diuretic drugs are used in the treatment of the conditions in which the retention of water and salt (NaCl) in the body severely interferes with normal function. Major clinical uses for diuretics include:

- Oedema in heart failure, nephrotic syndrome, hepatic cirrhosis
- Hypertension
- Acute renal failure
- Raised intracranial pressure (mannitol)
- Raised intraocular pressure (acetazolamide).

The complexities of the pharmacodynamic and pharmacokinetic processes of diuretics can, however, give rise to unwanted effects. Diuretic drugs act by:

- Inhibiting the reabsorption of Na^+ and Cl^- from the glomerular filtrate. Excretion of Na^+ and Cl^- ions increases, taking water with them.
- Opposing the antidiuretic action of aldosterone
- Increasing urine osmotic pressure to prevent tubular reabsorption of water
- Alkalinising the urine to promote excretion of bicarbonate, other ions and water.

Diuretics acting on the loop of Henle

Loop diuretics act on the loop of Henle (see Fig. 4.4). The main therapeutic example, furosemide, is a powerful diuretic, alleged to cause 'torrential urine flow'.

Pharmacodynamics

Loop diuretics promote Na^+ and Cl^- excretion by preventing reabsorption from urine in the ascending loop of Henle.

- Loop diuretics are actively secreted into the urine in the proximal convoluted tubule.
- Inhibition of the active symporter $Na^+/K^+/Cl^-$ ion pumps in the cell membrane of the ascending loop of Henle prevents the reabsorption of these ions.
- Urine passing into the distal convoluted and collection tubules is therefore hypertonic. The increased osmotic pressure prevents the reabsorption of water.
- 25% of glomerular filtrate passes out instead of the normal 1%, causing profuse diuresis.
- Increased Na^+ in the distal tubules increases the loss of K^+ and H^- ions there, which may lead to hypokalaemia and metabolic alkalosis.

Pharmacokinetics

Loop diuretics are well absorbed when administered orally. In an emergency, e.g. acute heart failure or cerebral oedema, administration could be directly into the bloodstream by intravenous injection. The drug molecules are bound to plasma proteins and secreted into the urine in the proximal renal tubules by active, carrier-mediated transport.

Furosemide is metabolised in the liver by conjugation with glucuronide. Other loop diuretics, e.g. bumetanide, are metabolised by cytochrome P450.

Unwanted side effects

The more common, unwanted side effects of loop diuretics include:

- Hypokalaemia due to potassium loss, which affects the contractility of heart muscle and may be life-threatening.

Hypokalaemia may be avoided by giving K^+ supplements, or by concomitant administration of a K^+ sparing diuretic
- Metabolic alkalosis due to H^- and Cl^- loss, which exacerbates hypokalaemia
- Sodium and water depletion, particularly in the elderly, leading to collapse due to hypotension and hypovolaemia (from hyponatraemia)
- Urinary incontinence due to 'torrential urine flow'.

Diuretics acting on the distal tubule

Diuretics acting on the distal renal tubule include the thiazide diuretics, of which bendroflumethiazide (bendrofluazide) is the most commonly prescribed. Less commonly prescribed thiazides include hydrochlorothiazide and newer ones such as indapamide. The mechanism of their action is similar to loop diuretics, but their diuretic action is less powerful.

Pharmacodynamics

Thiazide diuretics act at the luminal surface of the distal convoluted tubules:

- Inhibition of Na^+ and Cl^- reabsorption by inhibiting the Na^+/Cl^- pump (symporter)
- Potassium is lost to a significant extent
- Onset of diuresis is slower than loop diuretics, but duration of action is longer
- Diuretic effect is reduced with impaired renal function (as in elderly people).

Unwanted side effects

The unwanted side effects of thiazide diuretics are similar to those produced by loop diuretics:

- Hypokalaemia
- Glycosuria – with long-term administration, a dose-related, progressive hyperglycaemia occurs. This is related to chronically low intracellular K^+ concentration, which inhibits insulin synthesis. This effect is reversible over time after cessation of the drug.

Potassium sparing diuretics

The main potassium sparing diuretic is spironolactone, which only has a weak diuretic action. Its main usefulness is as an adjunct to loop diuretics.

Pharmacodynamics

Spironolactone acts as a competitive antagonist at aldosterone receptors in the cells of the distal convoluted tubules, inhibiting its antidiuretic effect by inhibiting the Na^+ retaining and the K^+ secreting actions of aldosterone, hence 'potassium sparing'.

Pharmacokinetics

Orally administered spironolactone is well absorbed, and is metabolised in the gastrointestinal tract and liver to active metabolite, canrenone, which has a long duration of action with a half-life of 16 hours. Its onset of action is slow, over several days.

Unwanted side effects

- Used alone, spironolactone can cause hyperkalaemia, which is life-threatening

- Long-term administration may lead to metabolic acidosis
- Gynaecomastia may occur, because the steroidal structure of spironolactone has an oestrogen effect.

Osmotic diuretics

Osmotic diuretics act by increasing the osmotic pressure of urine in the renal tubules to limit tubular reabsorption of water. Mannitol is a pharmacologically inert substance. It is administered intravenously and filtered, unchanged, at the glomerulus, with little or no tubular reabsorption, and excreted unchanged. The most important uses are:

- Cerebral oedema and raised intracranial pressure
- Acute glaucoma.

Unwanted side effects

- Expansion of the extracellular fluid volume by osmotic diuretics can precipitate heart failure and pulmonary oedema
- Side effects include headache, nausea and vomiting.

Diuretics acting on the proximal tubule

Drugs acting on the proximal tubules are not used as diuretics, except for acetazolamide, which is used for treating glaucoma. Acetazolamide inhibits carbonic anhydrase to increase the excretion of bicarbonate, together with Na^+, K^+ and water in the urine. The urine is alkaline, and there may be an accompanying metabolic acidosis.

HEPATOBILIARY EXCRETION AND ENTEROHEPATIC CIRCULATION

Drugs, and glucuronide conjugates formed in the liver, can be secreted into the **bile** by active transport processes similar to those found in the renal tubules for anions and cations. Basic drugs (e.g. atropine) and non-ionised molecules (e.g. digoxin) can also be secreted into bile. Biliary secretion becomes more important as the molecular weight exceeds 300. Drugs and their metabolites with molecular weight exceeding 300 are released into the alimentary tract where, depending on the drug or conjugate:

- Either the drug or conjugate is excreted via the **faeces**
- Or the bacterial flora of the lower intestine may hydrolyse the conjugated drug back to the original drug, which is then reabsorbed by the intestine (e.g. oestrogens, morphine). This is known as **enterohepatic circulation**.

ROUTES OF DRUG ADMINISTRATION

Choosing how any particular drug is administered depends on how quickly effective plasma concentrations must be achieved, and how the drug is absorbed into the systemic circulation, metabolised and excreted. The main routes of administration of a drug, and abbreviations for them, are:

- Oral (PO)
- Parenteral: intravenous (IV), intramuscular (IM), subcutaneous (SC)
- Buccal/sublingual
- Rectal (PR)
- Transdermal and topical (vaginal, nasal, ocular)
- Inhalation.

ORAL ADMINISTRATION

Oral drug administration is the most commonly used route. It is also the cheapest and most convenient. Its suitability for a specific drug depends on how well the drug is absorbed into the systemic circulation from the gastrointestinal lumen and on how it is metabolised. Oral administration may be used to produce local effects within the gastrointestinal tract or for systemic effects.

Factors affecting gastrointestinal absorption of a drug

The factors that affect absorption of a drug from the gastrointestinal lumen into the systemic circulation are:

- Drug formulation
- Physico-chemical properties
- Rate of passage through the gastrointestinal tract.

Physico-chemical properties of the drug, the medium and surface area

Absorption of orally administered drugs is influenced by:

- Its solubility in water and lipid
- The characteristics (e.g. pH) of gastrointestinal contents from which it has to be absorbed into the systemic circulation
- The available surface where absorption takes place.

Drug solubility

Orally administered drugs have to cross cell membranes in the gastrointestinal tract to be absorbed into the systemic circulation. As drugs exist in the ionised and non-ionised forms, the non-ionised lipid-soluble form moves across cell membranes much more readily than the water-soluble, ionised form. Highly acidic (ionised) and basic drugs are poorly absorbed from the gastrointestinal tract, and most of the dose is excreted in the faeces.

Acid–base considerations

As most drugs are weak acids or weak bases, they undergo pH partitioning between the lumen of the gastrointestinal tract and the mucosal cells. Acid drugs are least ionised in the stomach so that they are best absorbed there. Basic drugs are better absorbed in the small intestine, where the pH is higher. There is also a zone with neutral pH at the interface of the stomach contents and the gastric mucosa, which acts as a barrier limiting drug absorption.

Surface area for absorption

The **surface area** over which absorption can take place in the stomach is relatively small compared with the small intestine. The surface area in the small intestine is increased 600-fold by the presence of villi and microvilli so that the small intestine is the major site for absorption. This large area allows even ionised drugs to be absorbed.

The **time** taken for the drug to pass through the small intestine also influences absorption. Absorption increases the longer the drug stays in contact with the mucosal surface. Intestinal hurry, as in diarrhoea, will reduce absorption. Inflammatory bowel disease that destroys the villi will also prevent absorption.

Fate of drugs in the stomach

Apart from the high acidity of the gastric juices, the presence of food and other drugs could affect the eventual absorption of the drug (Clinical box 4.7):

- Formation of complexes with ions (tetracycline antibiotics and Ca^{2+}) or with food reduces absorption
- Gastric emptying determines the time that it takes for an oral dose of a drug to reach the small intestine where absorption takes place.
- Drug formulation
- The active drug in an oral preparation (tablet, capsule, etc.) is only a small proportion of the preparation's constituents. The rest is made up of ingredients that influence the speed and site of absorption: excipients, disintegrating agents, diluents, lubricants, etc. These ingredients and their proportions – the **formulation** – vary among manufacturers, but with the aim of ensuring similar effects.
- The formulation determines the rate at which a tablet or capsule disintegrates and dissolves. A drug cannot be absorbed until it is liberated into the gastrointestinal fluid to form a solution. Usually, this occurs rapidly, but there are special **modified-release** formulations that disintegrate more slowly to control the amount of drug available for absorption over time.
- Drugs may be affected by the acid gastric juices and need to be protected by having a special **acid-resistant** coating on the tablet/capsule (**enteric coated**). For example, mesalazine, used in the treatment of inflammatory bowel disease, is enteric coated to protect the drug from the action of acid gastric juices and is transported to the colon where it is released.

Clinical box 4.7	The stomach and drug administration schedules

When an administered drug forms an insoluble complex with food in the stomach, the drug is best given on an empty stomach, usually about 30 minutes before meals:
- For example, tetracyclines chelate with the Ca^{2+} or Mg^{2+} ions in antacids and in calcium-rich foods in the stomach to form a complex that is poorly absorbed in the small intestine. Tetracyclines are therefore better administered on an empty stomach. Dairy products (high in Ca^{2+}) should be avoided at the time the drug is taken.
  Gastric emptying can be slowed by:
- Meals that are high in fat or carbohydrate content
- Co-administration of anticholinergic drugs (e.g. atropine) or opioid analgesics (e.g. morphine).
  Gastric emptying can be hurried by:
- Reducing the temperature of food
- Fasting
- Drugs such as metoclopramide which increase gastric motility.
  Usually, when a drug is taken with a meal, absorption from the intestine is delayed due to delayed gastric emptying, but some foods may improve absorption. For example:
- Griseofulvin is absorbed better in the presence of fatty foods
- A higher plasma concentration of propranolol has been reported in patients after a meal.
  The enhanced absorption is probably due to increased postprandial blood flow to the intestines. These drugs should be taken with or immediately after a meal.

Metabolism of drugs in the gastrointestinal tract

How much of an orally administered drug actually enters the systemic circulation and exerts a therapeutic effect is called **bioavailability**. Because most drugs are, to some extent, metabolised in the gut and liver before reaching the systemic circulation, bioavailability is not the same as the amount administered. It is calculated by comparison with an intravenously administered equivalent dose.

Some orally administered drugs undergo metabolism in the gastrointestinal tract and are then transported to the liver by the hepatic portal vein for further metabolism before distribution throughout the body:

- The **lumen of the intestine** contains **digestive enzymes** that can split amides and esters
- The **colon** contains a large number of **aerobic and anaerobic bacteria** that possess enzymes capable of catalysing a number of reactions, including hydroxylation (hydrolysis) and reduction
- Phase I hydroxylation and phase II sulphate conjugation enzymes are also present in the intestines (see drug metabolism)
- P-glycoproteins 'block' absorption by extruding drug molecules into the intestinal lumen, and may be part of the 'first pass' mechanism (see above).

Drug metabolism in the intestines reduces bioavailability. A normal oral dose of drug may not be therapeutically effective if much of the dose were inactivated in the intestine or first metabolised by the liver before reaching the systemic circulation (**first pass metabolism**).

Bioavailability and bioequivalence

Although bioavailability indicates the proportion of orally administered drug that reaches the blood, it does *not* indicate the extent of absorption. Regulatory authorities that approve the use of drugs on humans use the concept of bioequivalence, which is a comparison of the generic drug with the new, proprietary product to ensure that the new product is as effective as the generic.

First pass metabolism

Even if the orally administered drugs were absorbed intact, first pass metabolism in the liver reduces bioavailability to a greater or lesser extent.

- Some drugs are completely inactivated by first pass metabolism and therefore cannot be administered orally (e.g. glyceryl trinitrate). An alternative route, or a specific drug design, e.g. pro-drug, may be needed to bypass first pass metabolism.
- A larger dose of drug may be needed for drugs that are not entirely inactivated by first pass metabolism to achieve a therapeutic effect (e.g. propranolol, aspirin, morphine).

Impact of liver disease on first pass metabolism

Patients needing long-term medication may have coexisting impairment of liver function:

- The drug is not extensively metabolised by the liver before entering the systemic circulation

- The usual dose of the drug could therefore become an overdose or toxic dose
- Care must therefore be taken when prescribing for patients with liver failure, e.g. elderly or patients with pre-existing liver disease.

PARENTERAL ADMINISTRATION

Parenteral administration is to give a drug by injection. This could be through a variety of methods including intravenous, intramuscular, subcutaneous or intrathecal (into the cerebrospinal fluid) routes.

Drugs are administered by injection:

- When effective plasma concentrations are needed rapidly.
- To bypass first pass metabolism.
- When administration by the oral route is not possible, as in severe vomiting. Also, some drugs are **acid labile** and are destroyed by the low pH of the stomach contents or denatured by proteolytic digestive enzymes (e.g. insulin).

Intravenous

The intravenous administration of a drug produces a rapid onset of action. A known concentration of drug is administered into the bloodstream, either as a **bolus** when the whole amount of drug is given as one dose, or by **infusion** when the total dose is given slowly over a period of time. Drugs that would otherwise act as irritants can be administered intravenously, because veins are insensitive and the drug is rapidly diluted by plasma, particularly if injected into a large forearm vein.

Factors that determine the rate of **systemic absorption** after intravenous injection are the solubility of the drug in interstitial fluid and intercellular pores (gap junctions) in the vascular endothelium that promote rapid diffusion, independent of the lipid solubility of the drug. **Toxicity** can be a problem because of the rapidity of drug administration and onset of therapeutic effect. It requires trained personnel. It is also expensive because of sterilisation requirements and storage costs.

Subcutaneous

Subcutaneous injection is when the drug is injected just under the skin (e.g. insulin). Absorption is relatively slow, but usually complete and can be improved by massage or heat at the site of injection. Highly ionised or high molecular weight drugs are absorbed by diffusion through large intercellular pores in the capillary endothelium. A vasoconstrictor may be co-administered to delay the absorption of a drug (e.g. epinephrine (adrenaline) and local anaesthetic agent), thereby prolonging its effect at the site of injection. Drugs that have irritant properties can cause local tissue damage if administered subcutaneously (e.g. thiopentone).

Intramuscular

Drugs administered intramuscularly are either specialised depot (the drug is in a solvent, or vehicle, that keeps it at the site of injection, to be absorbed gradually), or sustained release preparations. These are a suspension of the drug in a non-aqueous preparation called the **vehicle**; for example, fluphenazine decanoate used in the treatment of schizophrenia, depot progestogens used as a long-acting contraceptive.

Absorption from depot injection is sometimes erratic, especially for poorly soluble drugs. The vehicle may be absorbed faster than the drug causing precipitation of the drug at the injection site.

OTHER FORMS OF INJECTION

Other forms of injection are used to deliver drugs to their precise site of action. Trained personnel are needed to perform these techniques.

Intrathecal

Some drugs have to be delivered directly into the cerebrospinal fluid (CSF) because the blood–brain barrier prevents entry from the systemic circulation. This is done via an intrathecal injection – the drug is injected through the theca of the spinal cord into the CSF in the arachnoid space. A lumbar puncture is performed under local anaesthesia and the drug, for example a cytotoxic drug, is injected straight into the CSF.

Epidural

Epidural injections are delivered into the space surrounding the meninges (dura) and therefore not into the CSF. They are used as a form of local anaesthesia, producing selective nerve block. This can be temporary, using a local anaesthetic, for surgical procedures such as inguinal herniorrhaphy, childbirth and caesarean sections. More permanent nerve block, using phenol (which destroys the nerves), is sometimes used to relieve intractable pain.

Local injections into tendons/bursae

Cortisone injection directly into tendon insertions (tennis elbow, golfer's elbow) and bursae sometimes help to relieve pain, but delays healing.

Buccal/sublingual administration

Some drugs are taken as small tablets that are held in the mouth, in contact with the buccal mucosa (buccal) or under the tongue (sublingual) (Clinical box 4.8). This route facilitates rapid absorption of lipid-soluble drugs into the systemic circulation across the mucous membranes, thus avoiding first pass metabolism.

Rectal

The rectal route is useful for patients who are unable to take drugs orally because of vomiting and for younger children. When given as a suppository or enema, more than 50% of the drug absorbed via the rectum bypasses the liver and so the effect of first-pass metabolism is reduced. However, absorption is often incomplete and erratic, and it may also cause irritation of the rectal mucosa.

Topical/transdermal

Some drugs are formulated for direct application to the skin for **topical** cutaneous application when a local effect is needed. Some absorption through the skin (transdermal absorption) can, however, take place to give systemic effects.

Examples for choice of route for drug administration

Selecting the appropriate route for the administration of a drug depends on the therapeutic indication of the drug and its physico-chemical properties.

Glyceryl trinitrate (GTN), a drug widely used for the treatment of angina, is extensively inactivated by first pass metabolism in the liver, so that oral administration is contraindicated.

- For the relief of angina:
  - Oral tablet: GTN is inactivated by first-pass metabolism and so is not suitable for oral administration
  - Buccal/sublingual tablet or spray: because of its high lipid solubility, GTN is absorbed rapidly through mucous membranes; effects last 20–30 minutes, so it is used for rapid relief of angina attacks in the patient who has occasional angina attacks
  - Transdermal patch: GTN is absorbed more slowly through skin, so patches are used for prophylaxis in the patient who has frequent angina attacks
- For chest pain due to myocardial infarction: intravenous administration for rapid relief in emergency situation. When oral drug administration is impossible:
- Diazepam is given rectally to epileptic patients who are fitting continuously (status epilepticus).
- Prochlorperazine, an anti-emetic, is administered rectally for patients with intractable vomiting.
- Penicillin G, a broad-spectrum antibacterial drug, is destroyed by the low pH of the stomach contents. It has to be given by intramuscular injection. The formulation of penicillin V, however, is not acid labile, and can be given by mouth.
- Insulin is denatured by proteolytic digestive enzymes, therefore cannot be given orally. Insulin has to be administered subcutaneously. When oral administration leads to unwanted effects:
- Non-steroidal anti-inflammatory drugs have been formulated for topical application for a local action on joints via the skin. This is to avoid undesirable effects on the stomach – irritation, ulceration or bleeding.
- Timolol, a β-adrenergic antagonist, is formulated for direct application to the eye in the long-term treatment of glaucoma. Not only is the drug effective, it also avoids the troublesome side effects produced by the systemic action of β-adrenergic antagonists.

To produce local effects, some drugs are applied directly (topical application) to the mucous membranes of the conjunctiva, or vagina (PV).

Lipid-soluble drugs can be formulated as skin patches to allow absorption through the skin (dermis) for systemic effect, known as the **transdermal** route. The topical and transdermal routes of administration bypass first pass metabolism. Some drugs are formulated for topical application so that they can be absorbed through the skin to bypass possible adverse side effects on the gastrointestinal tract (Clinical box 4.8).

Intranasal administration

Some drugs are administered as a nasal spray, to be absorbed through the mucous membrane to act directly on the mucosa or on the pituitary gland. Examples include:

- Vasopressin used in the treatment of diabetes insipidus
- Bromocriptine used for the suppression of lactation, hyperprolactinaemic disorders and the downregulation of menstrual cycles in the treatment of infertility.

Inhalation

Gaseous and volatile drugs (e.g. the general anaesthetics nitrous oxide, halothane respectively) are administered by inhalation. Absorption of drugs by the lungs is rapid because of the large surface area within the lung and the rich blood supply to the relatively thin pulmonary epithelium.

In the treatment of lung disorders (e.g. asthma) drugs can be inhaled as a powder or an atomised solution of a drug, which enables a high concentration of drug to be delivered directly to the target structures, for example mast cells or bronchial muscle, without significant systemic side effects.

Drugs can also be formulated for inhalation in a way that deliberately reduces their absorption across the cell membrane, to reduce side effects. The physical characteristics of the formulation, i.e. size of the particle, also determine the effectiveness of the drug. Particles greater than 20 μm in diameter stay in the mouth and throat and are swallowed, but 2–6 μm diameter particles penetrate deep into the lungs to produce a rapid local effect as well as being absorbed to produce a systemic effect.

THE MATHEMATICS OF PHARMACOKINETICS

The mathematical basis of pharmacokinetics seeks to analyse the drug concentration in different parts of the body, over time from administration to arrival at the site of action. The mathematics is complicated, attempting to synthesise the four basic processes of drug absorption, distribution, metabolism and excretion. These processes affect:

- The amount of drug that arrives at the site of action
- The intensity of action
- The duration of action.

Information about these variables informs the choice of appropriate drug dose and dosing regimen. This is a very simplified account of mathematical concepts that are relevant for understanding the relationship between drug dosage and the time it takes for the drug to reach target tissue sites and to be eliminated. Textbooks of pharmacology will give more details of the mathematics.

FIRST-ORDER KINETICS

Most physiological processes follow first-order kinetics: for example, passive diffusion down a concentration gradient. When applied to the fate of drugs, first-order kinetics states that the rate of elimination of a drug is directly proportional to plasma concentration. If plasma drug concentration (C) is plotted against time, the reduction in drug concentration as it is eliminated describes an exponential curve (Fig. 4.5A). Using the logarithm of concentration ($\ln C$) gives a straight line (Fig. 4.5B). This gives the information on how long it takes for the drug to be eliminated from the time of administration. The angle of decline for the slope ($-k_e$) indicates how quickly the drug is eliminated.

Drug half-life

Drugs vary in the time that it takes for the body to eliminate them. An important parameter in first-order kinetics is the time taken for the plasma concentration of a single dose of drug to decrease by 50%, the **half-life** ($t\frac{1}{2}$). $t\frac{1}{2}$ is independent of drug concentration at zero time, and the slope of the logarithmic curve is characteristic of the first-order process.

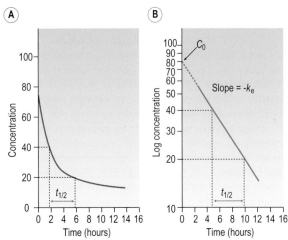

Fig. 4.5 **First order kinetics: plasma concentration curves for the distribution of a drug.** (A) An exponential curve is obtained when plotting concentration (arithmetic) versus time. (B) A straight line is obtained when plotting log concentration versus time. C_0, concentration at zero time; k_e, rate constant; $t\frac{1}{2}$, half-life.

The rate of decline for the log concentration curve (k), or slope, is specific for each particular drug, so that different drugs have different half-lives. It is a useful indicator of how long a drug remains in the body and allows for a dosing regimen to be established for any given drug (see below).

Drug clearance

Clearance is an estimate of the volume of plasma completely cleared of drug in a unit of time (e.g. mL/min), and is a measure of the ability of the organs of elimination to remove drugs from the body:

- The kidneys (renal clearance)
- The liver (hepatic clearance)
- Other organs, such as lungs.

Total body clearance is the sum of renal, hepatic and other clearances, measuring the time it takes for the body to be totally cleared of drug. It is a function of the volume of plasma cleared per minute, and the total apparent volume of distribution.

For drugs that follow first-order kinetics, clearance is constant over the therapeutic concentration range, so that a threefold increase in plasma concentration leads to a threefold increase in clearance.

Renal clearance

Renal clearance is important because it is the major process through which the body gets rid of foreign chemical compounds that might potentially be toxic. Renal clearance can be measured from the rate of excretion in the urine, or the amount of unchanged drug excreted in the urine over a fixed time period (e.g. 24 hours) (see also Ch. 14). Measuring renal clearance can be useful because:

- Comparing renal clearance with plasma clearance gives an indication of whether renal function is normal or impaired
- Hepatic clearance can be estimated from the difference between plasma and renal clearance to give an estimate of possible liver disease

- Comparing renal clearance with glomerular filtration rate gives an estimate of drug reabsorption or excretion by tubular secretion
- Changing the pH of urine can increase renal clearance (see Fig. 4.2).

ZERO-ORDER (NON-LINEAR OR SATURATION) KINETICS

At low drug concentrations, protein mediated processes for some drugs, e.g. enzymes, exhibit first-order kinetics. At high concentrations, however, binding sites on enzymes become saturated. The rate of reaction, e.g. drug elimination, can no longer respond to further increases in concentration, and can *only* proceed at a fixed maximum rate. The mathematics of this phenomenon is known as **zero-order kinetics**.

In zero-order kinetics, the rate of elimination of a drug is independent of the concentration of the drug (i.e. the drug is removed at a fixed amount per unit time). A plot of concentration against time gives a straight line (Fig. 4.6).

Consequences of zero-order kinetics

For zero-order kinetics, the decline in plasma drug levels is not exponential, unlike first-order kinetics, and therefore the duration of action is more dependent on the dose. The concept of half-life has no meaning. As the rate of elimination is constant, increasing the dose of the drug can result in a large and variable increase in plasma concentration. This can give exaggerated pharmacological responses and an increased risk of toxic effects.

Theoretically, if the rate of drug administration exceeds the rate of elimination then infinite accumulation of the drug would occur. However, this does not happen in practice because at high drug concentrations the relative contributions of other pathways of elimination (e.g. hepatic excretion) increase to achieve a steady state plasma concentration.

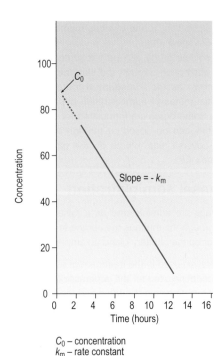

C_0 – concentration
k_m – rate constant

Fig. 4.6 **Time course of a hypothetical drug demonstrating zero-order kinetics.**

STEADY STATE AND MULTIPLE DOSING

Steady state concentration of drugs

A **steady state concentration** of the drug is reached when the plasma and tissue concentrations (including target tissue) reach equilibrium. Long-term drug therapy aims to achieve a constant steady state plasma concentration. When a drug is given intravenously, the time needed to reach steady state depends on the elimination half-life. The steady state concentration of a given drug varies markedly between patients, which can be further influenced by drugs that change the rate of metabolism, as in enzyme induction. Figure 4.7 shows an example of how the difference between a daily dose that gives therapeutic effects and one that gives toxic effects is very small.

Time needed to reach steady state plasma concentration

The decision about drug dosage and dosing regimen to achieve a therapeutically effective steady state concentration will depend on whether it follows first- or zero-order kinetics. A continuous intravenous infusion of a drug bypasses the absorption phase. The distribution phase is assumed to be constant, and, anyway, human tissue concentration cannot be measured easily. Therefore, elimination is the only measurable factor that affects the time needed for the drug to reach steady state plasma concentration. The rate of elimination is measured as the elimination half-life.

Figure 4.8A shows the log plasma concentration curve where steady state plasma concentration has been reached after several (usually five) elimination half-lives. However, the effect of oral administration of multiple doses will look different, if the elimination $t\frac{1}{2}$ is shorter than the absorption $t\frac{1}{2}$. The absorption phase now has an effect on the time to reach steady state. Figure 4.8B shows the time concentration graph of the logarithm of plasma concentration of repeated, fixed doses of a hypothetical, rapidly absorbed drug given at regular intervals.

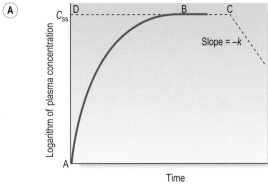

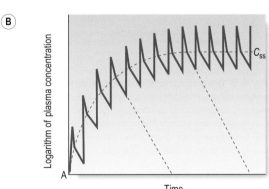

Fig. 4.8 **Steady state plasma concentrations after intravenous (IV) infusion and oral administration of a drug.** (A) Constant IV infusion (between A and C). Steady state concentration is reached at B. The steady state concentration Css is given by D. The slope on cessation of infusion C is the rate of elimination. (B) Regular oral therapy (——) compared with IV infusion (- - - - -) at the same dosage rate. The oral dose is rapidly absorbed and distributed followed by a slower elimination phase within each dosing interval. Cessation of therapy after any dose would produce the rate of elimination shown by the blue dotted slopes. Adapted with permission from Waller DG, Renwick AG, Hillier K 2001 Medical pharmacology and therapeutics. WB Saunders, Edinburgh.

- The rate of absorption will affect plasma concentration between doses
- Bioavailability of the drug (extent of absorption of the administered dose) will affect the steady state concentration
- Absorption has to be balanced by the rate of elimination, which is influenced by the function of the organs of elimination in the patient.

Safety margins of drugs: the difference between therapeutic and toxic doses

All drugs have some risk of toxicity. This risk always has to be taken into account in the context of disease severity. Patients have to be informed of this risk when being prescribed therapeutic agents, particularly those with a high risk of toxicity.

Therapeutic index

The **therapeutic index** is a useful indication of safety margins.

Therapeutic index (TI) = Dose giving toxicity / Dose giving therapeutic response

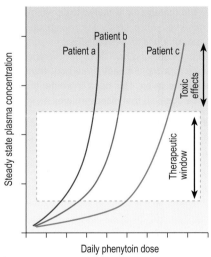

Fig. 4.7 **Steady state plasma concentrations as a function of the daily phenytoin dose.** Each curve represents a different patient receiving the same dose of phenytoin. In all three, initially the rise in plasma concentration is linear but it rises steeply to possibly produce toxic effects. The difference in the daily dose that produces therapeutic effects and the dose that produces toxic effects is small (very small in patients a and b), so that great care needs to be exercised when increasing daily dosage.

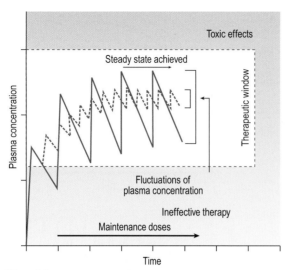

Fig. 4.9 Drug accumulation and steady state concentration. The diagram shows the effect of dividing the dose, and reducing the dosing intervals, on the accumulation and steady state concentration of a drug. (——) Oral dose given at unit intervals. (-----) Oral dose divided and given at half unit intervals.

Some drugs, such as benzodiazepines, have a therapeutic index of about 50, so that it would be difficult to be poisoned by benzodiazepines. Digoxin only has a therapeutic index of about 2, so that the dose difference between toxicity and therapeutic effect is very small.

Therapeutic window

The **therapeutic window** (see Fig. 4.9) refers to a range of responses in relation to rising plasma drug concentrations that varies from giving no therapeutic (subtherapeutic) to therapeutic to toxic responses. The therapeutic window is the range of plasma concentrations in which the patient is more likely to gain therapeutic benefit, with least risk of ineffective or adverse effects.

Multiple dosing

Very few drugs are administered as a single dose; most are administered serially with a fixed time interval between doses. The objective of repeat dosing is to achieve a therapeutically effective plasma drug concentration by accumulation and to maintain a steady state.

- If an intravenous dose (A) of a drug with a $t\frac{1}{2}$ of 2 h is administered to give a maximum plasma concentration of 10 units/mL, the plasma concentration will be 5 units/mL after 2 h.
- If a second dose (A) is administered at this time, the maximum plasma concentration will be 15 units/mL.
- After another 2 h the plasma concentration will be 7.5 units, an increase of 2.5 units in the lowest concentration.

The drug is accumulating in that the minimum concentration it reaches between half-life intervals, the peak plasma concentration, will gradually approach the maximal value of 10 units. At this stage the plasma concentration has reached a **steady state or plateau** (Css) because the amount of drug being eliminated from the body is approximately equal to the amount injected (See Fig. 4.8B).

The fluctuations between the maximum and minimum plasma concentration can be large. The time taken to reach the steady state is strictly dependent on the half-life of the drug and occurs within about five half-lives. A drug with a long half-life will take much longer to achieve a steady state than one with a short half-life. As a consequence, the final plasma concentration at which steady state occurs can be altered, as can the fluctuation between the maximum and minimum plasma concentrations, by altering:

- The time interval between doses
- The dose given, or
- Both.

Dosing at time intervals greater than half-life results in greater fluctuation in the plasma levels (*solid* line in Fig. 4.8).

Dosing at intervals less than half-life results in smaller fluctuation in plasma concentrations but the mean concentration at steady state is much higher (*dotted* line in Fig. 4.8). This can be achieved by halving the time intervals between doses.

Above the therapeutic window, toxic effects of the drug may be observed while below the therapeutic window the drug may not produce its desired effect.

If the drug has a long half-life or it is therapeutically desirable to achieve a rapid steady state concentration, a **loading dose** can be given. This dose is greater than the normal maintenance dose, so that disadvantages might be:

- Toxicity in a sensitive individual
- Delayed elimination (particularly after a toxic reaction).

PHARMACODYNAMICS

Pharmacodynamics is about how drugs work on living organisms: the qualitative and quantitative study of the biochemical and physiological effects of drugs on the body. Qualitative studies investigate the mechanisms of the action of drugs and endogenous molecules, while quantitative studies allow comparison of the relationship between drug **concentration** and **effect**. Quantitative studies include the measurement of drug effects at varying concentrations and this information is useful for estimating drug **potency** and **efficacy**.

DRUG TARGETS

For drugs to exert their pharmacological effect, they have to be bound to macromolecular components of a cell. The interaction of the drug molecule with a binding site on the cell elicits the therapeutic response from the cell. Because the amount of drug molecules relative to cellular macromolecules is small, binding has to be highly specific. Drugs are therefore designed to **target** specific macromolecules, most commonly proteins. Endogenous, naturally occurring, chemicals such as hormones and neurotransmitters act in the same way. There are four main regulatory proteins that are targets for drugs:

- Enzymes
- Carrier proteins (transporter)
- Ion channels
- Receptors.

Some specific classes of drugs target structural proteins and nucleic acids. For example, colchicine inhibits the assembly of the subunits that form microtubules, and anti-cancer drugs target DNA or RNA. Many drugs bind non-selectively to plasma proteins and other cell constituents without producing a biological response.

No drug is entirely specific in selecting its binding sites, giving rise to side effects if the drug binds to regulatory proteins that are not specific targets. For example, tricyclic antidepressant drugs are noted for producing the side effects of dry mouth and urine retention because they block receptors other than the monoamine transporters for which they were designed (see below, The autonomic nervous system). No drug is entirely without side effects.

In some texts, drug targets are sometimes referred to as receptors. Here, the term **receptor** will be used specifically for a protein molecule to which a drug or endogenous molecule binds selectively. The chemical substance, drug or naturally occurring molecule, is known as a **ligand** (tied or bound to the receptor). Binding of a ligand to a receptor may elicit a change in cellular function.

However, the binding of a ligand to a drug target does not necessarily induce a change in cell function: many proteins (enzymes, transporters and certain types of ion channel) do not act as receptors but do have **recognition sites** for ligands.

ENZYMES

Drugs may target enzymes as:

- Inhibitors – when normal enzyme action is inhibited
- False substrates – when an abnormal metabolite is produced
- Pro-drugs – when an inactive precursor is converted to an active drug by enzyme action.

Enzyme inhibitors

Enzyme **inhibitors** are drugs or their metabolites that inhibit enzyme activity. The inhibition may be:

- Reversible (e.g. anticholinesterase drugs such as neostigmine, the angiotensin converting enzyme inhibitor captopril)
- Irreversible (e.g. cyclo-oxygenase (COX) inhibitors such as aspirin): when the target enzyme is permanently altered so that a new enzyme has to be synthesised to replace the one bound to the drug.

The drugs produce their pharmacological effect by interacting with ligand recognition sites on enzymes by mimicking the substrate for that enzyme. The drug molecule may have a similar chemical structure to the natural substrate, competing with the substrate for recognition sites.

In non-competitive inhibition, the drug binds directly with the recognition site or to an allosteric site (another site on the enzyme to inhibit binding of the natural ligand), thereby inhibiting the action of the enzyme (Information box 4.7).

Information box 4.7	**Therapeutic uses of drugs that inhibit enzymes**

- Angiotensin-converting enzyme (ACE) inhibitors are used in the treatment of hypertension. The kidney plays a very important role in the regulation of blood pressure (see Ch. 14). Renin is secreted by the kidney in response to reduced renal perfusion and/or increased sympathetic activity, and converts angiotensinogen (produced by the liver) to angiotensin I. ACE then converts angiotensin I to angiotensin II, which is a powerful vasoconstrictor and has a role in hypertension. ACE inhibitors (inhibit the conversion of angiotensin I to angiotensin II, e.g. captopril) are now used extensively in the treatment of hypertension.
- Acetylcholinesterase (AChE) inhibitors: skeletal muscles contract through the stimulation of acetylcholine on neuromuscular junctions. Myasthenia gravis is a rare, autoimmune disorder in which the number of acetylcholine nicotinic receptors at the neuromuscular junction is greatly reduced, giving rise to the characteristic drooping eyelids (ptosis), rapid muscle fatigue on exertion and weakness. AChE is an endogenous enzyme that breaks down acetylcholine and terminates its action. The objective for the treatment of myasthenia gravis is to prolong the action of acetylcholine by inhibiting its breakdown by AChE. Neostigmine is a reversible, competitive inhibitor of AChE used in the treatment of myasthenia, although pyridostigmine is used more commonly because of longer duration of action and fewer side effects. Some poisons, such as nerve gases and insecticides, irreversibly inhibit AChE.
- Disulfiram is used as an adjunct in the treatment of alcohol dependence, as aversion therapy. Alcohol is metabolised to acetaldehyde by the enzyme alcohol dehydrogenase, then to acetic acid by aldehyde dehydrogenase. Disulfiram irreversibly inhibits aldehyde dehydrogenase so that acetaldehyde accumulates in the blood causing nausea, flushing of the face, palpitations and throbbing headaches among other symptoms – collectively called the **antabuse effect**. Some other drugs, such as metronidazole (treatment of anaerobic bacterial and protozoan infections), also inhibit acetaldehyde dehydrogenase to produce the antabuse effect if combined with alcohol. Patients prescribed metronidazole need to be warned against taking alcohol.
- Penicillin is a bactericidal antibiotic. In the last step in the synthesis of bacterial cell walls, an enzyme, transpeptidase, catalyses the 'transition state' reaction. This is the crucial step in bacterial cell wall synthesis. Penicillin is a synthetic analogue of the transition state and binds to transpeptidase, irreversibly inhibiting the enzyme. Bacterial cell wall synthesis is inhibited so that the bacteria are thin walled and fragile, destroyed by plasma osmotic pressure.

False substrates

Some drugs act as **false substrates**. The drug molecule is converted by endogenous enzymes to an abnormal substance that enters and disrupts normal metabolic pathways (Information box 4.8).

Pro-drugs

Inactive precursors of drugs, **pro-drugs**, can be converted by enzyme action to the active compound cortisone converted to active hydrocortisone. Some drugs are designed to exploit this characteristic. Conversely, therapeutically active drugs can be converted to toxic, reactive metabolites, e.g. paracetamol toxicity (see Information box 4.6).

CARRIER PROTEINS (TRANSPORTERS)

Carrier proteins, or transporters, transfer ions and small molecules that are not sufficiently lipid soluble across the cell membrane. ATP-dependent transporters, also called pumps, are the sites of action of a number of therapeutic agents. Transport-mediated responses are slower than ion-channel mediated ones.

ION CHANNELS

Charged ions cannot penetrate the lipid cell membrane and need ion channels to facilitate their diffusion across the membranes. Ion channels are large protein complexes that span the cell membrane. The intracellular concentration of important ions such as Na^+, Ca^{2+}, K^+ and Cl^- are controlled by the state of the channels, whether they are:

- Open, or activated, allowing selected ions to diffuse down a concentration gradient
- Closed, or inactivated and unresponsive to stimulus
- Rested, closed but opening in response to stimulus.

The electrochemical gradient of an ion between the intra- and extracellular compartments determines the direction and rate that the ion passes through the ion channel. Ion channel mediated responses are extremely fast, being measured in milliseconds. Drugs are developed and designed to target ion channels. Ion channels are classified according to:

- Their gating properties – many drugs target ion channels to exert a therapeutic effect by changing the status of the channel (i.e. open or closed).
- Their selectivity for specific ions – for example, cation channels are selectively permeable to Na^+, K^+ or Ca^{2+}, or all three. Anion channels would be permeable to Cl^-.

This property depends on the size of the ion channel and the difference in the amino acid sequence that lines it.
- The molecular structure of the ion channel.

The gating mechanisms of ion channels are:

- Voltage-gated – when the ion channel opens or closes in response to a change in the transmembrane electrochemical gradient
- Ligand-gated – when ion channels change status in response to the binding of a ligand to a receptor site incorporated into the channel structure. Ligand-gated channels are also known as **ionotropic receptors**.

Voltage-gated channels

Voltage-gated channels are therapeutically important ion channels. Voltage gating, as the name implies, is when ion channels selective for cations or anions open or close, due to a change in the transmembrane electrochemical potential. For example, a change in transmembrane potential in response to nerve impulses will cause different channels to open selectively to Na^+, Ca^{2+} or K^+. Na^+ and Ca^{2+} will diffuse into the cell, making the cytosol less negative and causing depolarisation of the membrane, and K^+ will diffuse out to make the cytoplasm more negative – repolarisation or hyperpolarisation.

Molecular structure of voltage-gated ion channels

Voltage-gated channels are made up of four subunits: an α subunit, a large glycoprotein (MW 270000), and smaller β, γ and δ glycoprotein subunits. Although not yet fully understood, different combinations of the subunits determine the selectivity of the subtypes of ion channels. The main channel forming subunit, known as the α1 subunit, is responsible for gating (Fig. 4.10A).

The α subunit of Na^+ and Ca^{2+} channels is a single polypeptide chain consisting of four homologous repeat domains (I–IV) that orientate themselves to form a pore (Fig. 4.10B). Each domain is made up of six transmembrane α helices (S1–S6). The polypeptide chain loops into the membrane to form the lining of the ion pore at the P-region, between S5 and S6. K^+ ion channels only have one domain (Fig. 4.10C). The S4 helix contains a set of positively charged amino acids (lysine and/or arginine) in a part of the protein that passes through the membrane. These charged molecules are thought to 'sense' the voltage across the membrane, causing the channel to either open or close.

Calcium channel antagonists

Calcium channel (Ca^{2+}) antagonists (blockers) were designed to target voltage-gated Ca^{2+} ion channels. Examples include nifedipine, amlodipine, verapamil and diltiazem. They are commonly prescribed for angina and hypertension.

Pharmacodynamics

The Ca^{2+} ion is essential for cardiac muscle contraction. Free Ca^{2+} ions have to enter the cardiac myocyte through voltage-gated Ca^{2+} channels or be released from intracellular stores before the muscle can contract. Ca^{2+} antagonists target the gating mechanism to inhibit Ca^{2+} influx. The effects include:

- Coronary artery dilatation to relieve or prevent the arterial spasm that reduces myocardial blood flow (ischaemia), causing the symptoms of angina

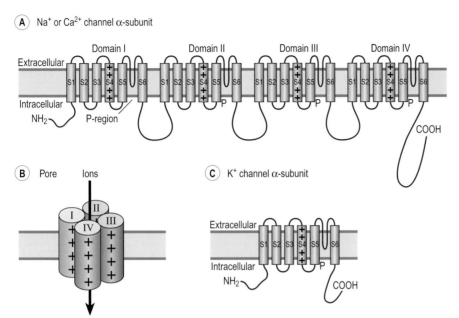

Fig. 4.10 **Voltage-gated ion channel.**

- Negative chronotropic effect by slowing the rate of firing at the SA node, and conduction in the AV node
- Peripheral arterial dilatation lowers peripheral resistance and blood pressure, reducing the work of the left ventricle and oxygen demand, thus relieving ischaemia.

Pharmacokinetics

The Ca^{2+} antagonists are well absorbed from the gastrointestinal tract, undergoing variable first pass metabolism by the liver. They have short half-lives, so the duration of action is relatively short. Attempts are made to prolong the duration of action by using modified-release formulations.

Unwanted side effects

- Heart block and bradycardia occur if administered with other negative inotropic drugs, e.g. digoxin, β-adrenergic antagonists
- Heart failure due to the reduced cardiac contractility in patients with poor ventricular function, e.g. elderly patients
- Symptoms due to arterial dilatation – ankle oedema, dizziness, flushing.

Ligand-gated channels

Ligand-gated channels are complex. They incorporate a receptor site that needs to be bound by a ligand (agonist) to open or by an antagonist to prevent the action of a ligand. Because a ligand-gated ion channel has a receptor recognition site incorporated into its molecular structure, the ion channel plus the recognition site is known as an **ionotropic receptor** (see below).

Ion channels as drug targets

Drugs are designed to block ion channel activity by one of two methods.

- They enter the channel during the open state and bind to a recognition site, for example the Na^+ channel and Ca^{2+} channel blockers

Information box 4.9	Example of use dependency and drug action on ion channels

Phenytoin is an important anti-epileptic drug despite having complex and sometimes serious side effects. Phenytoin produces use dependent block of voltage-gated Na^+ ion channels in neurons. It targets the abnormally fast firing neuronal tissue in the brain of patients suffering from epilepsy. Closing the ion channel prevents the influx of Na^+ into the neuron, thus 'damping down' the excessive neuronal discharge.

The unwanted effects of phenytoin are related to the effects of phenytoin on ion channels other than Na^+ channels. Its unpredictable toxicity is related to zero-order kinetics.

- They diffuse across the cell membrane and bind to an intracellular recognition site when the channel is in the inactivated state (e.g. lignocaine (lidocaine), a local anaesthetic).

The faster the ion channels 'cycle' through the open, inactive and rested states, the greater the blocking effect of the drugs will be. This is called use-dependency, a property exploited in therapeutics when the drug is designed to selectively act on ion channel cycles that are fast (Information box 4.9).

RECEPTORS

The majority of receptors targeted by drugs are transmembrane proteins involved in chemical signalling in cells. As most water soluble drugs (ligands) do not cross cell membranes, they have to exert their intracellular effect from an extracellular location. A **transmembrane receptor**, a protein that traverses the width of the cell membrane, is the means of signalling their 'message' to intracellular sites.

Ligands that activate receptors to send signals across the cell membrane are known as **first messengers**: they activate an intracellular **second messenger** system that causes changes in cell function.

A transmembrane receptor has a specific recognition site on the extracellular surface of the cell membrane for a given ligand – the **ligand binding domain**. The ligand–receptor interaction produces a small conformational change of the receptor protein, which in turn initiates a series of intracellular events via an intracellular **effector domain**. This is known as the **transduction mechanism**.

In a biological context, transduction means transforming a signal from one form to another. For example, light entering the eye (one form of signal) is transduced by rhodopsin, a protein in retinal rods, into nerve impulses (another form of signal) that are relayed to the brain. Transduction mechanisms can be the simple opening of an ion channel or the activation of a G protein (see below) by the effector domain, which in turn activates one of a number of enzymes, culminating in a physiological or biochemical response.

It is worth noting that some ligands are lipid soluble (e.g. steroid hormones, thyroid hormone). These readily diffuse through the cell membrane and bind to intracellular receptors to produce their effects, and so they do not need signal transduction.

Binding of a ligand to the receptor

A ligand is called a receptor **agonist** when it binds to a specific receptor, activates it and produces a cellular response. When a ligand binds to the receptor and produces no effect itself, but prevents the binding of an agonist acting at that receptor, it is a receptor **antagonist**.

- Binding is usually rapidly reversible, and the intensity and duration of the response depends on the continuing presence of the ligand
- The interaction between ligand and receptor involves a combination of weak, but readily reversible, chemical forces such as hydrogen bonds, ionic bonds and Van der Waals forces
- If the binding is **covalent**, the duration of the ligand–receptor association may be prolonged, if not irreversible
- The effect of irreversible binding can only be overcome, in the long term, by the synthesis of new receptors to replace those bound to the ligand

The number of receptors present in any cell is not static. There is a high turnover of receptors as they are continually formed and removed from the cell membrane. The number of receptors may be increased (**upregulation**) or decreased (**downregulation**) by drugs or disease. For example, during the treatment of infertility using artificial reproduction techniques, the woman's own ovulation cycle has to be suppressed so that ovulation can be stimulated by artificial means. A synthetic gonadotropin may be administered to inhibit the normal release of follicle-stimulating hormone and luteinising hormone, to 'downregulate' normal pituitary control over ovarian follicle development (see Ch. 10).

RECEPTOR CLASSIFICATION

Receptors were historically classified according to the drugs that act on them to produce a pharmacological response. For example, histamine receptors are activated by histamine, muscarinic receptors by muscarine and nicotinic receptors by nicotine.

Newer techniques in molecular biology, however, have identified many more new receptor subtypes and biochemical pathways. These techniques include molecular cloning, and studies of ligand binding and transduction pathways for receptor activation. The classification discussed below is only one system, at a point in time. As experimental data proliferate, systems for receptor classification are under constant review, and a useful summary is published annually.

Receptor classification based on structure and signal transduction

Receptors can be characterised in terms of their molecular structure and signal transduction mechanisms. There are four known superfamilies (Fig. 4.11):

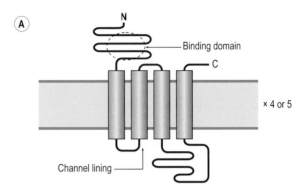

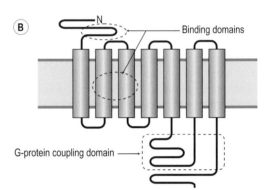

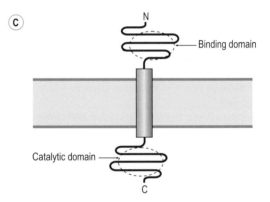

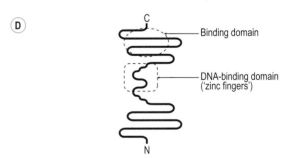

Fig. 4.11 **General structure of four receptor families.** (A) Type 1: ionotropic receptors. (B) Type 2: G protein-coupled receptors. (C) Type 3: kinase-linked receptors. (D) Type 4: nuclear receptors. Adapted with permission from Rang HP, Dale MM, Ritter JM, Moore PK 2012 Pharmacology, 7th edn. Churchill Livingstone, Edinburgh.

Type 1: **Ionotropic receptors** also termed **ligand-gated** or receptor-operated ion channels (Fig. 4.11A). These are membrane receptors coupled directly to an ion channel and are receptors on which 'fast' transmitters act. The tissue response occurs in a few milliseconds.

Type 2: **G protein-coupled receptors** (GPCR) also known as **metabotropic receptors** or 7 transmembrane spanning receptors (Fig. 4.11B). These are membrane receptors which are coupled to intracellular effector systems via a G protein. G proteins are so called because they interact with the guanine nucleotides GTP and GDP. The intracellular effector system is the second messenger (see below). The response to receptor activation occurs in 100 ms or seconds.

Type 3: **Enzyme-linked receptors** also termed kinase-linked receptors (Fig. 4.11C). These are membrane receptors that incorporate an intracellular protein kinase domain within their structure. Tissue response occurs in minutes.

Type 4: **Intracellular receptors** or DNA-linked nuclear receptors (Fig. 4.11D). These are receptors that regulate gene transcription and are located either in the cell cytoplasm or within the nucleus. The response to these receptors occurs in hours to days.

Ionotropic receptors (ligand-gated ion channels)

Ionotropic receptors are membrane bound proteins that are similar to other ion channels, but have a receptor binding (recognition) site on the extracellular domain. In some ionotropic receptors, the receptor protein is a G protein (see later).

Ionotropic receptors are usually the targets for 'fast' neurotransmitters (see below, The autonomic nervous system). Important examples include:

- Nicotinic receptors (stimulated by acetylcholine, nAChR): γ-amino-butyric acid A receptor (GABA$_A$-R), glycine receptor (Gly-R) and one subclass of the serotonin receptors (5-HT$_3$).
- Glutamate receptors (Glu-R).

Molecular structure of ionotropic receptors

The ionotropic receptor protein is a long peptide chain (Fig. 4.12A) that:

- Forms loops on the extracellular side of the cell membrane to produce the ligand binding site, known as the N-terminal.
- The protein then loops through the channels in the cell membrane a number of times. The lining of the ion channels is made up of four subunits: α, β, γ and δ.
- The subunits are membrane-bound proteins that congregate around a central, water-filled pore, thus forming a channel through the lipid bilayer of the cell membrane.
- The gating and ion-selective properties of ionotropic receptors are determined by the combinations of the subunits.

Nicotinic receptors (nAChR)

The ion channel in the nicotinic receptor is made with five subunits around the central pore (Fig. 4.12B). These are termed α (which is duplicated, i.e. there are two copies) β, γ

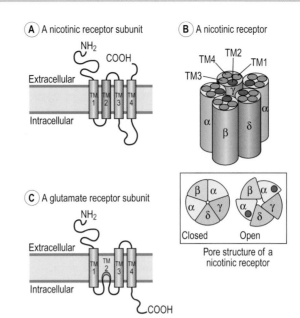

Fig. 4.12 **Molecular structure of ionotropic receptors.** TM, transmembrane.

and δ subunits. Each subunit consists of four transmembrane loops (TM1–4) (Fig. 4.12A). ACh is the ligand that activates the nicotinic receptor. There are two binding sites on the receptor and both have to be occupied by ACh before the channel pore will open.

GABA$_A$ receptor

The molecular structure of the GABA$_A$ receptor is similar to a nicotinic receptor. The α-subunit contains the extracellular binding site, which has a high affinity for GABA$_A$. The central pore (channel) is selective for anions, particularly Cl$^-$. Best examples of drugs that potentiate the binding of GABA$_A$ to its receptor are benzodiazepines and barbiturates.

Glutamate receptors

Glutamate is an excitatory amino acid neurotransmitter found in the central nervous system. There are two main classes of glutamate receptors (Fig. 4.12C): NMDA (N-methyl-D-aspartate), and non-NMDA receptors. The NMDA receptors are a family of ligand-gated ion channels that are also voltage dependent. For ions to flow, the receptor must bind glutamate or be depolarised. This receptor allows a significant influx of Ca^{2+}.

GPCR

GPCRs are a large family of transmembrane receptors. They are also known as metabotropic receptors because they initiate a chain of intracellular reactions known as the **second messenger system**. Over 250 GPCRs have been cloned.

Molecular structure

A GPCR protein is a single polypeptide chain, rather like a microscopic, very flexible electric wire (Fig. 4.13).

- The ligand binding site on the extracellular side of the cell membrane is a single polypeptide chain termed the N-terminal. The N-terminal is large, and extends into the extracellular space.
- From the N-terminal, the GPCR loops across the cell membrane seven times, the transmembrane domains of the receptor (TM1–7).

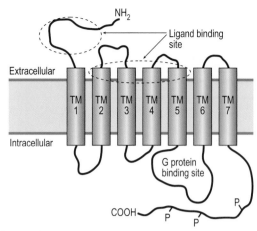

Fig. 4.13 **The molecular structure of a G protein-coupled (metabotropic) receptor.** Each of the seven transmembrane domains (TM1–7) is an α helix and consists of approximately 24 hydrophobic amino acids. Each domain is linked to the next one by an amino acid loop of varying length; three loops are intracellular and three are extracellular. The N-terminal extends into the extracellular space and the C-terminal extends into the intracellular space.

- After looping through the cell membrane, the GPCR terminates with the C-terminal on the intracellular side of the membrane.
- The loop connecting TM5 to TM6 contains the **G-protein coupling domain,** where the second messengers are produced.

GPCR (metabotropic receptors) and signal transduction mechanism

The major player in signal transduction by GPCRs is the **G protein.** G proteins are heterotrimers (trimers) consisting of three different subunits, α, β and γ. All three subunits are attached to the cell membrane by a fatty acid chain, coupled to the G protein. At the molecular level, the G protein is freely diffusible in the plane of the cell membrane, but bound to the intracellular surface. This allows the G protein to interact with a variety of enzymes and effectors in the cell in an apparently indiscriminate way.

However, ligands are particular about the receptors with which they interact. For example:

- The endogenous neuropeptides, which are large molecules, will only bind to the large GPCR N-terminal.
- Smaller neurotransmitters, norepinephrine and ACh, bind to the smaller terminals in the transmembrane domain. In fact, all the adrenoreceptor subtypes belong to the GPCR superfamily.
- Muscarinic ACh receptors and β-adrenergic receptors have opposing actions in cardiac muscle, yet the G proteins associated with the receptors can be selective.

G protein and signal transduction
When a ligand binds to a GPCR, through enzyme action:

- A change in conformation takes place in the αβγ trimer
- The trimer dissociates to α and βγ subunits

The α and βγ subunits are the 'active' forms of G protein that diffuse in the plane of the cell membrane and interact with various enzymes and ion channels, and initiate the production of second messengers.

Types of G protein
The specificity and selectivity of G protein is due to different characteristics in the α subunit, giving rise to three types that selectively produce different second messengers in the cell:

- G_s increases cAMP by activating the enzyme adenylate cyclase
- G_i (also G_o) inhibits adenylate cyclase
- G_q (also G_{12}) activates phospholipase C.

Second messenger systems

GPCRs control various cellular effector systems via the G protein. The G protein targets the following pathways to initiate the production of second messengers:

- **Adenylate cyclase** to synthesise cyclic adenosine monophosphate (cAMP) from ATP (adenosine triphosphate)
- **Guanylate cyclase** to synthesise cyclic guanosine monophosphate (cGMP)
- **Phospholipase C** catalyses the formation of inositol trisphosphate (IP_3) and diacylglycerol (DAG)
- **Phospholipase A_2** catalyses the production of arachidonic acid from membrane phospholipids, which is further metabolised to prostaglandins.

G proteins can also target ion channels, e.g. Ca^{2+}, K^+ (see below).

Cyclic nucleotide system
A variety of drugs are designed to relax vascular smooth muscle by targeting the cyclic nucleotide system to increase intracellular cAMP or cGMP. Inhibition of the phosphodiesterase (PDE) enzyme systems that inactivate cAMP and cGMP has similar effects on non-vascular smooth muscle.

Adenylate cyclase and cAMP Different drugs stimulate (drug A) or inhibit (drug B) production of the second messenger, depending on whether their receptor is linked to G_i or G_s (Fig. 4.14).

The synthesis of intracellular cAMP from ATP is a continuous process, catalysed by a membrane-bound enzyme, adenylate cyclase. cAMP is inactivated through hydrolysis by phosphodiesterases.

The cAMP formed from ATP activates **cAMP-dependent protein kinase** also known as **protein kinase A (PKA)**. PKA regulates a variety of cell functions including cell division and differentiation, muscle contraction, ion transport and energy metabolism.

Guanylate cyclase, cGMP and nitric oxide (NO) Two types of guanylate cyclase (membrane-bound and soluble) can synthesise cGMP from GTP in a reaction similar to the synthesis of cAMP from ATP.

- **Membrane-bound guanylate cyclase** is a transmembrane protein with a single α-helix domain, an extracellular binding site for neuropeptides (e.g. atrial natriuretic peptide), and a cytoplasmic **catalytic domain**. There are several isoforms of guanylate cyclase, each with a binding site for a distinct neuropeptide.
- **Soluble guanylate cyclase** is activated by nitric oxide (NO) to produce cGMP.

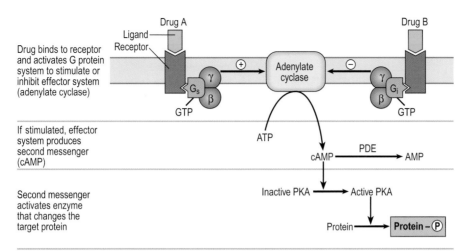

Fig. 4.14 **Action of drugs to stimulate or inhibit cAMP as a second messenger.** PDE, phosphodiesterases; PKA, protein kinase A.

cGMP exerts its effects by:

- Altering the activity of a number of phosphodiesterases
- Direct binding to ion channels
- Activating cGMP-dependent protein kinase (PKG).

Phosphodiesterases hydrolyse cGMP to GMP to terminate its action.

Phosphodiesterase inhibition Phosphodiesterases are inhibited by naturally occurring methylxanthines and xanthine drugs. Clinically important phosphodiesterase inhibitors include theophylline, theobromine and caffeine found in tea, cocoa and coffee. Methylxanthines cause bronchial smooth muscle relaxation. The second line asthma drug aminophylline is a theophylline derivative used to relieve bronchospasm when the response to β-adrenergic antagonists is poor. Side effects include those of CNS stimulation leading to wakefulness, alertness and tremor (c.f. excessive tea/coffee consumption).

Nitric oxide NO is derived from O_2 and L-arginine in a reaction catalysed by NO synthase to form NO and L-citrulline (Fig. 4.15). NO synthase is activated by Ca^{2+}-calmodulin complex (see below). NO is a gas which readily

diffuses from its site of synthesis, across the cytosol or cell membrane, to act on targets in the same cell or in nearby tissues (Information box 4.10).

Calcium

Calcium has a dual role as a carrier of electrical current and as a second messenger. The main mediator of Ca^{2+} action is the ubiquitous calcium-binding protein calmodulin. Calmodulin has no intrinsic enzymatic activity but has

---

Information box 4.10   Activation of cGMP by NO

Organic nitrates (e.g. glyceryl trinitrate and some longer acting nitrates) donate NO, which activates soluble guanylate cyclase to stimulate cGMP synthesis from GTP. They are used as therapeutic muscle relaxants in the treatment of angina.

Sodium nitroprusside, a NO donor, activates cGMP causing arterial and venous vasodilatation. Sodium nitroprusside:
- Is used in intensive care units to control hypertensive crisis
- Has to be given by IV administration.

Exposure to light converts nitroprusside to cyanide (poison!). The compound needs to be protected from light. Freshly made up intravenous solution is essential.

Sidenafil (Viagra) is a selective phosphodiesterase inhibitor. This inhibits the breakdown of cGMP, and releases NO to activate cGMP to increase penile erection.

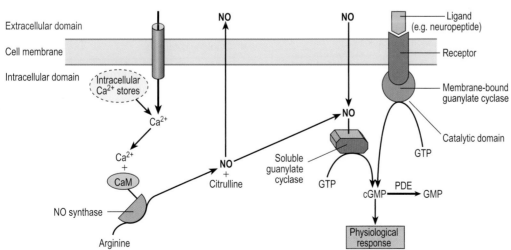

Fig. 4.15 **cGMP and nitric oxide (NO) as second messengers.** PDE, phosphodiesterases; cGMP, cyclic guanosine monophosphate; NO, nitric oxide; CaM, calmodulin.

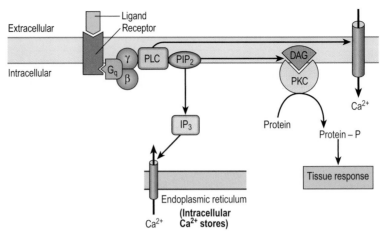

Fig. 4.16 **The inositol trisphosphate second messenger system IP₃ and DAG.** Protein - P, phosphorylated protein.

a central regulatory role by modulating the activity of various cellular targets. Ca^{2+}-calmodulin complex activates more than 20 enzymes including Ca^{2+}-ATPase, adenylate cyclase, cyclic nucleotide phosphodiesterases, nitric oxide synthase and several protein kinases. Ca^{2+} also affects proteins and enzymes independently of calmodulin, e.g. PKC, K^+ and IP_3 channels, calcium-binding proteins.

Phospholipase C
Phospholipase C (PLC) is a membrane-bound enzyme which, when activated by the binding of G protein, converts the membrane phospholipid, phosphatidylinositol 1,4-bisphosphate (PIP_2), into **inositol 1,4,5-trisphosphate (IP_3)** and **diacylglycerol (DAG)** (Fig. 4.16).

Inositol phosphates The main function of IP_3 is to control intracellular calcium. IP_3 is formed at the plasma membrane, diffuses into the cytoplasm and binds to IP_3 receptors on the membrane of endoplasmic reticulum to release intracellular Ca^{2+}. Activation of PLC also results in the influx of Ca^{2+} ions via Ca^{2+} ion channels. The IP_3 receptor, a macromolecular complex, thus functions as a Ca^{2+} channel as well as a receptor.

IP_3 is a transient signal, terminated by complete dephosphorylation back to inositol 1,4-bisphosphate, which is recycled into the phospholipid biosynthetic pathway (Clinical box 4.9).

DAG DAG is formed at the same time as IP_3, but unlike IP_3 is highly lipid-soluble and remains membrane bound. Its main effect is the activation of a protein kinase (PKC), which catalyses the phosphorylation of proteins.

- PKC is a cytosolic enzyme of which there are at least 13 different types with different tissue distribution and substrate specificities in terms of which proteins are phosphorylated

- PKC is involved in the transduction of a wide variety of processes including inflammation, ion transport, modulation of neurotransmitter release and smooth muscle contraction
- The action of DAG is rapidly terminated by conversion to phosphatidic acid and recycled to phospholipids
- Raised intracellular Ca^{2+} concentration, also stimulated by GPCRs, can also activate PKCs.

Phospholipase A₂ and eicosanoids
Receptor-mediated activation of phospholipase A₂ (PLA_2) results in the hydrolysis of PIP_2 to produce arachidonic acid and its metabolites (the eicosanoids: prostaglandins, leukotrienes etc.). These metabolites are released into the tissues as local hormones (e.g. insulin, glucagon).

Protein kinases in signal transduction

As a general rule, the protein kinases produced by the second messenger system have a central role in signal transduction. They control a number of different aspects of cell function, including:

- Enzymes, transport proteins
- Muscle contraction, to increase rate and force of cardiac muscle contraction, increase gut motility and secretion
- Energy metabolism via modulation of neurotransmitter release
- Ion transport via action on ion channels, particularly Ca^{2+} channels
- Cell division and differentiation
- Cytokine synthesis.

Amplification of transmembrane signals in signal transduction

The binding of a ligand to a GPCR activates a transmembrane signal that initiates a chain of events, which greatly amplifies the original signal to produce the tissue response.

Signal amplification takes place at a number of stages in a G protein-mediated signal:

- Ligand binding – at the point of binding, and as long as the ligand stays bound to the GPCR, as many as 20 G protein subunits will be activated
- Each G protein subunit will activate an effector enzyme, e.g. adenylate cyclase
- Each **effector** enzyme will produce a number of second messenger molecules

- Each second messenger will activate a number of second enzyme systems, e.g. protein kinase A
- The second enzyme system produces many molecules of a third enzyme system which activates numerous reactions to produce the tissue response (e.g. opening ion channels).

Speed of GPCR transmembrane signalling

GPCR transmembrane signalling is slow (100 ms to seconds) compared with ion channel signalling (2 ms). The advantages of GPCR signalling are that:

- A single GPCR class can initiate a variety of signals to produce a cumulative response
- A GPCR initiated signal can reach a cellular process that may be some distance from the receptor
- Diffusion of the second messengers can extend the signal transduction through the cell and into the nucleus to alter gene expression.

Termination of GPCR transmembrane signals

Metabolism of cyclic nucleotides by hydrolysis terminates the signal.

- IP_3 is dephosphorylated to inositol.
- DAG is converted to phosphatidic acid.
- Inositol and phosphatidic acid are recycled to generate PIP_2.

Ion channel modulation by G proteins

In addition to regulation by voltage changes and phosphorylation, ion channels can be modulated by G proteins:

- Indirectly through the second messenger system, e.g. via IP_3 or cAMP, to change channel status
- Via direct action by the G protein subunits, bypassing the second messenger system. For example, muscarinic ACh receptors have been shown to enhance membrane permeability to K^+ in cardiac muscle by the $\beta\gamma$ subunit of the G protein binding to the ion channel.

Enzyme-linked receptors (kinase-linked receptors)

Enzyme-linked, or kinase-linked, receptors are hormone receptors that are transmembrane proteins. They have an extracellular ligand-binding domain and an intracellular catalytic domain (see Fig. 4.12) that has enzyme activity when the ligand-binding domain is appropriately occupied.

The **extracellular ligand-binding domain** is very large because the endogenous ligands are large hormones such as insulin. The enzymic catalytic site of the intracellular domain is a protein kinase:

- **Tyrosine kinase,** which phosphorylates tyrosine (less commonly serine or threonine), or
- **Guanylate kinase**, which synthesises the second messenger cGMP (see above).

The peptides that are ligands for this type of receptor are hormones that promote cell growth and proliferation. They include insulin, insulin-like growth factor, platelet-derived growth factor, cytokines, leptin and atrial natriuretic peptide. These receptors are the focus of much research as drug targets for the treatment of cancers, obesity and disordered immunity and inflammation.

Intracellular receptors and nuclear receptors

Intracellular and nuclear receptors are proteins that are mostly in the nucleus, but may be free floating in the cytoplasm. They act on DNA to regulate the expression of specific genes to:

- Alter the genetic expression of enzymes
- Alter the genetic expression of cytokines
- Alter the genetic expression of receptor proteins.

Their action, therefore, initiates different patterns of protein synthesis to give different physiological effects. Nuclear receptors have a ligand-binding domain and a DNA binding domain known as 'zinc fingers' (see Fig. 4.11D). The ligands are all lipid-soluble compounds.

Unlike non-lipid-soluble compounds, lipophilic drugs and hormones do not need signal transduction by transmembrane receptors. They simply diffuse across the cell membrane to interact with nuclear and intracellular receptors.

In its inactive form, the intracellular receptor forms a complex with a protein called the heat shock protein (HSP90).

- The receptor dissociates from HSP on hormone binding, forming a receptor/hormone complex
- The receptor/hormone complex passes through pores in the nuclear membrane into the nucleus and interacts with hormone response elements (zinc fingers) on the DNA
- Binding of the receptor/hormone complex with hormone response elements usually activates genes, but sometimes inhibits the transcription of a specific mRNA.

Different steroid hormones (or drug analogues) induce or inhibit specific genes, which determines the pattern of DNA expression that is affected.

- Often the hormone response element requires two receptor/hormone complexes to form a dimer in order to alter gene expression
- Some receptor/hormone complexes bind to the same receptor/hormone complex to form homodimers
- Others bind with a different receptor/hormone complex to form heterodimers.

Selectivity for a specific DNA is the function of the **DNA binding domain** of the receptor, which is responsible for DNA binding and transcription; hormone specificity is the function of the **ligand-binding domain**.

Drugs that target nuclear and intracellular receptors

Most steroid hormone analogues (drugs) act as agonists for the endogenous hormone, but have better pharmacokinetic properties. Some are antagonists, blocking the binding of the endogenous hormone. With drugs that activate intracellular receptors, there is a delay of several hours to days before the onset of the pharmacological effect, because this type of signal transduction requires new protein synthesis.

Examples of drugs that target nuclear and intracellular receptors include sex hormones, mineralocorticoids, glucocorticoids, thyroid hormones, vitamin D and the retinoids (Clinical box 4.10).

There are, however, two classes of drugs used for treating diseases in humans that need special mention:

- Anti-cancer drugs
- Antibacterial drugs.

Anti-cancer drugs

The origins of cancer cells and the theories for oncogenesis are beyond the scope of this chapter (see Ch. 6). The majority of drugs used in the treatment of cancer, cytotoxic drugs, act by inhibiting DNA synthesis in the cancer cells. Their clinical use would therefore be most effective on rapidly dividing cells, but less effective on slow growing, solid tumours.

Toxic and side effects of cytotoxic drugs are related to their action on rapidly dividing human tissue. The tissues most likely to be affected include:

- Gastrointestinal tract – giving rise to the symptoms of anorexia, nausea, diarrhoea and mucosal ulceration
- Bone marrow – myelosuppression leads to anaemia, neutropenia and thrombocytopenia
- Hair follicles – partial or complete hair loss (alopecia)
- Reproductive organs – sterility, loss of libido
- Growing tissue in children – growth retardation, arrested sexual development, risk of second malignancy.

Antibacterial drugs

This is an extremely brief summary of antibacterial drugs. Textbooks of pharmacology and drug formularies should be consulted for more detailed classification. Antibacterial agents can be classified according to their mode of action on the invading microorganism:

- Inhibit bacterial cell wall synthesis so that the weak wall is ruptured by osmotic pressure, or activate enzymes that disrupt bacterial cell walls.
- Target bacterial DNA to inhibit bacterial cell division and growth.
- Inhibit bacterial protein synthesis. This is highly selective because bacterial protein is very different from human protein.
- Disrupt bacterial metabolism by blocking metabolic pathways.

Further classification of antibacterial agents is into whether the agent kills the bacteria (bacteriocidal), or merely stops it multiplying (bacteriostatic).

- **Bacteriocidal** drugs destroy the invading bacteria. They are more effective if the bacteria are not multiplying rapidly, and if the body's natural immune system is functioning normally.
- **Bacteriostatic** drugs are effective against rapidly multiplying bacteria, but rely on the immune system of the host to destroy the bacteria. They are much less effective in an immunocompromised patient.

The range of antibacterial action that the drug exhibits is also important when selecting the appropriate drug, known as the spectrum. A broad-spectrum antibacterial agent is effective against a wide variety of bacteria and protozoa, whereas a narrow-spectrum antibacterial agent is selective for specific bacteria.

Resistance of bacteria to antibacterial agents occurs when a safe dose of the drug is no longer effective against the microorganism. This occurs when:

- The microorganism produces enzymes that destroy the drug
- The microorganism modifies itself so that the drug can no longer penetrate bacterial cell membranes
- The microorganism changes its molecular structure so that the drug can no longer bind to bacterial receptors
- The microorganism finds alternate metabolic pathways to bypass the ones blocked by the drug.

Classification of some common antibacterial agents Table 4.4 sets out a classification of some commonly used antibacterial drugs.

THE SAFETY AND EFFECTIVENESS OF DRUGS

Safety and effectiveness are essential considerations before a drug can be used to treat patients. Regulating authorities, such as the Committee on the Safety of Medicines (CSM) in the UK, the Food and Drugs Administration (FDA) in the USA and the European Medicines Agency (EMEA), are responsible for the approval of drugs for human use. Laboratory testing on tissues, and animal experiments, provide evidence of safety and potential effectiveness to the point when controlled testing on human populations may be permitted.

The properties that contribute to the safety and effectiveness of drugs are those that are also likely to give rise to unwanted side effects and toxic effects. These properties are exhibited as:

- Specificity
- Selectivity
- Potency
- Efficacy.

The parameters for potency and efficacy are measured by dose–response curves in laboratory experiments. It should be noted that other variable factors affect the performance of a given drug, and observations in the laboratory are not necessarily replicated in vivo.

GRADED DOSE–RESPONSE CURVES

Dose–response curves are constructed by measuring target tissue response in relation to the concentration of the drug or dose. In an experimental setting, if a strip of smooth muscle is suspended in an organ bath, then a drug is added to the bath to elicit muscle contraction. The dose (concentration) of the drug needed to elicit the maximal response is measured. The measurement is based on a graded response, e.g. strength of muscle contraction.

The curve is produced by plotting the biological response on the ordinate (y) axis, and the drug concentration on the x axis.

Table 4.4   Classification of some commonly used antibacterial agents

Mode of action	Bacteriocidal or bacteriostatic	Spectrum	Antibacterial agent
Inhibits cell wall synthesis/ disrupts cell walls	Bacteriocidal	Broad	β-Lactams and penicillin and derivatives
	Bacteriocidal	Broad	Cephalosporins
	Bacteriocidal	Gram-negative bacteria	Other agents (glycopeptides, e.g. vancomycin)
	Bacteriocidal	Gram-negative organisms	Polymyxins, e.g. colistin
	Bacteriocidal on dividing cells, bacteriostatic on dormant cells	*Mycobacterium tuberculosis*	Isoniazid
Uncertain, probably on cell wall	Bacteriostatic	*Mycobacterium tuberculosis*	Ethambutol
Targets bacterial DNA	Bacteriocidal	Broad	Quinolones (fluoquinolone), e.g. ciprofloxacin
	Bacteriocidal	Anaerobic bacteria and protozoa	Metronidazole
	Bacteriocidal	Gram-negative cocci, *Escherichia coli*	Nitrofurantoin
	Bacteriocidal	Broad	Rifamycin, e.g. rifampicin
Inhibits bacterial protein synthesis	Bacteriostatic	Broad	Macrolides, e.g. erythromycin, azithromycin
	Bacteriocidal	Broad	Aminoglycosides, e.g. gentamicin, streptomycin
	Bacteriostatic	Broad	Tetracyclines
	Mainly bacteriostatic, bacteriocidal for some organisms	Broad	Chloramphenicol
	Bacteriostatic	Broad	Lincosamides, e.g. clindamycin
	Bacteriocidal	Gram-positive organisms	Fusidic acid
Inhibits bacterial metabolism	Bacteriostatic	Broad	Sulfonamides
	Bacteriostatic	Broad	Trimethoprim
	Bacteriocidal to dormant cells	*Mycobacterium tuberculosis* *Mycobacterium leprae*	Pyrazinamide
	Bacteriostatic		Dapsone

The resulting curve shows a rectangular hyperbola (Fig. 4.17A). By convention, the log of the dose (log[D]), giving a sigmoidal curve, is used for graded dose–response curves so that a wide range of concentrations can be displayed more easily (Fig. 4.17B). Both figures show the dose–response curve for a drug that is capable of a maximum response from the tissue.

The important features in a dose–response curve are:

- Increasing drug concentration produces an increasing response to reach a maximum that the tissue is capable of (E_{max})
- The drug concentration that produces 50% of the maximal response (EC_{50})
- The **slope** of the linear portion of the sigmoidal curve (between 20% and 80% in Fig. 4.17B).

CLASSIFICATION OF DRUGS ACCORDING TO PERFORMANCE

Drugs are classified according to the type of response they produce in tissues:

- **Agonists** are drugs that produce maximal response from tissues
- **Partial agonists** are drugs that are only able to produce submaximal response from tissues
- **Antagonists** reduce the effects of agonists by reducing their action.

Drug specificity

Most drugs bind to specific receptors: proteins that are drug targets have ligand **specificity**. Drugs with low specificity would bind to a series of different receptors, thereby producing a variety of side effects, e.g. chlorpromazine used in the treatment of schizophrenia.

Drug selectivity

Although many drugs are selective in binding to particular receptors, they tend to bind to different receptors to a greater or lesser degree, so that they may produce a variety of effects (Clinical box 4.11).

Drug potency

The **potency** of a drug depends on the strength of binding to its receptor targets – **receptor affinity**. Therefore:

- A drug has **high potency** if it has high receptor affinity. It will produce or block a tissue response at a low concentration.
- A drug with **low potency** has low receptor affinity. It will produce little or no response at low doses, and will need higher concentrations of drug to produce or block the tissue response.

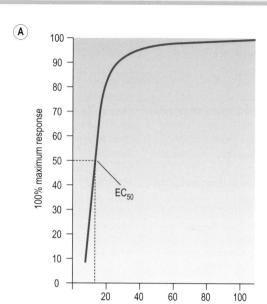

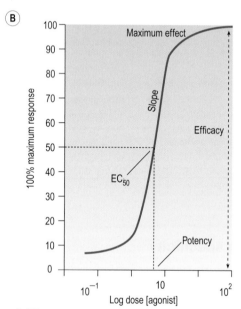

Fig. 4.17 **Graded dose-response curves for an agonist drug.**

Comparing potency between drugs

The concentration of a drug needed to produce 50% maximal response, EC_{50}, is used for comparing the potency of different drugs acting on the same receptors to produce similar therapeutic effects.

In Figure 4.18A, drugs A_1 and A_2 are both **agonists,** capable of producing maximal response. However, drug A_1 produces a maximal response at a lower concentration than drug A_2. Therefore, drug A_1 is more potent. Drug A_3, which is unable to produce a maximal response, is therefore a **partial agonist**.

The **potency ratio** is a comparative index of drug potency, and is derived by dividing the log EC_{50} of the test drug by the log EC_{50} of the comparator drug (Fig. 4.18B).

Drug efficacy

Efficacy is a measure of the ability of a drug, after receptor binding, to activate receptors, so that:

■ A **full agonist** is able to produce increasing responses with rising drug concentrations (doses) up to the maximal (drugs A_1 and A_2 in Fig. 4.18A)

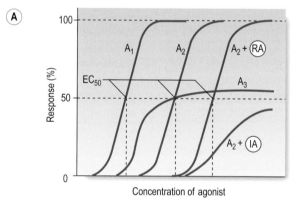

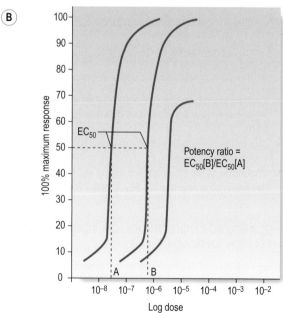

Fig. 4.18 **Dose-response curves for comparing potency.** RA, reversible antagonist; IA, irreversible antagonist. Fig. 4.18A adapted from Waller DG, Renwick AG, Hillier K 2001 Medical pharmacology and therapeutics. WB Saunders, Edinburgh.

Clinical box 4.11 **Examples of drug selectivity**

● The non-selective β-adrenergic antagonist, propranolol, binds equally to $β_1$- and $β_2$-adrenoceptors.
● The effect of propranolol binding to $β_1$-adrenoceptors would be to decrease heart rate and decrease the force of cardiac muscle contraction due to norepinephrine.
● Binding of propranolol to $β_2$-adrenoceptors, however, will block (antagonise) epinephrine induced relaxation of bronchial smooth muscle, causing bronchoconstriction and precipitating acute bronchospasm in patients with asthma and COPD (chronic obstructive pulmonary disease).
● A selective β-adrenergic antagonist, atenolol, would be less likely to have this effect on $β_2$-adrenoceptors as it would bind more selectively with $β_1$-adrenoceptors.
● A selective β-adrenergic antagonist, when indicated, should therefore be prescribed if patients have a history of asthma or COPD.

- A **partial agonist** also produces increasing response to rising drug concentration, but cannot reach the maximal response (drug A_3 in Fig. 4.18A)
- An **antagonist** drug is not shown in the figure, as it would produce a zero response, i.e. has no efficacy.

QUANTAL DOSE–RESPONSE CURVES

A **quantal response** is an all-or-none effect, such as death, and sometimes known as a **discontinuous** response. The outcome is a binary variable, 'yes' or 'no' to whether the specified response was observed. In animal experiments, the defined effect (e.g. death) will be produced in an increasing proportion of the experimental population as the dose of the drug increases. In humans, quantal responses to drugs are assayed on selected samples of the population. The relationship between the drug and the response is plotted as a graph of dose versus the number of subjects responding to that dose. As there will be individual variation in the response to the drug, the responses will follow the bell shaped, 'normal' distribution. The histogram is known as a **frequency distribution plot** (Fig. 4.19A). A more 'uniform' population will give a steeper curve.

The bell-shaped frequency distribution plot is transformed into a sigmoidal curve by plotting dose against the cumulative percentage of subjects responding to the drug – a **cumulative frequency distribution curve** or **quantal dose-effect curve** (Fig. 4.19B).

Quantal dose–effect curves to measure the safety of drugs

All drugs produce at least two effects – **therapeutic** and **toxic** (or **side**) effects. Therefore each drug can have at least two quantal dose–response curves – one for the therapeutic effect and one for the toxic effect (Fig. 4.19B).

- The dose of a drug that produces the desired therapeutic effect in 50% of the population is the **median effective dose** (ED_{50}).
- If the end point is death or toxicity, the median effective dose is called **the median lethal dose** (LD_{50}) or **the median toxic dose** (TD_{50}), respectively.
- The relative safety of a drug can be determined by dividing the TD_{50} or LD_{50} by ED_{50} to give the **therapeutic ratio**. The higher this ratio, the safer the drug.

FACTORS THAT AFFECT THE PERFORMANCE OF DRUGS

The factors that affect the specificity, selectivity, potency and efficacy of drugs relate to the nature of drug–receptor binding. A number of theories have been postulated in the attempt to quantify the relationship between a drug, or a natural ligand, and its receptors. These serve as a framework for interpreting experimental data. Advances in experimental techniques will uncover more and more surprises, so that some theories will be superseded.

Occupation theory

The binding of a drug to specific receptors to form a drug–receptor complex is governed by the Law of Mass Action, which states that the rate of any given chemical reaction is proportional to the product of the activities (or concentrations)

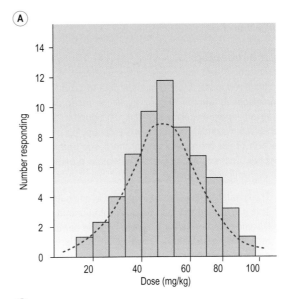

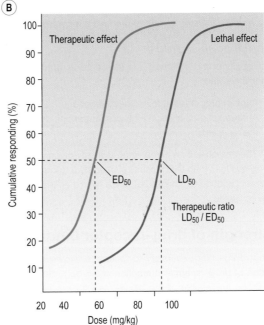

Fig. 4.19 Quantal dose–effect curves. In an experiment where a group of subjects were given an increasing dose until a required response was observed (e.g. pain relief), the results can be expressed as either: (A) a frequency distribution plot – each bar represents the minimum dose required for that number of subjects to respond (the broken line demonstrates a normal frequency distribution curve); or (B) a cumulative frequency distribution curve.

of the reactants. In pharmacology, the effect of an agonist drug is directly proportional to the number of receptors occupied by that drug, and the concentration of the drug.

Agonist drugs

The action of an agonist drug on specific receptors mimics that of its natural ligand, so that the action is additive. The dose of drug needed to produce a response depends on:

- The **affinity** of drug molecules for binding to receptor
- The proportion of receptor binding site occupied by the drug molecules – **receptor occupancy**
- The concentration of the drug – **dose**.

A full agonist can evoke a maximal tissue response at low concentrations and low occupancy.

Spare receptors

Some drugs need to occupy all the receptors to produce a maximal response. Most drugs are able to produce a maximal response without occupying all the receptors, so that there are **spare receptors**. Many full agonists are able to achieve a maximum response while occupying only a small fraction of the receptors, so that the tissue has a **receptor reserve**. The existence of spare receptors provides biological systems with flexibility:

- The greater the number of receptors in a tissue, the more able it is to respond to lower concentrations of drug
- If some receptors are inactivated or if the number of receptors decreases (downregulation), spare receptors can come into play.

The response will depend on the extent of receptor occupancy required to produce the maximum response. The spare receptors in a tissue are all equally capable of interacting with the effector system to produce a response.

Partial agonist drugs

The ability of a drug to activate a receptor is graded. Partial agonists show:

- Agonist properties at low concentrations
- Antagonist properties at high concentrations by blocking the receptors.

The response by a partial agonist at any given occupancy is always less than the maximal evoked by a full agonist, and cannot produce a maximal response even if all the receptors are occupied.

Strength of drug–receptor binding

Most drugs bind reversibly to receptors. However, the duration of drug–receptor interaction could be prolonged, and even be irreversible, if the binding is with covalent bonds. This has been discussed earlier in this section.

Receptor activation and efficacy

Receptors exist in a resting state or an activated state – the so-called 'two state model'. Drug molecules have a relative affinity for either the activated or the resting state.

- Agonists have a higher affinity for receptors in the activated state. The efficacy of the agonist will depend on its relative affinity for the receptors in the activated state, so that a higher affinity will give greater efficacy.
- Antagonists show no selectivity for receptors in either the activated or resting state. They simply block the effects of agonists, and have zero efficacy.
- Some agonists have a higher affinity for resting receptors, so that they produce a change that is the opposite of an agonist. These are known as **inverse agonists**.

Inverse agonists are said to have 'negative efficacy', tending to reduce the basal level of activity by the natural ligand. A further complication arises when normal antagonists at some tissue sites become agonists at other sites. The real role of inverse agonists in therapeutics is yet to be discovered.

Allosteric modulation of drug–receptor interaction

A drug sometimes interferes with the natural ligand/receptor interaction not by binding to the ligand/receptor site, but elsewhere on the receptor to decrease ligand/receptor binding. This is known as allosteric modulation.

Drug antagonism

A drug is classified as an antagonist when it binds to a receptor but produces no response. However, when two drugs that target the same receptor are present in the system, the effects on one may be reduced, or abolished by the other. An antagonist drug may block access to receptors by:

- An agonist drug, thus diminishing or abolishing the effects of the agonist
- A natural ligand, reducing or abolishing its effects.

Mechanisms of drug antagonism

Antagonist drugs block access to receptors by natural ligands and other drugs without activating the receptor (Clinical box 4.12). The mechanisms can be classified as follows:

- Chemical antagonism/drug sequestration
- Receptor antagonism
- Non-competitive antagonism
- Pharmacokinetic antagonism
- Physiological antagonism.

Clinical box 4.12 **Clinical application of drug antagonism: therapeutic examples**

Chemical antagonism
Chelating agents form a complex with the drug, reducing the concentration of free drug, e.g. dimercaprol chelates mercury to reduce the plasma concentration of mercury. Dimercaprol is used as an antidote for mercury poisoning.

Receptor antagonism
Irreversible, competitive receptor antagonists are usually used experimentally. They have few clinical applications (phenoxybenzamine is used in phaeochromocytoma). However, the irreversible, competitive enzyme inhibitors do have a clinical use (e.g. aspirin and cyclo-oxygenase; omeprazole and Na^+/K^+-ATPase pump).

Non-competitive antagonism
Verapamil and nifedipine, which are Ca^{2+} antagonists, non-specifically block the influx of Ca^{2+} into cells, and can block smooth muscle contraction produced by other drugs.

Pharmacokinetic antagonism
- Increasing the rate of renal excretion of aspirin by alkalising the urine with bicarbonate
- Enzyme induction to increase metabolism and reduce the effectiveness of other drugs: e.g. enzyme induction by rifampicin or barbiturates reduces the effectiveness of oral contraceptives and warfarin
- Reduction of gastric motility, e.g. atropine reduces absorption in the small intestine.

Physiological antagonism
Clinically important in the treatment of conditions such as asthma. The effectiveness of bronchodilators (e.g. salbutamol) is related to the degree of the airways constriction produced by histamines and prostaglandins (the greater the degree of bronchoconstriction the less effective the bronchodilator).

Chemical antagonism/drug sequestration

Chemical antagonism occurs when drugs combine in solution to produce an inactive product, reducing the plasma concentration of free drug. Examples include chelating agents used as antidotes in heavy metal poisoning.

Receptor antagonism

Receptor antagonism occurs when the drug blocks access to the receptor, and involves two important mechanisms (see Fig. 4.18A):

- Reversible competitive antagonism
- Irreversible (non-equilibrium) competitive antagonism.

Reversible competitive antagonism

Reversible competitive antagonism has been discussed in the context of how antagonists can displace agonists from receptor binding sites. However, because a potent full agonist would only need to bind on a small number of drug–receptor binding sites to achieve maximal response, unless all the binding sites are occupied by the antagonist, the effect of reversible, competitive antagonism can be overcome by increasing the drug concentration: the curve for A_2 merely shifts to the right, in the presence of a reversible antagonist.

Irreversible, competitive antagonism

Irreversible or non-equilibrium, competitive antagonism occurs when the antagonist dissociates very slowly or not at all from the receptor. Irreversible antagonists are chemically reactive compounds that bind to the receptor via covalent bonds. The synthesis of new receptor protein may be required to make antagonist free receptors available.

Because an irreversible antagonist reduces the total number of available receptors, increasing the drug concentration would not restore full agonist activity. Spare receptors may come to the rescue. In Figure 4.18A, the presence of the irreversible antagonist depresses the curve for A_2 so that it no longer reaches maximal response despite increasing agonist dose.

Non-competitive antagonism

Non-competitive antagonists block the chain of events leading to a tissue response at some point after the drug–receptor binding stage. As a rule, this turns a full agonist into a partial agonist.

Pharmacokinetic antagonism

Drugs that increase the rate of drug excretion or metabolism, or reduce the rate of absorption, may appear to act as antagonists by altering the pharmacokinetic parameters of the agonist.

Physiological antagonism

Physiological antagonism is an interaction between two drugs whose opposing actions (e.g. contraction and relaxation) via different receptors on the same tissue modulate each other's effect.

TOLERANCE, DESENSITISATION, TACHYPHYLAXIS

Receptors not only initiate physiological and biochemical responses but are themselves subject to regulatory controls. Continuous or repeated stimulation of receptors by an agonist can result in a diminished response.

Tolerance

Tolerance has occurred when the dose of a drug has to be increased to produce the same pharmacokinetic or pharmacodynamic effect, associated with continuous use over a prolonged period of time.

In **pharmacokinetic tolerance** the rate of drug metabolism changes primarily as a result of increased synthesis of hepatic microsomal enzymes (e.g. enzyme induction by barbiturates). Excretion of metabolised drug increases, and concentration of active drug in the blood, and subsequently at the drug's site of action, decreases. **Pharmacodynamic tolerance** results from changes within systems affected by the drug so that the same dose results in a reduced response. It can be due to receptor downregulation or reduced efficiency of receptor coupling to the signal transduction pathway.

Cross tolerance occurs when repeated use of a drug in a given class confers tolerance not only to its own actions but also to the actions of other drugs in that class (e.g. opioid analgesics).

Receptor desensitisation

Receptor **desensitisation** is a loss of receptor-activated response due to persistent exposure to an agonist. Desensitisation can occur within the course of a few minutes and is classified as short- or long-term:

- **Short-term desensitisation** is usually associated with phosphorylation of the receptor protein, followed by uncoupling from the signal pathway
- **Long-term desensitisation** usually involves changes in the regulation of gene expression of the receptor and other proteins in the signalling pathway.

Tachyphylaxis

Tachyphylaxis is a form of desensitisation due to depletion of an essential intermediate substance. For example, repeat administration of indirectly acting sympathomimetic amines (e.g. tyramine) over a short period of time results in a loss of pharmacological activity due to depletion of the vesicular pool of norepinephrine released by tyramine from the nerve terminals, and not to receptor desensitisation.

THE AUTONOMIC NERVOUS SYSTEM

The human nervous system is divided into the **central nervous system** (CNS) and **peripheral nervous system** (PNS). The PNS consists of the **motor (somatic)** and **autonomic nervous systems,** which are anatomically distinct (Fig. 4.20).

The autonomic nervous system (ANS) is further divided into the parasympathetic and sympathetic systems. The cell bodies of the parasympathetic and sympathetic **preganglionic** neurons are in the spinal cord; the preganglionic nerve fibres carry their messages to a series of parasympathetic and sympathetic **ganglia** outside the spinal cord. Autonomic ganglia contain the preganglionic nerve endings that synapse with the cell bodies of the postganglionic neurons. The ganglia act like junction boxes, where signals are relayed from the preganglionic nerve endings to the postganglionic cell bodies. The adrenal medulla functions as one big ganglion.

- In the parasympathetic system, the neurotransmitter at the short postganglionic neuron is acetylcholine, and the postsynaptic receptors stimulated by acetylcholine are muscarinic receptors.
- Nicotinic and muscarinic receptors are collectively known as **cholinergic** receptors and owe their names to historical experiments when their actions were reproduced by the injection of nicotine and muscarine. Muscarine is an extract of the poisonous toadstool *Amanita muscaria* (antidote is atropine).
- All sympathetic postganglionic nerves release norepinephrine at the **postganglionic** synapse, with the exception of sweat glands. Norepinephrine acts on **adrenergic** receptors.
- The postsynaptic transmitter for sweat glands is acetylcholine, which activates muscarinic receptors (see later).

NEUROTRANSMITTERS

Neurotransmitters are the chemical messengers that carry signals across synapses to stimulate postsynaptic receptors. They are synthesised in neuron terminals from precursors that are already present. There are systems for storage within the nerve terminals. The transmitters are released in response to neuronal stimulation to activate postsynaptic receptors, then removed by transport proteins or degraded to terminate their action. The most important neurotransmitters in the ANS are **acetylcholine** and **norepinephrine**.

- The neurotransmitter associated with all **preganglionic** neurons (parasympathetic and sympathetic) is acetylcholine, which stimulates postsynaptic nicotinic receptors at the ganglionic synapse.

FUNCTIONS OF THE AUTONOMIC NERVOUS SYSTEM

The ANS carries all motor outflow from the CNS to the major organs of the body, with the exception of the motor outflow to skeletal muscles. The parasympathetic and sympathetic systems are entirely linked to the CNS. Although part of the enteric nervous system receives autonomic input, most of the enteric system has local networks that are independent of the CNS. The ANS is not under voluntary control and regulates essential physiological processes such as:

- Rate (chronotropic) and force (inotropic) of contraction of heart muscle (Ch. 11)
- Secretions of exocrine glands: bronchial, salivary, sweat, etc.
- Vascular smooth muscle and thus blood pressure

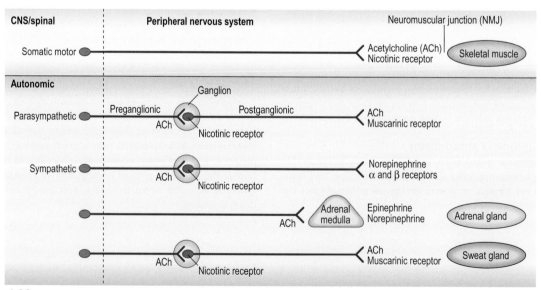

Fig. 4.20 **Simplified, diagrammatic representation of the anatomical and pharmacological subdivisions of the autonomic (peripheral) nervous system.** Somatic motor neurons convey signals from the spinal cord via efferent nerves to skeletal muscles. In the CNS, the cell body of each somatic motor neuron is in the spinal cord; the neuron terminates in close proximity to the effector muscle at a specialised site, the neuromuscular junction. The neurotransmitter released by the motor efferent at the neuromuscular junction is acetylcholine and the receptor stimulated by acetylcholine is a subclass of the nicotinic receptor.

- Smooth muscle contraction and relaxation: bronchial, enteric, eye, etc.
- Energy metabolism, e.g. hepatic glycogenolysis, skeletal muscle glycogenolysis, fat cell lipolysis, pancreatic insulin secretion (see Ch. 3)
- Some endocrine secretion (see Ch. 10).

The ANS is important pharmacologically because:

- It controls the functions of almost all the major human organ systems.
- The relative simplicity of the ANS in terms of receptor subtypes and the fact that there are only two main transmitters – acetylcholine and norepinephrine – make study of the chemical transmission relatively easy.
- The action of neurotransmitters can be mimicked and modified by drugs, which are synthetic analogues.
- Diseases with ANS dysfunction are common.

OVERVIEW OF THE AUTONOMIC NERVOUS SYSTEM

The ANS is subdivided into parasympathetic (cholinergic) and sympathetic (adrenergic) systems, which can be distinguished anatomically and functionally:

- **Parasympathetic system**: maintains essential bodily functions, controls the gastrointestinal tract (secretions and motility), and controls defaecation, urination and sexual function (genital erection). A complex system of neurons innervates and controls the function of glands, and smooth and cardiac muscles.
- **Sympathetic system**: primarily enables the body to adjust to stressful situations (exercise, fear, fight and flight) by acting to increase cardiac function, alter vascular tone (e.g. vasodilatation in skeletal muscle) and mobilise body energy stores.

At rest, most organs are under parasympathetic drive. This can be altered by increasing sympathetic drive when epinephrine is secreted by the adrenal medulla, as in the exercise, fear and flight responses. The two branches of the ANS often have opposing organ effects (physiological antagonism). Parasympathetic and sympathetic activity have to be coordinated for normal physiological function; for example, in defaecation, there is increased parasympathetic drive to the colonic smooth muscle to increase motility, at the same time as decreased sympathetic drive to relax the anal sphincter muscle.

There are, however, exceptions. For example, the two systems produce similar effects in the salivary glands. In some organs, only one or the other of the sympathetic or parasympathetic system is present:

- Sweat glands and most blood vessels only have sympathetic innervation.
- Ciliary muscles in the eye only have parasympathetic innervation.
- Bronchial muscle only has parasympathetic innervation (constriction).

THE PARASYMPATHETIC SYSTEM

Long preganglionic neurons terminate at a ganglionic site within or in close proximity to the effector tissue (see Fig. 4.22). Acetylcholine is the neurotransmitter that stimulates nicotinic receptors at the ganglionic synapse, and muscarinic receptors at the postganglionic synapse.

THE SYMPATHETIC SYSTEM

The sympathetic nervous system consists of short preganglionic neurons that terminate in the ganglionic **sympathetic chain** (see Fig. 4.22), where acetylcholine is the neurotransmitter stimulating nicotinic receptors. The postganglionic sympathetic neuron is long, synapses at the effector site and the neurotransmitter is norepinephrine. The receptors stimulated by norepinephrine are adrenergic receptors, consisting of α and β receptors.

Adrenal gland

The adrenal gland is innervated by a sympathetic preganglionic neuron and the acetylcholine that is released stimulates nicotinic receptors associated with **chromaffin cells** of the adrenal medulla, containing the hormones epinephrine and norepinephrine, which when released into the bloodstream stimulate adrenergic receptors.

Sweat glands

The innervation of sweat glands is an exception in that, although it is under sympathetic control, the postganglionic neuron of thermoregulatory sweat glands consists mainly of parasympathetic nerve fibres. Sympathetic stimulation results in the release of acetylcholine, activating muscarinic receptors. The pathways controlling nervous sweating (palms, armpits, etc.) release norepinephrine to activate α_1-adrenoceptors.

THE REFLEX ARC

In both the somatic and autonomic nervous systems, information from the periphery to the spinal cord and out to effector organs is relayed by simple reflex arcs. Although this chapter concerns the ANS, the somatic motor reflex arc is also described for comparison.

Autonomic motor reflex

The autonomic efferent pathway consists of two types of neuron – the pre- and postganglionic neurons in series (Fig. 4.21A). These neurons synapse in the autonomic ganglia. The autonomic reflex consists of:

- Visceral sensory afferent neurons conveying information from interoreceptors (e.g. chemoreceptors or mechanoreceptors).
- Visceral motor efferent neurons, which regulate visceral activity either by excitatory or inhibitory activity on the effector tissue (cardiac, smooth muscles, glands, etc.). The efferent output from the spinal cord is composed of a two-neuron pathway, consisting of a slow conducting, lightly myelinated preganglionic fibre and a non-myelinated postganglionic fibre.

Most nerve bundles are mixed nerves carrying both sensory and motor neurons in different proportions.

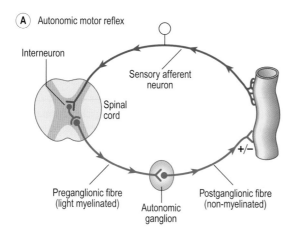

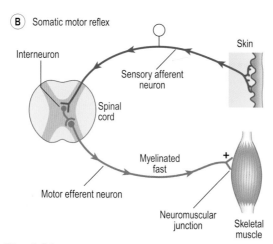

Fig. 4.21 **The reflex arc.**

Somatic motor reflex

The somatic nervous system regulates the voluntary control of skeletal muscle function (Fig. 4.21B). In contrast to the autonomic efferent pathway, which consists of two neurons, the somatic motor efferent consists of a single motor neuron. A simple somatic motor reflex arc is composed of:

- A sensory (afferent) neuron carrying information to the CNS from receptors, e.g. exteroreceptors (sight, sound, vision, taste, smell, pain, touch, thermal) and proprioceptors (muscle and joint position).
- A motor efferent neuron transmitting information from the CNS or spinal cord via a single motor nerve that is myelinated and fast conducting to the periphery. The absence of a ganglion body in the motor efferent increases the speed of conduction to the effector (skeletal) muscle to cause a contraction. The junction between the motor nerve and the skeletal muscle is the neuromuscular junction (NMJ).

ANATOMY OF THE AUTONOMIC NERVOUS SYSTEM

The cell bodies of the preganglionic neurons in the ANS lie in the CNS; their nerve terminals synapse with postganglionic neurons in the ganglia. Most of the parasympathetic ganglia

lie in or close to their effector organs (see also Ch. 8). The sympathetic ganglia are either paired, and lie on either side of the spinal cord to form the paravertebral, sympathetic chains, or are unpaired (single) and lie in the midline to form the prevertebral chain (Fig. 4.22).

The nerve supply to the gastrointestinal tract is more complex. Enteric neurons lie in the walls of the intestine. Some receive parasympathetic and sympathetic input, while others form a plexus of local reflex arcs (myenteric and submucosal) that function independently of the ANS.

THE PARASYMPATHETIC SYSTEM

The efferent parasympathetic pathway consists of cranial and sacral outflows. The cell bodies of cranial preganglionic neurons are in the brainstem. Preganglionic fibres synapse in ganglia that are close to the effector organ.

Nerve fibres from the sacral preganglionic cell bodies leave the spinal cord via the ventral roots of the spinal nerves S2–4 to synapse in scattered ganglia in the pelvis. Their postganglionic fibres innervate the distal colon, rectum, genitalia and urinary system.

THE SYMPATHETIC SYSTEM

The cell bodies of the preganglionic neurons are situated in the lateral grey horns of the 1st to 12th thoracic and 1st and 2nd lumbar segments of the spinal cord. The preganglionic fibres leave the spinal cord in the anterior roots of the spinal nerves. The ganglia of the postganglionic fibres of the sympathetic division are located at three sites:

- **Paravertebral ganglia** (sympathetic chain): 22 pairs of interconnected ganglia on either side of the spinal column. The output from any given segment of the thoracolumbar division of the spinal cord can stimulate a number of paravertebral ganglia. A single preganglionic fibre may travel through many ganglia and can synapse with up to 20 or more postganglionic sympathetic fibres. This accounts for the diffuse nature of the sympathetic response in humans. Postganglionic fibres innervate heart, sweat glands, pilomotor muscle as well as blood vessels of the skin and skeletal muscle.
- **Prevertebral ganglia**: the unpaired coeliac, superior and inferior mesenteric ganglia which are in the walls of the main branches of the abdominal aorta. Preganglionic fibres associated with these ganglia pass through the paravertebral ganglia before synapsing with the prevertebral ganglia to innervate the gastrointestinal and urinary tracts.
- **Terminal ganglia**: the inferior hypogastric plexus ganglia associated with the urinary and rectal areas, and the cervical ganglia (superior, middle and inferior) innervating the eye, salivary glands and blood vessels of the head and neck.

NEUROTRANSMITTERS AND RECEPTORS OF THE AUTONOMIC NERVOUS SYSTEM

Acetylcholine and norepinephrine are the major neurotransmitters of the ANS. Therapeutic manipulation of their effects is mainly aimed at modifying the concentration of neurotransmitters at their site of action (Information box 4.11):

Mammalian autonomic nervous system

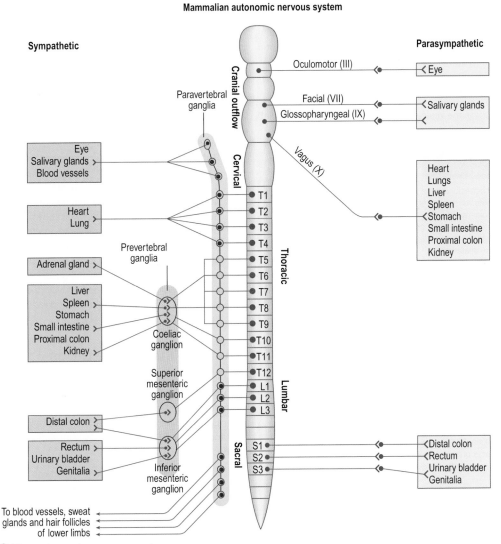

Fig. 4.22 **The autonomic nervous system.**

<table>
<tr><td>**Information box 4.11**</td><td>**Potential sites of drug targets in the ANS (see Fig. 4.20)**</td></tr>
</table>

Ganglion blockade:
- Postsynaptic ganglionic receptors (nicotinic receptors)
- Presynaptic receptors (auto- and hetero-receptors, see later)
- Muscarinic receptors at the postganglionic synapse
- α- and β-adrenergic receptors at the postganglionic synapse.
  The drug acts to facilitate or inhibit:
- Acetylcholine – synthesis, storage or release
- Norepinephrine – synthesis, storage or release.
  The earliest drugs that were found to affect the ANS were **ganglion-blocking** drugs. They blocked acetylcholine receptors in both parasympathetic and sympathetic ganglia. They now have restricted clinical use because of the mixed effects. For example, ganglion blockers used in the treatment of high blood pressure (hypertension) are now obsolete (except for specialised indications) due to:
- Sympathetic blockade causing vasodilatation, leading to hypotension
- Parasympathetic blockade causing the side effects of dry mouth, urine retention, blurred vision, impotence and constipation.

- Change rate of synthesis – increase or reduce concentration
- Change storage – deplete neurotransmitter

- Change rate of release – reduce concentration
- Block re-uptake (into presynaptic neuron) – increase concentration
- Block degradation of neurotransmitter – increase concentration
- Change number of receptors – up- or down-regulation.

PARASYMPATHETIC (CHOLINERGIC) SYSTEM

Acetylcholine (ACh) is the neurotransmitter at both pre- (nicotinic) and post- (muscarinic) ganglionic nerve terminals. The receptors are collectively known as cholinergic receptors (Fig. 4.23).

Synthesis of acetylcholine

ACh is synthesised from a precursor, choline, and acetyl-CoA (see Ch. 2) by the enzyme choline acetyltransferase (CAT). Choline is derived from the diet, ACh breakdown or synthesised by the liver and transported into the nerve terminal by a high affinity Na^+-choline co-transporter. Acetylcholine synthesis may be reduced by hemicholinium, a neuronal choline transporter inhibitor.

Storage of acetylcholine

Once synthesised, ACh is transported by a vesicular transporter to be stored in vesicles. The ACh vesicular transporter can be inhibited by vesamicol.

Release of acetylcholine

Acetylcholine in the vesicles is released into the synaptic cleft by Ca^{2+}-dependent exocytosis (Information box 4.12).

Information box 4.12	Inhibition of acetylcholine vesicular release

Substances that inhibit the influx of Ca^{2+} into nerve terminals prevent vesicular release of ACh (Fig. 4.23). Effects of inhibiting ACh vesicular release into the **synapse** include:
- Inhibition of sweating, giving symptoms of a dry, warm skin
- Inhibition of salivation with symptoms of dry mouth
- Pupillary dilatation.
  Inhibition of ACh vesicular release at the **neuromuscular junction** would lead to muscle paralysis:
- Aminoglycoside antibiotics such as streptomycin and neomycin block ACh vesicular release and occasionally produce muscle paralysis as an unwanted side effect.
- Botulism is a severe form of food poisoning with a high mortality rate, caused by the anaerobic bacillus *Clostridium botulinum*. *C. botulinum* can multiply in canned or preserved food, producing an exotoxin that inhibits the vesicular release of ACh. Blockade at the NMJ leads to voluntary muscle paralysis and fatal respiratory muscle paralysis. Botulinum poisoning also causes parasympathetic paralysis with symptoms of dry mouth and blurring of vision.
- β-Bungarotoxin is contained in the venom of a variety of cobras and the black widow spider, and has similar effects to botulism. The same venoms also contain α-bungarotoxin, which acts presynaptically, causing the rapid discharge of vesicular contents, followed by paralysis.

Parasympathetic synthesis and receptors

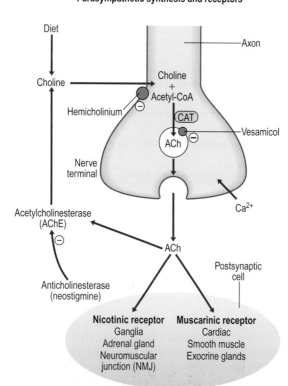

Fig. 4.23 **Synthesis, metabolism and receptors associated with parasympathetic nerve terminal.**

Inactivation of acetylcholine

ACh is rapidly hydrolysed by the enzyme **cholinesterase,** which is associated with the cholinergic synaptic membranes and also in a soluble form in plasma, to choline and acetic acid, which in turn is converted to water and CO_2.

There are two distinct types of the cholinesterase enzyme and they have different distributions and functions:

- **Acetylcholinesterase** is membrane bound and hydrolyses ACh released at cholinergic synapses.
- **Butyrylcholinesterase,** also known as pseudocholinesterase, is widely distributed in tissues such as brain, liver, gastrointestinal tract, and in the soluble form in plasma. The function of the synaptic membrane-bound form is not well known, but the soluble plasma enzyme inactivates a variety of circulating drugs including procaine, benzocaine (local anaesthetics) and suxamethonium (NMJ blocker). A subpopulation of patients is deficient in plasma pseudocholinesterase activity, resulting in prolonged activity of drugs such as suxamethonium, a muscle relaxant used during general anaesthesia for major surgery.

Anticholinesterase drugs

Anticholinesterase drugs are used therapeutically to increase cholinergic activity, but are also poisons. Anticholinesterase drugs may be reversible short- or medium-acting, or irreversible.

Blockade of cholinesterase enzymes results in increased autonomic activity but primarily with increased cholinergic effects:

- At the postganglionic nerve terminal with increased stimulation of muscarinic receptors (see below), enhancing synaptic cholinergic activity, causing excessive salivation, bradycardia, bronchospasm and hypotension
- By increasing NMJ activity with muscle fasciculation and twitching, and may result in a depolarisation block and paralysis
- Anticholinesterase drugs that cross the blood–brain barrier have central effects due to increased muscarinic receptor activation, leading to excitation and convulsions followed by unconsciousness and respiratory failure. The antidote is atropine.

Short-acting, reversible anticholinesterase

The ionic bond formed between short-acting, reversible anticholinesterases is rapidly reversible, and the duration of action of the drug is very brief, measured in seconds. Edrophonium is the only clinically important one, used primarily in the diagnosis of myasthenia gravis. Muscle strength temporarily improves after the injection of edrophonium in myasthenia gravis, but not other conditions with muscle weakness.

Medium-acting, reversible anticholinesterase

Medium-acting, reversible anticholinesterases are carbamyl, instead of acetyl, esters. The carbamyl ester takes longer to hydrolyse than edrophonium so that the action can be long-lasting, although reversible. Physostigmine and neostigmine are clinically important in the treatment of glaucoma, reversal of a competitive NMJ block and the treatment of myasthenia gravis.

Irreversible anticholinesterases (organophosphates)

Irreversible anticholinesterases are phosphorus compounds with a labile fluoride (e.g. dyflos) or an organic group (e.g. malathione, used in preparations for the treatment of head lice) that binds covalently to the cholinesterase enzyme. The phosphorylated enzyme is stable, with no appreciable hydrolysis so that a new enzyme has to be synthesised to restore cholinesterase activity, which may take several weeks (see Information box 4.13).

Information box 4.13	Chemical and biological weapons

Irreversible anticholinesterases were developed as nerve gases for chemical warfare and pesticides (e.g. sheep dip used by farmers). These compounds have high lipid solubility and are readily absorbed through mucous membranes and unbroken skin. Poisoning by these agents requires the antidote pralidoxime and hospitalisation. Pralidoxime reactivates the enzyme by attracting the phosphate group away from the active site on the enzyme. Reactivation has to be done in the first few hours, because the enzyme cannot be reactivated after prolonged binding to the organophosphate.

The Geneva Protocol of 1925 banned the use of chemical weapons. In 1971, the Biological Weapons Convention (BWC) completed work on the Convention on the Prohibition of the Development, Production, Stockpiling and Use of Chemical Weapons and on Their Destruction. This should have banned all production and use of these weapons. The BWC was opened for signatures and ratification by all nations in 1972, and was entered into force in 1975.

Cholinergic receptors

Acetylcholine, the neurotransmitter of the parasympathetic system, stimulates the two major classes of cholinergic receptor:

- Nicotinic receptors (nAChR)
- Muscarinic receptors (mAChR).

Nicotinic receptors

There are two subtypes of nicotinic receptor:

- N_M receptors, at the neuromuscular junction
- N_N receptors, at all autonomic ganglia, in the adrenal gland and in the CNS (neuronal nicotinic receptors).

The molecular structures of these receptors are similar. Both types are ligand-gated ion channels with varying selectivity for cations (Na^+, Ca^{2+}), which, when stimulated by ACh, produce rapid excitatory responses, owing to localised depolarisation of cell membranes. The differences between the two types are exploited pharmacologically. See Table 4.5 for examples and therapeutic effects.

Pharmacological effects of nicotinic receptor agonists

Acetylcholine and nicotine are N_N receptor agonists (Table 4.5). Stimulation of ganglionic N_N receptors by ACh causes complex peripheral responses due to generalised stimulation of all autonomic ganglia (i.e. increased sympathetic and parasympathetic activity). Ganglionic N_N stimulation also stimulates the adrenal medulla to release epinephrine and norepinephrine, **Nicotine** initially stimulates

Table 4.5	Examples of drugs acting at cholinergic receptors and their clinical uses			
Receptor	Agonists	Clinical uses	Antagonists	Clinical uses
Nicotinic (ganglionic)	Acetylcholine	None	Hexamethonium	
	Nicotine	None	Trimetaphan	Orthostatic hypotension in surgery
Nicotinic (NMJ)	Suxamethonium	Muscle relaxant (depolarising block)	Tubocurare	
			Pancuronium Atracurium	Muscle relaxants
Muscarinic	Acetylcholine	None	Atropine	Antispasmodic, causes CNS excitation, tachycardia
	Pilocarpine	Reduces intraocular pressure in glaucoma, contracts iris (smooth muscle)	Hyoscine	Anti-emetic, motion sickness
			Ipratropium	Bronchodilator (asthma, COPD)
			Trihexyphenidyl hydrochloride (benzhexol)	Anti-muscarinic action at NMJ: used to treat tremor and spasticity in Parkinsonism
			Tropicamide	Mydriatic: used to dilate pupils in ophthalmology
			Pirenzepine	Inhibits gastric secretions in peptic ulcers
	Carbachol Bethanechol	Stimulate smooth muscle contraction in bladder and intestinal tract	Oxybutynin Tolterodine	Inhibits bladder contraction, used to treat urinary incontinence

N_N in the autonomic ganglia but produces a depolarisation block with prolonged use (i.e. becomes antagonistic).

Suxamethonium has a similar structure to ACh (two Ach molecules attached together back to back) and acts as a N_M receptor agonist at the neuromuscular junction. In contrast to ACh, which is rapidly hydrolysed, suxamethonium remains at the NMJ for a long time. After initial stimulation of the NMJ leading to muscle twitching or fasciculation, muscle relaxation sets in due to depolarising block, when the muscle loses electrical excitability for the duration of the drug action.

Pharmacological effects of nicotinic receptor antagonists

The effect of blocking ganglionic nicotinic receptors results in a generalised decrease in postganglionic parasympathetic and sympathetic activity (see Table 4.5). The physiological response observed depends on which division of the ANS is dominant in any given organ. In the majority of organs the parasympathetic innervation is dominant (heart, eye, gastrointestinal tract, urinary tract, sweat glands, salivary glands). The vascular system is, however, solely under tonic sympathetic control and so ganglionic nicotinic receptor antagonists produce a fall in blood pressure, with ensuing postural hypotension. Some N_N antagonists, such as hexamethonium, have only experimental use but trimetaphan is used to lower blood pressure during surgery.

Drugs that act as N_M receptor antagonists, such as tubocurare, competitively block the action of ACh on N_M receptors at the NMJ. The effects of these drugs are mostly to produce motor paralysis of skeletal muscle. They have very little or no antagonistic action at neuronal N_N receptors and vice versa.

Muscarinic receptors

Molecular biology has identified five different subtypes of muscarinic receptors (M_1–M_5). Each subtype couples to a second messenger system through an intervening G protein. M_1, M_3 and M_5 receptor stimulation results in increased levels of the second messengers IP_3 and DAG whereas M_2 and M_4 receptor stimulation results in reduced cAMP levels. The important functions are those of M_{1-3}. The tissue distribution differs for each subtype:

- M_1 – act at autonomic ganglia (where they produce depolarisation of the cell membrane). Mainly located in the hippocampus and cerebral cortex and on the parietal cells (where they increase HCl release) and in the gastrointestinal tract.
- M_2 – also known as 'cardiac' receptors, cause slowing of the heart rate and a decrease in the force of contraction. Mainly located in the heart, gastrointestinal smooth muscle, and CNS, they are also presynaptic autoreceptors (see later).
- M_3 – also known as 'glandular' receptors, stimulate secretion of exocrine glands (salivary, gastric, etc.) and visceral smooth muscular contraction. Receptors in vascular endothelium cause vasodilatation and a fall in blood pressure.

Pharmacological effects of muscarinic receptor agonists

Stimulation of muscarinic receptors has the following effects (Table 4.5):

- **Cardiovascular**: slowing of heart rate (sino-atrial node), reduction in force of contraction (atria) and reduction in atrio-ventricular node conduction

- **Vascular endothelium**: mediation of the release of nitric oxide to produce vasodilatation
- **Smooth muscle**: contraction of bronchial and bladder smooth muscle
- **Gastrointestinal tract**: increase in smooth muscle tone, peristalsis and increasing gastric and pancreatic secretions
- **Exocrine glands**: increased sweating, lacrimation, salivation and bronchial secretions; induction of histamine release from histaminocytes; increased HCl secretion from gastric parietal cells
- **Eye**: contraction of pupillary muscle (constrictor pupillae) causing pupillary constriction in response to bright light, and contraction of ciliary muscles to change the shape of the lens in ocular accommodation.

Pharmacological effects of muscarinic receptor antagonists

Muscarinic receptor antagonists selectively block parasympathetic activity with the following effects (Table 4.5):

- **Inhibition of secretions**: causing dry mouth and skin (dry and warm to the touch due to lack of sweating), inhibition of mucociliary clearance in lungs
- **Heart**: initial slowing in rate (bradycardia) due to central stimulation, followed by tachycardia (vagus blocked and the sympathetic effect is unopposed)
- **Eye**: dilation of pupil (mydriasis), which becomes unresponsive to light; relaxation of ciliary muscles, resulting in loss of accommodation and blurred vision (cycloplegia)
- **CNS**: a dose-dependent excitatory effect (restlessness, disorientation), which can be reversed by physostigmine (anticholinesterase).

Table 4.5 shows some examples of muscarinic receptor agonists and therapeutic uses.

SYMPATHETIC (ADRENERGIC) SYSTEM

With the exception of sweat glands, norepinephrine is the principal postganglionic neurotransmitter in the sympathetic nervous system. Norepinephrine belongs to a group of neurotransmitters known as catecholamines. They have the biochemical structure of a benzene ring joined to two adjacent hydroxyl groups (catechol), which forms a complex with an amine. Both the catechol and the amine groups are receptor binding. The main catecholamines are norepinephrine, dopamine and epinephrine. Serotonin, or 5-HT, although not strictly a catecholamine, has catecholamine-like actions. Isoprenaline (US: isoproterenol) is a synthetic analogue of norepinephrine.

Sympathetic receptors are adrenergic, and drugs that activate adrenergic receptors (adrenergic agonists) are known as sympathomimetic amines, as they mimic the action of sympathetic stimuli.

Sympathomimetic amines

Sympathomimetic amines are developed by modifying the norepinephrine molecule. They may be directly or indirectly acting.

- **Directly acting sympathomimetic amines** have a direct action on adrenoceptors and mimic the action of norepinephrine and epinephrine

- **Indirectly acting sympathomimetic amines** may partially act weakly on adrenoceptors, but predominantly are taken into the nerve terminals by transporters, displacing norepinephrine, which is either metabolised by MAO/COMT enzymes (see below) or released into the synapse by a reverse neuronal transport system (see below) to act on postsynaptic receptors.

Norepinephrine (adrenaline) synthesis

The sympathetic ganglion contains the cell bodies of noradrenergic neurons, whose postganglionic nerve terminals end in numerous varicosities (swellings or boutons) that contain many synaptic vesicles. Tyrosine is converted to dopamine in the cytoplasm of the nerve terminals which is transported into the synaptic vesicles where it is converted to norepinephrine for storage and release. The last step in the catecholamine synthesis pathway is the catalysis of norepinephrine to epinephrine which only occurs in the adrenal medulla (see later). The carbon skeleton of norepinephrine comes from the metabolism of the essential amino acid tyrosine or its precursor, phenylalanine (Fig. 4.24). Phenylalanine is converted to tyrosine by phenylalanine hydroxylase.

Norepinephrine synthesis pathway

Norepinephrine is synthesised from L-tyrosine in adrenergic neurons. Tyrosine is converted to dopa (levodopa) by the enzyme tyrosine hydroxylase, which requires a pteridine cofactor (Fig. 4.24). The activity of tyrosine hydroxylase is **rate-limiting** for catecholamine synthesis (i.e. the slowest acting enzyme in the series involved in the synthesis of norepinephrine). Tyrosine hydroxylase activity can be regulated by a variety of signals within the nerve cell body or terminal:

- Increased cytoplasmic concentration of free norepinephrine inhibits the enzyme by competing for the cofactor, pteridine – known as **end-product inhibition**
- Increased phosphorylation of tyrosine hydroxylase by elevated cAMP levels results in an increased rate of conversion and/or affinity of the enzyme for the cofactor
- Increased intracellular Ca^{2+} levels due to increased neuronal activity increases the sensitivity of the enzyme
- Increased neuronal firing rates or depletion of neuronal transmitter stores results in increased tyrosine hydroxylase activity, as indicated by increased levels of mRNA for the enzyme
- Dephosphorylation of the enzyme by stimulating autoreceptors (α_2 resulting in reduced cAMP levels) reduces activity of tyrosine hydroxylase.

These changes in the synthesis and function of tyrosine hydroxylase, in response to neuronal activity, serve to maintain the rate of synthesis of norepinephrine relative to the requirement for the transmitter.

Dopa is rapidly converted to dopamine by the enzyme dopa decarboxylase. In dopaminergic neurons, this is the end of the synthetic pathway. In sympathetic neurons, a proportion of the dopamine that is formed in the cytoplasm of the nerve terminal is actively transported by a vesicular transporter into the storage vesicle, where it is converted to norepinephrine by the enzyme dopamine β-hydroxylase. The remainder of the dopamine is converted to the metabolite vanillyl mandelic acid (VMA) also known as homovanillic acid, which is excreted in the urine (see Clinical box 4.13 for examples of drugs targeting norepinephrine synthesis).

Sympathetic synthesis and receptors

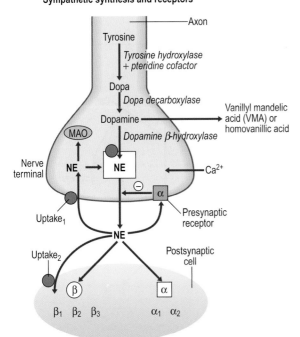

Fig. 4.24 **Synthesis and release of norepinephrine) from sympathetic neurons.** MAO, monoamine oxidase; NE, norepinephrine; α, α-adrenoceptor; β, β-adrenoceptor.

| Clinical box 4.13 | Examples of drugs acting on the synthetic sequence of norepinephrine |

- Phaeochromocytoma is a rare chromaffin cell tumour of the sympathetic nervous system, the vast majority arising in the adrenal medulla. Uncontrolled, intermittent oversecretion of norepinephrine leads to severe hypertension and hyperglycaemia. Tyrosine hydroxylase can be inhibited by α-methyltyrosine, which is used in the treatment of phaeochromocytoma. Measurement of urinary VMA is a useful screening test for phaeochromocytoma. A 24-hour urine collection is needed. Dietary vanilla and some drugs can interfere with the test.
- Administration of levodopa bypasses the rate limiting step in tyrosine hydrolysis, leading to the increased synthesis of dopamine. Levodopa is used in the treatment of Parkinsonism. Parkinson disease is the result of progressive degeneration of the substantia nigra in the brain resulting in dopamine deficiency, leading to neurohormonal imbalance in the basal ganglia. These centres initiate and modulate movement, so that dopamine deficiency would lead to the characteristic rigidity and tremor of idiopathic Parkinson disease. Levodopa is sometimes used in combination with a dopa-decarboxylase inhibitor, carbidopa, which inhibits the peripheral conversion of dopa to dopamine allowing more L-dopa to enter the CNS and be converted to dopamine.
- The antihypertensive drug, α-methyldopa (an analogue of levodopa), was developed as an inhibitor of dopa decarboxylase, thereby inhibiting norepinephrine synthesis. The hypotensive effect was thought to be due to the inhibition of norepinephrine synthesis. It was later found to have a presynaptic effect on the CNS to reduce sympathetic output.

Adrenal conversion of norepinephrine to epinephrine

Norepinephrine is further converted to epinephrine by the enzyme phenylethanolamine-*N*-methyl transferase in the adrenal medulla.

Norepinephrine storage

In the nerve terminal, cytoplasmic dopamine is actively taken into vesicles by a vesicular transporter and converted to norepinephrine. The vesicle is impermeable from inside to outside, under normal circumstances, preventing norepinephrine from leaking out. Inhibition of the vesicular transporter leads to the depletion of norepinephrine stores (Clinical box 4.14).

Norepinephrine release

Norepinephrine is released in response to sympathetic stimulation. The synaptic vesicles release their contents by Ca^{2+}-dependent exocytosis. Norepinephrine may be released by substances that are taken into the vesicles, where they displace norepinephrine into the cytoplasm. Norepinephrine is then released into the synapse by reversing neuronal uptake transport. Examples include tyramine, ephedrine and amphetamine. These substances are structurally related to norepinephrine, and are known as indirectly acting sympathomimetic amines (Clinical box 4.15). Prolonged, repeated use of these drugs produces diminishing responses (see Tolerance, desensitisation and tachyphylaxis, above).

Modulation of norepinephrine release

Norepinephrine release is modulated by substances that act on presynaptic receptors. Presynaptic modulation is an important control mechanism in the peripheral nervous system. A variety of nerve terminals are subject to this kind of control; different mediators can act on presynaptic terminals. For example, acetylcholine acting through presynaptic muscarinic receptors regulates cholinergic nerve terminals. Other presynaptic receptors include dopaminergic D_2 and serotinergic $5HT_{1D}$ receptors.

Presynaptic autoreceptors

Norepinephrine can modulate its own neuronal release by the stimulation of presynaptic **autoreceptors**. These autoreceptors can be either inhibitory or excitatory (Fig. 4.25).

- **α-Adrenergic receptors** are inhibitory receptors – reduce norepinephrine release.
- **$β_1$-Adrenoceptors** are excitatory autoreceptors – increase norepinephrine release.

Clinical box 4.14 **Example of a drug that interferes with norepinephrine storage**

Reserpine binds to the vesicular transporter with a slow rate of dissociation and a prolonged duration of action. Norepinephrine is depleted through non-replenishment of the vesicles. Although now obsolete, reserpine has been used in the treatment of hypertension in the past, exploiting its main action of depleting norepinephrine. It also depletes other important neurotransmitters such as dopamine and 5-HT, giving rise to the unwanted side effect of depression.

Clinical box 4.15 **Clinical importance of some indirectly acting sympathomimetics**

- Tyramine is contained in foods such as fermented cheeses (e.g. ripe Camembert), and food containing meat extracts (e.g. Marmite). Dietary tyramine is destroyed in the gut and liver by monoamine oxidase (MAO). This is prevented by MAO inhibition, so that eating food rich in tyramine could result in high concentrations of tyramine in the blood, stimulating excessive release of norepinephrine and leading to dangerous hypertension.
- Ephedrine is a drug developed as a nasal decongestant, contained in commercial nasal sprays for relieving the symptoms of the common cold. Ephedrine causes vasoconstriction in the nasal mucosa. The potential for ephedrine to release norepinephrine has led to its classification as a banned substance in competitive sport by the International Olympic Committee. Side effects include hypertension, cardiac arrhythmias and insomnia.
- Amphetamine and its derivatives: 3,4-methylenedioxymethamphetamine (MDMA, Ecstasy), methamphetamine (Speed) and dexamphetamine, act by releasing norepinephrine, dopamine and 5-HT from nerve terminals in the brain (see below). Central stimulant effects include wakefulness, euphoria, anorexia, schizophrenia-like behaviour and hallucinations. Peripheral sympathomimetic effects include hypertension, cardiac arrhythmias and death. Withdrawal causes depression, anxiety and craving. MDMA also causes a disturbance in thermal regulation, so that symptoms of heat stroke and dehydration occur after exertion, which has led to death. Dexamphetamine has been used occasionally for narcolepsy, and a related substance, methylphenidate hydrochloride (Ritalin), is used in conjunction with psychological remedial measures in the treatment of attention deficit hyperactivity disorder (ADHD).

Presynaptic heteroreceptors

There are other receptors involved in controlling norepinephrine release. For example, dopamine and acetycholine can also inhibit release of Norepinephrine by stimulating dopaminergic D_2 and cholinergic M_2 receptors respectively. These are called presynaptic heteroreceptors.

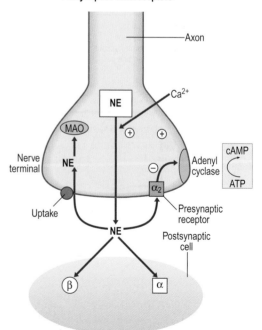

Fig. 4.25 Inhibition of norepinephrine release. MAO, monoamine oxidase; NE, norepinephrine; α, α-adrenoceptor; β, β-adrenoceptor.

Adrenergic neuron blocking drugs (ANBs)

ANBs act presynaptically on norepinephrine release. ANB drugs, such as guanethidine and bretylium, enter the vesicle and replace norepinephrine. This reduces the concentration of norepinephrine released by exocytosis in response to sympathetic stimulation. These drugs are hypotensive, but are obsolete because of their unpleasant side effects. The effects of ANBs can be reversed or prevented by uptake$_1$ inhibitors (e.g. cocaine, tricyclic antidepressants).

Termination of action of neuronally released norepinephrine

The action of neuronally released norepinephrine is terminated by its re-uptake from the synapse into the presynaptic nerve terminal by two specific transporters (Fig. 4.26):

- Neuronal uptake$_1$
- Extraneuronal uptake 2.

Neuronal uptake$_1$

Neuronal uptake$_1$ is the most important process for terminating the action of norepinephrine. About 70% of neuronally released norepinephrine is taken back into the nerve terminal, so that neuronal uptake can be considered as a mechanism of transmitter conservation. The uptake$_1$ transporter is a protein that is selective for the different types of neurotransmitter released from particular neurons, e.g. norepinephrine, dopamine, 5-HT. The more recently developed drugs exploit the differences between transporters so that the drugs are selective in their neuronal uptake inhibitory properties (Information

box 4.14). The uptake$_1$ transporter has a greater selectivity for norepinephrine than for epinephrine, so drugs that inhibit the transporter have no effect on the action of epinephrine. Other substrates for the transporter are dopamine and 5-HT.

Extraneuronal uptake$_2$

The uptake$_2$ transporter effects the re-uptake of epinephrine from the bloodstream into extraneuronal tissue. It is unaffected by the drugs that inhibit uptake$_1$. Although not of major clinical significance, uptake$_2$ is inhibited by corticosteroids. This may be relevant in the treatment of conditions such as asthma.

Metabolism of catecholamines

Norepinephrine is eliminated from the body by metabolic degradation. Two enzymes are important in the metabolism of catecholamines: the mitochondrial monoamine oxidase and cytoplasmic catechol-O-methyltransferase. Both are widely distributed in the body. The degradation of epinephrine, dopamine and 5-HT follow similar pathways.

Monoamine oxidase

Mitochondrial monoamine oxidase (MAO) mediates the oxidative deamination of Norepinephrine and other monoamines (dopamine, 5-HT). It is the main metabolic pathway for Norepinephrine and other catechol- and monoamines. Deamination produces:

- A corresponding acid – 3,4-dihydroxymandelic acid (DOMA), or
- A corresponding alcohol – dihydroxyphenylethylglycol (DOPEG).

The highest activity of MAO occurs in catecholamine containing nerve terminals. It is also active in 5-HT nerves, liver and intestinal mucosa. A number of dietary amines (e.g. tyramine) are detoxified by MAO in the intestine and liver.

There are two main forms of MAO: MAO-A and MAO-B. They have different distributions in the brain and peripheral organs:

- Both are found in neurons and astroglia of the CNS
- MAO-A – most abundant in placenta, liver and intestines
- MAO-B – found in platelets.

The isoforms differ in their substrate specificity: norepinephrine, epinephrine and 5-HT are substrates primarily for MAO-A; dopamine is substrate for both.

> **Information box 4.14** | **Examples of drugs with uptake$_1$ transporter inhibition as the primary action**
>
> - **Tricyclic antidepressants** exert their major action on the CNS. Blocking the action of uptake$_1$ increases norepinephrine concentration at the synapse. PNS effects, however, will give rise to the unwanted side effects of tachycardia and cardiac dysrhythmia.
> - **Cocaine** has a similar stimulant action to tricyclic antidepressants on the brain but causes excitement and euphoria, effects that make the drug liable to misuse. It also increases sympathetic transmissions leading to tachycardia and raised arterial pressure.
> - Other drugs that have an effect on norepinephrine synthesis, storage or release, may also have an uptake$_1$-blocking effect. Examples include amphetamine and guanethidine.

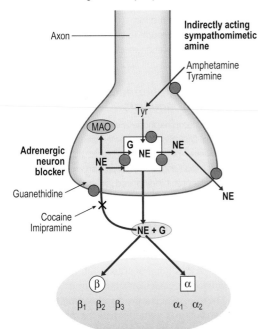

Fig. 4.26 Drugs and norepinephrine release. A diagrammatic representation of the site of action of an adrenergic neuron blocker (guanethidine), neuronal uptake$_1$ inhibitor (cocaine, imipramine) and indirectly acting sympathomimetic amines (tyramine, amphetamine). MAO, monoamine oxidase; NE, norepinephrine; α, α-adrenoceptor; β, β-adrenoceptor; G, guanethidine.

Clinical box 4.16 **Monoamine oxidase inhibitors**

MAOIs were developed to act as antidepressants by increasing the accumulation of neurotransmitters such as norepinephrine and 5-HT (serotonin). The original MAOIs were non-selective, and had many unwanted effects:

● Inhibition of the metabolism of other monoamine drugs administered at the same time (e.g. indirectly acting sympathomimetics in common cold and cough medicines): their accumulation, by not being degraded, increases their pressor effects and can lead to severe hypertension
● MAOI prevents the destruction of dietary tyramine, potentiating the hypertensive effect of tyramine in foods (abundant in cheese, fava beans, meat and vegetable extracts): this causes severe hypertension due to the release of norepinephrine by an indirect sympathomimetic effect.

The discovery of the two isoforms enabled the development of MAOIs that were selective for either MAO-A or MAO-B. MAO-A is abundant in the liver and gut, so inhibition of MAO-A is more likely to lead to the side effects due to interaction with tyramine. MAO-B is abundant in the extrapyramidal system in the brain, but not in gut or liver. The selective MAO-B inhibitor selegilin, which was developed for the treatment of Parkinsonism, does not have the interaction with tyramine containing foods and drugs.

MAOIs used for treating depression need to be prescribed with great caution and accompanying dietary advice. This is why they are used less frequently for depression than tricyclic antidepressants and selective serotonin re-uptake inhibitors (SSRIs).

MAO inhibitors (MAOIs) were developed to selectively inhibit either MAO-A or MAO-B to minimise side effects. Non-selective MAOI (phenelzine) is used in the treatment of depression and the selective MAO-B inhibitor (selegiline) is used to treat Parkinsonism (Clinical box 4.16).

Cytoplasmic COMT

Catechol-O-methyltransferase (COMT) is a widespread enzyme that occurs in neuronal and non-neuronal tissues. COMT is particularly active in the liver. It is an alternative, but relatively minor, pathway for inactivating norepinephrine and dopamine.

COMT methylates one of the catechol hydroxyl groups on the benzene ring to give a methoxy derivative (e.g. norepinephrine forms normetanephrine). It also methylates the deaminated products of catecholamines from MAO activity, DOMA and DOPEG, to produce the major urinary metabolites of VMA and 3-methoxy-4-hydoxyphenylglycol (MOPEG), respectively. VMA is the predominant metabolite of peripheral norepinephrine metabolism whereas MOPEG is the main metabolite associated with norepinephrine turnover in the CNS. Urinary VMA and MOPEG are useful indicators of the amount of norepinephrine released peripherally and centrally.

COMT inhibitors, e.g. entacapone, that block the degradation of levodopa, are used with levodopa in the treatment of Parkinson disease to prolong its action.

Adrenergic receptors

Adrenergic receptors (adrenoceptors) respond to stimulation by norepinephrine. It was originally thought that there were two types of adrenergic receptors: α and β types based on their pharmacological responses. It is now recognised that there are two main α-subtypes and three main β-subtypes. The different subtypes vary in their affinity for epinephrine and norepinephrine. All α- and β-adrenoceptors are G protein-coupled receptors and are linked through the G protein mechanism to a specific second messenger system.

α-Adrenoceptors

α-Adrenoceptors are subdivided into α_1 and α_2: α_1 are postsynaptic; α_2, although termed presynaptic, are also present postsynaptically. Each subtype has been further divided into three subtypes.

Clinically, the most important effects of α-adrenoceptors are on vascular smooth muscle. Generally, smooth muscle contracts in response to a stimulation, but gastrointestinal smooth muscle relaxes. Responses to α-adrenoceptor stimulation include:

■ α_1-Adrenoceptors: vasoconstriction, gastrointestinal muscle relaxation, salivation, hepatic glycogenolysis
■ α_2-Adrenoceptors: smooth muscle contraction, inhibition of norepinephrine release, inhibition of insulin release, platelet aggregation.

β-Adrenoceptors

The β-adrenoceptors have been divided into β_1, β_2, γ_3 and possibly β_4.

■ β_1-Adrenoceptors are located mainly in the heart but are also present in the gastrointestinal tract and presynaptically
■ β_2-Adrenoceptors are located on a number of tissues including bronchi, blood vessels, gastrointestinal tract and mast cells
■ β_3-Adrenoceptors are present in adipose tissue
■ Recent evidence suggests that there may be a β_4-adrenoceptor associated with cardiac tissue.

β-Adrenergic stimulation generally causes smooth muscle relaxation. The most important clinical effect is cardiac stimulation. Clinically important physiological effects in response to β-adrenoceptor activation include:

■ β_1-Adrenoceptors: increased heart rate and force of cardiac muscle contraction
■ β_2-Adrenoceptors: bronchodilation, vasodilation, visceral smooth muscle relaxation, hepatic glycogenolysis
■ β_3-Adrenoceptors: fat cell lipolysis.

Physiological and pharmacological effects of adrenoceptor agonists

Epinephrine and norepinephrine are not particularly selective in receptor binding. Directly and indirectly acting sympathomimetic drugs that activate, or drugs that block, adrenoceptors were developed by modifying the norepinephrine molecule. Their specificity for receptor binding and potency depends on their chemical structure, and this relationship is complex. The basic principles of receptor affinity and efficacy, and neuronal uptake and reaction with MAO and COMT, affect therapeutic response.

Cardiovascular and cardiac effects

Stimulating α- and β-adrenoceptors has a profound effect on both cardiac and vascular smooth muscle (Information box 4.15). These effects are the basis of drug therapy in angina, hypertension and some respiratory diseases. The net effect in the whole body will depend on the proportion of each class of receptor and the response at any given site.

Adrenoceptor agonists in cardiovascular disease

■ **Anaphylactic shock** (type I hypersensitivity) is a life-threatening condition. Epinephrine, a non-selective α-adrenoceptor agonist, is used in anaphylactic

Cardiac tissue contains predominantly β_1-adrenoceptors. Stimulation of β_1-adrenoceptor in the sino-atrial node results in increased rate (positive chronotropic) and increased force of myocardial contraction (positive inotropic).

In blood vessels, sympathetic nerve stimulation produces either α-adrenoceptor mediated vasoconstriction or β-adrenoceptor mediated vasodilatation in both the arterial and venous systems. Distribution of α- and β-adrenoceptors and their subclasses on vascular smooth muscle determines the response of any given vascular bed:

- Vasoconstriction in skin and mucous membranes because the vascular bed contains predominantly α_1- and α_2-adrenoceptors
- Coronary arteries dilate because β_2-adrenoceptors are dominant although α-adrenoceptors are present
- Increased peripheral resistance due to stimulation of α-adrenoceptors on arteries, arterioles and veins. Both subclasses of α-adrenoceptors produce vasoconstriction.

shock caused by hypersensitivity reactions to drugs (e.g. penicillin), allergens (e.g. nuts) and bee stings. A severe reaction results in airways obstruction from glossal and laryngeal oedema due to mucosal swelling, bronchospasm and cardiovascular collapse due to generalised vasodilatation. Epinephrine produces vasoconstriction by stimulation of α-adrenoceptors and β_2-adrenoceptor mediated bronchodilatation. Epinephrine is also used to restore cardiac rhythm in patients with **cardiac arrest**.

- The local vasoconstriction effect of epinephrine can be used to prolong the action of local anaesthetics (LA) by reducing tissue perfusion and preventing the dispersal of the LA.
- Non-selective β-agonists, e.g. isoprenaline, have positive chronotropic and positive inotropic effects on the heart. It is sometimes used in the treatment of cardiac dysrhythmias and in heart block while awaiting electrical pacing.
- The selective α_2-adrenoceptor agonist, clonidine, is used in the treatment of **hypertension**. Its action is thought to be primarily due to the activation of α_2-adrenoceptors in the lower brainstem resulting in a reduced sympathetic outflow to the periphery. Clonidine also has partial agonist effects.
- Dobutamine, a synthetic analogue of dopamine, is a selective β_2-adrenoceptor agonist, and a cardiac stimulant without vasoconstriction. It has a more pronounced inotropic than chronotropic effect on the heart so that tachycardia is less likely. It is useful in the treatment of impaired cardiac contractility due to **congestive heart failure** or **myocardial infarction**, and in open heart surgery.

Respiratory system

Although the respiratory system has very sparse sympathetic innervation it is populated by β_2-adrenoceptors. Circulating epinephrine and norepinephrine stimulate these receptors to produce relaxation of bronchial smooth muscle and maintain the patency of the airways. Stimulation of β_2-adrenoceptors decreases secretion by bronchial goblet cells and increases mucociliary clearance in the lumen of the airways. β_2-Adrenoceptor agonists also inhibit histamine release from mast cells.

Adrenoceptor agonists in respiratory disease

β_2-Adrenoceptor agonists are primarily used in the treatment of bronchospasm associated with asthma and chronic obstructive pulmonary disease (COPD).

- Selective β_2 agonists include salbutamol, terbutaline and salmeterol. Salbutamol by aerosol inhalation is still the mainstay of therapy but new longer acting agonists have been developed (salmeterol). Tachycardia and tremor have been reported as side effects. Chronic stimulation of β-adrenoceptors may result in receptor desensitisation, resulting in a reduced physiological response to subsequent β-adrenoceptor stimulation. The increase in reported asthma deaths in the 1960s was attributed to receptor desensitisation.
- β_2-Agonists can inhibit histamine release in the lung responding to allergic challenge.
- Selective α_1-agonists include ephedrine, phenylephrine and metazoline. They cause vasoconstriction and are used in nasal decongestants.

Gastrointestinal tract

Both α- and β-adrenoceptors cause gastrointestinal smooth muscle relaxation. The pyloric and ileocaecal sphincters are constricted by α-adrenoceptor stimulation. This effect often leads to chronic constipation in patients taking adrenoceptor agonists, particularly in elderly people. Administration of other drugs, such as a diuretic, can further exacerbate the problem.

Metabolism

Adrenoceptor stimulation mobilises energy stores for fuel metabolism.

- β_2-Adrenoceptor stimulation in the liver and muscle increases the conversion of glycogen and fats to glucose and fatty acids, causing a rise in plasma levels
- β_2-Adrenoceptor stimulation in adipose tissue results in increased lipolysis
- Insulin release is increased via stimulation of β_2-adrenoceptors but inhibited by α_2-adrenoceptor stimulation
- Glucagon release is activated by stimulation of β-adrenoceptors associated with the α cells of the pancreatic islets
- Anti-obesity drugs based on selective β_3-agonists are being developed.

Other effects

- β_2-Adrenoceptor stimulation in skeletal muscle increases the twitch tension of fast-contracting fibres, but shortens the active state of red, slow-contracting muscle. These two effects plus an increased discharge of muscle spindles are thought to be important in the production of tremor associated with β_2-adrenoceptor agonists (e.g. salbutamol).
- β_2-Agonists can cause long-term changes in skeletal muscle. Clenbuterol is a performance enhancing 'anabolic' drug that increases muscle bulk and force of contraction.

Adrenoceptor antagonists

Unlike adrenoceptor agonists, adrenoceptor antagonists are selective for either α- or β-adrenoceptors.

α-Adrenoceptor antagonists

α-Adrenoceptor antagonists may be selective or non-selective. Their main clinical uses are in treating hypertension.

■ Selective α_1-adrenoceptor antagonists, prazosin and the longer-acting doxazosin, are used in the treatment of essential hypertension as they produce less tachycardia than with phentolamine; they do not block the inhibitory presynaptic α_2-adrenoceptors.

■ Selective α_1-adrenoceptor antagonists are used in the treatment of urinary retention in benign prostatic hypertrophy. Tamsulosin causes relaxation of the smooth muscles of the bladder neck and prostate capsule.

■ Non-selective α-adrenoceptor antagonist, phenoxybenzamine, is used to treat hypertension associated with phaeochromocytoma. Phenoxybenzamine produces an irreversible antagonism and requires the synthesis of new receptor protein for cellular responsiveness to be restored. Phentolamine is a non-selective competitive antagonist at the α-adrenoceptor and is useful in the diagnosis of hypertension due to phaeochromocytoma. Neither of these drugs is used in the treatment of essential hypertension as the rapid fall in blood pressure due to inhibition of vascular α-adrenoceptors triggers reflex tachycardia, as well as increased norepinephrine release due to inhibition of the inhibitory autoreceptor in cardiac tissue to increase heart rate.

Unwanted side effects of α-adrenoceptor antagonists

■ Non-selective α-Adrenoceptor antagonists may cause tachycardia, cardiac dysrhythmia and increased gastric motility.

■ α-Adrenoceptor antagonists may cause impotence.

β-Adrenoceptor antagonists

β-Adrenoceptor antagonists can be classified according to a number of pharmacodynamic and pharmacokinetic properties.

■ **Selectivity**. β-Adrenoceptor antagonists are classified as non-specific (propranolol, alprenolol) or specific β_1-adrenoceptor antagonists (atenolol). The specificity of the latter group of drugs is dose-dependent (increase the dose and β_2-adrenoceptors will also be blocked).

■ **Membrane stabilising activity** (propranolol, alprenolol, oxprenolol, timolol). A number of β-adrenoceptor antagonists possess membrane stabilising effects. (Propranolol affects electrical conduction in the heart, similar to quinidine, but unrelated to its β-adrenoceptor antagonist properties. Propranolol increases atrio-ventricular conduction time and decreases spontaneous ectopics.)

■ **Intrinsic sympathomimetic activity**. Several β-adrenoceptor antagonists (pindolol, alprenolol) have initial agonist activity at β-adrenoceptors before exerting an antagonistic action, but their intrinsic activity is less than that for a full agonist such as isoprenaline. These partial agonists are said to have intrinsic sympathomimetic activity. Whether there is a therapeutic value for this property is debatable.

β-Adrenoceptor antagonists can also be classified according to their route of elimination, being either completely metabolised in the liver (alprenolol, propranolol, oxprenolol) or excreted predominantly unchanged (60–100%) by the kidneys (atenolol, sotalol). Care should be taken in patients with renal failure as these agents may accumulate.

Clinical uses of β-adrenoceptor antagonists

The β-adrenoceptor antagonists (β-blockers) are very important drugs used primarily for their effects on the cardiovascular system. The cardiovascular effects produced in humans are dependent on the degree of sympathetic activity. At rest, propranolol has little effect on heart rate, cardiac output or arterial pressure. During exercise, however, propranolol reduces heart rate and cardiac output, thereby reducing the exercise tolerance. In addition to the effect on the heart, skeletal muscle vasodilatation is also reduced.

Cardiovascular disease

A major role for β-adrenoceptor antagonists is in the treatment of **hypertension**. A fall in arterial pressure is only seen in hypertensive patients. The exact mechanism by which β-adrenoceptor antagonists produce their effect is complex and is probably a combination of the following effects:

■ Reduction in cardiac output.

■ Reduction in renin release from the juxtaglomerular apparatus in the kidney. The relationship between renin and hypertension is unclear. Pindolol has little or no effect on renin levels but is an effective antihypertensive agent.

■ Central action, which may reduce peripheral sympathetic activity. However, not all β-adrenoceptor antagonists enter the CNS in significant concentrations (e.g. timolol).

In the presence of β-adrenoceptor antagonists, coronary perfusion is slightly reduced. There is, however, a significant fall in cardiac O_2 consumption due to the reduction in heart rate and force of contraction, resulting in improved myocardial oxygenation. This effect is important in the treatment of **angina pectoris**.

Propranolol is also used in the treatment of **cardiac dysrhythmias**, due to its ability to slow heart rate and decrease atrial and atrio-ventricular node conduction. It has proved particularly useful as an adjunct in the treatment of atrial fibrillation due to thyrotoxicosis.

Randomised controlled clinical trials have shown that β-adrenoceptor antagonists may prolong survival in stable **cardiac failure**.

Migraine

The mechanisms underlying the classic symptoms of migraine – the premonitory aura, momentary loss of visual field and unilateral, severe headache and vomiting – are not well understood. Blood flow studies in patients during migraine attacks have shown changes in blood flow during the different phases, but no consistent pattern. Many theories have been postulated over decades. There is a strong suggestion that 5-HT deficiency is implicated in some way.

For an acute attack, if simple analgesics (e.g. aspirin, paracetamol) together with an anti-emetic is insufficient, then 5-HT agonists are effective:

■ Ergotamine is a 5-HT partial agonist.

■ Sumatriptan is a 5-HT agonist.

■ Newer proprietary compounds are said to be longer and faster acting.

β-Adrenoceptor antagonists (e.g. metoprolol, propranolol) are effective for prophylaxis.

Other clinical uses

- β-Blockers are used as adjuncts in the treatment of hyperthyroidism where tachycardia, atrial fibrillation and tremor are due to increased sympathetic activity
- Timolol is used in the treatment of glaucoma, as β-blockers reduce the production of aqueous humour
- β-Blockers are used to treat acute anxiety states to control symptoms due to excessive sympathetic drive such as tremor and palpitations.

Unwanted effects of β-adrenoceptor antagonists

Side effects of β-adrenoceptor antagonists are caused by receptor blockade:

- Bronchoconstriction – β-blockers cause bronchoconstriction in patients with asthma or chronic obstructive pulmonary diseases. Normal subjects are not affected.
- Cardiac failure – patients with heart disease may depend on sympathetic drive to maintain their cardiac output. Blocking this drive with β-blockers could precipitate cardiac failure.
- Bradycardia – antidysrhythmic drugs (e.g. verapamil) impair cardiac conduction. Concomitant administration of a β-blocker can further impair conduction leading to bradycardia, progressing to complete heart block (atrio-ventricular block).
- Hypoglycaemia – β-blockers reduce the early warning signs of hypoglycaemia, mediated by the sympathetic nervous system (e.g. tachycardia). Non-selective β-blockers may worsen the effects of hypoglycaemia by inhibiting sympathetic nervous system and epinephrine mediated glycogenolysis and lipolysis, prolonging the period of hypoglycaemia.
- Tiredness – β-blockers cause a reduction in cardiac output and muscle perfusion during exercise. This may account for the fatigue experienced by patients on this medication.
- Exacerbation of ischaemic heart disease – sudden cessation of long-term β-blockers can result in exacerbation of angina, increased ventricular arrhythmias, myocardial infarction and sudden death. These effects have been reported to be due to receptor supersensitivity which may be due to an increase in the number of β-adrenoceptors.
- Oculomucocutaneous syndrome – idiosyncratic reactions to practolol consisting of keratoconjunctivitis with scarring and loss of lacrimation, mucosal ulcerations in the nose and mouth, and rashes were reported, leading to its withdrawal from clinical use.

GENERAL ANAESTHETICS

General anaesthetics (GAs) enabled the development of modern surgical procedures, during which the patients need to be entirely unaware of all sensory input so that they are:

- Unconscious, therefore unaware and have no memory (amnesia) of the procedure
- Unresponsive to painful stimuli (analgesia)
- Immobile, with complete skeletal muscle relaxation and loss of reflexes.

In the distant past, alcohol was the only help available to patients during surgery, e.g. amputations. Ether and chloroform, now obsolete, were the first volatile anaesthetics in clinical use. 'Laughing gas' (nitrous oxide) was the first gaseous general anaesthetic, and is still in use today. Much progress has been made in the development of anaesthetic agents. The two most commonly used forms of general anaesthetic are:

- Inhaled anaesthetics, which may be volatile or gaseous
- Intravenous anaesthetics.

The administration of general anaesthetics needs to be controlled, to achieve **safe** blood and tissue concentrations that meet the main aims of unconsciousness, unresponsiveness to pain and immobility. Highly trained and skilled anaesthetists are required.

From the patient's viewpoint, rapid onset of anaesthesia and rapid recovery with minimal or no side effects would be most beneficial. Generally, a combination of the different forms of anaesthetics are used for surgery.

Inhaled anaesthetics

- Volatile anaesthetics are liquid at room temperature; they vaporise to produce enough partial pressure for inhalation. They are all non-flammable and non-explosive. (Examples: halogenated derivatives of ether, e.g. isoflurane, enflurane, sevoflurane; halogenated derivatives of alkanes, e.g. halothane, widely used.)
- Gaseous anaesthetics are simple gases. They may be explosive, and are usually administered in a mixture with air or oxygen. (Examples: the best example of a gaseous anaesthetic that is widely used is nitrous oxide (N_2O), administered as gas and air, and an effective obstetric analgesic during labour.)

Intravenous anaesthetics

Intravenous anaesthetics act much faster than inhaled agents.

- Barbiturates – e.g. thiopental, induces unconsciousness in 20 seconds
- Benzodiazepines – e.g. diazepam, midazolam act directly on GABA receptors
- Phenols – e.g. propofol
- Cyclohexanes – e.g. ketamine
- Opiates – e.g. fentanyl, remifentanil, used for sedation, analgesia and to reduce anxiety.

Because of their rapid action, intravenous GAs such as thiopental and propofol are used to induce unconsciousness before surgery, and anaesthesia is maintained by inhaled anaesthetics during surgery.

A combination of an opiate, e.g. fentanyl, and a dopamine antagonist, e.g. droperidol, is used to induce deep sedation and analgesia, **neuroleptanalgesia,** for minor surgical procedures such as endoscopy.

Pharmacodynamics of GAs

How GAs work is not well understood, as the agents can vary from simple gases to steroids. It is, however, generally agreed that, at the cellular level, GAs act on signal transmitters at the **synapse**, rather than at the neuron. Several theories have been proposed to explain the action of GAs, of which two are discussed here.

Lipid theory

At the turn of the twentieth century, Meyer and Overton independently described a relationship between lipid solubility of anaesthetics (i.e. olive oil:water partition) and their anaesthetic potency in which the more soluble the anaesthetic is in oil, the more potent it is. The Meyer-Overton hypothesis suggested that dissolving anaesthetic agents into cell membranes altered cell function. It does not, however, explain how the entry of an exogenous substance into the cell membrane can alter cell function.

Protein theory

Recent research in cell biology has found evidence to show that anaesthetic drugs target proteins, e.g. intracellular enzymes, ion channels and membrane receptors. The example of the effects of GAs on ion channels illustrates the molecular mechanisms leading to the inhibition of synaptic transmission.

Laboratory research has found evidence that inhibition of synaptic transmission may occur at three processes:

- Inhibition of neurotransmitter release
- Inhibition of the action of the neurotransmitter
- Inhibition of the excitability of the postsynaptic cell (e.g. muscle).

The effect of GAs on neurotransmitter release

The likely candidates are

- L-Glutamate (excitatory neurotransmitter acts via the ionotropic NMDA receptor, Na^+/Ca^{2+} channel) and GABA (inhibitory neurotransmitter acts via ionotropic GABA$_A$ – **Cl⁻ channel**) are likely candidates.
- Halothane and isoflurane modulate GABA$_A$, NMDA and non-NMDA receptor-mediated synaptic transmission.
- Volatile anaesthetics depress glutaminergic synaptic transmission by a direct action on the NMDA receptor and a reduction in presynaptic glutamine release. They also increase the uptake of glutamate by astrocytes. Astrocytes terminate glutaminergic transmission by removing released glutamate from the synaptic cleft.
- Thiopentone and propofol enhance effect of GABA at GABA$_A$ receptors.
- Ketamine reduces NMDA receptor-mediated responses of glutamate and enhances GABA$_A$ receptor-mediated responses.
- Intravenous and inhalational anaesthetics also modulate the presynaptic release or uptake of GABA.

It has not yet been possible to identify the 'target' postsynaptic cells that are affected by GAs. Increasing the concentration of anaesthetic eventually leads to suppression of all brain function, including all autonomic control, respiration and reflex motor activity.

Pharmacokinetics

Inhaled, volatile and gaseous GAs are absorbed through the alveoli into the bloodstream for distribution, and eliminated through the lungs. Intravenous anaesthetics bypass the absorption phase altogether, and are eliminated via hepatic metabolism and renal excretion. As both forms of anaesthetics are highly lipid-soluble, distribution by crossing the **blood–brain barrier** is no problem.

Inhaled anaesthetics

Inhaled anaesthetics are small, lipid-soluble molecules that easily permeate the alveolar membrane, and enter and leave the body via the lungs. Their kinetic behaviour is determined by:

- The rate of delivery from inspired air to the blood circulation – increasing alveolar ventilation (see Ch. 13) enables a faster equilibration between alveolar and blood concentration, whereas respiratory depression slows elimination.
- Solubility in blood
- The rate of delivery to brain
- Accumulation in fat and other tissues.

Elimination via metabolism is not problematic, except for the production of toxic metabolites.

The brain is well perfused, and the blood–brain barrier is readily permeable to GAs, so concentration in the brain rises rapidly, and equilibrium between the blood and brain is quickly achieved. Surgical anaesthesia is achieved when the patient no longer responds to pain, i.e. the first incision.

Halothane

Anaesthetic concentration in poorly perfused adipose tissue rises slowly, to equilibrate with blood concentration, and anaesthetic accumulates in the fat. At effective anaesthetic doses, halothane at equilibrium mostly accumulates in adipose tissue (95%), and is slowly released into the bloodstream after GA administration ceases. This prolongs the action of halothane to give the 'hangover' symptoms of drowsiness, confusion, amnesia and headache.

Hepatic metabolism of halothane produces bromide, trifluoroacetate and other metabolites that are hepatotoxic. Severe reactions can give rise to hepatic failure.

Nitrous oxide

Nitrous oxide (N_2O) was first used in the 1800s as a general anaesthetic to cause unconsciousness and analgesia. N_2O has a good analgesic effect but is of low potency and is therefore used in combination with other inhaled anaesthetics. It has the following properties:

- Although it has a low potency as an anaesthetic, it has a rapid onset of effect due to its low blood:gas partition coefficient and high inhaled concentration.
- Abrupt discontinuation results in a rapid transfer of N_2O from blood and tissues to the alveoli and a decrease in arterial tension of oxygen, i.e. diffusion hypoxia.
- Has a good analgesic property. Entonox (50%/50% with O_2) is used for pain control.
- By itself has minimal effects on respiratory drive, minimal skeletal muscle relaxation, minimal effects on the circulation.
- Causes euphoria.
- Anoxia will occur if it is used with less than 20% O_2.
- Thought to be free of adverse effects, but shown to oxidise cobalt in vitamin B$_{12}$, required for synthesis of methionine which is essential in DNA and protein synthesis, leading to anaemia if used repeatedly.

Intravenous anaesthetics

Intravenous anaesthetics are administered directly into the bloodstream, so the onset of anaesthesia is much faster than inhalation: the time for the blood to travel from the injection site in an arm vein to the brain. Metabolism and elimination are rapid, so the duration of action is short. Intravenous anaesthetics are commonly used for induction of anaesthesia.

Anaesthetic from the brain is redistributed to fat, and accumulates in fat so that highly lipid-soluble drugs like thiopental could have their action terminated by redistribution (see Information box 4.2), shortening the duration of action. Release of the drug from fat prolongs the hangover effects.

Unwanted effects

The unwanted effects of general anaesthetics are related to:

- 'Hangover' effects
- Respiratory and cardiac depression
- Muscarinic inhibition of secretions leading to dry mouth, dry hot skin and lack of bronchial secretions

- Toxic metabolites
- Hypotension due to the rapid action of intravenous anaesthetics
- Allergic reactions to intravenous anaesthetics.

Muscle relaxants

The use of muscle relaxants to produce immobility enables lighter levels of anaesthetics to be used. They are given as premedication, acting on N_M receptors at the NMJ.

- Suxamethonium is a N_M receptor agonist, but after initial stimulation of the NMJ it produces a depolarising block to paralyse the muscle
- Tubocurare and atracurium, derivatives of curare, the active ingredient in the poisoned arrows of South American Indians are competitive N_M receptor antagonists.

5

Human genetics

Denise Syndercombe Court and David P. Kelsell

Introduction	**155**
Historical background	155
Basis of modern genetics	156
The human genome	**157**
DNA and chromosomes	157
DNA and genes	166
DNA damage	168
Genes and development	169
Mediators of development	169
Patterning	170
Organogenesis	171
Human genetic variation	**172**
Polymorphisms	172
Modes of inheritance	**177**
Mendelian disorders	177
Polygenic or complex disease	**183**

Continuous effects models	184
Threshold effects models	184
Characteristics of multifactorial diseases	184
Tools to investigate polygenic diseases	186
Cancer genetics	**187**
Cancer as a multi-step genetic disease	187
Inheritance of cancer genes	187
Cancer genes	188
Identifying disease genes	**190**
Genome mapping	190
The human genome project	199
Genetic disease, diagnosis and therapy	**204**
Gene testing	204
Congenital disease	205
Pharmacogenomics	205
Genetic medicine	207

INTRODUCTION

HISTORICAL BACKGROUND

Genetics is a very new science, changing rapidly by the day with advances in technology. Although humans have long been aware of some form of heredity, the mechanisms have only recently become clear. Early philosophers talked about the male ripening the female, or seeds being produced in various organs to be transmitted to the child. In the early 18th century scientists were divided as to whether the sperm held the new child, the purpose of the female simply to provide the womb, or whether the egg held the child, already determined as male or female, growth being stimulated by the sperm.

The theory of **pangenesis** was a major early influence: pangenes were said to be developed in each organ and then passed to the child through blood. This is probably the origin of phrases such as 'royal blood' and 'blood line'. **Blending** was the most accepted theory at the time: a tall man and a short woman would tend to produce offspring of average height. This clearly did not always work, for example when two brown-eyed parents had blue-eyed children.

Although **Gregor Mendel**'s experiments, over 8 years in the late 19th century involving thousands of garden pea plants, were perhaps all too perfect, his crossing of plants with different characteristics laid the foundation for modern genetics. Describing the appearance of simple characteristics, he used mathematical principles to show that these traits were passed from parents to offspring through what

became to be known as genes. Four fundamental principles of modern genetics were illustrated by his experiments:

- Each parent contributes only one of a pair of factors (tall or short, wrinkled or smooth in Mendel's experiments) – or **alleles** – of each trait (plant size or seed shape) through a process of separation, or **segregation**, when the gametes are formed
- Factors can be **dominant**, while others can be hidden, or expressed when the dominant factor is not present (**recessive factor**), but remain unchanged when passed to their offspring (do not blend)
- Males and females contribute equally to their offspring
- Different traits are inherited independently of each other – **independent assortment**.

The later recognition of **chromosomes** (see below), leading to the chromosomal theory of inheritance, and understanding of the process of **meiosis** when gametes are formed (see below) helped to explain these observations during the early 20th century. Occasionally Mendel's prediction for what should be inherited in the next generation did not happen; these occurrences were described as **mutations**. Mendel's principles of inheritance and an acceptance of mutation provided scientific support for the theories put forward in **Charles Darwin**'s *On the origin of species* in 1869.

Although DNA had been isolated at about the same time as Darwin's publication, its recognition as the hereditary material, rather than a protein being responsible, was not proved until the 1950s. The publication in 1955 of the structure of DNA marked the start of modern molecular biology, to which the rest of this chapter is devoted.

BASIS OF MODERN GENETICS

The genetic code, located within DNA, provides the instructions for the complex development and organisation of the multicellular human. Genetics has become an essential component of medicine, extending our understanding of disease mechanisms to facilitate preventive, diagnostic, prognostic and therapeutic developments.

The understanding that disease can be caused by chromosomal abnormalities, or can be inherited, because of the segregation of mutant genes, has provided the impetus to the development of genomic medicine. Along with the association of specific gene mutations and disease comes a greater understanding of the molecular and cellular mechanisms required for normal human development and homeostasis. A key factor that has facilitated our current understanding of human genetics has been the technological developments that have enabled the complete sequencing of the human **genome** and led to the collection of vast amounts of data that can be 'mined' to produce useful information. Current sequencing technology can now sequence two individuals' genomes in 1 week.

- The **genome** is the complete collection of genetic material within an organism.

Three levels of genetic classification are used to enable the management of an enormous amount of information:

- **Genomics** – the DNA structure of genes and their localisation within the genome
- **Gene expression** – the mechanisms through which genes are 'switched on' and transcribed into **messenger RNA (mRNA)** to be translated into protein or other types of RNA
- **Proteomics** – the characterisation of biological processes from measurement of protein expression, localisation and post-translational modification.

These 'banks' of genetic data can be used to provide information for disease therapies. The variable responses to established drugs, and the effects of particular chemicals on gene transcription and protein expression (drug discovery), are collectively described as **pharmacogenomics**. The combination of pharmacogenomics and the traditional pharmaceutical sciences offers the potential for better and safer drugs and the ability to provide individualised therapies.

Profiling an individual's DNA for the presence of specific gene variants will enable the future understanding of the inherited basis of many **congenital** disorders (disorders present at birth) and the risk of developing particular **multifactorial** conditions (those with many causes) in later life, such as cancer and neurological disease. With more research, it is likely that our lifetime risks of developing a whole range of diseases could be predicted by our individual 'genetic barcode' and, of equal importance, what medicines and lifestyle changes will prevent the onset and early management of these diseases. Already commercial companies offer personal disease risk predictions but the evidence for the reliability of any estimates and usefulness of the information provided to an individual is presently limited.

Most human disorders have a genetic component that is either inherited in the **germline** or acquired through **somatic** mutation.

- The **germline** refers to the **gonadal** cells that become eggs or sperm, and also to the genetic material that comes from them.

- **Somatic** cells are those that come from the body, but not directly from the gonads. A particular genetic variant (often termed mutation) underlies the **monogenic** disorders.
- **Monogenic** disorders are those controlled by a single gene, in contrast with **polygenic** disorders. In **polygenic** diseases, a complex genetic interaction of several genes and environmental factors predisposes to or protects an individual from a particular disorder.

Genetic disorders can be classified in a number of ways:

- **Single gene disorders** – a mutation in a single gene leading to disease (e.g. cystic fibrosis)
- **Chromosomal disorders** – a change, gain, loss or exchange of chromosome elements (e.g. trisomy 21 – Down syndrome (see Clinical box 5.1)
- **Polygenic disorders** – due to the combined effects of many genes, or in combination with environmental factors (multifactorial) (e.g. neural tube defects)
- **Somatic disorders** – disorders of body (non-germline) cells, such as uncontrolled cell growth, or cancer.

Individuals who are affected, or are at risk of being affected, by genetic disorders are likely to be offered **genetic counselling** and prenatal diagnosis. This is when a trained professional provides information, risk assessment and support to patients and their families.

Along with the rapid developments that are coming with the sequencing of the human genome and the associated advances in analytical technologies, there is also a proliferation of ethical, legal and social questions that must be considered by governments. This means that individuals are increasingly faced with important decisions; it is the role of the genetic counsellor to provide information and support to help affected individuals make informed decisions.

Down syndrome can be screened for in early pregnancy through the measurement of various proteins and hormones that are characteristically altered in this condition. Women at high risk are normally offered an examination in early pregnancy that samples foetal cells and allows a detailed examination of all of the chromosomes. Small numbers of foetal cells

---

Clinical box 5.1   **Trisomy 21**

Trisomy 21 is seen in about 0.1% of live births, and produces the phenotype originally described by John Langdon Down in 1866. In 1959, it was recognised as being due to the presence of an extra copy of chromosome 21. The extra chromosome copy appears more often to originate from the mother and prevalence increases significantly with increasing maternal age from less than 1 in 1000 under the age of 30 years, to about 1 in 25 over the age of 45 years. Individuals with Down syndrome have distinctive facial features: a small head, a flat nose bridge, misshapen ears, a broad and short neck, and narrow upward slanting eyes. These are often accompanied by a variety of medical conditions including intellectual disability, congenital heart defects, gastrointestinal obstruction and leukaemia.

Trisomy 21 accounts for about 95% of cases of Down syndrome. The remaining 5% are due to other abnormalities:

- **Translocation and partial trisomy**: in this condition copies of parts of chromosome 21 are **translocated** to other chromosomes. Although there are no additional chromosomes in this case, there are still three copies of particular genes from chromosome 21 (partial trisomy).
- **Mosaics**: in which there is a mixture of cell lines in different tissues within one body, some displaying trisomy 21, others being normal.

escape into the maternal circulation and techniques that can separate and enrich these are now being developed; genome testing of these will offer diagnosis of a large number of congenital disorders in the future.

THE HUMAN GENOME

Genetic information is stored within **deoxyribonucleic acid** (**DNA**), its sequence providing the 'blueprint' for all the proteins in the body. The **Human Genome Project** (HGP, see below) began formally in 1990, and the identification of the entire human genome sequence was completed in 2003.

The information is arranged in genes that code for proteins. The genes are located on chromosomes. Forty-six chromosomes, arranged in 22 pairs of different chromosomes, plus two sex chromosomes, are found within each somatic cell in the body. The gametes (sperm or egg cells) contain just one sex chromosome and one of the pairs of each of the 22 **autosomal**, or non-sex, chromosomes.

DNA AND CHROMOSOMES

DNA is a double-stranded molecule (the **double helix**), the strands forming a twisted 'ladder' with sides of sugar and phosphate molecules forming strong phosphodiester bonds, connected by 'rungs' of nitrogenous bases, linked through weaker hydrogen bonds. The order of the nucleotide bases on the strand is called the DNA sequence; these specify the genetic instructions to produce and maintain an organism. There are four bases in DNA:

- Adenine (A)
- Cytosine (C)
- Guanine (G)
- Thymine (T).

The stands of DNA are joined by the specific pairing of these nucleotides: A with T, and C with G to form a double-helical structure. Each of the strands is therefore complementary to the other. Each strand has a 3′ ('3 prime') and a 5′ end and the complementary strand reverses these. There are 3 billion base pairs (bp) making up the human genome sequence. The majority of human DNA is packaged into different-sized chromosomes (Fig. 5.1) located within the nucleus of the cell, with an additional circular piece of **DNA** located in the **mitochondria**.

In a **diploid** human cell (having two sets of chromosomes), there are 46 chromosomes comprising 22 paired autosomal chromosomes (numbered 1–22). Each pair of chromosomes is homologous (very similar), and one of the pair is inherited from the father and the other from the mother (see Meiosis, below). The largest is known as chromosome 1 and consists of around 250 megabases (Mb) of DNA, chromosome 2 has 240 mb and then chromosomes descend in size to the smallest autosomes, 21 and 22, which have 55 mb and 60 mb of DNA, respectively. The remaining two are the sex chromosomes, which are not homologous and are called the X and Y chromosomes.

In the gametes (egg and sperm cells), the genome is **haploid**, carrying only one copy of the 23 chromosomes. The Y chromosome (60 mb of DNA) is much smaller than the X chromosome (140 mb of DNA) (see Fig. 5.2).

- Males have an X and a Y chromosome. The Y chromosome is inherited from the father and contains the primary genetic information for determining some of the male characteristics. The Y chromosome is much smaller than the X chromosome and has very few genes: for this reason there are not very many diseases associated with defects in the Y chromosome, compared with those associated with the X chromosome.
- Females have two X chromosomes, although only one of the two X chromosomes is transcriptionally active in order that female cells do not express twice as much of the X chromosome genes as male cells. This random inactivation of one of the female X chromosomes is termed **X-inactivation** (or **lyonisation**) and occurs via a chromosomal/gene silencing mechanism involving **methylation** in early embryogenesis. Once this occurs, the same X chromosome is inactivated in all somatic cells.

Chromosome karyotypes (Fig. 5.2)

Chromosome karyotyping is the process of visually examining the chromosomes, arranged in pairs, for gross abnormalities. To see chromosomes under the microscope, dividing somatic cells (such as white blood cells) are exposed to spindle toxins, such as colchicine, which arrest the cell cycle in **metaphase** when the chromosomes are more condensed and thus easiest to see.

Each chromosome has a constriction at the middle (**meta-centric**) or towards one end (**acrocentric**). This constriction is termed the **centromere** and joins the homologous chromosomes (**chromatids**) together during mitosis.

The centromere also divides the chromosome into two diagnostic parts, the shorter **p arm** and the longer **q arm**. The banding pattern seen across each chromosome is produced by nuclear staining that produces a characteristic light and dark banding pattern. The dark bands represent condensed supercoiled chromatin (**heterochromatin**) that is transcriptionally silent. The light-staining bands represent chromatin that is not so tightly coiled, and these are transcriptionally active regions of the chromosome. At the end of each chromosome arm are the **telomeres**, which do not contain any coding genes but numerous copies of the hexa-meric nucleotide sequence TTAGGG. Telomeres are thought to maintain the stability of the chromosome, promote complete DNA replication and aid chromosome pairing. Telomeres become progressively shorter as the cell divides and this has been linked to the regulation of cell longevity.

Mitochondrial DNA

The remaining DNA within the genome is packaged in circular DNA molecules (around 16.5 kb), found in the numerous mitochondria within the cytoplasm of the cell. The mitochondrial genome encodes 13 proteins, 22 **transfer RNA** (**tRNA**) and two **ribosomal RNA** (**rRNA**) molecules that are primarily involved in the generation of ATP to fulfil the cell's energy requirements. There can be hundreds of mitochondria within each cell. This DNA is always inherited from the mother, since at fertilisation only the nucleus of the sperm cell is transferred into the egg.

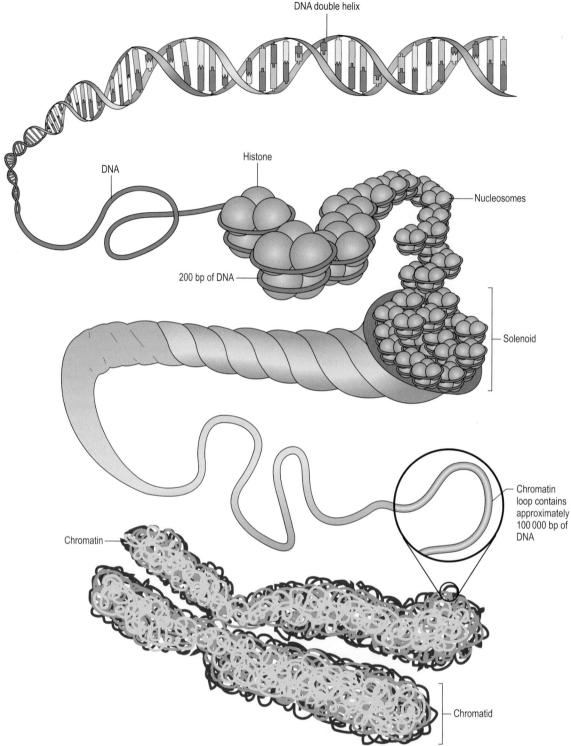

DNA double helix

DNA

Histone

Nucleosomes

200 bp of DNA

Solenoid

Chromatin loop contains approximately 100 000 bp of DNA

Chromatin

Chromatid

Fig. 5.1 **Organisation of DNA within a chromosome.** DNA strands are about 2 m in length and need careful packing to fit within a cell nucleus. The helical molecule is packaged into **nucleosomes** that consist of about 150 bp wrapped around a histone protein core, having a 'bead-on-a-string' appearance. Nucleosomes themselves wind in a helix, about six forming a **solenoid**. Solenoids in series are arranged in **chromatin loops**, each being about 100 kilobases (kb) in length. These chromatin loops pack themselves together in **chromatids** that form the familiar X-shaped chromosome, which has two short and two long arms. Redrawn from Jorde LB et al. 2009 Medical Genetics, 4th edn. Elsevier, Edinburgh, with permission.

Cell division

Human cell division occurs by two processes, **mitosis** and **meiosis**.

- In **mitosis** the entire DNA content of the cell is duplicated and the cell divides into two identical **diploid** daughter cells.

- **Meiosis** is a special form of cell division that maintains the correct number of chromosomes in the gamete cells. During fertilisation the egg and sperm cells merge to form a single cell with 23 pairs of chromosomes. To ensure that the gametes only have a single set of chromosomes, in meiosis the DNA content of the cell is halved and the daughter cells are referred to as being **haploid**.

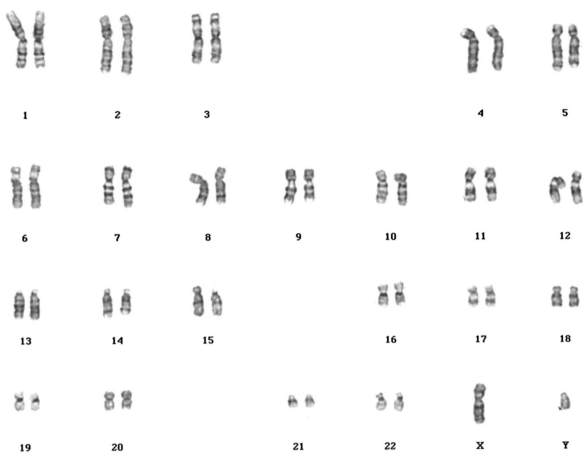

Fig. 5.2 **Human chromosome karyotype.** Paired human metaphase autosomes from a human male are shown from the largest to the smallest, followed by single X and Y chromosomes. The banding pattern is produced by Giemsa staining. Courtesy of Dr Debra Lillington.

The cell cycle

The cell cycle is the name given to the series of events by which cells duplicate their DNA and divide, in a process known as **mitosis**. This process is preceded by the longer **interphase** in which the cell prepares for the division, synthesising the necessary material (Fig. 5.3). DNA replication occurs once during each cell cycle and the process is tightly regulated to ensure that DNA is accurately copied and equally divided between the two daughter cells.

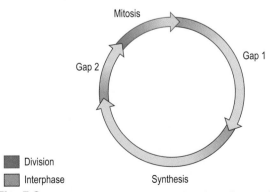

Fig. 5.3 **The cell cycle.** During the cell cycle, cells spend most of their time in interphase, during which synthesis of RNA and proteins occurs in the G1 (gap 1) phase. DNA is then replicated in the S (synthesis phase), and in G2 some DNA repair takes place and the cells, now containing 46 pairs of chromosomes, prepare to divide by mitosis.

The length of the cell cycle varies depending on the cell type: epithelial cells in the human gut may divide every 12 hours, whereas neurons and muscle cells lose their ability to divide altogether. Key molecules in this regulation are the **cyclin-dependent kinases** (**CDKs**) that are produced and destroyed at key points in the cell cycle. An understanding of these and other proteins is an important focus of research into the causes of cancer.

Interphase

The time from a cell completing mitosis to the beginning of the next mitosis is referred to as **interphase**. Cells can remain in a nascent stage, the **G0** phase, until stimulated to enter the cell cycle by a variety of agents, such as growth factors or intracellular messengers. Three stages follow:

- G1 (gap 1) phase:
  - The step between division and synthesis
  - Transcription factors activated
  - DNA synthesis initiated
- S phase (synthesis):
  - Chromosomes duplicated to form the 'sister' chromatids
  - Material may be exchanged between sister chromatids (**recombination**)
- G2 (gap 2) phase:
  - The step between synthesis and division
  - DNA repair
  - Preparation for mitosis.

Each cycle starts with 46 (a pair of 23) chromosomes, and ends with a duplicated set by the end of G2.

Mitosis (Fig. 5.4)

Mitosis is a continuous process during which the chromosomes, duplicated during interphase, are separated prior to the physical division of the cell into two daughter cells. The main physical events that occur during mitosis were first observed in the latter part of the 19th century and elucidated by Flemming in 1882. Flemming divided mitosis into four stages based on morphological changes in the nucleus and cytoplasm of the dividing cell:

- **Prophase**: chromosomes condense and become visible. Each duplicated chromosome comprises two chromatids lying side by side and attached at the **centromere**

(Fig. 5.5), held together by the SMC (structural maintenance of chromosome) protein, **cohesin**. A bipolar **mitotic spindle** starts to form outside the nucleus, radiating out from the **centrioles** lying at opposite sides of the cell.

- **Metaphase**: metaphase starts (**prometaphase**) with the disappearance of the nuclear membrane. Chromosomes become attached to the mitotic spindle via **kinetochore microtubules**. At the end of metaphase the chromosomes are aligned in a plate around the centre of the mitotic spindle apparatus, the **equatorial plane**. At this point the chromosomes are at their most condensed. Examination of chromosomes for clinical diagnostics is normally done on metaphase chromosomes.

- **Anaphase**: during anaphase the spindle fibres contract and sister chromatids are separated and

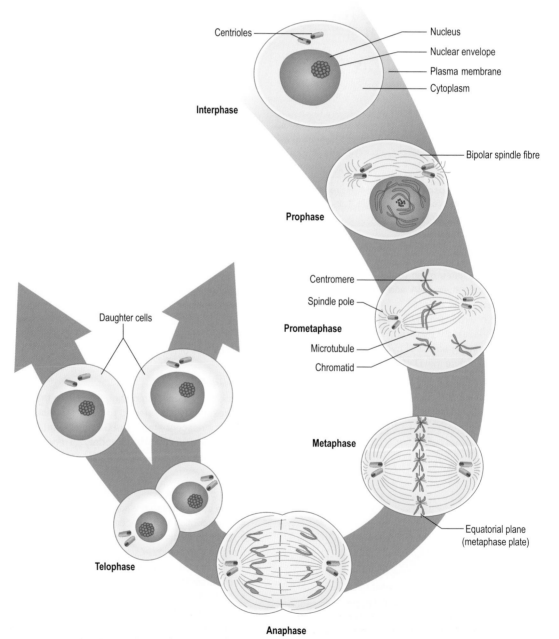

Fig. 5.4 **Mitosis.** A diploid cell undergoes mitosis to form two identical daughter cells. Redrawn from Jorde LB et al. 2009 Medical genetics, 4th edn. Elsevier, Edinburgh, with permission.

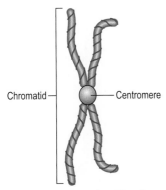

Fig. 5.5 **Chromosome structure.** The diagram shows a pair of sister chromatids joined at the centromere.

pulled apart, apparently from the centromere, towards opposite spindle poles. Cohesin molecules that held the chromatids together are dissolved with protease enzymes. This process typically lasts only a few minutes. At this point there will be 92 chromosomes, identical halves being located at opposite sides of the cell.

■ **Telophase**: the daughter chromatids lie at the spindle poles. The kinetochore microtubules disappear and a nuclear envelope forms around each group of daughter chromosomes.

■ **Cytokinesis**: cleavage of the cytoplasm starts during anaphase. The cell membrane around the centre of the cell is drawn in to form a cleavage furrow and then tightens until it reaches the remains of the mitotic spindle. This is known as the **midbody** and may persist for some time before it breaks to form the two daughter cells, each containing 46 chromosomes.

Meiosis

In meiosis (see Fig. 5.6) DNA replication is followed by two rounds of cell division and leads to the formation of four haploid cells, each containing a single set of chromosomes, i.e. half the normal chromosomal content. This process forms female egg cells or male sperm cells only. Like mitosis, each round of division in meiosis can be divided into four phases based on the nuclear and cell morphology.

The process begins with **interphase I**, in which, like mitosis, a single DNA strand duplicates to form a sister chromatid, joined with the other at the centromere. Because the cells are diploid for each chromatid, these are **homologues** (Fig. 5.7).

Meiosis I is the phase in which two haploid cells are produced from a single diploid cell. It is during this phase that genetic diversity takes place through cross-over (**recombination**).

■ **Prophase I**: this is a very different process from mitotic prophase and about 90% of meiotic time is spent in this phase. Female eggs are suspended in this stage at birth until puberty. Prophase I can be subdivided into five stages:

■ **Leptonema** (thin): the diploid chromosomes condense to form long thin threads. Each chromosome attaches by both ends via an attachment plaque to the nuclear envelope. Individual chromatids are not visible at this stage.

■ **Zygonema** (yoke shaped): **synapsis** or intimate pairing marks the beginning of zygonema. Synapsis

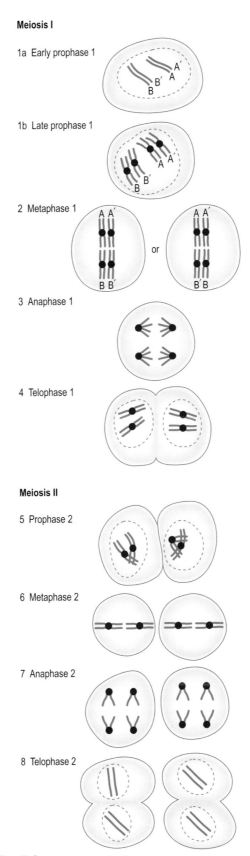

Meiosis I

1a Early prophase 1

1b Late prophase 1

2 Metaphase 1   or

3 Anaphase 1

4 Telophase 1

Meiosis II

5 Prophase 2

6 Metaphase 2

7 Anaphase 2

8 Telophase 2

Fig. 5.6 **Phases in meiosis.**

(pairing) starts when the homologous regions of the two chromosomes come together, starting a zipper-like process during which the two chromosomes become aligned side by side. This can also take

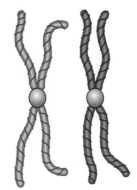

Fig. 5.7 **Diploid chromosomes:** homologous chromosomes, each containing paired sister chromatids.

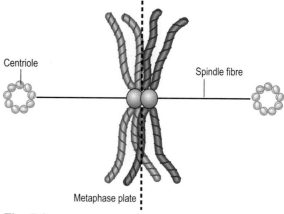

Fig. 5.9 **Metaphase I.** Spindle fibres form between centrioles at opposite sides of the cell and tetrads line up on the metaphase plate.

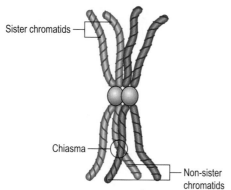

Fig. 5.8 **Tetrad chromosome formation.** The tetrad has four chromatids, with the non-sister chromatids joined at the **chiasma**.

place when an X chromosome is paired with a Y chromosome, but limited to the pseudoautosomal regions, PAR1 and PAR2, located at the tips of the short and long arms, respectively. Synapsis often starts at the nuclear membrane and proceeds inwards, but can also start in the centre of the chromosome and proceed out towards the ends. The paired chromosomes are known as **bivalents** (one from each parent) and have four chromatids. The whole is known as a **tetrad** (Fig. 5.8).

- **Pachynema** (thick): cells enter pachynema when all the chromosomes are aligned. This stage can last several days. Recombination nodules become visible, which are thought to result in an exchange of chromosomal material between the two non-sister chromatids.
- **Diplonema** (double): at this stage the two homologous chromosomes condense, to the position where the sister chromatids are visible, and start to move away from each other. Each tetrad remains attached at **chiasmata**, which are formed at the point where crossover has occurred. In oocytes, this stage can last for several months or years, but it only takes about 24 days in the human male. The chromosomes de-condense and RNA synthesis starts, to provide storage materials for the egg.
- **Diakinesis** (across): RNA synthesis ceases and chromosomes condense, thicken and detach from the nuclear membrane. The four chromatids can be clearly distinguished within each tetrad. Sister chromatids are joined at the centromere. Non-sister chromatids are joined by chiasmata.

- **Metaphase I**: in this phase spindles form between centrioles, at opposite **poles** of the cell, within the nuclear membrane, and the tetrads line up on the spindles on the equatorial plane (**metaphase plate**), with centromeres from the homologous chromosomes lying on opposite sides of the plate (Fig. 5.9).
- **Anaphase I**: the spindles pull the two homologous chromosomes apart, towards opposite ends of the cells. Unlike in mitosis, the chromosomes do not duplicate and so only half the original number will lie in each half of the cell, which will contain only one of a pair of autosomes (with crossed-over genetic material), and one sex chromosome (23 chromosomes in total).
- **Telophase I**: when the chromosomes reach the poles, a new nuclear membrane develops between each set of chromosomes (Fig. 5.10). Cytoplasmic division is about equal between the daughter cells in males, whereas in females there is unequal division. The daughter cell with the most cytoplasm goes on to form the egg, the other becoming a **polar body** that eventually degenerates.

Meiosis II is the phase in which each haploid cell produces two additional daughter haploid cells. Like in the previous phase, there are a number of similar stages:

- **Prophase II**: this is very similar to mitotic prophase, sister chromatids lying together, joined at the centromere, but the cell nucleus has only a haploid number of chromosomes.
- **Metaphase II**: spindle fibres line up the chromosomes on the equatorial plane.
- **Anaphase II**: this resembles mitotic anaphase – the centromeres split and sister chromatids are pulled towards separate poles. In meiosis, however, because of crossing over that has taken place in the first stage, the separated daughter cells may not be identical.
- **Telophase II**: this is like telophase I; nuclear membranes again form round each set of chromosomes. Again the cytoplasmic division is unequal in female gametes, keeping as much cytoplasm as possible with the true egg/future **zygote** (combination of the female and male gametes in a fertilised egg).

In females meiosis II takes place only during fertilisation, stimulated by the penetration of a sperm into the cell, with

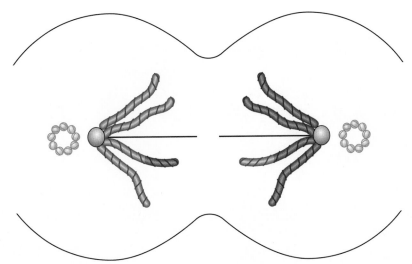

Fig. 5.10 **Telophase I.** The chromosomes reach the poles and a cytoplasmic membrane forms between the two halves.

the sperm nucleus uniting with the large egg nucleus to produce the zygote.

At the end of meiosis the result in males is four daughter haploid cells, two with 22 chromosomes plus an X chromosome and two with 22 chromosomes plus a Y chromsome, whereas in female cells, two daughter haploid cells plus two polar bodies will form. Occasionally, polar bodies formed in stage 1 can divide and there will be three polar bodies.

Chromosome abnormalities

Abnormalities in number

Defects in fertilisation or meiosis can result in an additional or reduced number of chromosomes being detected. The body is better able to deal with small excesses of genetic material than a deficit.

- **Polyploidy** occurs when an additional set of chromosomes is present; this always happens as a multiple of 23 chromosomes. **Triploidy** results in 69 chromosomes and **tetraploidy** leads to 92 chromosomes in each cell. These conditions are rarely compatible with life and triploidy is a common cause of spontaneous miscarriages.
- **Aneuploidy** occurs when a multiple of 23 chromosomes is not present. There can be a gain or loss of chromosomes, which can affect either autosomal or sex chromosomes. These conditions are usually caused by non-disjunction during meiosis and can lead to **monosomy** (one copy of a chromosome in a normally diploid cell) or **trisomy** (three copies of a chromosome in a normally diploid cell).
- **Autosomal monosomy** – is rarely compatible with life.
- **Autosomal trisomy** – trisomy 21 (Down syndrome) is the most common.
- **Sex chromosome monosomy** – because of normal X inactivation, the loss of a single X chromosome (Turner syndrome) is compatible with life. The surviving X chromosome is normally maternal in origin and often the result of non-disjunction as a result of meiotic errors producing X chromosomes with p arm deletions, or abnormal Y chromosomes in the male.
- **Sex chromosome trisomy** – XXY (Klinefelter syndrome), XXX (trisomy X) and XYY syndrome have fewer problems than the above.

Abnormalities in structure

Sometimes, as gametes are formed, structural alterations can occur – pieces can be lost, moved to another chromosome or duplicated. These events can be the result of homologous chromosomes failing to line up properly during meiosis, causing an unequal crossover, or chromosome breakage with an imperfect repair. The alterations that can occur are:

- **Translocations** – where genetic material is exchanged between different chromosomes (**reciprocal** translocation), or where the short arms of two chromosomes are lost and the long arms fuse at the centromere to make a single large chromosome (**Robertsonian** translocation). In the latter, although there is the overall loss of one chromosome, this is usually only seen in chromosomes where the amount of genetic material in the short arm is limited, such as in chromosomes 14 and 21.

  The **Philadelphia chromosome** involves a translocation between chromosomes 9 and 22, and is characteristically observed in chronic myeloid leukaemia (see Ch. 12).

- **Deletions** – a loss of genetic material can occur when breaks happen. Some of these deletions can lead to clinically important abnormalities:
- **Cri-du-chat** syndrome, so called because of the child's distinctive cry, occurs because of the loss of part of the short arm of chromosome 5.
- **Wolf–Hirschhorn** syndrome is because of the loss of part of the short arm of chromosome 4. This, and the previous example, are examples of a **microdeletion**.
- **Ring** chromosomes occur when there is a deletion at both ends of the chromosome and the ends join, forming a ring. This often leads to the loss of that chromosome, resulting in a monosomy. The formation of a ring X chromosome can be another cause of Turner syndrome.
- **WAGR** syndrome is due to a deletion of the p arm of chromosome 11, involving a series of genes, resulting in **W**ilms tumour (a kidney cancer), **a**niridia (no iris), **g**onad tumours or other genitourinary abnormalities, and **r**etardation. This is an example of a **contiguous gene syndrome**.
- High-resolution banding techniques and **fluorescence in situ hybridisation** (**FISH**) (see Information box 5.1, including Fig. 5.11), and more latterly gene array molecular technologies, have enabled many microdeletions to be described, and more are likely to follow.

Information box 5.1   Fluorescence in situ hybridisation (Fig. 5.11)

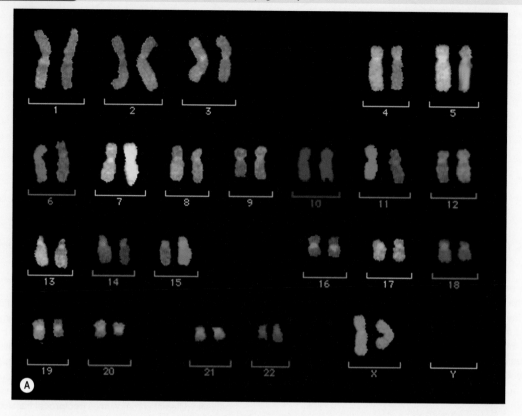

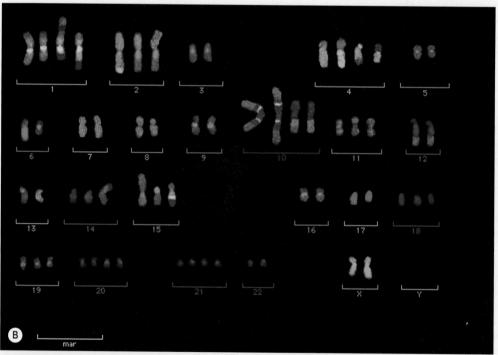

Fig. 5.11 **Fluorescence in situ hybridisation (FISH).** (**A**) M-FISH showing a normal human karyotype from a female. (**B**) M-FISH showing an abnormal human karyotype with duplications and translocations in a female.

Information box 5.1   Fluorescence in situ hybridisation—cont'd

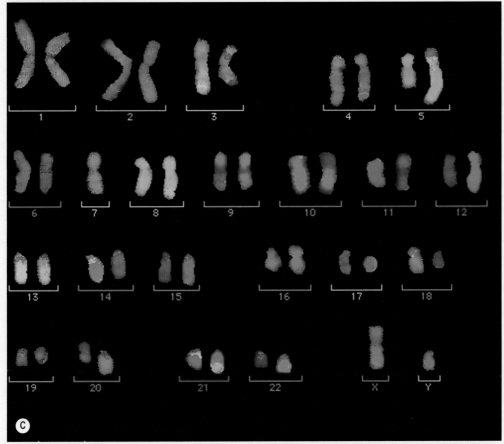

Fig. 5.11, cont'd **(C)** M-FISH showing an abnormal human karyotype with chromosome loss and translocations in a male. Courtesy of Dr Debra Lillington.

- FISH is a technique that has been developed to map (locate) particular regions of a chromosome, or even whole chromosomes, regardless of whether or not the cells are actively dividing. The technique requires the use of a piece of single-stranded DNA that matches the genetic sequence in the area of interest – the **probe**.
- Chromosomes prepared on a glass slide are **denatured** (the DNA complementary strands are separated) **in situ** (on the slide), allowing the probe DNA to **hybridise** (bind) to its complementary sequence on the separated strand. Fluorescent dyes are attached to the probes so that the results can be visualised under a fluorescence microscope.

- FISH can be used in different ways:
  - **Gene location**: the genetic sequence of every gene is known and a probe can be developed to show the chromosomal location of the gene. The technique is sensitive enough to identify deletions of very small amounts of DNA from a chromosome.
  - **Centromeric probes**: probes can be used to identify the repetitive sequence found around the centromere. This can be used to check the number of chromosomes.
  - **Spectral karyotyping**: this involves the use of a large number of probes, labelled with different coloured fluorescent dyes, in order to 'paint' a whole chromosome. This technique is particularly useful in detecting chromosomal translocations, in which a part of one chromosome is moved to another chromosome.

- **Duplications** – can occur as a result of unequal crossover, or in the children of someone with a reciprocal translocation.
- **Inversions** – this can happen when there are two breaks in the chromosome and the free portion rotates. These changes are said to be **pericentric** if they involve the centromere, **paracentric** if they do not. While these abnormalities may not have severe consequences, they can interfere with the normal meiotic process and therefore they are at higher risk of producing offspring with deletions or duplications. Occasionally, the inversion can be very serious and is the cause of almost 50% of

cases of severe haemophilia, where the inversion has interrupted the factor VIII gene, resulting in insufficient production of factor VIII for normal clotting processes (see Ch. 12).
- **Isochromosome** – chromosome pairs normally line up, joining and separating at the centromeres, but retaining their own long and short arms. An isochromosome occurs when the chromosomes split at the centromere to produce two chromosomes, one with only short arms, and the other with only long arms. Only isochromosomes involving the X chromosome appear to be compatible with life.

DNA AND GENES

Chromosomal DNA is located in the nucleus and is composed of regions that actively make proteins and those that are inactive. **Genes** are the active DNA sequences coding for proteins and are organised into:

- Regulatory regions (**promoters**, enhancer or repressor sequences)
- **Exons** – which encode the mRNA, and, in most cases, the protein
- **Introns** – which are not transcribed into proteins.

Some genes are only found at a single **locus** (chromosome location). They are called **single copy** genes and share little or no DNA sequence homology with other genes. Other genes are part of large **gene families**. These families have occurred due to gene duplication, and gene members therefore share a high degree of DNA (and amino acid) sequence homology. They often cluster at specific regions of the genome and have similar but distinct functions in different tissues.

Homeobox (HOX) genes

Genes can also be classified into gene families based on the presence of highly conserved **domains**, with the rest of the gene sequence sharing no homology at all with other family members. **Homeobox** (**HOX**) genes are examples of these.

HOX genes are associated in clusters on different chromosomes and control production of body parts. They are organised in similar ways throughout the animal kingdom and are arranged along chromosomes in an order that reflects the body parts that they control. While a specific HOX gene from a fly can be identical with one from another organism, such as the chicken, reflecting their common ancestry, a small mutation can lead to fundamental changes in morphology – called **homeotic mutations**. For example, additional fingers on the hand are the result of a mutation in a specific HOX gene.

Non-coding DNA (see Ch. 2)

Genes are also separated by repetitive non-coding regions. Despite not being used for making proteins, this DNA is not unimportant and has a number of gene regulatory functions.

Unlike human chromosomal DNA, all the mitochondrial DNA (mtDNA) sequence codes for proteins used to maintain their propogation and the functional aspects of oxidative phosphorylation. mtDNA is present in many copies in the mitochondria within the cytoplasm of most cells and is maternally inherited. Sperm contain very few mitochondria and so are overwhelmed by the female contribution, but there also seem to be regulatory mechanisms that inhibit their propagation.

Two processes are involved in making proteins:

- **Transcription** – in which DNA is transcribed (copied) into mRNA, which then leaves the nucleus
- **Translation** – in which mRNA is used to specify the amino acids required to make the relevant protein.

These processes take place in one direction only along a nucleic acid strand. Nucleic acids are arranged in sequence along a strand and each end is named after the number of carbon atoms in the nucleotide sugar ring at the end.

- The **5′** end has a 5-carbon deoxyribose ring
- The **3′** end has a hydroxyl group on the third carbon in the sugar ring.

The distinction between the two ends of the molecule is important because nucleic acid can only be synthesised in a 5′ to 3′ direction. By convention sequences are written in a 5′ to 3′ direction.

Transcription (Fig. 5.12)

The process of making mRNA is initiated when an RNA polymerase enzyme binds to a **promoter** site on the DNA. **Sigma factors** associated with the enzyme bind and are released on transcription. The availability of a particular sigma factor can also regulate transcription. The promoter region is a sequence of DNA close to, but outside, the gene. The position of the promoter determines which strand is used, because nucleotides can only be added to a 3′ end. Thus mRNA is only made in the 5′ to 3′ direction along the chromosome. Several different promoters can exist in different parts of the gene, allowing for slightly different proteins being produced in different locations in the body.

Transcription begins by the assembly of the basal transcription apparatus, involving transcription factors and associated proteins upstream of the start codon. In most promoters the assembly site is determined by the **TATA box** sequence. This is a conserved sequence of A:T pairs, usually located 25–35 bases upstream of the start codon. Other sequences are involved in determining the efficiency of the promoter, such as those found in the **CAAT box**, normally located further upstream. Many genes also have GC-rich regions, or **CpG islands**, upstream of the transcription start site. CpG islands are unmethylated regions of the genome that are associated with the 5′ ends of many genes.

The polymerase enzyme pulls the DNA strands apart, zipper-like, exposing the DNA bases. This provides a template (**antisense** strand), with the enzyme moving from the 3′ to 5′ direction along this template, producing a complementary copy (**sense** strand), which eventually becomes the mRNA. Note that this molecule is identical to the other of the DNA strands that have not been used as a template, except that the thymine base is replaced with a uracil base. As the enzyme progresses down the DNA strand, unwinding upstream and reannealing with the new RNA strand downstream of the

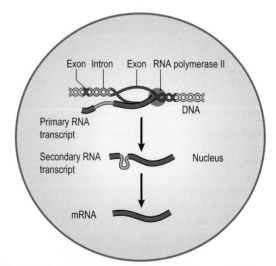

Fig. 5.12 **Transcription of DNA to messenger RNA (mRNA).** The enzyme RNA polymerase II moves along the DNA strand separating the strands and assembling a strand of mRNA nucleotides that are complementary to the DNA.

polymerase, this may be visible as a **transcription bubble** using specialised microscopy or spectroscopy.

To the 5′ end of the developing precursor mRNA molecule is added a modified guanine molecule – the **5′ cap**. This 'cap' appears both to protect the molecule from degradation by 5' nucleases as the modification makes it look like a functional 3' end and it acts as a marker for translation to begin. Transcription continues, through a sequence of exons and introns, until a **termination sequence** signals the end. Before mRNA leaves the nucleus introns are excised and the exons spliced together.

Splicing can also happen in different ways: intentionally, resulting in different proteins being produced, or unintentionally, resulting in a **mutation** (error), which can produce genetic disease. A large number of adenine sequences are added (**polyadenylation**) to the 3′ end – **polyA tail** – close to this termination sequence and, although transcription may continue, this tail is later lost. The mRNA finally separates from the polymerase enzyme and template DNA. Figure 5.13 illustrates the process. The sequence formed consists of a series of **codons** – three nucleotides that code for particular amino acids.

Regulation of transcription

The regulation of transcriptional processes is a vital component in the control of gene expression. Genes are normally transcribed in particular tissues at particular times, but typically only about 3–5% of genes are expressed at any given time. In addition, even though all cells have the same DNA sequence, only a few genes are actively transcribed in any one cell. For example, only nucleated red cell precursors transcribe globin, used in the production of haemoglobin. Other genes may be transcribed all the time, to maintain cell integrity (**housekeeping genes**), or at particular times to aid other processes. For example, RNA polymerase needs other proteins to stabilise the polymerase, to help it bind in order to initiate transcription.

Transcription can be modified by **enhancers**. These are sequences that do not interact with the relevant genes, and may not even lie close, but which bind to transcription factors, known as **activators**. The whole then binds to **coactivators**, increasing transcription. **Silencers** are analogous to enhancers but they repress transcription. The various transcription factors interact with their targets through **DNA-binding motifs**, particular protein configurations that fit with, interact and modify the secondary and tertiary structure of the target molecules. These are some characteristic motifs:

- Helix–turn–helix (hth):
    - Two α-helices lie in different planes, one fitting into the groove on the DNA molecule
- Zinc finger:
    - Zinc ions are used to stabilise protein secondary structure in the form of α-helices and β-sheets, enabling the α-helix to bind with DNA in the major groove
- Leucine zipper:
    - Two α-helices that form a y-shaped structure, being held together with amino acid side chains that also bind to the DNA molecule in the major groove.

Translation

This process takes place on ribosomes; mRNA provides the template, specifying the amino acid sequence, helped by molecules of **tRNA**. tRNA consists of about 80 nucleotides that have a clover-leaf structure (Fig. 5.14). There is at least one type of tRNA molecule for each amino acid, determined by the **anticodon** sequence in the loop of the molecule.

rRNA first binds to mRNA at the **start codon** at its 5′ end. This is the sequence adenine–uracil–guanine (AUG), which codes for the amino acid methionine. (See Table 2.16 for a list of codons.) Mitochondrial genomes using other start codons – often GUG. The tRNA that binds is determined by the nucleotide sequence of the mRNA: the three nucleotide codon binds to the complementary anticodon on the tRNA molecule. In the process, the ribosome provides specific enzymes (aminoacyl-tRNA synthetases) that pick up the specific amino acid and attaches it to the 3' acceptor end – matching the

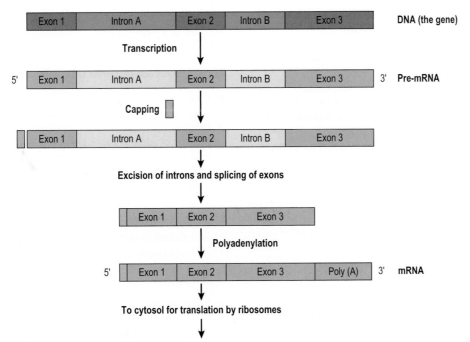

Fig. 5.13 **Production of messenger RNA (mRNA).** After transcription from the antisense DNA strand, the growing mRNA molecule is capped at the 5′ end, introns are spliced and the exons joined. mRNA produces a tail of adenine nucleotides (polyA tail) at the 3′ end.

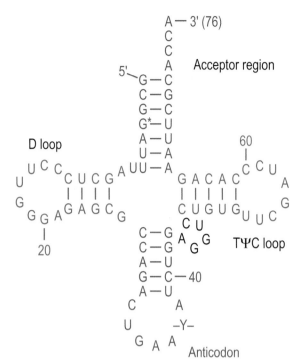

Fig. 5.14 **Structure of tRNA.** The diagram illustrates the secondary structure of the molecule which is composed of four base-paired stems and three non-base-paired loops: D loop (green); the anticodon (red); the TΨC loop (blue); as well as a variable region (black) and an acceptor region (purple). The 3' end always terminates with the sequence CCA, with the 3' hydroxyl of the ribose of the terminal A being the point of covalent attachment of specific amino acids, determined by the three nucleotide anticodon sequence.

codon in the mRNA molecule. Ribosomes move along the mRNA sequence in a 5′ to 3′ direction and also provide enzymes that make covalent bonds between each of the amino acids, in order to produce the growing polypeptide chain. Translation continues until reaching a **stop codon** (a nucleotide triplet, normally UAG, UAA or UGA).

DNA DAMAGE

DNA can be damaged by a variety of factors, such as X-rays, and a large number of chemicals, but damage can also occur naturally during replication. There are two main types of error: physical abnormalities, such as breaks in the DNA molecule, and **mutations**, where there is a change in the DNA sequence. This base change can alter the codon, and thus the amino acid and subsequent protein being produced. While damage may be repairable, mutations cannot be and are transmitted each time the cell replicates. Mutant cells will increase or decrease in frequency, dependent on the stability of the cell to survive. Although DNA damage and DNA mutation are different, they are linked because damage will often cause errors in DNA synthesis during repair or replication, producing a mutation.

DNA damage from environmental factors

- Radiation, from ultraviolet light (non-ionising), X-rays or gamma rays (ionizing) can damage DNA in various ways.

- UV light can directly damage the DNA by crosslinking adjacent thymine and cytosine bases, producing pyrimidine dimers, or can indirectly damage the DNA through the production of free radicals.
- Ionising radiation breaks the phosphate backbone by severing the bond between oxygen and phosphate groups. Mechanisms exist to attempt to fix the broken ends, by joining to other pieces of DNA within a cell – a translocation. Where the translocation breakpoint is within or near a gene then the function of the gene may be affected.
- Thermal damage increases the loss of purine bases from the DNA backbone (depurination)
- Human-made mutagenic chemicals, such as vinyl chloride, and other polycyclic aromatic hydrocarbons such as are found in smoke and tars, create a large number of different DNA adducts – changes to the DNA such as oxidation (from reactive oxygen species), alkylation (often methylation), and hydrolysis (deamination, depurination, depyrimidation) of bases, or DNA cross-linking, or bulky covalently attached compounds, all of which are associated with carcinogenesis
- Viruses
- Plant toxins.

Spontaneous damage (DNA replication mistakes)

During DNA replication, the polymerase very occasionally makes a mistake, about once every 100 000 000 bases, even after normal repair mechanisms. These errors may also be induced by the presence of reactive oxygen species produced from normal metabolic processes, such as during oxidative deamination.

Repair mechanisms

A series of genes are involved in producing enzymes that assist in repair mechanisms, recognising altered bases, excising them and replacing them. The process is highly efficient, correcting about 99.9% of errors.

Direct reversal of base damage

- Photolyase is activated by UV light and reverses the pyrimidine dimer formation induced by the light
- Common damage involves methylation of cytosine, guanine or adenine bases (alkylation) and sustained exposure to this damage produces an adaptive response in which alkylation repair enzymes are upregulated.

Breakage repair

Single-strand breaks

These are repaired using the base excision repair (BER), nucleoside excision repair (NER) and mismatch repair (MMR) mechanisms.

- **Base excision repair (BER).** First the **glycosylase** enzyme removes the damaged base and other enzymes (AP endonucleases) remove the phosphate in the backbone. This is followed by **DNA polymerase beta** (β) replacing the correct nucleotide; then **DNA ligase** enzymes mend the break.

■ the same chromosome, if there are duplicate copies of the gene on the same chromosome in opposite directions. The process involves **BRCA1** and **BRCA2**; mutations in the genes encoding these proteins predispose to breast and ovarian cancers.

Clinical box 5.2 | **Xeroderma pigmentosum**

Xeroderma pigmentosum (XP) is a rare inherited disease that predisposes individuals to skin lesions (dry skin and freckles) and an increased incidence of skin cancer. The areas affected are particularly those areas exposed to sunlight. Several genes have been implicated, all involved in nucleotide excision repair. Patients are advised to avoid ultraviolet light exposure.

- **Nucleotide excision repair (NER)**. (see Clinical box 5.2). Protein factors recognise large helix-affecting damage, such as pyrimdine dimer formation, and **transcription factor IIH** (also involved in normal transcription) unwinds the DNA to produce a 'bubble'. Cuts are made on the 3′ and 5′ side of the damage, removing a 'patch' of nucleotides. **DNA polymerases delta (δ) and epsilon (ε)** then synthesise the repair using the opposite strand as a template. Finally, DNA ligase binds the new piece into the backbone.
- **Mismatch repair (MMR)**. This process corrects mismatches of normal bases and uses enzymes involved in BER and NER. The **MSH2** protein recognises the mismatch and the **MLH1** protein cuts it out. DNA polymerase δ and ε repair the patch. Mutations in the genes *MSH2* and *MSH1* predispose to colon cancer and they are therefore referred to as **tumour suppressor genes**.

Double-strand breaks (DSBs)

When both strands of the double helix are broken this can result in genome rearrangements and is particularly hazardous to the cell. There are three main repair mechanisms for DSBs: non-homologous end joining (NHEJ), microhomology-mediated end joining (MMEJ) and homologous recombination.

- **Non-homologous end-joining (NHEJ)**. This process enables the direct joining of broken ends – the nucleotides involved do not have to be complementary. It uses short homologous DNA sequences (microhomologies) of 10 present in single-stranded overhangs on the ends of double stranded breaks. When the overhangs are compatible the repair is accurate, but otherwise there can be losses of nucleotides, potentially leading to translocations, such as the Philadelphia chromosome (see Ch. 12), or telomere fusions seen more frequently in tumour cells. Repair takes place in the G0/G1 and early S phase of the cell cycle.
- **Microhomology-mediated end joining (MMEJ)**. This mechanism is used in the S phase of the cycle, when NHEJ is inactive or unsuitable because of the deletions it would introduce; it involves a **Ku heterodimer protein** and a DNA-PK independent repair mechanism. It ligates the mismatched hanging strands and removes overhanging nucleotides (flaps) which are replaced with a short homology of complementary base pairs from the strands to fill in the gaps and to realign the molecule. Since the repair relies on microhomologous regions up or downstream from the break any important nucleotide sequences lost in the gaps can result in significant coding errors which may create oncogenes.
- **Homologous recombination**. Broken ends can also be repaired using information from:
    - the homologous chromosome in G1 phase
    - the sister chromatid from G2 phase

GENES AND DEVELOPMENT

The most common cause of infant death is due to a birth defect, and up to 3% of babies have a recognisable defect. Many of these defects are due to mutations in developmental genes. The prevalence of genetic abnormalities is even higher among foetuses that miscarry.

After fertilisation the developing ovum not only undergoes simple multiplication but changes to form different cell types, tissues and organs in a highly coordinated fashion. Understanding how cells with identical genes (**stem cells**) develop into different cell types has been studied through the discipline of developmental biology.

Many of the genes and pathways involved in human development are the same across a large range of species and the function of many of these genes has been elucidated using non-human organisms, such as the roundworm, fruit fly, zebrafish, frog and mouse. Many of these organisms have fast generation times thus facilitating the research by being able to examine a large number of events in a short period of time.

Embryo development begins with defining the major axes of the body: ventral/dorsal, anterior/posterior, medial/lateral, left/right. Cells then are differentiated and arranged spatially to form the tissues; organs and limbs are then formed through organogenesis. These processes are driven through the production of proteins that provide signals and switches.

MEDIATORS OF DEVELOPMENT

Developmental genes code for a variety of proteins with differing functions, for example signalling, DNA transcription and extracellular matrix components.

Signalling molecules

Signalling molecules allow interactions between cells. A protein is secreted by a cell and diffuses across the extracellular space to bind to a receptor on the target cell. These molecules are called **paracrine** signalling molecules and include:

- Fibroblast growth factor (FGF) family
- Hedgehog family
- Wingless (Wnt) family
- Transforming growth factor β (TGF-β).

Fibroblast growth factor and fibroblast growth factor receptor

The receptor for FGF (FGFR) is a glycoprotein consisting of peptides and immunoglobulin-type areas on the outside of the cell, with a protein that crosses the cell membrane and an intracellular **tyrosine kinase**. Different FGFs can bind to the receptor, leading to phosphorylation and activation of the tyrosine kinase. Many FGFs are involved in bone development, and mutations in the FGFR lead to a variety of skeletal problems in children (see Clinical box 5.3).

Sonic hedgehog

The hedgehog family of genes was called after a mutant form of hairy fruit fly. Vertebrates have similar forms, the most common of which is called **sonic hedgehog** (**SHH**), involved in specifying the body axis. *SHH* binds to its receptor, a transmembrane protein called **patched** (**PTC**), which suppresses transcription of **Wnt** and **TGF-β** and inhibits cell growth.

- PTC *somatic* mutations affect the regulation of cell differentiation and cause cancer, such as basal cell carcinoma.
- PTC *germline* mutations cause birth defects – rib anomalies, jaw cysts and cancer in later life – **Gorlin syndrome**.

Wingless (Wnt)

The **Wnt** genes were named after wingless mutant flies. A variety of different types are present in humans, and are involved in **dorsal/ventral axis** specification and development of various organs, binding to **frizzled** and low-density lipoprotein (LDL) receptors.

Wnt genes are involved in signalling processes throughout the cell and have been linked to the development of B cell and lymphoid malignancies. Different forms appear to act as both tumour suppressors and tumour activators in cancer formation. Mutations in **R-spondin** proteins that are involved in Wnt signalling have produced inherited defects such as **anonychia** (absence of nails) and sex reversal.

Transforming growth factor β

TGF-βs are a large number of related genes that are involved with bone formation through the production of **bone morphogenetic protein** (**BMP**).

DNA transcription factors

There are many families of transcription factors. These are genes that produce proteins that activate or repress other genes. They often share a common DNA-binding domain but have a wide variety of effects (**pleiotropy**).

Transcription factor genes are important in human development: HOX, SOX and T-box are important examples of these.

SOX family genes

There are a large number of **SOX** (**Sry-related HMG** (**high mobility group) box**) genes that are involved in neuronal development and sex determination. SOX genes have much in common with the *SRY* (**sex-determining region on the Y chromosome**) gene found on the human Y chromosome.

- *SRY* produces DNA-bending proteins that promote events leading to male differentiation through:
  - **Sertoli cell** differentiation (these cells are found in the testes and aid sperm development)
  - Production of **Müllerian-inhibitory factor** (embryonic Müllerian ducts develop into the female reproductive organs)
- *SRY* abnormalities can produce sex reversals:
  - XX males and XY females can be the result of a faulty crossover in meiosis between the X and Y chromosome, where the *SRY* gene is transferred to the X chromosome and the resultant affected offspring depends on the chromosome the father passes to his child
  - XY females can also be the result of a mutation in the *SRY* gene.

Extracellular matrix proteins

These are a large collection of molecules, including collagens and glycoproteins, that form the extracellular matrix and allow for cell migration.

A mutation in the **fibrillin** gene, responsible for the development of microfibrils in connective tissue, results in **Marfan syndrome**, with its multiple pleiotropic effects, leading to skeletal, cardiovascular and ocular defects.

PATTERNING

The position of organs and appendages is laid down in patterns defined during embryogenesis under the control of a series of genes. Important in this process are genes that specify the various body axes.

Most of the knowledge of pattern formation has come from experimentation with 'knockout' mice and tissue transplantations between regions in the early embryo (Fig. 5.15). Mutations in many of the early developmental genes are likely to be lethal in humans.

Anterior/posterior axis formation

The developing collection of cells in the fertilised ovum, or blastula, undergoes **gastrulation** in which the three embryonic layers, **ectoderm**, **mesoderm** and **endoderm**, are defined and an anterior/posterior thickening occurs, the **primitive streak**, under control of a series of **HOX** and other developmental genes.

There are a large number of HOX genes on different chromosomes and they are expressed at different times, in an order that specifies the positioning of cells and tissues along the anterior/posterior axis. A mutation in one of these genes results in the replacement of antennae by legs in the *Drosophila* fly; limb abnormalities have also been observed in humans.

Left/right axis formation

At the anterior end of the primitive streak lies the **node**, which is the source of the left-side-expressed **nodal** protein, stimulated by asymmetrical expression of **SHH** from the **notochord**.

Dorsal/ventral axis development

Bone morphogenic proteins (**BMPs**) are growth factors influencing the development of bone and cartilage, and are also important in the embryonic development of the heart and central nervous system.

- **BMP-4**, excreted from the dorsal notochord in the mesoderm, along with SHH proteins, from the ventral notochord, establishes the dorsal/ventral axis and stimulates development of the overlying ectoderm.

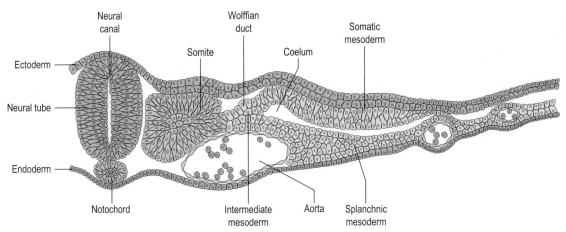

Fig. 5.15 **Cross-section of a chick embryo at 45 hours' incubation,** showing the principal anatomical features of the early embryo.

- **Noggin** and **chordin** are **morphogens** (proteins that govern pattern development) that spread from a node and are expressed in a concentration gradient across a tissue. They **inhibit** BMPs. Noggin is needed in embryonic development to form the neural plate that lies opposite the primitive streak, allowing it to develop into the neural tube and subsequently to form the brain and spinal cord.
- Noggin and chordin bind directly to BMP-4, inhibiting its ventralising signal, promoting dorsalisation in the mesoderm region that experiences high concentrations of the proteins. Noggin and chordin are thus important in defining the back, as opposed to the front, of the developing embryo.

ORGANOGENESIS

Organogenesis occurs after gastrulation and involves many of the same proteins, expressed differentially.

Neuronal development

FGFs influence differentiation of the neural plate into the spinal cord. Absence of FGF towards the anterior part of the neural tube allows brain tissue to generate. HOX genes further control the development of the forebrain, midbrain and hindbrain from the neural tube. FGFs are also important in the development of the skull bones and limb formation.

Neural crest cells, located on the lateral edges of the neural folds and formed from ectoderm, are induced by BMP, Wnt and FGF signalling to migrate through the extracellular matrix. They are very important in development and there are four major types:

- **Cranial** – important in development of tissues in the facial region
- **Vagal and sacral** – forming parasympathetic neurons involved in gut peristalsis and blood vessel dilation
  - **Hirschsprung disease** leads to severe constipation. It is commonly due to mutations in the **RET** (**rearranged during transfection**) gene that is important for neural crest cell migration into the distal bowel
- **Trunk** – forms two populations that influence the development of skin pigment cells and neurons of the sympathetic nervous system
- **Cardiac** – influencing the development of the great vessels supplying the heart.

The asymmetrical heart

While the developed heart shows left/right asymmetry, the embryonic heart is formed inverted and is bilaterally symmetrical. Various influences are needed to transform the heart tube into chambers and establish the asymmetry.

dHAND and **eHAND** are basic helix–loop–helix transcription factors that are expressed in different areas of the heart tube. Both factors are transcribed initially, but later dHAND predominates in the region due to become the right ventricle, and eHAND in the region that will become the left ventricle. This, along with the **right cardiac forward looping** produced by the **nodal** protein, changes the anterior/posterior orientation into the left/right asymmetry of the developed heart.

Organ formation

While the endoderm gives rise to the gastrointestinal tract, respiratory system, liver and pancreas, the mesoderm produces the circulatory, reproductive and urinary systems, the muscles and connective tissues, through complex interactions mediated by a variety of signalling molecules acting through complex interconnected networks.

Genes that are involved in the development of a particular organ are often also involved in the function of specialised cells within the organ; for example:

- Transcription of **insulin** from β-cells in the pancreas is stimulated by binding of **insulin promoter factor 1**.
- Mutations in the gene producing this factor prevent development of the pancreas.

Limb development

Much is known about genes that control limb development because, next to congenital heart defects, abnormalities of the limbs are the next most common birth defect. Many of the pathways and transcription controls involved in limb development are conserved throughout the animal kingdom, and experimentation in model organisms, such as *Drosophila*, has helped in understanding the processes involved.

Limbs develop from the **lateral plate mesoderm**, which leads to bone and cartilage development, and the **somatic mesoderm**, which produces the muscles, nerves and blood vessels. The **intermediate mesoderm**, close to the Wolffian duct, is thought to be the origin of the signal that induces

Thalidomide was marketed in the late 1950s as an anti-sickness drug given to women in early pregnancy. Use within a particular gestational window led to multiple birth effects, predominantly characterised by an absence of arms.

Thalidomide has been shown to increase the production of free radicals, leading to oxidative stress. **Nuclear factor κB**, an anti-apoptotic transcription factor, is redox sensitive and it is proposed that a species-selective failure to bind to its DNA promoter, because of oxidative damage, leads to a failure of expression of fibroblast growth factor 10 (**FGF10**), which in turn attenuates expression of **FGF8** in the apical ectodermal ridge, essential for limb development.

limb production from the **apical ectodermal ridge (AER)** structure in the ectoderm under control of FGF and Wnt signalling proteins. The protein **FGF8**, for example, is capable of producing a limb if transplanted into mesoderm tissue (see Clinical box 5.4).

The AER, destined to produce the skin covering of the limb, sustains the limb formation within the **progress zone** in the mesoderm, where the limb develops. Both the AER and the progress zone of the mesoderm are needed for limb development. These developmental axes are important:

- **Proximal/distal**. The length of time that cells spend in the progress zone will determine the proximal/distal axis. Removal of the AER will lead to a short limb with more distal elements, the actual elements depending on how late the AER influence was removed.
- **Anterior/posterior**. The AER provides signals to the **zone of polarising activity (ZPA)**, at the root of the limb bud, and establishes the anterior/posterior axis (thumb/little finger) in the limb bud. **FGF8 is** needed to maintain the expression of SHH from the ZPA, which guides the anterior/posterior patterning through the asymmetrical expression of various downstream genes.

Apoptosis leads to separation of the fingers, stimulated by BMP signalling; noggin blocks cell death within the digits.

HUMAN GENETIC VARIATION

POLYMORPHISMS

E.B. Ford was a British ecological geneticist who defined genetic polymorphism in 1940 as a 'type of variation in which individuals with sharply distinct qualities co-exist as normal members of a population …', stating that they occur 'in such proportions that the rarest of them cannot be maintained merely by recurrent mutation.'

Polymorphisms are all the result of mutational events:

- Mutations in the germline cells that produce the gametes are inherited mutations. Some of these will produce deleterious effects, leading to inherited diseases, while others will have no effect, and are therefore passed down the generations as a polymorphism that is maintained at a reasonable level, generally in more than 1% in the population.
- Mutations of somatic cells potentially result in cancer.

The different polymorphisms, or different sequences of DNA at a particular region (**locus**) of the genome, are referred to as **alleles** of a gene. Each person inherits half their DNA from one parent, and half from the other. Individuals sharing the same allele on both their chromosomes are said to be **homozygous** for that particular polymorphism; those having different alleles are therefore **heterozygous**.

Mutation or polymorphism?

The distinction between what is a pathogenic mutation and what is polymorphic variation is not always clear.

- A mutation can be defined as an alteration in the (normal) DNA sequence that affects protein function or expression
- A polymorphism is defined as a locus where two or more alleles have been seen at a frequency greater than 0.01 (or 1%) in the population.

This implies therefore that a polymorphism is a mutation that is compatible with life in its **heterozygous** form.

Types of mutational events leading to polymorphisms

At the nucleotide level polymorphisms can be a **single base substitution**, the insertion or deletion of one or more bases, or **repeat length** or **copy number polymorphisms** and rearrangements. They are present throughout the genome and can be subdivided into those that alter a protein sequence (**coding polymorphisms**) and those which do not (**non-coding polymorphisms**).

Single nucleotide polymorphisms

The most common type of polymorphism in the human genome is the **single nucleotide polymorphism** or **SNP**. Each SNP will have two, or occasionally three, alleles. Approximately 10 million SNPs have been identified with a minor allele frequency of greater than 0.5%. SNPs are not homogeneous across the genome; the greatest diversity is found at the **human lymphocyte antigen (HLA)** locus, the least on the sex chromosomes. Less than 1% of SNPs are predicted to result in changes in the composition of proteins and are therefore unlikely to be a major source of phenotypic variation. It is not currently known, however, to what extent SNPs in regulatory regions contribute towards phenotypic diversity.

Sequence variation that does not result in a change in the amino acid that is coded for are referred to as **silent** substitutions; those that produce an amino acid change, as **missense** mutations (e.g. **sickle cell disease** – see Clinical box 5.5), and those that produce **stop codons**, as **nonsense** mutations.

Deletions and insertions (Clinical box 5.6)

Deletions and insertions are defined as the loss or addition of one or more bases from a DNA sequence. Because of the three-nucleotide code for a single amino acid, loss of bases that are not multiples of three is more likely to produce major detrimental effects (**frameshift** mutations).

Sickle cell disease is an example of a **missense** mutation in which A is replaced by T at the seventeenth nucleotide of the β-chain haemoglobin gene. The normal GAG codon for glutamic acid thus becomes GTG, which encodes the amino acid valine. When it is present in two copies it results in the **sickling** (a sickle shape) of red blood cells. The consequences of this are numerous, and include severe anaemia and tissue and organ damage due to the accumulation of the rigid red cells in small blood vessels (see Ch. 12).

Clinical box 5.6   **Examples of deletions and insertions**

Cystic fibrosis is a common inherited autosomal recessive genetic disorder among Caucasians, affecting as many as 1 in 2000 in northern Europe, leading to fibrotic lesions throughout the body, but particularly affecting the lungs, pancreas and intestines. The most common mutation involves a three-base deletion that removes the amino acid phenylalanine from the **cystic fibrosis transmembrane regulator** (*CFTR*) gene sequence, although more than 1300 mutations have been described involving several different mutational types.

The gene codes for a chloride channel protein controlling the movement of chloride from the inside to the outside of the cell, and from sweat into the cytoplasm in the sweat glands. The mutant gene needs to be present in two copies (recessive), inherited from both parents, to produce the disease. *CFTR* mutations lead to the negatively charged chloride ions being trapped and this accumulation also prevents the movement of positively charged ions, such as sodium. The ions combine to form salt, which is found in large amounts within sweat glands in this condition. This forms the basis of the **sweat test** for cystic fibrosis. The salt imbalance leads to loss of water and results in thick obstructive secretions, including mucus within the lungs. The thick mucus is an ideal environment for bacterial infections.

Huntington disease results from increased numbers of repeated CAG (glutamine Q) sequences (polyQ) that produce a mutant Huntingtin protein (mHTT), which interferes with synaptic transmission in the brain. Neuronal transmission worsens with increasing size of the polyQ component.

PolyQ lengths involving more than 36 glutamines lead to increased neuronal death. An early age of onset and more rapid progression of the disease are associated with increased polyQ lengths. The autosomal dominant inheritance is also affected by 'dynamic' mutations, in which the number of repeats is not always exactly copied. The disease occurs at higher prevalence in the Afrikaner population of South Africa and is thought to be the result of a **founder** (see below), a Dutch man who arrived there in 1652 (see also Clinical box 5.7).

Fragile X syndrome results from stretches of CGG repeats in the X chromosome. Repeats can be many without obvious effect but the repeat stretch tends to get longer from generation to generation and several thousand repeats have been described. These very long repeats weaken the structure of the X chromosome and can lead to varied conditions including intellectual disability. Because females carry two X chromosomes, males are predominantly severely affected, though females can show variable clinical symptoms.

Sometimes the proteins produced are truncated, or not produced at all. These types of mutation are often associated with recessive diseases. A four-base pair insertion in the *HEXA* gene results in low activity of an essential lysosomal enzyme, leading to **Tay–Sachs disease** when inherited in a recessive fashion. The mutation is prevalent in Ashkenazi Jews and some French Canadians and leads to nerve cell deterioration early in life.

Some disorders are caused by insertions of nucleotides in multiples of three, preserving the **reading frame**. Several trinucleotide repeat diseases exist, such as **Huntington disease** (large numbers of CAG repeats leading to polyglutamination) and **fragile X syndrome** (CGG – arginine repeats).

Gene duplications

In meiosis, when the sister chromatids line up, if there is a slight mismatch this can result in an unequal crossover, which can result in two copies of a gene. For example:

- Families showing two copies of the **aldosterone** gene suffer from high blood pressure and are at increased risk of stroke.
- **Charcot–Marie–Tooth** disease arises from a duplication on chromosome 17. One of the genes involved produces a protein involved in myelin formation; demyelination is one characteristic of this disease.

The unequal crossover can also interrupt the promoter region of the gene (**promoter mutation**), which may result in different gene expression.

Consequences of genetic mutation

Not all genetic variation is detrimental to the organism. SNPs can have positive or negative effects, or can be neutral. **Sickle cell disease** in its homozygous state is almost always lethal and one would expect the allele to be selected against, and therefore be very rare in all populations. The sickle gene is, however, present in about 15% of the black population. In its heterozygous state it causes mild anaemia but confers resistance to malaria. Thus the heterozygous individual is at an advantage in populations where malaria is present (Fig. 5.16). Comparison of African Americans with Africans has shown that the sickle cell gene is much reduced in African Americans, indicating that the gene is being eliminated where there is absence of positive selection pressure. This is an example of a **balanced mutation**.

Duplications lie at the core of evolution. Within single organisms there are many genes with similar sequences (**paralogous genes**) that have resulted from repeated duplications of an ancestral gene. In contrast, **orthologous genes** are homologous genes in different species – these are likely to have descended from a common ancestor. For example, there is about a 99% similarity between human and chimpanzee DNA, with the differences mostly being seen in those influencing the nervous system.

Paralogous genes can be beneficial by providing for **redundancy**. Removing a gene (such as in **knockout** mice) sometimes has little effect because the function has been taken over by a paralogue. Over time one of a pair of duplicated genes can also mutate and acquire a new and advantageous function (**adaptive evolution**).

Founder effects

The **founder effect** was defined by Ernst Mayr as 'The establishment of a new population by a few original founders (in an extreme case, by a single fertilised female) which carry only a small fraction of the total genetic variation of the parental population', and is recognised when a particular polymorphism can be traced back to a single individual.

The reasons for this phenomenon are twofold. First, a particular area may become populated with a small number of individuals, with all subsequent generations originating from these people while the particular population remains isolated (Fig. 5.17). For example, many individuals living in Tristan da Cunha originate from the original British settlement in 1816.

The second reason concerns the origin of a particular set of Y chromosome polymorphisms. The male Y chromosome is passed without change (other than rare mutations) through the generations. Thus males with the same paternal ancestors are very likely to share identical Y chromosome polymorphism (known as a **haplotype**, as there is only one Y chromosome).

Genghis Khan and the founder effect

One particular Y chromosome haplotype is found in about 8% of the population in the former Mongolian Empire, and has spread throughout the world population. Although the success of this haplotype could be the result of it having some form of biological advantage, scientists have suggested that it could originate from the dynastic family of Genghis Khan and his male relatives in their predominance and subsequent spread of the Mongolian Empire across the whole of Asia.

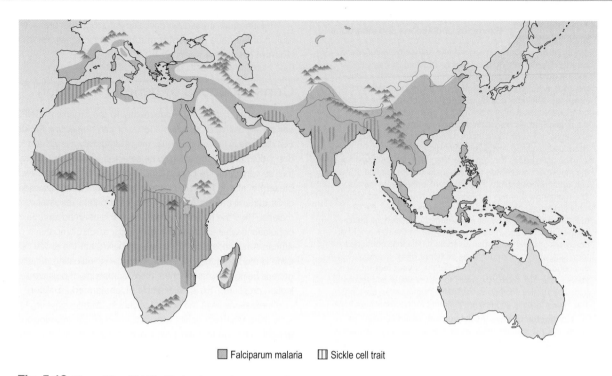

☐ Falciparum malaria   ☐ Sickle cell trait

Fig. 5.16 **Map of the Old World** showing regions where *Plasmodium falciparum* malaria and sickle cell trait are prevalent (Source: http://www.pearsonhighered.com/anthrosupersite/phys/databank/map2.18.html).

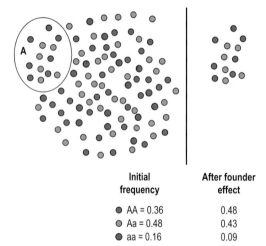

	Initial frequency	After founder effect
● AA = 0.36		0.48
● Aa = 0.48		0.43
● aa = 0.16		0.09

Fig. 5.17 **Founder effect.** The relative frequencies of the different phenotypes in the population are shown on the left of the diagram. A small subpopulation that has become separated (area A) from the main population is shown on the right. The phenotype frequencies in this new population differ from the original by chance alone and as long as the founder population remains relatively isolated the founder frequencies will be propagated.

Social norms were very different at the time and Khan's male descendants appeared to have sired many sons from a high number of associations with women.

Bottlenecks

Sometimes the same effect can be the result of a **bottleneck**, where only a few individuals pass through, or survive, and then expand later. The individuals who pass through the bottleneck may have some polymorphisms that are rare in the original population, but proportionately are not so rare in the second new population.

A bottleneck is one possible reason for the very different mitochondrial sequences seen when comparing African and non-African populations. African mitochondrial DNA shows high divergence, whereas non-African lineages appear to be less divergent and originate from an African branch. This supports an **out-of-Africa** origin of humans and suggests that there might also have been a bottleneck some 80 000 years ago, with a relatively small population thereafter populating the whole of Europe and Asia (Fig. 5.18).

Population drift

Population drift has also resulted in populations in different areas possessing different polymorphisms. This has led to phenotypic variation in humans with respect to their race or geographical origin. Figure 5.19 illustrates this over a limited number of generations within a small population. In practice drift is seen to be inversely proportional to population size and so the frequency differences that we observe between populations are likely to have taken place over a considerable period of time.

Drift may also be influenced by selection pressures and can lead to **fixation** where all, or virtually all, of the population presents only a single phenotype.

- Membrane associated transporter protein (MATP): the gene **MATP** is associated with the production of melanin (mutations in the gene are associated with albinism) and there is SNP in the gene that is fixed in individuals from northern Europe (Fig. 5.20).

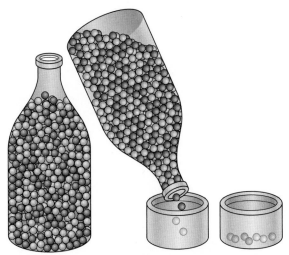

Fig. 5.18 Bottleneck effect. A 'bottleneck' that allows only a small proportion of the population through has the effect of reducing genetic variation in the new population. Bottlenecks could result from stringent conditions due to geography or climate.

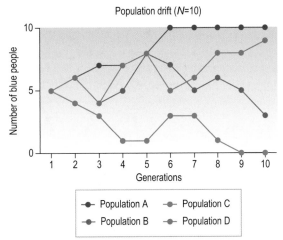

Fig. 5.19 Population drift. The graph illustrates the possible effects of drift on a small population that shows two phenotypes. For example, if sets of five blue people and five green people produce 10 offspring, the binomial theorem tells us that, on average, five will be blue. There will be some variation and it is quite possible that one of the sets will actually produce only four blue offspring (population C, for example). In the next generation of that set, on average, four will be blue. Not every set will produce four blue individuals: some, like population C, may have only three blue individuals; others may have more, or less. This results in **drift** of blue individuals. Eventually a population may end in **fixation**, with all individuals being all blue, or all green, as population A has after six generations (all blue people), and population C has after nine generations (all green people).

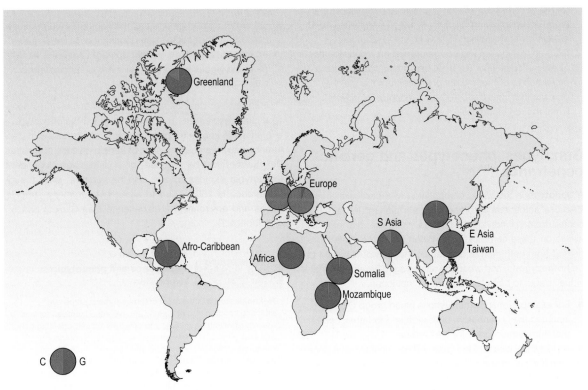

Fig. 5.20 Fixation in the *MATP* gene single nucleotide polymorphism (SNP). The C SNP (shown in blue) is almost universally found among white-skinned Europeans, although the G SNP (shown in red) does not identify individuals with a dark skin as the latter also predominates among the light-skinned south-east Asian populations.

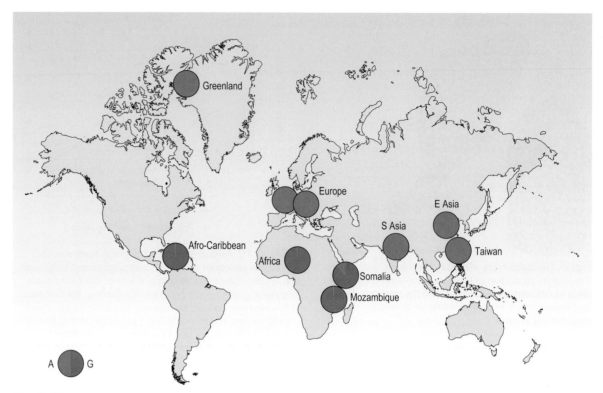

Fig. 5.21 **Fixation in the *DARC* gene single nucleotide polymorphism (SNP).** The G SNP (shown in red) is found among individuals of African origin that have originated from areas where malaria is prevalent. The more evident mixture of the two SNPs seen in the Somali population reflects the admixture in Somalia with the nearby Asian population.

- Duffy antigen receptor for chemokines (DARC): the ***DARC*** gene has a SNP that codes for a particular Duffy blood group polymorphism, Fy (a⁻b⁻), in which the DARC protein is not expressed. The G polymorphism has reached fixation among a large proportion of individuals of African origin (Fig. 5.21). Its predominance appears to be related to environmental pressure from the malarial parasite that uses the DARC as a receptor in order to infect the red blood cell.

Genotypes, phenotypes and genetic penetrance

A **genotype** is the allelic composition at a particular locus. Because autosomal chromosomes are present in pairs, inherited from an individual's parents, there are also pairs of alleles on these chromosomes. When the same allele is inherited from both mother and father, the individual is said to be **homozygous**, and when the alleles are different, the individual is said to be **heterozygous** at that locus.

- For example, an individual who is blood group O has inherited the O gene from both mother and father, and is therefore homozygous for the O allele.
- An individual who is blood group AB has inherited an A gene from one parent and a B gene from the other; therefore the individual is heterozygous for the A and B alleles.

Whereas the genotype details all the alleles present at a locus, the **phenotype** details the alleles that can be observed:

- For example, the *genotype* of someone who is blood group O is OO, whereas the *phenotype* is O.

- In blood group AB, both the genotype and phenotype are AB.
- Other ABO blood groups are more complicated because both the A and B alleles are dominant over the O allele. An individual who is blood group A (phenotype is A) may be homozygous with a genotype AA, or heterozygous with a genotype AO.

Sometimes, despite a particular genotype, the phenotype is not expressed. This extent to which the phenotype is expressed is known as **penetrance**, and alterations in penetrance can be a characteristic of certain disease processes. Penetrance may be reduced, or possibly age dependent. Phenotypic expression can also be variable, even though penetrance is 100%, due to allelic heterogeneity, modifier genes and environmental experience (see Clinical box 5.7 and Table 5.1).

Clinical box 5.7 | **Penetrance and phenotypic expression**

Retinoblastoma is the most common tumour of the eye affecting children and mutations are expressed through familial (usually affecting both eyes) and sporadic (usually affecting only one eye) origins. The retinoblastoma gene on chromosome 13 produces a protein that helps control the cell cycle. Mutations in this gene can lead to cell proliferation of the developing retinal cells (retinal blasts) found in the developing foetus. Thus the gene can be defined as a **tumour suppressor gene**.

The familial form has an autosomal dominant inheritance. The phenomenon of tumours skipping a generation has meant that the gene has a **reduced penetrance** (approximately 90%). Knudson, in 1971, hypothesised that the reason for the reduced penetrance was due to the fact that more than one mutation was needed to lead to proliferation (the **two-hit hypothesis**).

An individual possessing the mutant retinoblastoma gene does not experience proliferation in every retinoblast, even though the mutation is present in every cell, but the large number of retinal cells means that a sporadic mutation occurring in just one retinoblast, resulting in a double hit, is much more likely. Those individuals who do not, by chance, experience this second hit, remain free of disease, but still have a 50% chance of passing on the affected gene.

Huntington disease (Huntington's chorea) is an autosomal dominant disease described by George Huntington in 1872. It is a neurological disease that usually becomes apparent in middle age and leads to progressive loss of motor control and dementia. The disease normally has 100% penetrance (all who inherit the defect will be sufferers) but is an example of **age-dependent penetrance**. The famous American folk musician Woody Guthrie died of the disease in 1967. Until the molecular defect was identified, children of affected individuals could only wait to see if they had inherited the gene from their parent. The defect is due to a trinucleotide expansion of CAG repeats within the HD gene, resulting in an accumulation of a neuronal transport protein (**Huntingtin**) around neuronal nuclei, leading to neuronal death. Paternal transmission of the disease tends to result in a higher repeat instability (**anticipation**), resulting in even greater expansions and earlier onset.

Osteogenesis imperfecta (brittle bone disease) is due to an inherited defect in collagen production and leads to affected individuals being particularly vulnerable to bone fractures. Some individuals have many fractures, others have few, and the degree of severity can be different within the same family (**variable phenotypic expression**). Several reasons have been proposed for the varying severity of this disease:

- **Allelic heterogeneity**: different mutations within the procollagen molecule, which is then further cleaved to form collagen, can result in different disease severity, depending on the end of the molecule the mutations occur.
- **Gene modifiers**: even where genes are inherited, individuals may experience different disease severity. This is thought to be due to the presence of genes at a different loci that interact with the gene, changing its expression.
- **Environmental factors**: an event that results in a bone fracture can mean that the damaged area is much more vulnerable to subsequent trauma.

Table 5.1	Phenotype series associated with cardiovascular disease	
Phenotype	**Examples**
Healthy	Possessing none of the following
Possessing risk factors	Hyperlipidaemia, diabetes, smoking, hypertension, possession of certain haemostatic and inflammatory mediators
Subclinical disease	Coronary, carotid and peripheral atherosclerosis
Clinical complex disease	Coronary artery disease, peripheral vascular disease, stroke, death from cardiovascular disease, sudden death

MODES OF INHERITANCE

MENDELIAN DISORDERS

A **Mendelian disorder** is defined as a trait that is associated with one specific genotype, such as a mutation at a particular genetic locus. There are a number of different forms of single gene disorders, based on:

- The pattern of inheritance being either **dominant** or **recessive**
- Whether the mutation is **autosomal** or **sex linked**.

In reality, it is often very difficult to determine the mode of inheritance of the disorder in many families for a number of reasons (see below).

Autosomal dominant inheritance
(Figs 5.22 and 5.23)

Autosomal dominant disorders are seen in around 1 in every 200 individuals. The main characteristics of autosomal dominant inheritance are:

- Sex-independent – that is, it affects both sexes and can be transmitted by either sex
- One of the affected child's parents will also be affected with the same condition
- A child with an affected parent has a 50% chance of inheriting the disease genotype
- The mutant genotype, when present on only one of the autosomes, is sufficient to cause the disorder.

Dominance is when the expression of the wild-type (normal) allele is not sufficient to prevent the manifestation of the disorder and is normally associated with a **gain of function** (having a new function). Cellular mechanisms associated with dominant mutations are:

- Overproduction of a protein at the wrong time, or in the wrong place. For example, in **neurofibromatosis type II**, a deletion of a tumour suppressor gene leads to overgrowth of the Schwann cells that surround nerve cells. An example is an **acoustic neuroma**.

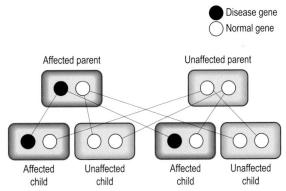

Fig. 5.22 **Principles of autosomal dominant inheritance.**

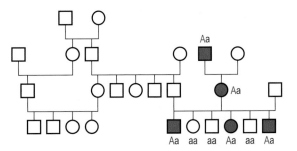

Fig. 5.23 **Pedigree illustrating the typical pattern in autosomal dominant disease inheritance.** Affected individuals are shown in solid red, with the normal gene being indicated by (a) and the disease gene by (A). Autosomal dominant inheritance typically results in the disease being seen in each generation, with about half the offspring being affected, regardless of their gender.

- **Dominant-negative effects**: the mutant protein inhibits the function of the normal protein produced by the wild type allele. For example, in **glucocorticoid resistance syndrome**, a mutation in the gene for GR decreases the activity of hGRα protein, which in turn leads to excessive secretion of androgen hormones.
- **Haplo-insufficiency** may also produce a dominant disorder. This occurs when loss of 50% of the protein product is not sufficient for normal function. For example, in **familial hypercholesterolaemia**, a gene mutation in the LDL receptor (*LDLR*) gene results in loss of half the receptors for transporting LDL, leading to a build-up in circulating cholesterol.
- **Anticipation** is seen in a small proportion of autosomal dominant disorders, including fragile X and Huntington disease. It describes the phenomenon seen when the disease becomes progressively more severe and has an earlier onset through each generation, related to an increase in trinucleotide repeats as the gene is transmitted. A critical expansion size has an adverse effect on the RNA and protein production that it is associated with. For example, in Huntington disease, greater than 36 CAG repeats within the Huntingtin gene are associated with the disease, but repeats of between 10 and 26 are present among normal individuals.

Autosomal recessive inheritance
(Figs 5.24 and 5.25)

Autosomal recessive disorders are more rare, being seen in about 1 in 500 individuals and may appear as a sporadic mutation. Only when another affected child is born is the genetic nature of the disease recognised (unless it is an already known recessive disorder). Characteristics of autosomal recessive disorders are:

- Sex independent
- The affected child inherits the disease gene from both parents (the child will be homozygous for the disease gene)
- The affected child's parents appear normal (the parents will be heterozygous **carriers**, carrying a normal and a disease gene)
- A child with carrier parents has a 25% chance of inheriting the disease genotype and a 25% chance of inheriting a normal genotype

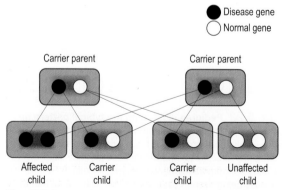

Fig. 5.24 **Principles of autosomal recessive inheritance.**

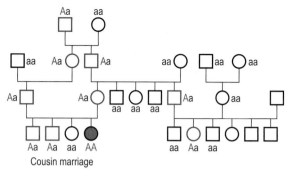

Fig. 5.25 **Pedigree illustrating the typical pattern in autosomal recessive disease inheritance.** The affected individual is shown in solid red, and carriers outlined in red, with the normal gene being indicated by (a) and the disease gene by (A). Autosomal recessive inheritance typically results in the disease being seen in siblings, regardless of their gender, but usually not in previous generations. Only about a quarter of the offspring of carrier parents are affected, and sibling expression is therefore only likely in larger families, although another 50% are carriers. In very rare disorders consanguinity is likely to be evident in the family.

- 50% of children of carrier parents will also be heterozygous carriers
- Offspring of consanguineous relationships are more likely to have an autosomal recessive disorder because the disease gene, if present, will be present at a higher frequency within a family.

Recessive disorders are often characterised by **loss-of-function** mutations. The mutation results in a complete loss of protein production, but in the heterozygous individual the protein continues to be produced at 50% of the normal level. Where this level continues to be sufficient for normal function (contrast this with haplo-insufficiency), heterozygous individuals will be unaffected.

For example, in **oculocutaneous albinism**, there is a defect in melanin production, caused by a mutation on chromosome 11 that results in a lack of expression of the protein tyrosinase. When no tyrosinase is produced (in the homozygous individual) the lack of melanin results in the pale skin, white hair and pink eyes associated with albinism.

Consanguinity and recessive disorders

The rate of transmission of recessive disorders increases dramatically with increased incidence of consanguineous matings, or relatively high frequency of recessive alleles in the population (such as might occur in areas with a small founder population). Its continuing presence within a population can also be due to heterozygote advantage, whereby recessive alleles are maintained in the population as they offer some selective advantage in the heterozygous form. For example, carriers of the **sickle cell** gene appear to be protected against malaria, and mutations in the **cystic fibrosis** gene are thought to offer some protection against cholera and other diarrhoeal diseases.

Sometimes recessive disorders appear to occur at a relatively high frequency in the population because mutations in a number of different genes result in clinically similar disorders, e.g. **non-syndromic sensorineural deafness**.

Coefficient of relationship

Related individuals are more likely to share mutant genes that have been inherited from a common ancestor. The **coefficient** of relationship (**COR**) provides a measure of the probability of related individuals sharing a gene.

As a parent will pass half of his or her genes to their children then we can say that the probability that the parent and child share a particular gene is 0.5. As there are two parents, each parent will have a 0.5 chance of sharing a particular gene with their child, but together they have a $0.5 + 0.5 = 1.0$ (certain) chance of sharing a particular gene with their child. This makes sense as all genes present in a child must have been inherited from one or other parent, unless there has been a mutational event.

The COR can be calculated using the formula:

$$COR = \left(\frac{1}{2}\right)^N$$

where N is the number of generation steps between individuals and a common ancestor.

For example, there are two generation steps between siblings through their common father:

$$COR = \left(\frac{1}{2}\right)^2 = \frac{1}{4}$$

and an additional two generation steps between siblings through their common mother.

Therefore the combined COR for siblings is $\frac{1}{4} + \frac{1}{4} = \frac{1}{2}$. In other words, siblings will share half their genes, on average. Probabilities for gene sharing between other related individuals can be calculated in the same fashion. Table 5.2 gives these probabilities down to second cousins.

Rare disorders and consanguinity

Cystic fibrosis is one of the most common autosomal recessive disorders affecting northern Europeans. About 4% of individuals (1 in 25) are carriers, leading to a prevalence of affected children in the population of around 1 in 2500.

- Chance of two individuals having the cystic fibrosis gene: $\frac{1}{25} \times \frac{1}{25} = \frac{1}{625}$
- Chance of both parents passing the cystic fibrosis gene to their children: $\frac{1}{2} \times \frac{1}{2} = \frac{1}{4}$
- Chance of a newborn child having cystic fibrosis: $\frac{1}{4} \times \frac{1}{625} = \frac{1}{2500}$

Someone who is a carrier has a 1 in 25 chance of mating with another carrier if he chooses a partner from the general population. If the carrier chooses his cousin as a partner, the chance that his cousin is also a carrier is 1 in 8 (from the COR calculation). Mating of cousins is therefore about three times more likely to result in a child with cystic fibrosis.

Table 5.2	Coefficient of relationship values
Relationship	**Coefficient of relationship (probability of gene sharing)**
Full siblings	$\frac{1}{2}$
Half siblings	$\frac{1}{4}$
Grandparents	$\frac{1}{4}$
Uncles/aunts	$\frac{1}{4}$
First cousins	$\frac{1}{8}$
Second cousins	$\frac{1}{16}$

Familial Mediterranean fever is a very rare autosomal recessive disorder where affected individuals suffer from acute fevers, but is generally seen only in a few restricted populations around the world. The highest number of cases are found in Israel where the frequency of cousin marriages approaches 50% among the Arabic population. A very rare autosomal recessive disorder therefore can become considerably more likely (in comparison with cystic fibrosis, for example) in a population with a high rate of consanguinity.

X-linked inheritance

The Y (male) chromosome is relatively gene-free and there are few disorders associated with mutations on the Y chromosome and these will only affect the males in the family. Those that have been described are associated with male infertility. However, there are a large number of **X-linked** disorders that can be inherited in either a dominant or a recessive manner.

Lyonisation

Proteins produced by genes on the X chromosome are expressed at similar levels in males and females, whereas it might be expected that, because females have two X chromosomes, they may produce double the amount of protein. In the 1960s, Mary Lyon hypothesised that one of the two X chromosomes is inactivated, and that this happens at random, sometimes affecting the paternally derived X chromosome, and sometimes the maternally derived X chromosome. This is known as **lyonisation** or the **Lyon hypothesis**. Evidence supporting the hypothesis came from an observation made in the 1940s of interphase nuclei which showed densely staining chromatin material in females, but not in males. These have become known as **Barr** bodies, named after their discoverer, Murray Barr. Individuals who have variable numbers of X chromosomes will also have more or fewer Barr bodies. XXY male individuals will have one Barr body, XXX females will have two Barr bodies and X females will have none.

Biochemical evidence of the phenomenon was shown when individual cells in females heterozygous for variants of glucose-6-phosphate dehydrogenase were shown to express just a single variant type. The inactivation takes place very early on after fertilisation and is not complete, spreading down the long arm of the X chromosome. It must also be reversible in cells destined to become egg cells, which will only carry a single set of chromosomes.

Males are thus **hemizygous** for X (because they only have a half representative in the pair) and females are **mosaics** for the X chromosome because they have two different populations of cells, some carrying active maternal X chromosomes, and others having active paternal X chromosomes.

Dominant X-linked inheritance
(Figs 5.26 and 5.27)

Dominant X-linked disorders can affect either sex, but predominantly affect females. This is because all female offspring of an affected male will inherit the mutation on the X, but male offspring will receive the affected man's Y chromosome and therefore be normal. Offspring of an affected female (carrier) will have a 50% chance of passing on the gene, to both males and females: hence the slight female imbalance.

Because a female will usually still have a normal X chromosome their disease may be milder. In certain conditions, males, having no normal X chromosome material, may die in

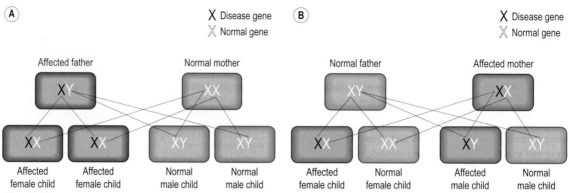

Fig. 5.26 (A) X-linked dominant inheritance with an affected father. When the father has the disease all of his female offspring will be affected, but males will be normal. **(B) X-linked dominant inheritance with an affected mother.** When the mother has the disease, half of her children will be affected, regardless of gender.

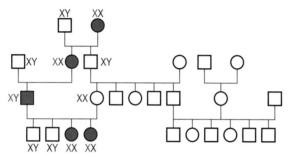

Fig. 5.27 **Pedigree illustrating X-linked dominant inheritance.** Affected individuals are show in solid red, with the normal X gene being shown in black, and the diseased X gene in red. X-linked dominant inheritance typically results in the disease being seen in each generation, like autosomal dominant disorders. In contrast, affected individuals are predominantly female. Males can only pass the disease to their daughters. Females pass the affected X chromosome to about half of their offspring, regardless of gender.

utero. Dominant X-linked diseases are much rarer than the recessive forms.

- **Incontinentia pigmenti** is a single gene disorder of the X chromosome due to mutations in NF-κB essential modulator (NEMO). The gene is also known as inhibitor of κ light polypeptide gene enhancer in B cells kinase gamma (IKBKG or IKK-gamma) and affects tissues derived from the embryonic ectoderm and neuroectoderm. As well as early skin involvement, which gets worse with age, there are often major

developmental and other nervous system problems. Female carriers of the gene for NEMO are only mildly affected. There appears to be selective apoptosis as part of the X-inactivation process, promoting the normal X chromosome containing cells. Males usually die in utero.
- **Hypophosphataemic rickets** is an X-linked disorder where the reduced amounts of inorganic phosphate lead to problems in bone ossification. The disorder is milder in females because of the random X inactivation, leaving some of the cells carrying the normal X chromosome.

Recessive X-linked inheritance (Figs 5.28 and 5.29)

Recessive X-linked disorders are more prevalent than the dominant forms and, in the vast majority of cases, affect only the male offspring. This is because males with the disease inherit an abnormal X chromosome from a female carrier (they are **hemizygous**), whereas females will generally only inherit one abnormal chromosome, the presence of the normal X chromosome being sufficient for normal life, despite having lower levels of the gene product. This leads to an inheritance that skips generations and is only evident in males.

Haemophilia A is the best known of the two haemophilic disorders, this one resulting from a defect in the factor VIII gene. Affected individuals produce very low levels (less than 1% normal) of factor VIII, which is a key component of the intrinsic clotting pathway. As well as severe external bleeds, sufferers experience bleeds into joints, resulting in joint deformities; intercranial bleeding used to be a common cause of early death before treatment options improved. Haemophilia

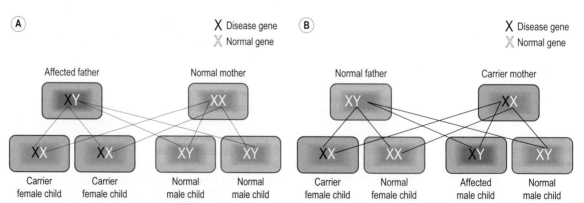

Fig. 5.28 **(A) X-linked recessive inheritance with an affected father. (B) X-linked recessive inheritance with an affected mother.**

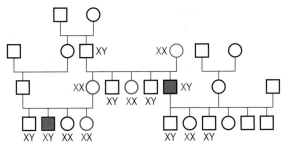

Fig. 5.29 **Typical X-linked recessive inheritance.**
Pedigree illustrating the typical pattern in X-linked recessive disease inheritance. Affected individuals are shown in solid red, and carriers outlined in red, with the normal gene being shown in black and the diseased gene in red. X-linked recessive inheritance typically results in the disease being seen in some males only, with a sporadic appearance within the family. While the disease may be evident among male siblings and other relatives, it would not be seen in the parents, as affected fathers can only pass the disease gene on to their daughters, who will be carriers. Carriers will have a 50% chance of passing the affected chromosome on to their male offspring, who will show the disease, and a 50% chance of passing it to their female offspring, who will also then be carriers.

A is found as a new, spontaneous, mutation in about one-third of cases.

Other examples of X-linked recessive disorders are haemophilia B, red-green colour blindness, fragile X syndrome and Duchenne's muscular dystrophy.

Haemophilia – the royal disease

One of Queen Victoria's nine children, Leopold, died at the age of 31, from an internal head bleed after a fall, possibly as a result of inheriting haemophilia. He was the only one of four sons to suffer from the disorder. The British Royal Family, which stems from Queen Victoria's first son, Edward, has therefore remained free of the disease. Before Leopold died he married and produced a daughter, an obligate carrier, Alice, and one of her sons developed haemophilia.

Prior to Leopold's birth there was no history of the disease in the family, and his disease could have resulted from a spontaneous mutation. Evidence that he inherited it from Queen Victoria, however, came from the marriages of two of Victoria's daughters, Alice and Beatrice.

- Alice married into the Prussian Royal Family and one of her sons, and three of her grandchildren, including the famous Alexei, son of Tsar Nicholas II of Russia, had the disease. Prince Philip, who was one of her great-grandchildren down a female line, would have been potentially vulnerable had the intervening females been carriers, but the disease has not developed in any male in that line. In 2007 the bones of the family members, murdered during the Russian revolution, were discovered, and in 2009, genetic analysis revealed a mutation, characteristic of haemophilia B, within bones believed to have been those of Alexei, his sister Anastasia and their mother, the Tsarina, Alexandra.
- Beatrice had two sons with the disease and her daughter married into the Spanish Royal Family, resulting in two more affected sons.

It is generally accepted that Queen Victoria received her carrier status as a new mutational event. Her father, Prince Edward, Duke of Kent and the fourth son of George III, was in his 50s at her conception, suggesting that his age may have been instrumental. Sperm are more vulnerable to mutations as they are continuously produced from a bank of primitive cells that may accumulate mutations with age; this is in contrast to egg cells which are essentially frozen in time until signalled to develop through fertilisation. This theory has not stopped historians from speculating that Victoria was the illegitimate child of a haemophilic man. It is also possible that Victoria inherited the disease from a carrier mother as several male children of her maternal antecedents died young.

Other modes of inheritance

Genomic imprinting

The expression of some mutant genes during development, and in diseases such as cancer, may be dependent on the parental origin. The imprinted gene from one parent is silenced and the non-imprinted gene is expressed. The mechanism that regulates the differential expression of two alleles of the same gene is termed **genomic imprinting**.

The imprinted locus follows a Mendelian pattern of inheritance. The first examples discovered were **Prader–Willi syndrome** and **Angelman syndrome**, the former related to loss of the paternally expressed gene and the latter to loss of the maternally expressed gene. The mutations are only expressed when they are passed through the gametogenesis process leading to the opposite sex. Both disorders are related to mutations found in the 15q11–q13 region of the genome. The region is about 5 Mb and consists of three regions:

- Distal – non-imprinted genes
- Central – maternally expressed genes
- Proximal – paternally expressed genes.

These regions appear to be under the control of an **imprinting centre** that modify the structure of the chromatin rather than the DNA sequence itself – **epigenetic mechanisms** – most commonly methylation and histone modifications (see Clinical box 5.8).

Clinical box 5.8 **Some clinical syndromes associated with gene deletion**

Prader–Willi syndrome (PWS) is a common microdeletion causing genetic obesity and associated with neuro-behavioural disorders. It is caused by transmission of a maternal imprinting mutation, but is only expressed when passed from a female ancestor through a male during the gametogenesis process. The normal loss of the maternal epigenotype during male gametogenesis does not happen (the maternal/paternal switch is blocked) and maternal imprinting will therefore be transmitted to half of the gametes. Those individuals who inherit the abnormal epigenotype develop PWS.

Angelman syndrome is characterised by particular behavioural features of intense happiness, associated with developmental delay, seizures, hyperactivity and severe intellectual disability. In most patients there is a large deletion in the maternally derived chromosome. It is caused by transmission of a paternal imprinting mutation when passed from a male ancestor through the female germline. It blocks the paternal/maternal switch, leading to the inheritance of an abnormal paternal epigenotype in about half the offspring, affected individuals developing Angelman syndrome.

DNA methylation involves the addition of a methyl group to cytosine nucleotides where cytosine is next to guanine – **CpG sites**. In mammals most CpG sites are methylated. **CpG islands** are stretches of genomic DNA rich in CpG sites and are found at a higher frequency in the promotor regions of genes and are unmethylated when the genes are expressed. There is also an asynchronous DNA replication that occurs in these gene clusters, with non-imprinted alleles replicating earlier. This phenomenon is seen in the female X chromosomes that are inactivated by the lyonisation process.

In some diseases, such as cancer, CpG islands can become hypermethylated leading to **transcriptional silencing** because the physical modification may mean that transcriptional protein can no longer be bound. Methylated DNA areas are associated with **methylated DNA binding proteins (MDBP)** and other proteins that create **heterochromatin** – compact inactive chromatin.

■ **Rett syndrome** is a neurodevelopmental disorder associated with loss of MDBP.

Both hypermethylation and **hypomethylation** is common in all cancers, although the patterns are very variable

Histone modifications, due to a large number of different chemical modifications, directly affect the structure of chromatin and regulate the binding of effector molecules and will influence not only transcription, but also DNA repair, replication and recombination.

Mitochondrial disorders

Although most genetic diseases are associated with nuclear DNA, mitochondrial mutations lead to a significant number of inherited disorders. A feature of **mtDNA** is that it has a much higher mutation rate than nuclear DNA (5–10 times higher).

Mitochondrial inheritance of a disorder produces unique inheritance patterns because it is passed only by the mother but can affect offspring of either sex. During fertilisation the sperm cell contributes only nuclear DNA, the MtDNA being that present in the material egg cell.

Mitochondria are membrane-bound cytoplasmic organelles present in large numbers in a single cell and are essential for cell metabolism in the production of ATP. mtDNA has 16 569 base pairs in a double-stranded circular molecule. It has no introns (redundant genetic code); about 93% is coding (compared with about 3% of nuclear DNA). Mitochondria are thought to have origins as aerobic bacteria enabling oxidative phosphorylation.

Disease expression of a mitochondrial mutation also depends on whether all the mitochondria in a cell are identical (**homoplasmy**) or whether different populations of mitochondria exist (**heteroplasmy**) and, when heteroplasmy exists, what proportion carries a mutation. Because of the random segregation of mitochondria in cell division this proportion can vary between mother and child, leading to **variable penetrance** (see Clinical box 5.9).

Mosaicism

Mosaicism is when more than one genotype contributes to the phenotype of an organism. An adult has approximately 10 trillion cells, and mutations occur at any given locus about once in every 50 000–1 000 000 cell divisions. It is, therefore, likely that we are all mosaics in some sense. The effect of these mutations will depend on how many cells are involved,

---

where the cells are, and which genes are affected. There are three types of mosaicism:

■ **Chromosomal mosaicism** occurs in all females, in that there is random, almost complete inactivation of one of the X chromosomes.

■ **Somatic cell mosaicism** is a mutation that can occur in any body cell, other than a germline cell, and may not be very apparent as it may only affect portions of the body. Somatic mutations that occur early in the embryonic process will have more wide-ranging phenotypic effects and can lead to gonadal mosaicism. Somatic cell mosaicism is a common event in the development of cancer; for example, cancer might be the result of mutation in a tumour suppressor gene. All subsequent cancer cells will retain this mutation.

■ **Gonadal mosaicism** occurs in the germ cells and may be present in a small or significant proportion of the germ cells. This form of mosaicism:

 ■ Leads to the observation of two or more affected children from normal parents with 'apparently' non-mutant genotypes. The pedigree would suggest an autosomal recessive inheritance.

 ■ Often occurs in very severe disorders that would normally result in impaired reproduction. Thus the only way the disorder can be transmitted is either by new mutation, or via a 'mosaic' germline from a phenotypically normal parent.

 ■ Is the cause of some incidences of osteogenesis imperfecta, epidermolysis bullosa, Ehlers–Danlos syndrome type IV and Duchenne's and Becker's muscular dystrophies.

Inborn errors of metabolism (see Ch. 3)

The term 'inborn errors of metabolism' was used by Sir Archibald Garrod in 1908 to describe the genetically inherited amino acid disorder **alkaptonuria**, or 'black urine disease'. Although individually rare, many disorders have been described, simply reflecting the vast numbers of metabolic reactions in the human, all of which have the potential for error. Overall they affect about 16 per 100 000 births and result in significant morbidity and mortality. They may present clinically in the prenatal environment, through to adulthood (see Clinical box 5.10).

Traditionally inborn errors of metabolism are thought of as Mendelian traits caused by single gene mutations, normally

---

Clinical box 5.10   **Primary carnitine deficiency**

Primary carnitine deficiency (see Ch. 3) is a rare inborn error of metabolism seen in at most 1 in 40 000 newborns, and often will result in sudden death. The defect here is not in an enzyme, but in a *transporter* protein. This lack of transporter results in significant metabolic changes that illustrate all of the consequences of altered metabolic flux.

Carnitine is a naturally occurring hydrophilic amino acid derivative produced within the kidneys and liver, and ingested through the diet. Carnitine is utilised in ATP production from fatty acids within mitochondria. This is facilitated through the following normal process:

1. Fatty acids in the cytosol are esterified with CoA (coenzyme A) to form acyl-CoA
2. Medium-chain fatty acids (8–10 carbon atoms in the chain) diffuse across the plasma membrane into the mitochondria
3. An oxidation step releases acetyl-CoA to enter the TCA (tricarboxylic acid) cycle and electron transport chain, releasing ketone bodies in the process
4. Longer-chain fatty acids require a **carnitine transporter**
5. This is facilitated through the carnitine palmitoyltransferase system in which CoA is exchanged for carnitine, which allows movement across the membrane
6. Within the mitochondrial matrix, carnitine is exchanged for CoA and the process proceeds as for medium-chain fatty acids, carnitine being transported back to be reused.

Primary carnitine deficiency is due to a mutation in the ***OCTN2*** gene that leads to a lack of the plasma membrane carnitine transporter.

The altered metabolic flux has considerable consequences:
- Carnitine cannot be transported from the cytosol and excess is lost in the urine:
  - Systemic secondary carnitine depletion means that this substrate is not available for use within muscle, leading to cardiac and skeletal myopathy.
- There is an excess of long-chain fatty acid substrate within the cytosol:
  - Excessive lipid accumulates in muscle, heart and liver
  - Accumulated long-chain acylcarnitines are believed to cause cardiac arrhythmias.
- There is a reduction in products downstream – the long-chain fatty acids are not available to produce energy, nor are sufficient ketone bodies produced:
  - Energy loss leads to weakness
  - Lack of ketone bodies leads to acute hypoketotic encephalopathy in the brain and liver.
- An imbalance in under-utilised CoA within the mitochondria leads to an accumulation of acyl-CoA:
  - Excess acyl-CoA interferes with all pathways requiring CoA – including the TCA cycle, amino acid oxidation and pyruvate oxidation
  - Acute hypoglycaemia, secondary to the above, contributes to the encephalopathy associated with hypoketosis.
- Excess long-chain fatty acids are diverted into other pathways and lead to secondary inhibition of the urea cycle enzymes, resulting in excess toxic ammonia. Ammonia is normally metabolised to urea by the urea cycle and excreted in urine. Where it accumulates in the blood it can lead to encephalopathy and death (see Ch. 3).

---

inherited in an autosomal recessive fashion; however, greater understanding of many of these diseases has shown that they are often a more complex interaction between genes and nutrients. The primary defect is best considered in relation to an alteration in **metabolic flux**. In the classical sense only one metabolite flux is involved but in a more complex disease more fluxes might be involved, all leading to a particular phenotype, typical of the disease. Any metabolic pathway can be affected and may affect any organ or system. For example, fatty acid metabolism defects can result in low blood glucose (hypoglycaemia), loss of muscle (rhabdomyolysis), changes affecting heart muscle (cardiomyopathy) and liver disease.

The pathogenic mechanism is normally associated with a loss of function or a gain of function, of an altered protein, generally an enzyme or transporter (Fig. 5.30). The actual genetic change can be of any type – point mutation, deletion, insertion, rearrangement – and affect different regions of the gene. The clinical consequence of the defect is related to the changed metabolic flux and can be due to:

- Toxicity of excess upstream substrate
- Lack of downstream product
- Feedback activation or inhibition of this or other pathways
- Diversion of the metabolite to other pathways, resulting in an alternative product.

Treatment of inborn errors of metabolism depends on the particular defect but these conditions can often be treated through diet, whether restriction of a substrate, replacement of the enzyme, or supplementation of downstream products. For example, phenylalanine is an essential amino acid that is normally metabolised by **phenylalanine hydroxylase**. Where there are mutations in this enzyme **phenylketonuria** (**PKU**) results. The amino acid accumulates and disrupts cellular processes in the brain, causing intellectual disability. Restriction of phenylalanine in the diet can ensure development of children with normal intelligence.

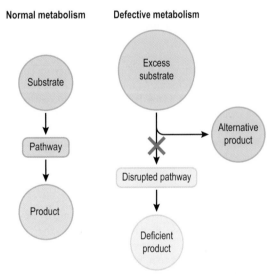

Fig. 5.30 Pathological mechanisms in inborn errors of metabolism. The defective enzyme or transporter within a metabolic pathway leads to a build-up of substances upstream and a loss of product downstream with clinical consequences being related to any potential toxicity of the excess material or alternative product, and effect of the lack of the intended product.

POLYGENIC OR COMPLEX DISEASE

The main genetic contribution to human disease is found in relation to much more complex genetic interactions between different genes. **Polygenic disease** is defined as a disease thought to be caused by the effects of two or more genes. When environmental factors are also thought

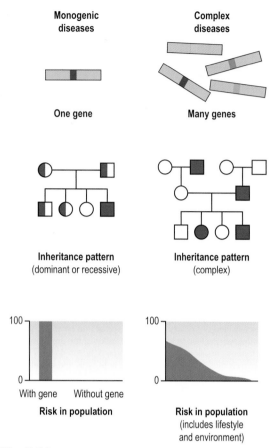

Fig. 5.31 Monogenic versus complex (polygenic) disorders.

- **Transcriptome** – the set of all active mRNA molecules (transcripts) expressed in a particular tissue under particular conditions
- **Proteome** – the set of all the proteins expressed in a particular tissue under particular conditions
- **Metabolome** – the set of metabolic pathways that are followed in a particular tissue under particular conditions.

THRESHOLD EFFECTS MODELS

Some diseases seem to be polygenic, but do not show the typical bell-shaped distribution with its associated severity of disease. Instead, disease symptoms seem to be related to a liability threshold within a distribution that must be passed before the disease is expressed. This threshold is sometimes different between the sexes, resulting in different risks between male and female siblings. An individual at the high end of the liability distribution is more likely to have more of the disease-causing genes and experience more of the environmental factors, and therefore be more likely to develop the disease. Conditions such as cleft palate, spina bifida, infantile autism (see Clinical box 5.11) and pyloric stenosis are considered to follow the threshold model of inheritance.

CHARACTERISTICS OF MULTIFACTORIAL DISEASES

Multifactorial diseases tend to show characteristic risks of the disease in family members, but there is no clear Mendelian pattern of inheritance and environmental factors can increase or decrease the risk of disease. It may occur more frequently in one gender and in particular ethnic groups, perhaps because they have more of the contributing 'bad' genes or are exposed to a more detrimental environment.

- Affected children may have apparently normal parents due to the variable penetrance of the disease genes, but parents who are related have children with a higher risk of disease. Although the parents may appear normal, they may have contributed some of the genes that are associated with an increased risk. For example, in cleft lip and palate, it may be that the parents have contributed some underactive genes that would be needed for normal development.
- There is often evidence that environmental factors influence the risk. For example, there is an association between nutritional deficiencies and maternal cigarette smoking and the cleft lip and palate birth defect. There is evidence from twin studies that risk is not simply associated with the genes that have been inherited (see **concordance** below).
- The risk in the family is higher if more than one family member is affected. This is because if you see more affected relatives, it is more likely that that these people have more risk factors (i.e. are at an extreme position on a liability distribution) than those in families that only have one affected family member.

to influence the expression of the disease, then its cause is said to be **multifactorial**. As a consequence the presence of a genetic variant in the family is not sufficient to lead to the disease, but this may significantly increase the risk to family members (Fig. 5.31). There are many examples of multifactorial diseases, **hypertension** and **diabetes** being two examples.

CONTINUOUS EFFECTS MODELS

Polygenic diseases are influenced by a series of different factors to varying degrees; therefore they do not exhibit simple inheritance patterns, which tends to suggest that a disease is either present or absent. Where the traits are expressed quantitatively they tend to follow a bell-shaped distribution. **Height**, for example, which is typical in this respect, may be influenced by a series of SNPs that collectively influence height. These genetic polymorphisms appear to act in an additive fashion, each adding or subtracting small amounts to the phenotype. They also interact with environmental factors, such as diet, to determine final height.

Diseases are often characterised by their phenotypes in series, from the healthy state, through a disease risk state and subclinical disease, ending with the clinical complex disease. Progression through the phenotypes is influenced by various environmental and genetic determinants. Clinical and scientific assessments can be used to define phenotypes. Phenotype determination is likely to become more sensitive over time with increasingly sensitive biomarkers and high-resolution imaging. Genetic tools offer more information by helping to define functional genomic phenotypes, such as:

- If the disease is severe in the patient then the risk in a family member is increased. This is because they are more likely also to have inherited some of the genetic factors that result in disease expression.
- The disease may occur more frequently in one gender than in the other, but is not a sex-linked disorder. The risk is higher in first-degree relatives of diseased individuals from the less commonly affected gender. This is because these affected individuals are likely to be from families with high liability.
- The risk decreases considerably as the degree of relationship decreases, because disease is the result of a combination of many genes and factors, all of which may not be uniformly present. This is unlike single gene disorders, where the risk is 50% in siblings and 25% in half-siblings, decreasing by half with each degree of distance.

Coronary artery disease has all the characteristics of a multifactorial disease. For example, coronary artery disease can occur in isolation, and also runs in families and shows no clear Mendelian inheritance pattern. The risk is greater in males and in African Americans, in comparison with females and Caucasians or Asians, and there are a number of environmental and other factors that increase the risk, including obesity, high blood pressure, high levels of LDL-cholesterol and type 2 diabetes.

Heritability

Heritability is an estimate the proportion of the variability in a trait that is due to genetic rather than environmental factors. Unlike single gene mutations, multifactorial diseases do not show complete heritability. For example, lipid levels vary across the population, but less so between family members. Assessments of heritability can be made by correlating biochemical levels in relatives of individuals with cardiovascular disease, in comparison with controls, such as spouse pairs. Different estimates of heritability are quoted in the literature. Table 5.3 presents these in terms of very high, high, median, low and very low heritability.

Complex diseases are influenced by both genetic and environmental factors and the balance between these affects how public health will target prevention. For example, where a disease has low heritability, such as lung cancer, changes in environmental exposure to tobacco smoke will be very important. In contrast, the environmental influences on the occurrence of breast cancer are not considered of importance in comparison with family history, because of the much higher heritability of breast cancer.

Genetic epidemiology

Multifactorial diseases may be caused by defects in one or more genes that seem to explain most of the disease seen, but influenced possibly by many other genes and environmental factors that have modifying influences. Twin and adoption studies are used to distinguish genetic and environmental influences. Identifying possible genes that may be involved is the role of genetic epidemiology (see Clinical box 5.12).

Twin studies

Monozygotic twins originate from one embryo and the individuals are identical. In contrast, **dizygotic** twins are produced after fertilisation of two eggs at the same time, so they are no different from full siblings. Any differences observed between monozygotic twins must be due to environmental factors. Same-sex dizygotic twins form good controls for epidemiological studies, as they are more likely also to have been exposed to identical environments, particularly in the womb, whereas the same cannot be said for siblings.

Concordance – inheritance of a genetic factor – is 100% in monozygotes, in whom a trait is determined only by genes. Dizygotic twins are expected to be **discordant** as they will only share about half of their genes. Concordance is measured as either a rate or a correlation coefficient, and the difference between these in monozygotic and dizygotic twins is used to calculate heritability. Where heritability is high there is a large difference between concordance rates in the different twin types.

Table 5.3	Examples of heritability estimates
Very high (>90%)	Bipolar affective disorder
	Autism
	Body fat percentage
	Fingerprints (ridge count)
	Idiopathic epilepsy
	Height
High (>65%)	Ankylosing spondylitis
	Asthma
	Body mass index
	Cleft lip or cleft palate
	Pyloric stenosis
	Schizophrenia
	Spina bifida
Median	Alcoholism
	Blood pressure
	Club foot
	IQ
	Multiple sclerosis
	Myocardial infarction (female)
Low (<35%)	Myocardial infarction (male)
	Peptic ulcer
Very low (<10%)	Contagious disease

Clinical box 5.12 **Heritability of diabetes**

Diabetes, in which the body fails to produce enough insulin, occurs in two main forms (see Ch. 3):
- Type 1 diabetes is due to an autoimmune destruction of the cells that produce insulin
- Type 2 diabetes occurs when there is an imbalance between the ability of the cell to produce insulin and the reduced effectiveness of insulin on a target tissue (insulin resistance).

Both forms of diabetes run in families. The risk for a sibling developing type 1 diabetes is between 10 and 100 times the risk in the general population, reflecting the high genetic contribution to this form of the disease.

Concordance is higher among monozygotic twins in type 2 diabetes, reflecting the high heritability. However, environmental factors are also thought to be important in this form of the disease. Low birthweight is associated with subsequent development of type 2 diabetes, but another explanation could be that there are genetic factors that explain both. Studies of identical twins, in which only one twin has developed type 2 diabetes, show that this twin is more likely to be of lower birthweight, supporting an environmental contribution.

Diabetes is increasing in prevalence, especially among the middle aged, and mirrors the increase in obesity worldwide, emphasising the influence of environmental factors in accelerating a disease process in a population that is already at risk. Genome-wide studies have already identified mutations within genes that point to an increased risk of type 2 diabetes. One of these is in the zinc transporter gene that is involved in regulating insulin secretion; this may help identify people at risk at an early stage.

Infectious diseases, such as measles, are not expected to be influenced by genetic factors (although genetic factors can influence the course of the infection). Both twin types have high concordance (because they both tend to share the infectious experience) and the concordance rates between them are quite similar, leading to very low estimates of heritability.

Biases in twin studies

Studies of twins were once thought to provide a perfect model in order to tease out genetic and environmental influences. However, problems exist:

- It is assumed that monozygotic twins and dizygotic twins will share the same environment, but monozygotic twins will tend to show higher concordance because they are:
  - Treated more similarly
  - More likely to seek similar environments or experiences.
- Because of the polygenic nature of many behavioural traits, and the fact that the genes tend to act synergistically, the absence of just one gene in a dizygotic twin pair may produce a marked difference in behaviour, significantly over-estimating the importance of the genetic contribution.
- Monozygotic twins are probably not completely identical, as there may be a small number of mutations (**single-nucleotide polymorphisms**, **SNPs**, nucleotide insertions or deletions – **indels**, or copy number variations – **CNVs**) that may have occurred early in the development of one or other of the twins. It has been suggested that a child has about 50 new mutations in the material originating from a parent; we would expect that identical twins will therefore have fewer.
- Uterine environments may vary among monozygotic twin pairs as they may or may not share amnions or chorions.

Because of the possible biases, studies of twins raised apart have been done. However, these also have problems:

- Sample sizes are small and so there may be a relatively high standard error of measurement (see Ch. 7)
- Recruitment bias may lead to volunteers with an interest in being twins
- Twins are likely to have contact before separation
- Separated twins are more likely to be placed in similar environments as social services aim to provide them with a background that reflects their heritage.

Adoption studies

In adoption studies, children with diseased parents, but brought up by adoptive parents who do not have the disease, can provide useful information. The likely genetic involvement of schizophrenia has been made more persuasive by the higher rates of disease among adoptive children of affected parents than in adoptive children of unaffected parents. Potential biases, however, also exist here:

- Prenatal environmental influence may be very strong
- Children may be adopted after several years, retaining a parental influence
- Children are likely to be placed in similar environments to those of their natural parents.

Association studies

Association studies make use of particular study design methodologies (see Ch. 7):

- **Case-control studies**: individuals with the disease of interest are collected and controls are selected from the same population, except that they do not have the disease. The frequencies of possible predictors (genotypes) in each group are then compared.
- **Prospective cohort studies**: a group (cohort) of individuals representative of the general population is selected and divided into two subgroups, depending on whether the individuals have a particular genotype of interest. The cohort is then followed over a defined period of time in order to see whether the individuals develop the disease of interest and the possible association evaluated.

TOOLS TO INVESTIGATE POLYGENIC DISEASES

Twin studies cannot identify the genes responsible for disease, but can only provide an assessment of the genetic involvement. A variety of other tools (see also Identifying disease genes) are used in order to provide a better understanding of these complex diseases. Information is gleaned from studies of candidate genes using:

- Information from single gene disorders
- Animal models
- Linkage analysis
- Expression profiles
- Whole genome-wide association studies.

Information from single gene disorders

The bulk of disease is polygenic and caused by the interactions of genes that are common in the population and the underlying environment. Diseases caused by mutations in single genes are rare and usually exhibit extreme phenotypes. Where these monogenic diseases produce phenotypes that are similar to the polygenic disease, this can give clues to the more complex form and can help elucidate pathways in the disease and provide ideas for therapeutic targets.

Animal models

Animals that are inbred to develop a form of human disease (**animal models**) may be useful in the investigation of the molecular basis of the disorder. For example, research in mice with alopecia, a skin condition resulting in hair loss in adults and thought to be a defect of T lymphocytes that act on hair follicles, has identified areas on chromosomes 8, 9, 15 and 17 as being associated with the condition.

Linkage studies

Linkage analysis looks for polymorphic areas of DNA or SNPs that are inherited along with a disease. **Microsatellites** are small pieces of DNA that are highly polymorphic. By using a selection of microsatellites across the genome, it may be possible to track a particular polymorphism within a family pedigree whose members have also developed the disease. This technique helps identify areas of a chromosome that are likely to contain the disease gene. One of the early discoveries using this methodology associated type 1 (insulin-dependent) diabetes with an area on chromosome 11, where the insulin gene is located.

Expression profiles

A large number of genes can be monitored in parallel using microarray technology, identifying clusters of genes that are over- or underexpressed in an **expression profile**. Although this technology can be used to study the whole genome, arrays can be customised to include sets of genes of interest.

Whole-genome association studies (WGAS)

Most disorders are influenced by a small number of genes spread across the genome that have major effects, but underlying these is a comprehensive catalogue of genes that influence linked pathways and can provide useful predictive biomarkers in the future. These genes may be identified by chance through SNP analysis, but this is usually only achieved with any significant success through the use of high-sensitivity **whole-genome association SNP arrays**. These studies have already identified a series of important SNPs involved in the development of type 2 diabetes, for example, but are currently being applied to a large number of diseases. Key to large amounts of information that comes from whole genome analyses is a robust **bioinformatics** approach undertaken in large populations (Information box 5.2).

Two main approaches are used in polygenic association studies:

- **Candidate gene** approach – chosen because of the lower cost, both in molecular and computation, and decreased complexity and time of analysis
- **Whole genome** approach – this method considers all possible variables but is inevitably more complex and more costly. WGAS is an example of this approach and is becoming more popular because of the reducing costs of this type of analysis. It is important in the investigation of polygenic diseases because if a gene effect is only seen in association with other genes it is unlikely that it will be selected as a candidate gene.

Information box 5.2	DNA databanks and the hunt for disease genes

An innovative approach to studying complex diseases has been set up by deCODE Genetics. This company, founded by an Icelander in 1996, engaged the Icelandic community as a genetic resource in the hunt for disease genes. This population offers a number of advantages over other populations:
- The population is large (about 275 000) and genetically homogeneous
- Genealogical information goes back 1000 years
- Good medical records are available
- The population is cooperative
- There is a large databank of DNA.

Over half of the adult Icelandic population have volunteered and the company has extended its research to include over half a million individuals from worldwide populations. The disease risk variants that they describe are all validated by replicating the link between the marker and risk of disease in multiple populations, thus raising the quality of the associations they report.

CANCER GENETICS

CANCER AS A MULTI-STEP GENETIC DISEASE

Cancer is a collection of disorders that share the common feature of uncontrolled cell growth, leading to the formation of a mass of cells known as a **neoplasm** or **tumour**. Malignant neoplasms have the ability to invade adjacent tissues and often **metastasise**, or spread, to more distant parts of the body, a process that is the cause of 90% of cancer deaths. There are more than 100 distinct types of cancer, and each is classified according to the tissue type they arise in. In some families an inherited disposition has been shown to play a role in cancer formation.

There is strong evidence that a cancer arises from a single cell, as a result of clonal expansion. The model that fits best is that of **multi-hit carcinogenesis** (Fig. 5.32). There are two classes of mutations that cause a normal cell to develop into a cancer cell:

- Mutation types that enhance cell proliferation, so that there are more cells harbouring the somatic mutation
- Mutations that make the genome more unstable, either at the DNA level or at the chromosomal level.

Cell growth and differentiation are normally regulated by a series of external signals:

- Growth factors transmit signals from other cells acting through:
    - Growth factor receptors, resulting in
    - Signal transduction molecules (protein kinases), which, through a series of phosphorylations, interact with
    - Nuclear transcription factors that regulate genes that influence cell growth and proliferation.

Although any mutations are rare, those that occur produce cells that fail to differentiate normally. Progressive mutations may lead to further deregulation and allow the cell, and its descendants, to escape the confines of normal cell regulation, leading to unrestricted growth.

INHERITANCE OF CANCER GENES

Mutations that occur in the germline may lead to cancers being seen more commonly within families. **Familial retinoblastoma** is a clear example of this. Many forms of breast and colon cancers also show evidence of a strong family history.

Colon cancer

Although most cases of colon cancer occur sporadically, about 25% show a family history of the disease. Particular genetic mutations have already been identified that account for about 8% of colorectal cancers (see Ch. 6):

- **Familial adenomatous polyposis** is due to germline mutations in the **APC** gene, which codes for a tumour suppressor protein
- **Hereditary non-polyposis colorectal cancer**, caused by germline mutations in **MMR** genes.

Most of the mutations that predispose to colorectal cancer are inherited in an autosomal dominant fashion.

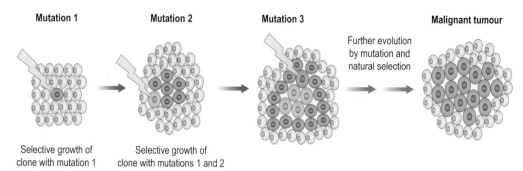

Fig. 5.32 **Multi-hit hypothesis of carcinogenesis.** Normal cells may experience a mutation after exposure to a genotoxic agent, or from random errors in DNA replication. Epigenetic influences may allow selective clonal growth of the mutated cell, which may also be more vulnerable to further mutating influences, forming a 'pre-cancerous' cell. Time and possible further epigenetic influences, enhancing the clonal expansion of altered cells, may result in some cells becoming cancerous, producing tumours of cells that lack the normal cellular mechanisms that inhibit uncontrolled proliferation.

CANCER GENES

A number of genes have been implicated in carcinogenesis. They have been identified as having an important inherited component and/or are somatically altered during tumour formation. Cancer genes can be divided into three main groups:

- **Tumour suppressors** – inhibit proliferation
- **Oncogenes** – activate cellular proliferation
- **DNA repair genes**.

Tumour suppressor genes

The loss of specific chromosomal regions is a common event in the majority of tumours. These deletions may result in loss of function of a gene or genes which are involved in the aetiology of the cancer. Such genes are termed **tumour suppressors** and their subsequent inactivation removes the gene's inhibitory role in the regulation of cell growth and differentiation.

For example, the **retinoblastoma gene** (*RB1*) normally produces a protein that interacts with components in the cell cycle, blocking the uncontrolled proliferation of cells.

- When the protein is active (unphosphorylated) it binds to a complex necessary for the cell cycle to enter into the S phase, therefore putting a 'brake' into the cycle
- When the protein is inactive (phosphorylated by a cyclin dependent kinase (**CDK**)) the cell cycle continues.

A 'loss-of-function' mutation in the *RB1* gene can lead to permanent inactivation, allowing cell division to continue uncontrolled. Other tumour suppressor genes may also produce inhibitors of CDK, preventing it from phosphorylating target proteins, providing a further brake in the cell cycle, or by inducing apoptosis.

Retinoblastoma and the two-hit theory of carcinogenesis

Knudson, in 1971, described the **two-hit theory of carcinogenesis** to explain the inheritance of **retinoblastoma**, the most common eye cancer in childhood. Retinoblastoma has two forms:

- Sporadic:
  - Parents are normal
  - No risk to offspring
  - Single tumour affecting only one eye.

The mutation rate for the retinoblastoma gene is 10^{-6} (1 in 1 000 000). If two events are needed for retinoblastoma then this will occur at a rate of 10^{-12}. There are around 10^8 retinoblasts in an individual, which would explain a sporadic rate of a single tumour in 1 in 10 000 cases, which is close to the observed rate of sporadic mutation.

- Inherited:
  - Parent is normally affected
  - 50% of offspring inherit the disease
  - Several tumours, affecting both eyes.

The multiple bilateral tumours are thought to be due to two mutations – **the two-hit theory**. A mutation to the retinoblastoma gene in the germline, if passed on to a child (50% chance), will show the mutation in every cell of the body (a **constitutional mutation**), including all retinoblasts. They will be heterozygous for the mutation. But not all of the retinoblasts form tumours and behave like recessive genes; providing the cell contains one normal allele then tumour suppression continues.

A second mutation, within any of the retinoblasts in embryonic life, can then result in loss of the normal chromosome. Any retinoblast that carries two abnormal chromosomes, a homozygote, will develop a retinoblastoma. With a 1 in 1 000 000 chance of a second mutation, one might expect around 100 retinoblasts to experience a second hit, resulting in multiple tumours occurring in both eyes. A small minority of individuals will not experience the second hit and so will not inherit the disease.

Inheritance will therefore tend to be autosomal dominant in relation to the disease (because individuals that inherit the gene from an affected parent will be affected) but recessive as far as the cell is concerned as the cell must be homozygous for the abnormal gene for the tumour to develop.

Loss of heterozygosity

Loss of heterozygosity (LOH) can be used to investigate inherited cancers. In situations where surrounding normal cells are heterozygous for a genetic polymorphic marker, but tend to be homozygous for the marker within a tumour, familial cancer involving tumour suppressor genes may be implicated (Fig. 5.33). An exception to this would be if the tumour suppressor gene is present on the X chromosome, affecting all males and putting females at risk if the mutation occurs on the X chromosome that is not inactivated. In the past, these genes have been identified using polymorphic microsatellite

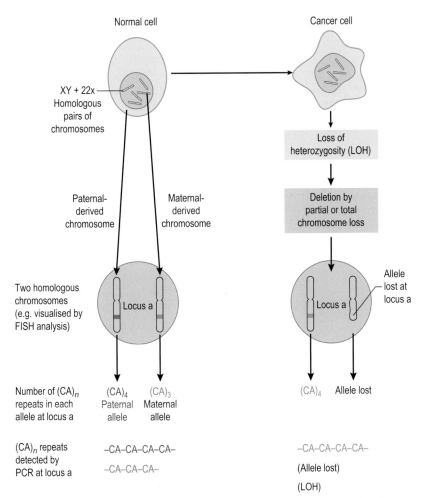

Fig. 5.33 **Loss of heterozygosity observed in cancer cells.** The normal cell is heterozygotic at locus a, showing two alleles with three and four repeats, respectively, one paternal in origin, the other maternal in origin. In the cancer cell the a locus on the maternally derived chromosome, for example, has been lost through a deletion, leaving only the paternal allele. Cells originating from the tumour will appear to be homozygous. PCR, polymerase chain reaction. Adapted from Fig. 2 in Caldos C, Pharoah PDP 1999 Molecular genetics and the assessment of human cancers. Expert Reviews in Molecular Medicine, Vol. 1: 1–19.

markers. The information provided by the HGP, however, has allowed high-resolution whole-genome SNP array analysis, which provides a more sensitive analysis to help rapidly identify important target genes in a given cancer (see also gene arrays, below).

Oncogenes

Proto-oncogenes are involved in normal cell growth regulation. Cells will not divide unless stimulated by a growth factor that binds to a receptor on the cell. For example EGF (epidermal growth factor) is stimulated by HER1 (human epidermal receptor 1 – also known as EGFR). The binding stimulates kinases that phosphorylate proteins that act as transcription factors, switching on genes, which may, in turn, stimulate cyclins to prepare a cell for mitosis. If a mutation occurs in any of genes involved in these steps, unregulated growth can occur: the mutated gene is said to be an **oncogene**, and the cell is said to be **transformed**. The presence of the single mutation in only one copy of the gene leading to the oncogene means that expression is **dominant** at the cellular level. Oncogenes promote cellular growth and proliferation and are thus characterised as **gain-of-function** mutations.

Unlike tumour suppressor genes, oncogenes are mainly found in sporadic tumours. The discovery of oncogenes has been helped through experimentation involving **retroviruses**, **transfection** and **tumour mapping** techniques.

Retroviruses

Oncogenes can also be induced through the action of a retrovirus. **Retroviruses** have an RNA genome and are common in animals. When they attack a cell the viral reverse transcriptase changes the viral RNA into DNA, integrating with the DNA of the host cell, referred to as **transduction**. The viral genome contains a powerful promoter of transcription that promotes the production of new viral particles and this will also give a growth advantage to the host cell – producing oncogenes and **transforming** the cell.

Studies of transforming retroviruses have identified many oncogenes involved in growth and proliferation. The **RAS** (rat sarcoma) oncogenes have been identified this way and are involved in about 25% of cancers.

Transfection

Transfection takes place when cellular proto-oncogenes are transferred from tumour cells into normal cells. Studies look at whether recipient cells are transformed as a result, and

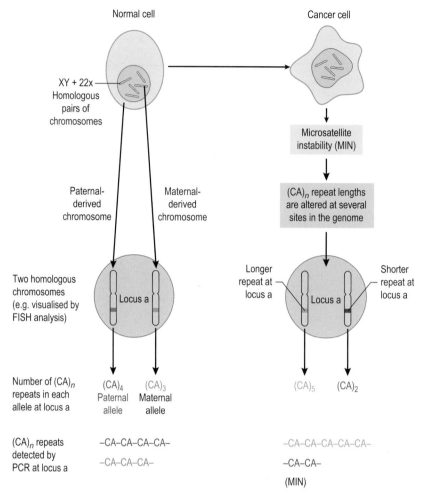

Fig. 5.34 Microsatellite instability in cancer cells. The normal cell is heterozygous at locus a has alleles with three and four repeats, respectively. In the cancer cell mutations in mismatch repair genes have led to an inability to repair nucleotide mismatches during DNA replication. This produces changes in the number of repeats observed (mlcrosatellite instability). Adapted from Fig. 2 in Caldos C, Pharoah PDP 1999 Molecular genetics and the assessment of human cancers. Expert Reviews in Molecular Medicine, Vol.1: 1–19.

what changes have taken place. The first study to be done transferred human bladder cancer cells into mouse cells; examination of the transformed mouse cells revealed a mutated RAS oncogene. The RAS protein product produced by the mutated gene remained in an active form, stimulating cell growth.

DNA repair genes

DNA repair genes exist to repair DNA to facilitate accurate DNA replication. In some inherited disorders and familial cancer syndromes, defects in these repair mechanisms lead to **genomic instability**. Genomic instability results in chromosomal abnormalities such as breaks, abnormal chromosome numbers and widespread mutations, these somatic changes often affecting genes important in proliferation and carcinogenesis.

Several gastric and breast cancer syndromes are known to have defects in the replication of short tandem repeat sequences (**microsatellite instability**). This indicates an **MMR** defect in which, for example, a single base change can lead to a DNA molecule where the base pairs are not complementary (Fig. 5.34). This replication error defect is caused by mutations in the MMR genes, leading to a cascade of secondary mutations in oncogenes, and tumour suppressor genes that give rise to cancer.

Genes that are likely to be involved in the genesis of cancer include growth factors and their receptors; many of these will be oncogenes or tumour suppressors. Identification of mutations and comparisons of gene expression between individuals with and without cancer, or between patients with different outcomes from cancer, are all vital techniques used in cancer research. This research has been facilitated using **gene arrays**, or gene 'chips'.

IDENTIFYING DISEASE GENES

GENOME MAPPING

Genome mapping is the first step in identifying the position of where disease genes are located on a chromosome. Mapping uses several techniques in order to find the chromosomal location of genes. Mapping can be:

- Physical to find the exact position of a gene on a chromosome, or
- Genetic, which uses studies of human pedigrees to locate the relative position on a chromosome.

Physical maps

Physical maps are where the distances between particular features are measured in real units, such as numbers of base pairs, rather than genetic distances. Just like an atlas, a map can display the information at different scales or resolution.

Low-resolution mapping

Karyotyping

An example of a **low-resolution** map is a human chromosome **karyotype**, seen with standard microscopy, with characteristic banding. Low-resolution mapping can only resolve differences that are several million base pairs apart. Examination of a chromosome karyotype can identify translocations, such as the Philadelphia chromosome, where there is an exchange of material between two chromosomes, and additions, or losses, of whole chromosomes, but deletions large enough to be visible by light microscopy are likely to be lethal.

Dosage mapping

Gene associations with deletions may be broadly mapped by **dosage mapping** when they are seen in association with reduced levels of their protein product.

Fluorescence in situ hybridisation (FISH)

FISH utilises complementary strands of DNA, labelled with a fluorescent marker to find out on which chromosome, and where on the chromosome, a particular sequence lies (Fig. 5.35). This technique is useful for areas of repetitive DNA, which is not suitable for cloning. When the probe used is a copy of the mRNA, this cDNA identifies the area that enables the gene protein production.

FISH may also reveal rearrangements in chromosomes associated with particular cancers. Many cases of chronic myeloid leukaemia are characterised by the presence of the Philadelphia chromosome, in which a translocation between chromosomes 9 and 22 activates the ABL proto-oncogene (see Ch. 12).

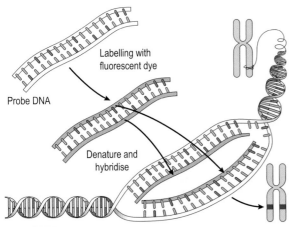

Fig. 5.35 Principle of fluorescence in situ hybridisation (FISH). Probes, complementary copies of the target DNA with a fluorescent marker, are hybridised with denatured metaphase chromosomes. The label indicates the position on the chromosome of the target DNA.

High-resolution mapping

Sanger sequencing

Sanger sequencing was developed by Frederick Sanger in 1977 and remains the gold standard for the detection of point mutations and small variants although the method is being taken over by '**next generation**' sequencing methods, particularly for large scale, whole genome work. It will not detect structural changes, however, and so its use in diagnosis is limited but it has been the core approach in genome sequencing. The process uses:

- A single stranded DNA template is annealed with a DNA primer
- DNA polymerase extends the chain adding deoxynucleotide trisphosphates (dNTPs) available in the reaction mixture
- The reaction process is divided into four with each replacing one of the four dNTPs (dATP, dGTP, dCTP or dTTP) with a modified dideoxy-NTP (ddNTP) that lacks the 3′ OH group necessary for phosphodiesterase bond formation, thus terminating the DNA strand elongation
- The ddNTP is labeled with a fluorescent or radioactive marker and its detection will reveal the particular ddNTP that has been incorporated as the next nucleotide in the sequence through examination of all four reactions
- Subsequent rounds that extend the DNA will reveal the sequence of nucelotides further along the template molecule.

Sequence tagged sites

Key tools in fine mapping of the human genome have been the use of **bacterial artificial chromosomes (BACs)** or **yeast artificial chromosomes (YACs)** in libraries. **Contig maps** contain all the DNA from within a predefined region of a chromosome, in series of DNA fragments that partially overlap so that a contiguous series is available for analysis. The overlap is defined with the use of **sequence tagged sites (STSs)**, which are sequences of DNA of known chromosome location used as signposts throughout the DNA.

In order to define the whole sequence of interest it was important to be able to order the fragments using STSs. Using primers to the STS sequences, if two clones each produce the same PCR product they have sequences that overlap. A series of different STSs are used with several clones to order the sequences they contain. Thus, analysing Table 5.4 shows that the clones are in the following sequence of STSs: B C E D A on the DNA (Fig. 5.36).

The sequences defined by the STSs form the contig map, from which the overlaps can be identified and the molecular sequence of the DNA discovered and recorded.

Table 5.4	Cloning sequence tagged sites				
CLONE	STSa	STSb	STSc	STSd	STSe
1	−	−	+	+	+
2	−	+	+	−	−
3	+	−	−	+	+
4	+	−	−	+	−

STS, sequence tagged site.

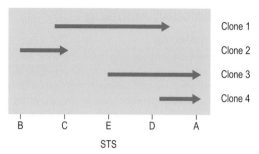

Fig. 5.36 Diagram showing order of sequences in clones according to the sequence tagged sites (STS). The order of overlapping DNA from each of the clone set can be defined by examining the PCR product shown in Table 5.4 and knowledge of the STS. Sequencing all of the clones in this order will provide information for the whole of the functional area under examination.

Cloning

Cloning provides a way of producing a large amount of material that can be sequenced using standard approaches. A primer is made to a known sequence in the area of the gene on a particular clone from a genomic library, and then a short complementary strand is synthesised. The complementary strand is then sequenced and its end used as the next primer. In this way it is possible to move down the chromosome (**chromosome walking**), systematically sequencing from between markers flanking the gene of interest (Fig. 5.37).

Cloning vectors are artificial circular DNA molecules (**plasmids**), derived from a variety of cellular types: bacteria, bacteriophages, yeast cells. These **BACs** or **YACs** are made by assembling all the essential parts of the natural bacterial or yeast chromosome and splicing in some human DNA

(Fig. 5.38). The artificial plasmid is put back into its parent cell, such as a bacterium, where it behaves as though it were a normal constituent of the cell. The plasmid is copied many times during each cell cycle. The result is a colony of cells, each containing a many copies (**clones**) of the human DNA fragment.

A **genomic library** is made by using restriction enzymes to break up genomic DNA and cloning these in vectors. These fragments will have fragments that overlap each other but will include all of the human genome: introns, exons, promoters, enhancers and non-coding (filler) DNA. A **cDNA library** is more limited as it contains only exons. It is made by taking mRNA and using the **reverse transcriptase** enzyme to produce cDNA to clone within a vector.

Bacteriophages can only carry small fragments of DNA, around 10–20 kb; in contrast YACs can hold 1000 kb of human DNA inserts. Use of different vectors allows the cloned DNA molecules to be made progressively smaller, until small enough to be sequenced. This technique, as well as providing material for sequencing, can also be used to produce large amounts of **recombinant** material for medical use – insulin (for treatment of diabetes) and erythropoietin (for treatment of renal failure) are produced in this way.

Positional cloning is the name given to the process of locating and cloning the disease gene once a process such as linkage has provided an approximate region on a chromosome. Various approaches can be used to help define the position of the gene within this sequence.

■ **Candidate genes**: these are possible disease-causing genes, identified because they produce a protein possibly associated with the disease profile and are therefore useful starting points to look for the gene.

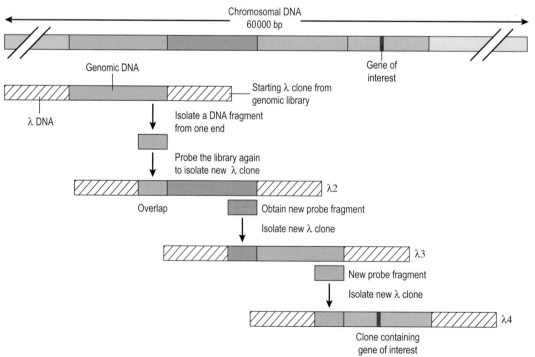

Fig. 5.37 Chromosome walking. The region of λ DNA containing the genomic DNA sequence where the sequencing will start is selected from a library made within a bacteriophage and used to make a complementary strand, which is sequenced. The end of this sequence, closer to the gene of interest, is used as a probe to find a new clone from the library which contains this short overlapping sequence. The process is repeated, sequencing each complementary strand until the gene has also been sequenced.

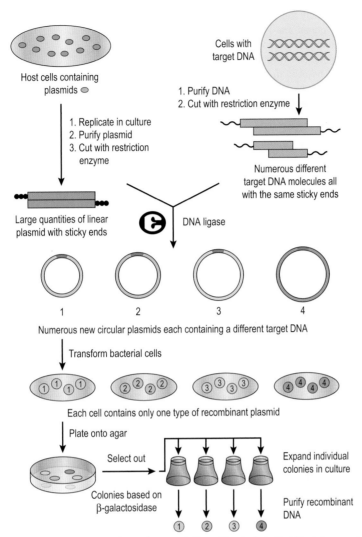

Fig. 5.38 DNA cloning using bacteria. One of the characteristics of bacteria is that the take up of plasmids is very inefficient and usually only one type of plasmid will enter each bacterium. Plating the bacteria onto agar will produce bacterial colonies, some of which will contain many copies of the original single plasmid, and particular piece of target DNA, originating from a single bacterium. Colonies that contain plasmids are selected using another molecular tool: the gene for β-galactosidase. This is a marker gene placed within the plasmid but designed so that, if DNA is inserted, the β-galactosidase gene becomes disrupted and non-functional. The normal gene product reacts with substrates in the culture to produce a coloured colony. Thus the *uncoloured* colonies will be those that contain the plasmid. In the diagram the 'uncoloured' plasmid-containing colonies are shown coloured to illustrate the different plasmid types containing the target DNA. Individual colonies can then be selected and separately cultured to produce large quantities of the target DNA. From Baynes J, Dominiczak M 2004 Medical biochemistry, 2nd edn. Elsevier, Edinburgh.

■ **Conserved sequences**: a large amount of DNA that codes for particular proteins required for life will be very similar (**highly conserved**) across species. This is because any mutational changes may be lethal to the organism. Over time, some mutations may provide an advantage to the species and be maintained over others – an evolutionary change.

In contrast, the non-coding DNA may undergo mutational change without it being lethal and so it is reasonable that non-coding DNA will be more variable, especially between different species. This characteristic can then be used to define coding sequences.

■ **GC islands**: GC dinucleotides are usually methylated, but in the 5′ end of many genes they are unmethylated. This may be to facilitate transcription. Identification of clusters of these unmethylated GC clusters (GC islands) may indicate the position of a gene.

■ **cDNA selection**: a sequence of DNA is inserted into a YAC, which is then hybridised to clones from a cDNA library. cDNA is coding only and so will only hybridise with **exon** sequences (DNA that codes for proteins in a gene).

■ **Trapping exons**: a sequence of DNA inserted into a vector that undergoes transcription will produce mRNA which is then processed to leave only exons. Therefore DNA containing exons will result in larger fragments after transcription than if there are no exons present.

■ **Expressed sequence tags** (**ESTs**): ESTs are short sequences of DNA clones taken from a cDNA library. Because cDNA originates from mRNA, the sequences must be expressed (protein-producing) regions of genes. These pieces are around 200–500 nucleotides long and are used as a tag with techniques such as FISH or radiation hybrid mapping. ESTs are normally sequences from each end of the cDNA molecule and can be synthesised quickly and cheaply.

ESTs have been used to identify the genes involved in Alzheimer disease. Candidate genes are examined for areas of the DNA that match with the ESTs. Then the identified genes can be examined for mutations in affected individuals. Further family studies must be used to validate the link. Scientists contribute ESTs for public use to a database, **dbEST**, which is part of the NIH **GenBank** gene sequence database.

Chromosomal comparative genomic hybridization (CGH) arrays

CGH arrays use a SNP-array approach to detect chromosomal and genomic rearrangements and deletions and offer greater sensitivity and specificity in comparison with FISH. The Database of Chromosomal Imbalance and Phenotype in Humans using Ensemble Resources (DECIPHER) and the International Standards for Cytogenomic Arrays Consortium (ISCA Consortium) are databases that are cataloguing these findings.

Genetic linkage and monogenic disease

Genetic linkage studies involve using families that have a number of diseased individuals and show evidence of Mendelian inheritance. These studies help identify disease genes by pinpointing the location of the disease-associated mutation in the genome. Linkage analysis depends on the presence of polymorphic markers near to the disease gene of interest. Until the variation in DNA sequences could be exploited there were very few polymorphic markers; those that existed (blood groups, red cell enzymes and serum protein polymorphisms) were of little use where they did not lie close to the gene of interest. The ability to utilise DNA has resulted in many more markers, and more polymorphic markers, including more than 10 million SNPs, becoming available for use as tools in the analytical process.

Linkage analysis has been used successfully to map numerous disease genes of either dominant or recessive inheritance with complete or variable penetrance and the density of the SNP map has added more power to the analysis. Genetic mapping of a disease or trait involves the identification of markers that are always inherited together. If the marker lies within the gene causing the disease then linkage will mean that the same marker allele will always be inherited along with disease. Figure 5.39 illustrates the principle of linkage mapping.

Genes that are physically very close to each other are rarely separated in this process and therefore sets of alleles are inherited as a block, or **haplotype**. The closer two genes are on a chromosome, the less likely they are to be separated during recombination in meiosis. This fact is used to provide a measure of closeness, measured in **centimorgans (cM)**. One cM is defined as a 1% recombination between two loci (a **recombination frequency** of 0.01). The maximum recombination possible is 50% (recombination frequency 0.5). Therefore loci that are more than 50 cM apart are considered to be unlinked.

Linkage disequilibrium

Linkage disequilibrium also looks at the association between a marker and a disease locus, but there are some fundamental differences. When the appearance of a particular

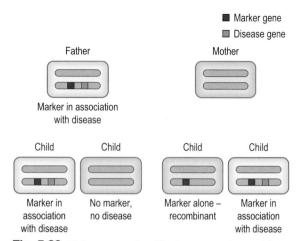

Fig. 5.39 Linkage mapping. The frequency of recombinant events between markers within a family pedigree provides a measure of relative proximity of the genes. The lower proportion of recombinants seen, the closer the marker is to the gene, and the higher the chance of linkage. The larger a family pedigree, the more accurate is the assessment.

marker allele is not influenced by the presence of the disease locus, this absence of association between the two loci is called **linkage equilibrium**. Some alleles, however, exhibit an association – **linkage disequilibrium**. This technique increases the resolution even further, down to 0.1 cM approximately.

The concept of linkage considers the locus, and recent recombination events, within a family pedigree. In contrast, linkage disequilibrium considers particular alleles seen within the population as a whole that co-segregate with a disease allele – an **association**. It is thus characterised by allele frequencies that do not match with those predicted by chance. As explained above, during meiosis, chromatids are formed from a pair of chromosomes and recombination occurs when parts of the chromatids exchange (cross over). Genes that are a long distance apart will tend to be separated in this process; those that are close together will tend to remain together (linked). The tighter the linkage, the longer the disequilibrium (association) will last.

During fertilisation, genetic material is swapped between paired chromosomes in the crossing-over process, known as **genetic recombination**. The position and frequency of crossover differs at each meiosis with, on average, one or two exchanges per chromosome per meiosis. Genetic recombination accounts for the differences seen between siblings.

LOD scores

An assessment of the strength of a particular recombination frequency is provided by comparing the likelihood that two loci are linked at a given recombination frequency versus the likelihood that they are not linked (recombination frequency 0.5). This likelihood is known as the **logarithm of the odds (LOD) score**. LOD scores with a likelihood ratio greater than 3.0 are said to be evidence of linkage; scores less than −2.0 are said to be evidence that the loci are not linked. Because LOD is a logarithm, a score of 3.0 means that the likelihood of linkage occurring at the particular genetic distance is 1000 times greater than there being no linkage.

Genetic linkage – a clinical example

One of the first chromosomal linkages identified in humans was between the locus for **nail–patella syndrome** (**NPS**) and the ABO blood group on chromosome 9. NPS is inherited as an autosomal dominant trait and individuals have abnormalities of nails and patella and other skeletal problems. Associated abnormalities of the basement membrane lead to renal problems, which are a significant cause of mortality among individuals with the disease.

Calculating the recombination frequency

The pedigree of a family with NPS (Fig. 5.40) allows one to make certain observations:

- All affected individuals have at least one parent with NPS, suggesting dominant inheritance
- Both males and females are similarly affected with NPS, suggesting an autosomal defect
- Of the 19 related individuals:
  - 10 are affected and 9 of these carry blood group B, suggesting that NPS is linked to ABO blood type
  - 9 are unaffected, but only 2 of these carry blood group B, suggesting that these 2 are recombinants
  - One affected individual is blood group O, suggesting that he too is a recombinant.

In the family there are 16 informative loci; 13 in the second generation, but only 3 in the third. The 2 children of the marriage with the group A woman have to be ignored; as the B group has not been transmitted, it is not possible to know whether recombination has taken place. Three in total are recombinant. The genetic distance can be calculated as follows:

$$\text{Genetic distance} = \frac{3}{16} \times 100 = 18.8 \text{ cM}$$

$$= 0.188 \text{ recombination frequency}$$

Calculating the LOD score

The example with NPS suggests that the genes for NPS and the ABO blood group may lie close together. The LOD score is calculated from:

$$\text{LOD} = \log \frac{\text{Probability of offspring with these genotypes if the genes are linked}}{\text{Probability of offspring with these genotypes if the genes are not linked}}$$

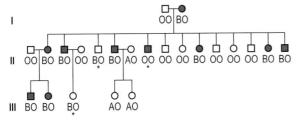

Nail–patella syndrome = ● or ■
Blood types = OO, BB, BO, AO

Fig. 5.40 Pedigree detailing nail-patella syndrome (NPS) phenotypes and ABO blood group genotypes. The pedigree shows a strong association between NPS and blood group B, suggesting that these genes are closely linked. Only three individuals show only blood group B, or have NPS, indicated with*. These individuals are the recombinants.

From the examined pedigree the following observations can be made:

- If the recombination frequency is 0.188, then the probability of seeing the recombination genotype is also said to be 0.188. But the chance of an individual child being a recombinant has to be half of this (0.094), as there are two parents and thus two parental types.
- The probability of no recombination is therefore 1 − 0.188 = 0.812, and the chance of an individual child not being a recombinant is therefore 0.406.
- As there are 3 recombinant and 13 non-recombinants in the pedigree examined, the chance of seeing the genotypes in the children of the NPS pedigree can be calculated by multiplying each separate and independent probabilities for each child. This is the top part of the equation (the probability of offspring with these genotypes if the genes are linked):

$$\left(0.406^{13}\right)\left(0.094^3\right) = 6.76 \times 10^{-9}$$

- If there is no linkage, then the recombination frequency is 0.5. It is 0.5 because there is a 50% chance of a particular allele being passed from a parent to child. The chance of possessing a particular genotype from a pair of parents is half of this (0.25).
- The probability of seeing the particular genotypes in the NPS pedigree can be calculated using the individual probabilities for each child. This is the bottom part of the equation (the probability of offspring with these genotypes if the genes are not linked):

$$0.25^{16} = 2.32 \times 10^{-10}$$

- The LOD score can be calculated as follows:

$$\text{LOD} = \log\left(\frac{6.76 \times 10^{-9}}{2.32 \times 10^{-10}}\right) = \log 29.05 = 1.46$$

- Note that the LOD score here has not reached the level of 3.0, the level where we can safely assume linkage, and therefore, from this family alone, it is not possible to be sure that the NPS and ABO blood group genes are linked, despite the pedigree appearing to be quite convincing in this respect. We can look at other families with NPS and calculate the LOD scores for each family. The LOD scores can then be added together, accumulating evidence until a convincing LOD score is achieved of either:
  - LOD > 3.0, supporting linkage
  - LOD < −2.0, against linkage.

LOD problems encountered in linkage studies

Locus heterogeneity

Locus heterogeneity is seen when mutations in different genes give rise to the same disease phenotype. This is more likely to be seen when a large number of families are examined. If evidence from several small families is used, rather than one or two large pedigrees, and locus heterogeneity is present, then simply combining LOD scores may suggest a lack of association.

Many diseases have been described that show locus heterogeneity, including **osteogenesis imperfecta type I**, which is due to mutations in genes on chromosome 7 and chromosome 17.

Incomplete penetrance

Even though an individual may have inherited a mutation in a susceptibility locus, other factors may affect the clinical presentation of the disease, such as environmental effects, chance and/or modifying gene loci, any of which may result in the individual appearing to be unaffected. This will cause a problem while doing linkage analysis as one cannot assume that unaffected people do not carry the disease allele.

Phenocopies

This occurs when individuals show the disease even though they are not carrying a susceptibility mutation. This sporadic disease may be explained by a non-inheritable occurrence, or by a distinct mutation in the same gene or a gene different from that inherited by the majority of affected cases in the family. For example, there is a very high rate of sporadic prostate cancer (a 1 in 5 lifetime risk in US males), thus making it difficult to find informative families for linkage analysis.

As long as the proportion of **phenocopies** to gene carriers in a family is low enough, linkage analysis models can cope with this problem. The same problem can occur if there has been a misdiagnosis. This underlies the importance of clinical confirmation of the affected status of each individual, which can be difficult in extended pedigrees.

Genetic linkage and polygenic disease

Many of the methods used in the techniques described below rely on the use of particular tools to manipulate DNA. Both restriction enzymes and the polymerase chain reaction (PCR) are utilised in many of the analytical processes to examine the DNA but these have been largely superseded by analysis of SNPs on array platforms. Now that the whole genome has been sequenced, many of these tools are now redundant. Nevertheless some key techniques have been described here as they provide an historical background to the complex nature of unravelling genetic material.

Restriction fragment length polymorphism

The endonuclease enzyme has the ability to cut DNA into separate pieces at a particular DNA sequence (**restriction site**). For example, the enzyme EcoR1 cuts DNA at GAATTC. If there is a mutation (base change, insertion or deletion) at the site (**restriction site polymorphism**), the enzyme will not cut the DNA. The cut, or uncut, fragments can be separated by placing the DNA in a gel and applying an electric current (**electrophoresis**). The charged DNA fragments will be pulled through the gel by the current, small fragments will move more easily and the fragments will be spread out by size.

The presence of a particular cut, or uncut, fragment is detected by using a DNA **probe**, which is a sequence of DNA that is complementary, and therefore binds, to the respective cut, or uncut, sequence type. Addition of a marker to the probe, such as a chemiluminescent tag, will mean that the relative position of the fragments on a gel can be detected when the gel is transferred to a membrane and then exposing the membrane to an X-ray film (**Southern blotting**). These polymorphisms are called **restriction fragment length polymorphisms** (**RFLPs**) and have provided many thousands of new polymorphic markers, enabling major advances in gene mapping in recent years.

RFLP linkage analysis was used in the detection of fragile X syndrome (see Clinical box 5.6).

Variable number of tandem repeats

Historically, RFLPs were not sufficiently polymorphic or abundant for fine mapping of the genome (although many SNPs could be regarded as RFLPs). There are areas of the DNA with sequences that are repeated, one after the other (in tandem). The number of repeats in any particular area of the genome varies considerably.

- **Minisatellites** or **variable number of tandem repeats** (**VNTRs**) have repeated sequences that are tens of base pairs long.
- **Microsatellites** or **short tandem repeats** (STRs) have repeated sequences that are much shorter – generally 2–6 base pairs.

A disadvantage of VNTRs is that they are found more often towards the ends of the chromosomes. Dinucleotide repeats (**CA repeat microsatellites**) – CACACACA ... – are found spread throughout the whole genome and the number of repeats is very polymorphic.

There are no restriction sites within the repeats and so the restriction enzymes cut outside the repeat region, but the resultant fragments are very small – too small to be seen using a DNA probe on a gel – and the relative difference in the numbers of repeats requires highly sensitive detection. These problems have been resolved in two ways:

- The small amount of DNA has been resolved by the use of the **PCR** (Fig. 5.41) in which a sequence of DNA is copied many times
- The resolution of small size differences, sometimes only by a single base, has been enabled by passing the fragments through very fine capillaries, and employing sensitive fluorescent probes in the PCR reaction that anneal to the DNA sequence just beyond the repeat region.

STRs have proven useful in linkage analysis because they are highly polymorphic and inherited in a Mendelian fashion. For example, variations in the number of repeats within an allele in the factor VIII gene have been used in the prenatal diagnosis of haemophilia A, and in the verification of female carrier status.

Single nucleotide polymorphisms

SNPs are simply those polymorphisms where a single base has changed. For example, one person may have a DNA base A, where another person might have a base C. There are estimated to be at least 10 million SNPs in the genome and many have been identified as part of the international HapMap project. SNPs that are close together will tend to be inherited together as a **haplotype** and most chromosome regions have only a few common haplotypes, with frequencies greater than 5%. Not all SNPs need to be analysed, however, as typing only a few SNPs (called tagging SNPs) can capture all the haplotype data for genetic association studies – they will define the haplotype.

Once possible disease-causing genes had been selected, scientists would verify the choice through:

- **Targeted allele-specific mutation screening**: identified genes are examined for mutations in affected individuals. This is usually performed by PCR amplification of the gene, followed by sequence analysis and is ideal for carrying out simple assays on common defined variants. For example, real-time PCR **TaqMan assays** can be

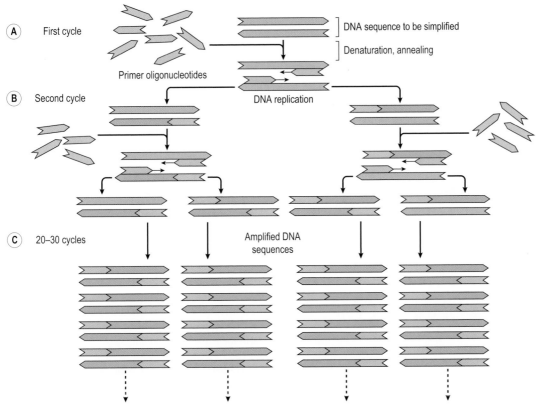

A First cycle

DNA sequence to be simplified

Denaturation, annealing

Primer oligonucleotides

DNA replication

B Second cycle

C 20–30 cycles

Amplified DNA sequences

Fig. 5.41 Diagrammatic representation of the polymerase chain reaction (PCR). PCR is a method of multiplying (**amplifying**) DNA. The process starts by heating the double-stranded DNA (in purple). Heating separates the two strands (**denaturation**) and allows **primers** (small pieces of DNA that are complementary to a specific location on the DNA) (in yellow) to stick (**anneal**) and provide a starting point for the DNA polymerase enzyme. A copy of each strand results (with new single-stranded DNA (in blue) and the new complementary strand pairs come together as the temperature is allowed to fall. At the end of the first cycle the DNA has doubled. Further heating and cooling sequences repeat the process. After 40 cycles, the DNA will have been amplified by about one trillion-fold.

used in genotyping to reveal the factor X Leiden mutation (see Ch. 12). The assay (Fig. 5.42) consists of:

- Taqman probes from Life Technologies are designed to bind between the primers and consist of a short primer with fluorescent reporter at one end and a fluorescent quencher at the other. **Fluorescence resonance energy transfer** (**FRET**) ensures that the light energy in the reporter is not released while the quencher is in close proximity.
- A primer designed to bind only to DNA carrying the mutant allele.
- A **minor grove binder** (**MGB**) designed to bind only to the normal (wild) DNA strand and block binding of the mutant-specific primer.
- **Taq polymerase** extends only the mutant-specific primer and continues until it meets and digests the **TaqMan** probe from the strand.
- The digestion disrupts the reporter and quencher and light energy released and detected, indicating the presence of a mutant allele.
- **Gene expression**: possible disease-causing genes are further verified by looking at tissue expression. This is done by a technique called **northern blotting**, in which purified mRNA from tissue is hybridised with a probe made from the gene. If the gene is the disease gene, it would be expected to hybridise with mRNA from the tissue known to be affected by the disease. For example, a gene responsible for osteoporosis will be more likely to be expressed in the bone-forming cells than in other tissues.

- **Family studies**: further validation and verification associating a particular disease with a gene may be done by examining affected families and control populations to look for consistent patterns (see also Clinical Box 5.13).

Genome microarrays

Gene arrays use a form of solid support, such as a glass slide or nylon membrane, onto which a collection of nucleic acids, specific for a particular gene, are **spotted**. These **target** nucleic acids are **probed** with fluorescently labelled nucleic acids extracted from a sample, and those that **hybridise** to the spot are detected through the fluorescent label. The advantage of using an array is that many thousands of targets can be examined in a single experiment. Arrays can be used in different ways for a number of different purposes:

- **Expression arrays**: these can be used to compare different RNAs from, for example:
  - Different tissues
  - Normal and tumour tissue
  - Treated and untreated cell cultures.
  RNA is converted to complementary DNA (cDNA) using reverse transcriptase before being hybridised onto the array.
- **SNP arrays**: the accumulation of large numbers of SNPs through worldwide projects, such as the HapMap project, and their availability within databases, has facilitated large numbers (up to 1 million) covering the majority of the human genome, to be spotted onto a single array offering a statistically very powerful approach

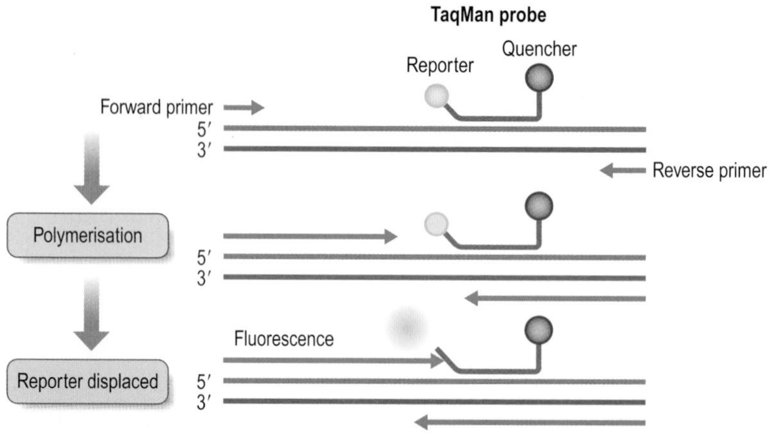

Fig. 5.42 **Principle of the TaqMan assay (Life Technologies).** The TaqMan probe is bound to the strand of DNA that is to be copied. The probe includes a reporter fluorophore and a quencher that inhibits fluorescence. As the polymerase reaction copies the strand from the 5′ end it displaces the fluorophore from the probe, which then fluoresces as it is no longer inhibited by the quencher molecule.

Clinical box 5.13 | **Some clinical conditions identified by linkage analysis**

Glutathione reductase is an important enzyme as it protects haemoglobin, red cell enzymes and cell membranes from oxidative damage. **Glutathione reductase deficiency** can lead to a haemolytic anaemia in patients. The gene was located on the short arm of chromosome 8 when a child with anaemia and a deletion on chromosome 8 was also shown to have about 50% of the normal glutathione reductase activity.

---

to the identification of SNPs that are associated with particular diseases, as well as identifying chromosomal alterations in tumours.

- **Copy number arrays**: copy number variation (CNV) is important in a number of different mechanisms and modern arrays include around 1 million known variants. Analysis of copy number has been used in:
  - Cancer – changes in copy number are associated with tumour initiation and progression, and analysis of copy number arrays can help identify new tumour suppressor genes and oncogenes.
  - Disease association – germline CNV is common but has also been associated with specific diseases and analysis of copy number is often done in association with SNP analysis.

Personal genomics

Private companies, such as 23andMe, Pathway Genomics and Navigenics, offer personal predictive and presymptomatic tests for a wide range of conditions that are increasingly being taken up by the public who may have limited understanding in interpretation of the results they obtain. Most of the SNP-based diagnostics that are offered are probabilistic, and not deterministic, in particular because they only identify a limited range of variants. Exome chips, covering all coding variants reported in patients and controls, may improve the assessment of relevant mutational load in the future.

Next generation sequencing (NGS)

NGS enables powerful parallel sequencing allowing efficient sequencing of the **whole genome** (**WGS**) or the coding regions targeted **whole exome sequencing** (**WES**). On the horizon are single molecule third and fourth generation se-

quencing, the latter probably using **nanopore technology** in which sequencing is done using conductance differences as DNA passes through holes just large enough to allow the DNA molecule to thread through.

NGS can also be used to detect methylation, splicing, small RNAs, allele-specific expression, haplotypes and gene rearrangements and so is likely to become the technology of the future. However, different sequencing platforms are variable in their accuracy. Confirmation of interesting variants identified with WGS or WES still favours Sanger sequencing in the probands and family members because of the method's superior accuracy. Table 5.5 summarises the differences in the currently available technologies.

Bioinformatic tools

Studying a whole genome will inevitably reveal rare alleles, which may or may not be important in the development of a disease. Analyses considering **additive effects** where collections of rare alleles can be incorporated and considered with other alleles are becoming important in association studies. The consideration of additive effects has led to the emergence of a new theory, **CDRV (common disease/rare variant)** as an alternative to **CDCV (common disease/common variant)** theory, and new bioinformatics methods have been developed to deal with this concept.

One of the main problems in analysing multiple hypotheses when dealing with whole genome data is the increased probability of associations by chance. New bioinformatics tools for polygenic association studies include:

- **PLINK** – looks for the transmission of genetic markers that are not linked in diseased patients, in comparison with healthy individuals
- **MDR** (multifactor dimensional reduction), in which a set of healthy and diseased individuals is used as a 'training' set to derive an algorithm of disease risk, which is then validated with a 'testing' set to define the accuracy of the method
- **MCMC** (Markov chain Monte Carlo) algorithm seeks to improve on the inefficiency of models where there are enormous numbers of comparisons, and **BEAM** (bayesian epistasis association mapping), **logistic regression** and **APSampler** provide different bioinformatics methods making use of MCMC but provide further sophistications that vary between them.

Table 5.5 Comparison of sequencing methods

	Sanger sequencing	Pyrosequencing[1]	Ion semiconductor (Ion Torrent™)[2]	Synthetic (Illumina®)[3]	SOLID (Life Technologies™) synthesis[4]	Single molecule real-time (Pacific Bio)[5]
Read length	400–900 bp	700 bp	200 bp	50–250 bp	50 + 50 bp	5000 bp
Accuracy	99.9%	99.9%	98%	98%	99.9%	87% single read, 99.99% consensus
Reads per run	Forward and reverse	1 million	5 million	3 billion	1.5 billion	50 000
Time per run	Hours	Day	Hours	Day/s	Week/s	Hours
Disadvantages	Expensive	Expensive	Errors	Expensive instrument	Slow	Expensive instrument
Advantages	Long reads	Fast and long read	Fast and cheap	Long read and cheap	Cheap	Moderate thoughput

[1]Attempts are made to bind nucleotides to a DNA sequence and the instrument detects successful binding with a peak of fluorescence. The height of the peak indicates how many nucleotides of the same type have been added and the sequence is inferred.
[2]Detects hydrogen ion release when a complementary dNTP is bound.
[3]Incorporates pyrosequencing for detection when synthesising on beads.
[4]Uses clonal fragments bound to magnetic beads with attached PCR products covalently bonded to glass slides. Fluorescently-labelled probes compete to ligate to the sequencing primer.
[5]Uses tiny cylindrical chambers that allow only one nucleotide to be present at a time. Individual dNTPs are fluorescently labelled on the phosphate, rather than on the base, and the label is cleaved, releasing fluorescence, when the polymerase acts to bind the particular dNTP, next in the sequence.

The advantages of increasingly affordable whole genome studies that can be conducted in large multicentre research groups outweigh the older approaches in terms of statistical power as well as in the greater homogeneity of the patient data and has allowed the development of a minimal subset of particular alleles as a marker of risk in particular diseases.

THE HUMAN GENOME PROJECT

Sequencing of human DNA was the aim of the **Human Genome Project** (**HGP**), which completed the analysis of one human genome for over $2.7 billion. The human genome has now been sequenced in a up to 100 individuals, including James Watson, and this information is available in public genome databases. The commercialisation of whole genome scanning is undergoing rapid expansion and advertised costs as low as $100 means that this is likely to become a high growth area.

The Human Genome Initiative was started by the US Department of Energy in 1986 and, with the National Institutes of Health, the HGP began in 1990, soon to be joined by major collaborators around the world. HGP's aim was to create a high-quality reference DNA sequence for the whole human genome, consisting of 3 million base pairs, and to identify all human genes. While scientists from China, France, Germany, the UK, Japan and the USA have all collaborated in the project, five institutions, four in the USA and one in the UK, were the most productive.

The working draft of the human genome sequence was announced in June 2000, accompanied by separate publications in 2001 from both the publicly funded HGP and the private company Celera Genomics. The project was declared complete in 2003, having sequenced about 99% of the human gene containing regions to an accuracy of 99.99%. Since then entire chromosome sequences have been published and the 1000 genomes project, published in 2010, revealed genetic variation within 1092 human genomes.

Can a DNA sequence be patented?

The potential power of information within the human genome has led companies to attempt to patent DNA sequences and a challenge to limit testing for mutations in the *BRCA1* and *BRCA2* genes (associated with high breast and cervical cancer risk) to one company was refused by the US Supreme Court in 2013. They declared that naturally occurring DNA sequences were not patentable, although they allowed the patenting of synthetic complementary DNA (cDNA). The decision has been welcomed by many because of the potential for lower cost genetic diagnostic testing in the future.

Beyond the sequence

In addition to sequencing each chromosome to a high level of quality scientists have been examining sequence variation at the level of single nucleotides (**SNPs**), as well as looking at variation in much larger chromosome segments and many of these are incorporated into the SNP microarrays discussed above. The **Single Nucleotide Polymorphisms Database** (**dbSNP**), hosted by the **National Center for Biotechnology** (**NCBI**) in collaboration with the **National Human Genome Research Institute** (**NHGRI**) holds information on more than 25 million polymorphisms: SNPs, indels, short tandem repeats (STRs), multinucleotide polymorphisms (MNPs) and other variants from a wide variety of organisms that will help the understanding of human evolution. For example:

- The **Japanese pufferfish** has the smallest known vertebrate genome, which makes it simpler to investigate; comparison with the human genome will help identify those genes that have been preserved over some 450 million years.
- The **sea squirt** is the smallest organism with a spinal cord and over 80% of its genes are also found in the human genome. It will be particularly useful for the investigation of the evolutionary aspects of the nervous system.

- The **Western clawed frog** is being used as the major vertebrate model for embryonic development and cellular mechanisms.

Microbes are the oldest and most prevalent organisms on earth. Many are now being sequenced as part of the **Human Microbiome Project**, launched in 2008. It is hoped that knowledge of their molecular structure will enable scientists to use them for pharmaceutical, industrial, agricultural and environmental purposes.

Research in animal disease models is likely to remain important in the investigation of the pathogenic potential of variants revealed as part of whole genome screens.

What the HGP has already told us

Sequencing the human genome has been a major achievement but it is only the tip of the iceberg. Much work remains to be done, not only so that we can discover much more about particular organisms but also so that we can gain a better understanding of the more complex interactions involved within and between different life systems. Early analysis has already produced useful information.

Statistics

- The human genome consists of over three billion nucleotide bases (A, C, T and G) and it is estimated that 99.9% of the order is identical between all individuals.
- The total number of genes is estimated to be around 25 000, with each gene being composed of around 3000 bases. The number of bases in a gene is very variable, however.
- The **dystrophin** gene is possibly the largest gene with 2.4 million bases. The highest number of genes on a chromosome are found on the largest chromosome 1 (over 3000), whereas the small Y chromosome has relatively few (less than 400).

Functions

The function of more than half of the genes is not yet known.

Structure

- About 50% of the human genome is composed of repetitive short sequences of nucleotides. These repeated regions do not code for proteins and may have no direct function, other than as a separator between the genes.
- While most of the gene-dense regions are rich in G and C nucleotides, the intervening gene-poor areas are characterised by being AT rich.

Variation

- The genetic sequence of different humans is very similar but a SNP occurs in about 1 in 1200 bases and there are about 10 million common SNPs. Mutations are about twice as common in the male germline.
- A second type of variation, copy number, has been shown to be a common occurrence.

Comparison with other species

- The structure of the human genome is much more random than in other organisms, whose genes are also more evenly spaced. Humans have the same protein families as worms, flies and plants but proteins involved in development and immunity are more prolific.
- Humans have about three times as many protein products as other organisms and about five times the number of repeat sequences as other organisms. The apparent evolutionary expansion of repeated sequences in humans over time seems to have halted about 50 million years ago, whereas the process seems to be continuing in rodents.

Using data from the HGP

The altruistic principles that have been embedded into the HGP, along with the ready worldwide access to information provided through the Internet, have ensured that genetic information has been made widely available to the whole scientific community. **GenBank** is a collection of all publicly available DNA sequences and is part of an international collaboration which includes the DNA DataBank of Japan (DDBJ), the European Molecular Biology Laboratory (EMBL) and NCBI.

Investigating the human genome

The **NCBI Human Map Viewer** can be accessed via a link on the NCBI website homepage (http://www.ncbi.nlm.nih.gov). As well as humans, the NCBI source also has maps of other mammals, other vertebrates, invertebrates, plants, fungi and protozoa. A particular gene can be entered as a search term and this will lead to a diagram of human chromosomes showing the gene location. Figure 5.43 shows a search for cystic fibrosis that identifies the *CFTR* gene on chromosome 7.

The **Online Mendelian Inheritance in Man (OMIM) database** (first online in 1985) contains information about all known Mendelian inheritance genes and focuses on the relationship between genotype and phenotype. In Figure 5.44 cystic fibrosis is shown at position 7q31.2, associated with the gene 602421 – cystic fibrosis conductance regulator (*CFTR*) gene. Other associated conditions are also detailed.

Also available is a wealth of information that has already been gathered about the gene such as the nucleotide sequence, SNPs, known biological evidence available in the literature and sequences that are orthologous with the mouse genome, along with a vast amount of other information that can be used by scientists wishing to research a particular gene.

Other databases are also available that can be used to provide similar information, such as the University of California, Santa Cruz (UCSC) browser and Ensemble.

Gene families

The molecular basis of a disease can also be investigated by examining **homologues**. These are genes that share a common evolutionary history and so will have a similar sequence. There are two kinds of homologues:

- **Orthologues** are genes with similar sequences in two different species that have evolved from a single gene in the last common ancestor

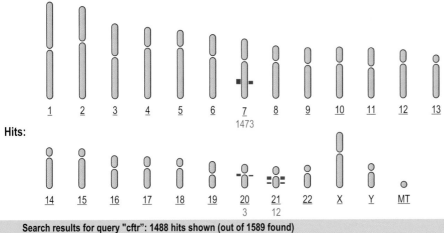

Hits:

Search results for query "cftr": 1488 hits shown (out of 1589 found)

Hits shown: 1-100   1 2 3 4 5 6 **7** 8 9 10 11 12 13 14 15 16 17 18 19 **20 21** 22 X Y

Chr	Assembly	Match	Map element	Type	Maps
7	reference	<u>all matches</u>			
		DB229645 TRACH3 Homo sapiens cDNA clone TRACH3022821 5-, mRNA...	<u>DB229645.1</u>	TRANSCRIPT	<u>HsRNA</u>
		Human cystic fibrosis mRNA...**CFTR**)	<u>M28668.1</u>	TRANSCRIPT	<u>HsRNA</u>
		H.sapiens **CFTR** mutation mRNA.	<u>X73053.1</u>	TRANSCRIPT	<u>HsRNA</u>

Fig. 5.43 **NCBI Human Map Viewer displaying information about cystic fibrosis** (www.ncbi.nlm.nih.gov/). A search for the cystic fibrosis gene *CFTR* has revealed references locating the gene on chromosome 7. In addition to the sequence found on chromosome 7, others are seen on chromosomes 20 and 21 which reveal genes that are associated with CFTR modification.

---

*602421

Cystic fibrosis transmembrane conductance regulator; CFTR

Alternative titles; symbols

ATP-BINDING CASSETTE, SUBFAMILY C, MEMBER 7; ABCC7

HGNC Approved Gene Symbol: CFTR

Cytogenetic location: *7q31.2*   **Genomic coordinates (GRCh37):** *7:117,120,016 - 117,308,718* (from NCBI)

Gene Phenotype Relationships

Location	Phenotype	Phenotype MIM number
7q31.2	Congenital bilateral absence of vas deferens	277180
	Cystic fibrosis	219700
	Sweat chloride elevation without CF	
	{Bronchiectasis with or without elevated sweat chloride 1, modifier of}	211400
	{Hypertrypsinemia, neonatal}	
	{Pancreatitis, idiopathic}	167800

Fig. 5.44 **Morbid information showing genes closely associated with the gene implicated in cystic fibrosis.** (www.ncbi.nlm.nih.gov/). OMIM (Online Mendelian Inheritance in Man) information showing gene relationships associated with the CFTR (cystic fibrosis transmembrane regulator) gene on chromosome 7.

■ **Paralogues** are genes with similar sequences within a single organism that have diverged because of gene duplication.

Figure 5.45 illustrates the differences.

Molecular phylogenetics

Phylogenetics examines the evolutionary relationship between organisms. These relationships are depicted in **phylogenetic trees**, the relative position of branches representing the evolutionary time point at which species split from their common ancestor. Trees can be **rooted**, where a common ancestor is identified, or **unrooted**, in which case the trees only show the relationships between the species.

Patterns of DNA, the nucleotide and protein sequences are used to build trees using the observed patterns. Gene trees can be compared with species trees. Branches in gene trees occur at mutational events, whereas branches in species trees occur at the point at which a new species is identified. Therefore the trees are unlikely to be identical. Figure 5.46 shows an evolutionary tree predicted from mutational changes observed in the cytochrome c gene and corresponds reasonably, but not completely, with that expected in the evolution of vertebrates.

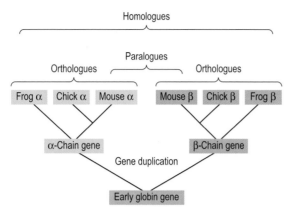

Fig. 5.45 **Different types of homologues.**

The **molecular clock hypothesis** assumes that mutations occur at a constant rate so that the difference between two sequences can be used to date the time of divergence. The rate of change however differs between organisms and so must be calibrated against fossil DNA.

Protein modelling

The nucleotide sequence is not sufficient on its own to be able to understand how the proteins that are encoded are structured. Scientists need to be able to determine the two-and three-dimensional structures of proteins in order to be able to understand how they function. Different techniques are used to investigate the structure of proteins.

X-ray crystallography

Proteins must first be made into crystals having a regular lattice structure, which is done by slow precipitation and can be very difficult. When an X-ray is passed through a crystal, the ray will be deflected and split, dependent on the angle of the crystal surfaces that the ray encounters. The intensity and relative positions of the deflected rays reflect the protein structure, and the information can be collected and used to produce a computer model of the protein.

Nuclear magnetic resonance

Nuclear magnetic resonance has the advantage over crystallography as the proteins can be examined in solution. However, the technique cannot be used to examine very large proteins. The protein molecules are placed in a magnetic field and excited by bombarding them with radio waves. This causes the nuclei to spin (resonate) in a particular direction. At a certain frequency the nucleus will flip over and this frequency is associated with protein structure.

Homology modelling

This technique uses the genome and computers to predict the structure of a protein. There are various databases that assist in this process, including:

- The **Protein Data Bank** (**PDB**), managed by the Worldwide Protein Data Bank (wwPDB) consortium
- The **Molecular Modeling DataBase** (**MMBD**), managed by the NCBI, also has a three-dimensional view of the protein structure
- **Clusters of orthologous groups** (**COGs**) attempts to classify proteins according to their phylogenetic, or

evolutionary, links and can be found within the EcoliWiki resource in the portal for *E. coli* research
- **Basic local alignment search tool** (**BLAST**) is a tool to search for homologous sequences over large databases and is maintained by the NCBI. Modifications of BLAST aid protein analysis
- **Vector alignment search tool** (**VAST**) is a tool to search for homologous protein structures available within the NCBI
- **Conserved Domain Database** (**CDD**), also held by the NCBI, is a database of protein building blocks that have been retained throughout the evolutionary process
- **GenBank**, from the NCBI, holds a large number of publically available information about proteins.

Model organisms

Although enormous progress has been made towards identifying the genetic changes underlying many human disorders, there are still a large number of inherited conditions for which the gene or genes responsible have yet to be found. Even in cases where the underlying genetic lesions are well established the mechanism of the disease is often poorly understood.

A large proportion of the human genome shares many common elements, even with seeming disparate species, such as flies. An understanding of both the differences and similarities is critical to our understanding of biological processes in humans. Model organisms are those non-human species that have been chosen for laboratory research because they have particular characteristics:

- Rapid development
- Short lifecycle
- Small adult size
- Ready availability.

In addition, it is obviously an advantage of having many scientists working on just a few representative species so that all the genetic information can be pooled and made available to the whole scientific community. Model organisms are found among mammals, non-mammals and plants.

Mammals as model organisms
The mouse
The mouse genome is the closest model organism to humans (approximately 99% of mouse genes are present in humans) and this has already been invaluable in genetic, developmental and immunological research. Knowledge of the mouse genome will assist in our understanding of the genetic mechanisms of disease. This is particularly so because experiments can be carried out in animals with a uniform genetic background in a controlled environment, helping to tease out the disease variability that occurs in humans because of the greater genetic variation and the variable effects of the environment on humans.

Mice are also very economic models as maintenance is inexpensive, sexual maturity is achieved after 6 weeks, gestation is only 20 days and they have litters of 10 or more pups. Mutant strains of mice – mice with particular disease characteristics that have been bred for laboratory use – are particularly useful for studying these diseases. Mutations can be readily induced in mice using *N*-ethyl-*N*-nitrosourea (ENU).

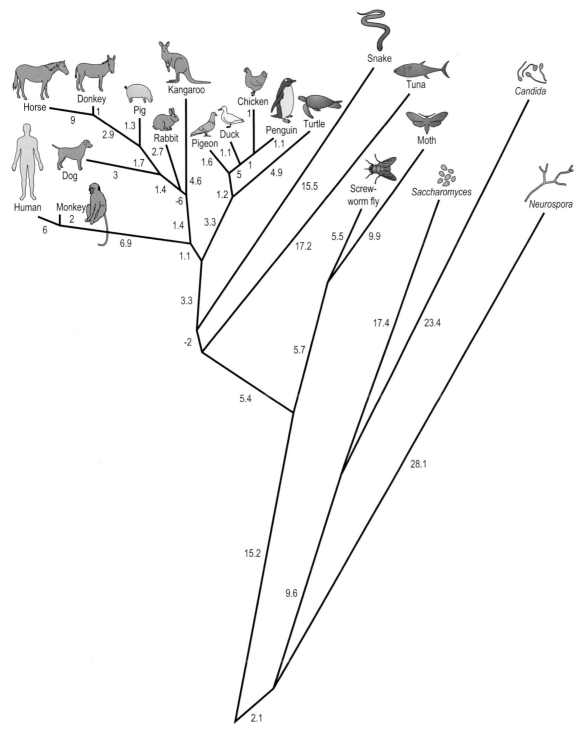

Fig. 5.46 A phylogenetic tree of 20 species developed by Walter Fitch and Emanuel Margoliash from observed changes in the cytochrome c gene between species. The numbers relate to the average corrected minimum number of nucleotide substitutions to produce the different proteins seen in each species. Adapted from Fitch WM, Margoliash E 1967 Construction of phylogenetic trees. Science 155 (3760): 279–284.

Transgenic mice have their genome altered artificially. DNA sequences developed in the laboratory are introduced into mouse embryos which are then placed into foster mice until birth. The changes produced by these designed mutations can be researched in the quest for an understanding of human disease. **Knockout mice** have specific genes altered by engineering a change sufficient to make the gene non-functional.

Non-mammals as model organisms

Retroviruses

Retroviruses are important because they are the causative agent of many serious diseases, such as acquired immune deficiency syndrome (AIDS). They are different from other viruses as their transmission is horizontal by infection, and vertical through the genome. The infective particle does this by converting its RNA to DNA and incorporating this into the host genome. Retroviruses are important organisms in the study of DNA replication, transcription and RNA processing.

Bacteria and other microbes

Microbes make up a high proportion of the earth mass and have survived longer than most other living organisms. Microbes are also extremely diverse and can survive in many environments. Knowledge of the various genomes will aid the understanding of medical, industrial and environmental processes.

Saccharomyces cerevisiae (baker's yeast)

This was the first eukaryotic organism to be fully sequenced (as early as 1996). It is easy to manipulate genetically and the Saccharomyces Gene Deletion Project aims to produce deletion mutant strains for each of its 6000 genes.

Archaea

Archaea are very primitive, having some genes in common with bacteria (prokaryotes) and some in common with later organisms (eukaryotes), in addition to genes not found anywhere else. Because these organisms can survive in extreme environments their study is useful for biotechnology and climate change and evolution.

Caenorhabditis elegans (round worm)

Caenorhabditis elegans is one the simplest multicellular organisms, comprising 959 cells with a full set of organs and a complex sensory system. The fate of each cell during the lifetime of the organism is known and its genome has been completely sequenced. The nematode can be rapidly grown and genetically modified.

Caenorhabditis elegans has approximately 20000 genes of which many are orthologues of human genes. Recently it was discovered that previously unknown genes in the insulin signalling pathway of the worm have human homologues and that human insulin can function in the worm insulin pathway. Thus *C. elegans* is a viable system in which to model disorders of the insulin pathway.

Drosophila (fruit fly)

Drosophila has been studied over many years and has a biological system of similar complexity to humans. The fly has many human homologues and its genetic system is easy to manipulate. Its short reproductive cycle and its exoskeleton make it easy to screen for developmental abnormalities. Its genome was sequenced in March 2000, which is a further advantage.

Danio rerio (zebrafish)

Danio rerio has many advantages as a model organism. It is small, easily grown, has a short lifecycle and produces hundreds of eggs. It is a vertebrate, but with half the genes of humans, making it invaluable in identification of key vertebrate genes. Mutations are easily induced and embryonic development can be observed through its transparent coat and the use of fluorescent markers.

A large number of cardiovascular mutations have been identified and more than 100 genes are known to be required for normal heart development and function. The mutant 'pickwick' (*pik*) zebrafish is associated with dilated cardiac myopathy, and mutations of the same gene in humans results in a similar disorder.

GENETIC DISEASE, DIAGNOSIS AND THERAPY

GENE TESTING

Gene tests are undertaken in various ways:

- Direct examination of the DNA molecule, looking for mutated sequences
- Biochemical tests for gene products – abnormal, or abnormal amounts of particular enzymes or proteins
- Examination of stained chromosomes, looking for abnormal structures.

 Gene tests may be used, for example:

- To identify **carriers** – individuals who are not affected because they carry only one copy of an aberrant gene that requires two copies for the disease (recessive) to be expressed
- To undertake prenatal testing
- To undertake presymptomatic or susceptibility testing
- To confirm diagnoses in symptomatic people.

 Genetic tests can provide useful information, enabling therapeutic actions to be taken to improve the life of individuals thus affected. Identification of individuals who are currently healthy, but who are at high risk of developing a life-threatening disease, is more problematic, since not everyone who tests positive will develop the disease.

Ethics

Until now genetic data has been used to confirm a diagnosis but in future this could change with individuals being sequenced to determine a set of variants which will need to be defined as to whether they are clinically important or not, and will be evaluated alongside other research data and databases such as the **Human Gene Mutation Database** (**HGMD**), **Clin Var** and **MutaDatabase**. A set of ranked categories from 'disease causing' to 'not disease causing' and 'variant of unknown clinical significance' has been proposed by the American College of Medical Geneticists. A problem that will be faced all too soon is the reporting of variants that have not been shown to be associated with any pathology, within a patient genome report, long before research is done that provides information on their diagnostic validity (see Ch. 7).

 The potential ethical issues associated with WES and WGS are considerable. While these have been widely discussed with participants in research in this area, there are important privacy issues that must be confronted before these approaches can be used in a clinical setting as they may reveal secondary information about disease risk that may not be welcome to the individual, or could be misused by third parties.

Genetic counselling

Genetic counsellors are health professionals with experience in the area of medical genetics, who are trained to provide information and support to families or individuals at risk of, or already affected by, genetic disease. The American Society of Human Genetics defines genetic counselling as 'A communication process which deals with human problems associated with the occurrence, or the risk of occurrence, of a genetic disorder in a family.' This process involves an attempt by one or more appropriately trained persons to help the individual or family to:

- Comprehend the medical facts, including the diagnosis, probable course of the disorder and the available management
- Appreciate the way heredity contributes to the disorder, and the risk of recurrence in specified relatives
- Understand the alternatives for dealing with the risk of recurrence
- Choose the course of action which seems to them appropriate in view of their risk, their family goals and their ethical and religious standards, and to act in accordance with that decision
- Make the best possible adjustment to the disorder in an affected family member and/or the risk of recurrence of that disorder.

Genetic counsellors often work as part of a multidisciplinary team that may include medical geneticists, physicians in the relevant specialty, nurses, psychologists, social workers and nutritionists. Support will also come from the primary care physician and disease support groups, the latter often set up by family members of sufferers.

CONGENITAL DISEASE

Congenital defects are those present, but not necessarily identified, at birth and are the most frequent cause of death in infants. Table 5.6 lists the most common congenital anomalies and their causes. Mostly there is no known reason for the malformation – this accounts for around 45% of all abnormalities, with multifactorial inheritance, familial causes and chromosome defects explaining a further 45%.

Different abnormalities can be defined as:

- **Malformation** – a primary defect due to abnormal development affecting part of the body, or an organ, such as a cleft lip
- **Dysplasia** – a primary defect of tissue formation, such as a vascular malformation
- **Sequence** – a primary defect that results in secondary structural changes, such as in oligohydramnios (reduced amniotic fluid) that leads to growth deficiencies, facial and limb deformities and pulmonary hypoplasia
- **Syndrome** – multiple primary malformations with a single cause, such as Down syndrome
- **Deformation** – change in body shape due to external sources affecting the developing foetus, such as a mechanical force
- **Disruption** – a change due to the breakdown of an originally normal development, such as a limb not developing properly because a vascular problem has limited the blood flow.

Teratogens

Teratogens are external agents that produce birth defects. There are some well-established teratogens, of which thalidomide is one of the best known. Others include alcohol, isotretinoin (prescribed in the treatment of acne), phenytoin (given to treat epilepsy), maternal infections (such as rubella), maternal disease (such as diabetes mellitus) and ionising radiation (see Clinical box 5.14).

Table 5.6	Some common congenital disorders
Congenital anomaly	**Cause**
Down syndrome	Chromosomal
Trisomy 13	Chromosomal
Trisomy 18	Chromosomal
Turner syndrome	Chromosomal
Prader–Willi syndrome	Microdeletion
William syndrome	Microdeletion
Neurofibromatosis type I	Single gene autosomal dominant
Marfan syndrome	Single gene autosomal dominant
Noonan syndrome	Single gene autosomal dominant
Achondroplasia	Single gene autosomal dominant
Osteogenesis imperfecta	Single gene; heterogeneous
Oligohydramnios sequence	Heterogeneous
VATER	Unknown
Cornelia de Lange syndrome	Unknown
Foetal alcohol syndrome	Excess alcohol

PHARMACOGENOMICS

No patients react in exactly the same way when given a drug and some will display dramatic differences when treated with a particular drug, or a particular dose of a drug, for the same condition.

- For example, **warfarin** is given to prevent thromboembolism but too little or too much can be life threatening and so it is important that patients are kept within the correct therapeutic window. Individuals, however, can vary over 20-fold in the amount they need to take on a daily basis and so need regular monitoring to achieve safe and effective anticoagulation. The reason for this difference relates to different mutations in the protein, vitamin K epoxide reductase, which is the target of warfarin.

If we could always predict which patients were going to react badly, or differently, from a study of their genetic make-up then modifications could be made to the drugs, or alternatives prescribed, before the adverse events.

Clinical box 5.14	Some birth defects caused by teratogens

Foetal alcohol syndrome is a preventable teratogenic congenital abnormality. High alcohol consumption in the first trimester leads to children showing several facial abnormalities with a small head and accompanied by developmental delay, heart defects and intellectual disability.

Neural tube defect (NTD) is a malformation of the developing neural tube that leads to anencephaly (normally fatal because most of the brain is absent), encephalocele (when the skull plates do not seal) and spina bifida (where the spinal column does not seal). Individuals with NTDs have significant problems, including hydrocephalus (accumulation of spinal fluid in the skull that compresses brain tissue), leg paralysis and urinary obstruction. Ingestion of 4 mg folate has been shown to reduce the risk of NTD by 70%, and it is recommended that all pregnant women, and those planning pregnancy, should take folic acid daily.

Pharmacogenomics is the study of the many different genes that determine drug behaviour. This is done by being able to define individual SNPs that predict a variable response to the particular drug. The hope for the future is that we will be able to provide treatment that is individualised to the individual. We must not lose sight, however, of the possibility that this personal genetic information will be misused and consideration of safeguards should be at the forefront of plans to utilise this approach more widely.

The best known examples of the potential of a pharmacogenomic approach are related to single gene traits that affect drug metabolism.

It is not only variations in drug metabolism that are observed; there is a growing collection of polymorphisms within genes that encode proteins involved in transporting and targeting drugs. Most of those that have been found are the ones that are easy to identify because they are associated with single genes and clearly recognisable effects. This is not how many drugs work, however, as multiple genes may be involved in determining the outcome of treatment. This has led to genome-wide approaches to identify genes that determine variant drug response.

■ For example, between-family metabolic responses to the antihypertensive drug debrisoquine were used to identify the *CYP2D6* gene in the action of this drug and polymorphisms identified that were responsible for this variation.

■ This gene has also been shown to be important in the metabolism of around 20% of described drugs, including sparteine and propafenone, both anti-arrhythmic drugs; amitriptyline, an antidepressant; and codeine, an analgesic. This knowledge could be utilised to benefit individuals.

Even where a single gene variant appears to have a strong effect on drug action, much of the variation in patient response remains unexplained by the polymorphism alone. The reasons for this are that there may be many other polymorphisms within genes that are important in cellular pathways that are involved in the interaction between the drug and its subsequent effect. It is not only the direct effect on the gene itself, but there may be polymorphisms within, for example, the promoter and enhancer regions that affect the expression of the gene.

Future studies are likely to identify polymorphisms that interact with each other in different ways.

■ For example, cytochrome P450 enzymes, including **CYP3A5**, are important in the metabolism of many drugs and a high expression of the latter enzyme, leading to more rapid drug metabolism, is seen more often in the black population.

■ In contrast, many of these same drugs are also metabolised faster if an individual possesses a particular p-glycoprotein polymorphism. These are more common among Caucasian individuals.

■ Customised treatment will have to consider all polymorphisms that alter a drug's metabolism. The identification of drugs that may have different efficacies in different racial groups may lead to questions of discrimination if some drugs are developed that benefit particular groups, even if no benefit ensues.

Any pharmacogenomics approach may be complicated by:

■ **False negatives** – where there are differences between the tissue used in research and the tissue of action in the body
■ **False positives** – simply because of the large number of areas that are being looked at, as areas will be identified by chance alone.

Identified regions in the genome will need to be confirmed through epidemiological association and biochemical functional studies, as well as in clinical models. The future hope for pharmacogenomics is the development of:

■ New drugs:
  ■ Genes identified with differing expression in cancer cells that are sensitive or resistant to anti-cancer drugs are candidates for the development of inhibitors of the gene product, reversing the drug-resistant phenotype.
  ■ For example, **imatinib** inhibits **BCR-ABL tyrosine kinase**, which is required for chronic myeloid leukaemia cell growth. Most CML patients respond well to imatinib but about 10% relapse because of mutations in the ABL kinase region.
  ■ Genetic and crystal structural information has allowed imatinib to be modified to improve binding, in the form of a new drug, **nilotinib**. Inevitably, however, different mutations are revealed that prevent nilotinib binding, requiring further research.
  ■ Development of drugs, or drug combinations, targeted to particular tissues to maximise therapeutic benefits and decrease damage in healthy cells.
■ Safer and better drugs:
  ■ Instead of the current 'trial and error' approach, where a patient is treated and switched to another therapy if the first one does not work, or has too many side effects, knowledge of the patient's genetic profile may allow the more appropriate treatment to be given from the start.
■ Appropriate drug dose:
  ■ Genetic response may be a better way to determine dose than a person's body mass in future.
■ Susceptibility to disease:
  ■ Most diseases are influenced by environmental factors and knowledge of risk may allow individuals to make important lifestyle changes and influence the timing of future drug therapies.
  ■ Genetic variants associated with increased or decreased risk of many common diseases are being identified.
  ■ **HIV** infection in humans requires chemokine receptors (CCR5 and CCR2) to effect entry of the virus into the target cells. About 10% of people carry a CCR2 polymorphism that significantly slows progression of the disease.
  ■ About 9% of Caucasian individuals have a deletion in the CCR5 gene that disrupts the receptor and makes the cells highly resistant to infection.
  ■ This knowledge has led to anti-HIV drugs being developed that interfere with the interaction between the normal CCR receptors and the virus.
■ Better drug discovery:
  ■ Many potentially useful drugs have been abandoned because of toxic side effects in some people. If this can be shown to be linked to polymorphic variations then individuals can be selected to receive, or not receive, the particular therapy.

- For example, abacavir, an anti-HIV drug, produces extreme hypersensitivity reactions in a minority of patients. This has been linked to possession of the HLA-B*5701 genotype and prospective screening of individuals has led to a significant reduction in side effects of abacavir.
- Lower healthcare costs:
  - The costs associated with getting a drug to market will be reduced if there is more information that allows the prediction of the likely response through knowledge of the genetic pathway involved.

Antibiotics and pharmacogenomics (Clinical boxes 5.15 and 5.16)

The increasing resistance of bacterial pathogens to the current antibiotics has led to the need for new ways of identifying potential antimicrobial compounds. Traditional methods of identifying such compounds have involved whole-cell screening assays, with selection based on antibacterial activity. More recently biochemical assays have been used to screen compounds for their ability to target enzymes or specific cellular pathways. Neither approach, however, has resulted in many new antibiotics being developed.

A more rational approach in the identification of potential antibiotic targets has come from genomic sequencing. The genomes of more than 100 bacteria have been sequenced and this allows the identification of proteins that are conserved across pathogens. This approach produces better information about the likely spectrum of activity of an antimicrobial agent against a particular protein, and is an unbiased approach. Comparison with the human genome also allows the identification of homologues that could present toxicity problems. Using currently available data, around 300 potential drug targets have been identified.

Evidence-based treatment

(see also Ch. 7)

We are some way off using pharmacogenomic approaches for making treatment decisions, despite there being clear candidates for their use. Current approaches in drug therapy use a trial and error approach, starting with a standard dose that will be modified by the results of biochemical tests or reporting of side effects. Changes in clinical practice will not come without proper randomised controlled studies that demonstrate a benefit in outcome. This will require a significant investment and there may be commercial pharmaceutical pressures that do not, necessarily, see the

---

Clinical box 5.15 — Examples of variation in drug metabolism associated with gene traits

Thiopurine-S-methyl-transferase (**TPMT**) breaks down drugs used as immunosuppressants, such as mercaptopurine and azathioprine. There are, however, polymorphic variants in the enzyme that result in TPMT not working. For those people who inherit two inactive variants and need to be treated with these drugs, the result will be an excess level of the drugs, leading to high toxicity that may be life-threatening. Knowledge of the type of TPMT polymorphism that an individual carries may allow lower doses of the drugs to be used effectively, without the danger of increased toxicity.

Clinical box 5.16 — Genomic sequencing and potential antibiotic targets

Peptide deformylase is a critical enzyme in the initiation of bacterial but not mammalian protein synthesis. Inhibiting the enzyme will lead to a reduction in bacterial growth and this therefore may provide a useful antibiotic target. Two compounds have been identified that inhibit the enzyme and show antibacterial activity with a potential for treating Gram-negative and Gram-positive infections.

---

advantage of the approach. Despite the costs of essential clinical trials, others will point to the high cost of providing an individual genetic profile, although this will be offset by the reduced ongoing need to monitor deleterious effects through biochemical tests, and cost is already being driven down through the introduction of SNP genotyping arrays.

GENETIC MEDICINE

Greater knowledge of the human genome means that there is hope for significant breakthroughs in the treatment of hereditary diseases. To date there has been considerable success with some diseases using metabolic manipulation or protein augmentation; genetic strategies being researched use stem cells, gene transfer and RNA modification.

Metabolic manipulation

Metabolic manipulation has been used extensively to treat inborn errors of metabolism, but may also be used to prevent complications of other therapies. Examples are:

- Diet modification:
  - **Galactosaemia**, caused by mutations in galactose-1-phosphate uridyl transferase, means that galactose cannot be converted to glucose and is metabolised to galactitol and galactonate. These metabolites lead to liver disease, intellectual disability and poor growth. Galactosaemia is the commonest disorder of carbohydrate metabolism and can be treated by restricting dietary galactose.
  - **Familial hypercholesterolaemia** can be treated with a low-cholesterol diet but this is best supplemented by drugs (**statins**) that inhibit hydroxymethylglutaryl co-enzyme A reductase.
- Protein substitution:
  - **Hydroxyurea** given to sufferers of **sickle cell anaemia** stimulates production of foetal haemoglobin, which lowers the proportion of the abnormal sickle haemoglobin, thus limiting the occurrence of sickle cell crisis.
- Treatment of toxic therapies:
  - The anaemia caused by **thalassaemia** is treated with repeated red cell transfusion. This leads to iron overload, leading to organ failure. **Desferrioxamine** chelates excess iron.
- Altering tertiary protein structure:
  - Genetic mutations may result in a mis-folding of a protein that prevents its normal function. Research is underway to look for molecules that will modify these proteins, or their target sites, in order for normal function to progress.

Protein augmentation

Individuals with absence of particular proteins can be treated through external purification of the protein and delivery back to the patient. Because there are problems with proteins reaching particular sites, such as the brain, these treatments are more simply used in diseases where the protein only needs to be available within the extracellular milieu.

- Extracellular augmentation:
  - **Cystic fibrosis** is due to mutation in the cystic fibrosis transmembrane receptor (**CFTR**) and leads to problems in sodium and chloride transport resulting in obstructive thick secretions and pancreatic insufficiency. Pancreatic enzymes are given as dietary supplements as part of the treatment.
- Intracellular augmentation:
  - **Lysosomal storage diseases**, such as **Tay–Sachs** disease, are produced by accumulations of substrates, such as sphingolipids, mucopolysaccharides, glycoproteins or glycolipids, which are not metabolised because of deficiencies in lysosomal enzymes. Excess substrate leads to cell, tissue and organ dysfunction. Enzymes need to be delivered across the cell membrane and this has been achieved, for example, by modifying the enzyme to accept markers that recognise and bind to mannose-6-phosphate within the **lysosomes** (organelles that contain enzymes that digest cellular waste, including worn-out organelles or engulfed viruses and bacteria).

Stem cell therapies

Stem cells are cells that have the ability to reproduce themselves and to differentiate along specialised lineages.

- **Embryonic stem cells** are derived from embryos in the blastocyst stage (around 100 cells) and are pluripotent
- **Somatic stem cells** are derived from organs and are already partially differentiated along the lineage of the tissue from which they originate.

Embryonic stem cell transplantation

The pluripotent nature of embryonic stem cells makes them attractive propositions for the delivery of genetic medicine, but science is not sufficiently advanced for trials to begin since human cells were first isolated and cultured only in 1998. Furthermore, there are considerable ethical considerations and public acceptability discussions to be had because of the requirement for 'unwanted' embryos. There are various ways in which it is proposed that embryonic stem cells are used:

- Cells may be differentiated in vitro and then transplanted to replace cells, or lineage-determined progenitors, in vivo.
- These cells could be used to deliver genes to alter phenotype through gene transfer.
- In vitro research can use embryonic stem cell lines carrying particular genetic disorders, derived originally from pre-implantation genetic diagnostic procedures. These form models of the disease so that pathogenesis can be studied and drug screening to be tested in vitro.

Immune rejection of material from unrelated donors may be overcome by integrating normal gene material from the patient into autologous cells, then replacing the nucleus of an unrelated donor egg by the genetically correct nucleus from the patient. The egg is stimulated to develop to the blastocyst stage and corrected autologous pluripotent stem cells are removed and transplanted into the patient. However, this simple-sounding process will depend on cells differentiating appropriately and being able to function properly when returned.

Haematopoietic stem cell transplantation

Bone marrow transplantation with haematopoietic stem cells has been used for many years to replace abnormal blood cell-forming lineages of the bone marrow in conditions such as leukaemia. This method has also been used to provide a presence of normal genes in diseases such as haemoglobinopathies, immunodeficiencies and lysosomal storage diseases.

Non-haematopoietic stem cell transplantation

Somatic stem cells have been identified in various organs and can be used to target particular deficiencies within the same lineage. Recent data demonstrate that these cells can be reprogrammed to pluripotent cells similar to embryonic stem cells by overexpressing (by gene transfer, see below) a number of transcription factors such as Oct4 and Sox2.

Neuronal ceroid lipofuscinosis (Batten disease) is due to a deficiency in **palmitoyl-protein thioesterase** and causes a neurodegeneration. Experiments in animals have shown that the transplantation of neural stem cells into the central nervous system produced engraftment of normally differentiated cells and a reduction in accumulated pathogenic substances.

Embryonic stem cells have been induced to produce **retinal pigment epithelial (RPE)** cells and clinical trials for safety of their use in patients with macular dystrophy are ongoing. Although no results have been published, there was a report in 2012 describing the outcomes in two patients whose eyesight had not deteriorated and who experienced no adverse effect. Stage I/II clinical trials for the use of RPE cells in severe myopia were approved in 2013.

Gene transfer

The principle of gene transfer is simply the introduction of a normal gene into the cells of an affected individual. Animal models have been quite successful but correction of human disorders is proving more difficult. Of the large number of trials already in place only a few have shown phenotype correction and clinical improvement. These include adenosine deaminase deficiency and X-linked severe combined immunodeficiency. There are two main methods to achieve transfer: ex vivo and in vivo.

Ex vivo approach

Cells from the relevant population are removed from the patient, modified genetically and replaced. This process is useful where the cells can be easily obtained, such as from within bone marrow, or the skin. For example:

- Transfer of factor VIII gene into autologous fibroblasts to treat haemophilia A
- Transfer of a 'suicide' gene into T lymphocytes to treat the graft-versus-host disease associated with non-autologous bone marrow transplantation.

In vivo approach

This involves direct transfer of the gene in vivo within a **vector**. If the abnormal phenotype is due to a secreted (extracellular) protein, then the transfer only needs to be sufficient, and to any site, to correct any clinical phenotype. Organs that prevent protein transfer, such as the brain and eye, will require direct delivery. If the protein works intracellularly, then the gene has to be transferred to sufficient numbers of the appropriate cells.

- Genes for transfer consist of cDNA with a promoter site, a stop site and a polyadenylation site, known as the **expression cassette**.
- The genes are placed within a vector which may be **viral**, or **non-viral**, the aim being to deliver them into the nucleus but not into a chromosome in non-dividing cells, as that will result in dilution of effect as the cells divide, or integrate the gene directly into the genome.
- **Viral vectors** include DNA-based adenoviruses, adeno-associated viruses, retroviruses and lentiviruses. Only retroviruses and lentiviruses allow permanent insertion of the gene into the genome.
- **Non-viral vectors** are normally circular plasmids that incorporate the expression cassette and an antibiotic resistance gene within a liposome that helps transfer across the plasma membrane. There are, however, no mechanisms to direct the plasmid into the nucleus, and no trials involving this method have proven successful to date.

RNA modification

This method targets mRNA in order to suppress it, or add functions. Delivery of these therapies is dependent on successful delivery and advances in research in gene transfer methodology.

Four approaches have been suggested to modify mRNA: antisense oligonucleotides, RNA interference (RNAi), trans-splicing and ribozymes.

- **Antisense oligonucleotides** are short single-stranded DNA sequences, complementary to the mRNA sequence. Once bound, ribonuclease in the cell is upregulated and this cleaves the mRNA strand, thus reducing expression of the protein that the mRNA codes for. Research to influence pre-mRNA in **Duchenne's muscular dystrophy** using antisense oligonucleotides to stimulate skipping of exons leads to removal of the mutant material and production of a truncated protein with some function.
- **RNAi** is a natural mechanism that works on a double-stranded mRNA loop and is thought to provide protection against viruses. The **Dicer** enzyme removes the loop and creates short double-sided fragments with a small 3′ overhang. One strand forms a complex and activates a ribonuclease silencing complex, which cleaves complementary sequence mRNA. If this is the mRNA associated with the disease process then expression will be reduced. This process will require significant development in the future. It needs to be able to continuously deliver enough RNAi, because it can only correct the phenotype of the cell it reaches, and would also need to be incorporated into a vector

to pass across plasma membranes. Combined gene transfer RNAi strategies have shown to work in a mouse model of **Huntington disease**, leading to improved phenotype.
- **Trans-splicing** involves correcting mutant pre-mRNA. The pre-mRNA exon is attacked by a trans-splicer pre-mRNA which has a normal exon and is delivered by a gene transfer vector. It has a 5′ tail that is complementary to the RNA strand lying 5′ of the mutant form exon, with which it hybridises. Spliceosomes remove the between-exon RNA and the normal exon is incorporated into the resultant mRNA. Animal models using this approach have been shown to correct **haemophilia A** and **cystic fibrosis**.
- **Ribozymes** are RNA constructs of the correct mRNA sequence, combined with an enzyme that recognises and cleaves the mutant mRNA, and allows ligation of the correct sequence. Specificity is provided by complementary flanking sequences. This process could replace mutant sequences, or reduce mutant mRNA levels. There are problems with ensuring efficient uptake into cells, and ribozymes are not very stable. In vitro studies using ribozymes have been shown to correct the mutation associated with **familial amyloidotic polyneuropathy**.

Future of genetic therapy

Some gene therapy trials have already been approved.

- Children born with **metachromatic leucodystrophy** have declining brain function. Bone marrow stem cells are removed and a modified virus is used to deliver correct DNA back to the patient.
- Other gene therapeutic trials are under way for Wiskott–Aldrich syndrome and adenosine deaminase deficiency, both of which lead to immune problems.

There are many challenges to be met before any genetic therapy can be used:

- Any treatment must be shown to be safe and effective.
- The rarity of individual diseases means that it will be difficult to conduct randomised controlled trials.
- Government advisory bodies will need to consider the public view of genetic therapy, and this may require education to allay fear.
- The development of genetic therapies will be very costly and impossible without the involvement of the pharmaceutical industry and there may not be sufficient financial incentives to take these processes forward.
- Use of embryonic stem cells is potentially more problematic. Some groups consider that use of blastocyst cells is the equivalent of a destruction of human life. Only since the inauguration of US President Barack Obama in 2009 has the US Food and Drug Administration approved the first clinical trial using human embryonic stem cells to treat patients paralysed through spinal cord injury. No official results have been published although preliminary results presented in 2011 reported no serious events, but also no changes to the spinal cord or neurological condition of the participants.

- In 2013 the **UK Human Fertilisation and Embryology Authority** (**HFEA**) approved the use of 'three parent' babies and the UK government will debate the proposal in 2014. Although pro-life groups have described the suggestion as 'macabre', the process is not as dramatic as the headlines suggest. The method seeks to avoid mitochondrial disease by transplanting the maternal nucleus from the disease affected 'mother' into an egg with its nucleus removed but containing healthy mitochondria. Akin to changing the cell's battery, the genetic material within chromosomes originates from the true parents.

Pathology and immunology

Denise Syndercombe Court, Paola Domizio and Armine M. Sefton

Introduction	212
INFECTION	**213**
Biological agents	**213**
Bacteria	**213**
Structure	214
Bacterial classification	215
Other bacterial surface features	215
Unusual types of bacteria	215
Replication	215
Viruses	**216**
Nucleocapsid structure	216
Host cell infection	216
Virus classification	217
Viruses and cancer	218
Fungi	**218**
Structure	218
Classification	219
Protozoa	**219**
Characteristics	219
Classification	219
Structure	220
Reproduction	220
Helminths	**222**
Classification	222
Replication	223
Prions	**223**
The symbiotic relationship between infectious agents and humans	**224**
Normal flora	224
Pathogens: successful biological infectious agents	**225**
How pathogens enter the host	225
How pathogens exploit their environments	227
The progress of a pathogenic infection	227
The pattern of disease	**231**
Local versus general infections	231
Persistence	231
Incubation period	231
Disease manifestation	231
Pandemics and epidemics	231
Prevention of infection by vaccination	231
IMMUNITY	**233**
The non-immunological defence system	**233**
Physical and functional barriers	233
Simple chemical and biological barriers	233
The immunological defence system	**233**
Detection and destruction of the invading immunogen	233

The innate immune system	234
The adaptive immune system	235
Antibodies	240
Complement	241
The cellular defences	244
Hypersensitivity	246
Tolerance	249
Autoimmune disease	249
Other substances important to the immune system	250
Inflammation and repair	**250**
Acute inflammation	250
Chronic inflammation	252
Repair	255
Lymphoid organs	**257**
Lymph nodes	257
The spleen	258
NEOPLASIA	**259**
Introduction	**259**
Growth, differentiation and development	259
Pathology of neoplasia	**263**
Epidemiology of neoplasia	263
Nomenclature and classification of neoplasms	263
Characteristics of benign and malignant neoplasms	265
Behaviour of malignant neoplasms	268
Effects of a neoplasm on the host	**269**
Local effects	269
Immunological effects	269
Metabolic effects	269
Paraneoplastic syndromes	**269**
Paraneoplastic endocrinopathies	270
Other types of paraneoplastic syndrome	270
Diagnosis, staging and prognosis of neoplasms	**270**
Diagnosis of neoplasms	270
Staging of neoplasms	271
Prognosis of neoplasms	272
Screening for malignancy	272
Carcinogenesis	**273**
Biology of neoplastic cells	273
Genes associated with cancer and oncogenesis	273
Chemical carcinogens	273
Infective carcinogens	273
Effects of radiation	274
Effects of hormones	274
Genes and inherited cancer syndromes	274
Host factors	274
Multistep theory of carcinogenesis	275

INTRODUCTION

Disease results from a failure of homeostasis within the body, which causes impaired function. Failure of homeostasis itself can be due to a multiplicity of causes, extrinsic and intrinsic, many of which are discussed in other areas of this book, and are summarised in Tables 6.1 and 6.2.

This chapter deals with biological agents that are the agents of infectious disease as well as the body's defence system, both immune and cellular, and the failure of cells to control their growth.

- Biological agents, such as bacteria and viruses, cause infections by entering the host body and are important causes of injury and damage. Often, but not always, specific organisms cause particular diseases. The defence system deals with the body's attempt to resist and repair injury. It includes inflammation, wound healing, non-immunological defence and the immune system.
- A disorder of cell growth, or neoplasia, is an abnormal proliferation of cells. Proliferation may be benign (non-progressive) or invasive (malignant).

Table 6.1	Extrinsic causes of disease	
Extrinsic factor	**Agent**	**Example**
Biological	Prion	Creutzfeldt–Jakob disease
	Bacteria	Urinary tract infection
	Viruses	Acquired immune deficiency syndrome
	Fungi	Candidiasis
	Protozoa	Malaria
	Helminths	Schistosomiasis
Chemical	Toxin	Bee sting
	Inflammatory substances	Asthma
	Poison	Tobacco smoke
Physical	Trauma	Fracture, laceration, crushed tissue
	Temperature	Burn, frostbite
	Radiation	Cancer
	Environment	Dehydration

Table 6.2	Intrinsic causes of disease	
Intrinsic factor	**Agent**	**Example**
Biochemical	Endocrine	Diabetes
	Nutritional	Obesity
	Metabolic	Phenylketonuria
Cellular	Autoimmune	Rheumatoid arthritis
	Degenerative	Alzheimer disease
	Uncontrolled cell division	Cancer
Genetic	Single gene	Sickle cell disease
	Multifactorial	Hypertension
Structural	Congenital	Heart malformation, spina bifida
	Acquired	Osteoarthritis

INFECTION

BIOLOGICAL AGENTS

The burden of infectious disease

Infectious disease is the cause of about 15–20% of deaths worldwide, but in low income countries this increases to about 40%. Figure 6.1 shows the top 10 causes of death in low income countries in 2008 and the overall percentage of deaths from each of these causes.

The variety of biological infectious agents

Organisms that cause infectious diseases can be grouped into seven major categories: bacteria, viruses, fungi, protozoa, helminths, arthropods and prions. Many are **microbes** that need a microscope to be visualised. Each has its own classification system. Early classification divided organisms into **prokaryotes** and **eukaryotes**.

Prokaryotes:

- Have no nuclear membrane
- Have DNA in the form of:
    - A single circular chromosome, forming a nucleoid
    - Plasmids, which are extracellular circular DNA molecules of varying size
- Have no membrane-bound organelles
- Have cytoplasm rich in ribosomes
- Transcription and translation can be carried out at the same time.

All **bacteria** are prokaryotes and they can be further subdivided into **eubacteria** (true bacteria) and **archaebacteria** (archaea). **Archaea** are prokaryotes, because they have no nucleus, but have introns within their genes and their ribosomal RNA (rRNA) sequence is similar to that found in eukaryotes. They were originally discovered in extreme temperature and chemical environments, but none are known pathogens and they will not be discussed further. **Viruses** have genetic material, but no other cellular characteristics, and depend on other cells for their survival. **Prions** are collections of protein molecules and are not considered living organisms. **Fungi, protozoa** and **helminths** are eukaryotes.

Eukaryotes:

- Have a separate nucleus
- DNA is carried on several chromosomes within the nucleus
- Have membrane-bound organelles – mitochondria, ribosomes on endoplasmic reticulum, Golgi apparatus and lysosomes
- Transcription requires movement of messenger RNA (mRNA) from the nucleus to the cytoplasm
- Translation takes place on ribosomes.

BACTERIA

Bacteria are a large group of ubiquitous unicellular microorganisms. They form much of the world's biomass and are vital components of the living world. Most, when they invade the human body, are destroyed by our immune system; some are beneficial, but others are harmful to humans and are described as **pathogens**. Each organism can be further classified according to various characteristics and described as a species, within a genus. For example bacteria can be grouped according to how they stain, what their shape is, whether they need oxygen and how they group or reproduce.

Information box 6.1	General characteristics of bacteria

- Prokaryotes – contain DNA and RNA
- No nuclear membrane or membrane-bound intracellular organelles such as mitochondria, Golgi apparatus or endoplasmic reticulum
- Have ribosomes for protein synthesis but these are different structurally from eukaryotic ribosomes
- Have a plasma membrane, like eukaryotes
- Most also have a cell wall, which gives bacteria their distinctive shapes
- Divide by binary fission, but can exchange genetic material.

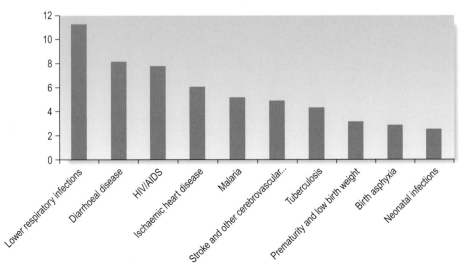

Fig. 6.1 **The top 10 causes of death in 2008 in low-income countries and % of deaths caused by each.** Data from WHO 2011, Factsheet 310, 'The top ten causes of death'.

The main cellular features of bacteria are illustrated in Figure 6.2.

Cytoplasm

Within the bacterial cytoplasm are:

- **The genome**: a single circular chromosome, plus or minus **plasmids**, which are independently replicating fragments of circular, double-stranded DNA. The chromosome is located in the **nucleoid** but there is no nuclear membrane. The genetic material is coiled and supercoiled, under the control of the enzymes DNA gyrase and DNA topoisomerase. The DNA lacks introns and extragenic sequences, such as are found in eukaryotes – it is just a continuous coding sequence of genes.
- **Bacterial mRNA**: is transcribed from DNA as in animal cells. There is no editing. Ribosomes can begin translation at one end of an mRNA molecule before the other end has been fully transcribed.
- **Ribosomes**: often a string of ribosomes is joined by a single mRNA molecule. Bacterial ribosomes are different from eukaryotic ribosomes:
  - Bacterial ribosomes are 70 S, and are composed of a 30 S portion and a 50 S portion
  - 'S' refers to **Svedberg units**, which relate to how a particle behaves under ultracentrifugation
  - Eukaryotic ribosomes are 80 S, although they do have 70 S ribosomes in their mitochondria.
- **Granules** – some bacteria have granules containing stored nutrients.
- **Mesosome** – an invagination of the cell membrane, involved in cell division.
- **Other constituents** – proteins, carbohydrates, messenger and transfer RNA, amino acids, etc.

Cell membrane (plasma membrane)

This is a phospholipid bilayer with embedded protein molecules and structures, similar to eukaryotic membranes. The membrane has four important features:

- Pores to control the entrance and exit of substances, such as nutrients, waste products and toxins

- Respiratory enzymes on the inner surface
- Enzymes involved in cell wall synthesis on the outer surface
- Is involved in binary fission.

Entry and exit of molecules through the membrane is controlled by permeases through a variety of mechanisms:

- Carrier-mediated down a concentration gradient
- Phosphorylation-linked transport
- Active transport.

Cell wall

This important structure surrounds the bacterium outside the plasma membrane. Animal cells do not have cell walls. The cell wall is strong, protects the bacterium from lysis in hypotonic solutions and from some physical trauma, and controls the access of some chemicals to the cell membrane. Different groups of bacteria have differently structured walls, determining the shape of the bacterium. They also cluster in different ways. Non-motile bacteria often stick to each other after replication.

- If they always divide in the same plane, they will end up forming long chains, like streptococci
- If they divide in different planes, they form clusters, e.g. staphylococci
- Some bacteria stick together more firmly forming long filamentous threads, such as those seen in *Actinomyces* or *Streptomyces* cultures.

The main bacterial forms are:

- Spherical (coccus) – cocci often occur in long chains (**streptococci**), in pairs (**diplococci**) or in clusters like grapes (**staphylococci**).
- Rod shaped (bacillus).
- Comma shaped (vibrios).
- Spiral (spirochaetes) – spirochaetes are long thin spiral-shaped bacteria with an outer membrane. Between the cell wall and the outer membrane are 'internal flagella': filaments running the length of the bacterium. They are motile through a spinning action and the filaments flex the bacterium to achieve this.

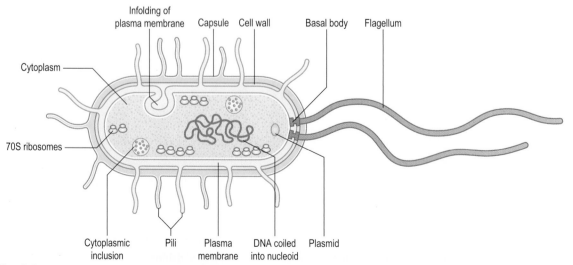

Fig. 6.2 **Illustration of a generalised bacterium.**

BACTERIAL CLASSIFICATION

Gram staining, invented by a Danish scientist in 1884, remains the standard method for classifying bacteria dependent on the structure of the cell wall. Gram staining of a heat-fixed smear of bacteria is used to separate them into **Gram positive** or **Gram negative**. The process has four stages:

- Primary staining with crystal violet (CV) which penetrates the cell wall and plasma membrane, staining the cells purple.
- A mordant, Gram's iodine (I), is added and forms a complex with the crystal violet (CV-I).
- Adding alcohol or acetone interacts with the cell membrane lipids, removing the outer layer and exposing the peptidoglycan layer. This layer is very thin in Gram-negative bacteria and the CV-I complexes are readily washed away. In contrast, the multilayered structure of Gram-positive bacteria retains the purple stain.
- Counterstaining with basic fuchsin gives a red colour to the otherwise decolourised Gram-negative bacteria.

Some bacteria, e.g. *Mycobacterium tuberculosis*, responsible for tuberculosis, also have fatty acids and waxes within the cell walls, making it very difficult for materials to pass through the wall. While this means that they are very slow at dividing it also means they do not take up the Gram stain. Ziehl–Neelsen staining method uses an acid to allow fuchsin to penetrate the cell wall and colour the bacteria, making them visible under the microscope (see Clinical box 6.1).

OTHER BACTERIAL SURFACE FEATURES

- Some bacteria form **endospores** – tough, spherical forms that resist extremes of temperature. Spore formation is triggered by adverse environmental conditions. In this form they remain dormant, with the ability to survive for many years.
  - Inhalation of endospores of *Bacillus anthracis* can lead to **anthrax.**
  - Contamination of wounds with endospores from *Clostridium tetani* leads to **tetanus**.
- Bacteria sometimes have extra material (**capsule**) outside the cells wall (Gram positive) or outside the outer membrane (Gram negative), composed of carbohydrates and/or proteins. This material hides the antigenic proteins, making them more resistant to host cell phagocytosis.
- **Flagella** are whip-like structures that move, making the bacterium motile and allowing them to respond to chemical stimulants. They are completely different from eukaryotic flagella in both structure and function.
- **Pili (fimbriae)** are long thin stiff structures, enabling bacteria to adhere to the cells of the host through specialised molecules, **adhesins**. Adhesins of *Escherichia coli* allow these bacteria to interact with fucose and mannose molecules on the intestinal epithelial cells. Although the pili are immunogenic their antigens can change (**antigenic variation**), leading to avoidance of immune recognition.

UNUSUAL TYPES OF BACTERIA

- **Chlamydia** are small Gram-negative bacteria, difficult to see, which can only divide within host cells. They have

Clinical box 6.1   Tuberculosis

Tuberculosis is an infectious, airborne disease caused by *Mycobacterium tuberculosis* (less commonly *M. bovis,*). Primary tuberculosis develops in response to the first infection by *M. tuberculosis*. This is usually subpleural, in the upper part of the lower lobe or the lower part of the upper lobe surrounded by the lobar fissure, known as the Ghon focus. The hilar lymph nodes draining the area may also be affected, and together with the primary lesion are known as the Ghon, or primary, complex. A delayed hypersensitivity reaction, an immune response, then takes place over 3–8 weeks after the initial infection, with exudate formation, and aggregations of neutrophils which are replaced by macrophages that react with T lymphocytes to form granulomas. The bacteria are not eliminated, but cell necrosis occurs to form the caseous (like soft white cheese) centre of the granuloma (tubercle) with variable amount of fibrosis. The caseous lesions heal completely, and may be calcified so that they are visible on X-ray. Some of these lesions still contain active tubercle bacilli that are dormant, but may be re-activated (usually years later) if the host immune system is compromised (e.g. in diabetes, immunosuppression, AIDS or malnutrition). Post-primary tuberculosis may then develop if the bacteria enter the bloodstream and disseminate to other foci in the body causing infection. The commonest site of post-primary tuberculosis is the lungs. Other sites include lymph nodes, the brain, skin, gastrointestinal tract and kidneys. Diffuse blood-borne dissemination results in miliary tuberculosis, which is fatal without treatment.

A positive tuberculin test, an intradermal injection of a purified protein derivative of *M. tuberculosis* (tuberculin/PPD), indicates the development of cell immunity. The Mantoux test is used for testing in individual patients, and the Heaf test is used for population screening. The vaccine bacille–Calmette–Guérin (BCG), a live attenuated vaccine made from a bovine strain of tuberculosis (*M. bovis*), is effective in reducing the risk of developing tuberculosis. The public health policy of vaccination for school children in the UK had almost eradicated the disease. The AIDS pandemic, however, has led to the re-emergence of tuberculosis, particularly in the developing world where poverty and malnutrition combined with limitation of access to medicines compound the problem.

Successful treatment of tuberculosis entails continuous self-administration of a combination of anti-tuberculous drugs, rifampicin and isoniazid (see Ch. 4), over at least 6 months. A lack of compliance, misuse of therapy and inadequate treatment have led to the emergence of multidrug-resistant tuberculosis (MDR-TB). Direct supervision in special clinics – directly observed therapy short course (DOTS) – improves compliance. Hospitalisation for treatment may sometimes be necessary for persistently uncooperative patients or those with severe disease or social indications.

a 'lifecycle' with two forms: the **elementary body** and the **reticulate body**. Both forms have a cell wall and an outer membrane. They are reminiscent of viruses, in that they have to replicate in a host cell, but they encode all of their own material, obtaining only nutrients from the host.
- **Rickettsia** can also only replicate within a host cell, but they lack the special structures and lifecycle of chlamydia. They are just small fastidious bacteria with Gram-negative structure.
- **Mycoplasma** have no cell wall, are very small and of no definite shape.

REPLICATION

The rate at which bacteria grow and divide depends mainly on the nutritional environment. *Escherichia coli*, in a rich nutrient, can divide several times in an hour, others, due to structural differences, may only divide once every 24 hours.

Bacteria when placed in a new environment grow according to a characteristic pattern:

- **Lag phase** – adjustment to the environment
- **Exponential phase** – rapid growth with constant doubling rate
- **Stationary phase** – induced as nutrients are depleted and toxic products accumulate
- **Death phase** – cell growth declines and the cells die.

Bacteria divide by binary fission. The circular chromosome replicates by using a DNA-dependent DNA polymerase, with the help of **DNA gyrase** and **DNA topoisomerase** to facilitate uncoiling. The plasmids (if any) replicate independently of the chromosome. The chromosomes attach to the plasma membrane on opposite sides of the mesosome, and binary fission takes place, dividing the cytoplasm where the mesosome invaginates.

Bacteria do not form gametes, but DNA can be exchanged between them by various methods:

- **Conjugation**: a conjugation tube forms between two bacteria, made by an outgrowth of the cell wall. Plasmids pass from one bacterium to the other along the tube.
- **Transduction**: bacteriophage viruses (complex DNA viruses) infect bacteria and replicate in the usual viral fashion. The new virions may incorporate bacterial genes from the chromosome or from plasmids, and transfer them to other bacteria.
- **Transformation**: bacteria can pick up naked DNA molecules and transcribe and translate the genes thereon. This is useful in the laboratory, but it is not certain if it occurs outside.

DNA can also move within the genome of a single bacterium: to a different place in the chromosome, from the chromosome to a plasmid, or from a plasmid to the chromosome. This is mediated by **transposons**: sequences of DNA that can loop out and in again to the main DNA strand. This ensures that any gene can be transferred by conjugation.

VIRUSES (see Information box 6.2)

The origin of viruses is unknown, but because they are dependent on host cells it seems unlikely that they are some form of precursor to life in its cellular form.

Viruses are metabolically inert; although they have genetic material they can only use this information to reproduce within host cells where they are assisted by enzymes and ribosomes from the infected cell. Outside the cell they are in the form of virus particles, or **virions**, and may lie within body fluids, within the body tissues or outside the body within the environment. Virions may sometimes be in the form of a nucleocapsid, but sometimes this may be surrounded by an outer envelope which is normally a lipid bilayer of host origin. These different forms influence how viruses survive and are transmitted.

Information box 6.2	**General features of viruses**

- Dependent on a living cell (obligate intracellular pathogen)
- Nucleic acid core (DNA or RNA, and rarely both) with protein coat (the nucleocapsid)
- 10–300 nm in size
- Circular, elongated or segmented
- Surface binding protein to attach to cell.

NUCLEOCAPSID STRUCTURE

Genomic material

This may be DNA or RNA, single stranded or double stranded. It can be linear or circular and may, or may not, use enzymes that copy the viral genome once it enters the host cell. In addition, single-stranded RNA may be:

- **Sense** – used directly as mRNA to translate viral protein
- **Antisense** – the complementary strand must be produced within the host cell to be used as mRNA.

Capsid

The capsid is a protein shell made up of numerous subunits (**capsomeres**) that give the virus a particular shape. There are three main shapes:

- **Helical** – in which the capsomeres assemble around the genome to form a tubular capsid. Most human pathogenic viruses have an envelope, e.g. the **paramyxovirus** family.
- **Polyhedral** – in which the capsid forms a geometrical shape with a central cavity. **Icosahedral** viruses have 20 faces and are a common form, e.g. the **adenovirus**. Sometimes these too are enveloped, such as the **herpesvirus**.
- **Complex** forms are larger and more varied in their structure. The **bacteriophage**, for example, has an icosahedral head and helical tail and can have a hexagonal base with protein fibres coming from it. Other complex viruses are very different in form; the **poxvirus** may show an ovoid or brick shape.

HOST CELL INFECTION

Viruses enter the human body in a variety of ways:

- Inhalation – through infected droplets
- Ingestion – from contaminated food or drink, or from saliva
- Inoculation – through injection, trauma exposure or insect bites
- Transplacentally
- Sexual intercourse.

Viruses normally infect only one or a small range of species and, once within the body, the continued success of the virus will depend on its ability to attach to the host cell and then replicate. Although replication varies, there are six basic stages (Figure 6.3):

- **Attachment**: specific receptors on the host cell bind with the viral capsid, e.g.:
  - HIV binds to human T cells through its surface protein **gp120** interacting with **CD4**, a glycoprotein found on the surface of T cells
  - Influenza virus binds to **sialic acid** found on the surface of red cells and mucous membrane cells.
- **Penetration**: this can happen in two main ways in human infections:
  - **Fusion**: attachment to the receptor causes a change in the viral envelope allowing the membranes to fuse.
  - **Viropexis**: the virus is taken up in an endocytic vesicle and the virus enters the cytoplasm. If the virus has an envelope this fuses with the vesicle membrane, like the above process but this time from within the cell.

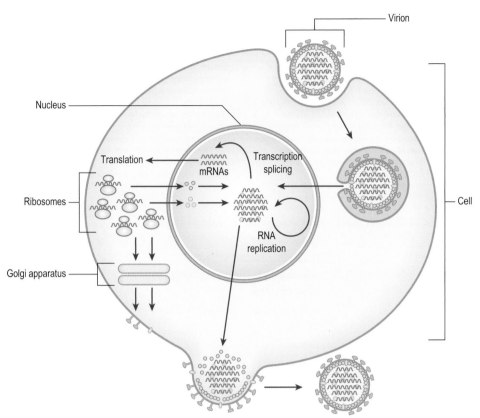

Fig. 6.3 **Viral replication.**

- **Uncoating**: enzymes from the virus or host degrade the capsid and release the genomic material into the host cell cytoplasm.
- **Replication**: this is a complex process and depends on the genomic material made available. The **Baltimore classification** proposes seven different schemes to deal with the different genomic structures. Important enzymes in these processes are:
  - **DNA-dependent DNA polymerase** which makes a complementary strand of DNA, converting a single strand into a double strand. Some viruses use the human enzyme, others use their own.
  - **DNA-dependent RNA polymerase** which uses viral DNA to produce mRNA, which can then be translated into proteins and other enzymes on host ribosomes. There are human and viral forms of this enzyme and different viruses will use different ones.
  - **RNA-dependent DNA polymerase** (**reverse transcriptase**) which makes a complementary strand of DNA from RNA strands. Humans do not have this enzyme and so these viruses (e.g. retroviruses) must use their own.
  - **RNA-dependent RNA polymerase** makes a complementary strand of RNA. Again humans do not have this enzyme, which must therefore be provided within the virion.
- **Assembly**: some of the mRNA produced through the above enzymes acting on the viral genomic material is translated on host ribosomes into viral proteins which, with replicated viral genomic material, are assembled into new nucleocapsids. This may be followed by modification (or maturation) of the viral protein, which may take place after the virus has been released from the host cell, such as in HIV.

- **Release**: although some viruses are released through lysis of the host cell, enveloped viruses **bud** off. New virions accumulate near the cell membrane which then envelopes them and then forms a bud which breaks off from the host cell, releasing the virions into the environment.

Viruses differ in how long they infect the host cell. Some are only present within the cell for a few days (such as that producing the common cold), others may be present for a long time producing a chronic infection (e.g. hepatitis B, although more commonly this causes an acute infection which then clears) and some may infect but not replicate for years, resulting in a chronic latent infection (such as HIV, or the chickenpox virus when it results in shingles). They also differ in their seriousness: Ebola, SARS (severe acute respiratory syndrome) and avian influenza are recognised as being very serious infections whereas the common cold virus and herpes simplex virus type 1 (producing cold sores) are not serious human infections (see also Clinical box 6.2).

VIRUS CLASSIFICATION

Although very varied, viruses are distinct from all other organisms. In biology a species is a population whose members can interbreed to form fertile offspring. Viruses do not undergo sexual reproduction; nevertheless the concept of species is still used, differentiating between them according to structure and genome sequence. Groupings within a species are called **strains** or **serotypes**, produced as a result of mutations that occur when the viral material undergoes replication. Table 6.3 gives examples of the classification of various clinically important viruses.

HIV is the cause of the acquired immunedeficiency syndrome (AIDS). The infection may be sexually transmitted, vertically transmitted from mother to baby, acquired through transfusion of contaminated blood, blood products and organ donation, or via intravenous drug misuse. Symptoms include fever, lymphadenopathy, sore throat, mucosal ulcers, joint and muscle pains and occasionally a transient rash. There is usually an incubation period of 2–3 weeks followed by HIV conversion lasting about 6 weeks after exposure, before symptoms develop. Clinical manifestations of AIDS cover a wide spectrum, and are related to either the direct effects of HIV infection or to immunodeficiency.

HIV infection directly affects nearly all the body systems, including neurological complications, eye disease, skin and mucous membrane complications, haematological complications and diseases relating to the gastrointestinal, renal, respiratory and endocrine systems and the heart. Immunodeficiency increases the risk of all types of infections, including tuberculosis, candidiasis, herpes simplex, pneumonias (those caused by *Pneumocystis jiroveci* in particular), cytomegalovirus, toxoplasmosis and septicaemias. Tumours, such as lymphomas and Kaposi's sarcoma, may also develop.

The introduction of highly active anti-retroviral therapy (HAART) has improved prognosis greatly, to the extent that AIDS has become a chronic disease in the developed world.

Table 6.3   **Examples of clinically important viruses and their classification**

Species	Baltimore class	Shape	Envelope
Adenovirus	Double-stranded DNA (dsDNA)	Icosahedral	No envelope
Ebola, Marburg	Antisense single-stranded RNA (−ssRNA)	Complex	Enveloped
Hepatitis A, poliovirus	Sense (+) ssRNA	Icosahedral	No envelope
Hepatitis B	dsDNA and single-stranded DNA (ssDNA)	Icosahedral	Enveloped
Hepatitis C	+ssRNA	Icosahedral	Enveloped
Herpes simplex, Epstein–Barr virus, cytomegalovirus, varicella zoster	dsDNA	Icosahedral	Enveloped
Human immunodeficiency virus (HIV)	+ssRNA	Icosahedral	Enveloped
Influenza	−ssRNA	Helical	Enveloped
Measles, mumps	−ssRNA	Helical	Enveloped
Papillomavirus	ssDNA	Icosahedral	No envelope
Rabies	−ssRNA	Helical	Enveloped
Rotavirus	dsRNA	Icosahedral	No envelope
Rubella	+ssRNA	Icosahedral	Enveloped
Smallpox	dsDNA	Complex	Enveloped

Table 6.4   **Viruses associated with particular human cancers**

Virus	Cancer
Epstein–Barr	Burkitt's lymphoma
	Nasopharyngeal carcinoma
Hepatitis B and C	Liver cancer
Human papilloma	Cervical cancer
	Skin cancer
HTLV-1 (human T cell lymphotrophic virus)	T cell leukaemia
HSV-2 (herpes simplex virus)	Cervical cancer

- Possess DNA and RNA and have a nuclear membrane
- Have complicated membrane-bound intracellular organelles: mitochondria, Golgi, endoplasmic reticulum
- Have a cell wall outside the cytoplasm, different from bacterial cell walls
- Can grow as filaments (**hyphae**) forming a mesh (**mycelium**)
- Can be **syncytial** – having multiple nuclei in the same cytoplasm
- May grow as single cells (**yeasts**) which divide asexually
- Replicate asexually (**budding**) and sexually, with gamete formation.

VIRUSES AND CANCER

Both RNA and DNA viral infections are associated with certain cancers and can lead to a malignant transformation in cells. Sometimes it is believed that other agents (**cofactors**) may also be implicated, such as malaria influencing Burkitt's lymphoma, or ultraviolet light stimulating skin cancer. Generally, but not always, the viral genome has been isolated within the cancer cells. Table 6.4 lists some viruses that are associated with particular human cancers.

FUNGI (see Information box 6.3)

Fungi are multinucleate or multicellular organisms and are eukaryotes, but quite distinct from plants and animals.

STRUCTURE

Fungal cells are eukaryotes, possessing a DNA genome, organised in linear chromosomes, with introns and extragenic material. There are no plasmids.

- The **chromosomes** are in a nucleus, with a nuclear membrane and nucleolus.
- There are **ribosomes** typical of eukaryotes having mitochondria, endoplasmic reticulum, Golgi material, etc. within the cytoplasm.
- Around the cytoplasm is a **cell membrane** which differs from those of other groups in using **ergosterol** instead of cholesterol. This is the main feature exploited by antifungal therapy.

- Outside the cell membrane is a **cell wall**; although different from bacterial cell walls it stains Gram positive. There is sometimes a **capsule** outside this.

There are two main forms that fungi can take: yeasts and mycelia. Some species can take both forms:

- **Yeasts** are individual cells, which divide by budding or binary fission
- **Mycelia** are long threads, in some cases divided by septa into cells, in others existing as syncytia.

CLASSIFICATION

There are over 250 000 species of fungi, which are classified by mycologists into four phyla according to the mode of sexual reproduction, or lack of it. Fewer than 200 species are pathogenic in humans. The mycologist's classification is not much use to the medical practitioner, and a strictly pragmatic classification is used instead, with the fungi being divided into groups depending on where the infection takes place:

- Superficial infection of the skin or hair
- Infection of the nails or subcutaneous layers of the skin
- Systemic infections.

The first two groups generally produce mild infections. Systemic infections may be life-threatening and are often seen as opportunistic infections in patients who are immunocompromised.

Fungi enter the human body through inhalation, or through wounds, but others are part of the normal flora and only cause problems in individuals whose normal body defences are reduced. Table 6.5 lists some of the important fungal infections in humans.

PROTOZOA (see Information box 6.4)

Protozoa are single-celled animals, some of which cause infections in humans. While the disease may be a direct consequence of the infection, frequently the symptoms are the result of the immune response to the infection.

| Information box 6.4 | General characteristics of protozoa |

- Are unicellular eukaryotic organisms, with DNA, RNA and a nuclear membrane
- Possess complicated membrane-bound intracellular organelles: mitochondria, Golgi apparatus, endoplasmic reticulum, etc.
- May form cysts with thick walls outside the plasma membrane, different from fungal or bacterial walls
- May have complicated lifecycles
- Replicate asexually (binary fission), and sexually, with gamete formation.

CHARACTERISTICS

Protozoa form the bulk of the biomass and play a vital role in ecology. They can grow up to 1 mm in size and are easily seen under a microscope. They are predators of bacteria and microfungi, absorbing food through their cell membranes and digesting the food in vacuoles. Protozoa have complex lifecycles. Some alternate between growth, as **trophozoites**, and dormancy, as **cysts**. Cysts allow protozoa to survive extremes of environmental conditions outside the host.

Some protozoa are important parasites of humans, infecting them in an opportunistic fashion, or are only important in the immunocompromised. The AIDS epidemic has meant that new important human parasites have come to light. Parasitic protozoa can infect all major tissues and organs either as **intracellular** or **extracellular** parasites and are most prevalent in hot countries.

CLASSIFICATION

Although originally protozoa were classified according to their movement ability, as human parasites it is more useful to classify them according to their intracellular or extracellular location.

- **Intracellular** parasites obtain nutrients from the host by direct uptake or by ingestion of cytoplasm. They infect a wide variety of cells – epithelial cells, red cell, muscle cells, brain cells, macrophages. They are

Table 6.5	Examples of fungal infections in humans		
Type	**Region of infection**	**Disease**	**Characteristics**
Superficial	Hair cells, dead skin	Tinea nigra	Produces brown macules on the hands or feet
Cutaneous	Epidermis	Tinea (ringworm)	Raised red area of skin, often looking like a ring, rapidly spread by contact
Subcutaneous	Dermis	Mycetoma	Caused by actinomycetes entering into abrasions and producing a granulomatous disfiguring infection of the skin
Systemic	Internal organs	Histoplasmosis	Fungal infection usually affecting the lungs through inhalation
Opportunistic	Internal organs	Cryptococcosis	Produces a type of meningitis in immunocompromised people. Normally found in soil and harmless otherwise
		Candidiasis	A yeast infection generally symptomatic in superficial infections (e.g. thrush) but systemic infections occur in the immunocompromised
		Aspergillosis	The fungus is found widely and used in industrial applications (such as production of citric acid) but produces an aspergillosis infection of the lungs in immunocompromised patients and others with poor respiratory function
		Pneumocystis pneumonia (PCP)	Produces pneumonia in immunocompromised people but rare otherwise

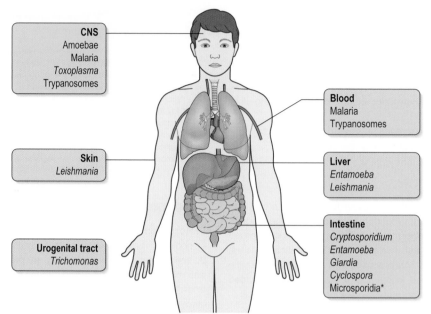

Fig. 6.4 **The occurrence of protozoan parasites in the body.** *Can also occur at other sites. CNS, central nervous system.

normally transmitted by insects (e.g. **malaria**), but can also be acquired through ingestion or in utero (e.g. ***Toxoplasma***).

■ **Extracellular** parasites obtain nutrients directly, or by ingesting host cells. This latter action can have serious implication, such as where the **malarial parasite** ruptures the infected human red cells. They are found in various locations – blood, intestine, urinogenital tract – and are normally transmitted by ingestion of cysts in contaminated food and water. Other mechanisms are possible: insect vectors transmit **trypanosomes**, and *Trichomonas vaginalis* is transmitted through sexual activity.

Figure 6.4 shows the main sites of parasitic infections in the human body.

STRUCTURE

As single cell organisms protozoa vary in size from 2 μm up to 1 mm and have evolved in different ways in order to evade immune detection of their plasma membrane.

■ Intracellular species, when within the cell, are removed from attack by antibodies, complement and phagocytes. In order to survive within macrophages (such as in **leishmaniasis**) they have developed a range of mechanisms to evade or inactivate harmful intracellular enzymes, reactive oxygen species and nitrogen metabolites. Because their antigens may be expressed at the surface of the host cell, this has offered opportunities for therapeutic intervention.

■ Extracellular species evade recognition through changes in their cell membrane, or through their fight against body responses:
  ■ **Amoebae** consume complement at the cell surface
  ■ **Malarial parasites** have polymorphic surface antigens
  ■ **Trypanosomes** undergo repeated antigenic variation, changing their surface antigens.

REPRODUCTION

In humans, reproduction of parasites is usually asexual, through binary division in trophozoite stages, which involves multiple divisions. Sexual reproduction is usually only seen within insect vectors but ***Cryptosporidium*** undergoes sexual and asexual reproduction in humans.

The complex nature of staged reproduction is illustrated by the lifecycle of the **malarial parasite** (Fig. 6.5) (see also Clinical box 6.3). The lifecycle of the malarial parasite involves a human and a mosquito host which is prevalent in tropical regions. In 2010 malaria caused an estimated 655 000 deaths of which 81% were in Africa and about 91% of these deaths in Africa were in children under 5 years old.

In the human host:

1. During a blood meal an infected ***Anopheles*** mosquito injects **sporozoites** into the human
2. **Sporozoites** infect liver cells and grow into **schizonts**, which mature, rupture and release **merozoites** (**exo-erythrocytic schizogony**)
3. **Merozoites** infect red cells and undergo asexual reproduction, producing **ring stage trophozoites** that mature again into schizonts, rupturing to release more merozoites (**erythrocytic schizogony**)
4. Rupturing of the red cell produces the clinical manifestations of the human disease. Some parasites differentiate into male and female **gametocytes** (**sexual erythrocytic stage**).

In the mosquito host (sporogenic cycle):

1. During a blood meal the *Anopheles* mosquito ingests gametocytes from an infected human host
2. In the mosquito stomach the male and female gametocytes fuse to make **zygotes**
3. Zygotes become motile and elongate as **ookinetes**, invading the midgut, and develop into **oocysts**
4. Oocysts develop and grow, rupturing to release **sporozoites**, which travel to the mosquito salivary glands
5. Sporozoites are injected into the human host with mosquito saliva during a blood meal.

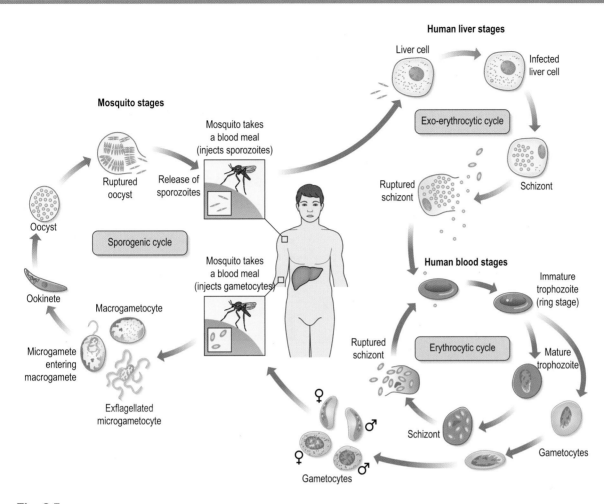

Human liver stages

Liver cell

Infected liver cell

Exo-erythrocytic cycle

Schizont

Ruptured schizont

Mosquito stages

Ruptured oocyst

Release of sporozoites

Mosquito takes a blood meal (injects sporozoites)

Oocyst

Sporogenic cycle

Ookinete

Microgamete entering macrogamete

Macrogametocyte

Exflagellated microgametocyte

Mosquito takes a blood meal (injects gametocytes)

Human blood stages

Immature trophozoite (ring stage)

Mature trophozoite

Erythrocytic cycle

Ruptured schizont

Schizont

Gametocytes

♀ ♂

♀ ♂

Gametocytes

Fig. 6.5 **Lifecycle of the malarial parasite.**

Clinical box 6.3 **Malaria**

Malaria is a parasitic, protozoal infection caused by *Plasmodium falciparum, P. vivax, P. ovale* or *P. malariae* in humans. The disease is transmitted by a vector, the female anopheline mosquito, but may also be transmitted by transfusion of contaminated blood and blood products. When the mosquito bites an infected individual, gametocytes, the sexual form of the malaria parasite, enter the insect. During an incubation period of 1–3 weeks in the mosquito stomach, fertilisation takes place and the infective malaria sporozoites develop and migrate to the salivary glands to be inoculated into the next victim bitten by the mosquito. Malaria then develops in non-immune individuals with fever, general malaise and sometimes gastrointestinal symptoms. The fever is usually severe with body temperature reaching up to 41°C, sweating and rigors.

Once the immature parasites have entered the circulation, those that are not destroyed by the immune system are taken up by the liver where they multiply in the hepatocytes (merozoites). The hepatocytes rupture after a few days to release merozoites into the bloodstream where they invade the red cells and multiply

and form new merozoites. The red cells then rupture, releasing the new merozoites which infect more red cells. Some species attack young red cells and reticulocytes. The subsequent course of the disease depends on the infecting *Plasmodium* species. Widespread organ damage may occur due to haemolytic anaemia resulting from the rupture of red cells, cytokine release and impaired microcirculation (*P. falciparum*). Cerebral, renal, metabolic, respiratory and endocrine complications may also occur. The genetic variation that resulted in the sickle cell gene evolved owing to the increased malaria resistance conferred by sickle cell disease (see Ch. 12).

Treatment of malaria with chloroquine or quinine is usually effective, but widespread resistant strains of *Plasmodium* have emerged. Personal protection (malaria prophylaxis) when travelling to endemic areas is preferable. Vector eradication is necessary, but not always feasible or desirable (e.g. use of insecticides). Protection from mosquito bites with treated bed nets is also effective.

There are four main parasites that produce malaria, and the disease caused by each is usually characterised by the frequency of the fevers produced by the reproductive stages in the human. Fevers tend to occur at 2-day (tertian) or 3-day (quartan) intervals.

- *Plasmodium vivax* (**tertian**):
  - Prevalent in Asia, Latin America and some parts of Africa.
  - Has a dormant phase in which **hypnozoites** persist in the liver and result in relapses, weeks or years later.

- Generally the disease caused is non-fatal, but it can result in **splenomegaly** (enlarged spleen) which can cause complications that lead to death.
- *Plasmodium falciparum* (**tertian**):
  - The most dangerous malarial parasite, accounting for the majority of deaths.
  - Prevalent in sub-Saharan Africa.
  - Trophozoites and gametocytes are often seen in the peripheral blood, unlike in other species.

- Individuals with the abnormal **sickle cell** haemoglobin are relatively protected from *P. falciparum* infection. Merozoites normally interact with red cells through two PfEMP-1 (*Plasmodium falciparum* erythrocyte membrane protein 1) dependent interactions. These proteins are impaired in individuals with sickle cell haemoglobin, explaining why sickle cell disease has not been lost from the tropical world through natural selection.
- *Plasmodium ovale* (**tertian**):
  - Rarer than *P. vivax* and *P. falciparum*, it is found in west Africa and the extremes of south-east Asia.
  - Like *P. vivax* it can produce hypnozoites in the liver, allowing relapses.
- *Plasmodium malariae* (**quartan**):
  - Rare but found worldwide.
  - Produces a benign or chronic long-lasting disease.

HELMINTHS (see Information box 6.5)

Helminths are eukaryotic parasitic worms that live within and obtain nutrients from their hosts.

Worms are complex and often large organisms. Although the infecting larval forms are usually small (100–200 µm), the adults can be several metres in length. Infections are more common in warm countries, in children and in people working closely with animals because of the association with food. Intestinal infections, in particular, are seen worldwide, but worms can live in other tissues. Transmission can occur in four main ways (Fig. 6.6):

- Faecal–oral – ingesting infective eggs or larvae from an infected human host
- Intermediate – ingesting infective larvae from another infected host, such as eating uncooked infected meat
- Active – when larval stages penetrate the skin
- Bite – when insects suck blood – relatively uncommon.

CLASSIFICATION

There are three main groups of helminths important in human infections:

- Tapeworms (Cestodes)
- Flukes (Trematodes)
- Roundworms (Nematodes).

Information box 6.5	General characteristics of helminths

- Multicellular eukaryotic organisms, with DNA, RNA and a nuclear membrane
- Lack backbones, notochords and jointed exoskeletons: they are 'worms' in common parlance
- May form cysts with thick walls around the whole organism
- May have complicated lifecycles, with different forms in different hosts
- Replicate asexually and sexually, with gamete formation.

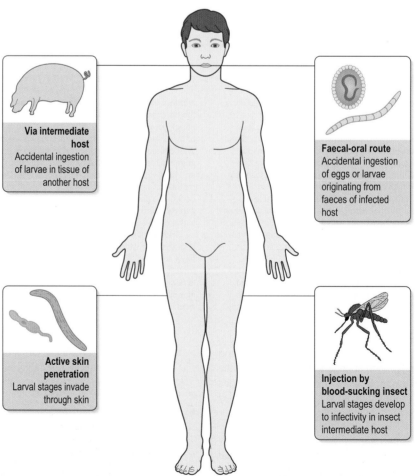

Via intermediate host
Accidental ingestion of larvae in tissue of another host

Faecal-oral route
Accidental ingestion of eggs or larvae originating from faeces of infected host

Active skin penetration
Larval stages invade through skin

Injection by blood-sucking insect
Larval stages develop to infectivity in insect intermediate host

Fig. 6.6 **How helminth parasites enter the body.**

Schistosomiasis is an important helminth parasitic infection in humans. Also known as **bilharzia**, the disease is spread in water contaminated with infected freshwater snails. Common in many tropical developing countries it particularly affects children who may be playing or swimming in the water. Although it is not fatal, it produces a chronic disease that damages other organs and can impair development in children, and can increase the risk of some cancers.

- Flukes are mainly hermaphrodites that release larva from intermediate hosts, such as fish, crustaceans or vegetation, which are subsequently ingested
- Schistosomes, whose larvae released from snails penetrate the skin, have separate sexes (see also Clinical box 6.4)
- Tapeworms have replicated reproductive organs along their body (**strobila**) that break off when filled with mature eggs, passing out through the faeces.

Flukes and roundworms feed on human tissues and the contents of the host intestine. Tapeworms have no digestive system and must absorb digested nutrients from their host. Both tapeworms and flukes have complex plasma membranes with mechanisms to protect themselves from a host attack. They release large amounts of soluble antigenic material that plays an important role in the disease and subsequent immunity. Nematodes have a collagenous cuticle in the adult form, which makes them less vulnerable to immune attack.

Humans may also be infected by larvae from other hosts. *Toxocara canis* is a dog parasite that can also infect humans.

REPLICATION

Most helminths replicate outside the host. In the intestine sexual reproduction produces eggs which are released in the faeces and return to the human host as adults through faeces or injection.

- Nematodes:
  - Can develop to maturity within a single host. The *Strongyloides* nematode also hatches its eggs within the intestine producing an **autoinfection**
  - Have separate sexes
  - Some mature in the intestine: *Ascaris,* hookworms, *Strongyloides, Trichinella*
  - Some mature in deep tissues: filarial worms.
- Flukes and tapeworms:
  - Must pass through an intermediate host or hosts

PRIONS

Prions were named by the American neurologist, Stanley Prusiner, when he defined them as: '**pro**teinaceous **in**fectious particles that lack nucleic acid'. The unlikely concept of an infectious agent that lacks nucleic acid has meant that there continue to be scientists who believe that they could be acting with other agents, such as slow-acting viruses.

PrP^C is a normal protein found in cell membranes and consists of amino acids in a mainly α-helical structure. There is some evidence that the protein is involved in the maintenance of long-term memory within the part of the brain known as the **hippocampus**. **PrP^{SC}** is an atypical form in which a large proportion of the α-helical structure is replaced by a different type of secondary structure, the β-sheet. Its amino acid sequence is, however, no different from the normal form, although there are sequence differences in the protein between species. This sequence difference is thought to be the reason for resistance to cross-species infectivity.

An isoform of PrP^C appears to catalyse its transformation into the abnormal form, PrP^{SC}, resulting in a different structure and attracting, through aggregation, free proteins, to form **amyloid** that accumulates and is deposited locally in the tissues. Over 20 different strains of the infective agent have been described, resulting in variable incubation periods and pathology. It is thought that these strains arise through a conformational change that occurs on crossing between the species (see Clinical box 6.5).

Five different human prion diseases have been identified, including Creutzfeldt–Jakob disease (CJD), variant CJD (vCJD) and kuru.

Creutzfeldt–Jakob disease (CJD). Classic CJD is a fatal neurodegenerative disease that occurs sporadically in about 1 in 1 000 000 people each year, although inherited forms caused by a mutation in the prion gene also exist. It is more common with increasing age and patients experience dementia and show early neurological abnormalities. Sections of brain tissue have a 'sponge-like' appearance. Transmission has been shown within human growth hormone, through corneal implants and on surgical instruments.

Variant CJD (vCJD). This was first described in 1996 and has a different clinical presentation from CJD, patients typically being young adults displaying marked behavioural symptoms and a marked accumulation of the abnormal protein.

There is strong evidence that vCJD is causally linked to ongoing outbreaks of **bovine spongiform encephalopathy (BSE, or 'mad cow disease')** which is a prion disease occurring in cattle. BSE began in the 1970s after cattle were fed with a bone meal food probably from sheep infected with **scrapie**, another prion disease. BSE became more common in the UK when calves were fed with BSE-infected bovine material. By the end of 2005 more than 35 000 herds of cattle had been affected.

vCJD was linked to the BSE outbreak during which individuals ate beef contaminated with central nervous system material from infected cattle. Until the end of 2007, 166 patients had been identified in the UK, 163 of whom died, with a peak in deaths in 2000. Although many individuals may carry the infection, only those who are homozygous for amino acid methionine at position 129 in the *PRNP* gene have so far been infected by this route. Although there are measures to prevent potentially infected tissues from entering the human and animal food chains, reducing the disease incidence, more recent cases have been associated with blood transfusions from individuals who themselves subsequently developed vCJD, suggesting that blood donation is a relatively efficient transmission route.

Kuru, meaning 'trembling in fear', was a fatal disease that occurred in the Fore people of Papua New Guinea in the 1950s and was associated with cannibalistic rituals in which the people ate human brain tissue. It is very similar to vCJD and is thought to have originated from scrapie-infected sheep.

THE SYMBIOTIC RELATIONSHIP BETWEEN INFECTIOUS AGENTS AND HUMANS

An infectious agent may be able to live completely independently of its potential host, but usually it has to form some association with it. These associations are called **symbiosis**.

- **Parasitism** is when one member of the association gains an advantage, and the other is harmed. The harm ranges from some disadvantage without overt disease, to overt disease which may be lethal.
- **Commensalism** is where one member of the association gains an advantage, and the other is left unaffected. *Bacteroides* species are present in large numbers in the large intestine.
- **Mutualism** is where both members of the association gain an advantage, the popular meaning of symbiosis. *Bacteroides* infection in cattle rumen provides fatty acids as a nutrient for the host.

When an infectious agent causes disease it is acting as a pathogen. However, there are many infectious agents that can exist in a commensal or even mutualistic relationship with their host, and only become pathogenic in some special circumstances.

NORMAL FLORA

The **normal flora** consist of microorganisms, mostly bacteria, present on many of the body surfaces in the normal healthy individual.

The whole body is normally sterile immediately before birth, but the surfaces rapidly become colonised after delivery. The skin, mouth, upper respiratory tract, gastrointestinal tract and genitourinary tract acquire a variety of microorganisms from the environment and from contact with other people. Bacteria form a major component of faeces. Secretions such as saliva, sebum and tears are normally sterile within the glands but become contaminated as soon as they reach the mucous membrane or skin surface. Blood, cerebrospinal fluid, lymph, bones, joints and all internal organs are normally sterile in health.

Establishment of microorganisms at particular sites depends on several factors, including exposure of the site, availability of suitable receptor sites and ability of organisms to adhere to target receptor sites, to compete for nutrients and to evade or withstand host defence mechanisms. Figure 6.7 illustrates microorganisms found within the body as normal flora.

Normal flora offer humans several benefits:

- Colonisation leads to resistance to more virulent bacteria.
- Microorganisms may digest nutrients in the bowel (more important in animals).

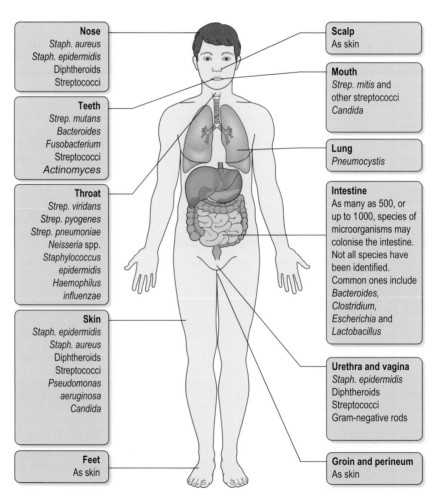

Nose
Staph. aureus
Staph. epidermidis
Diphtheroids
Streptococci

Teeth
Strep. mutans
Bacteroides
Fusobacterium
Streptococci
Actinomyces

Throat
Strep. viridans
Strep. pyogenes
Strep. pneumoniae
Neisseria spp.
Staphylococcus epidermidis
Haemophilus influenzae

Skin
Staph. epidermidis
Staph. aureus
Diphtheroids
Streptococci
Pseudomonas aeruginosa
Candida

Feet
As skin

Scalp
As skin

Mouth
Strep. mitis and other streptococci
Candida

Lung
Pneumocystis

Intestine
As many as 500, or up to 1000, species of microorganisms may colonise the intestine. Not all species have been identified. Common ones include *Bacteroides*, *Clostridium*, *Escherichia* and *Lactobacillus*

Urethra and vagina
Staph. epidermidis
Diphtheroids
Streptococci
Gram-negative rods

Groin and perineum
As skin

Fig. 6.7 **Examples of organisms that occur as members of the normal flora and their location on the body.**

- Presence of the normal flora also resists other colonisation attempts through:
  - Competition for receptor sites involved in adhesion
  - Competition for essential nutrients for growth
  - Creation of unfavourable micro-environments that discourage colonisation.
- Lactobacilli in the vagina produce acid from glycogen and maintain low pH which is unsuitable for many exogenous bacteria and *Candida.*
- Production of inhibitory substances. Some staphylococci on the skin produce antibiotics, which inhibit other bacteria.

Different groups of bacteria that are adapted to live as normal flora are found in different sites: the mouth, the gastrointestinal tract, the nose and oropharynx, the skin, the vagina. There are no simple criteria such as morphology, staining, biochemical characteristics or growth requirements that distinguish normal flora from pathogens. The normal flora may be disrupted through a variety of mechanisms:

- Suppression by antimicrobial agents allowing overgrowth with resistant organisms
- Changes in general health or immunity
- Hormonal changes
- Local trauma.

Particular sites of normal flora may be affected in certain circumstances, allowing overgrowth by more virulent organisms:

- Mouth:
  - Dietary changes
  - Reduction in salivary secretion
  - Dental disease, dental treatments and oral hygiene
- Gastrointestinal tract:
  - Dietary changes
  - Gut disorders
- Female genital tract:
  - Menstrual cycle
  - Pregnancy
  - Intrauterine contraceptive device
- Skin
  - Use of soaps, cosmetics, antiseptics
  - Moisture – wet or dry
- Respiratory tract
  - Viral infections
  - Secondary bacterial infections
  - Damage to ciliated epithelial cell function (through smoking, for example).

Sometimes organisms which are part of a person's normal flora can act as pathogens. This tends to occur when there is:

- Breakdown in the local epithelium because of trauma (e.g. surgery) or other infection
- Introduction to an unusual site (e.g. gut organisms in the urinary tract, possibly introduced by medical interventions such as catheterisation)
- Alteration in balance of normal flora (e.g. use of antimicrobial drugs can also lead to suppression of *Lactobacillus* in the vagina, encouraging *Candida* growth)
- Immunodeficiency.

PATHOGENS: SUCCESSFUL BIOLOGICAL INFECTIOUS AGENTS

HOW PATHOGENS ENTER THE HOST

Microorganisms, in order to become pathogens, must attach to, or penetrate the **body surface** – a series of surfaces (Fig. 6.8) that is extensive, offering considerable opportunities for its penetration. All these surfaces offer a portal for entry and all are covered by some kind of epithelium; the keratinised stratified squamous epithelium of the skin is the toughest. Epithelia have both innate and adaptive immune mechanisms in place and are capable of mounting an immunological response (see below). For example:

- IgA in mucous membranes blocks pathogenic adhesion
- Lysozyme attacks bacterial peptidoglycan.

The epithelial surfaces are more easily breached if defence mechanisms are impaired. In untreated or uncontrolled diabetes mellitus, which impairs phagocyte activity, there is increased glucose available for pathogens, predisposing the patient to infection, especially of the skin and urinary tract. In AIDS, depletion of CD4 T lymphocytes and infection of dendritic cells allow opportunistic infections to gain access (see below). Other mechanisms that allow, or protect from, entry are described below.

Skin

The skin is a tough, multilayered membrane rendered waterproof by keratin, and more resistant to pathogenic invasion than internal membranes.

- Sebum from sebaceous glands has antibacterial action
- Clothing helps maintain integrity.

Some agents can penetrate intact skin:

- **Arthropods**: some pathogens have adapted to a lifecycle that is dependent on biting arthropods (e.g. mosquitos,

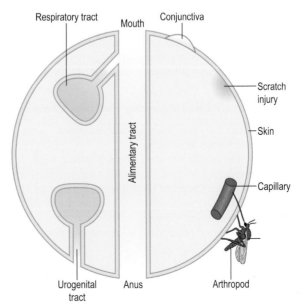

Fig. 6.8 **Body surfaces which are sites of infection and shedding.**

flies, fleas, bugs, ticks and mites), penetrating the skin when they feed on human blood.

- **Needles**: any mechanism in which needles are introduced into patients (taking blood, setting up intravenous access, blood transfusion) may introduce a pathogen. A patient may be infected locally by skin flora, staff may be infected, or the agent that is being transmitted may carry a pathogen. Good hygiene, screening of donated blood and education of intravenous drug users can reduce this.
- **Surgical wounds** allow entry of any contaminating pathogens in much the same way. *Staphylococcus aureus* is a particular problem because of antibiotic resistance.
- **Abrasions and wounds**: apparently intact skin often allows entry through minor cuts and abrasions leading to conditions such as warts, from the **papillomavirus**, or impetigo from *Staph aureus*.
- **Animal bites** enable a large variety of bacteria to infect the tissues. For example, **rabies** virus is present in the saliva of infected animals, and is passed on via bites.
- **Wounds of violence and war** allow infection by a wide variety of contaminating bacteria. Foreign bodies in tissues are associated with local anoxia, encouraging the growth of anaerobic bacteria.
- **Intact skin** can be penetrated by some larvae.

Respiratory tract

This is particularly vulnerable because it is a very large area of moist living cells which are exposed to pathogens that may be present in inspired air, or through the lachrymal duct in the eye. The fact that the barrier between air and circulation in the alveoli is only one cell thick makes the potential for infection high. The respiratory system offers various defences:

- Hairs in the nose trap large foreign particles
- Sneeze and cough reflexes expel foreign bodies, excess mucus and infected secretions
- Mucus, produced by goblet cells and subepithelial mucous glands, contains IgA and lysozymes and traps foreign particles
- Cilia in the pharynx help remove particles so they can be swallowed (mucociliary escalator)
- Alveolar macrophages phagocytose and destroy small particles.

Other environmental factors may break these defences:

- Conditions that inhibit the mucociliary escalator – such as cystic fibrosis, or smoking
- Anatomical defects that allow mucus to collect, e.g. bronchiectasis
- Foreign bodies that might block bronchi, e.g. peanut inhalation
- Drugs that suppress the cough reflex
- Inhalation of food or vomit in the unconscious person.

Gastrointestinal tract

This is vulnerable because, in order to absorb nutrients, it has a very large surface area which is constantly being exposed to the environment through food and drink, which might be contaminated (see Clinical box 6.6).

Clinical box 6.6 **Bacterial causes of food poisoning**

Food poisoning (gastroenteritis) may be defined as 'usually either infectious or toxic in nature, caused by agents that enter the body through the ingestion of food (or water)'. Diarrhoeal diseases are among the leading causes of death in children under the age of 5 years, particularly in the developing world. Bacteria cause gastroenteritis in three possible ways, sometimes a mixture of all three:

- By adherence to specific receptors in the intestinal mucosa prior to invasion, to produce secretory diarrhoea as the direct result of adhesion.
- By invasion of the intestinal epithelium to produce bloody diarrhoea with abdominal pain (dysentery). Common infecting agents include *Campylobacter*, *Shigella*, *Salmonella* and enteroinvasive *Escherichia coli*.
- By producing toxins that cause excessive fluid loss into the intestinal lumen, causing profuse, watery diarrhoea. Organisms include *Salmonella*, *Vibrio cholerae*, verotoxin-producing *E. coli*, *Bacillus cereus*, *Staphylococcus aureus*, *Clostridium difficile*, *C. botulinum* and *C. tetani*.

The gastrointestinal tract defends itself through:

- Stratified squamous epithelium in the mouth and oesophagus, which is less easy to penetrate than the simple epithelium found below the stomach
- Low pH in the stomach and bile, both of which kill many pathogens
- Mucus traps microbes and impedes their transport
- IgA in saliva and digestive juices blocks the adherence of pathogens, and lysozyme attacks bacterial cell walls
- Normal flora in the small and large intestine compete with pathogens
- The vomiting reflex and diarrhoea void damaging contents through refection and increased turnover of gut epithelium.

Urogenital tract

Pathogens may pass up the urethra or vagina. Sexual intercourse is frequently involved. There are various defence mechanisms, which vary according to male or female anatomy:

- In the **urinary tract** the flow of urine, complete emptying of the bladder and functional integrity of the epithelium are important to resisting infection
- In the **vagina** normal flora are important, competing with pathogens and maintaining an acid pH.

Most **urinary tract infections** come from the outside, via the urethra (**ascending**). Females are much more vulnerable because they have a shorter urethra and are more exposed through sexual intercourse, which can breach the intact epithelium. The entire urinary tract can also be infected through other routes: for example, renal abscess, renal tuberculosis and bladder schistosomiasis offer opportunity for infection to enter the urinary tract other than the usual route, through the urethra.

The eyes

- The conjunctiva of the eye is formed of stratified, but not keratinised, epithelium and is protected by tears (containing lysozyme and IgA) and the cleansing action of the lids
- **During childbirth**, neonates' conjunctivae are vulnerable to infections of the mother's cervix or vagina, such as those caused by *Neisseria gonorrhoeae* or *Chlamydia trachomatis*
- The naso-lachrymal duct offers a possible route of infection from the eye to the upper respiratory tract.

Placenta

A variety of pathogens may cross from an infected mother to the foetus across the placenta, such as rubella and hepatitis B viruses (although the latter much more commonly causes infection during delivery).

Childbirth

Childbirth offers further opportunities for exposing a newborn infant to infections through a variety of portals described above and it may not always be possible to determine which.

HOW PATHOGENS EXPLOIT THEIR ENVIRONMENTS

Pathogens are successful because they exploit the environments provided by a host, whether living within or outside cells. All pathogens need a supply of metabolic material, although viruses (which lack nuclei) need nuclear synthesis. This means that viruses can only live within host cells. Other organisms may flourish inside or outside the cell, or both, taking their nutrients from the cytoplasmic or extracellular fluid. The larger pathogens, such as **nematodes**, are almost always extracellular and some may gain their nutrients by ingesting host cells.

- **Intracellular pathogens**, while being vulnerable to intracellular killing mechanisms, are protected from many of the host defence mechanisms, as well as from therapeutic agents. The pathogens may also live within the same cells that are responsible for the host immune reaction, reducing the ability of the host to mount a defence against the infecting organisms. To succeed, however, these organisms must have an extracellular phase as they pass between cells, and this offers opportunities for host and therapeutic attack. Any attack, intracellular or extracellular, makes the host cells vulnerable and many will die, leading to tissue damage.
- **Extracellular pathogens** are exposed continuously to the host cellular defence mechanism. For this reason they tend to be larger and more complex: they are able to move rapidly and reproduce faster than others. They may also have a structure that means, for example, that they are not vulnerable to mechanisms such as phagocytosis. The **helminths** (worms) are typical of these organisms.

THE PROGRESS OF A PATHOGENIC INFECTION

Adhesion

Almost all pathogens have to adhere to host cells. The cells at the portal of entry are often the first target, but adhesion is essential later in dissemination round the body. Pathogens that are injected into the host do not have to adhere in order to invade, but they will probably have to adhere later.

- **Bacteria** exhibit various different adherence mechanisms:
  - **Non-specific** adherence: hydrophobic molecules in walls, capsules and slime all adhere non-specifically to host cells.
  - **Specific** adherence: many bacteria have adhesins, either on the cell wall, outer membrane or other wall structures, which bind to molecules on host cells.
  - Carbohydrates, such as D-mannose, sialic acid and blood group carbohydrates.
  - Proteins, e.g. fibronectin.
- **Viruses** have docking proteins, e.g. haemagglutinins on the influenza virus. This may be at the portal of entry, or, if they are injected in some way, they may travel to a site where they can bind.
- **Helminths** may have specialised mouth parts, such as found in the tapeworm or the hookworm, which enable the organism to be retained within the bowel.

Invasion

Some pathogens do not invade, but continue to adhere to the epithelium at the portal of entry, e.g. skin fungi, *Vibrio cholerae*. Others may invade the portal of entry, and spread no further, while others do spread further. Invasion may take the pathogen into the host's cells, or between the cells into the extracellular spaces, or both. It usually follows adhesion, but a pathogen may invade by being injected.

- **Bacteria**: may move between cells, through the intercellular junctions, e.g. *Salmonella* spp., while others may invade the cells to which they have adhered. This can lead to host cell involvement:
  - host cell actin polymerisation may be induced, leading to pseudopod formation and bacterial engulfment within a vacuole, and
  - the vacuole disintegrates and the bacterium lies free within the cytoplasm.
- **Viruses**: all viruses must invade (infect) a cell to reproduce after adhesion via the docking protein. Many viruses enter cells on mucous membranes and remain localised to the epithelium with disease developing within a few days. There is little or no invasion of underlying tissue, and the virus is shed directly to the exterior. These local infections offer only short-term immunity. Influenza viruses, rhinoviruses and, in the gastrointestinal tract, rotaviruses are all viruses of this type.
- **Fungi**: use enzymes to break down ground substance and matrix of epithelia and connective tissue.

Host organ dissemination

- **Bacteria** can be disseminated through:
  - Tissues, aided by enzymes such as collagenase, hyaluronidase and streptokinase.
  - Blood through which bacteria can reach any tissue or organ. A **bacteraemia** is the presence of live bacteria in the blood; when the bacteria multiply in the blood this produces septicaemia.

(See also Clinical boxes 6.7 and 6.8.)

Viruses that have the capacity to invade subepithelial tissues may enter the lymphatic system.

- If the virus is quickly inactivated by macrophages from the lymph node sinuses, the immune response is initiated, resulting in a regional **lymphadenopathy**, but the infection does not progress.

Clinical box 6.7 **Meningitis**

Meningitis, an inflammation of the meninges, is an important public health issue that is often potentially preventable. It is more prevalent in developing nations. Viral meningitis is commoner than bacterial meningitis but is usually self-limiting in the UK with the exception of *Herpes* meningo-encephalitis.

The main bacterial causes of acute bacterial meningitis in people who have not been immunized are:

- *Haemophilus influenzae* B (in children under 5 years)
- *Neisseria meningitidis*
- *Streptococcus pneumoniae*
- Other bacterial causes include *Mycobacterium tuberculosis*, *Listeria monocytogenes* (in the immunocompromised) and Group B streptococci and *E. coli* in neonates.

Clinically, the classic triad of fever, headache and neck stiffness should give rise to suspicion of meningitis. A petechial rash may precede the symptoms, septicaemic shock may develop, and death may ensue. Bacteraemia may lead to multisystem/multiorgan infection.

The capsular polysaccharides of *N. meningitides* that inhibit destruction and clearance (phagocytosis) by the host defence mechanisms have been used to produce vaccines (meningococcal conjugate C vaccine), which were introduced into the UK's routine vaccination of children programme in 1999. *Haemophilus influenzae* B (Hib) vaccine and a polyvalent pneumococcal vaccine are also available.

Clinical box 6.8 **Multisystem bacterial infection: *Escherichia coli***

Some bacteria target specific organs or systems, but other bacterial infections can lead to multisystem disease. One example is *E. coli*, which has an enterohaemorrhagic form (serotype 0157:H7), also known as verotoxin-producing *E. coli* (VTEC). The enteroinvasive form of *E. coli* causes bacillary dysentery, but VTEC not only causes bloody diarrhoea but also secretes a toxin that affects vascular endothelial cells in the bowel and kidneys, when the patient may develop thrombocytopenic purpura and/or haemolytic uraemic syndrome (HUS). Administration of antibiotics may exacerbate HUS by increasing toxin production.

- If the virus is not inactivated, particularly if it can survive or replicate in macrophages or lymphocytes, the particles are passed through the lymph nodes into the bloodstream.
- The virus is likely to be distributed to distant parts of the body and establish infection in the reticuloendothelial system (the **primary viraemia – an** asymptomatic event during the incubation period).
- Following a period of replication in distant sites, such as liver and spleen, large amounts of progeny virus may be released into the bloodstream, leading to the onset of clinical effect of a **systemic viral infection**, which can spread to other organs.
- If the virus lodges in skin capillaries, a rash may be a prominent feature, such as is seen in measles and chickenpox.
- The nature of viraemia depends on the virus. Those carried in monocytes or lymphocytes are more protected and can be disseminated more widely.

Survival within the host

As soon as a pathogen reaches the portal of entry, it encounters the defence system. The **non-immune aspect** includes the integrity of the epithelium, chemical defences and normal flora. Agents of the innate and adaptive immune systems may be present at the portal, and will be further encountered

Clinical box 6.9 **Versatility of microorganisms: example *Helicobacter pylori***

In order to invade the host, microorganisms have to evade normal protective physical or chemical barriers. One example is *H. pylori*, a Gram-negative spiral organism that causes gastritis and peptic ulcers, and is a predisposing factor for gastric cancers. *H. pylori* infects 50–90% of the world population with the highest prevalence in developing countries with poorer hygiene. In order to attach to and colonise the human gastric mucosa, *H. pylori* has to survive in the extreme acidic environment and overcome the mucous secretions in the stomach. This is facilitated by its motility and the secretion of the enzymes urease and catalase.

if the pathogen invades or is disseminated. Survival of the pathogen depends on circumventing the defence system, which it does in several ways (see also Clinical box 6.9):

- Stress survival:
  - Host defences may damage the pathogen by denaturing proteins.
  - **Chaperonins** (heat shock proteins) protect against denaturing of other proteins.
  - **Free radicals**, such as superoxide and hydroxyl radicals, and hydrogen peroxide damage and kill pathogens. They may be produced by the pathogen's aerobic metabolism, or by host defences.
- Scavenge for nutrients:
  - Some nutrients, sugars, amino acids and fatty acids are freely available, but iron, in the form of Fe^{3+}, is not. This form of iron is important for bacterial survival and its inaccessibility is part of the non-specific defence provided by the body.
  - Bacterial siderophores bind iron avidly and capture it for the bacterium.
  - Fungi use sophisticated mechanisms to acquire nutrients as saprophytes.
- Shelter:
  - If the pathogen can enter host cells it will be protected from **antibody** attack. All viruses replicate within host cells, and some bacteria, fungi and protozoa shelter within cells.
  - Some survive within phagocytes, either by escaping from the phagosome into the cytoplasm, preventing phagosome-lysosome fusion (e.g. **toxoplasmosis**), or by being tough and resisting the phagocytic enzymes and radicals (e.g. *M. tuberculosis*).
  - When bacteria or virions are released from the cell they are fully exposed to the immune system, but viruses or bacteria that pass directly from one cell to another minimise this exposure.
  - Some pathogens survive in sites where the immune system is poorly represented, such as the lens of the eye, which can become infected in congenital rubella infection.
  - The pathogen is not completely protected from the immune system. The infected cell will present pathogen-derived antigens on class I human leucocyte antigen (HLA) molecules, and can be killed by CD8 T lymphocytes, destroying the shelter (see below).
  - Some viruses, however, can suppress the expression of HLA molecules (e.g. cytomegalovirus). Latent infections by viruses will not generate any viral proteins.

- **Stealth**: sometimes the pathogen is fully exposed but avoids a lethal encounter through disguise or deception. This can be done in a variety of ways:
  - **Shielding**: bacteria, for example, may have structures outside their cell walls, such as capsules and slime, which prevent recognition and subsequent phagocytosis and complement activation that would destroy them.
  - **Active action**: bacteria may also possess protein A, which blocks binding of the Fc portion of the antibody to its receptor, thus blocking **opsonisation**, the process through which a pathogen is prepared for phagocytosis.
  - IgA proteases within bacteria can also cleave IgA, which mediates transport of immune complexes across epithelial cells.
- **Antigenic variation**: some pathogens mutate and thus change their antigens. This may happen during an infection of a single individual, such as in **African trypanosomiasis**, or it may happen between outbreaks, such as in **influenza**, so that the pathogen remains one step ahead.
- **Antigenic mimicry** or adsorption of host protein: for example, *S. aureus* adsorbs fibrin and IgG.
- **Ineffective antibody**: many pathogens elicit an antibody response, but it is ineffective because it is acting on unimportant determinants. Sometimes the antibody produced may even help the pathogen by enabling uptake into phagocytes where it can survive.
- **Forming a stronghold**: pathogens may create some form of sanctuary where the immune system cannot reach them, or which is too strong to be destroyed. For example:
  - Coagulase: for example, *S. aureus* causes coagulation of plasma proteins around the bacterium, hindering the immune system.
  - Abscesses are surrounded by fibrosis, isolating the contents.
  - Some helminths form cysts that are too tough to be destroyed.

Attacking the host

Inhibition or death of cells of the immune system, and damage or death of other cells, can inhibit the defence system (see also Clinical box 6.9).

- **Bacteria** make a variety of toxins, which make the patient ill, and promote bacterial survival by killing cells of the defence system, or by killing other cells and disabling tissue function, which indirectly damages defence:
  - **Exotoxins** are substances produced by bacteria with a variety of functions
  - **Pore-forming** proteins lyse cells by assembling into pores in the cell membrane
  - Enzymes with **phospholipase** activity lyse cells by destroying part of the membranes
  - Toxins can enter cells and **inhibit protein synthesis**, e.g. **diphtheria** toxin
  - Toxins can also enter cells and **deregulate** their metabolism, e.g. cholera toxin stimulates adenylate cyclase in the gut epithelium, leading to massive electrolyte efflux, and copious watery diarrhoea (see Clinical box 6.10)
  - Toxins **stimulate nerves**, e.g. **staphylococcal enterotoxins**, which act on gut nerves, which signal to the brain to cause vomiting

---

Clinical box 6.10　The virulence of microorganisms: example *Staphylococcus aureus*

Microorganisms can produce disease by direct invasion of tissues or by producing toxins. The bacterium *S. aureus* is a good example.

Diseases produced by invasion include:

- Skin infections such as impetigo, boils and cellulitis
- Bone infections such as osteomyelitis
- Brain abscesses, meningitis
- Pneumonia, lung abscesses.

Diseases produced by the toxins include:

- Staphylococcal food poisoning (enterotoxin B)
- Scalded skin syndrome
- Toxic shock syndrome (most commonly due to retained vaginal tampons).

Clinical box 6.11　Septic shock

Bacterial endotoxins in the bloodstream due to severe infection promote the release of pro-inflammatory factors such as tumour necrosis factor (TNF) from phagocytic and non-phagocytic cells that mediate a systemic inflammatory response. At the same time, compensatory anti-inflammatory cytokines are released. This is part of the normal defence mechanism in response to the challenge of exogenous infection. However, when this response is disseminated due to overwhelming infection, shock and widespread tissue damage can occur, known as septic shock, which is clinically characterised by fever, hypotension and intravascular coagulation, and is potentially fatal. The initial overwhelming inflammatory response may be followed by immune suppression. Gram-negative bacteria that produce endotoxins are more likely to have this effect, mediated by the release of TNF.

- Toxins also act as **superantigens**, activating many T lymphocytes, with the release of many cytokines, especially tumour necrosis factor (TNF), causing shock (see also Clinical box 6.11).

Endotoxins are lipopolysaccharides from the cell wall, produced by Gram-negative bacteria in large quantities, particularly in Gram-negative septicaemia. They stimulate macrophages to release cytokines, especially TNF and interleukin (IL) 1. They also initiate intrinsic coagulation and alternative complement cascades that can lead to fever, hypotension, shock, disseminated intravascular coagulation, organ failure through poor perfusion, and death.

Some bacteria and protozoans **disable the phagocyte response** by living within phagocytes.

Viruses often kill the cells which they infect, and if they are cells of the immune system this will promote their own survival. For example, HIV infects CD4-positive T cells and causes profound immunosuppression.

Exit

For a microorganism to be successful, it must leave the body and be transmitted to a fresh host. Most microbes leave from the body surfaces, but some have to be extracted by vectors. Examples of exit mechanisms are the:

- Gastrointestinal tract through faeces, vomit or anal intercourse
- Respiratory tract through coughing and sneezing producing droplets
- Genitourinary tract through sexual intercourse or in urine

- Conjunctival fluids entering water, such as when swimming, or going onto the hand
- Skin surfaces through touching or shedding of bacteria on skin
- Through normally intact skin by insect vectors, needles, donating infected blood, blood splashing after wounding.

Transmission

The ability of an organism to transmit its infection once it has exited the host depends on three main factors:

- The number of organisms shed and the route of shedding
- Its stability and survival outside the host within a wide variety of environments
- The number of organisms needed to infect a fresh host.

Infections are transmitted through a variety of routes and these are the focus for many public health initiatives (Fig. 6.9). Transmission can also be described, not only by the route, but by the mechanism:

- **Vertical transmission** occurs when infection is spread from mother to foetus, or breastfed infant:
  - The rubella virus, for example, if present in the mother's blood, crosses the placenta, infecting the foetus, which will not be protected because of the lack of ability to produce antibodies.
  - During delivery, abrasions and wounds from the birth process can breach the skin, or infectious agents can enter through the conjunctiva or mucous membranes. Hepatitis B and streptococcal infections are both examples of this type of transmission.
  - During breastfeeding, if the infectious agent is present within breast milk, this may infect the child. Human lymphotropic virus 1 (HTLV-1) and HIV can both be spread in this way.
- **Horizontal transmission** occurs between individuals or between species, other than mother and offspring in utero or at or around the time of birth. The transmission may be:
  - **Direct** – when the transmitter and recipient are close: for example, through infected skin or other **surface contact** with a portal of entry, or inhaled **droplet infection** from a sneeze.
  - **Indirect** – where the transmitter and recipient can be distant from each other. Several mechanisms are possible and involve some form of vehicle. For example: food – such as *Salmonella* being transmitted through eggs; water – sewage can infect water, and cholera can be transmitted this way; fomites – any agents that retain an infective agent, such as cytomegalovirus surviving on toys; surgical instruments – before the days of sterilisation, or if sterilisation fails (prions are not inactivated by heat sterilisation), or through needle-stick injury; and transfusion of infected blood – the transmission of HIV to individuals with haemophilia through factor VIII concentrate prepared from pools of individuals, some

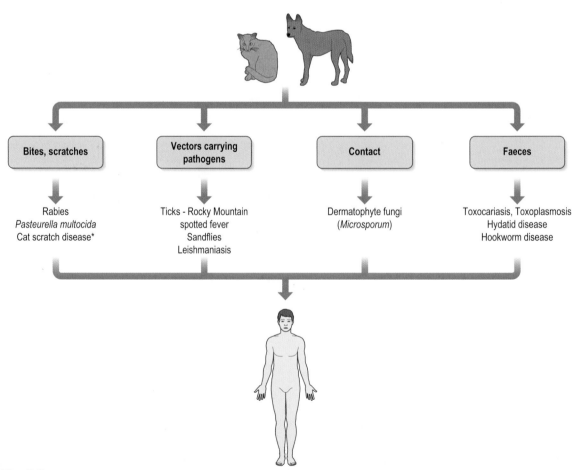

Fig. 6.9 **Zoonoses transmitted from dogs and cats.** *A benign infection, with skin lesions and lymphadenopathy, shown to be due to infection with bacteria of the *Bartonella* or *Afipia* species.

of whom were later found to have HIV, is an example of how large number of people were adversely affected by therapeutic intervention.

- **Vectors**, such as mosquitos, that transmit malaria or yellow fever, and the tsetse fly that transmits trypanosomes.
- **Airborne**: such as dust from dried smallpox crusts, or water droplets from air conditioning transmitting Legionnaires disease.

THE PATTERN OF DISEASE

The disease experienced by a person will depend on the infecting agent, the status of the patient, the circumstances of the infection and its subsequent treatment. Treatment of microbial infections is too big a subject for this chapter and the reader should consult a specialist textbook on microbiology. Distinctions can be drawn between the various patterns, however, which help in describing what is observed.

LOCAL VERSUS GENERAL INFECTIONS

- Some viruses cause **local infection** at the portal and replicate, but do not spread
- In some cases there is limited replication at the portal and the infection spreads to the local lymph nodes for a further cycle of replication, spreading subsequently to a target tissue, resulting in a **general infection**.

PERSISTENCE

- Some virus infections cause local or general infections but these do not persist
- Those that persist, with continuous viral production, lead to a **chronic infection** (e.g. HIV and hepatitis C infections)
- Those that persist for long periods without virus production, but which can be reactivated, are called **latent infections** (e.g. herpes infection).

INCUBATION PERIOD

This is the time between infection and disease manifestation and can be short, medium, long or very long.

DISEASE MANIFESTATION

Sometimes diseases may first become evident as a result of a **prodromal** illness, or become evident because of the appearance of specific symptoms which may or may not continue over time. Fever is a common feature of infections (see Clinical box 6.12).

PANDEMICS AND EPIDEMICS

Human pandemics have been recorded throughout history. Many, but not all (e.g. the Black Death, which was caused by a bacterium, *Yersinia pestis*) have been caused by viruses.

- An **epidemic** is when the frequency of an infection or disease increases above the normal (**endemic**) levels.

Clinical box 6.12 Fever in response to infection

In healthy human beings, inflammatory cytokines are released to combat bacterial or viral infections. These cytokines stimulate the hypothalamic thermoregulatory centre in the brain to increase prostaglandin (PGE2) synthesis, leading to an increase in body temperature (fever). Fever has an inhibiting effect on bacterial and viral proliferation, and thus a beneficial effect on the course of infection. The use of salicylates and non-steroidal anti-inflammatory drugs (NSAIDs) to reduce fever is based on their inhibitory effect on prostaglandin synthesis.

- A **prodromal illness** is one that produces non-specific symptoms, usually due to the release of cytokines, which usually occurs at the end of the incubation period of viral infections. For example, fever, malaise, myalgia, abdominal pain, anorexia and bowel disturbance may be observed several days before the patient becomes jaundiced in hepatitis B infection.
- **Acute** disease starts suddenly, lasts a few hours or days, and then ends in death or the person recovers (such as the bubonic plague, or the common cold, respectively). Some diseases have a more insidious onset (**subacute**), while others are **chronic**, lasting many years. The same disease can produce all of these patterns. For example, osteomyelitis can have an acute onset, but can then last a long time and eventually lead to death. Pulmonary tuberculosis has an insidious onset but it too leads to a chronic disease, which without effective treatment culminates in death.
- **Self-limiting** diseases are those in which the person recovers without treatment.

Clinical box 6.13 Influenza

Influenza is caused by a virus of the orthomyxovirus family, not to be confused with the common cold which is caused by a rhinovirus. The clinical features and normal course of the two conditions are also different, where influenza is more debilitating and has potentially more long-lasting complications, such as the postviral or chronic fatigue syndrome. After an incubation period of 2–3 days, influenza presents with an acute onset of fever, muscle pains, severe headache and sore throat. Secondary lower respiratory tract bacterial infection can occur due to *Streptococcus pneumoniae* and *Staphylococcus aureus*.

The influenza virus has two main forms, A and B. Influenza A has the ability to develop antigenic variants at irregular intervals and was the cause of the 1918 pandemic. A major change in the antigenic makeup of influenza A led to the emergence of the Hong Kong influenza type H3N2 in 1968, the avian H5N1 strain in 1997 and 'swine flu' in 2008.

- A **pandemic** is a 'global' epidemic. The first recorded pandemic was thought to be smallpox in 430 BC, to be followed over the intervening years by outbreaks of bubonic plague (the Black Death) and, more recently, cholera. In the twentieth century, it was the viral infection influenza which produced three pandemics. The first, 'Spanish' flu, was estimated to have killed over 40 000 000 people and was followed by 'Asian' flu in 1957 and 'Hong Kong' flu in 1968. Pandemics occur when a new virus emerges (see also Clinical box 6.13).

PREVENTION OF INFECTION BY VACCINATION

History

Vaccination is the administration of antigenic material to a person in order to make them immune to a disease. It first became known about in Britain in the eighteenth century when Lady Mary Wortley Montagu wrote about the practice of people inoculating themselves with fluid from people suffering from smallpox when she was in Turkey and used it on her children. Edward Jenner (1749–1823) is regarded as the founder of modern vaccination: milkmaids who had been exposed to cowpox (vaccinia) were resistant to smallpox infection and he tested this hypothesis by experimenting on a young boy, first infecting him with cowpox. Subsequent inoculation with smallpox failed to produce the latter disease. Vaccines can be made to provide protection against both viruses and some bacteria and there is a great deal of effort being made to produce vaccines to prevent malaria.

Aim of vaccination

The best that can be hoped for is that vaccination should be used so that a disease is eradicated. Smallpox was reported as being eradicated in 1977 and polio is close to being eradicated. Sometimes vaccination is used to prevent the symptoms of a disease, such as avoiding toxins produced by tetanus, or attempting to block transmission of a disease, such as malaria.

Types of vaccines

- **Live attenuated**: these are the most successful vaccines and consist of live virus particles that are less virulent (attenuated), perhaps by passing them through cell lines, or adapting the virus to work best at low temperatures. Polio (Sabin), measles, mumps, rubella and yellow fever are all examples of diseases that are treated with live attenuated vaccines.
- **Inactivated**: inactivated viruses have been killed by a process such as heat, or exposure to formaldehyde. The virus capsid is still recognised by the immune system, thus protecting the individual, but because there is no replication an individual will need booster injections over time. Polio (Salk), rabies, hepatitis A and influenza are examples of these types of vaccine.
- **Subunit**: these vaccines use parts of the virus, such as the capsid, or surface coat, or other viral proteins. This is not always very successful because the proteins are readily denatured and any antibodies that are produced may bind to the denatured protein, but not the viral protein itself. A development of this idea has led to **recombinant** vaccines in which the relevant protein gene is placed into another virus. Vaccination with the second virus will lead to expression of the harmful virus protein, stimulating antibody production protecting the patient from the harmful infection. Hepatitis B vaccination is an example of this type of vaccination.

Table 6.6 summarises the advantages and disadvantages of the different types of vaccine.

Table 6.6	**Advantages and disadvantages of different types of vaccine**	
	Advantages	**Disadvantages**
Live attenuated	Most successful as they produce all features of the infection in a mild form and protect over many years. Attenuated strains may pass into the population, further protecting people	May revert to a more virulent form
		Produce severe disease in immunocompromised patients
		Hypersensitivity to proteins from the attenuation process, such as chicken eggs
		Danger of passing on animal viruses
Inactivated	Present no hazard as they are killed	Short acting
Subunit	Non-hazardous as they do not contain whole virus	May only stimulate B cells, producing only a primary response, rather than producing the longer antigenic memory that is the result of T cell activation
		T cell activation may vary between people, depending on their inheritance of different polymorphisms of the class II human lymphocyte antigens (HLA-D)

IMMUNITY

Everybody, to stay healthy, tries to keep other life forms outside. We are surrounded by a large variety of organisms, from viruses to insects, many of which try to subvert our cells, or live in our bowel, eat our food, frolic in our tissue spaces, breed in our bladders or brains, or lay their eggs under our skin. It has been known for a long time that such invaders are associated with disease. Koch, in 1890, defined four criteria that needed to be fulfilled to establish a causal relationship between a microbe and a disease (**Koch's postulates**). He later abandoned the italicised part of the first postulate, because of the finding that asymptomatic carriers existed.

Koch's postulates (the italicised part now having been abandoned):

- The microorganism must be found in abundance in all organisms suffering from the disease, *but not in healthy organisms*
- The microorganisms must be isolated from a diseased organism and grown in pure culture
- The cultured microorganisms should cause disease when introduced into healthy organisms
- The microorganisms must be re-isolated from the inoculated, diseased experimental host and identified as being identical to the original specific causative agent.

To keep these infecting organisms away, the body has defence mechanisms, which may be classified as:

- Non-immunological
- Immunological – innate or adaptive.

THE NON-IMMUNOLOGICAL DEFENCE SYSTEM

The body has various barriers, which have been more fully discussed in the previous section. Some examples are given here.

PHYSICAL AND FUNCTIONAL BARRIERS

- The skin acts as a barrier, preventing microorganisms entering the body fluids
- The upward flow of mucus in the bronchi, propelled by the cilia, washes out microorganisms (see Ch. 13, the mucociliary escalator)
- Complete emptying of the bladder and the inhibition of urine flow up the ureters both inhibit infection of the urinary tract (see Ch. 14, Clinical box 14.17).

SIMPLE CHEMICAL AND BIOLOGICAL BARRIERS

- There is a low pH in the stomach and vagina. If the pH of the stomach rises, for example, infections of the bowel are more frequent.
- The skin is constantly anointed with **sebum**, an oily secretion from the sebaceous glands which contains chemicals that do no harm to the human host, but are not liked by many pathogens.
- There is significant growth of bacteria in the lumen of the bowel, in the vagina and on the surface of the skin in the form of **normal flora**, which inhibit the growth of pathogens.

THE IMMUNOLOGICAL DEFENCE SYSTEM

Destructive agents, in the form of specialised cells and molecules – lymphocytes, macrophages, antibodies and complement – form the body's immunological defence mechanisms. To be successful they must be able to distinguish friend from foe – to recognise **non-self** – and to be able to tell the difference between **damaged** and **undamaged** tissue.

Activation of some of these cells and molecules is called an **immune response**. Some other definitions that will be useful at this point are:

- **Immunogen** – anything that provokes an immune response.
- **Antigen** – anything that is recognised by the cells and molecules of the immune response.
- Agents of the defence system recognise antigens through receptors and recognition sites. The part of the antigen that is recognised is called a **determinant**.
- A **receptor** is a molecule or complex of molecules which has at least one recognition site, the molecular feature recognised being the determinant. Receptors are normally present on the surface of cells.

DETECTION AND DESTRUCTION OF THE INVADING IMMUNOGEN

The immune system needs:

- To detect the presence of **non-self** and, usually, to destroy and/or eliminate the invader
- To leave undamaged, as much as possible, the body's own components (**self**)
- Sometimes to allow **toleration** of some non-self substances where an aggressive immune response serves no useful purpose.

It does this by acting through receptors and antigenic determinants and applying mechanisms that assist in destruction of the immunogen.

Receptors

The recognition site on the receptor binds to the determinant not only because of their respective shapes, but also because of electrostatic forces. There are different types of receptor that aid in the detection of the invader and subsequent healing processes.

- **Antigen receptors** recognise determinants that are present on non-self substances, such as **pathogen associated molecular patterns** (**PAMPs**) which may be related to substances, such as lipoproteins, present in pathogen cell walls, but are scarce or absent on self – distinguishing **self** and **non-self**.

- **Scavenger receptors** recognise determinants or features characteristic of dead or denatured material, but scarce or absent on healthy tissue – distinguishing **damaged** and **healthy** tissue. They also act as **pathogen recognition receptors** (**PRR**), triggering an immune response when bound.

Some elements of the defence system distinguish between these forms by recognising determinants characteristic of healthy self tissues. Cells and molecules of the immune system also interact and cooperate with each other through specialised receptors and determinants, such as:

- Receptors on macrophages for antibodies
- Interactions within the complement cascade.

Receptors can be specific or non-specific.

- A receptor is said to be very specific if it binds only to one particular kind of determinant. Some receptors are more specific than others.
- A receptor that is **non-specific** might, for example, bind to a variety of determinants with strong negative charges, because of its strong positive charge, in spite of there being differences in their shapes.

Specificity, on the other hand, is a different concept and refers to the identity of the determinant which it recognises. For example, the specificity of one receptor might be a determinant on *S. aureus,* and the specificity of another a determinant on tetanus toxoid. A **cross-reaction** occurs when a receptor binds to more than one kind of antigen. This may be because the same determinant is present on different antigens and the receptor is acting in a specific fashion, or because the receptor is acting in a non-specific way, binding to determinants of different shapes, as described above.

There are many different classes of receptors, for example scavenger receptors A (SR-A) through to SR-F bind to different forms of low density lipoprotein (LDL):

- SR-A1 and SR-A2 on macrophages pick up excess LDL within blood vessels
- SR-A and SR-B (also known as CD36) on macrophages bind to pathogens, such as *E. coli*, through collagen recognition sites. They act in two main ways:
  - The macrophage engulfs the bacteria in a phagosome. Lysosomes fuse and release their acidic destructive content.
  - They act as co-receptors with **toll like receptors** (**TLR**), binding to pathogen cell walls and releasing **transcription factor** (**TF**) which travels to the nucleus to instruct production of cytokines that attract more immune cells.

Antigens

Antigens are usually polypeptides or polysaccharides, sometimes with other chemical groups attached. The determinant size is probably only between three and 10 peptides or saccharides in length. Individual molecules may have several determinants recognisable by the receptors of the defence system. This allows tissues, cells (live or dead), cell fragments, molecular aggregates or single protein molecules

(of eukaryotic, prokaryotic, viral or artificial origin) to be recognised, simply through the presence of a determinant that is foreign to the body.

Agents of destruction

Identification must be followed by destruction and elimination of the invader. The defence mechanism does this by acting through cells that use phagocytosis, lytic enzymes and strong oxidising agents, both inside and outside the cells. Some cells kill other cells by opening ion channels in their cell membranes. An important factor is that the destruction should be as localised as possible to minimise damage to healthy tissue.

While it is important that **self** is not a target of destruction, there are many molecules that are foreign, but not dangerous. There is evidence that the defence system can specifically **tolerate** such potential antigens. For example, pollen antigens probably cross the lung mucosa but do not produce significant damage: an inappropriate aggressive immune response might result in damage also to self.

Cells that are part of the immune response communicate with each other through:

- Cell surface molecules – cells touching each other may communicate through structures that allow them to fit or bind together to mediate communication
- Secreted molecules, or mediators – such as hormones, cytokines or lymphokines
  - Hormones are products of specialised endocrine cells
  - Cytokines are polypeptides
  - Lymphokines are cytokines secreted by, or acting on, lymphocytes.

In general, a cell must express a receptor for a mediator to be influenced by it: usually on the cell surface, but sometimes in the nucleus.

- In **autocrine** activity a mediator acts on the cell that secreted it
- In **paracrine** activity a mediator diffuses from the secreting cell to neighbouring cells and acts on them
- In **endocrine** activity the mediator is carried by the circulation all over the body, and acts on cells remote from those that secreted it.

THE INNATE IMMUNE SYSTEM

The innate immune system is the first line of defence and involves several different types of cells – macrophages, dendritic cells and mast cells – and other substances – chemical mediators and complement proteins. These components cannot readily distinguish self and non-self but, nevertheless, provide elements that protect the body. For example, all **lysozyme** molecules are the same and have the same specificity of attack, which is different from other defending molecules, such as **mannose-binding lectins** (**MBL**). There are several other soluble factors that assist in the body defence:

- Lysosomes act by damaging bacterial cell walls, but do no harm to eukaryotic cells, which lack a cell wall.
- MBL acts through recognition of particular carbohydrate patterns found on the surface of many pathogenic microorganisms.
- **C-reactive protein** (**CRP**) binds to phosphorylcholine on bacteria, enhancing phagocytosis and assisting in **complement** binding.

- The **complement pathway** is a cascade system of enzymes reminiscent of the clotting pathway and is triggered by certain foreign chemical configurations found in endotoxins, and bacterial and fungal cell walls, or by antigen/antibody complexes. It culminates in the activation of enzymes destructive to foreign organisms. It also produces chemotactic substances and adherent factors that promote the phagocytosis. It also acts to discriminate self and non-self as it is only stimulated by foreign material.
- **Chemotactic factors** are chemical substances that direct the movement of cells – human or invading – to particular locations.

All body cells play their part in the innate immune system. Any cell that is damaged or undergoes necrosis may release mediators, or material such as heat shock proteins that signal the damage to neighbouring cells. Many cells that are virally infected signal the fact by releasing mediators (**interferons**, IFNs).

Basophils in blood and **mast cells** in tissues are motile and chemotactic, but not phagocytic. They are activated directly by physical and chemical stimuli, and also by nerves (collateral branches of afferent sensory nerves, which can detect damage through their receptors), complement and receptors, allowing them to interact with the **adaptive** immune system. **Phagocytes**, such as neutrophils, monocytes/macrophages, dendritic cells and eosinophils, deploy a variety of cell surface receptors which can detect non-self and damaged tissues. Some are also used in cooperation with other parts of the immune system. Examples of the different types of receptors are:

- **TLRs –** molecules which in various combinations in the cell wall, sometimes in heterodimers, recognise microbial molecules and components, such as cell wall lipoproteins, virus RNA and DNA (on the endosomes) and material released from damaged self cells (**heat shock proteins**) and dead self material. They are signalling receptors that bind to pathogenic material and form a cascade of events leading to production of transcription factors for various cytokines, including IFN, **nuclear factor kappa enhancer of B cells**, (**NF-κB**) and **activator protein-1** (**AP-1**) for example.
- **Collectins –** proteins which recognise sugar groups characteristic of microbes, e.g. the mannose receptor.
- **CD14 –** a receptor for lipopolysaccharide, a component of Gram-negative bacterial cell walls. When an antigen engages these receptors, the cell will attempt to phagocytose and destroy it in the lysosomes. CD14 also assists TLRs.
- **C3b and Fc receptors –** mediate cooperation with complement and antibodies, respectively.

All these phagocytes can degrade the material that they phagocytose, and if they phagocytose microbes they are often able to kill them. These mechanisms involve enzymes, free radicals and exclusion of nutrients from the phagosome. The phagocytes, however, retain no memory of the attack to protect the body against repeat incursions. Secretion of mediators is an important function of phagocytes, mediating the recruitment of more phagocytes and inflammatory changes.

In summary, the innate immune system uses a relatively small number of receptors and recognition sites that detect components common on microorganisms, but not found within the human body. These mechanisms do not recognise all determinants and successful pathogens hide these. The body needs a more sophisticated defence mechanism to deal with these – the **adaptive immune system**.

THE ADAPTIVE IMMUNE SYSTEM

When the innate immune system fails to resolve an infection, the adaptive immune system comes into action. In contrast, but in co-operation with the innate immune system, the adaptive immune system initiates and uses specific memory of the infection. This system is provided through the **lymphocytes**. There are different forms of lymphocytes: B lymphocytes, T lymphocytes and null lymphocytes. T lymphocytes can be further divided into:

- **CD4-positive** (**helper T cells**) to promote the immune response
- **CD8-positive** (**cytotoxic T cells**) to destroy pathogens.

Figure 6.10 summarises the differences between these two systems of body defence. Any one lymphocyte, and its **clone** from division of a single naïve progenitor cell, will have receptors which are **specific** for an antigen, but different lymphocytes will have different specificities. After recognising an antigen the lymphocyte will divide to form a clone, which is generally stable. The body may produce receptors on lymphocytes specific for self components but these are deleted or inactivated, probably through **clonal deletion**. Thus lymphocytes are produced that have receptors for many different non-self specificities, producing a comprehensive defence system.

T lymphocytes

T lymphocytes originate in the bone marrow, but undergo further development in the **thymus** before they are mature. The receptors are formed of four subunits (two alpha and two beta chains) and consist of a constant region, which defines the T cell type, and a variable region which recognises specific **epitopes** (antigen receptors) on pathogens, but which are *not* antibody. The receptors on the surface of any single T lymphocyte all have the same specificity, as to single B lymphocytes.

T cells are activated through the innate immune system. Macrophages that have engulfed pathogens will degrade the organisms and selected epitopes to present to the T cells. The receptors on T lymphocytes are known as **complementarity determining regions** (**CDRs**). Highly variable, these regions interact with an **MHC** (**major histocompatibility complex**)–peptide complex to activate the lymphocytes. **HLA** refers to a subset of MHC genes that encode for cell surface antigen-presenting proteins.)

Terminology
CD nomenclature
CD stands for **cluster of differentiation**. This is a classification system for the different antigenic determinants found on cells.

- Each cell surface molecule on a T lymphocyte must be recognised by a cluster of monoclonal antibodies developed in the laboratory before it is assigned a CD number.
- The surface molecules are different on different cells and so act as markers of differentiation. The different CD complexes are given a number to differentiate them.

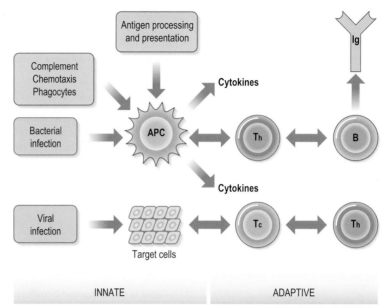

Fig. 6.10 **Innate and adaptive immunity.** Th, helper T cell; Tc, cytotoxic T cell; B, B cell; Ig, immunoglobulin; APC, antigen-presenting cell.

Major histocompatibility complex (MHC)

The MHC region is located on chromosome 6 and consists of about 140 genes, many having immunological functions. Proteins produced from fragmented microorganisms bind to various MHC molecules. The MHC molecule can be divided into three groups: class I, class II and class III.

- **MHC class I** molecules are present on the surface of virtually every cell. They present antigen fragments to T lymphocytes and bind to **CD8** receptors on cytotoxic T cells.
- **MHC class II** molecules are found mainly on macrophages and B cells and present antigen to helper T cells, binding to the **CD4** receptor.
- **MHC class III** genes encode for other immune components, such as complement, or cytokines such as **TNF**.

Human leucocyte antigen (HLA)

HLA antigens are classified into nine divisions:

- HLA-A, HLA-B and HLA-C all belong to MHC class I
- HLA-D consists of six genes, all belonging to MHC class II.

The HLA molecules, class I and II, are both two-chain glycoproteins. Class I molecules have a single transmembrane chain whereas class II molecules have two transmembrane chains. Both classes have an antigen-presenting groove where oligopeptides bind (Fig. 6.11).

Interactions with T lymphocytes

The interaction of a T cell receptor with an MHC receptor indicates the presence of a cell with a foreign particle, such as an intracellular microbe. The binding stimulates the T lymphocytes, which become activated and release various cytokines, depending on what type of lymphocyte has been stimulated.

- Most **CD8 T lymphocytes** (having CD8 receptors) are **cytotoxic**. They recognise specific antigens associated with intracellular pathogens, like viruses, when presented. This recognition activates them and

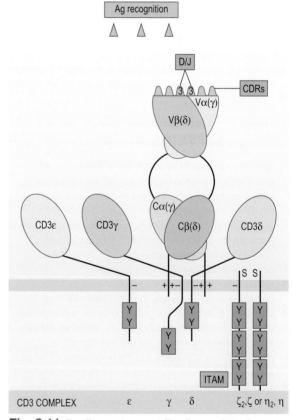

Fig. 6.11 **T cell receptor on αβ T cells consists of an α- and a β-chain, each composed of a variable (V) and a constant (C) domain resembling the immunoglobulin Fab antigen-binding fragment in structure.** The highly variable complementarity determining regions (CDRs) on the variable domains contact the MHC–peptide antigen complex. This produces a signal that is transduced by the invariant CD3 complex composed of γ, δ, ϵ and ζ or η chains, through their cytoplasmic immune receptor tyrosine-based activation motifs (ITAM), which contact protein tyrosine kinases. $\gamma\delta$ T cells have receptors composed of γ and δ chains. Ag, antigen. From Goering R et al. 2008 Mims' medical microbiology, 4th edn. Mosby, Edinburgh, with permission.

also stimulates neighbouring cells. The activated cell induces signals that promote apoptosis of the infecting cells.

- **CD4 T lymphocytes** (having CD4 receptors) have a **helper function**. When a helper T lymphocyte encounters an antigen of the correct specificity, correctly presented, it responds by dividing and secreting cytokines. These lymphocytes cannot eliminate or kill antigen but the secreted cytokines initiate events that do.
  - CD4 cells have high affinity receptors for the viral gp120 glycoprotein, allowing HIV antigens to bind, along with a co-receptor, the CCR5 β-cytokine, activating these cells in an attempt to respond to the invasion. Around 1% of individuals have deletions in the *CCR5* gene which provides resistance to the infection. The subsequent failure of the immune response leads to a decline in CD4 counts, and their level is used as a measure of the patient's immune health and potential vulnerability in the fight against secondary infections.

T lymphocytes cannot respond to antigen: it has to be presented to them by HLA molecules on cells such as dendritic cells, macrophages, B lymphocytes or other cells (**antigen-presenting cells (APCs)**; Fig. 6.12). There are two possible sources for the antigen presented by APCs:

- **Exogenous antigen** – an antigen taken in by the APC. It may be self or non-self.
- **Endogenous antigen** – an antigen manufactured within the APC. It may be self (coded for by the APC's own genes) or non-self (derived from an intracellular pathogen infecting the cell).

There are various cells that act to present antigens:

- **B lymphocytes** recognise exogenous antigen (determinant) through their antigen receptors (antibodies). Unless there are many copies of the determinant on the same antigen molecule, the B lymphocyte cannot respond immediately. Instead, it endocytoses the antigen, processes (cuts) it into peptides, which it presents, on **class II HLA** molecules, to **helper CD4 T lymphocytes**.
  - MHC class II molecules leave the endoplasmic reticulum (ER) in an **endosome** with their peptide binding site blocked by the **Li protein**.
  - The endosome then fuses with a lysosome and Li is broken down by the acidic material to leave bound **class II invariant chain peptide (CLIP)**, preventing self-peptides from binding.

- **HLA-DM** is a molecular chaperone intracellular protein and breaks down CLIP, controlling what peptides can bind to the molecule.
  - The MHC class II molecule, now with its foreign peptide bound, fuses to the presenting cell membrane.
  - T helper cells with their CD4 receptors check that this is an MHC class II molecule and the T cell receptors check for specificity with the presented epitope, binding and leading to cell mediated or humoral responses through cytokine production or presentation and activation of B cells through specific B cell receptors.
  - The B lymphocyte can now form a clone; antibody production follows after receiving 'permission' from helper T cells.

- **Macrophages** also pick up antigens because they have various surface receptors for foreign determinants. Although they can become activated and destroy what they have phagocytosed, in order to become fully activated they must process and present antigen in a similar way to the B lymphocytes, the released cytokines activating the macrophage.

- **All nucleated cells** can become infected by viruses or other intracellular pathogens, which are then shielded from antibodies and macrophages while they remain in the host cells. However, cells process a sample of these proteins (endogenous antigen), and present the resulting peptides (on class I HLA molecules) to **cytotoxic CD8 T lymphocytes** which, if activated, can kill that cell.
  - Endogenous antigens that have entered the cell are processed in cylindrical proteasomes to form peptides that enter the ER through (**transporter associated with antigen processing, TAP**) transport channels.
  - MHC class I has four subunits (2α and 2β), the $β_2$ subunit being stabilized with calnexin. The latter protein dissociates and other proteins, including calreticulin, and **endoplasmic resident reticulum proteins (ERPs)**, are needed to bind to allow the antigenic peptides to bind to the class I molecule.
  - The MHC class I molecule then leaves the ER in an endosome and presents on the surface of the infected macrophage.
  - T cytotoxic cells with their CD8 receptors check that this is an MHC class I molecule and the T cell receptors check for specificity with the presented epitope, allowing binding to take place, activates the cell and leads to cell death.

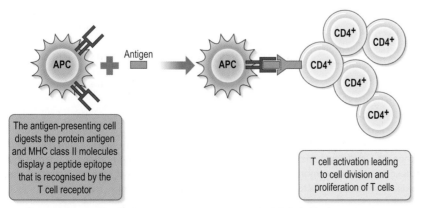

Fig. 6.12 **Antigen presentation to T cells by antigen-presenting cells (APCs).** MHC, major histocompatibility complex.

- **Dendritic cells** are derived from blood cell precursors. Within different tissues the dendritic cells differentiate and become active, taking up and presenting antigens to MHC molecules. The activated cells migrate to lymphoid tissue where they act as APCs and interact with other cells to produce cytokines.

  - **Langerhans cells** are specialised dendritic cells that can activate 'virgin' T cells. They are not themselves seeking to be activated through presenting antigen, but appear to be a determinant of T lymphocyte activation. The potential importance of these cells in HIV patients has been recently recognised. Dendritic cells can take up HIV via specific receptors. While they may have a role mopping up viral particles, they may also provide a reservoir of HIV.

Antigen recognition

Mature T lymphocytes are released from the thymus bearing antigen receptors. Each cell has many thousands of receptors and all on a single cell have the same specificity, but they are derived from the same set of genes by random genetic rearrangement. It is thought that the maturation in the thymus deletes any self recognition and commits the cells to either the CD4 or CD8 lineage.

T lymphocytes also have other receptors. CD3 is a molecular complex on all T lymphocytes. When antigen is recognised, a conformational change takes place in the lymphocyte which enables particular activation events to take place.

The HLA molecule is on the APC and presents an oligopeptide antigen bound within the groove of the molecule. The size of the oligopeptide differs between the two classes.

- **Class I HLA** molecules (on most nucleated cells) present **endogenous** antigen to **CD8** cytotoxic T lymphocytes.
- **Class II HLA** molecules (on B lymphocytes and macrophages) present **exogenous** antigen to **CD4** helper T lymphocytes.

A mnemonic

Extra Help for you **too = Exogenous** antigen, **Help**er T lymphocytes which are CD**4**, and recognise antigen presented on class **II** HLA molecules.

It should be noted that there is not a 100% correlation between function and CD4/CD8 status; thus CD4 cells are not always helper cells, nor CD8 cells always cytotoxic cells. CD4 T cells that can activate macrophages, but cannot help B cells, are called **T helper 1 (Th1)** cells, and CD4 T cells that can help B cells but cannot activate macrophages are called **T helper 2 (Th2)** cells. CD4 T cells that retain both patterns of cytokine secretion are called **Th0** cells.

T cell activation and killing

Once antigen has been recognised, the T cell may be activated, or remain unresponsive (**anergic**). Various factors encourage activation:

- **Antigen presentation by dendritic cells**, probably because of their ability to stimulate 'virgin' T cells. T cells are likely to become anergic if their initial exposure to antigen is not through a dendritic cell.
- **Past memory**. Once a T lymphocyte has been activated, it and its mitotic descendants are memory cells, activation is more likely on re-exposure to the antigen, whatever the APC is.

- **Adhesion molecules**. There are several pairs of adhesion molecules that are important in T cell activation. For example, all T cells have CD2 molecules on their surface which interact with CD58 on APCs, promoting adherence and transmitting activation signals (positive or negative) to the T cell.
- **IL-1** is a polypeptide cytokine, secreted by APCs during antigen presentation. It lowers the activation threshold of CD4 T cells.

Once activated, the CD4 T cells, in particular, respond by expressing receptors for **IL-2**. IL-2 binds to receptors which continue activation, producing more cytokines which are different, dependent on the type of T lymphocyte. If there is insufficient IL-2, or if some of the other factors are lacking (dendritic cells, adhesion molecules, etc.), then the cells become anergic. CD8 T cells probably do not make enough IL-2 to induce activation without help from neighbouring CD4 T cells. Table 6.7 compares the different cytokines released by activated CD4 and CD8 T cells and their actions.

Cell killing can take place in two ways:

- **Perforin** in the granules produces ion channels in the target cell membrane followed by osmotic lysis.
- Release of **TNF** interacts with receptors on the target cell and initiates programmed cell death (**apoptosis**).

The T cell can thus lead to the death of many cells, but is undamaged by this process.

Switching off activated T cells

Continued antigen presence continues to stimulate the T cells and so, when the antigen disappears, the stimulus to release the activating cytokines is 's**witched off'**. Other substances appear to assist in this process:

- **Transforming growth factor** β (**TGF-β**) controls proliferation and cell differentiation and is released by many cells. Some cells not only secrete TGF-β, but also have TGF-β receptors, which mean that this substance can suppress surrounding cells non-specifically (**autocrine signalling**)
- **Hydrocortisone**, a steroid hormone, interferes in various ways with antigen presentation
- T cells might specifically suppress each other, not responding to consumed cytokines.

B lymphocytes

B lymphocytes originate from the bone marrow with receptors for specific antigen on their surface (**antibodies**) produced through somatic recombination and circulate through blood and lymph to B cell areas in lymphoid tissues. Antibodies are glycoproteins with a characteristic structure – two heavy chains and two light chains. Any one B lymphocyte has antibodies all of the same specificity.

When antigen interacts with the antibodies on the surface of a B lymphocyte, the cell responds by dividing. Some of the progeny change their appearance and become **plasma cells**, which continually **secrete antibody**, others become memory cells. Antibodies cannot themselves destroy or eliminate non-self or antigen, but they interact with other agents that do, such as the classical complement pathway, null cells, macrophages, neutrophils, mast cells and eosinophils.

Table 6.7 Cytokines released by CD4 and CD8 activated T lymphocytes

Cytokine	CD4 cell	CD8 cell	Functions
Interleukin 2 (IL-2)	✓	Low	Maintains T cell activation Increases natural killer cell activity Help CD8 cytotoxic T cells Facilitates B cell antibody production
IL-3	✓	✗	Growth factor for pluripotent stem cells
IL-4	✓	✗	B cell growth factor promoting proliferation, antibody secretion and switch to IgE Mast cell growth factor Weak macrophage activator
IL-5	✓	✗	B cell growth factor Growth factor and activator of eosinophils IgA production
IL-6	✓	✗	B cell growth factor and promotes antibody secretion Haemopoeitic stem cell differentiation Stimulates acute phase protein release from liver
IL-8	✓	✓	Chemotaxis and activation of neutrophils, monocytes, eosinophils, basophils
IL-9	✓	✗	Stimulates mast cells Potentiates IgM, IgG, IgE
IL-10	✓	✓	Activates B cells Stimulates macrophages to produce cytokines Inhibits Th1 cytokines (IFN-γ, lymphotoxin alpha (previously TNF-β), IL-2) Stimulates Th2 cells
IL-12	✓	✗	Differentiates lymphocytes into cytotoxic T cells Inhibits IL-10 Stimulate NK cells to produce IFN-γ, lymphotoxin alpha (TNF-β)
IL-13	✓	✗	Stimulates B cells to produce IgE Inhibits Th1 cells Inhibits macrophage cytokine production
IL-14	✓	✗	Controls B cell profileration Inhibits Ig production
IL-16	✗	✓	CD4 cell chemoattractant
IL-21	✓	✗	CD8 activator and proliferator Augments NK cell cytotoxicity
α-Interferon	✓	✓	Activates macrophages Induces cells to become antiviral Amplifies TNF activity Increased expression of class I and class II HLA molecules
Granulocyte-monocyte colony-stimulating factor (GM-CSF)	✓	✗	Stimulates growth and differentiation of monocytes and granulocyte precursors
Migration inhibitory factor	✓	✗	Retains macrophages and activates them
Perforin	✗	✓	Pore forming protein, producing apoptosis with granzyme (a serine protease). Similar to complement protein C9
Transforming growth factor β (TGF-β)	✓	✓	Switches off activated T cells
Tumour necrosis factor (TNF) (previously TNF-α) (cachectin)	✓	✓	Kills some tumour cells and some virally infected cells, amplified by TNF Increased expression of class I and class II HLA molecules Can activate eosinophils, neutrophils and macrophages

B cell activation

The first step in B cell activation is when the surface antibody binds to an antigen of the correct specificity. If the antigen is **T independent**, then this is sufficient to activate the B lymphocyte. T-independent antigens have many copies of the same determinant, cross-linked on the surface of the B cell, providing a strong enough signal to exceed the activation threshold. The capsule of **pneumococcus** is a clinically significant T-independent antigen. Most antigens do not have this repetitious structure and are **T-dependent antigens**. In this latter case the B lymphocyte must present the antigen to a helper T lymphocyte of the correct specificity:

1. The B cell endocytoses and processes the antigen
2. Fragments of processed antigen are presented to the T cell on the B cell surface, in association with class II HLA molecules

3. The helper T cell responds by secreting lymphokines – B cell growth factors (IL-2, IL-4, IL-5 and IL-6) which push the B lymphocyte over the activation threshold.

IL-1 from nearby macrophages can also contribute to the activation by reducing the activation threshold of B cells and helper T cells.

Antigen may also be trapped on the surface of macrophages or follicular dendritic cells in lymphoid tissue, making it more available to B cells (called **antigen presentation**). Antigen processing and HLA molecules are *not* involved. This antigen retention may be essential to the persistence of memory B cells. Following activation, B lymphocytes get bigger (**blast transformation**) and become **centroblasts**, differentiating through somatic hypermutation in the **dark zone** of the germinal centres of the lymph nodes. Some members of this expanded clone differentiate to form **plasma cells**, which secrete the antibody into the surroundings.

Plasma cells are short lived, so for the clone to survive, some members must remain as B lymphocytes, eventually to become memory cells. Immediately following the first activation, the B cell membership of the emerging clone will express IgM only, and the descendant plasma cells will secrete IgM. However, over time, individual B cells from the clone may move into the **light zone** of the germinal centre as **centrocytes** and switch production to a different immunoglobulin class in a process known as **class switching**, followed by clonal expansion. Plasma cells descended from such a B cell will then secrete antibody of the new class. If the antigen exposure is repeated or prolonged, most of the B cells concerned will switch away from IgM antibody production. This class switching can only occur with T lymphocyte help.

B cell response

Primary responses, to an antigen never encountered before, are measured by detectable specific antibody in the serum that occurs after about 5 days, peaking after about 9 days. Initially the response is mainly IgM, but IgG may reach a comparable concentration after about 11 days. Antibody levels are often low again by about 3 weeks.

The **secondary response** to this same antigen is much more rapid, becoming evident in about 3 days and resulting in a higher peak of specific antibody concentration. The majority of the antibody is IgG and of a higher affinity. The plateau of response is longer and antibody production has a much slower decline (Fig. 6.13).

Antibodies may neutralise viruses and toxins by binding to active sites, but they cannot themselves destroy non-self. Instead they:

- Prepare antigens for phagocytosis (opsonisation – any molecule that allows cells to come together, such as coating negatively charged molecules on the membrane surface)

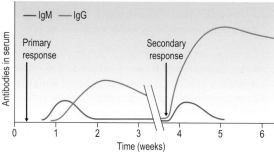

Fig. 6.13 **Pattern of antibody production after initial and second exposure.**

- Interact with killer cells
- Trigger the classical complement pathway.

All these processes lead to the destruction of non-self.

Switching off B cells

B cells may be switched off in several ways. Possible mechanisms include:

- Disappearance of antigen because of successful defence
- Withdrawal of T cell help through suppression
- Negative feedback from immune complexes.

Null lymphocytes

These cells do not make antibodies or produce T cell receptors but have a variety of inhibitory and activating receptors. The outcome depends on the balance of activation of the different receptors. They kill some neoplastic and virally infected cells through two different mechanisms, both promoting apoptosis:

- **Natural killer (NK) activity** acts through recognising and inhibiting normal healthy cells, allowing the killing of cells without self (MHC class I) markers (innate immunity).
- **Killer activity.** Null cells also bear receptors that enable them to interact with antibody that has bound to other cells (Fc receptors). Here it is the antibody that discriminates between non-self and self.

ANTIBODIES

Antibodies are glycoproteins. They are the antigen receptors on the surface of B lymphocytes and are secreted by plasma cells. Plasma cells are B lymphocytes that are in their final antibody-secreting phase. Each receptor binds a specific antigenic determinant, and all antibodies produced by a particular plasma cell clone have the same specificity as the antigen binding site. Between them, the many millions of plasma cells produce an enormous range of specificities.

Figure 6.14 illustrates the structure of a typical immunoglobulin molecule, or antibody. Each antibody has two identical light chains and two identical heavy chains.

- Each light chain consists of two domains: one **variable region** domain, and one **constant region** domain.
- Each heavy chain has one variable region domain, and either three or four constant region domains.

Variable regions have very wide variation between clones. In contrast, the constant regions are more or less the same between clones.

Light chains come in two types – lambda (λ) and kappa (κ) – but only one type of light chain is present per antibody, determined by the constant region domain. **Heavy chains** come in five different classes: alpha (α), delta (δ), epsilon (ε), gamma (γ) and mu (μ), determined by the constant region domains of the heavy chain. The type of heavy chain determines the class of antibody – IgA, IgD, IgE, IgG and IgM, respectively (Fig. 6.15). Subclasses have also been defined. The λ and ε chains have four constant region domains; the remainder have three constant and a **hinge** region, which probably gives more flexibility to α, δ and ε chains.

- The **specificity**, determined by the variable region domains, is almost fixed, as is the type of light chain.
- The **class**, determined by the heavy chain constant regions is not fixed. A given clone can (and well may)

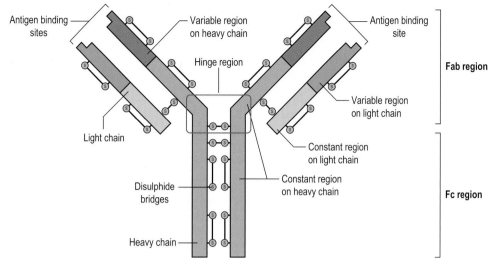

Fig. 6.14 **Generic structure of immunoglobulins.**

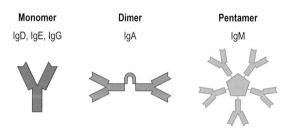

Fig. 6.15 **The different antibody complex shapes.**

produce antibodies of all the different classes and subclasses. Even so, each plasma cell is probably committed to a single class.

The 'arms' of the antibody form the **fragment, antigen binding (Fab) region**, composed of a constant and a variable domain from each heavy and light chain. At the tip is the **antigen-binding site**. The base region, composed of two heavy chains that contribute two or three constant domains, is called the **fragment crystallisable (Fc) region**. This region is involved in modulating the **immune** cell activity by binding to specific proteins. The Fc region also binds to other cell receptors and molecules, such as **complement**, enabling various responses such as opsonisation and lysis of cells.

- Fc receptors for IgG on phagocytes and null lymphocytes are of low affinity, so these cells will only bind onto immune complexes where multiple Fc portions are available in an array, minimising the opportunity for the complex to dissociate by chance.
- Mast cells have a high affinity Fc receptor for IgE, so they are able to bind individual IgE molecules effectively.

Antibody complexes

While IgD, IgE and IgG exist as monomers, IgA forms a dimer, and IgM a pentamer (Fig. 6.15).

Antibody functions

Antibodies can be described according to their strength. **Affinity** refers to the strength of the antibody–antigenic determinant bond. **Avidity**, in contrast, is the strength of

attachment between an antibody and antigen – different because antibodies have at least two antigen-combining sites and antigens may have many different determinants of the relevant specificity.

The different antibody classes have different functions, described below and summarised in Table 6.8.

- **Blocking and neutralisation**: IgG, IgM and IgA are all present at significant concentration, and if they are specific for the appropriate molecule they may block the binding of microbes and toxins to human tissue.
- **Complement fixation**: IgM and IgG subclasses 1, 2 and 3 fix complement (C3b is bound to the pathogen membrane).
- **Opsonisation and killer activity**:
  - IgG mediates opsonisation and phagocytosis of bound antigen by neutrophils, macrophages, monocytes, dendritic cells and eosinophils, all of which possess Fc receptors for IgG.
  - IgG also mediates killer activity by null lymphocytes, which possess Fc receptors for IgG.
  - IgE mediates phagocytosis by eosinophils, which possess Fc receptors for IgE.
- **Mast cell activation**. Mast cells possess Fc receptors for IgE leading to granulation and release of mediators.

COMPLEMENT

The complement system is a triggered enzyme cascade. Their main aim is to destroy an invading pathogen through:

- Opsonisation – coating the pathogen with a protein that is recognised by macrophages, enabling phagocytosis
- Producing a **membrane attack complex (MAC)** which makes a hole in the pathogen cell membrane and causes cell lysis
- Enhancing the inflammatory process.

The complement proteins are produced in the liver and are soluble, circulating in inactive forms, the first member of the series, once activated, activating the next. Each molecule can activate several molecules of the next component of the series, so the reaction is amplified. There is a complex collection

Table 6.8	Functions of the different antibody classes		
Class	**Serum concentration (g/L)**	**Functions**	**Comments**
IgM	0.6–2.0	Blocks binding of toxins and adherence of microbes	In secretions and on surface of B cells
		Activates classical complement pathway	Destroys pathogens in early stages of B cell-mediated immunity
		First antibody to appear in the immune response	
IgG	8.0–16	Blocks binding of toxins and adherence of microbes	Provides majority of antibody-based immunity
		Subclasses 1, 2 and 3 activate classical complement pathway	Can cross the placenta to protect the foetus
		Opsonises antigen for phagocytic cells	
		Mediates killer activity of null cells	
IgA	1.5–4.0	Blocks binding of toxins and adherence of microbes	Mucosal linings
		Transported across mucous membranes, including gut	Saliva, tears, breast milk
		Has a secretory piece to protect against digestion	
IgD	0.03	Function unclear but may act as an antigen receptor on virgin B cells. Very low concentration	
IgE	0.0003	Low serum concentration because adsorbed onto mast cells	Involved in allergy, triggering release of histamine from mast cells and basophils
		Cross-linking of IgE on mast cells by antigen mediates degranulation	Provides protection against parasitic worms
		Opsonisation of antigen for eosinophils	

of factors and controlling molecules that make up the complement system and include: C factors (C1 through to C9), factor B, factor D, properdin, mannose binding lectin (MBL), ficolin and MBL associated serine proteases (MASP-1 and MASP-2)

Activation of a component is often achieved by splitting, and the two products that result are labelled with the suffixes **a** and **b**: thus C4 is split into C4a and C4b. The larger fragment generally gets the suffix b and this is also usually the active part. Difficulty arises with the nomenclature of the C2 subunits because C2a and C2b are similar in size and, historically, C2a was the active unit. There has been a move to change C2a to C2b, because 'b' otherwise stands for the functional part, but there is no consensus on this and people working in complement genetics continue to use C2a to stand for the active part.

The aim of the complement cascade is to activate C3 by splitting it into C3a and C3b:

- C3a is a chemotactic agent which enhances the inflammatory process
- C3b binds and coats the cell membrane (**opsonisation**)
- C3b initiates the formation of a lytic structure (the **MAC**).

There are three pathways leading to activation of C3: the **classical pathway**, the **lectin pathway** and the **alternative pathway**:

- The classical pathway is triggered by the interaction of an antibody with an antigenic determinant
- The lectin pathway is triggered by some bacterial cell walls, fungal cell walls and some endotoxins, and does not depend on a pathogen-binding protein.

Both pathways form a C3 convertase enzyme to activate C3. The presence of C3b then activates a third pathway, the

alternative pathway, which forms a different type of C3 convertase enzyme.

The classical and lectin pathways
(Fig. 6.16)

The classical pathway is triggered when the **C1q** part of the **C1 complex** (C1q, C1r and C1s) binds to IgM or IgG complexed with antigen, or when C1 binds directly to a pathogen.

C1q has a bunched form (Fig. 6.17) and each of the six subunits can bind to a constant region domain on the immunoglobulin. It is necessary for several of the subunits to bind for the pathway to be triggered; this ensures that activation does not simply occur when C1q happens to meet a circulating immunoglobulin molecule. Although a single IgM, in contrast to IgG, can initiate the pathway, because of its pentameric structure, the site to which the C1q binds is only revealed when most of IgM antigen-binding sites are actively binding antigen.

Activation leads to conformational changes in C1q, activating C1r and then C1s, cleaving it. C1r and C1s are controlled by a circulating **C1 inhibitor**, raising the triggering threshold.

- **Angioneurotic oedema** is due to a deficiency of C1 inhibitor so that triggering the complement cascade can lead to a dermal and submucosal oedema that can be life-threatening if the airway in involved
- The C1 complex splits C4, and then C2 and the subunits C4b and C2a form a complex, **C4b2a**
- C4b2a (also called **C3 convertase**) cleaves C3 into **C3a** and **C3b**. C3a is chemotactic for leucocytes and C3b joins with C3 convertase to make **C3/C5 convertase** (**C4b2a3b**) which breaks down more C3 and also interacts with C5, initiating the lytic sequence.

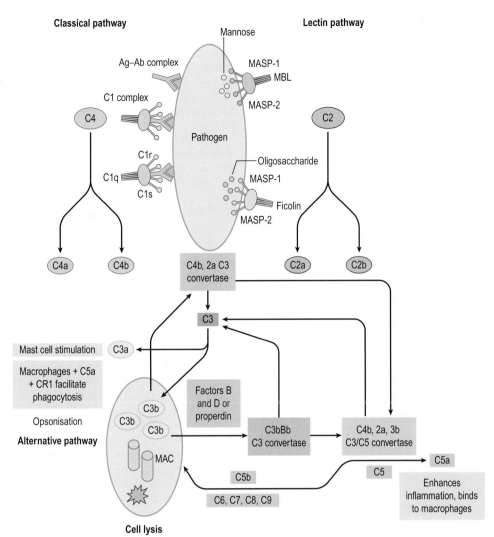

Fig. 6.16 **The complement pathways.** The complement cascade in which C3 convertase is formed through the classical or lectin pathways, splitting C3 into C3a and C3b. C3a stimulates mast cells to enhance the inflammatory response, attracting leucocytes and increasing vascular permeability. C3b binds to the pathogen membrane and activates the alternative pathway producing a different C3 convertase with factors B and D or properdin. Bound C3b and C3 convertase produce a C3/C5 convertase which amplifies the cascade in a feedback mechanism and breaks down C5 to form C5a and C5b. C5b activates other complement proteins and together they form the MAC which forms a channel in the membrane leading to osmotic lysis of the pathogen. CR1, complement receptor 1; MAC, membrane attack complex; MBL, mannose binding lectin; MASP, MBL associated serine protease.

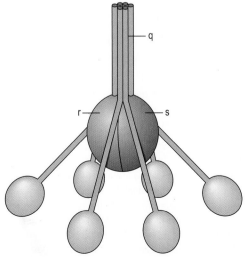

Fig. 6.17 **Structure of the C1 complex.**

The alternative pathway (Fig. 6.16)

The alternative pathway is activated when circulating C3 is cleaved.

■ C3b production simulates the alternative pathway. It binds to the pathogen membrane and, with factor B, factor D, or with properdin, produces another C3 convertase (C3bBb).

Factors that inhibit the alternative pathway

Some factors control the alternative pathway:

■ C3b is inactivated by factors H and I in the blood, and the proteins **DAF (decay accelerating factor)** and **MCP (monocyte chemotactic protein**, CD46) on cell surfaces
■ DAF and factor H compete with factor B for C3b
■ MCP and factor I (**C3b inactivator**) together cleave C3b.

Factors that encourage positive feedback of the alternative pathway

In addition to any disturbance of the presence of membrane factors DAF and MCP, or of circulating factors H and I, activation of **properdin** binds and stabilises C3b, protecting it from factors H and I.

The central role of C3

C3 is central to both the classical and alternative pathways and is the most abundant. It contributes to innate immunity and a deficiency of C3 leads to a susceptibility to bacterial infections. C3 cleavage results in:

- The activation of the lytic sequence through release of C3b
- Release of C3a, which interacts with other complement proteins to stimulate mast cells that can enhance the inflammatory response, or release histamine which increases permeability
- Opsonisation:
  - C3b molecules bind to the pathogen surface through thioester bonds
  - Macrophages have receptors for C5a, released on cleavage of C5 (see below), which aids the **CR1 (complement receptor 1)** to bind to the C3b molecules on the pathogen, facilitating phagocytosis.

The lytic sequence (Fig. 6.16)

C3b and C3 convertase produce the C3/C5 convertase (C4b2a3b).

- C3/C5 convertase cleaves more C3 to produce more C3a and C3b
- C3/C5 convertase cleaves C5 to produce **C5a** and **C5b**.

Release of **C5a**, which binds to specific macrophage receptors, aids opsonisation, and enhances the inflammatory response through chemotactic action, and activates mast cells

Release of **C5b**. C5b has a cell membrane binding site and normally attaches to the cell which has the activating complex attached to it. **Bystander lysis** may occur because sometimes innocent bystander cells may be affected and lysed. This is an important factor in **hypersensitivity** as, for example, if platelets are the innocent cells, their destruction and degranulation can lead to activation of the clotting system and lead to a thrombosis.

- **C5b** also binds to C6 and C7, to form **C5b, 6, 7** and then C8 and multiples of C9 are bound, forming the **MAC (C5,6,7,8(C9))**.
- C8 and C9 have hydrophobic components that incorporate into the membrane lipid but making, at the same time, an ion channel. This channel allows water to move, but not protein. As a result water enters osmotically and the cell is lysed.

THE CELLULAR DEFENCES

Basophils and mast cells

Basophils are derived from the pluripotent stem cell in bone marrow via precursors (see Ch. 12). Found in blood, basophils move into tissue during inflammation. **Mast** cells are also derived from the pluripotent bone marrow stem cell,

and although there are many differences, certain similarities suggest that, although related, their roots are not particularly close and that one is not the precursor of the other. Mast cells are distributed throughout the tissues. They are heterogeneous, those in mucous membranes being different from those in connective tissue, but they have much in common with basophils and what follows generally applies to both cell types.

Both cells are rich in granules that contain **histamine** and other substances that are released by degranulation. The cells are also involved in the manufacture of leukotrienes, prostaglandins and other substances.

Mast cell activation

A number of different mechanisms lead to activation of mast cells and subsequent release of active components:

- **IgE meeting its antigen**: mast cells have Fc receptors for IgE molecules. The cells' different antigen-binding sites are exposed on the surface and bind to any antigen they encounter in the circulation. As the antibody sites become filled with antigen so the complexes become cross-linked and the mast cell degranulates. Helper T lymphocytes are required as IgE production is under their control. Even if the antigen is T independent, class switching to IgE can only take place with helper T lymphocyte approval through presentation by APCs. It is not known how helper T lymphocytes decide which specificities of B lymphocyte should switch to IgE but IL-4, secreted by Th2 T cells, is involved.
- **C5a and C3a components of complement** are chemotactic and cause mast cell degranulation.
- **Neurological factors**. Mast cells are frequently found near nerve endings. The neurotransmitter **substance P**, involved in pain recognition, activates mast cells.
- **Physical stimuli** such as pressure, heat/cold and products of tissue damage, possibly mediated through IL-8 cytokines.
- **Certain chemicals** can stimulate mast cells directly, for example substances in foods.

Substances released by mast cells

- **Histamine**: this is not chemotactic. Its release produces powerful and visible changes through acting on:
  - H_1 **receptors** (blocked by antihistamines such as chlorphenamine) and slightly on
  - H_2 **receptors** (blocked by cimetidine and ranitidine)

  to:

  - Increase venule permeability
  - Cause some arteriolar dilatation
  - Contract smooth muscle.

  This results in a local increase in blood flow and oedema. In the skin, the consequences can be seen as a weal (swelling) and flare (erythema), which appear within a few minutes of histamine release, peak within 30 minutes and are often accompanied by itching.

- **Leukotrienes**: these are metabolites of arachidonic acid and increase permeability of post-capillary venules over a longer period than histamine. They also contract smooth muscle and are chemotactic for various phagocytic cells. Macrophages and polymorphonuclear cells also produce leukotrienes, whereas these cells do not make histamine.

- **Other prostaglandins** from arachidonic acid: these are made in the cell membrane and released on degranulation. Many other cells also produce various prostaglandins that are released by the action of IL-1 and as a result of tissue damage. They act to:
  - Dilate arterioles, increasing local blood flow
  - Induce pain (by blocking **glycine**, which suppresses the transmission of pain signals in the dorsal root ganglion)
  - Cause fever (through their action on the hypothalamus).
- **Cytokines**: these include TNF, IL-1, IL-4, IL-5, IL-6, IL-3 and granulocyte-macrophage colony-stimulating factor (GM-CSF).

Neutrophils

Neutrophil granulocytes are circulating white cells that play an important role in the body's defence system. Along with eosinophils and basophils, these granulated cells originate from the same precursor in bone marrow and are part of the myeloid series of white cells. On their surface are class I HLA molecules, but not class II, which means that they cannot present antigen. They also have Fc and C3b receptors.

Neutrophils are the most common and most dynamic of all the polymorphs with large numbers being made rapidly available from bone marrow when stimulated by **chemotactic factors**, released from activated endothelium, mast cells and macrophages at sites of damage. Cell surface receptors on the neutrophils enable detection and movement up a concentration gradient, enabling their rapid relocation of these cells to the site of damage. Various chemical signals encourage neutrophil chemotaxis and include:

- Complement breakdown products, especially C5a
- Secretory products of inflammatory cells (polymorphs and macrophages) such as leukotrienes, platelet-activating factor (PAF) and IL-8
- Oligopeptides that contain a formylated amino acid, products of prokaryote metabolism.

Response to these may indicate the capacity of neutrophils to recognise non-self.

Role of neutrophils in inflammation
Movement to site of damage
Neutrophils form the bulk of the early acute inflammatory cellular infiltrate at the site of damage and generally arrive before monocytes. In response to chemotactic agents they adhere to the endothelium of local capillaries and venules, and then their pseudopodia squeeze between the endothelial cells and dissolve basement membrane in order to move into the tissue space (**diapedesis**).

Phagocytosis
Neutrophils and other polymorphs have receptors for antibody (Fc receptors) and for C3b. Material coated with these opsonins is phagocytosed, if not too big. Some other material, e.g. latex beads, can be phagocytosed without the aid of opsonins, perhaps indicating an ability of polymorphs to recognise the non-living. Polymorphs are activated mainly by:

- Either C5a and the engagement Fc or C3b receptors
- Or PAF and *N*-formylated peptides – metabolites from microorganisms.

Activation produces a **respiratory burst** in which oxygen is consumed and large quantities of reactive oxygen species (e.g. hydrogen peroxide) are released. Enzymic catalysis of the superoxide and subsequent products produces **hypochloric acid** (chlorous bleach), which is a potent killer of microorganisms and results in **degranulation**, releasing enzymes both into and outside the phagosome. These include proteases and hydrolases, myeloperoxidase, lysozyme and proteins:

- **Myeloperoxidase** is bactericidal in the presence of hydrogen peroxide and halide
- **Lysozyme** breaks the bond between muramic acid and *N*-acetylglucosamine (key bacterial cell wall components)
- **Lactoferrin** (binds iron) and **vitamin B$_{12}$-binding protein** deprive bacteria of important nutrients.

The neutrophil response is continued through release of leukotrienes and PAF, which attract more polymorphs and macrophages and contract smooth muscle. Leukotrienes increase local vessel permeability and prostaglandin release dilates local arterioles and induces the pain and fever associated with inflammation.

Monocytes and macrophages

Monocytes are circulating white cells derived from precursors in the bone marrow, becoming macrophages when they leave the circulation. Like neutrophils they are chemotactic, although with a slower response, and have Fc and C3b receptors. In contrast they have both class I and class II HLA molecules and therefore they can present antigen.

Macrophages and monocytes respond to the following chemotactic agents:

- C5a and (much more weakly) C3a
- Leukotrienes (from mast cells, polymorphs and macrophages)
- The IL-8 group cytokines, from other macrophages, and activated CD4 T cells
- Products of tissue damage (denatured proteins, etc.)
- Some non-self substances (e.g. formylated peptides, typical bacterial products).

Migration inhibition factor (**MIF**), released from activated helper T cells, prevents macrophages migrating away.

Role of macrophages in inflammation
Macrophages are versatile cells and act as the main scavengers of old cells and debris. Producing a wide variety of substances, they are important agents in the inflammatory response and are also the main APCs in the fight against pathogens. They are activated by a variety of agents including:

- **Macrophage-activating factors** (**MAFs**) from activated helper T cells are the most efficacious and include IFN, MIF and TNF
- Non-self substances engaging macrophage receptors
- Chemotaxins (the least efficacious).

Phagocytosis is initiated when cell surface receptors are engaged (see The central role of C3, above), leading to expression of class II HLA molecules and triggering of the respiratory burst, induced by MAF. Cytokines also assist in antigen presentation to T helper cells, enabling antibody production. Antibodies coating the pathogen make it easier for the macrophage to stick and phagocytose the foreign body.

Activation also leads to the lysosomes being filled with strong oxidising agents (superoxide radicals), destructive enzymes (including those specifically to attack bacteria, such as lysozyme) and antibacterial agents (such as vitamin B_{12}-binding protein and iron-binding lactoferrin, removing substances needed by bacteria for their growth).

Highly activated macrophages may have their 'index of suspicion of non-self' raised sufficiently to attempt to destroy most neighbouring substances and cells discharging the content of the lysosomes outside the cell. Not all macrophage products are destructive. α_1-Antitrypsin and α_2-macroglobulin neutralise destructive proteases and also release factors that promote repair and cell division.

Macrophages may help cancer cells proliferate through their attraction to hypoxic tumour cells. TNF released by the macrophage activates a transcription factor, **nuclear factor-κB (NF-κB)**, which enters the cancer cell and produces substances that inhibit apoptosis.

A functioning macrophage

Pneumocystis carinii (*jiroveci*) is a protozoon to which we are exposed continuously. The immune system, with assistance from macrophages, ensures that healthy people are not affected. People with pure B cell deficiencies are also not affected. Macrophages on their own do not become sufficiently activated but interaction with the helper T cell is key. Individuals who are T cell deficient can experience life-threatening pneumonia as a result of exposure to *P. carinii* (see Clinical box 6.2).

A struggling macrophage

Mycobacterium tuberculosis is phagocytosed by macrophages but is not killed. This is because macrophages lack a receptor for a particular component in the tough mycobacterial cell wall which inhibits the usual lysosome–phagosome fusion. This ensures that bacteria are retained within the cell, producing a prolonged chronic response that leads to widespread tissue damage; this **delayed-type hypersensitivity (type 4 hypersensitivity)** encourages the development of granulomas.

Eosinophils

Eosinophils are derived from the same precursors as neutrophils in the bone marrow and circulate as white cells in the blood. Precursor differentiation into eosinophils depends on particular stimulation from IL-3 and IL-5. Like neutrophils they are phagocytic, chemotactic, have Fc and C3b receptors and class I, but not class II, HLA molecules. They differ particularly in their granule content.

Eosinophils may be activated by engagement of Fc or C3b receptors with specific IgG and C3b molecules, by formylated peptides (metabolites from microorganisms) and by cytokines (including IL-3 and IL-5).

Role of eosinophils in inflammation

Eosinophils have special roles in combating helminth parasitic incursion (such as in schistosomiasis) and are also important in the mechanisms involved in the control of allergy. They are less effective than neutrophils in destroying bacteria but play a role in fighting viral infections and in the removal of fibrin, deposited as part of the inflammatory process.

Toxins are released into phagosomes or, in the case of helminths, onto the surface of the parasite to which the eosinophil is attached. These toxins include:

- Superoxides from the respiratory burst
- **Eosinophil cationic protein** and **major basic protein**.

  These are toxic to helminths.

- Peroxidases and neurotoxins (with antiviral activity).

Red cells

Some red cells have receptors for C3b and carry immune complexes that contain C3b, to be phagocytosed in the liver or spleen.

Platelets

While platelets are mainly involved in haemostasis, they are also involved in the inflammatory process where they interact with other cells through secretion of various inflammatory mediators. Substances released from the lytic sequence of complement activation and PAF from activated neutrophils stimulate the aggregation and degranulation of bystanding platelets, bringing about a local thrombosis. Platelets also have Fc receptors for IgG and so bind to antigen via specific antibody. They also secrete PAF and IL-8. While filarial and other worms release prostaglandins that inhibit platelet aggregation, the interaction between platelets and the parasite can induce cytotoxicity.

HYPERSENSITIVITY

Hypersensitivity refers to the undesirable side effects of the normal immune response, whether or not that response is directed against self or non-self. There are five types of hypersensitivity (Table 6.9).

Table 6.9 Types of hypersensitivity and their manifestation

Type	Synonyms	Mediator	Examples
1	Allergic, immediate	IgE	Asthma; anaphylaxis; urticaria
2	Cytotoxic, antibody dependent	IgM or IgG (and complement)	Autoimmune haemolytic anaemia (AIHA), idiopathic thrombocytopenic purpura (ITP), haemolytic disease of the newborn
3	Immune complex	IgG (and complement)	Systemic lupus erythematosus (SLE), polyarteritis nodosa
4	Delayed type, antibody independent	T cells	BCG vaccination, transplant organ rejection, contact dermatitis
5	Subtype 2	IgM or IgG (and complement)	Graves disease; myasthenia gravis

Type 1 hypersensitivity

The interaction between antigen and IgE results in mast cell degranulation and the release of histamines, leukotrienes, prostaglandins and other substances that cause symptoms within minutes. Figure 6.18 summarises the process.

Local exposure can result in:

- **Hay fever** (due to pollen antigens)
- **Asthma** (pollens, house dust mite, fungal spores)
- Local **urticaria** (insect bites and stings).

In highly sensitised people, antigen exposure, trivial in most people, causes massive mast cell degranulation, with systemic effects: anaphylaxis, general urticaria, angioneurotic oedema of skin and mucosa, asthma, hay fever, gastrointestinal symptoms. Individuals who are **atopic** have an increased predisposition to form IgE antibodies against common environmental antigens, leading to conditions such as asthma or eczema (see Clinical box 6.14). These conditions have a strong inherited component.

The **Prausnitz–Kustner (PK)** experiment showed that type 1 (immediate) hypersensitivity could be transferred by serum. Prausnitz was hypersensitive to a certain antigen and he injected this antigen into Kustner's skin. Subsequent injection of serum from Prausnitz injected into Kushner's skin showed an immediate flare and weal, mediated by specific IgE in the transfused serum. Other stimuli can lead to a type 1-like hypersensitivity resulting from mast cell degranulation:

- Heat/cold/pressure leading to urticaria
- Food allergy – although some foods may act as antigens for IgE, the effect is probably due to direct activation of mast cells from chemicals in the food
- Complement mediated – often mixed with type 2 or type 3 hypersensitivity.

Type 2 hypersensitivity

(see Clinical box 6.15)

This occurs when antibodies attach to determinants on self structures (auto-antibodies). The tissues are damaged by classical complement activation, phagocytosis and/or killer activity. Although originally used to describe antibodies against blood cells, it now includes antibodies against other tissues that mediate damage. For example, **Goodpasture syndrome**, in which antibodies develop against basement membrane in kidney and lung.

Type 3 hypersensitivity

Antigen–antibody immune complexes, with or without complement, cause damage to neighbouring tissue. The antigen may be self, e.g. nuclear constituents as in systemic lupus erythematosus (SLE), or non-self, e.g. streptococci. Effects can be local or systemic.

- **Local form**: the Arthus reaction. In this model of the reaction, an individual is thoroughly immunised against an antigen, producing high titres of IgG. Antigen is then injected subcutaneously, producing localised inflammation of the skin, peaking several hours later. Clinically, inhaled fungal spores can cause **extrinsic allergic alveolitis** (farmer's lung).
- **Systemic form**: serum sickness. Experimentally, when a large quantity of foreign (horse) serum is injected intravenously, antibodies build up. When the concentration equals that of the antigen, immune complexes precipitate resulting in rashes, joint pain, fever, lymphadenopathy and hypotension, for example. Clinical examples are **SLE**, **glomerulonephritis**, **Henoch–Schönlein purpura**, and **polyarteritis nodosa**, but often the causative antigen is unclear (see Clinical box 6.15).

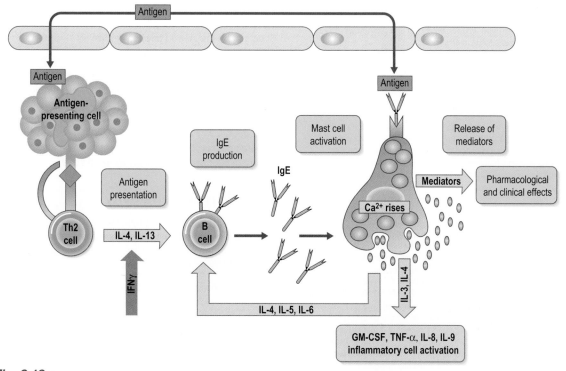

Fig. 6.18 **Type 1 hypersensitivity.** See text for abbreviations.

Clinical box 6.14   Asthma

Asthma is essentially an inflammatory disease of the airways, which is as yet poorly understood, but thought to be a type 1 hypersensitivity reaction (see also Ch. 13) exacerbated by an imbalance of the Th1/Th2 cytokines. The inflammation is due to an immune response to allergens (e.g. pollen, house dust mite faecal particles, fungal spores and some chemicals).

Bronchial hyper-responsiveness in asthma is caused by an attempt to compensate for airflow obstruction due to airway inflammation through hyperventilation, but this is limited when tidal volume approaches the lung dead airspace volume. A ventilation/perfusion mismatch leads to vasoconstriction and both lead to an uneven distribution of air and alveolar hypoxia. Initially hypercarbia is prevented and carbon dioxide easily removed leading to a reduction in $PaCO_2$ and respiratory alkalosis, but with the worsening obstruction and increased ventilation/perfusion mismatch, carbon dioxide is retained as it becomes more difficult to breathe out, leading to hyperinflation of the lungs. This, and the increased oxygen consumption associated with the extra work of breathing, and increased cardiac output, leads to metabolic acidosis and respiratory failure leads to respiratory acidosis. Airway remodelling also takes place with hypertrophy of bronchial smooth muscle, transformation of fibroblasts into myofibroblasts and collagen deposition.

The **airway inflammation** appears to be driven by an imbalance in cytokine production. Th1 lymphocytes normally produce IL-2 and IFN-α which initiates a cellular immune response, imitated early after birth in response to environmental allergens. Th2 lymphocytes, in contrast, stimulate a variety of cytokines (IL-4, IL-5, IL-6, IL-9 and IL-13). IL-4 and IL-13 stimulate IgE and this and other cytokines lead to stimulation of mast cells, basophils and eosinophils that produce histamine and prostaglandins that mediate the subsequent inflammation and remodeling processes:

- Lymphocytes and dendritic cells: dendritic cells take up and present allergens to the lymphocytes, stimulating the Th1 and Th2 lymphocytes to produce and release cytokines that promote the migration and activation of mast cells and eosinophils. It is hypothesised that environmental 'hygiene' may

be responsible for the Th1/Th2 imbalance resulting in increased prevalence of asthma in westernised populations. Lymphocyte and macrophage activity is inhibited by corticosteroids, but not γ-adrenoceptor agonists.

- Mast cells, stimulated by IL-4 and IL-9, release histamine, prostaglandin D2 and leukotriene C4, powerful mediators that act on bronchial smooth muscle and blood vessels to cause the immediate bronchial constriction in asthma. Here, the β-adrenoceptor agonists (e.g. salbutamol, salmeterol) used in the treatment of asthma inhibit mast cell mediator release, but have no effect on airway inflammation (or hyper-responsiveness). Mast cell activation is inhibited by the anti-inflammatory agents sodium cromoglycate and nedocromil sodium. In susceptible patients, the inadvertent administration of drugs that inhibit prostaglandin synthesis leads to an overproduction of leukotrienes by eosinophils (e.g. aspirin, NSAIDs), and the administration of non-selective β-adrenoceptor antagonists (blockers) may thus precipitate an acute asthma attack. Basophils are stimulated by IL-3.

- Eosinophils congregate at the airways under the influence of eosinophilopoietic cytokines (IL-3, IL-5) and chemokines. When activated, the eosinophils release leukotriene C4 and other proteins (enhanced by cytokines and chemokines) that are toxic to the bronchial epithelium, triggering airway inflammation, where oedema and increased exudative secretions obstruct the airways. Inhaled or oral corticosteroids (the preventive and rescue treatments for asthma) inhibit eosinophil activation and decrease their number. Leukotriene receptor antagonists may also be effective in reducing inflammation. Eosinophil activation is also prevented by sodium cromoglycate and nedocromil sodium.

Airway remodelling in chronic asthma, the structures of bronchial epithelium and smooth muscle are altered. When combined with the ongoing effects of inflammatory cells and mediators, the normal function is impaired. Damage to the epithelium causes thickening of the airway wall and makes it more vulnerable to infection. Hyperplasia of the bronchial smooth muscles increases hyper-responsiveness.

Clinical box 6.15   Disordered immunological response to bacterial infection

Disease can result from disordered immunological responses to apparently minor bacterial infections. Examples include rheumatic fever (type 2 hypersensitivity) and glomerulonephritis (type 3 hypersensitivity) in children.

- **Rheumatic fever** is a complication of throat infection by a group A streptococcus (sore throat, scarlet fever) in children (aged 5–15). Although the precise mechanism is unclear, it is thought to be the result of a type 2 hypersensitivity reaction in genetically vulnerable individuals, leading to an autoimmune response triggered by molecular mimicry between bacterial cell wall M proteins and cardiac myosin and laminin. All the tissues of the heart may be affected leading to pancarditis, but consequent damage to the heart valves is common. Associated inflammation of the synovial membranes of joints (flitting arthritis), subcutaneous nodules (Aschoff's nodules) and erythema marginatum may be present during the acute stage of the disease. Owing to the widespread prescription of antibiotics in the developed world, rheumatic heart disease is now rare, but it still occurs in developing nations.

- **Post-streptococcal glomerulonephritis** (PSGN): PSGN is thought to be due to a type 3 hypersensitivity reaction where immune complexes formed to combat a bacterial infection infiltrate the glomerular basement membrane. Activation of the complement cascade then destroys the basement membrane. A child may develop an acute nephritic syndrome, with proteinuria, oedema and hypertension (see Ch. 14), 2–3 weeks (the time taken for development of the immune complex) after a streptococcal infection (Lancefield group A β-haemolytic streptococcus). Treatment with dietary salt and protein restriction, diuretics, antihypertensives and dialysis may be necessary. Prognosis is usually good.

Type 4 hypersensitivity

This is damage associated with the interaction between activated helper T cells and activated macrophages, or activated cytotoxic T cells and NK cells (**delayed type hypersensitivity**). It cannot be transferred through serum.

- BCG vaccination (injection of attenuated *M. bovis:* the causative agent of bovine tuberculosis and a relatively uncommon cause of human tuberculosis) in people who have previously been exposed to tuberculosis produces a lesion that is maximal after more than 2 days.

- Granulomas, T cell infiltrates, contact dermatitis and organ rejection are probably all results of this.

Type 5 hypersensitivity

This is a subtype of type 2 hypersensitivity – instead of the antibodies acting against cell surface components, this definition is used to describe situations when the antibodies act against cell receptors. For example:

- **Graves disease**, where antibody to thyroid stimulating hormone receptors stimulates the thyroid, causing thyrotoxicosis

- **Myasthenia gravis** in which antibodies develop to acetylcholine receptors in postsynaptic neuromuscular junction, resulting in muscle weakness and fatigue.

TOLERANCE

Tolerance is a specific immune non-reactivity against a certain substance. Individuals should be tolerant of their own body components (**self-tolerance**). Experiments in newborn mice show that foreign antigens introduced within a few hours of birth are usually tolerated while the antigen persists (**neonatal tolerance**). In humans the exposure probably happens when the foetus is only a few months old. Particular immunisation schedules in adults may induce tolerance, rather than immunity (**acquired tolerance**). Variations in solubility, route of delivery, or concentration of antigen, and the ability of the person to launch a response are all factors that influence the development of tolerance.

Tolerance mechanisms

There are three main cellular mechanisms that lead to toleration.

Clonal deletion (central tolerance)

Clonal deletion occurs when developing B cells and T cells recognise self-antigen while in the bone marrow or thymus and are deleted before they become fully immunocompetent. Initiated in foetal life it will continue throughout life as new lymphocytes are produced.

Anergy

If a mature T cell or B cell recognises antigen in certain unfavourable circumstances, it will become anergic, or frozen, temporarily but not permanently refractory to activation.

- T cell anergy can occur in the absence of dendritic cells at the first encounter with antigen
- B cell anergy may occur in the absence of T cell help.

Acquired tolerance

Acquired tolerance is where there is a specific non-reactivity to an antigen which would normally lead to an immune response. For example, in pregnancy, the foetus must be tolerated by the mother. There are several hypotheses that have been suggested to explain this phenomenon: Eu-FEDS is the best known.

- **Eu-FEDS (eutherian fetoembryonic defence system)** hypothesis states that glycoproteins and carbohydrate present in the reproductive system and expressed on gametes (for example α-**fetoprotein** and **CA125**) suppress the immune response that would otherwise reject sperm and eggs. The latter do not carry any HLA antigens allowing them to be recognised as self and so there must be another mechanism. Support for this model comes from the apparent acquisition of these substances by invading pathogens. The profile of the main oligosaccharides linked to CA125 and the major surface glycoprotein of HIV-1 (gp12) almost perfectly overlap.

The ability to produce acquired immunity is an important aim of medical treatment in organ transplantation. **Oral tolerance** is important as the gut mucosa will be exposed to a variety of foreign antigens in food. **Inflammatory bowel disease** may be the result of a failure in oral tolerance (see Clinical box 6.16).

Clinical box 6.16 **Inflammatory bowel disease**

Crohns disease (CD) and **ulcerative colitis** (UC) are the major recognised forms of inflammatory bowel disease. CD can affect any part of the gastrointestinal tract (including oral manifestations), whereas UC affects the colon. Clinically, they both present with diarrhoea, abdominal pain and weight loss (malnutrition), but a diagnostic distinction is important because they are managed differently. Clinical, radiological and histological information give the diagnostic clues. Extra-gastrointestinal manifestations include inflammatory arthritis.

Immunologically, the inflammatory process in CD and UC is similar. It is thought that susceptible patients have defects in the genetic regulation of the immune response so that both specific and non-specific inflammatory responses to endogenous antigens in the intestinal lumen are exaggerated. In CD, macrophages and Th1 lymphocytes are upregulated leading to an excess of pro-inflammatory mediators such as cytokines (interleukins IL-12 and tumour necrosis factor α). In UC, the Th2 lymphocyte response is altered with excess production of interleukins (IL-5 and IL-10) and IgG and IgE. Activation of neutrophils, eosinophils, mast cells and fibroblasts leads to excess chemokine production, which can result in tissue damage, ulceration and inflammation in the wall of the bowel.

AUTOIMMUNE DISEASE

Autoimmune disease is a disease resulting from **autoreactivity**. Autoreactivity, a response to self, is common, but does not necessarily lead to autoimmune disease. There are also many diseases characterised by a lymphocyte/macrophage inflammatory infiltrate that have no detectable infection. They are often called 'autoimmune', meaning that they are caused by some breakdown in self-tolerance. This is often unproven. Examples of such conditions are where there is:

- **Covert viral infection** and the viral antigens manufactured by the body's cells are the targets of the immune response. No breakdown in self-tolerance is necessary.
- **Chronic tissue destruction** provokes a chronic inflammatory infiltrate, and this might be called 'autoimmune' if the real mechanism of tissue destruction is not detected.
- Examples of true autoimmune disease are where there is a breakdown in B cell or T cell self-tolerance.

B cell self-tolerance breakdown

Autoreactive B cells that escape clonal deletion in the bone marrow and enter the circulation may avoid anergy in two ways:

- **Recognition of mixed self/non-self material.** Foreign infective material may have some determinants that resemble self which the autoreactive B cells process. The material will also have non-self determinants and presentation of these may gain help from a self-tolerant helper T cell population. For example, autoimmune disease can be initiated artificially by injecting self tissue in **Freund's adjuvant** (a suspension of mycobacteria in an oily suspension) which can lead to the production of particular immunoglobulins.
- **Autoreactive B cells** may receive help from autoreactive T cells.

T cell self-tolerance breakdown

This may also allow breakdown of self-tolerance among B cells. There are several theories as to how this might happen:

- **Release of material from a privileged site.** Some structures, like the lens of the eye, contain self material that is not accessible to the immune system, and is only released in minute quantities and so there will have been no deletion or anergy of lymphocyte clones. A substantial release of this material, perhaps as a result of injury, may result in an autoimmune response against it.
- **Unusual expression of HLA molecules and/or other ligands.** If a specialised cell only expresses class I HLA molecules, for example, along with few other immunologically important adhesion molecules or ligands, T cells may not be deleted or anergised against peptides made only in that cell type. These active peptides become 'immunologically invisible'.
- **Cross-reaction of microbial peptide with uncommon self-peptide.** If a microbial peptide cross-reacts with an immunologically invisible self-peptide, or with a self-peptide that has elicited anergy but not deletion, then it may elicit an immune response. As it is the HLA molecules that present self and foreign peptides, and different HLA alleles select different peptides, then the HLA alleles that an individual possesses may determine whether or not an immune response is elicited.
- **Loss of suppression.** If autoreactive cells are being suppressed by other T cells, then this might change if the suppressing cells are eliminated, or the cytokine profile changes, as it might during a microbial infection.

OTHER SUBSTANCES IMPORTANT TO THE IMMUNE SYSTEM

Interferons

IFNs are natural proteins or glycoproteins that have non-specific antiviral activity acting through cellular metabolic processes involving synthesis of RNA and protein. There are three major classes of IFN, which depend on the type of receptor. Some are produced by virally infected cells and activated macrophages, others may be produced by activated T lymphocytes.

IFNs have an antiviral effect, repress cell growth (of both normal and tumour cells) and regulate the immune system through signals induced when they interact with cell surface receptors. They increase NK activity, increase expression of HLA molecules (synergistically with TNF) and are the main macrophage activator. Binding of IFNs to special receptors on the cell surface induces an **antiviral state**. They act by triggering a process in the cell that:

- Inhibits viral replication
- Upregulates class I HLA molecules, thus increasing presentation of molecules to cytotoxic T cells
- Increases activity of p53, a transcription factor that induced apoptosis of the infected cells.

Tumour necrosis factor

TNF is a polypeptide made by activated macrophages and activated lymphocytes. Its primary role is in the regulation of immunity. It activates and **enhances the ability of phagocytes** to destroy microbes and also **acts on vascular endothelium** to allow leucocytes to move out of the circulation.

TNF is also involved in the induction of **apoptosis** of tumour cells and virally infected cells, assisted by IFNs, and also interacts with cell surface receptors (different from IFN receptors) to elicit an antiviral state. Increased production of TNF has significant side effects. Chronically high levels are seen in malignancy, producing **cachexia**. Cachexia is an unwanted loss of weight and loss of appetite seen in some conditions, particularly end-stage cancer. Cachexia was named after a substance, cachectin, now called TNF. Acutely high levels produce shock (fever, hypotension, metabolic acidosis, disseminated intravascular coagulation (DIC) and diarrhoea).

Acute phase proteins

Acute phase proteins are secreted by liver cells. They increase or decrease in concentration in response to inflammatory processes. Those that increase in concentration act to destroy or inhibit microbe growth (e.g. CRP) or provide negative feedback (e.g. α_2-macroglobulin – a damage limitation agent).

Transforming growth factor-β

Transforming growth factor-β (TGF-β) is secreted by almost all cells in an inactive form but can be activated by proteases. Activated T cells and activated macrophages secrete the active form, which has a wide range of effects, positive and negative, on cell growth. It causes the growth of new blood vessels and inhibits T cell proliferation. It also induces **apoptosis** through two pathways:

- **SMAD** is a class of proteins that are altered and form complexes through TGF-β interacting with cell receptors. The complex enters the cell nucleus, where it acts as a transcription factor inducing apoptosis.
- **DAXX** (death domain-associated protein) plays a major role in apoptosis. It is involved with TGF-β as it interacts with its receptor. Binding of TGF-β induces the main DAXX apoptotic pathway.

INFLAMMATION AND REPAIR

ACUTE INFLAMMATION

Inflammation is the reaction of a vascularised living tissue to local injury (see also Clinical box 6.17) Its aim is to:

- Contain and isolate the injury
- Destroy invading microbes and neutralise toxins
- Heal and repair the damage.

There are five main signs of acute infection: **heat**, **redness**, **pain**, **swelling** and **loss of function**. These are the result of vascular and cellular events.

Vascular events

Substances released as part of the inflammatory response produce transient and rapid **vasoconstriction** of arterioles, followed by **vasodilation**, causing increased flow of blood through downstream capillaries. The increase in permeability leads to an **extravascular exudate**.

- An **exudate** is a fluid with a high protein content, approaching that of plasma. The combination of the increased intravascular hydrostatic pressure (because of the vasodilation) and reduced or absent osmotic gradient (because of the leakage of protein) contribute to the increased volume of the exudate.
- **Pus** is inflammatory exudate rich in leucocytes, especially neutrophils, living and dead, together with microorganisms.

Cellular events

Leucocytes need to move from the circulation to the site of infection (**extravasation**). They do this through a series of processes. In leaky capillaries, they **marginate**, moving to the vessel wall, **roll** along the endothelium and **adhere** to the wall. **Diapedesis (transmigration)** follows, in which the leucocytes insert pseudopodia through the endothelium at or near the intercellular junctions, then pass through the basement membrane into the tissues. Endothelial cells and leucocytes express mutually recognising adhesion molecules that are necessary for rolling, adhesion and diapedesis.

The leucocytes then **migrate** through the tissues, induced by **chemotaxis**, moving within tissues up concentration gradients of various chemicals and mediators, leading them to the site of the inflammation.

Phagocytosis and killing of microbes

A phagocyte must **bind** to material that is to be phagocytosed through its own receptors that recognise dead/denatured or non-self material, or use special receptor molecules that have been made by other cells in the body and are already bound to the microbe, such as acute phase proteins, complement or antibodies. The phagocyte extends pseudopodia around the material producing a vacuole, or **phagosome**.

Intracellular **lysosomal granules** fuse with the phagosome, introducing enzymes such as lysozyme, proteases and hydrolases that can destroy the cell. Other agents are also involved

which are dependent on the **respiratory burst**: by generating NADPH, the phagocyte can generate toxic superoxides.

Initiation of the inflammatory response

In the **plasma** there are three 'cascade systems' of proteins that help to mediate the inflammatory response:

- The **coagulation system** is activated in tissue damage by both intrinsic and extrinsic pathways, culminating in the production of fibrin which helps to contain the infection. When fibrin is broken down its degradation products act as chemotactic factors for leucocytes and increase endothelial permeability, bringing more cells to the site of the damage and increasing the blood flow in the area.
- The **kinin system**, activated through coagulation factor XII, culminates in the production of bradykinin. Bradykinin leads to vasodilation and sensitises sensory nociceptor peripheral terminals, reducing the pain threshold and allowing pain to be experienced.
- The **complement system** is activated by foreign substances. C3a and C5a activate leucocytes to express adhesion molecules. They are also chemotactic for leucocytes and activate mast cells. C3b also acts as a receptor for phagocytes. The system produces products that lyse microbes and cells.

In the **tissues**, various cells, especially **mast cells**, produce important **mediators of inflammation**. Figure 6.19 shows the pathways that lead to the production of various inflammatory mediators. **Mast cells** are scattered throughout the tissues, especially near epithelia and blood vessels, and are important sources of mediators. They can be activated:

- Directly by **tissue damage** and agents causing tissue damage

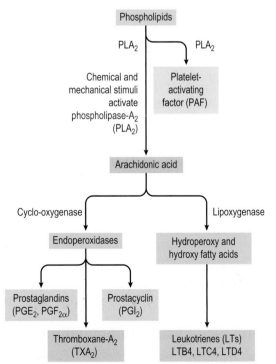

Fig. 6.19 **Inflammatory mediators derived 'de novo' from cell membrane phospholipids.**

- Through **nerves**, including the branch axons of sensory nerves, which secrete substance P
- Through the action of **C3a** and **C5a**, derived from complement.

Through foreign substances interacting with **IgE**. Activated mast cells produce important mediators:

- **Histamine** causes arteriolar dilatation and an increase in vascular permeability.
- **Leukotrienes** cause an increase in vascular permeability and are chemotactic for leucocytes.
- **Prostaglandins** cause arteriolar dilatation and pain.
- **PAF** causes activation and aggregation of platelets, increases vascular permeability, activates leucocytes to express adhesion molecules, and is chemotactic for leucocytes.

Many body cells produce **prostaglandins** and **chemokines** when damaged, or exposed to the products of tissue damage, e.g. denatured proteins.

- Chemokines activate **leucocytes** to express adhesion molecules, and they are chemotactic for leucocytes.
- **Macrophages** resident in uninflamed tissue become activated if exposed to the products of tissue damage or microbial products. They secrete **prostaglandins**, **chemokines**, **IL-1** and **TNF**, causing endothelial cells to express adhesion molecules; TNF increases vascular permeability.
- **Endothelial cells** are activated by direct damage, by IL-1 and TNF, and by interacting with activated leucocytes in the lumen. Once activated, expression of adhesion molecules increases, permeability increases, and thrombosis is promoted, which prevents spread of infection. Endothelial cells also secrete **chemokines** and **nitric oxide**, which is toxic to microbes and cells, and is a powerful vasodilator.

Systemic effects of acute inflammation

Fever occurs through resetting the hypothalamic thermostat at a higher level. IL-1 and TNF release prostaglandins in the hypothalamus and prostaglandins act directly on the thermostat. Fever helps infection, but if the temperature increases too much it can lead to fitting and death. **Acute phase proteins** are released from the liver, stimulated by IL-1, some of which interact with microbes and aid phagocytosis.

Colony-stimulating factors stimulate the release of more leucocytes by the bone marrow causing a **raised white cell count**. Feelings of **malaise**, **lethargy** and **sleepiness** are due to cytokines acting on the brain, preventing behavioural excesses that might enhance the damage. Acute inflammation can also cause damage to self. The main dangers are through:

- The release of destructive lysosomal contents
- The action of complement
- Swelling in a confined space (e.g. brain)
- The excessive release of cytokines causing hyperpyrexia, shock and death.

Outcome of acute inflammation

Acute inflammation may be resolved in several ways. Resolution is the best outcome, the tissue returning to the state before the damage took place. Often, however, organisation and repair processes that lay down fibrous tissue lead to scarring. Abscesses can also form, in which pus remains trapped in the tissues and may, with time, become organised and persist as a chronic inflammation. Outcomes can be more serious. Local damage can result in death because important structures are involved, e.g. in meningitis. Uncontrolled infection may lead to septicaemia and excessive cytokine release can cause hyperpyrexia, shock and death.

CHRONIC INFLAMMATION

Chronic inflammation differs from acute inflammation in various ways:

- Longer time span (months/years rather than days/weeks)
- Tissue destruction, inflammation and healing all happen simultaneously
- The predominant inflammatory cells are different – macrophages, lymphocytes and plasma cells predominate, rather than polymorphonuclear leucocytes.

Initiation of chronic inflammation

Chronic inflammation can occur after, or in the absence of, an acute inflammatory process. An example of the former, where an initial acute inflammation does not resolve, is found in **chronic osteomyelitis**. In this disease there is an initial acute infection due to blood-borne bacteria seeding in the bone, possibly at the site of minor damage. Resolution is impaired because the tissues are rigid: pressure builds up, pus cannot drain, the blood supply is impaired and pus tracks under the periosteum, further impairing the blood supply. Some bone dies and acts as a foreign body, continuing the stimulation.

Chronic inflammation also occurs where an initial phase of acute inflammation is absent or not severe. This occurs if:

- A non-degradable foreign substance is present in the tissues (e.g. talc, asbestos or silica) (see also Clinical box 6.18)

Clinical box 6.18	**Lung diseases associated with inhaled foreign bodies**

A number of lung diseases are associated with inflammation due to occupational exposure to foreign bodies, giving rise to health and safety issues. These conditions may be caused by acute or chronic inflammation or allergy. They include:

- Acute bronchitis from inhalation of noxious, irritant gases such as chlorine, sulphur dioxide and ammonia.
- Widespread pulmonary fibrosis from inhalation of mineral dusts, such as pneumoconiosis (miner's lung) from inhalation of coal dust, localised pulmonary fibrosis due to asbestosis from inhaling asbestos among shipbuilders and from the use of asbestos in insulation material in houses and even domestic appliances, and silicosis in glass foundry workers, stonemasons and sand blasters.
- Occupational asthma and chronic obstructive pulmonary disease, due to inhalation of varnishes and paint sprays, cement dust, enzyme washing powders and allergens from flour and grain.
- Cryptogenic fibrosing alveolitis (idiopathic pulmonary fibrosis) of unknown aetiology may occasionally be associated with exposure to wood or metal dust. Some patients, however, may have autoimmune disease.
- Allergic alveolitis (extrinsic) is associated with exposure to moulds and fungal spores, e.g. farmer's lung (mould from hay or vegetables), bird fancier's lung (bird feathers and excreta), and cheese washer's, mushroom worker's and wine maker's lungs.
- Cancers associated with exposure to industrial substances such as asbestos (mesothelioma) and radon (miners).

There is a persistent pathogen, often intracellular (e.g. viruses or mycobacteria)
An immune response is made in the absence of any apparent pathogen – an **autoimmune** reaction.

Manifestation of chronic infection

The principal signs of acute inflammation (redness, heat, swelling, pain, loss of function) and inflammatory exudates are often less marked in a chronic infection. The tissues are infiltrated by many cells. In chronic infections this infiltration tends to be macrophages, with or without lymphocytes and plasma cells. In acute inflammation neutrophils predominate. Repair takes place through:

- New vessel formation
- Fibroblast accumulation
- Laying down intercellular matrix including collagen
- Remodelling.

The repair has special features:

- **Granulomas**. If there is non-degradable foreign matter, or persistent pathogenic presence, these special histological features may occur.
- **Eosinophils**, specialised phagocytes for fighting helminths, increase in these infections.

Granulomas

Granulomas differ in appearance depending on the cause. They are roughly spherical and macrophages are the essential ingredient. Granulomas have a distinctive architecture:

- A central zone of **necrosis** – not present in all granulomas.
- A zone rich in **macrophages** and cells derived from macrophages. If there is no necrosis, this will be in the centre; if there is central necrosis, the macrophages surround it. Macrophages may adopt an elongated shape to form **epithelioid cells**, or may join together to form **giant** cells.
- A zone of mainly **lymphocytes** and **plasma cells** develops surrounding the macrophages. These are not always present: they are scanty or absent in granulomas caused by non-degradable foreign material.

Old granulomas may become infiltrated with **fibroblasts** and **collagen**, ending as a fibrous scar. They may **calcify**.

Stimulants of granulomas

Foreign body granulomas are caused by non-degradable foreign substance within tissues, such as talc or asbestos.

- In granulomas there is no central necrosis and few or no lymphocytes, because there is no protein, carbohydrate or lipid antigen. Instead there are collections of **macrophages**, and **foreign body giant cells**, formed from macrophages, with nuclei scattered throughout the cytoplasm.
- Macrophages secrete IL-1, TNF and IFN-α, which are involved in the formation of the granuloma, and of giant cells. In the longer term they stimulate **fibrosis**. In conditions such as silica inhalation, granulomas develop widely throughout the lung tissue. The subsequent widespread fibrosis impairs lung function.

Tuberculosis

Mycobacterium tuberculosis most commonly enters the body by inhalation into the lungs, or through the gut by swallowing (see Clinical box 6.1).

- After an initial neutrophil infiltrate, the mycobacteria are taken up by macrophages. Mycobacterial antigens are presented to T lymphocytes and the macrophages become strongly activated.
- Mycobacteria are resistant to this killing process, and the contents of lysozymes spill out and damage surrounding tissues before many mycobacteria are killed.
- Granulomas form, with a central zone of necrosis (caseous 'cheesy' necrosis).
- Beyond the granuloma is a macrophage-rich zone, containing epithelioid cells and **Langerhans giant cells**, surrounded by lymphocytes (T cells, B cells and plasma cells).

It is the secretion of cytokines, particularly IFN-α, which fully activates the macrophages. If the infection is contained, then the granulomas may eventually fibrose and calcify, though they may still contain viable mycobacteria.

Schistosomiasis

This is an important helminth infection with a complicated lifecycle. The adult forms live in mesenteric or bladder veins (depending on species), and the eggs are shed and may accumulate in the liver or bladder wall. Granulomas form around these, with eosinophils as well as macrophages and lymphocytes surrounding them.

Many other **bacteria**, **fungi** and **helminths** induce granuloma formation, though only a few have central necrosis. The details differ from pathogen to pathogen.

Other granulomatous conditions

Sarcoidosis an immune system disorder of unknown origin and involves granuloma formation, mainly in the lungs. The granulomas are similar to those in tuberculosis, but with no central necrosis (see Clinical box 6.19). **Crohn disease** affects the gut. The granulomatous chronic inflammation affects all layers of the bowel wall, with a lymphocytic infiltrate, and granulomas develop, similar to those in sarcoid, with no central necrosis (see Clinical box 6.16). **Rheumatoid arthritis** is a complicated disease, with many manifestations, including subcutaneous nodules at pressure points (at the elbows, for example) called rheumatoid nodules. These nodules manifest a central zone of fibrinoid necrosis, surrounded by a palisade of epithelioid cells, further surrounded by lymphocytes (see Clinical box 6.20).

Clinical box 6.19 Sarcoidosis

Sarcoidosis is a granulomatous multisystem condition of unknown aetiology most often presenting as lung disease. Genetic and environmental factors, atypical mycobacterial, fungal and viral infections have been proposed as risk factors, but none has been proven. Diagnosis is commonly made on routine chest X-ray, which shows bilateral hilar lymph node enlargement and pulmonary infiltration. Ocular, neurological and skin (erythema nodosum) lesions may also be present. Myocardial sarcoidosis leads to cardiac failure. Rarely, hypercalcaemia may be present. Young adults are more often affected, and, African Americans appear to experience a more severe course of the disease. The condition may resolve spontaneously, and, although controversial, corticosteroids may be used for treatment. Respiratory functions tests are used to monitor progression.

Clinical box 6.20 **Inflammatory arthritis**

Inflammatory arthritis is characterised by synovial membrane inflammation that ultimately leads to destruction of the joint. The large variety of inflammatory arthritides may roughly be divided into rheumatoid factor (RF)-seropositive (principally **rheumatoid arthritis**) and RF-seronegative types. Depending on the eventual condition, the initial inflammatory process is 'triggered' by an antigen that is sometimes infective (bacterial or viral) but not necessarily targeted at synovial membranes alone, but is often unknown. Other organs may be affected. **Molecular mimicry**, the phenomenon where antibodies against molecules of the attacking organism (antigen) mistakenly recognise similar host molecules for foreign molecules, sets off an autoimmune response when the antibodies destroy 'self' molecules and tissues. Once initiated, persistence of the condition (like most autoimmune diseases) is usually associated with genetic factors.

    Rheumatoid arthritis (RA) is the commonest autoimmune inflammatory arthritis. It is a multisystem disease, but predominantly affects synovial membranes where inflammatory cytokines cause synovitis. Typically, symptoms and signs begin symmetrically (sometimes asymmetrically) in small, peripheral joints (fingers, toes, wrists); multiple joints may be affected. Presentation is variable, and may begin in early childhood. Non-articular manifestations may occur, including fibrosing alveolitis and other pulmonary manifestations, vasculitis, pericarditis, neuropathies, scleritis and episcleritis affecting the eyes, amyloidosis of the kidneys and anaemia, and other organs in the reticuloendothelial system may be affected (e.g. Felty syndrome: splenomegaly and neutropenia).

- The triggering antigen is unknown; it has been postulated that abnormal glycosylation of immunoglobulins leads to antigen mimicry: the RFs are the circulating autoantibodies where the Fc part of IgG is the antigen. A high RF titre is diagnostic of RA, and patients are said to be seropositive. Potential bacterial and slow virus infections have also been suggested, but unproven.
- Molecular inflammatory mediators include tumour necrosis factor (TNF), interleukins (the rationale for using TNF and IL-1 blockers to treat RA) and some growth factors.
- The persistence of synovial (and other) inflammation is thought to be related to continuing T cell activation. The genetic association with chronic inflammation is better understood than the triggering mechanism for RA. Defects in the genes that regulate the immune response are thought to be responsible for the persistence of the inflammatory response. For example, HLA-DR4 (and some other genes have been identified) is associated with a poor prognosis for RA (see also Ch. 5).

    Seronegative spondylarthritis includes ankylosing spondylitis, reactive arthritis (e.g. Reiter syndrome), crystal arthritis (e.g. gout), psoriatic arthropathy and enteropathic arthritis associated with inflammatory bowel disease.

There are a number of diseases with **no apparent pathogen or foreign body** that manifest chronic inflammation. Some of them involve granuloma formation.

Granulomas and granulation tissue

Granulomas and **granulation tissue** have similar names. This is not a coincidence. They both play a part in chronic inflammation. Granulation tissue is the result of new vessel formation and fibrous connective tissue that replaces a fibrin clot as part of the tissue repair process. Both involve macrophages and fibroblasts, albeit in different roles, and both may end as fibrous scars. There are important differences, however, in:

- **Purpose**: granulation tissue repairs pre-existing defects. Granulomas destroy or isolate foreign material, but they may cause tissue destruction in the process.
- **Components**: new vessel formation is an important part of granulation tissue, but plays no part in granulomas.

- **Fibroblasts**: play an essential role in granulation tissue. In granulomas they are only sometimes involved at the end in healing.
- **Activity of macrophages**: in granulation tissue macrophages clear debris and fibrin, and direct new vessel formation and fibroblast accumulation through secretion of growth factors. In granulomas macrophages are trying to kill, eliminate or isolate microbes and foreign material through release of their lysosomal contents and cytokine secretion.

Complications of chronic inflammation

There are many complications of chronic inflammation that are the result of the immediate response to the inflammatory processes, or of longer-term changes to tissues.

- Consequences of fibrosis: contractures, stretching of tissues, and diffuse fibrosis in tissues (such as in the lungs) may compromise function. The lumens of nearby arteries and arterioles may be narrowed or blocked by fibrosis: endarteritis obliterans.
- Constitutional effects: fevers, sweating, anorexia, weight loss and chronic malaise are all symptoms of chronic inflammation.
- Anaemia of chronic disease.
- **Amyloid** formation: this is extracellular deposition in various organs (especially in the kidneys, liver, thyroid, adrenal glands and lymphoid tissue) of an acute phase protein, **serum amyloid associated protein** secreted by the liver. The tertiary structure of amyloid usually involves β-pleated sheets which form into long thin fibres (**fibrils**). Amyloid deposition can result in death through failure of the organs concerned (see also Clinical box 6.21)

Clinical box 6.21 **Amyloidosis**

Amyloidosis refers to a condition where amyloid protein is deposited in the tissues of various organs. The precise mechanisms are as yet unclear, and much research effort is given to it. The tendency to amyloid deposition may be secondary to chronic inflammation (acquired) or inherited. Amyloid deposits can only be identified histologically on tissue biopsy, which is not always feasible or possible (e.g. brain biopsy). Specific clinical signs and symptoms of amyloidosis related to chronic inflammation are few and uncommon, so that clinical suspicion related to some important clinical conditions need to be confirmed by tissue biopsy.

- Cerebral and cerebrovascular: amyloid deposits in the brain have been found in Alzheimer disease, Down syndrome, prion diseases (e.g. transmissible spongiform encephalopathies), Parkinson disease. Cerebrovascular amyloidosis, although rare, can present as recurrent cerebral haemorrhages.
- Cardiomyopathies: the commonest form of restrictive cardiomyopathy is associated with amyloidosis.
- Type 2 diabetes: amyloid deposits have been found in the pancreas of some cases of type 2 diabetes.
- Chronic inflammatory conditions: e.g. inflammatory bowel disease, rheumatoid arthritis.
- Chronic infections: e.g. tuberculosis, osteomyelitis, bronchiectasis.
- Dialysis amyloidosis: amyloid protein is not adequately cleared by dialysis, and is deposited in a variety of organs giving rise to dysfunction and/or debilitating symptoms: e.g. carpal tunnel syndrome, bone cysts and fractures, gastrointestinal bleeds, joint stiffness and pain.
- Renal and hepatic failure due to amyloid deposits is associated with amyloidosis elsewhere in the body. There may be renal and liver (hepatomegaly) enlargement and treatment of the underlying condition is essential.

- Reduction in growth, especially seen in children, is mediated by:
  - Increased energy requirements of inflammation
  - The influence of cytokines on cell division and on the systems that control growth.

Outcomes of chronic inflammation

The various outcomes of a chronic inflammatory process are **resolution** (rarely complete), **repair** (almost always present, culminating in fibrosis) or **persistence**. Chronic inflammation can persist indefinitely, even until death, to which it may contribute through tissue destruction, fibrosis, and amyloid deposition.

REPAIR

If tissue is lost through damage, there are four possible outcomes: regeneration, repair (healing) with fibrosis, persistence of a gap, immediate death, or some combination of these.

Regeneration

Regeneration implies that the tissues grow back to look the same as they did before the damage, in contrast to **resolution** in which acute inflammatory changes ebb away, leaving the tissue the same as it was before. If acute inflammation leads to some cell death and then the tissue returns to its former appearance, the combination of *regeneration* and *resolution* is called **restitution**.

Only labile and stable cells can regenerate. **Labile cells**, such as epithelial cells and bone marrow stem cells, are dividing all the time; **stable cells** only divide intermittently but can divide faster if the cells need to be replaced. **Permanent cells**, such as neurons, cardiac and skeletal muscle cells, cannot regenerate. Even if the constituent cells are labile or stable, the tissue or organ may not be able to regenerate, because the architecture cannot be rebuilt. For example:

- If a burn kills epithelial skin cells, the basal cells can regenerate more basal cells, but if the destruction penetrates through the basement membrane into the dermis over a significant area, the original structure cannot be achieved, and there will be fibrotic repair.
- In lungs, alveolar cells, and in the kidneys, renal tubular cells, can regenerate, but only if the basement membrane remains intact.

There are only three organs which can regenerate all the cell types, and the structure: the liver, bone and bone marrow.

Liver

If some liver tissue is excised or destroyed, it can be regenerated from the remaining tissue. If liver cells scattered throughout the liver are destroyed they can also be replaced. Although this regeneration can occur repeatedly, after many such episodes, some fibrous tissue gets laid down. This distorts the structure with regeneration creating nodules of new tissue, surrounded by fibrous tissue, known as **cirrhosis** (see Ch. 15).

Bone

Regeneration of bone is limited to a particular situation – where there has been a **fracture**. Following the fracture of a bone, there is bleeding at the fracture site, and clot forms. The bleeding lifts the periosteum, allowing the clot to extend around the bone fragments.

As part of the **healing** process that occurs in all tissues, neutrophils and then macrophages move into the clot and remove the debris. New blood vessel formation follows, fibroblasts accumulate and collagen is deposited forming **granulation tissue**. This is well developed as early as 4 days after the fracture. Differing from wound healing, cartilage cells now appear within the granulation tissue and islands of cartilage form, initially mostly round the outside of the bone where the periosteum has been elevated. The fractured ends of the bone are united by a fusiform sleeve of granulation tissue and cartilage, the **provisional callus**.

About a week after the fracture, calcification starts within the cartilage, and new osteoblasts appear, which produce new seams of osteoid. Over the next week calcification of the callus occurs prolifically, both subperiosteal and within the marrow cavity. It forms **fibrocartilaginous callus**, and then **bony callus**, which is mostly woven rather than lamellar bone, bulging out around the fracture site and extending into the marrow cavity.

The callus is then remodelled by osteoclasts and osteoblasts working together, guided by the stresses on the bone. By 7 weeks the bone is once again lamellar, and the normal architecture and strength is restored. Fractures in bone will not always heal perfectly. This will depend on factors such as the blood supply, relative movement and subsequent placement of the bone ends, relative splintering of the bone and presence of infection. The final result may be an angulation, twisting or shortening of a limb.

The regeneration of granulation tissue in bone is unique. In all other tissues the presence of granulation tissue leads to repair, with fibrous tissue, rather than regeneration.

Bone marrow

All the elements of blood and bone marrow are derived from pluripotent bone marrow stem cells, which divide constantly to produce all the derived cells (see Ch. 12). If blood or bone marrow is removed in haemorrhage or donation, the rate of replication increases to make up the loss. If there is extensive haemorrhage or destruction of blood cells, the marrow may colonise bone spaces previously unused. Bone marrow is semi-liquid and its cellular constituents are motile; thus when new marrow is laid down the structure is easily achieved. If regeneration cannot take place, there may be **repair**.

Repair

The body repairs itself through regeneration of dermal and epidermal tissue. It does this by initiating a complex cascade of different biochemical processes: inflammation, proliferation and remodelling.

Inflammation

The first response in inflammatory repair is **blood clotting**, in which platelets are activated by contact with subendothelium. They aggregate to form a platelet plug and this is strengthened by production of fibrin, either as a result of activation of the clotting cascade, or directly as a result of thrombin released from platelets when the damage is minor, catalysing fibrin production from plasma fibrinogen. Fibrin cross links with plasma fibronectin, forming a structural support until collagen is deposited.

In addition to producing the platelet plug, **platelets** release a variety of factors, such as serotonin, prostaglandins, thromboxane and histamine, which increase blood vessel permeability and stimulate cell proliferation and migration to the site of damage. Initial **vasoconstriction**, to reduce blood flow, is followed by **vasodilation** that assists in facilitating the movement of leucocytes to the area and through the vessel wall locally into the local tissue.

Neutrophils arrive at the site within an hour by chemotaxis. They phagocytose debris and any bacteria and secrete proteases that break down damaged tissues. **Macrophages** follow, removing dead neutrophils, assisted by **helper T cells** that secrete cytokines to maintain the inflammatory process. The macrophages attract cells involved in the proliferative process that follows, stimulating **angiogenesis** and the creation of **granulation tissue**, used as a foundation for a new **extracellular matrix** (**ECM**) in the next phase.

Proliferation

As the granulation tissue gets laid down, columns of **endothelial cells** grow in from the nearest intact capillaries, attracted by released growth factors and relative local hypoxia. These columns are initially solid, but then they hollow out to form new, patent, fragile, leaky capillaries which loop into the macrophage-infested clot, then loop back, so that blood can flow through: **angiogenesis** or **neovascularisation**. As the tissue becomes perfused so the angiogenic stimulation declines.

If the wound is a simple incision and the edges can be brought together, basal epithelial cells of the skin proliferate and meet at the surface of the wound, while granulation tissue forms in the clot underneath. This is healing by **primary intention**. If there is a large wound space this is filled by a mass of granulation tissue and the epithelial basal cells grow across the top. This is termed healing by **secondary intention**.

Fibroblasts begin to enter the wound as the inflammatory phase is ending. Fibroblasts are the main cells in the wound from about 1–4 weeks, migrating there from normal tissue, forming part of the granulation tissue laid down in the wound. They add glycoproteins, glycosaminoglycans and other substances to form a provisional **ECM**. Growth factors, such as **platelet-derived growth factor** (**PDGF**), TGF-β and fibronectin, stimulate the development of a more permanent ECM. The production and deposition of **collagen** by fibroblasts is important in the healing process, strengthening the repairing tissues. Collagen is also broken down by collagenases. Initially collagen predominates until production of more has no added benefit.

Once the open wound has been sealed, **re-epithelialisation** takes place with epithelial cells migrating in sheets across the wound from the outer edge, meeting in the centre. This process takes much longer if the basement membrane has also been penetrated. The faster the process, the less likely there is to be a scar. **Keratinocytes** (the main epidermal cell) migrate to the site and anchor to the ECM with transmembrane proteins. They secrete **plasminogen activator**, which activates **plasmin** to dissolve the fibrin scab. New epithelial cells follow, growing from the edge of the wound and replacing the keratinocytes. Cells re-establish desmosomes and anchor to the basement membrane. **Basal cells**, lying at the base of the epidermis, divide and differentiate to form the different strata found in normal skin.

Around 1–3 weeks after the wound is initiated the fibroblasts differentiate into **myofibroblasts** (smooth muscle cells) and the repair begins to **contract**, pulling in from the wound edge and laying down more collagen to reinforce the structure. As the provisional ECM breaks down so hyaluronic acid (a glycosaminoglycan which is a main component of the ECM) decreases, its place taken by chondroitin sulphate (a sulphated glycosaminoglycan which attaches to protein in the ECM where it forms proteoglycans and becomes the main component of the ECM), triggering the fibroblasts to stop proliferating, and the contraction phase ends.

Remodelling

As this phase of the healing process starts the macrophages will have phagocytosed all of the fibrin and moved away. Type III collagen, prevalent in the proliferation phase, is replaced by the stronger type I collagen. The new blood vessels are no longer needed and are removed by apoptosis, changing the tissue colour from pink to white. This is now **fibrous tissue**. As collagen fibres are resorted and new ones laid down there is a cross-linking and increase in fibre size. This causes the fibrous tissue to shrink and strengthen, producing a **fibrous scar**. The larger the wound, the more myofibroblasts form, and the potential for contraction is increased. Sometimes the contraction is substantial, reducing the size of the wound by more than 50%. This phase can continue for longer than 1 year after the initial wound.

Repair complications

Following a wound, granulation tissue may grow too exuberantly, and when fibrosis takes place the scar is thick and bulges out above the level of the skin: **keloid** formation. This is seen more commonly in people of African origin. **Contractures** occur when scars contract as part of remodelling, distorting the surrounding structures. This can lead to restriction of movement, or disfigurement. Sometimes, internally, important structures may be entrapped or squeezed. **Stretching** of the scar occurs if it is under constant strain after remodelling has taken place.

Repair following operations within the peritoneal cavity may leave bands of fibrous tissue round which the bowel may become entangled – **adhesions**. These can be very painful for the patient where nerves are involved. Sometimes there is neither regeneration nor repair, and a **cavity** persists in the tissues. It may be filled with pus, forming an **abscess**, or with fluid, forming a **cyst**. These may become organised later but, otherwise, the tissue is less bulky than normal. This can happen in skeletal muscle if a significant number of fibres have been destroyed.

The **brain** is a special case. Neurons do not regenerate, and granulation tissue is not formed. Instead, there is proliferation of astroglia: **gliosis**, without new vessel formation or fibroblast ingrowth. This often does not fill the space left by the damage, leaving a fluid-filled cavity. Problems also occur if **peripheral nerves** are damaged. Neurons cannot divide, and if a neuron dies it cannot be replaced. Schwann cells, however, can divide and damaging the axon does not usually kill the neuron. If a nerve is crushed, but the endoneurial channels are preserved, the axons peripheral to the injury will die, but will grow back down the appropriate channels. If a nerve is severed, the axons will try to regrow, but may not find the appropriate, or any, endoneurial channel.

Factors that hamper tissue repair
(see also Clinical box 6.22)

Healing is a complex process that marshals many resources in order to repair damaged tissue. It is not unexpected, therefore, that there is a long list of factors that may lead to the

Clinical box 6.22   Ulcers

An ulcer (from Latin *ulcus*) is produced by the shedding (sloughing) of necrotic tissue from the surface of an organ. The tissue necrosis is the consequence of an inflammatory response to injury (e.g. skin abrasions, lacerations or burns), ischaemia or infection, and the sloughing results in a surface defect (an ulcer) from excavation of the slough. Secondary bacterial infection exacerbates the condition. Ulcers may be acute or chronic. Healing takes place from the base of the ulcer by granulation, new vessel formation and laying down of new fibrous connective tissue. Ulcers can form on the surface of any mucous membrane, e.g. mouth ulcers, peptic ulcers, colonic, bronchial and others. The skin, however, is the largest organ of the body where ulceration may be relatively common in vulnerable patients, such as people with diabetes, other circulatory problems or compromised immune systems.

Common skin ulcers encountered in the community include venous or arterial ulcers (mostly on the lower limbs) and pressure (decubitus) ulcers mainly in elderly, bed-bound and immobile patients. Distinction between venous and arterial ulcers needs to be made because the underlying conditions that led to the ulceration are different, and healing requires different management strategies.

Venous ulcers occur mainly in the lower legs. Although the precise mechanism is uncertain, it is postulated that incompetence of venous valves (e.g. varicose veins) give rise to venous hypertension (increased blood pressure in the veins), which can exceed arterial blood pressure, resulting in the failure of tissue perfusion and transudation of inflammatory mediators into extravascular tissues with consequent tissue necrosis in the skin and ulcer formation. Logically, compression and elevating the leg would lower the venous pressure below arterial pressure to improve tissue perfusion and thus help healing.

Arterial ulcers are caused by ischaemia of the affected tissues. Narrowing of medium to small arteries by atherosclerosis (peripheral vascular disease), intravascular coagulation (as in thalassaemia or sickle cell disease) and vasculitis are some examples. Leg ulcers in diabetes mellitus may be due to atherosclerosis or be neurogenic, where sensory loss due to peripheral neuropathy increases the risk of injury, but often a mixture of both. Here, good glycaemic control is essential.

---

process taking much longer than expected and not having a perfect outcome. Some of the more important factors that can delay the process are:

- A poor blood supply
- Poor nutrition: protein, calories, vitamins (especially vitamin C) and zinc
- The presence of infection
- The presence of a foreign body
- Movement: wounds heal better if closed as well as possible, then not disturbed
- Low numbers of white cells
- Steroid therapy (anti-inflammatory)
- Radiation and cytotoxic therapy (inhibit cell division)
- Diabetes mellitus, which impairs white cell function
- Rare genetic defects of white cell function, affecting extravasation, chemotaxis, phagocytosis and the respiratory burst.

LYMPHOID ORGANS

LYMPH NODES

Lymph nodes are found throughout the body and form part of the lymphatic system. Several hundred are distributed around the body with clusters in the neck, chest, abdomen,

under the arms and in the groin. They are important organs in the successful functioning of the immune system as they act as traps for foreign material.

Naïve lymphocytes enter the nodes through specialised venules and are stored in the lymph nodes where they are exposed to antigen delivered to the site on macrophages and other specialised cells. B lymphocytes proliferate in the area as they respond to the need to produce antibodies. This is often experienced by the patient as a swollen gland.

Structure

Figure 6.20 illustrates the structure of a lymph node. Nodes range in size from a few millimetres to about 2 cm in the healthy individual. It is a kidney-shaped organ with a surrounding **fibrous capsule**. Inside the node, the fibrous capsular material extends in as collagenous **trabeculae** that divide up the outer part of the internal space.

Lymph circulates through the node, entering through **afferent lymph vessels** that penetrate the capsule and open into the **subcapsular sinus**. Underneath the sinus lies the **cortex** on the outside, which surrounds the **medulla**, the latter opening into the medullary sinus at the **hilum**. The **efferent lymph vessel** drains lymph from this sinus, leaving the node at the hilum

Afferent and efferent lymph vessels

The **afferent vessels** collect lymph from other lymph nodes or from tissue spaces where it has drained from blood vessels. The vessels have valves that prevent back flow. Lymph leaves the node via the **efferent lymphatic vessel** travelling to more lymph nodes and eventually draining into the large lymph ducts and central subclavian vein.

Cortex

The **cortex** consists mainly of B cells, particularly in the outer zones. The cells are arranged in **follicles**. The **primary follicle** contains B cells, follicular dendritic cells, tingible body macrophages and a few helper T cells, but no cytotoxic T cells.

- **Follicular dendritic cells** are unique to follicles and unlike any other dendritic cells, even those also found in lymph nodes. They retain antigen and are recognised by particular antibodies.
- **Tingible body macrophages** are different from other macrophages (tissue macrophages). They possess CD4 but not CD2 or CD3 and have unique cytoplasmic tingible bodies.

Secondary follicles in the cortex are like the primary follicles except they also contain a **germinal centre**. This is an area of B cell proliferation, stimulated by contact with an antigen, and is surrounded by a **mantle zone** of quiescent B cells with surface IgD and IgM. Areas between the follicles are filled with mixtures of T cells and B cells. Deeper in the cortex is the **paracortex** in which T cells predominate, with helper T cells, cytotoxic T cells and many interdigitating dendritic cells.

Medulla

The medulla is composed of **sinuses** with intervening **medullary cords** of lymphoid tissue, mainly plasma cells and tissue macrophages.

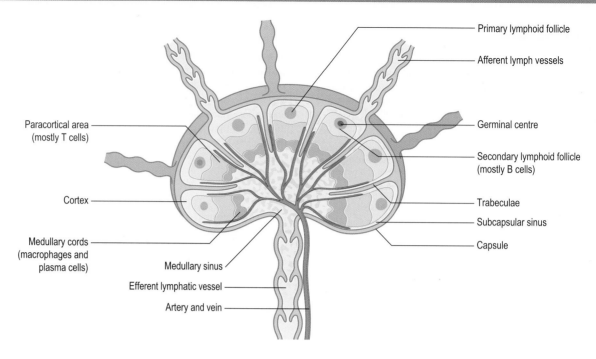

Fig. 6.20 **Schematic drawing of a section through a lymph node.**

Labels (clockwise from top right):
- Primary lymphoid follicle
- Afferent lymph vessels
- Germinal centre
- Secondary lymphoid follicle (mostly B cells)
- Trabeculae
- Subcapsular sinus
- Capsule
- Artery and vein
- Efferent lymphatic vessel
- Medullary sinus
- Medullary cords (macrophages and plasma cells)
- Cortex
- Paracortical area (mostly T cells)

Reticular network and sinuses

Fine fibres form a **reticular network** within the nodes, providing the support for the tightly packed follicles of lymphocytes, along with the dendritic cells and macrophages. The reticular cells are lined with endothelial cells which enable a smooth flow of lymph. The meshwork provides a large contact surface with the lymph node cells (macrophages and lymphocytes) enabling an efficient filtering process and an easy exchange of material with blood flowing through **high endothelial (post-capillary) venules** in the paracortex.

Blood is supplied to the lymph node though an artery and vein that enters through the hilum. Lymphocytes continuously circulate between the blood and the nodes, entering through the venules and moving into the sinuses by diapedesis. Lymph flows in through afferent vessels into the macrophage-lined **subcapsular sinus**. This sinus is continuous with **cortical sinuses** that are found on either side of the trabeculae and joins with the **medullary sinuses**, which are also lined with macrophages, into which the lymph drains before leaving the node through the efferent vessel at the hilum. Antigens and immune cells carried in the lymph are phagocytosed by the sinus wall macrophages and presented to lymphocytes within follicles. The number and composition of the follicles change when exposed to antigen as they form a **germinal centre**. Plasma cells, producing antibody, are formed and migrate to the medullary cords.

THE SPLEEN

The spleen functions in a similar way to lymph nodes, filtering blood instead of lymph. It is located in the abdomen, under the ribcage and above the stomach. It has two main regions: red pulp and white pulp (Fig. 6.21).

Red pulp is so called because it is mostly composed of sinuses filled with blood. The sinuses are lined by macrophages and phagocytes that filter the blood, removing material, including effete red cells. **White pulp** is composed of

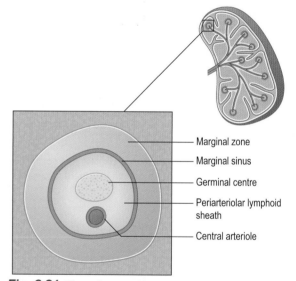

Fig. 6.21 **The spleen and its main functional regions.**

Labels:
- Marginal zone
- Marginal sinus
- Germinal centre
- Periarteriolar lymphoid sheath
- Central arteriole

follicles rich in B cells and **periarticular lymphoid sheaths** rich in T cells. After antigen stimulation, germinal centres form in the follicles. The sheaths form a cuff around arterioles with the B cells at the periphery in the follicles, the whole sheath being surrounded by a marginal zone of macrophages. Blood flows into the sheaths from arterioles via capillaries and can also leave through capillaries, passing into the red pulp.

In addition to its filtration and immune response roles, the spleen is also an important haemopoetic organ. It is the primary site of haematopoiesis in the foetus although the bone marrow takes over this function after birth. Nevertheless it retains the ability to produce lymphocytes and is an important storage area for all blood cells. The spleen is also the site of production of opsonins and properdin, both of which enhance phagocytosis.

NEOPLASIA

INTRODUCTION

GROWTH, DIFFERENTIATION AND DEVELOPMENT

Changes in cell growth and differentiation are implemented by the switching on and off of genes. This can be a normal event in response to certain stimuli, or can be abnormal, leading to defective growth and differentiation. The interaction of cellular signals and gene expression permeates all biology, and its discussion is not limited to this section. Most chapters discuss this material, especially Chapter 5.

The cell cycle

The cell cycle is discussed in detail in Chapters 2 and 5, and consists of two processes of cell division: mitosis and meiosis.

- **Mitosis** takes place in dividing somatic cells, where the entire DNA content of the cell is duplicated in distinct physical stages to produce two identical daughter cells, known as diploid cells (see Fig. 5.4).
- **Meiosis** occurs in germ cells, producing daughter cells with half the DNA content, where the entire chromosome complement is halved, known as haploid cells (see Fig. 5.6). The process is divided into stages depending on nuclear and cell morphology.

Between the end of one phase of mitosis or meiosis and the beginning of the next is the interphase. The cell cycle is driven through its stages by **cyclin-dependent kinases** (CDKs) that phosphorylate specific proteins. The CDK molecules and cyclins are specific for each stage of the cell cycle.

Control of cell proliferation

During the quiescent, G0 (gap) phase in **interphase**, the cells are dormant until activated by a variety of stimuli towards cell growth, differentiation or proliferation. These stimuli are receptor-mediated actions of various growth factors from other cells transmitted via intracellular second messengers to the nucleus, where interaction with nuclear transcription factors initiates DNA synthesis, which in turn will initiate another phase of mitosis or meiosis. These nuclear transcription factors regulate the genes that control cell growth and proliferation (see Ch. 5).

In cancers, a common feature is uncontrolled cell proliferation leading to the formation of a tumour or **neoplasm**, a 'new growth'. Mutations in the genes that control cell proliferation can lead to the development of cancer cells for normal cells by:

- Enhancing cell proliferation so that there are more cells with the mutant gene
- Loss of the ability to repair minor abnormalities in the gene thereby destabilising the genome at DNA or chromosome levels.

Cell death

Cells die either through **necrosis** or **apoptosis**:

- **Necrotic cell death** occurs as the result of external injury, such as hypoxia due to the sudden reduction in blood flow to tissues (embolism, thrombosis, infarction), or toxins which may be externally administered chemicals or endogenous (e.g. free radicals). The cell disintegrates as the result of damage to its normal physiology, and sets off an inflammatory response.
- **Apoptosis** is 'programmed' physiological cell death when specific genes are activated to cause the cell to die. Apoptosis is necessary for normal physiology, which may occur with ageing (as with shedding the superficial layer of skin or the epithelial lining of the gastrointestinal tract), the removal of apparently healthy but superfluous cells, tissue and organ formation in embryogenesis, wound healing and many other examples. Apoptosis also occurs as the result of injury by external agents such as viruses, toxins and genetic mutation. This does not, however, lead to an inflammatory response.

In the treatment of cancers, the aim of radiotherapy or chemotherapy is to trigger the cancer cell's apoptotic pathway.

Variation in cell growth and differentiation

Cellular growth and proliferation can vary under physiological and pathological influences.

Increased growth

Increased growth occurs in a tissue or organ due to increased functional demand. It can be the result of **hyperplasia**, **hypertrophy** or a **combination** of both. Hyperplasia is an increase in cell number by cell division, while hypertrophy is an increase in cell size without cell division. Both lead to an increase in the size of an affected tissue or organ. In tissues that cannot divide, such as cardiac muscle, hypertrophy is the only adaptive response possible.

The stimuli for hyperplasia and hypertrophy are very similar and include hormones, growth factors and work against resistance. Both hyperplasia and hypertrophy can occur as a normal physiological response (Clinical Box 6.23) or they can be 'pathological', which usually results in clinical consequences (Clinical Box 6.24).

Clinical box 6.23 | **Examples of physiological hyperplasia and hypertrophy**

Physiological hyperplasia
- The breast undergoes hyperplasia during puberty, pregnancy and lactation, stimulated by hormones such as oestrogens, progesterone and prolactin
- Red cell precursors in the bone marrow undergo hyperplasia at high altitude, in response to erythropoietin release stimulated by hypoxia
- The thyroid undergoes hyperplasia in puberty and pregnancy, stimulated by increased metabolic demand.

Physiological hypertrophy
- Skeletal muscle undergoes hypertrophy stimulated by increased muscle activity on exercise
- Cardiac muscle undergoes hypertrophy stimulated by sustained outflow increase in athletes
- The myometrium undergoes hypertrophy in pregnancy stimulated by oestrogens.

Pathological hyperplasia
- The prostate undergoes hyperplasia, stimulated by relative oestrogen excess in elderly men. This causes the syndrome of urinary outflow obstruction.
- The adrenal cortex undergoes hyperplasia in response to adrenocorticotropic hormone (ACTH) produced by either a pituitary adenoma or as a paraneoplastic syndrome by a small cell bronchial carcinoma. This results in Cushing syndrome.
- The thyroid undergoes hyperplasia in Graves disease, stimulated by auto-antibodies.
- The parathyroid undergoes hyperplasia in chronic renal failure, stimulated by hypocalcaemia.
- The endometrium undergoes hyperplasia as a result of excess oestrogen exposure. This results in abnormal uterine bleeding.

Pathological hypertrophy
- Left ventricular myocardium undergoes hypertrophy in systemic hypertension and aortic valve disease due to increased outflow pressure (Fig. 6.22)
- Right ventricular myocardium undergoes hypertrophy in conditions such as pulmonary hypertension and pulmonary valve disease, also due to increased outflow pressure
- Arterial smooth muscle undergoes hypertrophy in hypertension due to increased work against resistance.

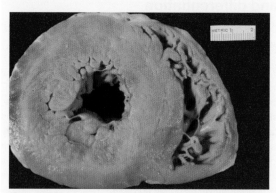

Fig. 6.22 **Cross-section through a heart showing concentric hypertrophy of the left ventricle.**

Decreased growth

A tissue or organ can be reduced in size either as a result of developmental failure, or as a consequence of atrophy. **Atrophy** is a decrease in cell size and/or number in a previously normal tissue or organ. Decrease in cell number is mediated by apoptosis, decrease in cell size by a reduction in cell growth. As with hyperplasia and hypertrophy, atrophy can be a normal physiological event (Clinical Box 6.25) or it can be pathological (Clinical Box 6.26).

Abnormal differentiation

Under certain conditions, mature tissues can differentiate abnormally, undergoing metaplasia, dysplasia or both. **Dysplasia**, which literally means disordered growth, is used in two contexts. The more common usage is to describe the abnormal maturation that often occurs before the development of malignancy but it can also be used to describe abnormalities of developmental differentiation.

- In the embryo and foetus, the notochord and branchial clefts undergo atrophy
- In the neonate, the umbilical vessels and ductus arteriosus undergo atrophy
- In early adulthood, the thymus undergoes atrophy
- In old age the uterus, testes, brain and bone all atrophy (Fig. 6.23).

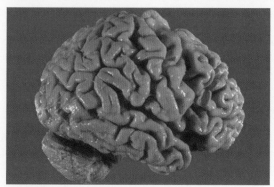

Fig. 6.23 **Atrophy of the brain in old age.** There is widespread shrinkage of gyri with widening of sulci.

- In immobilised patients, loss of function causes muscle atrophy and osteoporosis
- In patients with nerve transection or poliomyelitis, loss of innervation causes muscle atrophy
- In patients with peripheral vascular disease or bed-bound patients, reduction in blood supply causes skin atrophy or pressure sores
- In patients with hypopituitarism, loss of hormonal stimulation causes atrophy of the adrenal cortex, thyroid and gonads
- In patients on corticosteroid therapy, prolonged use causes skin atrophy.

Metaplasia

Metaplasia is defined as the transformation of one fully differentiated cell type into another. It is an adaptive response to environmental stress, usually chronic irritation or inflammation, as the metaplastic tissues are better able to withstand the adverse environmental changes than their normal counterparts. Metaplasia is caused by activation and/or depression (activation by unblocking a repressor) of groups of genes involved in the maintenance of cellular differentiation. Unlike dysplasia and neoplasia, there is no intrinsic gene defect; therefore metaplasia is reversible. Metaplasia per se does not progress to neoplasia, but because the metaplastic tissues are less genetically stable than their normal counterparts, they are prone to undergo further transformation to dysplasia and neoplasia. Metaplasia can affect epithelial or connective tissue cells.

Epithelial metaplasia
Epithelial metaplasia can be:

- Squamous – when there is transformation to squamous epithelium (Clinical box 6.27)
- Glandular – when there is transformation to glandular epithelium (Clinical box 6.28).

Connective tissue metaplasia
Connective tissue (mesenchymal) metaplasia is much less common than epithelial metaplasia. The main type involves

Clinical box 6.27 Examples of squamous metaplasia

- Ciliated pseudostratified columnar epithelium of the respiratory tract changing to squamous epithelium as a result of mucosal damage caused by smoking, bronchiectasis or chronic bronchitis
- Simple columnar epithelium of the endocervix changing to squamous epithelium due to changes of pH, injury or chronic inflammation
- Transitional cell epithelium of the bladder changing to squamous epithelium secondary to chronic inflammation caused by long-standing schistosomal infection or bladder calculi.

Clinical box 6.28 Examples of glandular metaplasia

- Stratified squamous epithelium of the oesophagus changing to simple columnar epithelium as a result of mucosal damage caused by gastro-oesophageal reflux. This is termed Barrett's oesophagus (Fig. 6.24).
- Simple columnar epithelium of the stomach changing to intestinal epithelium due to persistent chronic inflammation caused by *Helicobacter pylori* infection. In this example, one type of glandular epithelium (simple columnar) transforms into another (intestinal).

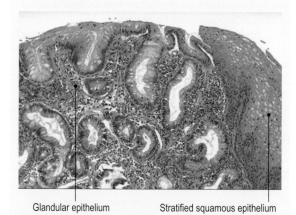

Glandular epithelium   Stratified squamous epithelium

Fig. 6.24 **Oesophageal biopsy showing glandular metaplasia of stratified squamous oesophageal epithelium (Barrett's oesophagus).**

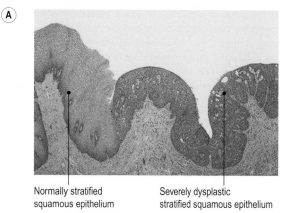

Normally stratified squamous epithelium   Severely dysplastic stratified squamous epithelium

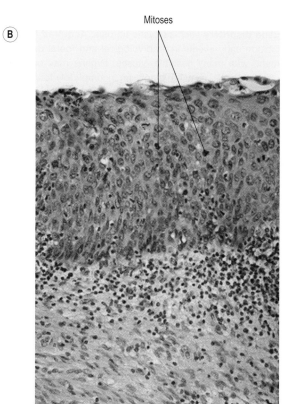

Mitoses

Fig. 6.25 **Cervical biopsy.** (A) Low-power view of a cervical biopsy sample showing an abrupt change between normal stratified squamous epithelium on the left and severely dysplastic squamous epithelium on the right. (B) High-power view of cervical biopsy sample showing severe dysplasia of the stratified squamous epithelium (equivalent to CIN 3 or carcinoma in situ). There are several mitoses visible and the nuclei are enlarged, hyperchromatic and atypical throughout the entire thickness of the epithelium.

formation of cartilage or bone in old scars, known as chondroid and osseous metaplasia, respectively, such as tuberculous scars in the lungs, in atheromatous plaques and in chronically damaged muscle. The term **myeloid metaplasia** is sometimes used to describe extramedullary haemopoiesis that occurs in the spleen, liver and lymph nodes in patients with myeloproliferative diseases.

Dysplasia

In this context, **dysplasia** refers to a failure of normal maturation that occurs prior to the development of malignancy. Dysplasia is often preceded by metaplasia, but in contrast to metaplasia it is usually irreversible. The features of dysplasia are more easily recognised in epithelia than in mesenchymal or other tissues. Such features include nuclear enlargement and atypia, loss of nuclear polarity and increased mitoses (Fig. 6.25). Nowadays, the term intraepithelial neoplasia is commonly used instead of dysplasia, reflecting the fact that this is a premalignant process. The term is most often applied to stratified epithelia, for example **cervical intraepithelial**

neoplasia (**CIN**) and **anal intraepithelial neoplasia** (**AIN**), though pathologists are trained to recognise the changes even in glandular epithelia.

In the most severe form of intraepithelial neoplasia, the entire epithelium is replaced by cells showing all the features of malignancy, but the basement membrane separating the epithelium from the underlying stroma has not yet been breached. This pre-invasive lesion is termed **carcinoma in situ** (Fig. 6.25B). The prognosis of carcinoma in situ is much better than that of invasive carcinoma because the neoplasm is not yet capable of metastasis. Detection of carcinomas at the stage of carcinoma in situ or intraepithelial neoplasia forms the basis of the breast and cervical cancer screening programmes. Other screening programmes to detect dysplasia before the development of invasive malignancy include screening for colonic mucosal dysplasia in patients with long-standing ulcerative colitis and screening for glandular dysplasia in patients with Barrett's oesophagus.

Defects of development

Failure to achieve normal development occurs because of a wide spectrum of disorders including inherited genetic defects, acquired lesions and environmental events. **Inherited genetic defects** include chromosomal abnormalities, such as Down syndrome or Edward syndrome, which affect many aspects of development, and **single gene disorders** such as cystic fibrosis. **Acquired lesions** include early events in embryological and foetal development, with many possible causes. Organs may be completely absent, as in renal aplasia, incompletely formed, as in spina bifida, renal hypoplasia and cleft palate, or wrongly sited, as in situs inversus. In some cases there may be extra tissues, as in polydactyly.

Environmental events affecting the embryo or foetus include maternal illness or placental dysfunction, birth hypoxia causing central nervous system damage, and infections or injuries in childhood that can have serious sequelae, such as meningitis. Malnutrition during infancy and childhood, and child neglect or cruelty, will also have an adverse effect on development.

Anomalies of organ development

Anomalies of organ development can occur at any stage during development but often begin during foetal life, when the structure concerned is being formed.

Aplasia (or agenesis) is the complete failure to develop an organ or structure. Examples include:

- Di George syndrome, when the thymus (and sometimes parathyroid glands) is absent due to defective development of the third and fourth branchial arches
- Renal aplasia, when one or both kidneys are completely absent due to failure of development of the metanephric blastema
- Anencephaly, when there is absence of the cerebrum and often the cerebellum due to failure of development of the neural tube.

Hypoplasia is the failure in development of the normal size and/or shape of an organ. Examples include:

- Thalidomide-induced limb hypoplasia
- Failure of neuromuscular development after poliomyelitis, resulting in a hypoplastic limb
- Failure of normal development of the acetabulum due to hypoplasia of the osseous nuclei, resulting in congenital dislocation of the hip.

Atresia is the failure in development of a normal lumen or orifice in the body. These conditions are always congenital. Examples include:

- Oesophageal atresia, in which the lumen of the oesophagus is narrow or absent. This is often associated with tracheo-oesophageal fistula
- Biliary atresia, in which there is obliteration of the biliary system leading to obstructive jaundice.

Dysplasia (or dysgenesis) used in this context is the failure of normal differentiation of an organ, often with the retention of primitive embryological structures. Examples include:

- Cystic renal dysplasia, in which islands of mesenchyme and/or cartilage are present within the kidney and cysts develop, possibly because of obstruction
- Fibrous dysplasia of bone, in which there are irregular masses of woven bone embedded in vascular fibrous tissue affecting predominantly the ribs, femur, tibia and skull.

Tumour-like developmental lesions

Some developmental abnormalities form tumour-like masses that can be difficult to distinguish from true neoplasms. Though they are usually present from childhood, such lesions may not present until later in life or may only be discovered incidentally.

Heterotopia is the displacement of part of an organ from its normal position. Examples include:

- Endometriosis, in which islands of endometrium are found outside the endometrial cavity
- Rests of pancreatic tissue in the wall of the stomach
- Foci of gastric tissue lining a Meckel's diverticulum.

Choristoma is a particular type of heterotopia in which one or more histologically mature tissues form a discrete mass at an abnormal site. An example is conjunctival choristoma, arising in the eye, which often contains masses of cartilage, bone, smooth muscle and adipose tissue. **Hamartoma** is a tumour-like malformation composed of mature tissues native to the organ in which the lesion arises. Hamartomas represent the borderline between developmental lesions and neoplasms. Like neoplasms, the tissues in a hamartoma are haphazardly organised and grow excessively but, unlike neoplasms, they do not proliferate autonomously. Examples of hamartomas are:

- Bronchial hamartoma, composed of bronchial epithelium and cartilage
- Juvenile polyp composed of an overgrowth of lamina propria
- Peutz–Jeghers polyp, composed of an overgrowth of muscularis mucosae (Fig. 6.26)
- Bile duct hamartoma, composed of haphazardly organised bile ductules
- Telangiectasia, composed of haphazardly organised, dilated blood vessels.

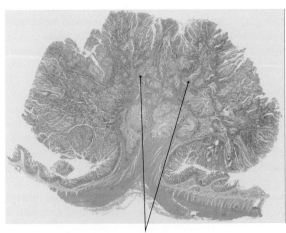

Overgrowth of muscularis mucosae

Fig. 6.26 **Peutz–Jeghers' polyp in the ileum.**

There has been disagreement in the literature as to whether lesions such as haemangiomas, lymphangiomas and pigmented naevi represent benign neoplasms or hamartomas. Though they are not neoplastic per se, in some cases hamartomas contain defective tumour suppressor genes and are consequently at higher risk of developing malignancy than are normal tissues. This is particularly true when hamartomas occur as part of clinical syndromes, such as Peutz–Jeghers syndrome and tuberous sclerosis.

PATHOLOGY OF NEOPLASIA

Neoplasm literally means new growth but the usual definition is 'a mass formed by the autonomous proliferation of cells that persists after cessation of the stimulus that provoked the change'. The word tumour has come to be used synonymously with neoplasm despite the fact that the literal meaning of tumour is 'abnormal swelling'. Compared with their normal counterparts neoplastic cells have disordered phenotype, function and behaviour. They can also have a damaging effect on the host – the more disordered the cells, the greater the adverse effect.

Benign neoplasms show the least cytological variation from their parent tissue, they do not invade surrounding structures and are not usually harmful to the host. Malignant neoplasms, on the other hand, usually show substantial cytological changes, they invade surrounding tissues and are frequently harmful to the host. The word cancer is synonymous with malignant neoplasm.

EPIDEMIOLOGY OF NEOPLASIA

Malignant neoplasms cause 28% of all deaths in the UK (157 275 deaths in 2010). Bronchial carcinoma is the most common cause of death from neoplasia, accounting for 22% of cases, followed by carcinoma of the colorectum (10% of cases). Although carcinoma of the breast is rare in men, the high incidence in women means that it is the third most common cause of death from malignancy in all persons (7% of cases). Carcinomas of the lung, large bowel, breast and prostate together account for almost half (46%) of all deaths from malignancy (Fig. 6.27).

Death rates from malignancy rise with increasing age, more than 75% of deaths occurring in persons aged 65 and over. Although there are fewer deaths from malignancy in people under 65 years, the proportion of deaths from malignancy in this group is greater (38%) than in the population as a whole. This proportion is even higher for women, in whom almost half (47%) of deaths in the under 65 age group are due to malignancy compared with 31% of deaths in men of the same age.

Despite the increasing incidence of malignant neoplasms in the UK, overall mortality from malignancy is decreasing. Between 1996 and 2005 the age standardised mortality rates for all malignancies fell by 15% for men and 10% for women. The largest falls were seen for carcinomas of the cervix, stomach, lung, bladder, breast and large bowel, largely due to earlier diagnosis and better treatment. In contrast, death rates from a few malignancies have increased in the past 10 years, particularly carcinomas of the liver, kidney, uterus and malignant melanoma. This rise has been linked to increased exposure to predisposing factors, such as ultraviolet radiation leading to malignant melanoma.

NOMENCLATURE AND CLASSIFICATION OF NEOPLASMS

Neoplasms are named according to whether they are benign or malignant, and also by their cell of origin (**histogenesis**). Accurate classification of neoplasms is vitally important for tailoring treatment and assessing prognosis. The major histogenetic categories of neoplasm are:

- Epithelial neoplasms, derived from epithelia or glandular structures
- Mesenchymal neoplasms, derived from tissues descended from mesenchyme: muscle, fibroblasts, bone, cartilage, fat, etc.
- Haemopoietic neoplasms, derived from cells descended from the pluripotent bone marrow stem cell
- Nervous system neoplasms, derived from cells of the central and peripheral nervous system
- Primitive embryonal neoplasms, derived from immature cells
- Germ cell neoplasms, derived from germ cells in the ovary and testis.

All neoplasms have the 'surname' -oma, though it should not be forgotten that several other non-neoplastic lesions have similar ending names, e.g. hamartoma, haematoma, granuloma. The 'forename' of neoplasms depends on the specific tissue of origin, as described below.

Epithelial neoplasms

Benign epithelial neoplasms are either **adenomas** or **papillomas**. Adenomas are derived from glandular or secretory epithelium, such as that of the gastrointestinal tract, breast and endocrine glands, while papillomas originate from non-glandular epithelium, such as stratified squamous or transitional cell epithelium (Table 6.10).

All malignant epithelial neoplasms have the suffix carcinoma. Carcinomas of glandular or secretory epithelium are termed adenocarcinomas, while those of non-glandular epithelium are named according to their cell of origin, e.g. squamous cell carcinoma, transitional cell carcinoma, basal cell carcinoma (Table 6.11).

Carcinoma in situ is a term used to designate an early, pre-invasive phase in the development of epithelial malignancy. It is closely related to epithelial dysplasia and is discussed more fully above.

Mesenchymal neoplasms

All benign **mesenchymal neoplasms** end in -oma and are prefixed by the name that indicates the cell or tissue of origin (e.g. leiomyo- for smooth muscle, rhabdomyo- for striated muscle). Malignant mesenchymal neoplasms keep the same prefix but the ending becomes -sarcoma (Table 6.11).

Haemopoietic neoplasms

Haemopoietic neoplasms arise in the bone marrow and lymph nodes. The features that allow distinction between

The 20 Most Common Causes of Cancer Death: 2010

Number of Deaths, UK

Cancer Site	Male	Female	Persons
Lung	19410	15449	34859
Bowel*	8705	7308	16013
Breast	77	11556	11633
Prostate	10721		10721
Pancreas	3872	4029	7901
Oesophagus	5105	2505	7610
Stomach	3102	1858	4960
Bladder	3294	1613	4907
Leukaemia	2526	1978	4504
Non-Hodgkin Lymphoma	2402	2050	4452
Ovary		4295	4295
Kidney	2451	1611	4062
Brain and Central Nervous System	2253	1636	3889
Liver	2249	1540	3789
Other Digestive Organs	1615	1540	3155
Myeloma	1355	1278	2633
Mesothelioma	1896	389	2285
Malignant Melanoma	1266	937	2203
Oral	1323	662	1985
Uterus		1937	1937
Other Sites**	8859	10623	19482
All Cancers (C00-C97)	82481	74794	157275

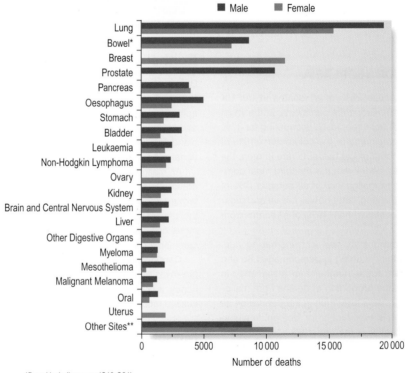

*Bowel including anus (C18-C21)

**8% of all female cancer deaths and 6% of all male cancer deaths are registered without specification of the primary site

Fig. 6.27 **Mortality from the 20 most common cancers in the UK, 2010.** Adapted with permission from CRC UK.

benign and malignant neoplasms are not so easily applicable to haemopoietic neoplasms since, apart from lymphomas, they rarely form solid masses. While some neoplasms behave less aggressively than others, it is difficult to classify any of them as truly benign. There are four main groups of haemopoietic neoplasms:

- Leukaemias, derived from myeloid (white blood cell) precursors
- Myeloproliferative disorders, derived from myeloid cells, with differentiation to mature forms. This group of neoplasms includes thrombocythaemia, polycythaemia rubra vera and myelofibrosis

Table 6.10   Nomenclature of epithelial neoplasms

Epithelial cell type/ normal tissue	Benign neoplasm	Malignant neoplasm
Stratified squamous, e.g. skin	Squamous cell papilloma	Squamous cell carcinoma
Basal cell, e.g. skin	Basal cell papilloma	Basal cell carcinoma
Transitional cell, e.g. urogenital tract	Transitional cell papilloma	Transitional cell carcinoma
Glandular, e.g. gastrointestinal tract	Adenoma	Adenocarcinoma

Table 6.11   Nomenclature of mesenchymal neoplasms

Cell type or normal tissue	Benign neoplasm	Malignant neoplasm
Fibroblast	Fibroma	Fibrosarcoma
Fat	Lipoma	Liposarcoma
Striated muscle	Rhabdomyoma	Rhabdomyosarcoma
Smooth muscle	Leiomyoma	Leiomyosarcoma
Cartilage	Chondroma	Chondrosarcoma
Bone	Osteoma	Osteosarcoma
Endothelium	Haemangioma	Angiosarcoma

- Myeloma, derived from plasma cells in the bone marrow
- Lymphomas, derived from B and T lymphocytes or their precursors.

The -oma suffix of lymphoma and myeloma should not lead to the assumption that these are benign neoplasms.

Nervous system neoplasms

As with epithelial and mesenchymal lesions, neoplasms of the nervous system are classified according to their cell of origin (Table 6.12). The nomenclature does not differentiate between benign and malignant; for example, **gliomas** are always malignant, while **meningiomas** and **schwannomas** are usually benign. In order to distinguish the small number of meningiomas and schwannomas that show atypical cytology and/or aggressive behaviour, the word 'malignant' is used as a 'forename', e.g. malignant schwannoma. Gliomas and meningiomas arise only in the central nervous system whereas schwannomas can arise in both the central and peripheral nervous systems.

Primitive embryonal neoplasms

These neoplasms arise from primitive cells and so resemble the embryonic form of the tissue in which they arise. They end in -blastoma and are prefixed by the name of the cell or tissue of origin (Table 6.13). All are malignant and occur in children below the age of 5.

Germ cell neoplasms

Neoplasms derived from germ cells are called **teratomas**, from the Greek for 'little monster'. Reflecting the pluripotent nature of germ cells, teratomas have the capacity to differentiate into tissues from any of the three germ cell

Table 6.12   Nomenclature of nervous system neoplasms

Cell type	Neoplasm
Glial cell	Glioma
Arachnoid cell	Meningioma
Nerve sheath cell	Schwannoma, neurofibroma

Table 6.13   Nomenclature of embryonal neoplasms

Cell type/normal tissue	Malignant neoplasm
Kidney	Nephroblastoma
Liver	Hepatoblastoma
Primitive neuroectodermal cell	Medulloblastoma
Neural tissue	Neuroblastoma
Retina	Retinoblastoma

layers (ectoderm, mesoderm and endoderm) and often contain derivatives of all three layers admixed haphazardly. Teratomas can be benign or malignant depending on the degree of differentiation of their component tissues. In benign teratomas, the tissues are mature and easily recognised. Such teratomas are common in the ovary, where they are often cystic and contain teeth, hair, cartilage, skin and sebaceous material. In malignant teratomas, the tissues are immature and resemble foetal or embryonic tissues; these teratomas are more common in the testis.

CHARACTERISTICS OF BENIGN AND MALIGNANT NEOPLASMS

All solid neoplasms, whether benign or malignant, are composed of neoplastic cells and variable amounts of supporting connective tissue (stroma). The neoplastic cells of individual neoplasms differ in the extent to which their morphology, growth pattern and synthetic activity resembles that of their parent tissue. Those that closely resemble their parent tissue continue to synthesise and secrete cell products such as mucin, keratin and collagen so that the histogenesis of the neoplasm is easily recognisable. Neoplasms that bear little resemblance to their parent tissue are often difficult to classify histogenetically.

The stromal component of neoplasms provides not only mechanical support but also nutrition to the neoplastic cells. Fibroblasts and myofibroblasts are the predominant cells found in stroma, though chronic inflammatory cells are also common. Neoplasms that contain many stromal fibroblasts are rich in collagen and are consequently firm and rigid to the touch; such neoplasms are said to show a desmoplastic reaction. Myofibroblasts are contractile, so neoplasms that have abundant myofibroblasts show puckering and retraction of adjacent tissues.

Neoplasms produce their own vascular supply (a process known as angiogenesis) by elaboration of angiogenic factors such as fibroblast growth factor, TGF-α, epidermal growth factor, PDGF and vascular endothelial growth factor. The signal for angiogenesis probably results from the same genetic events that underlie formation of the tumour itself. Lack of vascular supply causes tumour necrosis and infarction.

Macroscopic features and growth pattern

Benign neoplasms are mostly slow growing, always remain localised and never spread to distant sites. They grow by expansion and typically have a pushing margin that does not infiltrate adjacent tissues (Fig. 6.28). In solid organs, benign neoplasms are well circumscribed and often encapsulated (Fig. 6.29). Their cut surface can be soft or firm, but is not usually rock-hard; necrosis is rare. Benign neoplasms that arise in mucosal surfaces such as the bowel or skin usually take the form of a polyp, which may be pedunculated (with a stalk), sessile (without a stalk) or papillary (with seaweed-like fronds).

Malignant neoplasms are mostly fast growing, invasive and commonly spread to distant sites through the process of metastasis (see below). They grow by destroying adjacent tissues and have an infiltrative margin (Fig. 6.28). In solid organs, malignant neoplasms are typically poorly circumscribed and tethered to surrounding tissues – the exception being malignant mesenchymal neoplasms, which can sometimes be circumscribed. The cut surface is often heterogeneous with areas of haemorrhage and necrosis. Some malignant neoplasms, breast carcinomas in particular, have a rock-hard (scirrhous) surface and show spiculate extensions of neoplasm into the peritumoral tissues (Fig. 6.30). This growth pattern, which has been likened to the way a crab runs along the sand, gave rise to the word 'cancer' (Latin for crab).

Malignant neoplasms that arise in mucosal surfaces can be exophytic and fungating or endophytic and ulcerating (Fig. 6.31). In addition, those that occur in the bowel can be 'annular stenosing', which means that they involve the whole circumference, causing luminal obstruction, or they can be 'diffuse and infiltrating' with little intraluminal growth. Even neoplasms that do not have a predominant ulcerating growth pattern can show areas of surface ulceration leading to blood loss.

Histological features

Histological features that distinguish neoplasms from their parent tissue include:

- Loss of normal architecture
- Loss of cell cohesion
- Nuclear pleomorphism (variability in size and shape)
- Nuclear enlargement with increased nuclear:cytoplasmic ratio
- Increased mitotic activity.

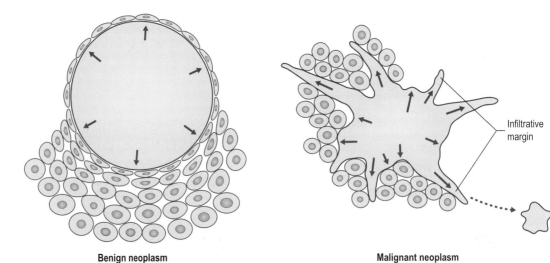

Benign neoplasm   **Malignant neoplasm**

Infiltrative margin

Fig. 6.28 **Growth patterns of benign and malignant neoplasms.**

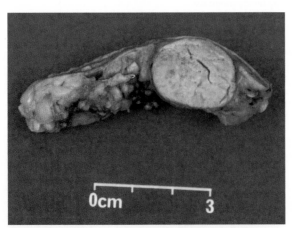

Fig. 6.29 **Benign neoplasm of the adrenal cortex showing a well-circumscribed margin.** The cut surface is homogeneous and lacks necrosis.

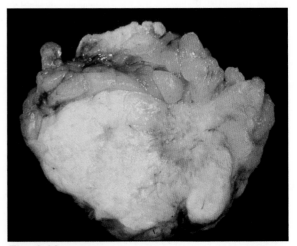

Fig. 6.30 **Lumpectomy from the right breast showing a poorly circumscribed spiculate mass tethered to the surrounding tissues.**

In malignant neoplasms the extent and severity of these changes is greater than in their benign counterparts (Fig. 6.32). Consequently, malignant tumours show less resemblance to their tissue of origin than do benign neoplasms. The main features used in distinguishing benign from malignant neoplasms are listed in Table 6.14.

Differentiation and grade of malignant neoplasms

The extent to which the morphology, growth pattern and synthetic activity of a malignant neoplasm resemble that of its parent tissue determines its differentiation. Neoplasms that closely resemble their parent tissue are termed well differentiated while those that show little resemblance are known as poorly differentiated (Fig. 6.33). Some neoplasms are so poorly

Fig. 6.31 Macroscopic appearance of neoplasms arising in mucosal surfaces.

Exophytic fungating neoplasm

Exophytic neoplasm with surface ulceration

Exophytic (ulcerating) neoplasm

Diffuse infiltrating neoplasm

Table 6.14	Characteristic features of benign and malignant neoplasms	
Feature	**Benign neoplasm**	**Malignant neoplasm**
Macroscopic appearance	Well circumscribed, often encapsulated	Poorly circumscribed, rarely encapsulated
Cut surface	Homogeneous	Heterogeneous
Margin	Blunt, pushing	Infiltrative, invasive
Nuclear:cytoplasmic ratio	Usually normal	Often high
Nuclear pleomorphism	Uncommon	Common
Necrosis	Uncommon	Often present
Mitotic rate	Very low, normal mitoses	Usually high, abnormal mitoses frequent
Metastases	Never	Often

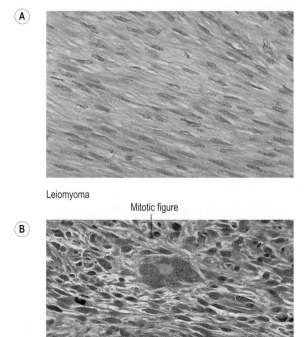

Leiomyoma

Mitotic figure

Leiomyosarcoma

Fig. 6.32 **High-power photomicrographs contrasting (A) a leiomyoma with (B) a leiomyosarcoma.** In the leiomyosarcoma, the nuclei are much more atypical; there is pleomorphism, hyperchromatism and multinucleation. Mitotic figures are easily visible.

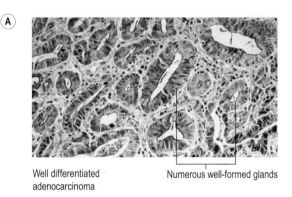

Well differentiated adenocarcinoma   Numerous well-formed glands

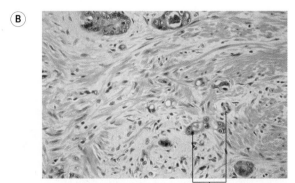

Poorly differentiated adenocarcinoma   Scanty poorly-formed glands

Fig. 6.33 **High-power photomicrographs comparing (A) a well-differentiated with (B) a poorly differentiated adenocarcinoma.** In the former there are many well-formed glands whereas the latter contains only a few poorly formed glands.

differentiated that it is impossible to establish their cell of origin at all; such neoplasms are termed anaplastic. Because benign neoplasms tend to resemble their parent tissue closely, it is convention not to assign a differentiation to them.

The differentiation of a malignant neoplasm is useful not only in determining the histogenesis of the neoplasm but also in assigning a grade. The grade of a malignant neoplasm is a reflection of its histological features and is correlated with behaviour. High-grade neoplasms tend to be poorly differentiated and behave aggressively while low-grade neoplasms are usually well differentiated and behave less aggressively. Consequently, the grade of a malignant neoplasm is important in deciding which treatment to offer a patient and also gives an indication of prognosis.

BEHAVIOUR OF MALIGNANT NEOPLASMS

The distinction of benign from malignant neoplasms is usually possible on morphological criteria alone. In a few cases, however, the distinction can be difficult or even impossible. In such neoplasms, the defining feature of malignancy is the ability of the neoplasm to invade locally and/or metastasise. Benign neoplasms never undergo local invasion or metastasis.

Local invasion

Secretion of collagenases and elastases by neoplastic cells facilitates growth into surrounding connective tissue, vessels and nerves (see Clinical box 6.29). This results in the poorly circumscribed margin typical of malignant neoplasms and also causes fixation of the tissues, pain and haemorrhage in the host.

Metastasis

Metastasis is secondary growth of a neoplasm at one or more locations distant from the primary site (Fig. 6.34). It only occurs with malignant neoplasms. Spread may occur:

- Via lymphatics
- Via blood vessels
- Across coelomic cavities
- Within cerebrospinal fluid
- Through implantation of neoplastic cells following biopsy or surgery.

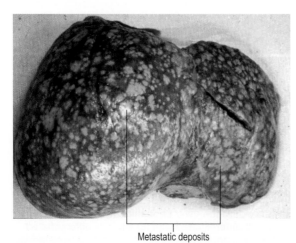

Metastatic deposits

Fig. 6.34 **A liver full of metastatic deposits from a primary carcinoma of the colon.**

Patterns and sites of metastasis

The route of metastasis taken by a neoplasm and the eventual site of metastasis can be predicted according to the type of neoplasm, its location and its drainage pathways. Typically, carcinomas first metastasise via lymphatics to regional lymph nodes and only via the bloodstream later in the disease. Sarcomas characteristically metastasise via the bloodstream early in their course, usually to the lung.

Some tumours (prostate, lung, thyroid, kidney and breast) metastasise preferentially to bone. Certain sites of metastases are preferred by individual malignancies, for example prostatic carcinoma metastasises to the skeleton, serous adenocarcinoma of the ovary metastasises to the peritoneum, bronchial carcinoma metastasises to adrenal and brain, and neuroblastoma metastasises to the liver. The reasons for this specificity are obscure but may be related to chemoattractants produced by the involved organ or to adhesion molecules produced by the neoplasm, which 'fit best' with a ligand on the epithelial cells of a particular organ.

Clonal evolution

Additional mutations frequently occur within monoclonal malignant neoplasms, resulting in subclones that differ from the original phenotype in terms of metastatic ability, proliferative activity and resistance to therapeutic agents. This is known as clonal evolution and results in **tumour heterogeneity**.

Clinical box 6.29	Mechanism of invasion and metastasis

Metastasis is a complex process involving the following sequence of events, shown diagrammatically in Figure 6.35:
1. Detachment of neoplastic cells from each other (through downregulation of cadherin expression)
2. Attachment to ECM via specific receptors
3. Degradation of the ECM through secretion of collagenases and proteases
4. Locomotion through the ECM via secretion of motility factors
5. Vascular intravasation
6. Interaction of tumour cells with host lymphocytes
7. Formation of tumour embolus
8. Adhesion to endothelium at a distant site via adhesion molecules
9. Vascular extravasation
10. Regrowth of the metastatic clone.

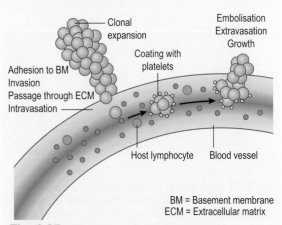

Fig. 6.35 **The stages involved in metastasis.**

EFFECTS OF A NEOPLASM ON THE HOST

Neoplasms do not benefit the host. Indeed, many malignant neoplasms shorten the lifespan of the host significantly. Even benign neoplasms, which are not usually harmful to the host, can sometimes have serious consequences.

The multitude of clinical effects produced by a neoplasm can be classified into local effects, metabolic effects, immunological effects or the effects of metastases. Some malignant neoplasms cause symptom complexes that cannot be explained by local or distant spread or by hormone production from the tissue in which the neoplasm has arisen. Such complexes are called paraneoplastic syndromes. The specific effects of a neoplasm on the host will depend on its histological type, its site of origin and its behaviour.

LOCAL EFFECTS

Neoplasms occupy space alongside normal tissues, which can lead to pressure effects or obstruction. In a large organ such as the liver, pressure effects are usually minimal, but if the neoplasm is close to a vital structure or there is little space for expansion, the consequences of even a benign neoplasm can be life-threatening. For example, a meningioma arising in the cranium can cause raised intracranial pressure, as there is no room for the underlying brain to expand. An adenoma arising in a main bronchus can cause the bronchus to become obstructed leading to bronchiectasis or atelectasis in the distal lung.

Malignant neoplasms infiltrate the adjacent normal tissues due to secretion of collagenases and proteases, thus destroying their structure and interfering with their function. Invasion of nerves around the neoplasm often causes considerable pain, while erosion of blood vessels causes local haemorrhage. Ulceration of neoplasms arising in mucosal surfaces can cause significant blood loss. Consequently, malignant neoplasms of the gastrointestinal tract are often associated with iron deficiency anaemia. Some malignancies, such as basal cell carcinoma of the skin, cause substantial local destruction with significant disfigurement, but rarely metastasise.

IMMUNOLOGICAL EFFECTS

Many neoplasms, particularly malignant ones, stimulate an immunological response in the host. Lymphoid infiltrates, usually cytotoxic T lymphocytes, are present at the invasive margin of many malignant neoplasms. Indeed, lack of such an infiltrate is often a poor prognostic factor. Infiltration of a malignant neoplasm by host NK cells can (very rarely) lead to spontaneous regression.

Certain malignant neoplasms, particularly of haemopoietic origin, cause downregulation of the immune system. This can lead to relative immunodeficiency, which is later compounded by the effects of chemotherapy. The consequence of this immune depression for the patient is predisposition to infection, particularly with opportunistic organisms. Haemopoietic neoplasms can also stimulate other immunological processes such as auto-antibody formation against erythrocytes, resulting in haemolytic anaemia. Formation of auto-antibodies against the acetylcholine receptor occurs with some thymomas, resulting in myasthenia gravis. Some malignancies, particularly bronchial carcinoma and melanoma, cause immune complexes to be formed, which, when deposited in the glomerular basement membrane, lead to membranous glomerulonephritis.

METABOLIC EFFECTS

Most malignant neoplasms disrupt the host's normal metabolic function to some degree, though the severity of the disruption varies from minimal to profound. The metabolic effects can be specific to individual neoplasms, usually resulting from hormone secretion, or non-specific resulting from release of cytokines and other metabolic products.

Specific metabolic effects

Neoplasms that arise in endocrine organs are (not surprisingly) associated with hormonal effects. Benign neoplasms produce such effects, as do well-differentiated malignant neoplasms that retain the synthetic activity of their parent tissue. Examples include acromegaly, resulting from secretion of growth hormone by a pituitary adenoma, and Cushing syndrome, resulting from secretion of cortisol by an adrenocortical adenoma or well-differentiated carcinoma. Some neoplasms that arise in non-endocrine organs can also produce hormones, surprising in view of the fact that their parent tissue does not normally do so. This 'inappropriate' hormone secretion is discussed fully in the section on paraneoplastic syndromes below.

Substantial necrosis within a malignant neoplasm, which can occur spontaneously but which more usually occurs following treatment with chemotherapy, results in the breakdown of neoplastic cells. The purine component of nuclear DNA is broken down to uric acid, so the net result of extensive tumour necrosis is the generation of large amounts of uric acid. Unless this hyperuricaemia is prevented by the use of prophylactic treatment, the likelihood of developing clinical gout is high.

General metabolic effects

Weight loss, anorexia and weakness are common in patients with advanced malignancy. This state of catabolism, debilitation and poor nutrition is known as **cancer cachexia** and is the source of considerable distress since affected patients are often little more than 'skin and bone'. The probable cause of cancer cachexia is secretion of cytokines such as TNF, IL-1 and IFN-γ, either by the neoplasm or by reactive host cells, though the underlying metabolic changes are obscure. Other causes of anorexia and weight loss in patients with malignancy include intractable pain, depression and side effects of chemotherapy.

PARANEOPLASTIC SYNDROMES

As outlined above, **paraneoplastic syndrome**s are symptom complexes that cannot be explained by local or distant spread of the neoplasm or by hormone production from the tissue in which the neoplasm has arisen. They are associated with 5–10% of malignant neoplasms but not with benign neoplasms. Their recognition is important as they can cause significant clinical problems and in a small number of patients they may be the presenting feature of the neoplasm. The most common type of paraneoplastic syndrome is endocrinological,

Table 6.15	Paraneoplastic endocrinopathies	
Clinical syndrome	**Most common tumour type**	**Causal mechanism**
Cushing syndrome	Small cell anaplastic carcinoma of the lung; pancreatic carcinoma	Production of adrenocorticotropic hormone
Hypercalcaemia	Squamous cell carcinoma of the lung; adenocarcinoma of the breast; renal cell carcinoma	Production of parathyroid-hormone-related peptide or cytokines TGF-α, TNF and IL-1
Polycythaemia	Cerebellar haemangioblastoma; hepatocellular carcinoma	Production of erythropoietin
Hyponatraemia	Small cell anaplastic carcinoma of the lung	Production of vasopressin

TGF, transforming growth factor; TNF, tumour necrosis factor; IL, interleukin.

Table 6.16	Other types of paraneoplastic syndrome	
Clinical syndrome	**Most common tumour type**	**Causal mechanism**
Eaton–Lambert myasthenic syndrome	Bronchial carcinoma (all types)	? Immunological
Clubbing	Bronchial carcinoma (all types)	Unknown
Hypertrophic osteoarthropathy	Bronchial carcinoma (all types)	Unknown
Acanthosis nigricans	Gastric carcinoma; bronchial carcinoma (all types)	? Immunological
Dermatomyositis	Adenocarcinoma of the breast; bronchial carcinoma (all types)	? Immunological
Migratory thrombophlebitis	Pancreatic carcinoma; bronchial carcinoma (all types)	Tumour products that activate clotting
Non-bacterial thrombotic (marantic) endocarditis	Advanced malignancy	Hypercoagulability

though haematological, neurological, dermatological and rheumatological syndromes are also recognised.

PARANEOPLASTIC ENDOCRINOPATHIES

Some malignant neoplasms that arise in non-endocrine organs secrete hormones, even though their parent tissue does not normally do so. One of the most common examples is the production of adrenocorticotropic hormone (ACTH) by about 10% of small cell anaplastic carcinomas of the bronchus. The ACTH secreted by the neoplastic cells stimulates the adrenal glands to produce cortisol, resulting in Cushing syndrome. Because the lung does not normally produce ACTH, when neoplasms that arise from the lung do so, the ACTH production is termed 'ectopic' or 'inappropriate' and the Cushing syndrome is termed 'paraneoplastic'.

Another common example is the production of parathyroid-hormone-related peptide by squamous cell carcinoma of the bronchus and adenocarcinoma of the breast. This results in non-metastatic hypercalcaemia. Other types of paraneoplastic endocrinopathy are listed in Table 6.15.

OTHER TYPES OF PARANEOPLASTIC SYNDROME

The most common examples of non-endocrine paraneoplastic syndromes are finger clubbing and hypertrophic osteoarthropathy. The former is hypertrophy of the soft tissues under the nail bed and the latter is subperiosteal new bone formation presenting with pain in the wrist and arm. Both of these usually occur in patients with bronchial carcinoma. A fuller list is given in Table 6.16.

DIAGNOSIS, STAGING AND PROGNOSIS OF NEOPLASMS

There may be a strong clinical suspicion that a patient is harbouring a neoplasm from the history and clinical examination. Systematic investigation, however, is needed to confirm the suspicion, assess the neoplasm to formulate treatment, and attempt to predict the future course of events (prognosis).

DIAGNOSIS OF NEOPLASMS

The presence of a neoplasm can be suspected clinically, radiologically or by the use of tumour markers (see below) but ultimately, diagnosis depends on visualising the neoplastic cells under the microscope. Histology (the study of tissues) and cytology (the study of cells) are the cornerstones of microscopic diagnosis. Biopsies for histological examination can be obtained by the use of cutting needles, which produce core biopsies, or by the use of forceps during endoscopic procedures. If the neoplasm is inaccessible externally, a laparoscopy or open operation is necessary to obtain diagnostic tissue.

Samples for cytological examination can be obtained by aspiration of a cystic or solid mass with a thin needle (known as fine needle aspiration cytology) or by retrieving cells shed from a luminal surface or into a cavity (known as exfoliative cytology). Examples of the former include aspiration of a breast or thyroid lump; examples of the latter include cervical smear (Fig. 6.36), bronchial brushing, sputum cytology and examination of ascitic fluid.

Cells and tissues must be stained in order to be visible microscopically. Most neoplasms can be diagnosed by the use of routine stains alone, haematoxylin and eosin (H&E) for histology and Papanicolaou stain for cytology. Histochemical stains are useful for demonstrating substances such as mucin, which do not stain with H&E. Immunohistochemistry, which uses labelled antibodies to detect specific antigens, is particularly useful for determining the histogenesis of a neoplasm when this is not apparent on H&E- or Papanicolaou-stained sections. Molecular biological methods such as in situ hybridisation and polymerase chain reaction are used in the diagnosis of haemopoietic neoplasms.

Tumour markers

Tumour markers are compounds (proteins, antigens or hormones) that can be detected in higher than normal amounts in the blood, urine or tissues of patients with certain types of malignant neoplasm. A tumour marker can be produced by the tumour itself or by the body in response to the neoplasm. The main uses of tumour markers are in:

- Screening for malignancy, either random screening of general populations (e.g. PSA) or targeted screening of high-risk populations (e.g. CA125)
- Diagnosis of suspected malignancy

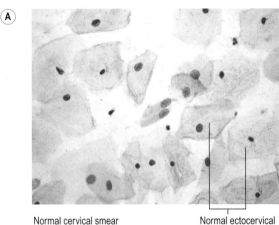

Normal cervical smear   Normal ectocervical squamous cells

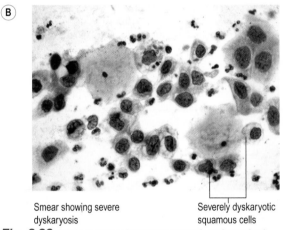

Smear showing severe dyskaryosis   Severely dyskaryotic squamous cells

Fig. 6.36 **High-power photomicrographs of cervical smears.** (A) A normal smear; (B) a smear showing severe dyskaryosis.

- Assessment of prognosis (e.g. HER-2)
- Allocation of patients to therapeutic subgroups (e.g. HER-2)
- Detection of recurrence following completion of therapy (e.g. carcinoembryonic antigen).

A diagnosis of malignancy should not be based on the presence of a raised tumour marker alone. Not only are none of the available markers specific to a particular malignancy but most marker levels can also be raised secondary to benign conditions, leading to false-positive results. False negatives are common because not every malignancy will cause elevated levels of its associated tumour marker, particularly in the early stages.

The most frequently used tumour markers are listed in Table 6.17.

STAGING OF NEOPLASMS

Staging is an indication of how far a malignant neoplasm has spread. The stage of an individual neoplasm is determined using several modalities – clinical assessment, imaging and histopathological assessment of the resected neoplasm. The purpose of staging is to decide which treatment to offer a patient and to give an indication of prognosis.

The first staging system to be widely applied was **Dukes' system** for colorectal carcinoma, first described by Cuthbert Dukes in 1932. This uses only histopathological analysis of the resected neoplasm to place a carcinoma into one of three staging groups:

- Dukes' A – invasion into, but not through, the bowel wall
- Dukes' B – invasion through the bowel wall into the mesentery without lymph node metastases
- Dukes' C – invasion of any part of the bowel wall with lymph node metastases.

Dukes' stage D was added later to describe carcinomas with distant metastases.

Nowadays, the most widely used staging system is the **TNM** (Tumour, Node, Metastasis) system based on the size or local extent of the primary tumour (represented by T), the number and site of involved lymph nodes (represented by N) and the presence or absence of extranodal metastases (represented by M). The TNM score is

Table 6.17	**Frequently used tumour markers**		
Tumour marker	**Compound**	**Primary malignancy**	**False positives**
α-Fetoprotein (AFP)	Protein produced by the yolk sac and foetal liver	Hepatocellular carcinoma; germ cell neoplasms of the testis and ovary	Cirrhosis; hepatitis; inflammatory bowel disease
β-Human chorionic gonadotropin (β-HCG)	Peptide hormone produced by trophoblast cells in the placenta	Hydatidiform mole; choriocarcinoma; germ cell neoplasms of the testis and ovary	Pregnancy
Carcinoembryonic antigen (CEA)	Glycoprotein found on the apical surface of normal intestinal epithelium	Adenocarcinoma of the colon and rectum; some adenocarcinomas of the stomach, pancreas, breast and thyroid	Pancreatitis; hepatitis; inflammatory bowel disease; biliary obstruction
CA125	Cell surface glycoprotein found on mesothelial cells	Adenocarcinoma of the ovary; some adenocarcinomas of the breast and pancreas	Pregnancy; endometriosis; pelvic inflammatory disease
Calcitonin	Hormone secreted by C-cells of the thyroid	Medullary carcinoma of the thyroid	
HER-2	Cell surface receptor	Adenocarcinoma of the breast – used to predict response to therapy	
Prostate-specific antigen (PSA)	Serine protease secreted into seminal fluid by prostate gland	Adenocarcinoma of the prostate	Benign prostatic hyperplasia; prostatitis

Clinical box 6.30   TNM staging for adenocarcinoma of the breast

Stage 0: carcinoma in situ, where there is no local invasion of surrounding normal tissues.

Stage 1: T<2 cm, has not metastasised to the axillary lymph nodes (N=0) and there are no metastases to other sites (M=0).

Stage 2: is considered in two categories:

- Stage 2A where:
  - T<2 cm, N positive, but nodes are not stuck together, M=0
  - T<5 cm, N=0, M=0, **or**
  - T=0 (i.e. presence of tumour not detected in the breast), N positive but not stuck, M=0.
- Stage 2B where:
  - T<5 cm, N positive but not stuck to each other, M=0
  - T>5 cm, N=0, M=0.

Stage 3 breast cancer is in three categories:

- Stage 3A where:
  - T=0, axillary N positive and stuck together, M=0, **or**
  - T<5 cm, axillary N positive and stuck to each other, M=0, **or**
  - T>5 cm, axillary N positive and may be stuck together, M=0.
- Stage 3B where:
  - T attached to skin or chest wall, N positive or negative, M=0.
- Stage 3C where:
  - T=any size, axillary and other (neck, internal mammary), N positive, M=0.

Stage 4 where:

- T=any size
- N positive or negative
- M positive to distant sites.

denoted as Tx Ny Mz where x, y, and z are numbers allocated according to specified criteria for each neoplasm site. An example of the TNM system for staging of adenocarcinoma of the breast is shown in Clinical box 6.30. For some neoplasms, particularly gynaecological malignancies, staging groups (e.g. stage I–IV) are used instead of the TNM system.

PROGNOSIS OF NEOPLASMS

The prognosis for a patient with malignancy is given in terms of the 5-year survival rate. Neoplasms with good prognosis usually have a 5-year survival of 80% or greater while those with poor prognosis have a 5-year survival of 20% or less. The main indicators of prognosis are the type of neoplasm, its grade and its stage at presentation. Some types of neoplasm, for example small cell anaplastic carcinoma of the bronchus, behave aggressively and have a poor prognosis irrespective of stage. Others, such as seminoma of the testis, have a good prognosis, even if they present at a high stage.

As discussed above, the grade of a neoplasm is based on an assessment of its histological features and differentiation. The histological features most useful in assigning a grade are mitotic activity, nuclear size and nuclear pleomorphism. High-grade neoplasms behave more aggressively and so have a worse prognosis than low-grade neoplasms. For most neoplasms, the greater the stage, the worse the prognosis. For example, Dukes' stage A colorectal carcinoma has a 5-year survival of 80–90% while a Dukes' stage C neoplasm has a 5-year survival of 30%.

Prognostic factors in pathology reports

Every pathology report on a malignant neoplasm should include an indication of the type and grade of a neoplasm, and (if appropriate) the stage. In addition, the pathologist should report on other factors that have also been shown to give prognostic information. These include completeness of excision, presence or absence of vascular invasion and presence or absence of premalignant lesions in adjacent tissues.

SCREENING FOR MALIGNANCY

From the foregoing discussion, it is evident that if a malignant neoplasm can be diagnosed early, the chances of successful treatment and cure will be maximised. This is best achieved by screening asymptomatic individuals in the population at risk with the aim of detecting neoplasms at the premalignant stage or, in the unfortunate event that a malignancy has already developed, before it has had the chance to metastasise. The criteria for a screening test have already been described (see pp. 326–327).

In the UK, the NHS funds three national screening programmes:

- The Breast Screening Programme, which screens women aged 47–73 using mammography every 3 years. When a suspicious lesion is detected, this is followed up by clinical examination, ultrasound, and cytology or needle biopsy.
- The Cervical Screening Programme, which screens women aged 25–64 by cervical smear every 3–5 years. When a severe abnormality is detected, further investigation by colposcopy and biopsy is offered.
- The Bowel Cancer Screening Programme, which screens all men and women aged 60–74 using faecal occult blood testing (FOBT) every 2 years. Individuals who test positive are offered further investigation by colonoscopy. In the near future, this screening programme will be expanded to offer all men and women aged 55 a one-off flexible sigmoidoscopy, in addition to FOBT.

There is currently no organised screening programme for prostate cancer but an informed choice programme, Prostate Cancer Risk Management, has been introduced. The aim of this programme is to ensure that men who are concerned about the risk of prostate cancer receive clear and balanced information about the advantages and disadvantages of measuring serum levels of the tumour marker PSA. Trials are also well advanced of a screening programme for ovarian carcinoma using ultrasound and/or the tumour marker CA125.

Other screening strategies involve targeting specific populations at high risk of developing malignancy, for example patients with Barrett's oesophagus and longstanding ulcerative colitis. Patients with these diseases are at high risk of developing adenocarcinoma of the oesophagus and colorectum respectively. Though there is no national screening programme for these patients, because the risk of developing malignancy is so high, local screening programmes for the detection of epithelial dysplasia have been developed in most regions.

Screening programmes have considerable financial and organisational implications, so the cost–benefit analysis is continually under review. The reasons why screening programmes may not be as effective as anticipated are beyond the scope of this discussion, but there is no doubt that results are improving as experience grows. Ultimately, the success of screening programmes will depend on public education and investment of sufficient resources.

Why do patients die from neoplasia?

Evolution has not yet managed to create a symbiotic relationship between malignant neoplasms and their host, with the result that many malignancies remain fatal. Preventing death from malignancy is one of the main challenges to medicine in the 21st century. There is no single reason why malignant neoplasms are so harmful. Death can occur from a number of factors related to the behaviour of the neoplasm or to the effects of therapy:

- Widespread disease in multiple organ sites (**carcinomatosis**)
- Metastatic disease in vital sites such as the brain, lung or heart
- Immunosuppression, either due to the neoplasm or to chemotherapy, leading to opportunistic infections
- Organ failure
- Haemorrhage exacerbated by anaemia and thrombocytopenia
- Late second malignancies, either due to inherited genetic abnormalities in the patient or to the effects of previous therapy.

Benign neoplasms do not generally cause significant harm to the host, though rarely they can be fatal. The most common neoplasms that cause death of the host are meningiomas, due to pressure effects inside the cranium, and insulinomas of the pancreas, which can cause profound hypoglycaemia and coma.

CARCINOGENESIS

Carcinogenesis is the process by which a normal cell becomes a cancer cell. Cancer cells are characterised by uncontrolled proliferation, invasion of adjacent tissues and often metastasis or spread to distant organs. Transformation of normal cells into cancer cells may be triggered by:

- Alteration of the genes that control cell proliferation and differentiation: gene mutation caused by mutagens
- Alteration of gene expressions by changes in the chemical structure of DNA (e.g. DNA methylation) where there is no gene mutation, known as the epigenetic theory for carcinogenesis.
- Cancers are classified according to the type of tissue from which they originate (see above).

BIOLOGY OF NEOPLASTIC CELLS

Multiple genetic changes take place over time before a normal cell becomes cancerous. During the pre-neoplastic stage (precursor), the cells appear different from normal, with variable sizes of nuclei, variable shapes and increased numbers of dividing cells. Dysplasia is characteristic of premalignant cells, and classified as carcinoma in situ when severe (see above). There is evidence to suggest that a cancer can arise from a single cell due to clonal expansion or clonal evolution (see Ch. 5 and above), when the aberrant gene due to damaged DNA enhances the cell's survival and reproduction despite the disorderly growth that would normally lead to apoptosis. Progressive gene mutations lead to properties of neoplastic cells that may be summarised as follows:

- Deregulation of normal cell growth and loss of sensitivity to anti-growth signals leading to unchecked cell proliferation
- Cell proliferation continues because cancer cells do not respond to the normal stimuli leading to apoptosis (genetic errors, ageing and external anti-growth signals)
- Ability to sustain growth beyond its blood supply
- Ability to invade surrounding tissues and metastasise to distant sites
- Inability to repair genetic errors with an increased mutation rate (genomic instability).

GENES ASSOCIATED WITH CANCER AND ONCOGENESIS

Three main groups of changes in genes that control cell proliferation and death, involving specific target genes, have been implicated in carcinogenesis (see Ch. 5):

- Oncogenes are normally silent (proto-oncogenes), but may gain expression in excessively high levels, or be genetically altered to activate cell proliferation through chemical messengers (hormones) between cells, the signal conducted to the nucleus causing an alteration in gene transcription that promote mitosis. Oncogenes also inhibit cell death.
- Inactivation (loss of function mutation) of tumour suppression genes that inhibit cell proliferation or promote cell death by deletion of specific chromosomal regions (alleles). Mutations in tumour suppression genes in germ cells may be inherited (hereditary cancer syndromes).
- Defects in DNA repair genes lead to genomic instability, resulting in chromosomal abnormalities with widespread mutations in genes that affect cell proliferation and accelerate carcinogenesis.

CHEMICAL CARCINOGENS

Chemical carcinogens may be mutagenic (causing mutation in genes) or non-mutagenic. The best researched mutagenic carcinogen is tobacco smoke – linked to cancers in many sites, particularly lung cancer. Asbestos is also mutagenic and associated with mesothelioma of the lung. Alcohol is not mutagenic, but is a chemical carcinogen that stimulates the rate of mitosis, reducing the time available for DNA repair and increasing the risk of genetic error (**aneuploidy**, see Ch. 5).

INFECTIVE CARCINOGENS

Epidemiological data suggest that viruses may be the second most important cause of human cancers (second to tobacco). Some viruses (acutely transforming viruses) carry an active viral oncogene that acutely transforms an infected cell into a cancer cell. Slowly transforming viruses insert a virus genome near a host proto-oncogene leading to upregulation of cell growth so that the proto-oncogene is transformed to an oncogene, inducing uncontrolled cell proliferation (see Ch. 5).

The main viruses associated with human cancers are the human papillomavirus (HPV) (cervical cancer), and hepatitis B and C viruses (liver cancer). The combination of alcoholic cirrhosis and chronic viral hepatitis represents the highest risk for liver cancer. Some virus infections, such as HIV infection, are associated with defects in immunity, which in turn is a possible aetiology for cancer. Kaposi's sarcoma and non-Hodgkin's lymphoma are associated with AIDS. It has also been postulated that the link between HPV and anal and cervical cancer is immunodeficiency. Some bacteria have a link with cancer, e.g. *H. pylori,* a bacterium that causes peptic ulceration, is linked to stomach cancer.

EFFECTS OF RADIATION

Ionising radiation occurs as electromagnetic rays (X-rays, γ-rays) or as particles (α- and β-particles). Exposure to ionising radiation has known associations with the development of cancer. Some occupations have a higher risk than others depending on the nature of the work and environment, with implications for health and safety at work. For example, ionising radiation from radon (radon 222), a naturally occurring gas usually found in enclosed underground spaces, is recognised as a cause of lung cancer.

Non-ionising radiation, of which ultraviolet rays from the sun is best known, can also cause cancers. Prolonged exposure to ultraviolet radiation has a known association with skin cancers.

EFFECTS OF HORMONES

Some hormones stimulate excessive cell proliferation, acting as a non-mutagenic carcinogen. Examples include excessive oestrogen secretion and endometrial cancer.

GENES AND INHERITED CANCER SYNDROMES

Although most cancers occur sporadically, there are some well-described cancer syndromes that have an hereditary component (see Ch. 5), including:

- Inherited genetic mutations associated with increased risk of breast and ovarian cancers (*BRCA1* and *BRCA2*)
- Familial adenomatous polyposis (FAP) and hereditary non-polyposis colorectal cancer
- Retinoblastoma
- Increased risk of leukaemia in people with Down syndrome (trisomy 21).

The development of genetic techniques for diagnosing hereditary cancer syndromes is clearly important for affected people and their families.

HOST FACTORS

The lifestyle and behaviours of individuals may increase their risk of exposure to carcinogens, so that modification of these factors may give a better chance for avoiding the

development of cancers. The major potentially modifiable risk factors for carcinogenesis related to lifestyle include:

- Smoking tobacco
- Excess intake of alcohol
- Inadequate dietary intake of fibre as fruit and vegetables
- Limited physical exercise
- Obesity.

These bear a remarkable resemblance to risk factors for coronary heart disease. Other behavioural factors include:

- Prolonged exposure to ultraviolet radiation
- HPV infection
- Intravenous drug use (increasing the risk of hepatitis B and C)
- Unprotected sexual intercourse.

The above host risk factors may be amenable to targeted health education or strategies for prevention such as vaccination against HPV infection. Other risk factors that may be related to the environment, such as the risk of exposure to ionising radiation, could be reduced through health and safety controls.

Some cancer risk factors are not modifiable, as in the hereditary cancer syndromes. Here, the possibility of early diagnosis using genetic techniques could be important, particularly if the technology for gene therapy becomes a practical reality.

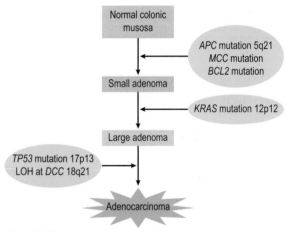

Fig. 6.37 Adenoma-carcinoma sequence for colorectal cancer. *APC,* the adenomatosis polyposis coli gene, a tumour suppressor gene mutated (inactivated) in people with familial adenomatous polyposis and early onset colorectal cancer; *MCC,* mutated in colorectal cancers, a colorectal tumour suppressor gene that inhibits cell proliferation, inactivated in colorectal cancer; *BCL2,* a gene that promotes apoptosis, loss of function mutation occurs in response to carcinogens in intestinal lumen; *KRAS,* a proto-oncogene mutated to oncogene; *p53,* a tumour suppressor gene that encodes the transcription factor p53 in response to DNA damage, delays DNA synthesis (S phase of cell cycle) to allow time for DNA repair. Loss of function mutation in colorectal cancer; *DCC,* deleted in colorectal carcinoma (cancer), a tumour suppressor gene. DCC is also the protein product of DCC (interchangeable name), a single transmembrane receptor; LOH, loss of heterozygosity.

MULTISTEP THEORY OF CARCINOGENESIS
(see also Ch. 5, Cancer genetics)

Many neoplasms progress from normality to malignancy in a stepwise fashion. This usually starts with histologically invisible changes followed by the development of dysplasia or a benign neoplasm such as an adenoma. This can then develop into a locally invasive malignancy, which eventually acquires the ability to metastasise. Each of these steps is associated with changes in proto-oncogenes and/or tumour suppressor genes and, in an established malignancy, with clonal evolution.

This model of tumour progression is well illustrated by the adenoma–carcinoma sequence, which occurs in the development of colorectal adenocarcinoma (Fig. 6.37). The changes from normal to cancer cells begin in the epithelial stem cells at the bottom of the colorectal crypts.

In sporadic colorectal cancer, epigenetic changes take place in response to carcinogens in the lumen so that the cells escape the control of normal signalling for cell proliferation, apoptosis and DNA repair. The presence of the mutated adenomatosis polyposis coli (*APC*) gene in hereditary colorectal cancer syndrome is responsible for the changes in hereditary colorectal cancer. Premalignant lesions, small adenomata, form, and further exposure to luminal carcinogens leads to mutations in pro-oncogenes, such as *KRAS*, to oncogenes, when the cells no longer respond to appropriate signalling. Large adenomata form, to eventually become malignant through further mutations in tumour suppressor genes (e.g. *p53*). Clonal evolution, when the cells acquire the ability to proliferate despite the normal controls for cell growth and cell death, then enables the cells to invade local tissues and to metastasise.

7

Epidemiology: science for the art of medicine

Jeannette Naish and Denise Syndercombe Court

Introduction	277	An overview of epidemiological enquiry	296
The epidemiological approach	**277**	**Investigation by review**	**319**
Epidemiology as the detective	277	Meta-analysis	319
Patterns of life and death	280	**Health education and promotion**	**321**
Epidemiological enquiry	**291**	Health education	321
Some basic concepts in epidemiology	291	Prevention	323

INTRODUCTION

The term **epidemiology** has its roots in Greek words meaning, very roughly, 'a discourse about something visited on the people'. While it is clearly a close cousin of 'epidemic', it is important to understand how the two relate to each other. **Epidemic**, though commonly understood to mean an outbreak of infectious disease, is more strictly defined as the prevalence of a disease among populations or groups of people at a particular time, and produced by special causes not usually present in the affected locality. The realm of epidemiology, however, is wider and more complex than the mere study of epidemics.

In clinical medicine, the focus is on the individual, on the **symptoms** and **signs** of the illness, on its diagnosis, and on subsequent decisions about therapy. Epidemiology, on the other hand, investigates patterns of disease among populations or groups of people, in order to understand causation and determine appropriate responses. Definitions and explanations of many of the terms that are used throughout the chapter are given in Table 7.1.

THE EPIDEMIOLOGICAL APPROACH

In diagnosing and managing the illness of particular patients, clinicians rely not only on their own experience, but also on knowledge and understanding derived from other clinicians' observations of patients with similar signs, symptoms and laboratory findings. For example, the observation of groups of children with **whooping cough** led to the understanding of how this disease develops (Information box 7.1).

The selection of effective treatments depends on an understanding of how similar patients fared on different treatments in the past. Epidemiology provides a scientific framework for understanding how health problems occur, how diseases behave and whether interventions are effective. In a clinical context, epidemiology also provides a better understanding of the issues that can inform further research to develop more effective strategies to reduce disease incidence (see below) and improve health.

Information box 7.1 **Whooping cough**

Whooping cough begins with symptoms similar to a common cold. After an incubation period of 7–10 days, an irritating cough progresses to spasms, or paroxysms, of coughing, sometimes accompanied by a characteristic 'whoop', particularly in young children. The coughing spasms may be followed by vomiting, and could last for 2–3 months – hence the term '100-day cough'. Severe complications such as dehydration, brain damage or death may occur, particularly in infants under 6 months old. The disease is transmitted by droplets and is highly infectious. Diagnosis is usually made from the history and symptoms, but may be confirmed by isolating *Bordetella pertussis* from the sputum. The problem for clinicians can be that their own direct experience of whooping cough is limited, so that they will need to draw on the collective story. The rarer the condition, the more important this is.

EPIDEMIOLOGY AS THE DETECTIVE

By careful and accurate descriptions of observed phenomena and by logical comparisons of these phenomena, epidemiology seeks to describe the natural progression of disease and epidemics, and identify factors that may have a causal relationship with diseases. This knowledge contributes to the understanding of how diseases and epidemics arise so that strategies for controlling and preventing epidemics and for treating disease may be formulated.

The Broad Street pump

In 1855, Dr John Snow published his treatise on the mode of communication of **cholera** (Greek *cholé bilea;* highly infectious disease characterised by profuse vomiting and diarrhoea). The 'cholera morbus' was first described near Jessore, India, in 1817. In 1823, it had spread to Russia; by 1831 it was in Hamburg, and the first case in east London was identified on 12 February 1832. In contrast, **H1N1 (influenza A, or swine flu) virus** emerged in the spring of 2009 and within 1 month cases had been reported in 48 countries with up to 90 million people being affected in 74 countries worldwide before the **pandemic** was over, reflecting its person to person transmission and global human movement.

Variously called 'Asiatic', 'spasmodic', 'malignant', 'contagious' and 'blue', cholera was also confused with 'common' or 'English' cholera, dysentery and food poisoning. Although the

Table 7.1	Terms used in epidemiology
Allele	Genes exist in different allelic forms defined by differences in nucleotide sequence
Allocation concealment	The inability to predict or discover the potential random allocation group until the point of assignment
Alternative hypothesis (H_1)	A statement that is different from the null hypothesis and that is true if the null hypothesis is false
Bias	A systematic difference between the observed and the true effect
Binary data	Have two possible values. For example yes or no, up or down. These data are represented mathematically by the binomial distribution
Case–control study	A study where diseased individuals (cases) are identified and compared with individuals who are as similar as possible as the cases except that they do not have the disease (controls)
Clinical trial	An experiment involving humans used to evaluate a new treatment in relation to a particular clinical outcome
Cohort study	A study in which a group of individuals without the outcome of interest (disease) is followed over time (usually prospectively) to investigate the effect of their exposure to a risk factor on outcomes in future
Collinearity	When two factors are very strongly associated
Confidence interval	A range in which we are confident (to a specified extent) that the true population parameter lies
Confounding	Occurs when we are looking at a relationship between two factors and a third factor (the confounding variable) masks or exaggerates the observed relationship between the two because that third factor is associated with *both* the other factors
Contingency table	A table which contains frequencies in 'cells'
Correlation coefficient	The extent of the relationship of the points to a straight line
Crude rate	A measure made without adjustment for other factors, such as age, that otherwise may be misleading
Degrees of freedom	A measure of how many numbers in the table are free to vary without affecting the totals. In a 2×2 table, provided the totals remain the same, only one number at a time is free to vary. As soon as this number is changed in *one* cell, the numbers in the other cells are forced to change. There is therefore *one* degree of freedom in a 2×2 table
Fisher's exact test	A method that evaluates all possible tables with the same totals as if the null hypothesis was true
Histogram	A graphical display of frequencies in separate categories of data. Frequencies are represented as bars, the area under the bar denotes the frequency (unlike bar charts where the height of the bar denotes the frequency). (Greek origin: *histos,* upright as in a vertical ship's mast, *gramma* a record or writing)
Incidence	Measure of the number of *new* cases of a disease, occurring during a specified period of time in a specified location
Interdecile range	The central 80% of the ordered data (between the 10ths, or 10th percentile and 90th percentile)
Interquartile range	The central 50% of the ordered data (between the quarters or 25th percentile and 75th percentile)
Kappa	The proportion of agreement in a classification beyond that due to chance in relation to the potential agreement beyond chance, where a value of 1 implies perfect agreement and a value of 0 no better than chance alone
Likelihood ratio (LR)	A ratio of two likelihoods, for example a ratio of the chances of getting a particular test result in those having and those not having the disease
Matching	A process of selecting individuals who are similar in characteristics known to be associated with the outcome but which are not of interest. Most common are age and sex which are known to be associated with many diseases
Mean or arithmetic mean	A measure of the centre of the data obtained by summing the individual values and dividing the total by the number of data points
Median (or 50th percentile)	When data are put into rank order the median divides the data into two equal parts. For example, if there are 9 data points the 5th in rank order will be the median, four datum points being below, and four above. If there are 10 datum points then the 5th and 6th, in rank order, will be in the middle. Traditionally, the median of those two numbers is given by their mean
Minimisation	Selection of an individual based on minimising the chance that the selection will unbalance the group for a particular factor
Mode	The item that is the most common in the data set
Null hypothesis (H_0)	A statement that assumes no difference or effect
One-tailed	Where the alternative hypothesis specifies a direction to the effect
Outcome or dependent variable	The characteristic or outcome of interest that is affected by one or more variables
Percentile	Division of ordered data into 100 equal parts. The median is the 50th percentile
PPV or positive predictive value of a test	The probability of actually having the condition when the test for the condition is positive. Sometimes referred to as the OAPR (odds of being affected given a positive test result)
Predictor or independent variable	An attribute that can have an effect on the outcome
Prevalence	Measure of the number of *existing* cases of a disease at a particular point in time (point prevalence) or over a specified period of time (period prevalence), in a particular place, divided by the total population

Table 7.1	Terms used in epidemiology—cont'd
Prospective study	One where individuals are followed forward in time
Random	Selection of a subject or item from a population such that the chance of being selected is the same for all subjects or items within that population
Randomised controlled trial	A clinical trial in which individuals are allocated to the different treatment groups in a randomised fashion
Retrospective study	A study in which what has happened in the past to individuals enrolled in the study is investigated
Sample	A subgroup of a population being studied
Sampling frame	A list of all individuals within a population
Scattergram	Plot of one variable against another with each pair of measurements represented by a point
Selection bias	Bias that occurs when the individuals being studied are not representative of the population of interest
Sensitivity	The proportion of people *with* a disease who are correctly identified by the diagnostic test (true positives). Sometimes referred to as the 'detection rate'. If a test is not 100% sensitive then there will be false positive results
Sign	Manifestation of a target disorder perceived by the clinician during an examination
Specificity	The proportion of people *without* a disease who are correctly identified by the diagnostic test (true negatives). If a test is not 100% specific then there will be false negative results
Standard deviation	A measure of the spread of numerical (continuous or discrete) data
Standard error	A measure of how precise the summary statistic is. The standard error of a proportion is a measure of how sure we are about an observed proportion
Standardise	To adjust a rate to allow comparison between different populations
Standardised mortality ratio (SMR)	Ratio between observed and expected number of an event (such as death) multiplied by 100 and computed by indirect standardisation
Stratification	Selection of a subgroup that has similar characteristics
Symptom	Manifestation of a target disorder perceived by the patient, spontaneously or on questioning
t-Distribution	A continuous distribution with a shape similar to the normal distribution. It is used to make inferences about means
Two-tailed	A test in which the alternative hypothesis does not specify a direction to the effect

general populace believed the disease to be contagious, its exact nature was much debated among the medical profession. A large proportion actually thought that the disease did not spread from person to person but could arise spontaneously, as a result of bad air. The popular *London Medical Gazette* agreed that there was a serious problem but simply discussed its prevention and cure, rather than the origin of cholera or its causes.

John Snow was prompted to study 'The most terrible outbreak of cholera which ever occurred in this kingdom'. This took place in Broad Street, Golden Square, in the centre of London's West End in 1854. Within the space of 10 days more than 500 people had died and most others had fled the area (Table 7.2).

Snow had already published a report suggesting that cholera was spread by contaminated water. Cholera, he noted, 'always commences with disturbances of the functions of the alimentary canal', and he suggested that it was spread by a poison passed from victim to victim through sewage-tainted water. Neither the authorities nor other members of the medical profession were persuaded by his theories, but the 1854 outbreak gave him a further opportunity to prove his thesis.

Since most of the deaths appeared to have occurred close to the water pump in Broad Street, Snow took the view that this was the source of the problem. He examined the water and at first saw nothing suspicious, but over a few days noted that the quality of the water varied, and that it seemed to have small white flocculent particles floating in it. At this point he decided to undertake a systematic survey of the deaths in the vicinity. Eighty-three deaths, mapped according to place of residence, had occurred within 3 days at the beginning of September in the three sub-districts that surrounded the Broad Street pump (Fig. 7.1).

In virtually all cases the Broad Street pump was the closest to the victims' home. Where this was not so, affected individuals were regular users of the Broad Street pump in preference to others closer to where they lived. Only two cases were exceptions to this pattern and these might in any case have been examples of the low incidence of cholera that was normally to be expected in London at this time. Within the area, however, were industries, breweries and workhouses where the workers were generally shown not to have developed the disease. Snow questioned the owners and found that each establishment had its own separate source of water, or, in the case of the brewery, the workmen only drank the malt liquor, made using deep well water. The pump had a reputation for 'better' water and 'was widely used for mixing with spirits in all the public houses around. It was used likewise at dining-rooms and coffee-shops'.

After presenting his evidence, Dr Snow persuaded the authorities to remove the pump handle, after which no new cases of cholera were reported. The pump well was examined, but there was no defect that would suggest the reason for the contamination of the water, and the local sewer was too far away. The whitish particles that Snow saw were examined under the microscope by Dr Arthur H. Hassall, a contemporary physician, who thought they were just decomposition of another matter. The water, however, even when clear, smelt offensive and Dr Hassall noted 'a great number of very minute oval animalcules in the water', which he declared to be of no importance.

Table 7.2	Reported attacks of cholera in Broad Street, Golden Square in Soho, in the West End of London, published by John Snow in 1854; 545 deaths occurred between 1 and 11 September		
Month	Date	Number of fatal attacks	Deaths
August	19	1	1
	20	1	0
	21	1	2
	22	1	0
	23	1	0
	24	1	2
	25	1	0
	26	1	0
	27	1	1
	28	1	0
	29	1	1
	30	6	2
	31	56	3
September	1	143	70
	2	116	127
	3	54	76
	4	46	71
	5	36	45
	6	20	37
	7	28	32
	8	12	30
	9	11	24
	10	5	18
	11	5	15
	12	1	6
	13	3	13
	14	0	6
	15	1	8
	16	4	6
	17	2	5
	18	3	2
	19	0	3
	20	0	0
	21	2	0
	22	1	2
	23	1	3
	24	1	0
	25	1	0
	26	1	2
	27	1	0
	28	0	2
	29	0	1
	30	0	0
Date unknown		45	0
Total		616	616

It would be some years before the agent, the bacterium *Vibrio cholerae,* was formally identified, but Snow did unearth the probable cause of the outbreak. Just before the epidemic, a child living in Broad Street had been taken ill with symptoms of cholera. The nappies had been steeped in water to be washed, and the water was subsequently tipped into a leaking cesspool, just 3 ft from the Broad Street well.

PATTERNS OF LIFE AND DEATH

In order to understand the 'health' of populations, observation and recording of events relating to ill health or death provide the information that is needed. These events arise naturally, rather than as the result of experimentation; for example, to see if a vaccination programme for whooping cough actually reduces the incidence of whooping cough. Descriptions of the information (data, statistics) collected through observation are the cornerstone of public health, where:

- **Morbidity** refers to the incidence (see below) of a disease or all diseases in a population. Newspaper headlines that tell us that more than 130 000 people will be diagnosed with colon cancer tell us little unless put into a context – over what period of time, and in what sized population?
- **Mortality** refers to the death rate in a population, which may be from all causes, i.e. the ratio of all deaths to the total population, or for a specific population, for example infant mortality rate refers to the ratio of the number of deaths of infants under 1 year of age to the total number of live births in a population in a particular year, or for a specific condition.

Descriptive studies

The essential components of descriptive epidemiology are concerned with **people**, **time** and **place**. Epidemiological methods are used to make inferences based on descriptions of groups of *people,* or populations, rather than individual patients. These groups have shared characteristics, which could be geographically defined (e.g. living within 2 km of pylons or nuclear power stations, or living in the vicinity of the Broad Street pump); defined by a common condition (such as coronary heart disease, childhood leukaemia, cholera); associated with possession, or lack, of a particular gene (such as in Alzheimer disease) or share personal attributes such as age, sex, racial origins, occupation, social class or lifestyle behaviour (e.g. tobacco smoking, alcohol consumption). Such characteristics may be used to identify and investigate differences in patterns of disease, and generate hypotheses about causal association, evaluate the effectiveness of treatment, plan health service provision or ask further questions.

Descriptive studies use collected information to examine a population, either at a single point in time, or over a period of time, looking at long-term trends, cyclical change or the kinds of sudden change associated with epidemics (see Information box 7.2).

Measuring disease occurrence

Epidemiological methods make it possible to estimate the risk within a group of people of the disease developing. To define disease occurrence, two important concepts are used: **incidence** and **prevalence**.

Disease incidence

Incidence is concerned with new cases of disease. The number of events (e.g. heart attacks) that are new cases occurring during the specified time (5 years) in a defined population (e.g. overweight male smokers aged 45–55), and resident in a particular geographical location is referred to as the **incidence**.

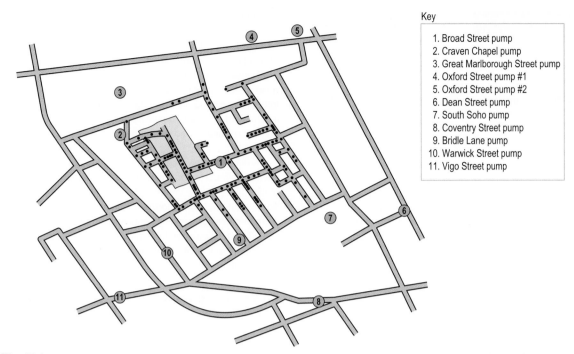

Fig. 7.1 Map of deaths in Soho showing that reported deaths from cholera clustered around the Broad Street pump.

Key

1. Broad Street pump
2. Craven Chapel pump
3. Great Marlborough Street pump
4. Oxford Street pump #1
5. Oxford Street pump #2
6. Dean Street pump
7. South Soho pump
8. Coventry Street pump
9. Bridle Lane pump
10. Warwick Street pump
11. Vigo Street pump

| Information box 7.2 | An epidemic of birth defects |

Birth defects are distressing, but thankfully rare. A single example can appear to a clinician to be nothing more than an isolated and random occurrence. The following story illustrates the importance of clinicians reporting unusual events such as these in order to contribute to a broader epidemiological understanding.

Thalidomide (α-phthalimido-glutarimide) was produced by the German company Chemie Grüenthal and supplied under the name Distaval in the UK, originally as an anticonvulsant, but later as a sedative, and was widely prescribed to women to combat symptoms common in early pregnancy. An apparent advantage – that overdoses did not result in death – led to its wide promotion, not only as a sedative, but in combination with other drugs for a wide range of common medical conditions.

In Germany, where thalidomide was available over the counter, two apparently similar cases of **amelia**, an unusual congenital absence of long bones in a limb or limbs, were first reported at a paediatric meeting in 1960. A year later, a clinician described 13 cases that had been referred to him over the previous 10 months, describing a variety of severe malformations seen in these children and remarking that the occurrences had the appearance of an epidemic. By the end of 1961 Lenz had reported that a common factor in these cases was that the mother had taken thalidomide. The same suggestion was reported from Australia and later confirmed throughout many Western countries. Fewer cases were seen in the USA because, as a result of early side effect reports from Europe, the drug had not been passed for general use there. Thalidomide was withdrawn from use in the UK in November 1961.

Disease prevalence

Prevalence is concerned with the number of people having the problem at one time and is another way of measuring disease occurrence. It is the total number of people with the disease (heart attack, new or old) over the specified time (5 years) in the population (overweight male smokers aged 45–55).

Rates and relationship between incidence and prevalence

A simple count of the kind described above does not really describe the size of the problem, however, since the same number will have different significance in populations of different sizes. Five cases in 50 are clearly very different from 5 in 5000. This is why it is more useful to think in terms of rates:

$$\frac{\text{Number of new events}}{\text{Population at risk of event in a specified time period}} = \text{incidence rate}$$

Prevalence is related to both the incidence and duration of a disease. A chronic condition such as rheumatoid arthritis would have few new cases in a year (low incidence) but a higher total number of cases (high prevalence), as there will be many more cases diagnosed in previous years. Prevalence of a particular condition therefore varies with incidence and the likely duration of the condition:

$$\text{Prevalence} = \text{incidence} \times \text{duration}$$

Measuring disease outcome

With the exception of death, which is usually unequivocal, measuring health outcomes can be difficult because of individual differences in the understanding of health-related terms. The assessment of causes of death and the diagnosis of stroke are just two examples that may be recorded differently by different clinicians. In these circumstances, different estimates of disease incidence may simply reflect differences in definition rather than in the frequency of events. This means that case definition becomes important when collecting information, so that there is unequivocal shared understanding of the way a case is defined. A case of high blood pressure, for example, may be defined as 'a person with an average blood pressure >140/90 mmHg from three readings over a period of no more than 2 years'.

If patterns of morbidity and mortality are to be established, the collection of data needs to be reliable and accurate, and this is not without its difficulties (see Information box 7.3). Much data depends on clinicians' vigilance, recording of observations and diligence in notification. Mandatory systems for reporting disease, birth and death are in place in all developed nations. The World Health Organization (WHO) publishes and updates morbidity and mortality information worldwide (http://www.who.int/en/). In the UK, some notifications of disease are required by law, while others are voluntary. Other types of data result from large-scale surveys and government initiatives such as the General Household Survey and the UK decennial population census. With increasing cost, decreasing compliance and the need for more regular updates, the census delivered in 2011 in the UK is likely to be the last and will be replaced by projects that aggregate information from existing records. Individual clinicians are mainly involved with reporting on births, congenital anomalies, abortions, deaths, cancers, communicable diseases and adverse drug reactions. This information is vitally important for understanding the trends and patterns of diseases, and, in the UK, it is also used to monitor the performance of the National Health Service (NHS).

Births and deaths

The civil registration of births and deaths is compulsory in the UK, as in many countries, where someone (usually parent or relative) has to register the event with local registrars. Births have to be registered within 42 days in England, Wales and Northern Ireland, and 21 days in Scotland. Other information required in birth registration includes the date and place of birth and occupation of the father, mother, or both parents depending on circumstances.

Deaths have to be reported within 7 days. Infants born dead after 24 weeks' gestation are registered as **stillbirths**. Infants born alive who die have to be registered as both a birth and a death. Death certificates are filled in by the attending doctor, who has to give accurate details of each death.

Terminations of pregnancy under the 1967 Abortion Act have to be reported on a prescribed form to the chief medical officers of England, Wales and Scotland within 7 days. The Act does not apply in Northern Ireland (where termination is permitted only in very exceptional circumstances, although a 2013 consultation seeks to modify the guidance). Data are published by the Office of National Statistics (ONS) (www.ons.gov.uk).

Confidential enquiries

Enquiries into deaths in some special categories are made through **confidential enquiries**, when information from anonymised case notes and reports from the professionals who looked after the deceased are reviewed by panels of relevant experts. Unlike audit, patient details are critically reviewed anonymously, and findings about the standards of care are published. The panels try to determine whether the deaths were 'avoidable', whether the quality of care given was of an acceptable standard and whether lessons can be learned. In the past, there was no attempt to compare the standards of care between regions or to establish a contemporary standard of care.

National level confidential enquiries include:

- Centre for Maternal and Child Enquiries (CMACE), previously the Confidential Enquiry into Maternal and Child Health (CEMACH), prior to 2011 – a system for maternal and perinatal mortality surveillance to identify avoidable factors with the aim to improve health care for mothers and babies. This replaced the Confidential Enquiry into Stillbirths and Death in Infancy (CESDI) and the Confidential Enquiry into Maternal Deaths (CEMD) in 2003.
- The National Confidential Enquiry into Suicide and Homicide by People with Mental Illness.
- The National Confidential Enquiry into Patient Outcome and Death (NCEPOD) aims to maintain and improve standards or medical and surgical care for the benefit of the public through undertaking and publishing the findings of confidential surveys and research.

Disease surveillance

Collecting data on the incidence of some specific conditions relies on general practice consultations or hospital admissions. Asthma is a good example in which accurate diagnosis (case definition) and coding are important, and a universally agreed system of case definition and coding is very useful. For example the **International Classification of Diseases (ICD)** classifies asthma into extrinsic, intrinsic, chronic obstructive, exercise induced, cough variant and unspecified, each with associated severity codes. Specific notification or registration systems are in place for monitoring cancers, congenital anomalies and communicable diseases.

Cancer registration

Cancer registration is voluntary and undertaken by regional centres across the UK. The United Kingdom Association of Cancer Registries (UKACR) brings together 11 different registries. The national system tries to record information on every patient with a diagnosis of cancer. Topics include diagnosis, tumour stage, treatment, place of treatment, consultant and place of death. Data are published by the Office for National Statistics (ONS), giving direct and indirect measures of incidence, mortality and survival. Cancer registration data are also used for epidemiological research into healthcare outcomes.

Congenital anomalies notification

Notification of **congenital anomalies** is also voluntary. The National Congenital Anomaly System (NCAS) was closed in 2010 because of perceived under-reporting in comparison with other registries and has been replaced by the **British Isles Network of Congenital Anomaly Registers (BINOCAR)**, part of the EUROCAT network, collating information about birth congenital anomaly prevalence and associated foetal, neonatal and perinatal mortality, in addition to prenatal diagnosis and any subsequent terminations of pregnancy.

Communicable disease surveillance

Notification of infectious diseases was first established in the UK in the late 19th century, when it was based on clinical suspicion and the reports of alert clinicians, with or without microbiological confirmation. Now there is a statutory requirement to notify certain infectious diseases (Information box 7.4). The list of diseases changes over time.

The Communicable Disease Surveillance Centre (CDSC) of the Public Health Laboratory Service (PHLS) was set up in 1977 before it become the Health Protection Agency (HPA – www.hpa.org.uk), now part of **Public Health England**, responsible for the administration of the notification system, working closely with public health agencies in the rest of the UK (see Information box 7.5).

Notification of infectious diseases

In the UK, **communicable disease surveillance** relies on notification of new cases by clinicians, and on information

---

Information box 7.4	**Diseases notifiable (to Local Authority Proper Officers) under the Health Protection (Notification) Regulations 2010**

Acute encephalitis	Leprosy
Acute infectious hepatitis	Malaria
Acute meningitis	Measles
Acute poliomyelitis	Meningococcal
Anthrax	septicaemia
Botulism	Mumps
Brucellosis	Plague
Cholera	Rabies
Diphtheria	Rubella
Enteric fever (typhoid or	SARS
paratyphoid)	Scarlet fever
Food poisoning	Smallpox
Haemolytic uraemic	Tetanus
syndrome	Tuberculosis
Infectious bloody diarrhoea	Typhus
Invasive group A	Viral haemorrhagic fever
streptococcal disease	Whooping cough
Legionnaire disease	Yellow fever

Source: Public Health England.

Information box 7.5	**Aims of communicable disease surveillance**

The objectives for communicable disease surveillance are to:
- Identify risk factors and their distribution
- Monitor levels of infection
- Inform targeting of health promotion and monitor its effects
- Monitor effects of prevention and treatment
- Forecast care needs
- Allow comparison with other countries
- Increase professional and public awareness
- Inform policy makers and service providers
- Detect new problems promptly.

---

from a network of microbiological laboratories which, since 1939, have been required to report to a national centre. A network of about 100 sentinel general practices return data on communicable and respiratory diseases to the Royal College of General Practitioners' (RCGP) Research and Surveillance Centre (RSC). The RSC publishes weekly and annual prevalence reports. The diagnoses are made clinically, without laboratory confirmation, using 'diagnostic guidelines' provided by the RCGP. These are not strict diagnostic criteria, but do represent an attempt to achieve some standardisation in the diagnoses. Important conditions include influenza-like illnesses and food- and waterborne conditions. The data are shared with the HPA and Department of Health (Information box 7.6). Information on influenza in this context can be found on the Public Health England (HPA) website (www.hpa.org.uk). The HPA also collects data from the microbiology laboratories in district and other general hospitals.

Examining data from different sources

Putting data from different sources together can be very informative. For example, in the early 1980s in the UK, when the public health policy of rubella immunisation of 11-year-old schoolgirls had been in operation for about 12 years, the first cohort of immunised girls were having their first babies. However, notification of congenital rubella remained high, as did therapeutic abortions on the grounds of rubella in the first trimester. Rubella infection in the early stage of pregnancy results in foetal damage in about 90% of infants, and the lack of a major policy effect was disappointing. Immunisation of girls only, and not boys, had allowed the disease to continue to circulate. The partial immunisation of the population raises the average age at which the unvaccinated catch the disease, causing those women who had missed immunisation, or who were poorly protected, to remain vulnerable. With the introduction of the measles, mumps and rubella (MMR) vaccine in 1988, the policy was changed and MMR is now given to girls and boys at 12 months and three years or soon after.

Infectious disease surveillance and information sources

Most developed countries have systems for reporting and monitoring communicable diseases. The WHO was established on 7 April 1948 by the United Nations. The objective was to enable all peoples of the world to attain the highest level of health – defined as a state of complete physical, mental and social well-being, and not merely the absence of disease or infirmity. The WHO vision is that every country should have the means to identify, verify and respond to epidemics and emerging infectious diseases as they arise, in order to minimise their impact on the health and economies of all nations. Globalisation, climate change, the growth of huge

---

Information box 7.6 | **Communicable and respiratory diseases in England and Wales reported by the RCGP weekly returns service**

Water- and foodborne disorders
- Infectious intestinal disease
- Viral hepatitis
- Non-infective enteritis and colitis

Environmentally sensitive disorders
- Asthma
- Hayfever/allergic rhinitis
- Respiratory and chest symptoms
- Conjunctival disorders

Respiratory infections
- Acute bronchitis
- Common cold
- Influenza-like illness
- Acute laryngitis/tracheitis
- Pleurisy
- Pneumonia/pneumonitis
- Respiratory system diseases
- Acute sinusitis
- Strep sore throat, scarletina and peritonsillar abscess
- Acute tonsillitis/pharyngitis
- Upper respiratory tract infections
- Whooping cough
- Infectious mononucleosis
- Lower respiratory tract infections
- Acute otitis media

Vaccine sensitive disorders
- Measles
- Mumps
- Rubella

Skin contagions
- Bullous dermatoses
- Chickenpox
- Herpes simplex
- Herpes zoster
- Infections of skin and subcutaneous tissue
- Scabies
- Other skin and integumental tissue symptoms
- Impetigo

Nervous system disorders
- Peripheral nervous system disorders
- Meningitis/encephalitis
- Nervous and musculoskeletal symptoms

Genitourinary system disorders
- Urinary tract infection/cystitis
- Sexually transmitted and other genital infections

(Source: Royal College of General Practitioners)

---

cities and the explosive increase in international travel are increasing the potential for rapid spread of infections.

Global infectious disease surveillance

The WHO Department of Communicable Disease Surveillance and Response (CSR), now called **Global Alert and Response (GAR)**, was set up in 2001 with three strategic aims: containing known risks, responding to the unexpected and improving preparedness.

GAR's core function is to:

- Develop a global operational platform for communicable disease response and provide regional office support in the event of a major disease outbreak
- Support states in their capacity to respond to epidemics in order to meet the requirements of the **International Health Regulations (IHR)** 2005, including provision of laboratory capacity, early disease warning and response
- Support national and international training programmes for IHR

- Support states in the preparation and response to pandemic and seasonal influenza and to develop standardised approaches for other major epidemic diseases such as meningitis, yellow fever and plague
- Strengthen biosafety and biosecurity readiness for dangerous and emerging pathogen outbreaks, such as SARS (severe acute respiratory syndrome) and viral haemorrhagic fevers.

These strategic aims underpin all public health strategies for the surveillance, prevention and control of infectious diseases. IHR is the only global regulatory framework agreed by the international community to support surveillance of global infections. Its website publishes health statistics on a wide variety of infectious diseases worldwide (http://www.who.int/ihr).

Special surveillance systems

The UK has a **special surveillance system** for acquired immune deficiency syndrome (AIDS). Genitourinary specialists, dermatologists and microbiologists supply confidential reports to the HPA which has developed the HIC and AIDS Reporting System (HARS). The Health Protection Agency has developed a dataset, the HIV and AIDS Reporting System (HARS) to improve data collection and quality of care.

Similar surveillance and monitoring systems are in place across Europe and in North America.

Monitoring adverse reaction to drugs

A system for monitoring adverse reactions to medicines is in place in most countries. In the UK, a **Yellow Card** is used to report all suspected reactions to new medicines, and serious suspected reactions to established medicines; even if the reaction is already well recognised, or the causal association is uncertain. The system is administered by the **Medicines and Healthcare Products Regulatory Agency (MHRA)** in association with the Commission on Human Medicine (CHM).

Measures for health of populations

Mortality and morbidity statistics are published by the WHO, and mortality statistics such as child (deaths in children under the age of 5 years) and infant (deaths under 1 year of age) mortality rates are used as measures of the health of nations, using comparisons between high-, medium- and low-income countries.

Mortality and life expectancy

The ONS in the UK regularly publishes mortality statistics that are used extensively for monitoring the health of populations. They are also used in resource allocation, in planning and monitoring services, and in describing and monitoring patterns of disease. For example, the number of deaths from AIDS and influenza epidemics is used to monitor the patterns of those conditions.

Mortality rates are often used as proxy measures for morbidity in the population; for example, using deaths from suicide to monitor psychiatric morbidity and the effectiveness of health interventions on mental health. The appropriateness of the way measures of performance are chosen and applied is open to debate. Mortality statistics are derived from notification and civil registration of death, where the doctor performs the vital role of death certification. Accuracy and standardisation of case definitions are clearly essential.

Years of life lost refers to the number of years of life lost due to premature death, taking age 85 as the 'cut-off', and years of working life lost is the number of years of life lost if death occurs before the end of working life, taken as age 65. These statistics are useful in comparing mortality in different parts of the world and in evaluating the effectiveness of policy and service innovations (e.g. accident prevention, legislation for compulsory car seat belts).

Other official statistics relating to health outcomes include life expectancy, maternal and perinatal mortality, child and infant mortality, communicable disease surveillance, cancer registration, congenital abnormalities and abortion notifications.

Morbidity

True morbidity, in terms of incidence and prevalence, is often difficult to measure. Service activity, such as **Hospital Episode Statistics** (**HES**), is sometimes used as another proxy measure for morbidity, or to assess the need for services.

The population census and health surveys

General measures of health (and sickness) are obtained from the population census held to date every 10 years in the UK, and from a variety of health surveys. The General Household Survey (GHS) is an annual survey of a stratified random sample (see below) of households, carried out by the ONS since 1971 and the GHS is now part of the **Integrated Household Survey** (**IHS**). The survey aims for a sample of 17 000–20 000 different households every year, and is intended as a continuous longitudinal survey which can detect trends. Financial constraints have meant that there are some years missing. A large range of questions are asked, covering health and sickness (including long-standing illness or disability, acute illness and general health), lifestyle and health behaviours. Additional questions have been included on mental health.

Some other health surveys have focused on specific conditions, such as cardiovascular disease. The annual Health Survey for England was commissioned by the Department of Health and started in 1991, aiming to monitor progress on *Health of the Nation* targets in obesity and high blood pressure but now has a different focus annually. A large number of other surveys from the ONS cover a wide variety of health associated topics, general practice, psychiatry and other subjects, such as the health of prisoners and health inequalities.

Measures for quality of life (QALYs)

With the aim of measuring health in terms of 'quality of life', a series of instruments for measuring socio-medical indicators of positive health and well-being have been developed. The Nottingham Health Profile was among the first and has been well validated.

Health inequalities

There are clear differences in health as measured by death rates, or incidence and prevalence for particular diseases. For example, there were 34 million people living with AIDS worldwide at the end of the year 2011, an increase of 16% which reflects both the increased number of new infections and the increased access to antiretroviral therapy. More than 23 million were, however, from sub-Saharan Africa and these people bear an inordinate share of the global HIV burden (Fig. 7.2). Deaths from HIV have decreased worldwide and was 1.7 million in 2011. Although the number of people dying in sub-Saharan Africa has declined by 32% between 2005 and 2011, this area still accounted for 70% of the deaths in 2011.

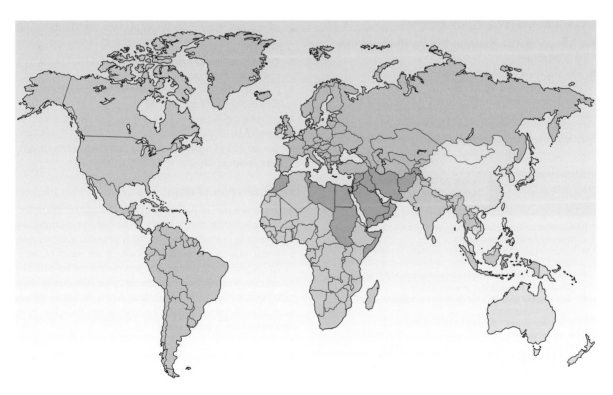

Prevalence (%) by WHO region

Western Pacific: 0.1 [0.1–0.1]	Europe: 0.4 [0.4–0.5]
Eastern Mediterranean: 0.2 [0.1–0.3]	Americas: 0.5 [0.4–0.6]
South-East Asia: 03 [0.2-0.4]	Africa: 4.6 [4.4–4.8] **Global prevalence: 0.8% [0.7-0.8]**

Fig. 7.2 **Global variation in health outcomes.** Human immunodeficiency virus (HIV) prevalence in 2011.
http://www.who.int/gho/hiv/en/

There are many factors that could contribute to this wide-ranging variation. As a general rule, consideration of the impact of social, economic, environmental and political influences, as well as access to medicines and medical services, on the health of populations gives an indication of how improvements might be achieved. Not all these factors are amenable to medical intervention.

Health inequalities in the UK

Since the passing of the New Poor Law Act in 1834 in the UK, there has been much interest in the patterns of health and disease, led by the General Register Office, which was founded in 1837. The Poor Law Commissioners commented on the 'filthy, close and crowded' housing, the 'want of drainage' and the 'putrefying matter' where the 'industrious poor are obliged to take their abode'.

Socio-economic differentials in health still persist today, and the UK government launched a number of initiatives to reduce polarisation in society. The Social Exclusion Unit Report (2001) *A New Commitment to Neighbourhood Renewal* aimed to ensure that 'within 10–20 years, no-one should be seriously disadvantaged by where they live'. Throughout the UK, strategies have been developed for the improvement of health, with the reduction on inequalities within different regions being an important integral part of the proposals: *The NHS Plan* for England, *Toward a Healthier Scotland, Better Health Better Wales* and, from Northern Ireland, *Investing for Health.*

The decennial supplement produced by National Statistics, *Geographic Variations in Health* (2001), reviewed the position, looking at regional and social inequalities. The key findings are given in Information box 7.7. **Right Care** is the UK NHS quality, innovation, productivity and prevention programme launched in 2010 to maximise:

- The value that the patient derives from their own care and treatment
- The value the whole population derives from the investment in their healthcare.

For example, through publishing the *NHS Atlas of Variation*, they aim to reveal variations in health care systems that can be used by commissioners to address inequalities.

Information box 7.7	*Geographic Variations in Health*, 2001 in the UK – key findings

- Age-standardised mortality is higher in Scotland, Wales and Northern Ireland than in England
- Within England age-standardised mortality is higher in the north
- Variation in health between local authorities within regions is greater than the variation between regions
- High levels of area deprivation produce higher levels of mortality in relation to:
  - Ischaemic heart disease
  - Lung cancer
  - Stroke
  - Infant deaths and stillbirths
- High levels of area deprivation produce increased incidence of:
  - Lung cancer
  - Teenage pregnancy
- Social class differences make a larger contribution to male mortality variation than region of residence but the latter is still an important determinant of mortality among those in Social Class V
- London has the highest rate of mortality from infectious and respiratory diseases.

Changes in health outcomes over time

Although mortality rates are generally declining, reviewing the changes over time has shown that the areas where health is poorer show the lowest reduction in mortality. Certain areas stand out as unchanged over many years. Examples are the high infant mortality in urban districts, such as Whitechapel in 2003 and in 1964, and similarly, low levels of life expectancy in Manchester and Liverpool in 1911–1912 and in 1995–1997.

In 2009 the House of Commons Health Committee reported on health inequalities in the UK. Although they found that health of all groups had improved over the previous 10 years, the gap between the social classes had also widened, by 4% in men and 11% in women, due to the greater health improvement seen amongst the rich.

Since 1950, deaths from heart disease, stroke and infectious diseases have all declined greatly. Not so cancer, which in 2008 was the most common cause of death in the UK. While improvements in treatment have led to reductions in mortality for some cancers over the preceding 10 years, the incidence of some cancers appears to have increased considerably (Fig. 7.3 and Information box 7.8).

In 2008 death from cancer in the UK was higher than average in the developed regions of the world: lung cancer accounted for about one in four cancer deaths in males, and about one in five cancer deaths in females. Prostate cancer was responsible for 12% (compared with 6%) of male cancer deaths worldwide and breast cancer deaths at 16% in females was also higher than the rest of the world.

The National Strategy for Cancer (Improving Outcomes: a Strategy for Cancer) was published in 2011, with its aim of improving health outcomes for people with cancer. The main aims of the strategy are to:

- Promote lifestyle changes to reduce cases of preventable cancers
- Increase uptake of cancer screening and introducing new and effective screening programmes
- Increase early diagnosis to improve the scope for successful treatment
- Improve patient experience and support for cancer survivors
- Ensure that all patients have the best possible treatment, care and support.

Interpretation of data

An important part of the study of epidemiology is the understanding and detection of **bias** (see below). For example, are the increases in incidence or mortality of certain cancers over time real, due to improved diagnosis, or the result of better cancer registration? While births and deaths are collected by national registration and considered to be high-quality data, much else is of very poor or variable quality, including factors such as registration of cause of death where there has been little regulation over the years.

Data inadequacies

The inadequacy, incompleteness and inaccuracy of much available data have already been referred to. For example, abortion statistics may be influenced by non-residents moving into temporary accommodation, or policy differences in different parts of the UK. Administrative boundary changes and postal code changes also produce problems of data interpretation over time. The latter is being improved with the use of map grid referencing.

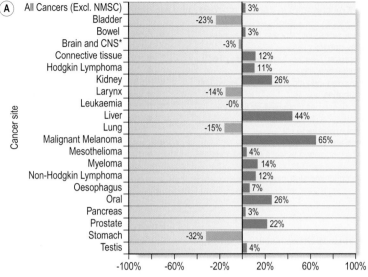

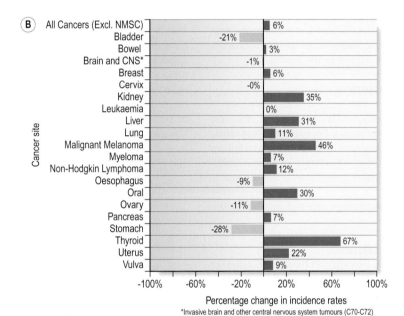

Fig. 7.3 **(A) Percentage change in age-standardised incidence of cancers by sex and site, UK 1999–2001 compared with 2008–2010. (B) Percentage change in age-standardised mortality from cancers by sex and site, UK 1999–2001 compared with 2008-2010.** Data from Cancer Research 2012 Cancer Incidence in the UK, 2010.

Information box 7.8 | **Key changes in cancer mortality and incidence 2000–2010**

Key changes in cancer mortality 2000–2010
- Mortality has *decreased* for about half of the most common cancers, including male lung, bowel, female breast and prostate cancers
- Stomach cancer mortality has *decreased* by about 34% due to:
  - Decline in *Helicobacter pylori* prevalence
  - Increase in dietary fresh foods
  - Improvements in diagnosis
- Cervical cancer mortality has *decreased* by 28% due to:
  - Screening
- Prostate cancer mortality has *decreased* by 11% due to:
  - Screening with prostate-specific antigen (PSA) testing
  - Better treatments

- Liver cancer mortality has *increased* by about 36%
- Digestive organ cancer mortality has *increased* by about 23%
- Uterine cancer mortality has *increased* by about 14%
- Malignant melanoma mortality has *increased* by 18% in males and 5% in females.

Key changes in cancer incidence 2000–2010
- Stomach cancer incidence has *decreased* by about 30%, for the same reasons as mortality has decreased
- Lung and laryngeal cancer incidence in males has *decreased* by about 15% due to:
  - Reduced alcohol and tobacco use
  - Reduced environmental exposure to tobacco smoke

Continued

| **Information box 7.8** | **Key changes in cancer mortality and incidence 2000–2010—cont'd** |

- Ovarian and oesophageal cancer incidence in females has *decreased* by about 10% due to:
  - In ovarian cancer, improved lifestyle, increased use of oral contraceptives and breastfeeding
  - In oesophageal cancer, reduced alcohol and increased fruit and vegetable consumption
- Malignant melanoma incidence has *increased* by 65% (males) and 4% (females) due to:
  - Increased recreational exposure to UV
  - Increased surveillance and better diagnosis
- Liver cancer incidence has *increased* by 44% (males) and 31% females) due to:
  - Liver cirrhosis from alcohol and viral infections

- Kidney cancer incidence has *increased* by 26% (males) and 36% (females) due to:
  - Obesity
  - Continuing cigarette smoking
- Prostate cancer incidence has *increased* by 22% due to:
  - Increased rate of diagnosis due to PSA testing
- Thyroid cancer incidence in females has *increased* by 67% due to:
  - Increased breast cancer incidence and subsequent treatment
- Mesothelioma incidence in females has *increased* by 24% due to:
  - Secondary exposure through handling of asbestos-contaminated work clothes (the disease has an estimated 40-year latency and the incidence is expected to increase).

Clustering

Clustering of risk factors in areas where health outcomes are poor may encourage the suggestion that one causes the other. The strong association, or **collinearity**, may in fact be due to clustering. Areas where health outcomes are poor are usually areas of multiple deprivation. Careful analysis of the data is required before one can conclude that specific deprivation might cause one or more of the poor outcomes. For example, sick people are more likely to be out of work and hence poorer than those who are well, so they may end up living in poor areas because of their ill health, rather than the reverse.

Socio-economic factors

It has been suggested that geographical differences in health are simply a reflection of a concentration of people of a lower socio-economic status. For example, large differences in infant mortality are seen between those with fathers in Social Class V and those with fathers in Social Class I. Mortality rates are also higher among men in Social Class V. In Africa, inequality and a lack of social cohesion, rather than relative poverty, are closely correlated with higher HIV prevalence.

Health-related behaviours

Epidemiologists are also interested in the contribution that health-related behaviour and the environment make to disease variation. Geographical variation in behaviour that affects health may produce different regional outcomes. Smoking is a good example, as areas with high incidence of lung cancer and high mortality correspond with areas of low social status, where individuals are more likely to be smokers. Less clear is the influence of physical activity, which varies with social status and shows a north–south divide in England.

Healthcare facilities

The aim of the NHS, established in 1946, was to have healthcare facilities evenly spread throughout the population. In the 1970s, Tudor Hart saw that those most in need of healthcare were the least likely to receive it, and proposed the 'inverse care law' that led to the introduction in 1976 of formula resourcing. This should have made things equitable. Nevertheless, expansion of private services remains concentrated in the south of England and poverty and poor educational skills both reduce appropriate access. While there is a policy of active shifting of resources to more deprived areas of the UK, this has not led to any closing of the gap and people within more deprived areas have significantly lower life and disability-free life expectations.

Environmental factors

Environmental factors are also likely to produce different geographical patterns in, for example, the incidence of various congenital anomalies. Ischaemic heart disease has been shown to be correlated with rainfall, water hardness, temperature, manual employment and car ownership, but questions about the environmental contribution to disease have proved controversial as in, for example, the role of electric power lines in the incidence of leukaemia. In contrast, atmospheric pollution is strongly associated with excess mortality from respiratory disease. The industrialisation of Britain resulted in a major increase in air pollution, when smoke from coal burning mixed with mist and fog to produce smog, which then contributed to increased mortality and morbidity (Fig. 7.4). While air pollution is no longer so obvious, long-term exposure to fine particulate emissions in London was said to contribute

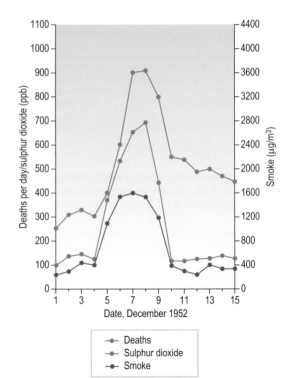

Fig. 7.4 **Deaths associated with pollution.** On 4 December 1952 an anti-cyclone formed and smog settled over London. The levels of sulphur dioxide were seven times that of normal, and the smoke three times of normal. Four thousand deaths occurred in under a week and peaked at the time of greatest pollution. Data from Reports of Public Health Medicine Subject 95, HMSO, London, 1954 (available at: www.doc.mmu.ac.uk).

significantly to more than 4000 deaths in 2008 and pollution in the UK was worse than in any other EU member state. The introduction of the Congestion Charging Zone (CCZ) in London in 2003 seemed to offer a unique opportunity to assess potential improvements in health outcomes, with hypothesised significant reductions in air pollutants. However, the hoped for reductions have not been achieved and any effect of the CCZ on pollutant levels has been confounded by other concurrent broader regional pollutant and weather changes and the increased use of diesel powered vehicles.

Migration

When health differences at a single point in time are considered, another effect that needs to be taken into account is that of migration (see Information box 7.9). A 'healthy migrant effect' has been observed: this occurs because younger people in good health and with, consequently, lower mortality rates, tend to move longer distances and into more affluent areas or countries. This can affect the average mortality rate of the area they move into. When migrants become ill, they may return home to die, and it is the place of death, not the place where they became ill, that is registered. Migration effects may obscure real health differences caused by locality and disadvantage. Migration may also influence birth rates and fertility.

Genetic factors and international migration also probably play an important part in disease incidence, producing pockets of the inherited haemoglobinopathies in the UK, for example. International migration has had much to do with the increased prevalence of tuberculosis (TB). London houses the highest proportion of TB sufferers in the UK, with particularly high rates in Newham and Brent – the rate in those not born in the UK being about 10 times that of those born here.

Standardisation of rates

When comparing prevalence or incidence of death or diseases in populations from different communities, geographical areas or time periods, the results may be misleading, as differences in overall (**crude**) rates may be due to differences in the age and sex structure of the populations.

One way to standardise rates would be by comparing rates in age bands of, say, 10 years, but this is laborious and cumbersome, and does not give a summary rate. The more usual way is to **standardise** the rates for age and sex. This would be the rate for a population of a specific age and sex structure. It must be borne in mind that standardised rates are simply mathematical manipulations, undertaken to allow comparison, and the resultant numbers are not the same as the crude rates.

There are two ways of standardising rates – direct and indirect (Information boxes 7.10 and 7.11). Both have the same objective – to get round the problem of different (age and/or

---

Information box 7.9 | **Example of confusing factors in migration: confounding**

Unless we have appropriate knowledge about our population makeup and the way it changes over time, our understanding can be confused. For example, in a study of native American Indians in 1988, a very strong **negative** association was seen between a particular genetic haplotype (Gm3;5.13.14) and non-insulin dependent diabetes. This might lead to speculation that **absence** of this haplotype is a risk factor for the disease; but in fact, although the haplotype is very common among the Caucasian population, it was rare among American Indians. Migrant populations (in this case the Caucasians) have mixed with the native population over time and once the genetic admixture is taken into account, the particular relationship between the Gm haplotype and not having diabetes disappears. What has happened in this example is a phenomenon known as **confounding**. The study does also illustrate, however, that there is likely to be another genetic component present in American Indians that increases their susceptibility to diabetes.

Information box 7.10 | **An example of direct standardisation**

The crude death rate for England and Wales in 1949 was 12.24 per 1000 and in 1979 was 12.41 per 1000. Is it possible that health advances have made no impact on the rate of death or are differences in the population age structure over time giving a false impression? In order to examine this we can use direct standardisation and calculate what the likely death rate would have been in 1949 (study population) if the population had the same age structure as that of 1979 (standard population). In other words, apply the rate in the study population to calculate the rate for the standard population. The age-standardised death rate for 1949, based on the 1979 population structure, can be calculated from the totals in Table 7.3. Numbers in italics in the Table are those calculated.

$$\text{Age-standardised 1949 death rate per 1000} = \text{Expected deaths/population in 1000s}$$
$$= 339868.4/23202 \times 1000$$
$$= 14.65 \text{ per } 1000$$

Thus it seems that the death rate has fallen between 1949 (standardised at 14.65 deaths per 1000) and 1979 (actual 12.41 deaths per 1000).

Table 7.3 | **Death rate in 1949 if the population had the same age structure as in 1979**

Age group (years)	Deaths (1949)	Population in 1000s (1949)	Crude death rate per 1000 (1949)	Population in 1000s (1979)	Expected deaths
	A	B	A/B	C	C × A/B
0–9	17 643	3417	5.16	3339	17 229.2
10–19	2345	2869	0.82	4063	3331.7
20–29	5031	3339	1.51	3534	5336.3
30–39	6839	3189	2.14	3326	7117.6
40–49	16 062	3178	5.05	2020	10 201.0
50–59	32 097	2335	13.75	2924	40 205.0
60–69	60 580	1727	35.08	2257	79 175.6
70–79	77 127	957	80.59	1384	111 536.6
80+	42 218	228	185.17	355	65 735.4
Total	25 9942	21 239	12.24	23 202	339 868.4

Information box 7.11   An example of indirect standardisation

In 1988, 516 men were diagnosed with stomach cancer in Wales. Since Wales had a male population of 1.39 million at that time, the crude incidence rate of the disease in that region was 372 per million of the male population. We may wish to compare that figure with incidence in the whole of the UK. Table 7.4 shows how to estimate the expected incidence of stomach cancer in Wales, if Wales was experiencing the same incidence as the UK as a whole, i.e. applying the rate in the standard population to the rate in the study population.

The incidence we would expect in Wales, if Wales were experiencing the same rate as the whole UK, is 402 per million of the population. This can be directly compared with what has been observed.

$$\text{Age} - \text{standardised} = \text{Observed rate/expected rate}$$
$$\text{incidence ratio} \quad = 516/402.07$$
$$= 1.28$$
$$\text{Standardised mortality ratio} = 1.28 \times 100 = 128$$

A ratio of 1.28 implies that the risk of stomach cancer in Welsh men is 1.28 times the risk in men in the UK in general. This could also be expressed as a 28% increase in risk.

Table 7.4   Incidence of stomach cancer in Wales in 1988 if the incidence was the same as in UK as a whole

Age group (years)	Incidence per million in reference population (UK)	Population of Wales in millions	Expected incidence per million
	A	B	A × B
0–24	0	0.5	0
25–34	5	0.19	0.95
35–44	42	0.16	6.72
45–54	182	0.16	29.12
55–64	558	0.15	83.70
65–74	1478	0.11	162.58
75 +	2380	0.05	119.00
Total			402.07

sex) structures when comparing populations. Comparisons are normally made using a reference, or **standard** population.

Direct method of standardisation

This involves looking at the age-specific (death) rates in the *study* population and applying these rates to the same age groups in the *standard* population (Information box 7.10 and Table 7.3). In our example we could then calculate the number of deaths we would expect to see in England and Wales if the country was experiencing the same death rate as in the study populations. This number divided by the number of deaths actually seen in England and Wales (the standard population) multiplied by 100 is the **comparative mortality index** (**CMI**). Results greater than 100 imply a higher death rate than expected in the study population than in the standard population.

Indirect method of standardisation

This is slightly different from the direct method and takes the age-specific (death) rate of the standard population and applies it to the same age groups in the study population to calculate expected deaths. The ratio of observed deaths to expected, multiplied by 100 gives us the **standardised mortality ratio** (**SMR**). Again values above 100 imply the death rate in the study population is higher than the death rate in the standard population.

Table 7.5 shows that, in 1971, the death rate was higher in Bournemouth than in the country as a whole. Bournemouth is a coastal resort in the south of England, which has a large elderly population, so it is not unreasonable to suppose that this may be the cause of the increased death rate. Only by adjusting the numbers in Table 7.5 to take the different age

Table 7.5   Is Bournemouth bad for your health?

	Bournemouth	England and Wales
Deaths per 1000 people in 1971	17.4	11.1
Standardised mortality ratio 1971	87.4	100

structures into account can we make an attempt to answer the question (see Information box 7.11 and Table 7.4). In our example we could calculate the number of deaths we would expect to see in Bournemouth if the people there were experiencing the national death rates for England and Wales in 1971. When we do this we would expect to see 1664 deaths, but in fact only 1454 deaths actually occurred. This difference is expressed as the:

$$\text{SMR} = (\text{number of observed deaths/expected}$$
$$\text{number of deaths}) \times 100$$
$$= (1454/1664) \times 100$$
$$= 87.4$$

If the SMR were equal to 100 it would mean that the expected mortality rate in the study population was the same as the reference population. Because the SMR is less than 100, as it is in Bournemouth, this means that Bournemouth has a comparatively low mortality rate even though the actual death rate is higher. The true association between death and living in Bournemouth has been confounded by the age structure of the population. The indirect method (SMR) is the one more commonly used when comparing mortality in different geographical areas.

Choice of method for standardisation

Why do we need both ways of standardising? Each has its advantages and disadvantages. If we wanted to compare the death rates in two study populations, one of which has an elderly population and the other a relatively young population, then it is best to take a ratio of the two CMIs obtained from the direct method. Ratios of SMRs can be misleading in this situation.

The direct method has a disadvantage when the study group is small – because the numbers of people in the different age groups may be very small. Applying the death rates from these small groups to a large population can mean that a small change in the numbers of deaths in the study population can produce a large variation in calculated numbers of deaths from one year to the next. This increases the possibility of error in the measurement. For example, if in one year you were to observe just one death in 50 people in the 20–25-year age group, and in the next you observed two or three deaths in the same group, you might put that down to a chance finding and not be too concerned. But the increase is from a 2% death rate to 4% or 6%. Applying these proportions to a large population produces large differences in expected deaths, which may be very misleading. Using the indirect method is better, because we apply the death rate in the standard large population to the smaller study population.

Sometimes it is just not possible to use the direct method. In our example we would need to know not only the number of people who had died in Bournemouth, but also the number of people who had died within each of the age groups that we used for the standardisation. This sort of information is generally available for the standard population but is more difficult to find easily or collect for a small study population.

The **SMR** can be calculated for all causes of death, or for a specific cause (e.g. cancers), or for a particular age (e.g. >65), or for an occupational group. A similar principle can be applied to activities such as hospital admissions, in which case the index becomes a standardised admission ratio (SAR).

EPIDEMIOLOGICAL ENQUIRY

As has been discussed, analyses that use routinely collected data may not give accurate results. We can, however, also undertake specific studies for specific purposes, which include understanding the natural history of diseases, some causes of disease and the effectiveness of interventions. A variety of methods are used, each selected to answer a specific research question. Understanding the principles underlying the epidemiological approach not only enables a critical appraisal of research evidence, as when reading research papers in the medical journals, but also helps towards understanding research methods.

SOME BASIC CONCEPTS IN EPIDEMIOLOGY

Some basic concepts used in epidemiology have already been discussed, e.g. incidence and prevalence, standardised mortality and morbidity rates. Other important basic concepts concern the distribution of data collected for epidemiological enquiry and statistical methods employed for analysing the data. The meaning of basic concepts rather than the mathematical calculations will be discussed.

The distribution of data

The distribution of actual data can be represented by a **histogram**. Distributions can be symmetrical, e.g. height, where the tails of the distribution are symmetrical (Fig. 7.5A). Some distributions are asymmetrical, where there are more instances of extreme values at either small values (negative skew) or high values (positive skew) (Fig. 7.5B). Adult weight is positively skewed, in that the proportion of very heavy people is greater and further away from the most common value than is the proportion of very thin (light) people. Gestational age is negatively skewed, most babies being born at 39 or 40 weeks, very few born after 42 weeks, but a high proportion born below 36 weeks. Most distributions are unimodal in that they have only one peak, but Figure 7.5C is bimodal (two peaks). Only very rarely are distributions U-shaped.

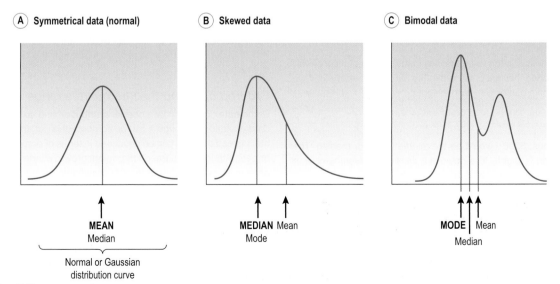

Fig. 7.5 **Data distributions and measures of centre.** The most appropriate measure of centre is shown in bold capital letters for each of the distributions.

The normal or Gaussian distribution curve

Frequency distributions can be thought of as smoothed curves through the appropriate large sample histogram. The **Gaussian (or normal) distribution curve** is bell shaped, symmetrical with certain fixed properties. Its shape is uniquely defined by the mean and standard deviation of the data. Figure 7.5A is an example of a Gaussian distribution, and adult height is very close to a Gaussian distribution. Much of theoretical statistics is based on the properties of the Gaussian distribution.

Some numerical data vary continuously, such as the height and weight of growing children, and are known as **continuous variables**. Other numerical data are **discontinuous**, such as the numbers of people in defined populations. The numbers of people are variable, but differ at different points in time.

Measures of centre

In describing data, the concept of 'average', or **centre**, is important. Commonly used to mean 'normal', 'regular' or 'middling', for statistical purposes 'average' needs to be more precisely defined. There are three main measures of average that are useful: the **mean**, the **median** and the **mode**. The best one to use in describing the data will depend on the shape of the data. In making the choice of which measure to use, it is very important to look at the data graphically. Because the mean is better than median (because it is a summary of a greater amount of information), and median is better than mode for statistical analysis, medians tend to be used only for quite skewed data while mode would be restricted to bimodal or other oddly shaped distributions.

The mean

The mean of the data, sometimes called the arithmetic mean, is what we normally think of when we say 'average'. The mean of a set of values is found by adding up all of them and dividing by the total number in the set. The mathematical formula for this is:

$$\bar{x} = \left(\sum x_i\right)/n$$

where $\bar{x}$ is the mean, x_i is one of the observations in the set, Σ means the sum of all the individual values, and n is the number of observations in the set. The mean is best used for data that are unimodal and not strongly skewed (Fig. 7.5A).

The median

The median is the value that lies in the middle of a set of values, once they are put in order (Fig. 7.5B). For example, if we have five babies with birth weights:

> 3100 g, 3300 g, 3100 g, 3200 g and 3800 g
> The order would be: 3100, 3100, 3200, 3300, 3800 g

Thus, 3200 g would be the middle value, or median. The median is slightly less obvious if there is an even number in the set. For example, if the set of birth weights were:

> 3100, 3100, 3200, 3300, 3300, 3800 g

There are two middle values, 3200 and 3300. In this case the arithmetic mean of the two middle numbers is calculated to give the median = 3250 g. The median is sometimes also referred to as the 50th percentile since half the data will lie at or below it, and half at or above. The median is best used for data that has a substantial skew, or for data where the measurements are ordered (**ordinal data**) rather than arithmetical

(e.g. pain scores). In this type of data the difference between adjacent categories is not usually the same (e.g. the difference between mild and moderate is almost certainly not the same as between moderate and severe).

The mode

The mode represents the observation that is the most frequent. In Figure 7.5C, there are two peaks, and the mode is the higher peak. In this case, however, the distribution would be better described as **bimodal** and it would not be appropriate to simply report the first peak. The mode is often used when dealing with data that are in categories and cannot be put into an order (**categorical data**). For example: among the four blood groups O, A, B and AB, blood group A is the modal category in London because it occurs more frequently in this population.

Data from surveys about attitudes often use what is known as the **Likert scale**, which is a three to five point scale of responses that ranges from 'strongly disagree' to 'no idea' to 'strongly agree.' Medians can be used with these type of data as they are ordinal (ranked and ordered), and if the data can be sensibly aggregated, means are sometimes used.

Measures of spread: standard deviation from the mean

In describing data, if the distribution is symmetrical enough to be described by the mean then it is appropriate to describe the variability – a measure of spread of data from the mean – by the **standard deviation** (SD). The standard deviation is arrived at using a formula (which it is not necessary to describe here, especially since every scientific calculator has a key to provide that number when a set of data are entered). Where data are normal (Gaussian), 95% of the data will lie between the mean ± 1.96 times the SD. For practical purpose we can usually assume that for data that are approximately Gaussian, about 95% will lie within the mean ± 2 SD. This is often the range that is considered 'normal' in clinical medicine, i.e. not of concern or not unusual (see Information box 7.12, Fig. 7.6).

Outliers

Sometimes, an isolated value will stand out from the rest of the data set. This is known as an outlier and checks are needed to see whether this is a mistake in measurement or transcription, or even consistent with life. If wrong it can be excluded, but if it is real then other methods of dealing with the data may be required, particularly if the data set is small.

Ordered data and the interquartile range

Some data do not follow a normal distribution and so a standard deviation (although it can be computed) is not appropriate. Instead the data can be described in terms of percentiles, or percentage points. Paediatric weight growth charts are examples of skewed data (Fig. 7.7), Paediatric height growth charts are presented in the same way but the data are more normally distributed at the different ages.

Various measures of spread such as the **interquartile range** or the **interdecile range** can be calculated from data. A **box and whisker plot** is a useful way of illustrating the data distribution (Fig. 7.8). The diagram provides a simple way of describing the data in some detail. It can be seen that there is a wide range of gestational ages at the lower end, with 50% of gestational ages ranging between 32 and 40 weeks,

Information box 7.12 | Standard deviation of normal platelet counts

The normal range for blood platelet count is 150–400 × 10^9/L. A useful property of the normal distribution is that about 95% of observations lie within the range mean ± 2 SD. (Actually it is 1.96 SD but we are using 2 here because it is very close and simple to calculate.) This range is known as the 95% reference range (Fig. 7.6). In order to produce this range we take a sample that is representative of the population and use that to provide our assessment of mean and SD.

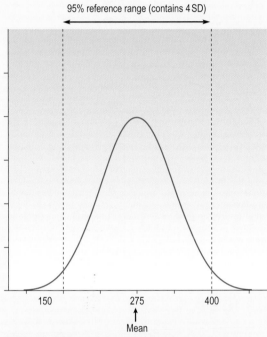

Fig. 7.6 **Distribution of *all* platelet counts in a normal population.** 95% of the platelets lie within the mean ± 2 SD, where SD is the standard deviation. The range 150–400 (×10^9/L) is referred to as the reference (or normal) range of platelet counts in the population and individuals would normally be expected to have a platelet count within this range. The value of the standard deviation of the sample should be contrasted with the standard deviation shown in Figure 7.9.

whereas at the top end the data are very tight, with 50% of gestational ages being between 40 and 41 weeks, showing a very skewed distribution.

How accurate is the distribution summary?

Measurements in epidemiology are usually taken from samples of the population, as it would be too difficult to take measurements from the whole population. But even when the whole population is measured we are often interested in how representative it is of an unknown underlying rate. An estimated mean from one sample is unlikely to be the true mean in the population. However, if we could take an infinite number of random samples of the same size from the population, the distribution of the potential sample means will be normal or Gaussian with a mean equal to the true mean, provided that the sample size is not too small for distributions that are not Gaussian. The standard deviation of the distribution of

potential sample means is the **standard error** (SE) of the mean (SEM). The standard error represents the uncertainty in the sample mean as a representative of the true mean (Fig. 7.9).

While in clinical medicine we may be interested in an individual measurement, in epidemiology we are often more concerned with the true, i.e. population or underlying, mean. We can never find the true mean because people are dying and being born every second, so we have to find a way of estimating where the true mean might lie. We could take the means of a number of samples of data, thus creating a set of means, and calculate the mean and standard deviation of the means. However, it is possible to estimate the standard error from one sample and from that infer the range in which the true mean is likely to lie.

Because the distribution of all potential sample means of given size is normal with a standard deviation equal to the standard error, 95% of all sample means will lie within the true mean ± 1.96 × SE. The one sample mean that we have calculated is within the true mean ± 1.96 × SE with 95% probability, hence the sample mean ± 1.96 SE will include the true mean with 95% probability. The sample mean ± 1.96 SE is referred to as the **95% confidence interval** (Information box 7.13) of the mean.

Standard errors and hence confidence intervals can be calculated for most summary measures including difference in means, proportions, differences in relative risks, odds ratios and SMRs.

Differences in **non-symmetrical** distributions are often better described by mean differences and 95% confidence intervals of mean differences rather than differences in medians. For example, it is more sensible to describe gestational age by median and percentiles, but if describing the difference in gestational age for babies born alive between 1970 and 2000, it would be better to describe this by a mean difference in gestational age.

Contingency tables

Some data cannot be expressed numerically but have to be grouped into descriptive categories. If a variable has only two values it is known as binary (e.g. dead/alive) and if there are more it is known as categorical data (e.g. blood group A, B, O or AB). If we are interested in comparing proportions that died by blood group, we would construct a **contingency table** where each cell in the table contains the number in each of the mutually exclusive categories. The percentages and differences can also be shown but it is the *number* of cases in each cell which is used to calculate statistical significance using a chi-squared test (see below). A commonly encountered form is the 2 × 2 contingency table (Table 7.6).

Some statistical concepts used in epidemiological enquiry (hypothesis tests and *p* values)

The purpose of clinical epidemiological enquiry is to reach a plausible and valid conclusion from observations, most often about cause and effect, which contributes to the body of knowledge about disease so that strategies for disease prevention and management may be formulated. This necessitates the generation of a theory, or **hypothesis**, about a disease, e.g. what caused it and how it progresses, before further hypotheses for what constitutes effective management and prevention can be developed. The **validity**, or truth, of the

Name.. Date of birth...................... Reg. No................

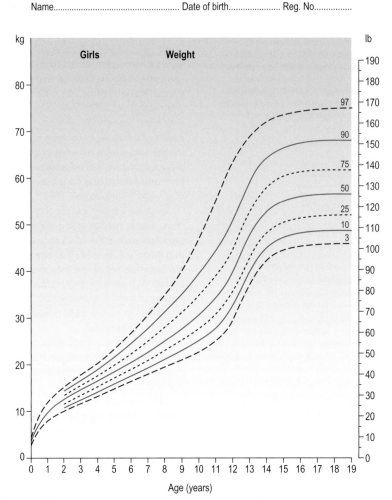

Fig. 7.7 **Growth centile chart for girls, showing weights for girls aged up to 19 years.** Weights lying between the 3rd and 97th centiles are considered 'normal', with the 50th centile considered the 'median' or average. The girls' weight is measured at different ages, beginning at birth. Growth in weight is considered 'normal' as long as a child stays on the centile at which she was born.

hypotheses is tested employing good study design and valid statistical methods, both of which are employed to limit the possibility of the results being affected by bias. When carried out logically and carefully, according to Sir Austin Bradford Hill, statistical analysis is 'an aid to clear thinking with regard to the meaning and limitations of the original records'. Hypotheses are difficult to prove as being true or false, but whether they are considered to be acceptable or not is based on the available evidence, and tested by statistical analysis.

Hypothesis tests

Statistical tests involve the examination of two alternative hypotheses. The **null hypothesis H0** is one that assumes no effect in the population. For example, if we wanted to examine the prevalence of smoking in teenagers and see if there is a difference between girls and boys, the null hypothesis might be:

- H0: there is no difference in smoking rates between teenage girls and teenage boys in the population.

An **alternative hypothesis H1** is what holds if the null hypothesis is not true. Different alternative hypotheses can be examined. For example:

- H1: smoking rates are higher in teenage boys than in teenage girls in the population.

This hypothesis only considers a change in one direction and would not examine the possibility that smoking rates were lower in the boys than in the girls, so it would not allow us to discover whether smoking were more prevalent in the girls. The statistical test that is undertaken in such a case is said to be **one-tailed**. However, we are rarely sure that a difference will only ever be seen in one direction, and it is always advisable to construct an alternative hypothesis to allow for that possibility by undertaking a **two-tailed** test. For example:

- H1: there is a difference in smoking rates between teenage boys and girls in the population.

Evaluating these two hypotheses involves looking at the evidence for each in order to obtain a test statistic. The particular statistic will depend on the type of test done, but generally the larger its absolute value (ignoring whether the number is positive or negative), i.e. the bigger the difference, the stronger the evidence against the null hypothesis.

Tests of probability: p values and confidence intervals

Probability is a concept inherent to all descriptive and comparative statistics. The only way to say that there is likely to be a difference (i.e. we reject the null hypothesis) is by finding that it is unlikely that the results from the study are consistent with there being no effect in the populations (i.e. the null hypothesis

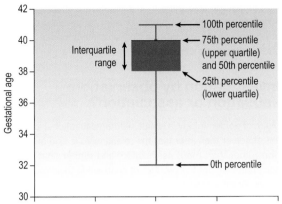

Fig. 7.8 Box and whisker plot of gestational age at birth. This figure relates to a set of gestational ages of 100 live births. The data are put into rank order, where the shortest gestation is 32 weeks (0th percentile) and the longest is 41 weeks (100th percentile). The middle 50% of births occur between 38 and 40 weeks, between the 25th and 75th percentiles – also known as the interquartile range, which by convention is shown as a box. The median, or 50th percentile, is shown as a horizontal line across the box (40 weeks' gestation); 25% of births occur between 32 and 38 weeks (0th to 25th percentile) and 25% between 40 and 41 weeks' gestation (75th to 100th percentile). These ranges are shown as lines, or whiskers, above and below the box. In this particular example, the 75th percentile (upper quartile) and 50th percentile (median) occur in the same place (and so we cannot see the median line within the box). This simply means that 25% of births occurred at 40 weeks in the data set.

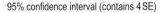

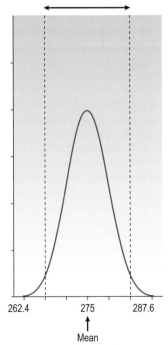

Fig. 7.9 The *sampling* distribution of mean platelet counts in a normal population. 95% of sample means lie within the mean ± 2 SE, where SE is the standard error. In a normal population you would expect that the mean platelet count is between 262.4 and 287.6 ($\times 10^9$/L). Note that in this figure, in comparison with Figure 7.6 above, the mean is the same, but the range is considerably reduced because the distribution relates to what the average might be, not what platelet count an individual healthy person might have.

Information box 7.13	Calculating confidence intervals

Confidence intervals are calculated from the standard error. The formula for estimating the standard error from one sample is:

$$SE = SD/\sqrt{n},$$ where n is the number of observations.

The 95% confidence interval, the parameters (limits) of the range of means in which the true mean lies, is the sample mean ± two standard errors (rounding up 1.96 to 2).

For example, if the sample we took to find the normal range of platelet counts consisted of 100 people, with a mean of 275 and SD of 63, then we can calculate the SE and 95% confidence interval (CI) as follows:

$$SE = 63\sqrt{100} = 6.3$$
$$95\% \ CI = 275 \pm 2 \times 6.3 = 262.4 \text{ to } 287.6.$$

Table 7.6	A 2 × 2 contingency table

Characteristic	Group 1	Group 2	Total
Present	a	b	a+b
Absent	c	d	c+d
Total	a+c	b+d	a+b+c+d

One subcategory of characteristics is tabulated in rows, e.g. brown eyes (present or absent). Another subcategory of characteristics is tabulated in columns, e.g. Asian (Group 1), Caucasian (Group 2). The letters *a–d* represent numbers or observations, not percentages or proportions, and each letter is in a **cell**. Any data in the column under the heading 'Total', as well the bottom row, would be called **marginal totals**.

---

is true). It is of course always possible that we obtained this 'unlikely' result if the null hypothesis is true (often referred to as by chance). This probability is known as the ***p* value**.

- By convention, if the probability of getting the result we saw (or one more extreme) if the null hypothesis is true is <0.05 (<1 in 20), we infer that there is a real effect.
- If $p < 0.05$, we *reject* the null hypothesis and say that the result is statistically significant – unlikely to be due to chance. Further evaluation of the hypothesis can then be done.
- By convention, if the probability of getting this result if the null hypothesis is true is ≥0.05, we say the result is not statistically significant.
- If $p \geq 0.05$ (no *statistically* significant difference between one set of observations and the other) this does not necessarily mean that the null hypothesis is true, but it cannot be rejected.

All test statistics have a mathematical probability function that describes the distribution of possible test results from a series of observations. Commonly used distributions (cited in medical journal articles) are those of the normal (Gaussian) and associated t-distribution (see below t-tests) and the χ^2 (chi-squared, pronounced ki-squared) distribution (see below χ^2 tests). Examination of where the test statistic value lies in relation to the appropriate distribution provides the probability of the test result, or one more extreme, occurring if there is no difference in the populations, or the p value.

An alternative to calculating the p value to establish the probability that a particular observation arose by chance or not, is to calculate a **confidence interval** (see above). Because it gives information about where the 'true or underlying' result lies, it is used to assess whether or not clinical importance can be established for the range of possible results. It also gives information about the precision of the observations. The narrower the confidence interval, the more precise is the observation.

AN OVERVIEW OF EPIDEMIOLOGICAL ENQUIRY

To understand how disease occurs and progresses, observation of people at a particular point in time or over longer periods of time is required to see what factors are associated with incidence of disease. These are known as **observational studies**, the cornerstone of epidemiology (see Information box 7.14).

Information box 7.14 | **Observational studies and experimental studies used in epidemiology and clinical medicine**

The designs for **observational studies** include:

- **Cross-sectional** studies: these are carried out with a defined population at a point in time at a specified geographical location. The information (data) of interest about individuals in the selected population is carefully collected, then analysed using the appropriate statistical method (see below). The conclusions are usually descriptions of population characteristics, such as 'at a moment in time, in the London Borough of Tower Hamlets (or Brooklyn New York), there are more cigarette smokers among teenage boys than girls'. **Surveys** are a form of cross-sectional study.
- **Case–control** studies: these compare two groups of people – those with disease (the **cases**) with those without disease (the **controls**), to investigate potential causes for the disease. The groups have to be carefully matched to avoid the results being dominated by known associations with incidence such as age and sex (e.g. teenage boys). The data collected might lead to conclusions such as 'cigarette smokers are more likely to develop lung cancer than non-smokers'. The **retrospective-type of case–control study** looks at the relevant histories of the individuals comprising the study population, to identify factors known as **risk factors**. These are factors that may be associated with the development of disease. Occasionally, matched cases and controls are taken from cohort studies (see below) for analysis. As in such a study (nested case–control study) data will have been collected prospectively, it will be a **prospective study**.
- **Cohort studies**: these identify a group of individuals at some risk of the disease(s) of interest (e.g. civil servants, newborn infants), at a particular time (e.g. 1984) and a specified place (e.g. England and Wales, Whitehall in London). The individuals in this group, known as the **cohort**, are then followed up over time, i.e. **prospectively**, to record the incidence of disease as well as measuring, at the start and intervening periods in the study, potential risk factors. The follow-up period varies, and could be very long, for up to 15–40 years or more, and thus these studies are costly. The purpose would be to identify factors in the individuals' lives that may have a causal association with disease. An example of the kind of conclusions that can be drawn from a cohort study is 'civil servants of a lower administrative grade are more likely to develop ischaemic heart disease and chronic bronchitis'.
- An **experimental study** design is adopted for investigating the effectiveness of an intervention, be it a pharmaceutical therapy, surgical procedure or population vaccination or screening programme to prevent disease. Preventive programmes, however, are less commonly subject to experiment for establishing effectiveness.
- The **randomised controlled trial (RCT)** is an experimental clinical trial to see if a new intervention is more effective than an established one or no intervention if none currently exists. Individuals, usually patients, are selected according to particular characteristics and randomly assigned to the experimental group (new intervention) or the control group (established or no intervention), then followed up over time to compare the effects in the two groups. Here, **randomisation** has a very specific meaning (see below).

Studies are also done to investigate the effectiveness of a procedure, such as a particular surgical procedure. These are **experiments**, rather than simple observations of process and are known as **clinical trials**.

Investigation by observation: causation or association?

Much of epidemiology is about inferring causation. How does the observer then infer that the relationship is one of **causation** rather than mere association, and further, that the association was not the product of chance? In the words of Sir Austin Bradford Hill, in 1977:

The interpretation of statistical data turns, it should be seen, not so much on the technical methods of analysis but on the application of common sense to figures and on elementary rules of logic.

It is unlikely that absolute proof of cause and effect can be found statistically, and what needs to be demonstrated is the most reasonable interpretation of the association. Some basic questions have to be addressed:

- Is the difference observed in the two groups a real difference, or did it occur by chance?
- If we are satisfied that the difference was not by chance, then what inferences can be drawn from this difference?

The first question is relatively straightforward. Statistical tests of significance could be applied to the numbers for each sample to show whether the results were due to chance, or were 'significant' (see above). However, a statistically significant difference is not necessarily a sufficiently important difference from which to draw inferences about causality or about the effectiveness of clinical interventions. The second question is very much more complex and difficult, and cannot be simply answered with statistical tests. Bradford Hill formulated a set of nine criteria for inferring causation; these were modified by Nicholas Wald in 1996 (Information box 7.15).

It would serve the reader well to consider these criteria when presented with assertions such as 'whooping cough vaccination causes brain damage' or 'MMR [measles, mumps, rubella] vaccine causes autism in children' as media headlines. (Autism is a condition starting in childhood with symptoms of delayed speech and communication being typically noticed between the first and second birthday.) It would be impossible to gather irrefutable evidence for (or against) a causal hypothesis, although a 2012 systematic review of MMR vaccine exposure studies, which included a variety of different types of studies involving several million children, failed to find a significant link with autism and other conditions. The evidence can, however, help us to decide whether there is any other explanation that is more likely than cause and effect.

Observational studies

Observations of a population may take place either at a particular *point in time,* or over a *period of time.* The monitoring of changes in disease patterns and behaviour over time (say 15 or 50 years) could yield clues to the aetiology and the impact of prevention. In a clinical context, knowledge of the incubation period of an infectious disease can help in its diagnosis, although we cannot always know when the exposure took place. Observation of other factors over time may, however, help the diagnosis, as in the example of whooping cough at the beginning of this chapter.

Information box 7.15 | **Criteria and evidence for inferring causality between an exposure and a disease***

Essential criteria

- A real association between exposure and the disease; that is, an association that is unlikely to be due to chance
- The exposure precedes the occurrence of the disease (*temporal relationship of the observed association*)
- The association cannot be reasonably explained by bias (e.g. through systematic measurement error) or through the effect of one or more confounding factors
- The causal explanation makes good biological sense (*biological plausibility depending on the biological knowledge of the day; coherence of the evidence with generally known facts about the natural history and biology of the disease*).

Additional evidence

- Strength of the association: a relative risk as high as 3 or 4 is less likely to be due to bias than a relative risk of 2 or less (*strength of the association; the relative incidence of the condition investigated in the populations contrasted must show a pronounced excess in the exposed population*)
- Consistency in the evidence from several studies that is unlikely to share the same bias (*consistency of the observed association repeatedly observed by different people, in different places, different circumstances and times*)
- Demonstration of a dose-response relationship between the exposure and disease in studies of individuals (*the association reveals a biological gradient*)
- The demonstration of reversibility; elimination or reduction in the intensity of exposure is associated with a reduction in the risk of disease
- The distribution and frequency of the disease in different places and in different groups and over time follows the distribution and intensity of exposure (as for additional evidence 2)
- Support from animal or in vitro experimental evidence (*evidence from experimental or semi-experimental evidence, which can include experimental evidence from humans*).

Other Bradford Hill criteria

- *Specificity of the observed association:* it would be preferable if the association were limited to specific people in particular places and particular types of disease. However, as diseases may have more than one cause, a specificity in the magnitude of the association would strongly support a causal relationship.
- *Reasoning by analogy:* in some circumstances, such as the known association of congenital amelia with the administration of thalidomide during early pregnancy, similar, but slighter, evidence about another drug may be acceptable.

*Original Sir Austin Bradford Hill concepts are in *italics*.

Where the observations took place could also be important. Differences in incidence or prevalence may be observed between countries (e.g. the prevalence of malaria) or within a country (e.g. higher prevalence of coronary heart disease in the north of England), giving further clues to the risk factors associated with particular conditions. The effect of population interventions, such as a vaccination programme, on disease incidence could be monitored. One example is immunisation against whooping cough (Fig. 7.10).

The variation in the distribution of risk factors could suggest explanations for the difference in disease patterns, and may also suggest a hypothesis for causation. Here, attention to the criteria for inferring causation is extremely important. For example, differences in the rates of type 2 diabetes between South Asian and indigenous white people in the UK could suggest genetic factors for developing the disease, whereas variation in rates between South Asian people living in the UK and those living in rural communities in South Asia might suggest environmental and lifestyle associations. The identification of risk factors is useful in the development of strategies to reduce disease and promote health, but conclusions drawn must be supported by evidence conforming to the criteria for inferring causation.

Cross-sectional studies

The commonest types of cross-sectional study are health surveys that collect data from a defined population in a particular way at a particular point in time. Table 7.7 sets out the design of cross-sectional studies that are commonly carried out and their uses.

Sampling for cross-sectional studies

A **sample** of the population is collected for a health survey, and this can be done by various means. Such studies are susceptible to a variety of biases, depending on the survey method used. For the results of a study to be useful, it is important that the sample should be representative of the population of interest. Although desirable, a truly random sample of the population is almost impossible to obtain and deliberate efforts must be made to ensure that the sample is as similar as possible to the population of interest. The way the sample was chosen must be described explicitly. For convenience, systematic sampling is often used in field studies – perhaps by collecting every 10th person in an alphabetical list. Lists that are compiled in other ways, such as the electoral roll, may also be used.

Sometimes a group of people will be selected instead of individuals. An example would be the General Household Survey carried out by the ONS. This has the advantage of concentrating fieldwork in a particular area, thus making the study cheaper and simpler. The assumption is made that people in a group are there for reasons unconnected with the reason for the study – although that of course might not be the case. Undertaking a survey is not without its problems. The minimisation of bias is an essential step in the design of any study that aims to infer causation (Information box 7.16).

Interpreting the data from cross-sectional studies

Often we will be interested, not just in making observations about one set of data, but also in making comparisons between different sets. The scientist first addresses the question: is the difference observed in the two groups a real difference, or did it occur by chance, using the process outlined below?

- The data are examined first, to determine the type of distribution.
- Statistical tests are then rigorously applied to ensure that the observed differences did not arise by chance (see probability above). We may be examining differences in proportions observed in different groups, but could also be looking at differences in the average value (mean) of a particular measurement.
- If the values are to be assessed more formally, then hypothesis tests and calculation of test statistics are required (see above).
- Only then may conclusions be drawn.

Case–control studies

The classic epidemiological enquiry is by observation. The examples of John Snow's Broad Street pump and cholera, and the thalidomide story were both case–control

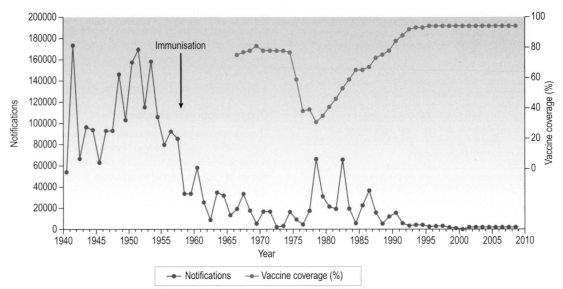

Fig. 7.10 **Notifications and immunisation rates for whooping cough for England and Wales 1940–2009.** The policy for immunising babies against whooping cough was initiated in the UK in 1958. The graph shows the incidence of whooping cough in England and Wales from 1940 to 2009, and how this came down once an immunisation programme was instituted. However, there was a 'scare' in 1974 that the whooping cough vaccine could cause brain damage, resulting in a dramatic fall in immunisation rate from over 80% coverage to below 30%. This was attended by a rise in whooping cough notifications. As the immunisation coverage improved, the incidence of whooping cough reduced. Data from Public Health England, Disease facts: whooping cough. www.hpa.org.uk.

Table 7.7	Cross-sectional study design					
Study type	Time	Definition	Past action	Starting point	Future action	Typical use for study
Cross-sectional	Present	Observation	None	Collect all information	None	Prevalence; current health status; reference ranges
Repeated cross-sectional	Present and future (longitudinal)	Observation	None	Collect all information	Collect all information again on several occasions	Changes over time

Information box 7.16   **Problems with data collection by survey: bias**

Bias in samples collected by survey can occur in several ways:
- Not using proper random selection. Volunteers are likely not to be representative of the population.
- Not being able to identify certain groups within the population sampled. Some people are hard to identify or include, for example: people who do not often leave their homes, people without official residences, children frequently absent from school.
- Selecting people who will not cooperate. Loss of information from large numbers of selected people will result in the study being unrepresentative and therefore meaningless. Leaving them out is not an answer but the process should be one that is most likely to engage their cooperation in the study.
- Replacing people in surveys. If people originally selected cannot be found, or refuse to cooperate, replacement with others who are more easily traceable or are more compliant will result in bias.
- Using an out-of-date list (sampling frame). Populations may change over time. For example, where there is movement in and out of a local authority, the area may change its demographic characteristics significantly, but an out-of-date list will not reflect this.

retrospective. By painstaking inquiry, the observer in each case found that appreciably more patients than unaffected people had consumed (or were exposed to) a particular substance.

Selecting the sample for case–control studies

In selecting a sample for a case–control study, as for *any* study, careful attention must be paid to the possibility of introducing bias, which would affect the ultimate outcome (see Information box 7.17).

A case–control study involves a comparison of the rate of exposure to a potential risk factor in groups with a disease with the rate of exposure in a group that is disease free. Cases are identified first, then suitable controls are selected. Ideally, in order to concentrate on a particular factor, the controls need to be as similar as possible to the cases in every respect (**specificity**, as referred to in the criteria for causation), except that they do not have the disease. Often this is achieved by rules which would result in cases being able to be controls if they did not have the disease, and vice versa. This selection also involves **matching** individuals, or groups, identifying and matching people for factors such as age, sex, ethnicity, etc., who have the potential to become cases, but without reference to the risk factor. However, care must be taken not to overmatch, in case the matching variable is associated with the factor of interest. Having

studies. **Case–control studies** may look back into the histories of affected persons (cases) and unaffected persons (controls) for evidence of exposure to the substance in question (Table 7.8). In other words, they are

Table 7.8 Case–control study design

Study type	Time	Definition	Past action	Starting point	Future action	Typical use for study
Case–control	Present and past (longitudinal retrospective)	Observation	Record risk factor exposure	Collect cases and controls	None	Aetiology; rare disease aetiology

Information box 7.17 — Potential biases in case–control studies

Minimising bias in studies designed to infer causation is extremely important. While it might be impossible to eliminate all bias, careful reflection about the potential sources of bias would help to avoid bias in the study design.

- Selection bias:
  - Control selection: although controls are matched with cases, differences may sometimes be present that render them atypical. One reason could be overmatching: for a chest physician studying the relationship between smoking and lung cancer, the easiest source of controls may be other patients without lung cancer in his or her care. These controls, however, are likely to be patients who have other conditions related to smoking. Community controls are preferable but not so easy to recruit.
  - Case selection: a disease may vary in its causes and its association with other diseases. For example, lung cancer in a particular person may or may not have been caused by smoking, and may be accompanied by other conditions (co-morbidity). This will influence the extent to which any conclusions from the study can be generalised: a study based, for example, on elderly people without any co-morbid conditions is unlikely to be of wide value.
- Recall bias: in retrospective case–control studies, cases are more likely to recall the risk factors to which they have been exposed. The controls, on the other hand, may under-report their exposure. The discrepancy is likely to lead to bias. Historical information may also be inaccurate; while not biasing the results it will increase uncertainty.
- Ascertainment bias: also known as 'detection bias', ascertainment bias can occur when there is an association between an individual characteristic and the likelihood of detecting the event. For example, women taking the contraceptive pill may have more frequent cervical smears, so that cervical cancer may be detected sooner in this group.

identified individuals we then enquire as to their exposure to that factor in the past (temporality). For example, if there is a group of cases of gastroenteritis after a wedding party, and a particular food preparation is suspected to be the cause, we would want to select our controls from the people who attended the party but did not suffer from gastroenteritis, since they had the potential to become cases, but without taking into account what they ate when they were selected. We then see whether eating a particular food at the party was associated with people who become ill after the party.

Case–control studies have a number of practical advantages, principally because they are done at one point in time and so are quick and cheap. They are, however, difficult to do properly and there are a number of inherent biases that are difficult to overcome (Information box 7.16). Nevertheless where a condition is rare, this may be the only type of study that can be done that affords a sufficiently large number of cases. The study strength can be increased in particularly rare conditions by having more than one control for each case.

Analysing and interpreting data from case–control studies

The basic questions that need to be addressed by research studies are reiterated here:

- Is the difference observed in the two groups a real difference, or did it occur by chance? This question is about hypothesis testing.
- If we are satisfied that the difference was not by chance, then what inferences can be drawn from this difference? (This requires understanding of potential confounders and biases.)

Again, the data must be examined to look at the distribution, and the appropriate statistical tests applied to test the probability that the observed differences arose by chance.

The seminal work of Doll and Hill in 1950 and later Doll and Peto in 1994 (the British Doctors' Study) are classic examples of investigation by observation. The scientific rigour and principles inherent in these studies apply to all studies seeking to demonstrate cause and effect, and should always be borne in mind when considering claims of causality. Here the criteria for inferring causation are used to help distinguish probable cause from a chance association.

Strength of the association

The stronger the association, the more likely it is to be causal. The original study of cigarette smoking and lung cancer by Doll and Hill (1950) was a case–control study. A sample of patients in hospital with lung cancer (cases) was matched with patients without lung cancer (controls). Their case notes were reviewed for factors that may have influenced the development of carcinoma of the lung, and the subjects were interviewed about other social, environmental and occupational factors. A significant difference in whether the participants smoked cigarettes was found when comparing the groups with and without lung cancer ($p < 0.05$) (Table 7.9).

Doll and Hill showed that cigarette smokers were 14 times more at risk of developing lung cancer than non-smokers. Despite this large difference, a causal relationship between cigarette smoking and lung cancer cannot yet be presumed from this evidence alone, as many other factors need to be considered.

Results of observational studies can be expressed in the form of a comparison of risks (see Information box 7.18).

In a case–control study, cases and controls are selected according to outcome (given in the columns) and the

Table 7.9 Case–control study: lung cancer and

Exposure	Disease status		Total
	Cases (lung cancer)	Controls (no cancer)	
Cigarette smokers	647 a	b 622	1269
$a+b$			
Non-smokers	c	d	$c+d$
	2	27	29
Total	649 $a+c$	649 $b+d$	1298 $a+b+c+d$

influence of various exposures (in the rows) is then investigated (from Table 7.9):

Odds of outcome (lung cancer) in smokers is a/b

Odds of outcome (lung cancer) in non-smokers is c/d

Odds ratio (OR) of outcome in smokers compared with non-smokers is:

$$\frac{a/b}{c/d}$$

$$\frac{a \times d}{b \times c}$$

In this example the OR $= (647 \times 27)/(622 \times 2) = 14$.

When the outcome that defines the cases is rare, then $a/(a+b)$ (calculated when working out a risk) will be similar to a/b (calculated when working out odds) and so we can use the odds as an estimate of **relative risk** and interpret it in the same way as relative risk (see below). Otherwise, as in the case of the calculated example, we have to get to grips with odds. In tossing a coin, for example, the risk or chance of getting a head is 0.5, or 50%, whereas the odds are 1, or 50:50. An interest in betting often helps. In this above case the odds are 14 to 1, providing an OR of 14.

Consistency of findings

Has the observed association been found by different observers, in different places and at different times? The same association between a causal agent and the disease should be observed in studies in different populations. If no such association is seen, it is important to compare methodologies in conflicting studies, and to know whether the selection of cases would have resulted in similar people being in all the separate studies.

At the time that Doll and Hill found the strong association in their sample between smoking and lung cancer, an Advisory Committee to the Surgeon-General of the United States Public Health Service reported the same finding in 29 retrospective and seven prospective studies. It was then justifiably inferred that this association was a true one.

Specificity of the association

In 1951, Doll and Hill began a 20-year prospective study, extended for another 30 years, of smoking and mortality in male British doctors (Doll and Peto 1994), a **cohort study** (see below). Questionnaires on smoking habit were sent to all male doctors on the medical register at the time, and the respondents became the cohort for the study (34 440 men).

| **Information box 7.18** | **Comparing risks (odds ratio and relative risk)** |

When estimating the risk of a particular outcome (e.g. developing a disease), the concepts of **odds ratio** or **relative risk** are used. People who have been exposed to risk factors (such as cigarette smoking, excessive alcohol consumption), or who possess particular defining characteristics (e.g. employment, raised serum cholesterol) are compared to those without such exposure or characteristics. These statistics (summary statistics) are calculated from study data.

- In **case–control studies**, the outcome is already known, since cases are selected according to outcome, such as death or having lung cancer, and the influence of various exposures, the risk (e.g. smoking, alcohol) is then investigated.
- Risk is assessed using the concept of **odds**, referring to the likelihood, or odds, of developing a disease if exposed to a 'risk' factor. For example, if 4 people (cases and controls) have been exposed to a risk and 3 develop the disease and 1 does not, then the odds of disease in the exposed group are 3:1.
- Groups are compared by calculating the **odds ratio (OR)**. If, for example, there are another 20 people who have not been exposed to the risk, but 4 of them develop the disease (and 16 do not), then the odds of disease in the non-exposed group are 4:16, or 1:4. The odds ratio is calculated as:

OR = Odds in exposed group/Odds in non-exposed group (see also Table 7.9)

$= (3/1)/(4/16)$

$= 12$

- It is important to be aware that in these studies the number of selected controls can be varied and the assessment of risk OR does not change. (Indeed, for rare outcomes, it would be usual to increase the number of controls several-fold in order to minimise bias and to have more precision for confidence intervals.) In the above example, there are 7 cases in total and 17 controls. If there were twice as many controls (34) then we would expect twice as many to have been exposed to the risk.

OR $= (3/2)/(4/32) = 12$ (identical to that above)

- In **cohort studies**, subjects are selected according to a defining characteristic, such as exposure to a factor, and subsequent outcomes (e.g. disease, death) are then investigated. The cohort is a defined (exposed) population. There is no concept of 'control' here, since the investigation is to observe the

incidence of an outcome, such as heart disease, in this defined population. The overall number of people in the cohort (denominator) is more or less fixed (depending on loss to follow-up).

- Risk in this population is the proportion of people with the defining characteristic who develop the disease, and is compared with the proportion of people who develop the disease without the defining characteristic, known as the **relative risk** (**RR**).
- For example, suppose in a cohort of 24 people, 4 have been exposed and 3 of them subsequently develop the disease then the proportion of people who develop the disease in the exposed group is 3/4.
- If, in the group of 20 people who have not been exposed, 4 of these subsequently develop the disease, then the proportion of diseased people in the non-exposed group is 4/20.

The RR $= (3/4)/(4/20) = 3.75$

- Note that if one applied relative risk calculations to the two case–control calculations above then very different estimates of risk would be obtained in the two situations.
- Relative risk does not provide an indication of the extent of a problem and calculation of the **absolute risk reduction** (**ARR**) or **absolute risk increase** (**ARI**) can be useful.
- **Absolute risk reduction** (**ARR**) is defined as the difference in proportions between the populations with and without the defining characteristics who develop the outcome. While this could lead to a *reduced* risk, looking at it in reverse would mean an *increase* in risk.
- In 1995 the UK Committee on Safety of Medicines reported a doubled risk (RR $= 2$) of deep vein thrombosis in women taking the third generation contraceptive pill (containing desogestrel and gestodene) in comparison with the second generation pill. As a result many women stopped taking the pill; there was a large increase in unwanted pregnancies and the number of legal abortions increased by about 6000, remaining at that level for the next 6 months.
- Although the risk had doubled with the use of the new pill, the actual risk had increased (ARI) by about 15 cases of deep vein thrombosis in every 100 000 women per year. This number of adverse events due to women continuing on the third generation pill is clearly very low in comparison with the marked increase in unwanted pregnancies.

Observations on mortality began in 1951, finishing in 2001. Details about doctors' deaths were obtained from the Registrar General and death notifications to the General Medical Council. Further follow-up questionnaires were sent in 1956, 1966 and 1972, including questions about stopping smoking (more doctors joined the study as they joined the medical register after 1951). During the first 20 years, 10 072 men died. The death rate for smokers was higher than non-smokers, but from a number of causes of death (heart disease, other cancers, Parkinson disease, cirrhosis, etc.). Smoking was not *specifically* associated with lung diseases or cancers. By looking at the associations in age-standardised death rate for each cause of death, the excess in deaths among smokers was estimated. The magnitude of the excess mortality in cigarette smokers by cause of death (between 22% and 52%) led to the inference that deaths from cancer of the lung, oesophagus or other respiratory sites, chronic bronchitis and emphysema and pulmonary heart disease (cor pulmonale) were caused by cigarette smoking.

The observed association between smoking and many diseases other than lung cancer warrants more detailed examination. For example, mortality from cirrhosis of the liver was five times greater in current cigarette smokers than in non-smokers, but adjustment for a potential confounder in this association (alcohol) accounts for the excess deaths. Alcohol consumption may also be confounding the association between smoking and ischaemic heart disease in a different way. Alcohol, in moderation, appears to be associated with a reduced risk of ischaemic heart disease and so its action as a confounder is to mask what is probably a higher risk of ischaemic heart disease in smokers.

Relationship in time

It may seem obvious that there needs to be a temporal aspect in the observed association, since, in order to demonstrate causality, the exposure needs to precede the effect. This temporal relationship is not always easily observed, particularly in chronic, slowly developing conditions, and where multiple environmental factors could contribute to the development of disease. The prospective nature of a cohort study aims to avoid this difficulty.

In the 40-year follow-up of the British Doctors' Study, the excess mortality in smokers was almost twice as high in the second half of the study as in the first half (Fig. 7.11).

This seems to be due to an improvement in survival in non-smokers, probably because of preventive measures, therapeutic improvements and environmental changes in the intervening years that have not been translated into improvements in smokers. Another reason for the non-improvement in smokers may be that those smokers who reached middle or old age in the 1970s and 1980s had a longer history of cigarette consumption than those who reached middle or old age in the 1950s and 1960s. Now we know that about 50% of persistent smokers are killed by their habit, and about 25% still while in middle age.

The biological gradient

The evidence for a causal relationship between cigarette smoking and lung cancer can be strengthened by demonstrating a biological gradient, or dose–response curve. In the study this was shown by dividing the data into categories for those who had never smoked, and those who smoked 1–14, 15–24, and more than 25 cigarettes per day. Doll and Peto (1994) demonstrated that with the exception of 4 out of over 20 conditions positively associated with smoking, mortality increased progressively from light to moderate to heavy smokers (Fig. 7.12).

Demonstration of reversibility

What effect did removal of the hazard have, if any? The smoking and mortality cohort study demonstrated this effect beautifully. As the study progressed, some doctors in the cohort stopped smoking, and after a period the rate of death from lung cancer in this group dropped compared with those who continued smoking, but the rate of death from some other cancers did not, underlining the causal relationship between cigarette smoking and lung cancer (Fig. 7.13). The statistical methods used for analysing effects over time are usually correlation and regression, with multivariable analyses when more than one predictor (independent variable) is studied (see below). Follow-up of the British Doctors' Study has shown that stopping smoking at age 50 halves the risk of death from smoking, and stopping at age 30 virtually eliminates it (Fig. 7.14).

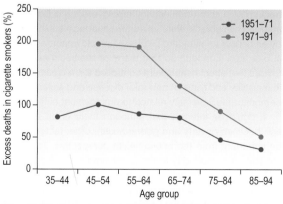

Fig. 7.11 **Excess age-specific mortality in cigarette smokers in first half of study compared with second half.** Data from Doll R, Peto R 1994 Mortality in relation to smoking: 40 years' observation on British male doctors. BMJ 309: 910–11.

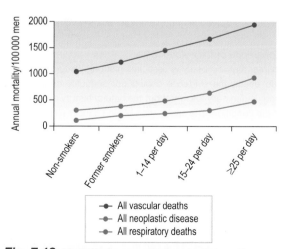

Fig. 7.12 **Mortality in non-smokers and cigarette smokers.** Analysis of data such as this may involve the use of a test for trend, such as a modification of the χ^2 test. Data from Doll R, Peto R 1994 Mortality in relation to smoking: 40 years' observation on British male doctors. BMJ 309: 910–11.

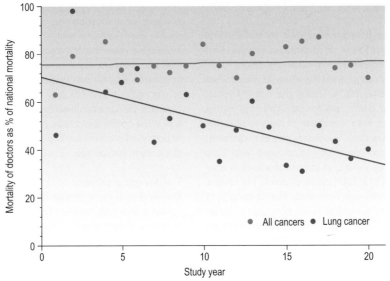

Fig. 7.13 **Trends in deaths of male doctors certified 1951–1971.** The doctors in the cohort reduced their cigarette consumption considerably; deaths from lung cancer grew less common, but not from other cancers. Data from Doll R, Peto R 1994 Mortality in relation to smoking: 40 years' observation on British male doctors. BMJ 309: 910–11.

Biological plausibility

The evidence for causation is more acceptable if it is biologically plausible. This depends on the currently available biological knowledge, which is added to continually. Even where an observed association may be new to science, if the causal explanation makes biological sense it may deserve serious consideration.

Smoking tobacco causes cancer not only of tissues of the upper respiratory tract and lungs with which the smoke has direct contact, but also of the oesophagus, bladder and pancreas. Tobacco smoke contains many carcinogens that induce oxidative damage (see Ch. 16) to DNA, and many of these carcinogens also interact with DNA, forming DNA adducts that modify proteins and DNA itself, with potential mutagenic consequences. Techniques to demonstrate their presence have led to their detection in blood and in tissues not in direct contact with cigarette smoke, but associated with smoke-induced cancer. Increased levels of protein adducts have been found in non-smokers exposed to tobacco smoke, compared with those not so exposed.

Coherence of the evidence

To infer that an observed association strongly suggests cause and effect, the evidence should not seriously conflict with what is generally known about the natural history and biology of the condition. The association of lung cancer with cigarette smoking was coherent with the increase over time of cigarette smoking and the rise in deaths from lung cancer among men. We are now seeing more women smoking, and in almost all developed countries lung cancer rates in women have increased.

Cohort studies

The other main category of observation is the **cohort** study. This starts with an unaffected sample of the population: a cohort. Each member of the cohort is characterised by a number of features and enquiry made at intervals over a period of time to see if a particular outcome has occurred. The association between a feature and outcome can then be examined (Table 7.10). An example of a cohort study is the Whitehall I study described below.

Selecting the sample for cohort studies

A cohort is a group of people selected according to shared defining characteristics in terms of people, time and place, such as all babies born in 1942 in England and Wales (birth cohort), male civil servants aged 40–64 in 1967 working within 2 miles of Whitehall in London. The cohort is selected knowing that some people will be exposed to various hazards and others not. While selecting a particular occupational group can be useful as an aid to long-term follow-up, it will also mean that the cohort may not reflect the average health in the population. In addition, any cohort will be slightly healthier than the general population because it is composed of people who are free of disease on entry. Like any other study, it is important to be aware of bias (see Information box 7.19). When reading reports of cohort (and other) studies, the reader should always think about whether the investigators had done their best to minimise bias when they designed and carried out the study.

The Whitehall studies

The Whitehall studies (Whitehall I in1984 and Whitehall II in 1991) conducted by Marmot et al. were **prospective** cohort studies aiming to see whether disease occurred more frequently in some civil service employment grades than in others. The subjects were all non-manual workers, not 'poor by any absolute standard', in stable employment, and living in one area (London), so that many of the socio-economic factors that affect health were controlled for. A clear gradient in mortality and rates of non-fatal disease and sickness was demonstrated, inversely related to employment category.

It could be inferred that although there is an association between poverty and poorer health, other factors might be important from the public health perspective. To reduce mortality and morbidity in the lower employment grades to a level comparable with those in the higher grades would need strategies to address early environment, social environment, job design and the consequences of differences in income, as well as to encourage healthy behaviours. This kind of study does not help with the treatment of coronary heart disease, but can identify risk factors that may be amenable to modification as a preventive measure.

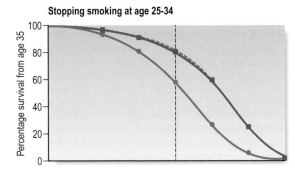

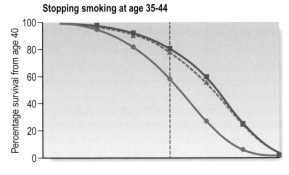

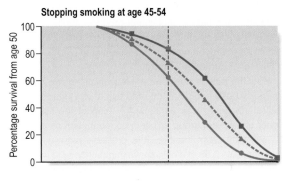

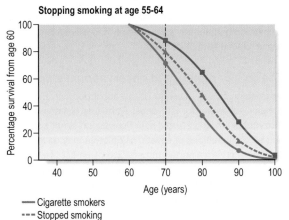

Cigarette smokers
--- Stopped smoking
Non-smokers

Fig. 7.14 **Effects on survival of stopping smoking cigarettes, at age 25–34 (effect from age 35), age 35–44 (effect from age 40), age 45–54 (effect from age 50), and age 55–64 (effect from age 60).** Data from Doll P, et al. 2004 Mortality in relation to smoking: 50 years' observations on male British doctors. www.bmj.com/content/328/7455/1519.

A well-designed and conducted cohort study provides the most valid evidence among the observational study types because it makes it possible to separate out prior causes from present associated factors, and although both suffer from potential confounding it is usually less likely to be biased than a case–control study. It can also be used to study several outcomes of the exposure to the same potential risk factor. Also, because the cohort is derived from the population, risk can be quantified (see Table 7.11).

Assembling the cohort

The Whitehall I study began in 1967, when a very large (17 530) cohort of male civil servants aged 40–64 and working in various departments within 2 miles of Whitehall in London were invited to participate in the study, and classified according to employment grade. At the start of the study, they were surveyed about their family and past medical history (specifically in relation to cardiorespiratory disease), lifestyle (including smoking history) and symptoms of diabetes. They also attended a screening examination, where blood pressure, height and weight were recorded, and a two-lead electrocardiogram (ECG) was taken.

The prospective follow-up

The assembled cohort of male civil servants was subsequently followed up for 10 years. Annual screening for illness and physical examination were undertaken and mortality was recorded.

It was found that there was a steep inverse relationship between employment grade and mortality. Compared with the highest administrative grade, the lowest grade had three times the mortality rate, not only from coronary heart disease but also from a range of other causes, and from all causes combined. The difference was partly accounted for by smoking, diet and other lifestyle gradients within each factor. Differences in height (higher grades were taller), relating to environmental factors in early childhood, suggested that early life may affect adult death rates, though height also has a genetic component.

Whitehall II

Twenty years later in 1985, a new, very large (10 314) cohort of civil servants aged 35–55 was established, this time including women, and followed up for 3 years. The inverse association between employment grade and morbidity, angina, ECG evidence of ischaemic heart disease and symptoms of chronic bronchitis, remained. Self-perceived health status and symptoms were worse in the lower employment grades. There were employment gradient differences in lifestyle (as in smoking, diet and exercise) and in factors affected by early life (reflected in height), and in social position, social support and circumstances at work (monotony, hostility, low control and low satisfaction).

Analysing and interpreting data from cohort studies

Because some of the factors of interest will be confounded by other factors, depending on the outcome, either multivariable regression or multivariable logistic regression will be used to analyse the data (see below). As for case–control studies, the strength of the association between exposure to risk factors and developing disease needs to be explored in cohort studies before any inference of causation may be attempted (Information box 7.19).

Table 7.10	Cohort study design					
Study type	Time	Description	Past action	Starting point	Future action	Typical use for study
Cohort	Present and future (longitudinal prospective)	Observation	None	Define cohort and assess risk factors	Observe outcomes	Aetiology; prognosis

Table 7.11	Cohort study: initial cholesterol level		
Characteristic	Death from coronary heart disease at 10 years		Total
	Yes	No	
Cholesterol at or above median	421 a	8530 b	8951 $a+b$
Cholesterol below median	c 282	d 8485	$c+d$ 8767
Total	703 $a+c$	17015 $b+d$	17718 $a+b+c+d$

Information box 7.19   Potential biases in cohort studies

- **Selection of subjects**: the sampling frame, the population from which the cohort was drawn, can give rise to bias, especially if a high-risk group is chosen and the expected length of follow-up is intended to be short. If the study outcome was death, then a hospital patient-based selection will be biased towards those patients likely to be at higher risk of death. More optimistic results for some conditions may be observed because the sample will not include individuals who have already died.
- **Association does not imply causation**: evidence for causation needs to be assessed against a number of criteria to be convincing (see above, Inferring causation). Various biases can be introduced, but in particular, potential confounders need to be considered. For example, if an association is observed between drinking alcohol and the subsequent development of lung cancer, smoking is associated with both the outcome (lung cancer) because it *is* a risk factor for lung cancer, and the possible risk factor (alcohol) because they tend to occur together in restaurants and bars. Reanalysis of the data adjusting for the confounder (smoking) reveals no association between alcohol and lung cancer.
- **Expense**: even with common diseases, large populations need to be studied to detect significant differences in outcome between exposed and non-exposed groups. If the incubation period for a disease is long, many years of study may be required.
- **Loss to follow-up**: it is not unusual to be unable to record the outcome for every individual in a cohort, given that this may occur several years after inception of the study. Large numbers lost to follow-up, particularly if associated with a predictor, can produce significant bias. Studies need to be designed carefully so that this effect is minimised. It may be possible to provide ways in which some basic information can still be collected, such as information from death certificates.
- **Changes over time**: analytical methods and diagnostic criteria change over time, and information collected early in the study may not be comparable with later information. Individuals may change their exposure to risk over time by changing their occupation or lifestyle.
- **Surveillance**: this should be the same for all participants; if a group thought to be at high risk is studied more intensively, the outcome of interest may be detected earlier, and falsely associated with the risk.

Part of the Whitehall study of male civil servants in London examined the effect of cholesterol levels on the risk of death from coronary heart disease. Data in Table 7.11 have been extracted from this study.

$$\text{Relative risk (RR)} = \frac{a/a+b}{c/c+d}$$

The risk of death in the subsequent 10 years in those with above average cholesterol levels is $421/8951 = 0.047$ whereas the risk in those with below average cholesterol levels is $282/8767 = 0.032$, providing a relative risk of $0.047/0.032 = 1.47$.

To interpret relative risk, if the risk (of death from coronary heart disease) in the lower cholesterol group was the same as that in the higher cholesterol group, then the ratio of the two risks (RR) would be 1.0. If being in the higher cholesterol group doubled the risk of death then RR would be 2.0. In the Whitehall study the relative risk is 1.47, meaning that the risk of death in the higher cholesterol group is about 1.5 times greater than the risk in the lower cholesterol group. We could also say that the risk was around 50% higher (150% − 100%) in the higher cholesterol group.

How the ratio is analysed will influence the way a risk is interpreted. We could say that the risk of death in the lower cholesterol group was $0.032/0.047 = 0.68$ of the risk in the higher cholesterol group. While a concept such as doubling the risk may seem intuitive, it is probably more difficult to conceptualise 0.68 of a risk, so we might choose to invert the equation as above. Alternatively, we could talk about a 32% reduction in risk (100%–68%), or a 32% benefit. Although, in the mathematical context, 'risk' does not necessarily imply something bad, for the sake of clarity it is often useful to talk about relative benefit instead.

The role of genetics in observational studies

Possession of the ε4 **allele** of the apolipoprotein E gene is a major risk factor for late-onset Alzheimer disease and homozygotes are at a 20-fold risk. Possession is not sufficient, and so combinations of several risk factors may be involved.

When determining the importance of an association between the gene and the disease we must also be aware of the various biases that occur when this kind of study is undertaken. **Selection bias** may occur in clinical or autopsy series of patients with Alzheimer disease and misclassification may influence population studies. A further problem is that many people suffering from Alzheimer disease are at a higher risk of dying because of their age. Bias can also occur when, for example, geneticists identify disease-associated genes within single blood samples. Since a **statistically significant** interaction will be found in about 1 in 20 comparisons by chance alone, false positives will abound.

Association between genotype and risk factor

In the early stages of studying the prevalence of Alzheimer disease, a strong association was found between presence of $ApoE_4$ and vascular factors that indicate the presence of atherosclerosis. It was thus thought possible that the gene may exert its effect because of its possible role in the latter disease. When a later prospective study was done, this association with atherosclerosis was no longer evident. Confusion also arose between different populations, no relationship being seen in a Japanese autopsy series, while a clinical study in Americans showed an association. Differences in ethnicity and age of the many groups being studied, and also in the associations found, further add to the difficulties that epidemiologists face when trying to find the causes of a disease and this field will become more complex in the future with greater knowledge about individual genomes (see Ch. 5).

Interaction with environmental factors

A second example illustrates the interaction between genetic makeup and environmental factors. Colorectal cancer in Japanese migrants to the USA is among the highest in the world, and considerably higher than in the indigenous Japanese. Between 1880 and 1920, a large Japanese workforce was imported into Hawaii to work on the sugar plantations. Unlike the example involving Native American Indians and the immigrant Caucasian population, the Japanese did not mix, and today, people of true Japanese descent form about 30% of the Hawaiian population. Could the rise in incidence of the disease be due to their exposure to American lifestyle factors, or could there have been some form of change to their genetic susceptibility to the disease? These later migrants have, however, retained many of the elements of their ethnic diet, and although their fat intake is consistently lower than that of the Caucasian American population, their beef intake was higher.

Figure 7.15 illustrates the importance of possession of both a family history (genetic factor) and eating a large amount of red meat (environmental factor) in a study conducted by Marchand in 1999. The possible reason for this interaction lies in the high prevalence of a 'fast' acetylator *N*-acetyltransferase (*NAT2*) gene, present in 90% of the Japanese population compared with 45% of Caucasians. When meat is cooked at a high temperature or for a long time, the burning of the creatine/creatinine produces heterocyclic amines (HCA), which have been found to be carcinogenic. In order to be toxic, however, HCA needs to be activated; two genes are involved and one of them is *NAT2*.

Investigation by experiment

When selecting the most appropriate and effective treatment or intervention, the clinician needs to know how these worked previously for similar patients. New treatments will need rigorous testing to see how effective they are and whether they cause harm. Experimental intervention of some kind is required, followed by observation of the effects of intervention. **Clinical trials** are the usual method of study.

- The intervention is administered to the experimental group
- The outcomes are observed and compared with those in a control group, which is not given the intervention
- The experiment has to be conducted in such a way that any difference that might be observed between the two groups is real, and not due to chance.

Once a difference has been observed, the next important question is whether the experimental treatment is the most likely cause of the difference: the two groups must, therefore, be similar in characteristics that could have a bearing on their condition at the start of the trial. A further question is whether, apart from the experimental treatment, the groups are treated in the same way. If a difference in the two groups is observed, and this difference is deemed not to have occurred by chance (is statistically significant), it may be inferred that the difference was the outcome of the intervention.

Medical treatment and surgical procedures are not the only interventions that can be tested experimentally. In public health policy, for example, some preventive action is taken as the result of an observed association. Does such action, in fact, prevent, or at least reduce, risk or frequency of associated events? In this context, experimental trials could be the means of testing for cause and effect.

Evaluation of clinical effectiveness: RCTs

To illustrate the processes for evaluating clinical effectiveness of a medical treatment, the Scandinavian Simvastatin Survival Study (4S), a randomised trial of cholesterol lowering in 4444 patients with coronary heart disease published in 1994, is used as an example. This study was a major milestone in cardiovascular treatment. The effectiveness of drug treatment to lower serum cholesterol concentration, in order to improve survival for people with coronary heart disease, had been in question because of insufficient clinical evidence of benefit. The 4S trial was a study of secondary prevention of the complications of established coronary heart disease, by the use of a drug that is known to reduce serum cholesterol. An RCT was done.

Selecting the sample: experimental and control groups

The first task here is to define the population of interest; what is meant by people with established coronary heart disease? The inclusion criteria for the 4S trial were men or women aged between 35 and 70 years, with a history of angina or acute myocardial infarct. There were also some exclusion criteria, which addressed the likelihood of pregnancy, severe disease or co-morbidity. Here, the idea is to eliminate, or at least minimise, bias and reduce any unknown risk to potentially

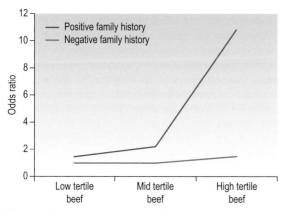

Fig. 7.15 Beef intake and colorectal cancer in people of Japanese origin, resident in Hawaii. A strong family history of colorectal cancer in the migrants increased the risk of disease (odds ratio of 3.0), and the Japanese migrants were found consistently to eat more red meat than the local Caucasian population. Data from Marchand LL 1999 Combined influence of genetic and dietary factors on colorectal cancer incidence in Japanese Americans. Journal of the National Cancer Institute Monographs 26: 101–105.

Information box 7.20 | **Potential bias in clinical trials 1: planning stage**

As with observation studies, introducing bias during the planning stage of an RCT must be avoided as far as possible. Factors that could affect the eventual outcomes of the trial may be introduced during the planning stage when selecting the sample.

- **Inclusion and exclusion criteria**: these need to be clear and unambiguous so that there is no possibility of excluding patients after randomisation is performed. The criteria need to be applied before randomisation to avoid any deliberate or inadvertent attempt to exclude or include once the result of randomisation is known.
- **Informed consent**: this should be taken before randomisation for ethical reasons and to minimise the chance of patients leaving the study once randomisation is known.
- **Allocation concealment**: if the researcher is aware of which group (treatment or control) subjects will be allocated to, subjects may be allocated to the treatment group in order to gain access to the new treatment. This may be an unconscious action, but nonetheless the result will be biased. The converse could also happen. It can be avoided by the randomisation being performed by a third party and the analysis being performed on the group according to how they were randomised.
- **Study sample size**: to ensure that any difference in outcome detected between the treatment and control groups reaches statistical significance, the power of the study to demonstrate this difference depends on calculating a large enough sample to do this (see below). A sample that is too small, or is underpowered, is unlikely to show a significant result even if, in truth, there is one, thus biasing the study. Medical literature is full of studies that suggest there is no difference between two treatments when the study samples have not been large enough to reveal a difference in effect by as much as 25%. Similarly, there must be a large number of negative studies that have not made it to publication because they did not show a positive effect that was statistically significant (**publication bias**).
- **Control treatment and blinding**: as far as possible the control treatment should be as similar to the intervention in looks, taste and follow-up from the health professionals in the study so that any 'inherent' placebo effects of taking a tablet are as similar as possible in both groups. If either the patient or the health professional is unblinded, this knowledge can affect the placebo effect, or the attitude of, or interpretation of results by the health professionals. Any of these could introduce bias between the groups.

- The first principle is that the study should be preceded by a careful assessment of risk and benefits and states that the interests of the subject must always prevail over the interests of science and society
- Secondly, a potential subject, or their legal guardian, must be adequately informed of the aims, methods, possible benefits, potential hazards and possible discomforts of the proposed intervention.

Sometimes it is difficult to provide an adequate definition of the risk, as for example during pregnancy. Some subjects, such as those with mental disability, may not be legally competent. However, such people are more likely to meet exclusion criteria and will therefore rarely be represented in these experiments. Sometimes important experiments are difficult to get approval for, because the study patients might be unconscious; the Corticosteroid Randomisation after Significant Head Injury (CRASH) trial is an example and illustrates the importance of being able to conduct these trials in the people who will be exposed to the treatment.

The CRASH trial
Many people with head injury die, or are severely disabled, some as a result of the pressure within the skull due to swelling. Steroids are known to reduce swelling, but the available evidence of benefit of steroids in this group of patients was unclear, and that available often from poorly conducted studies. Getting approval to do studies in individuals who may be unconscious is problematic although this study was finally approved and over 10 000 adults with head injury were randomised to receive steroid infusions, or a placebo. The study showed, importantly, that the risk of death was increased in the corticosteroid group and no benefit was shown in those who survived.

Another ethical consideration is that of coercion. This could be bribery, if the 'volunteers' to the trial were paid excessive sums of money to take part, or, in the case of a family doctor inviting a patient to take part in a trial, consent could be influenced by the relationship between the patient and doctor, or consideration that any existing treatment might be withheld if consent was refused.

Achieving similar groups for comparison: randomisation to minimise bias
Only when the participants have been selected according to the inclusion and exclusion criteria and given informed consent can they be allocated to either the control or intervention group. The best method of ensuring that the two groups are as similar as possible for both known and unknown characteristics is random allocation. This is done using a random numbers table or a computer program (see Information box 7.21). The only reason the groups may differ is then chance.

vulnerable patients (pregnant or co-morbid) (see Information box 7.20). Patients were recruited from 94 centres. In many cases, participants became eligible for a trial when they were first diagnosed with a problem or disease (incident cases). This resulted in patients being recruited over a period of time and then followed up for either a specific period of time or until a specific time point.

Ethical considerations during the planning stage of clinical trials
The major ethical considerations when inviting patients to volunteer to take part in a clinical trial are:

- Respect for the autonomy of the volunteer
- No harm must be done to the volunteer.

Volunteers must consent to participate, but informed consent cannot be given without having all the information needed to understand the issues involved in the study, and the information must be fully understood and considered.

The Declaration of Helsinki (World Medical Association 1960, revised 1975) outlines the ethical considerations when undertaking clinical research.

Selecting the sample for the 4S trial
In the 4S trial, potential subjects fulfilling the selection criteria were invited to take part and be screened for exclusion criteria. After final informed consent was obtained, they were randomly assigned to the treatment group taking 20 mg of simvastatin, or to the control group taking placebo. In this process, **allocation concealment** was provided so that it was impossible to predict the group an individual would have been randomised to until the point of randomisation. Because patients have already fulfilled the selection criteria

Information box 7.21   Random allocation

Only when volunteers have been selected, and informed consent is given, can subjects be allocated. A variety of methods are employed for allocating subjects to treatment or control groups in an RCT:

- **Simple random**: random, in this context, does not mean haphazard. Subjects are selected so that every individual has the same chance, or probability, of being chosen. A simple method could be by tossing a coin, but usually a computer is used.
- **Blocking**: blocking, also known as restricted randomisation, is done to ensure that the numbers are balanced between different treatment groups, and kept balanced at all times throughout the life of the study to increase the **power** (see below). To facilitate this, subjects are allocated in two small 'blocks' in random order, ensuring that each block contains a balance of the treatments. In a block of six used to allocate treatments A and B, each block will contain three subjects receiving treatment A and three receiving treatment B, and the order in which they are allocated will be randomised.
- **Stratified**: to overcome chance differences in important predictive characteristics arising from simple randomisation, subjects are defined by common characteristics which affect the outcome, e.g. cancer stage, and are then randomised within each stage to ensure similar proportions of cancer stage within the treatment and control groups. This is known as **stratification**. This is particularly useful for relatively small or multicentre studies where randomisation is usually stratified by the centre. **Minimisation** is another statistical technique that can be used to achieve very similar groups.
- **Cluster randomisation**: it may be impossible to randomise individual subjects, for example in a study of a particular health promotion, when outcomes may be biased by **contamination** (see below). In these cases groups of people (families, schools, GP practices, hospitals, etc.) are identified, and each group (or cluster) is randomised to be in the intervention group or the control group.

and consented, there is no opportunity to bias the selection process by leaving people out, as there would be if the randomisation details were available earlier. In the 4S study, a further refinement in randomisation was added by stratifying the subjects for geographical area and history of previous myocardial infarction. The eventual sample was almost perfectly balanced, and at the start of the trial the two groups were very similar.

Baseline characteristics for randomised patients are usually shown in the first table in reports of randomised clinical trials. Sometimes statistical tests are also done to indicate that the groups are balanced, though this should not be necessary if the patients have been properly randomised, and it should be remembered that in any series of statistical tests about 1 in 20 comparisons will be statistically different by chance alone ($p = 0.05$).

Calculating sample size

The size of a sample is chosen during the planning stage of a trial and is not an educated guess. Logical thinking at this stage of a study is needed:

- First, a decision has to be made about how large a difference needs to be detected between the treatment and control groups to show that the experimental treatment is more effective than the old or no treatment. In the case of opinion or attitude surveys, the difference would be in the proportions of people agreeing or disagreeing with something.
- The study needs to be large enough to have a strong likelihood of showing a statistically significant difference

if the true effect is the one decided on. This likelihood is known as the **power** of the study.

- Knowing the required effect, the power and the p value that is to be taken as statistically significant, the sample size can be calculated.
- Usually the p value is 0.05 and the power would be at least 80% although 90% is often used.
- With the sample size required for an 80% power calculation, we can be 80% certain that p will be <0.05 if the underlying effect is that used in the calculations.

Some idea of the likely difference in clinical outcomes between the two groups is needed before a power calculation for sample size can be undertaken. In practice, it may not be possible to know what this difference will be, unless there is information from a pilot or other studies. Past experience could give an idea of what the outcome in the untreated, control group should be from the natural history of the disease. A decision then needs to be made about what constitutes a clinically important change in outcome. For example, the 4S study was planned to detect a 30% reduction in total mortality in the treatment group. The numbers required to give a 'statistically significant' result were then calculated using a 'power calculation' (see below). The research protocol specified 4400 patients to be followed up until there were 440 deaths.

Power calculations

To estimate the number of subjects needed in a trial, a power calculation is used. Before doing the power calculation you will have to decide what is to be achieved by the trial – what you want to measure as the main outcome (see below). This may be categorical, for example how many subjects are dead or alive at the end of the study (Information box 7.22), or numerical, for example the change in blood pressure measured in mmHg (Information box 7.23). Power calculations may be applied for sample sizes for surveys as well as clinical trials.

You will also need to decide what sorts of results you would expect from the standard treatment. For example, you may know that not giving treatment results in about 10% of patients dying each year, or that the standard treatment lowers mean systolic blood pressure by 5 mmHg. In the latter situation we also need to know how much the change in blood pressure can vary between individuals (measured by the standard deviation); publications may provide relevant information.

Although mathematical formulae can be used to decide the number of subjects needed, it is simpler to use the nomogram developed by Altman (1982) (Fig. 7.16), or talk to a statistician. There are also computer packages that can do power calculations.

Measuring the outcomes during a trial

As well as bias in the planning stage of clinical trials, events that occur during the trial can also distort the eventual findings. Information box 7.24 outlines some potential biases during a trial.

'Blinding' to avoid bias during a trial

To minimise **bias**, the subjects in each group to which they are allocated are **blinded**, so that they are not aware of whether the tablet they receive contains the active drug or the dummy. A trial in which the patient is blind to the treatment given is a **single-blind** trial.

Information box 7.22   **Example of a power calculation 1: using proportions**

In the Medical Research Council/British Heart Foundation Heart Protection Study of cholesterol lowering with simvastatin in high-risk patients (age 40–80 years with coronary disease, or occlusive arterial disease, or diabetes) it was estimated that around 1500 out of 20 000 similar patients would die from coronary causes within 5 years. The aim of the study was to see whether this cholesterol lowering therapy could reduce coronary mortality by around 25%. A high level of power (90%) and a high level of statistical significance (p <0.01) were set in order that the study should stand a high chance of being successful and convincing.

For this the standardised difference was calculated:

$$\text{Standardised difference} = \frac{p_{control} - p_{simvastatin}}{\sqrt{\bar{p}(1-\bar{p})}}$$

where $p_{control}$ is the proportion of deaths expected in the control group (1500/20 000 = 0.075), and $p_{simvastatin}$ is the proportion of deaths expected in the treatment group (25% less, i.e. 1125/20 000 = 0.056) and p is the average of the two proportions (0.066)

$$= \frac{0.075 - 0.056}{\sqrt{0.066 \times 0.934}} = 0.076$$

Look at Figure 7.16. Draw a line between the standardised difference (0.076) and a power of 0.9, reading off the sample size (N) on the significance level 0.01 line. The nomogram gives a sample size of around 7000 in total so the researchers' plan to randomise over 20 000 patients gave them confidence not only to detect a 25% reduction in coronary deaths, but also to detect less pronounced differences associated with other non-coronary deaths or serious events.

Information box 7.23   **Example of a power calculation 2: using means**

The aim of a randomised clinical trial for a new antihypertensive drug is to demonstrate that the new drug can lower systolic blood pressure by more than 10 mmHg in comparison with the standard treatment. Looking at published data we discover that the standard deviation of average systolic blood pressure is about 15 mmHg. We need to be sure that if a difference of 10 mmHg is found between the treated and control groups, the difference is measured at the 5% level of significance or lower, so the significance level is set at 0.05, with 80% certainty (80% power).

To use the nomogram we calculate a **standardised difference**:

$$\text{Standardised difference} = \text{clinically relevant difference/}$$
$$\text{standard deviation}$$
$$= 10 / 15$$
$$= 0.67$$

On Figure 7.16, draw a line between the standardised difference (0.67) and a power of 0.8, reading off the sample size (N) on the significance level 0.05 line. This gives a total sample size of about 70 subjects, 35 per group. Increasing the power of the study (the ability to detect a real difference) will increase the number of people needed for the study, as will reducing the size of the difference we want to be able to detect.

The researcher (the doctor) could also introduce bias by favouring (or not) the treatment group; for example, by assuming that someone not receiving an active treatment (in the placebo group) is more likely to experience a cardiac event. For this reason, the researcher also needs to be blinded to the nature of the tablet given to the patient, and the 4S trial was a **double-blind** trial in this sense. Studies that have not been double-blinded, in comparison with those that have, have shown an overestimate of benefit of up to 17%. In the event that the patient is experiencing harm, the blinding is broken to establish the cause of this harm.

In some trials, for example in a trial of the effectiveness of a surgical procedure, it would be impossible to blind the patient who has to consent to the procedure or the surgeon who has to perform the procedure. It is therefore necessary to conceal the patient allocation from the observer, who takes measurements during the follow-up period, as to whether the subject had one or other procedure under investigation. For example, in a trial of myringotomy versus grommets in children with impaired hearing as a consequence of 'glue ear', the follow-up audiometry would be performed by a technician 'blind' to the procedure the child received.

Outcomes of interest: end-point definition

There are few unequivocal objective health outcomes. How the patient feels must be subjective, and might depend on a whole series of factors not necessarily related to disease. It is important that outcome measures provide a valid assessment of the effects of intervention, and are not determined by what is easily measurable.

The duration of follow-up will also affect outcome, because treatment effects, whether beneficial or harmful, may not be evident if the follow-up is too brief. For example, the drug clofibrate, known to reduce serum cholesterol levels in those patients who had high levels, was used in a clinical trial published by the Committee of Principal Investigators, to examine its benefit in the primary prevention of ischaemic heart disease. The earlier publication in 1978 revealed that fewer people in the clofibrate group experienced non-fatal heart attacks, but the later follow-on publication from 1980 revealed that mortality from all causes was higher in the clofibrate group, underlining the importance of considering all relevant outcomes (in this case death from all causes) and for continuing a trial for long enough to reveal these differences, or at least undertaking follow-up studies to find out whether an apparently promising treatment might be detrimental.

Defining outcomes is made easier if the research question is clearly focused. The question in the 4S trial was 'Does a reduction in serum cholesterol concentration reduce the incidence of complications in people with coronary heart disease?'. The primary end-point was total mortality, secondary end-point was defined as 'major coronary events', and tertiary end-points included any coronary event and related atherosclerosis events such as stroke. The effective follow-up time for the 4S study was calculated in the power of the study as when 440 deaths had occurred. Median follow-up was 5.4 years, and both subjects and controls had the same regimen of tests, such as annual electrocardiogram, observations and so on.

Ethical principles during a trial: stopping a trial and interim analyses

It has already been mentioned that trials that are too small are unethical. In addition, many people would consider a trial unethical if it had not been properly planned and organised. Furthermore, it is a fundamental principle that patients should not be exposed to any treatment if it is known to be harmful. The Declaration of Helsinki states that 'Doctors should cease any investigation if the hazards are found to outweigh the potential benefits'.

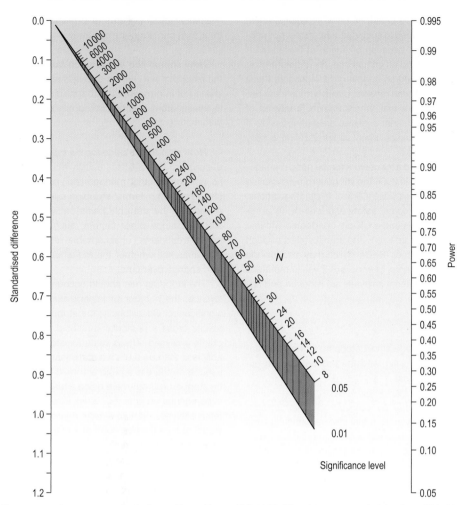

Fig. 7.16 **Nomogram for power calculations.** From Altman DG 1982. How large a sample? In: Gore SM, Altman DG, eds. Statistics in practice. British Medical Association, London, pp 6–8, with permission.

Information box 7.24   **Potential bias in clinical trials 2: during the trial**

Care should be taken when making observations during a trial. Bias may be introduced during the process of a clinical trial, which needs to be avoided.

- **The placebo effect**: the mere fact of taking a tablet (which could be a dummy, and therefore a **placebo**) can give a subject a sense of psychological well-being. Spontaneous events can also occur as part of the natural history of the disease. The placebo effect can account for up to 30% improvement in symptoms in some studies. Unpleasant effects can be ascribed to placebos, as in the 4S trial, where roughly the same number in the placebo group as in the treatment group stopped taking the tablets because they thought they were having adverse effects from the tablets.

- **Contamination**: individuals in the control group may intentionally or inadvertently receive the experimental intervention. This is more common in health education interventions, where news of a particular health-orientated approach being tested in one GP practice may become known throughout the community and be taken up by others who were within a control group. The bias will be towards the null, making it more difficult to detect a difference between the two groups.

- **Compliance**: subjects may not always comply with the allocated treatments in a trial, and this also occurs in the population at large. It is usual when planning the size of the study to take account of the proportion who may not comply with treatment and the proportion who may drop out (i.e. not have outcome measures). If non-compliance is larger than expected, the study may be compromised.

- **Intervention bias**: if a particular treatment is thought to have possible adverse effects in a particular subgroup of participants, it may be tempting to follow these subjects more carefully, thus adding an additional difference between the groups, beyond the experimental treatment. Bias may also occur in double-blinded trials in cases where it is possible to detect an active treatment because of an observable systemic effect. Both of these biases can make the two groups appear more different than they really are.

- **Cross-over**: if a particular treatment appears to be too aggressive for a particular subject then a medical decision might be made to treat them according to the other therapy. Depending on whether the new treatment is generally better or worse than the standard treatment, crossing over may bias either towards the null or towards a false impression of a difference (this is why we do intention-to-treat analysis).

- **Loss to follow-up**: loss to follow-up occurs when a subject who enters the trial moves away or otherwise cannot be traced, so that they are unavailable for outcome assessment. This is more likely to occur in longer studies. Subjects in studies involving patients who are seriously ill (e.g. acute leukaemia) are more accessible for assessment than subjects in studies of primary prevention, where they are well and not so motivated to continue treatment. In such cases more rigorous ways of maximising follow-up should be introduced into the study methodology at the design stage. (This is why all-cause mortality is usually an end-point, because provided permission to access these data was part of the inclusion criteria, it is generally possible to find out if someone has died or not, even if they are lost to follow-up.)

Unfortunately, there are probably many situations where trials have not been stopped in such circumstances, not necessarily by intention, but because of a lack of understanding of the principles behind an ethical trial. An understanding of the reasons for stopping an ongoing trial highlights these principles (see below). These reasons may become clear before the planned end of a trial, where **interim analyses** of the data can be useful. Interim analyses are only possible if follow-up is fairly long or recruitment is spread over a fairly long period.

In 2001 the EU adopted a framework for the good management of clinical trials and in 2004 the UK government passed the UK Medicines for Human Use (Clinical Trials) Regulations, intended to 'protect the rights, safety and well-being of research participants'. Trials in the UK are conducted within a Research Governance Framework and administered through Research Ethics Committees (RECs) which may also include data monitoring requirements. Members of these committees will determine whether interim analyses are required and approve any stopping rules.

Interim analyses

If decisions are to be made about stopping a trial, the reasons must be clear and valid, and the process should not bias the outcome of the trial.

What outcomes should be considered in an interim analysis? Outcomes relevant to a trial involve gathering large amounts of data about death, cause of death, morbidity, change in biochemical measurements, patient satisfaction, etc. If the interim analysis includes an assessment of all this information, the risk is increased of finding statistical differences between the treatments by chance alone. It may therefore be appropriate to have a p value much below 0.05 for each of them, otherwise multiple comparisons arising from the different outcomes would not be appropriate (because it would be desirable for all or most of them to be significant). The addition of an interim analysis itself increases the chance of getting $p < 0.05$ from 1 in 20 to 1 in 10. The reason that many outcomes are not considered at interim analyses initially (but they would be if it appears likely that the trial might have to be stopped) is probably because it is important to do it quickly after the appropriate time or number of patients have been followed up for long enough.

In any comparison, a difference is considered to exist (be statistically significant) if it is likely to occur less than 5% of the time by chance alone ($p < 0.05$ or less than 1 in 20 occasions). This definition of statistical significance implies that in about 1 in 20 comparisons, a difference considered to be significant will occur by chance alone. Doing an interim analysis doubles the chance of getting a significant result to 1 in 10 so smaller p values would be used before stopping a trial.

How should the information be obtained? Usually, the data are collated and analysed and presented by the trial statistician to the Data Monitoring and Ethics Committee (DMEC), blinded so the DMEC does not know if the results indicate better or worse outcomes.

In managing an interim analysis, it is important to have made a plan and then to keep to it. It is difficult not to be influenced when, for example, researchers in multicentre trials send in unscheduled and possibly incomplete information about patients who have died, or suffered bad side effects, as a result of one arm of a clinical trial. Only by a proper evaluation of all patients at a planned interim time in their treatment can doubt be avoided.

How should the information be treated? It is vital that the results of any interim analyses are kept confidential. The leaking of information about possible differences may result in investigators or subjects dropping out, or lead to a fall-off in recruitment.

How should the decision be made to stop a trial? The decision to stop a trial is usually made by the DMEC set up as part of the trial management process. The committee should set up a formal stopping rule, although that will not necessarily be the only basis on which the trial might be stopped, since other factors, such as cost, acceptability, newer treatments, unacceptable rate of side effects, etc., may influence whether the trial should continue, and might also change over time.

The stopping rule should account for the size of the difference, the number of interim analyses and its statistical significance. Occasionally, the stopping rule will apply if the results cross a particular threshold for the number of data points analysed. The p value for stopping will be considerably less than $p = 0.05$. If a statistical difference of $p < 0.05$ is used, then there is around a 1 in 20 chance that the trial will be stopped without there being a real difference between the experimental treatments – a risk that increases with more interim analyses. Setting a more rigorous p value (e.g. <0.005) would reduce the likelihood of a trial being stopped because of a false-positive result.

Measuring outcomes: follow-up

Subjects in the study have to be carefully followed up to observe the effects of intervention. All the patients entered into the trial have to be properly accounted for and attributed at the end. If patients cannot be traced they will be 'lost to follow-up', and it will be impossible to tell what outcomes they may have experienced, whichever group they were allocated to (see Information box 7.24).

Analysing and interpreting the results

When analysing the results of a clinical trial, particularly one that has a long follow-up period, all subjects have to be accounted for. The results may be biased by what happened to certain patients (Information box 7.24). To avoid distortion of the final result, patients are analysed by **intention-to-treat**, and it is important for the reader of reports of clinical trials to know that this was undertaken.

Analysis by intention-to-treat

Some patients in the treatment group may stop taking the tablets because of adverse effects, or illness severity may require that a subject in the control group has to take active treatment. In which group should these patients be accounted for? For example, in a trial of two different revascularisation procedures for coronary heart disease (the Randomised Intervention Treatment of Angina (RITA) trial, 1989), some patients assigned to one procedure had to undergo the other because of disease severity.

The statistical analysis for randomised clinical trials works by comparing outcomes between patients receiving the experimental intervention and patients not receiving the experimental intervention. **Intention-to-treat** analysis means that all patients are analysed in the group to which they were originally assigned. Therefore, those patients who were intended for the treatment group, but failed to complete treatment are included in the treatment group. While this may seem obtuse, any other action will bias the result because it breaks the randomisation.

At the start of the 4S trial, the subjects in each group were well balanced and similar. The patients who stopped taking the tablets may have been more (or less) severely ill than the ones who completed the trial. Leaving them out of the treatment group, or putting them with the controls, would have introduced bias by distorting the profile of the treatment group and consequently the outcomes. The same applies if patients in the control group were analysed in the treatment group for some reason.

Another good reason for analysis by intention-to-treat is that, in real life, there will be some patients who stop taking tablets because of side effects (nausea, other gastrointestinal upset, etc.) so that retaining them in the analysis would be a more realistic reflection of what would happen in a practical way (pragmatic approach). The data for the 4S trial were analysed by intention-to-treat.

Sensitivity analysis

A **sensitivity analysis** should be done to determine whether the loss to follow-up is likely to bias the results. Subjects lost to follow-up are likely to be different from those who remain available, and research has shown that their prognosis is probably also different. If a study loses a large proportion of its subjects (say over 20%), or if the loss is significantly unbalanced, then the resultant study can either be importantly biased, or the certainty of the observations sufficiently compromised to limit the value of the study. The relative importance of the loss can be investigated by undertaking a sensitivity analysis, consisting of:

- An analysis based on a reasonable, possible poor outcome for the missing individuals
- An analysis based on a reasonable, possible good outcome.

If the conclusions derived from the two analyses are different, then it is clear that the loss to follow-up has been so large that the study is no longer valid.

Measures of treatment effect

Various methods can be used to describe the results; these are illustrated in Table 7.12. The quoting of a relative risk reduction alone can be misleading because it does not take into account the baseline risk. The absolute reduction in risk is sometimes a more useful concept. Converting an absolute risk reduction into a number needed to treat is useful because it provides a whole number, rather than a decimal proportion, that is easier to remember.

Statistical significance

It must be remembered that the nature of statistical significance being set at the $p = 0.05$ level means that there is a 5% chance of obtaining a p value <0.05 where there is truly no difference. This also highlights the importance of not over-interpreting significant differences where large numbers of comparisons have been made. Statistical methods exist to help in the interpretation where there are multiple comparisons.

Statistical significance, or not, does not necessarily imply that the result obtained is important, or not, clinically. For example, a small but statistically significant difference in blood pressure may be so small as to not be clinically important, either in terms of the size of the difference or other clinical endpoints. In contrast, a large and potentially important clinical difference, which does not reach statistical significance, suggests that the study may have been underpowered. Careful examination of the position of the 95% confidence interval in relation to the point of no difference can help in the interpretation (Fig. 7.17).

Clinical significance: the number needed to treat

Whether a statistically significant finding has clinical meaning is largely dependent on the clinician's common sense. There is, however, a test that can give some clues: the **number needed to treat** (NNT). With reference to the 4S trial and its primary outcome, it means 'How many patients with established ischaemic heart disease (IHD) do we need to treat with simvastatin for 5 years in order to avoid (or defer) one death?' In practice, this number is the inverse of the **absolute** reduction in risk. Table 7.13 uses data about deaths taken from the 4S trial, showing that this number is 30. The smaller the NNT is, the more effective the treatment.

The confidence interval for NNT from the 4S trial, however, ranges from 20 to 64. The sorts of issues that a clinician (or a public health director) with a prescribing budget might think about include:

- Does the number needed to treat (30) to avoid one coronary death, give sufficient benefit to *my* patients with IHD?
- From the result of the 4S trial, I will need to treat 30 patients with IHD for 5 years to prevent or avoid one death (without considering the prevalence of IHD in my area).
- Given the confidence interval, at best I will have to treat 20 patients with IHD for 5 years to avoid, or defer, one death. At worst, it will be 64.
- Should I include the prescription of simvastatin in my treatment protocol for the secondary prevention of ischaemic heart disease? In addition to the proven benefit of the treatment I will need to consider the increase in my prescribing budget, which will also depend on the prevalence of IHD in my population. The Health Protection Study Collaborative reported in 2006 that costs were less than £2500 per life year gained across a wide age range, which has led to the wide use of this treatment within the adult population.

Table 7.12	Calculations for treatment effect						
Control event rate (CER)	Experimental event rate (EER)	Relative risk (RR)	Relative risk reduction (RRR)	Absolute risk (AR)	Absolute risk reduction (ARR)	Number needed to treat (NNT)
Event/control numbers	Event/ experimental numbers	EER/CER	|CER − EER|/ CER or (1 − RR)	EER for experimental group; CER for control group	|CER − EER|	1/ARR rounded to the next whole number quoting associated time

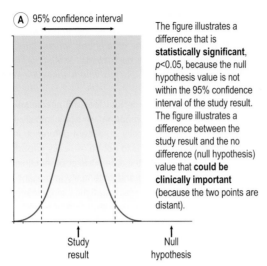

(A) 95% confidence interval

The figure illustrates a difference that is **statistically significant**, *p*<0.05, because the null hypothesis value is not within the 95% confidence interval of the study result. The figure illustrates a difference between the study result and the no difference (null hypothesis) value that **could be clinically important** (because the two points are distant).

Study result   Null hypothesis

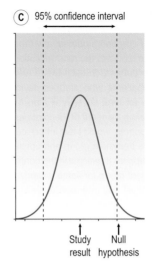

(C) 95% confidence interval

The figure illustrates a difference that is **statistically significant**, *p*<0.05, because the null hypothesis value is outside the 95% confidence interval of the study result. The figure illustrates a difference between the study result and the no difference (null hypothesis) value that **may, or may not, be clinically important** (depending on the context).

Study result   Null hypothesis

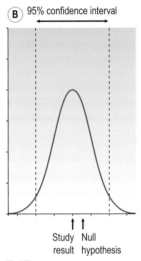

(B) 95% confidence interval

The figure illustrates a difference that is not **statistically significant**, *p*>0.05, because the null hypothesis value is within the 95% confidence interval of the study result. The figure illustrates a difference between the study result and the no difference (null hypothesis) value that **may not, be clinically important** (because the two points are close).

Study result   Null hypothesis

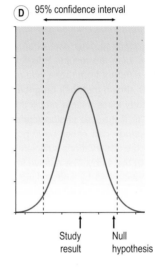

(D) 95% confidence interval

The figure illustrates a difference that is **not statistically significant**, *p*>0.05, because the null hypothesis value is within the 95% confidence interval of the study result. The figure illustrates a difference between the study result and the no difference (null hypothesis) value that **may, or may not, be clinically important** (depending on the context).

Study result   Null hypothesis

Fig. 7.17 **Clinical and statistical significance.**

Table 7.13	Results from 4S trial		
	Simvastatin		**Placebo**
No. of patients	2221		2223
No. of deaths	182		256
Death rate (absolute risk, AR)	8.2% (experimental event rate)		11.5% (control event rate) 95% CI
Absolute reduction in risk (ARR)		3.3%	1.6–5.1%
Number needed to treat (NNT)		100 + ARR = 30	20–64
Relative risk (RR)		8.2% + 11.5% = 0.71	0.58–0.85
Relative risk reduction (RRR)		1 − RR = 0.29 (or 29%)	15–41%

Data from the Scandinavian Simvastatin Survival Study Group. Randomised trial of cholesterol lowering in 4444 patients with coronary heart disease: the Scandinavian Simvastatin Survival Study (4S). Lancet 1994: 344: 1389–1399.

Interpreting the results

Evidence of the effectiveness of treatment (or any intervention) has to be evaluated based on:

■ Whether there was an effect that did not happen by chance, i.e. a reduction in the risk of death (or some other outcome of interest) in the treated group
■ How large the effect was clinically and statistically (magnitude of the difference)
■ Whether the results apply to patients generally (i.e. 'my patients'), or only to a highly selected group of subjects in the experiment

■ Whether the likely benefits of the new treatment are worth the potential harms and costs.

Tests of significance

The same statistical concepts apply to experimental studies as to observational studies (see above). From Table 7.13, showing death rates in the 4S trial, the difference in the risk of death (relative risk) within 5 years (median follow-up study period) of subjects taking simvastatin compared with those taking placebo is 0.71 (a value of 1 would indicate no reduction in risk). It can be said with 95% confidence that this falls within the range of 0.58 to 0.85 (confidence interval) reflecting the 'true' relative risk. While reporting the risk of death in the simvastatin group being 0.71 of that in the group taking placebo, a more easily understandable explanation would be to say that risk was reduced by an average of 29% $(1 - 0.71 = 0.29)$ in the simvastatin group.

The range of estimates for a confidence interval could be wide or narrow. If the confidence interval is wide, then the result is less conclusive. In the above example, if the range of values for relative risk (a ratio) included 1, then we would say that there was no statistical reduction in risk. Similarly, if in comparing the effect of two interventions and the result was expressed as a difference in rates, the range of possible differences included 0, there would be no statistical difference. This is sometimes referred to as the 'precision' of the result and the size of the sample has an effect, with larger samples giving more precise results (narrower confidence intervals).

The observed effect in a sample (a result) could happen by chance, and not as the outcome of an intervention. In the 4S trial, the probability (p) that the relative risk of 0.70 was a chance observation was 0.0003. The result was therefore highly significant, very probably related to the treatment with simvastatin, and not a chance finding.

Presenting the results

Having decided that the result of the study is statistically important, and relatively precise, there is a need to consider whether the result is clinically important enough to use the treatment generally for all patients with established coronary heart disease. Although the relative risk reduction (RRR) is more commonly cited, and here the RRR is 29%, it is worth thinking about absolute risk reduction (ARR) (Table 7.13). In clinical terms, the reduction in the risk of death related to coronary heart disease if the patient takes simvastatin in the required dose for at least 5 years is 3.3%.

The 'numbers needed to treat' (NNT) calculation is sometimes presented as a measure of the clinical significance of the effects of intervention, and has already been discussed. The smaller number suggests more effective treatment. Comparison of NNTs for different treatments, or in different patient groups, can be educative. For example, using drugs to lower blood pressure over 18 months where the starting diastolic blood pressure is between 115 mmHg and 129 mmHg has an NNT of <5 in the prevention of death, stroke or heart attack, whereas providing the same treatment for those with a diastolic blood pressure between 90 mmHg and 109 mmHg for over 5 years has an NNT of >100.

We do not always want to refer to a risk reduction. It may be important to refer to a risk increase (where an experimental treatment is detrimental) and it may then be more appropriate to quote a number needed to harm (NNH). Other ways of wording the comparison can be used in order to express the result effectively and 'benefit' is often used instead of 'risk' in certain circumstances. Nevertheless the formulae remain the same, even though the interpretation differs.

Dissemination

Publishing the results of any clinical trial, positive or negative, is vital, otherwise patients may end up being harmed. The current best evidence shows, however, that trials that report significant results are 2.4 times more likely to be published. Negative results are as important as positive results and efforts through open-access policies seek to address this problem, offering to publish all trials, regardless of results.

Although there are requirements to register clinical trials of new drugs, there are still also many unanswered questions about the efficacy of drugs within trials completed before 2007. Additionally, although there is also a requirement in the US FDA Amendment Act (2007) for the results of all trials to be provided to the register, evidence from a study in 2012 shows that only about 20% have complied with the regulations. **Publication bias** is a major problem in medical research because information about the true effect of any treatment may be hidden. While randomised controlled clinical trials are vital to prove the efficacy of any treatment, so is the knowledge of ineffective treatment so that patients are not further harmed by continuing experimentation through a lack of information.

Statistical assessment of data

There will be occasions when the data for a study do not follow a 'normal' distribution. Such data may be able to be ordered (ordinal data) or ranked. All of these data, whatever their distribution, are **quantitative** – the measurement being given in numerical format.

- **Parametric** statistical tests are done on data that follow a particular mathematical distribution. The 'normal' distribution is one such example. Statistical tests are used to compare sets of data. Parametric tests are the most powerful statistical tests because they use all of the information in the numbers.
- **Non-parametric** statistical tests are used when the data do not follow a particular distribution but can be ordered.

Some data are **qualitative**, describing, for example, the frequency of an observation within a category – **categorical data**. The frequency of particular blood groups is one such example. Sometimes it may be possible to order the categories in order to provide more detailed information. Numbers of responses within categories of pain can be better analysed if the categories are also ordered in degrees of severity.

Choosing a statistical test

Different types of data will need to be analysed by different statistical tests and the flow charts above can be used to help decide which test is the most appropriate.

Looking for differences in quantitative data
(Fig. 7.18)

- **Independent** data comes from sets of data that are not linked – e.g. the heights of men and women.
- **Paired** (**dependent**) data comes from sets of data that are linked – e.g. measurements of blood pressure in women, ante-natal and post-natal.

Both parametric (where the data are normally distributed) and non-parametric tests (where the data are skewed or is simply ranked) are shown in Figure 7.18. Sometimes it may be possible to mathematically transform skewed data so that parametric tests can still be used.

Statistical tests also need to be capable of being modified in order to deal with comparisons between more than two groups.

Comparing differences - data in categories

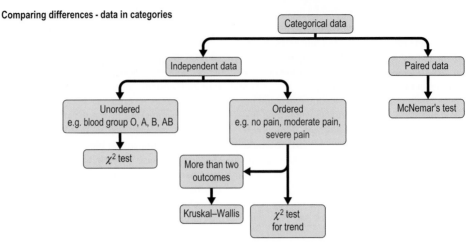

Fig. 7.18 Statistical analysis of quantitative data.

Comparing differences - quantitative data

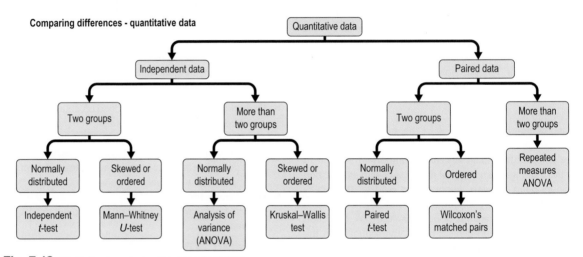

Fig. 7.19 Statistical analysis of categorical data.

Looking for differences in categorical data
(Fig. 7.19)

Categorical data can also be independent or dependent. For example the reporting of pain in two groups, treated or untreated, would be independent, whereas the reporting of pain in two groups, before and after treatment, would be described as paired data, because the two measurements would be linked by coming from one person.

Looking for patterns in data (Fig. 7.20)

Sometimes we are interested in looking for patterns or associations within the data and different tests can be applied depending on the type of data. For example we may want

to see if there is an association between current and past smoking, and lung cancer. Where we want to examine associations between sets of data that are continuous, e.g. height and weight, it is more powerful to use all of the data, rather than dividing the data into categories.

Degrees of freedom

In statistical tests of significance, such as the χ^2 test or the t-test, the concept of **degrees of freedom** is used. In a contingency table, the degree of freedom refers to the minimum number of cells in the table that need to be measured in order to complete the other cells. It is assumed that the totals for the rows and columns are known (Information box 7.25).

Looking at relationships

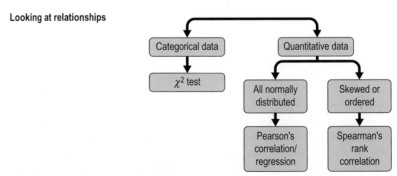

Fig. 7.20 Statistical analysis of association.

<table>
<tr><td colspan="2">Information box 7.25 An example of degrees of freedom</td></tr>
</table>

Information box 7.25 An example of degrees of freedom

This example is of fictitious data of a survey of 100 men and 100 women asking which of them would be more likely to use a particular product for cleaning carpets, to which the answers were 'yes', 'no' and 'don't know' (Table 7.14).

Assuming we know the totals in Table 7.14, we need to be told all except a minimum of any two of the numbers within the table in order to calculate the remainder. For example, in the samples of individuals questioned, if the observed numbers of 'yes' and 'no' were known, then the 'don't knows' calculated by simple subtraction must be:

Sample A : 100 − 32 − 12 = 56
Sample B : 100 − 25 − 15 = 60

We say that the Table has 'two degrees of freedom'. If a table has R cells in rows and C cells in columns then the degrees of freedom (df) can be calculated from:

$$df = (R - 1) \times (C - 1)$$

In the above example, df = (3 − 1) × (2 − 1) = 2
In a set of data divided into two independent groups, one would need to know all of the data except one in each group (df = 2). Where data are paired and the total is known, then all of the data must be known except one data point (df = 1).

Table 7.14 Contingency table of the survey data

Characteristic	Answers			Total
Sex	Yes	No	Don't know	
Male (A)	32	12	56	100
Female (B)	25	15	60	100
Total	57	27	116	200

The t-test

A *t*-test is employed to evaluate a difference in means, and is particularly important for small samples of fewer than 30 observations, because the measured standard deviation may not be very close to the population standard deviation and hence the calculated standard error of the mean may be inaccurate. The *p* value and 95% confidence intervals calculated from *t*-tests allow for this uncertainty.

Depending on the nature of the data being compared, slightly different statistical techniques are employed:

- An **independent group *t*-test** is used if different groups are being evaluated, for example to see if there is a difference in mean blood pressure between men and women at a particular point in time and, if a difference has been observed, is that just due to chance, or is there a real difference between the two populations.
- A **paired *t*-test** is used when the individuals being observed are matched for characteristics, e.g. age, sex, or when the same individuals are observed over a period of time. For example we may be interested in whether there is a difference in blood pressure before and after dietary advice to lower blood pressure and, if a difference has been seen, is that due to chance or is the difference likely to be real.

The procedure to calculate a *t*-test will not be given here but it is useful to understand the basic principles of all statistical tests which simply contrast a summary statistic, such as a mean, with the error in that summary statistic. For example in a *t*-test:

- *t*-statistic = difference in means between the two groups/standard error in the difference in means.

Most statistical software can calculate the appropriate *t*-statistic much less laboriously and more accurately than by hand.

Evaluating probability for *t*-values

To look up the *p* value or to calculate the 95% confidence interval requires knowing the degrees of freedom. For the paired test it is the number of pairs minus 1, for an unpaired test it is the total number of data points minus 2. For each degree of freedom, the *t*-statistic will correspond to a specific *p* value. The *p* value will be larger for the same *t*-statistic with smaller degrees of freedom.

The distribution can be shown as a graph (Fig. 7.21). The larger the degrees of freedom, the more closely does it resemble a Gaussian distribution. The *p* values are typically looked up in tables.

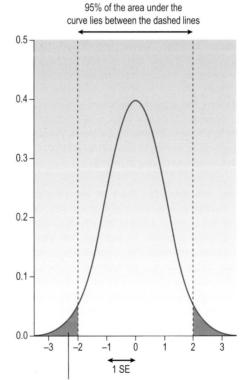

95% of the area under the curve lies between the dashed lines

1 SE

2.5% of area under the curve is found in each tail of the curve. The two 'tails', one positive and one negative, cover 5% of the distribution

Fig. 7.21 The t-distribution. The *t*-distribution is statistically derived from tables of *t*-values calculated from numerous sample means to approximate what would happen in a universal population of means. The centre, 0, is the 'true' mean. Each vertical dashed represents 1.96 standard errors from the centre (mean). The area of the curve of *t*-values within about 2 (actually 1.96) standard errors from the mean covers 95% of all means, if they were taken from samples of the universal population. The areas of the curve outside 2 standard errors are known as 'tails', covering 2.5% of all the *t*-values in each, 5% of the total.

The *t*-distribution differs from the Gaussian or normal distribution in that the proportion of points that lie within the central 95% varies according to the degrees of freedom. Hence the 95% confidence interval for results with 5 degrees of freedom would be much wider than a confidence interval of 10 degrees of freedom. The larger the study, and hence the larger the degrees of freedom, the more sure we will be about where the true value might lie within the confidence interval we have given, as that interval will increasingly narrow. When we do a *t*-test calculation and get a value for *t*, we see where the value for *t* lies on the *t*-distribution for the particular degree of freedom, according to our test. The *t*-distribution has a value of 0 at the centre.

The *p* value is the probability of the particular *t* value, or something further away from 0, by chance alone, if in truth there is no difference. On the *t*-distribution curve the *p* value is given by the area under the curve that is further away from the centre and beyond the *t* value. The larger the *t* value is, the further away from the centre it will lie and the smaller will be the area under the curve beyond it, and thus the lower the *p* value, or the less likely it is that what we have seen is due to chance.

When the degrees of freedom are large (above a sample size of about 30) then the *t*-distribution becomes more like the normal distribution in that 95% of all estimates of the mean will lie within the mean $\pm$ 1.96 standard errors (**the 95% confidence interval**). As we have discussed above, with smaller samples the number we need to multiply the standard error by will increase and the 95% confidence interval will increase.

Whatever the actual *t*-distribution we use, a *t* value that falls into one of the two tails outside the confidence interval is unlikely to be due to chance. By convention we say that if the probability of something happening is less than 5% ($p < 0.05$) then it is unlikely to be due to chance.

One- and two-tailed tests of significance From the above discussion, it is clear that *t* values may be positive or negative (Fig. 7.21). In a trial of the effects of a new drug for lowering blood pressure, for example, the effect could be beneficial or detrimental. As in calculating *p* values for the Gaussian distribution, we are interested in the probability of a result as extreme or more extreme in either direction, so *p* value corresponds to the proportion under the curve for values greater than $+t$ and less then $-t$. This is known as a **two-tailed** test of significance and is the conventionally used approach.

Very occasionally, however, we are only interested in either a positive or a negative difference in effect. For example, although we may be interested in the beneficial effects of a drug and are looking to get a large *t* value that lies within the 5% ($p < 0.05$) area in one tail of the curve (a one-tailed test) then this would be equivalent to the 90% confidence interval for the two-tailed test and a lower *t* value would be needed to declare that the treatment was effective, in comparison with using a two-tailed test. There will be situations, therefore, where statistical significance could be declared using a one-sided test, but not two-sided, and this must be made clear and the significance of the result must be reported as being **one-tailed**. Rarely, however, should we be doing a one-sided test. Even though we may only be expecting beneficial effects of a drug, clearly if the drug had the opposite effect and the *t* value was in the opposite tail of the distribution, should we not think that was also important?

Criteria for applying the *t*-test
Certain criteria must be met if a *t*-test is to be used:

- The spread of the data in the two groups (the **variance**) should be similar and similarly shaped, although there are special *t*-tests for when the variances are known to be different.
- If the groups are small (degrees of freedom <15) the separate groups (in independent tests) or the differences (in paired tests) should have an approximately normal distribution. Sometimes the data are skewed (asymmetrical) but often a mathematical transformation, such as taking logs of the data and using those values in the test, will make it suitable for a *t*-test. If the data cannot be made relatively 'normal' then other tests based on the rank ordering of data should be used, such as the Mann–Whitney *U*-test (for independent samples) and the Wilcoxon Matched Pairs test (for paired samples).
- If the samples are large, it is not necessary that the distributions are near normal, but for purposes of interpretation it is often better to use simple transformations to make the data more normal.

The χ^2 test
We might often be interested to see if people with particular attributes, for example having blue or brown eyes, might be differentiated in some other way, e.g. more or less likely to develop heart disease. We will need to randomly select a sample of people with blue eyes and another with brown eyes (a **predictor variable**), and then ascertain the proportions in the samples that have heart disease (an **outcome variable**). These (binary) data are best displayed in a contingency table. Such data do not follow a normal distribution curve when plotted graphically, and are said to follow the χ^2 distribution (Fig. 7.22). The χ^2 distribution is equivalent to the *t*-distribution squared so only has positive values. As the number of degrees of freedom increases it approaches the squared Gaussian distribution (see Fig. 7.21).

Even if eye colour and high blood pressure were not associated (null hypothesis), by chance there are likely to be differences in the proportions of people with heart disease in the two samples (Information box 7.26, Comparing proportions). The χ^2 test was developed to test the null hypothesis for this type of enquiry, and is usually applied to a contingency table.

The purpose of the χ^2 test is to:

- Establish whether the proportions of outcome in each category of predictor are inconsistent with each other. For example, does blood group differ by ethnicity
- A non-significant *p* value would imply that we cannot tell whether the proportions are the same or not
- A significant *p* value would imply that the proportions are unlikely to be the same in each predictor but cannot tell us which pair of groups might be different
- A χ^2 test is not appropriate if the outcome or predictor data are ordered.

There is a simple formula for calculating the follow-up value for 2×2 tables, but most statistical packages will also give information such as confidence intervals of differences in proportions and are therefore to be preferred.

Evaluating probability for χ^2 values
Once the χ^2 statistic has been calculated, the value is evaluated for probability at the 5% level ($p < 0.05$) for

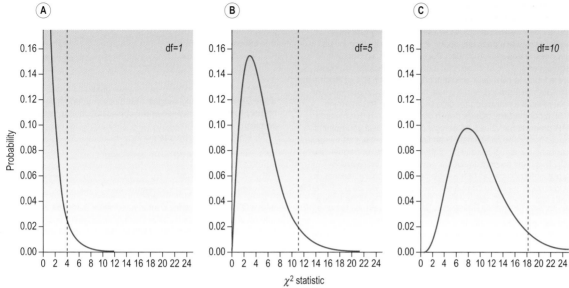

Fig. 7.22 The χ^2 **distribution.** (A) Data from a 2 ×2 contingency table and (B, C) data from tables with greater numbers of cells within the table. The *dashed lines* show the point on the distribution where the *p* <0.05 value lies. The area under the curve to the right of the line is 5% of the total area under the curve in each distribution. The *p* value is best obtained from χ^2 tables that show *p* values for different degrees of freedom. For example, from a table of the χ^2 distribution (A), a χ^2 value of 3.84 with 1 degree of freedom (shown by the *dashed line*) has a *p* value of 0.05 and, for any value larger than 3.84 (*p* <0.05), we can say that the distribution of numbers in the table is unlikely to have arisen by chance. A χ^2 value that is smaller than 3.84 will be not statistically significant (*p* >0.05). Looking up a table for χ^2 distributions, in part B, a χ^2 value of more than 11.07 with 5 degrees of freedom, gives *p* <0.05, statistically significant. The degree of freedom in any table is calculated as: df = (number of cells in rows − 1) × (number of cells in columns − 1).

statistical significance. The *p* values for χ^2 values are displayed in tables, adjusted for degrees of freedom. These are the proportions to the right of the *dashed* line shown in the χ^2 distribution (Fig. 7.22).

Criteria for applying the χ^2 test

There are certain criteria that must be met if the χ^2 test is to be used:

- Each individual studied must be in one cell and only one cell
- Cells must contain frequencies (numbers of observations), not percentages or proportions
- No cell should have an expected value of less than 5 (it does not matter what the observed value is). If this condition cannot be met a **Fisher's exact test** can be used.

Linear association: correlation and regression

In any investigation of the relationship between two variables it is important to produce a **scattergram** of the two measurements that usually come from an individual. Scattergrams can show:

- Whether there is any linear relationship between the variables
- Whether a straight line can be roughly drawn between the lines
- If a more complex form, such as a curve, is more appropriate.

In order to obtain valid results from the simple linear regression or correlation each data point on the scattergram must be independent (i.e. usually from separate individuals) and have the same weight (e.g. to have each point representing different sized towns would be wrong).

Correlation and regression are mathematically related but are used for different purposes.

- **Correlation** is used to measure the linear association between two variables whereas regression is used to predict one variable (**outcome** or **dependent variable**) from the other (**predictor** or **independent variable**).
- **Regression** is usually more appropriate than correlation. If we are interested in prediction, conventionally the predictor or independent variable is plotted on the x axis and the dependent or outcome variable is plotted on the y axis.

Because they are mathematically related, a correlation and linear regression on the same data points will give the same *p* value.

In analysing the data the **correlation coefficient (r)** measures degree, or strength, of the linear relationship between two variables, and can range from −1, where all the points lie on a straight line which slopes downwards, to 0, where there is no linear relationship at all (as in Fig. 7.23A) to +1 where all the points are on an upward sloping line (Fig. 7.23C). It is always important to look at the distributions graphically because an apparently strong correlation may disappear once it becomes evident that this is the result of an outlier in the scattergram, or due to different subgroups within the data. Linear regression of an outcome or dependent variable (*y*) with a single predictor or independent variable (*x*) produces a prediction equation of the form:

$$y = a + bx$$

where *y* is the predicted value of the outcome variable, *a* is the predicted value at *x* = 0, and *b* is the predicted change in *y* for a unit change in *x* (this is the slope of the line of best fit).

Figure 7.23C is a plot of car speed on the x axis against particle emission in the environment from a study in an urban

Information box 7.26 Comparing proportions

Quite often we will want to know whether the proportions of individuals with a particular characteristic are the same in two separate (independent) groups. For example, in a group of adolescents, 12% of those from a white European background were found to be regular smokers compared with 8% of those from an Asian background, and it would be of interest to see whether that reflects a real important difference. In order to determine this, a contingency table is drawn containing the different values. The proportional value (percentage) on its own tells you nothing about how good an estimate is and so it is essential that the table contains the actual observed numbers of people, or frequencies (O). This must be done in such a way that each individual is represented in one cell of the table only. If two characteristics in two groups are being compared, then the table will be a 2 × 2 table with four cells and marginal totals (Table 7.15). From the table it is possible to calculate the expected frequencies (E) given these values.

The proportion of regular smokers altogether in the study (the **prevalence**) is:

$(a + b)/n = 55/505 = 0.109$ (10.9%)

As there are 344 white Europeans in the study, if there were no difference between the two racial groups we would *expect* to see, in the regular smokers' cell: $344 \times 0.109 = 37.9$.

The expected numbers are those given in brackets in the table, and the same reasoning can be used to work out the expected values for each of the cells. It will become evident when doing this that a simple way of thinking about the calculations is to use the formula:

$$\text{Expected value}(E) = \begin{bmatrix} \text{Row total } (a+b \text{ or } c+d) \times \\ \text{column total } (a+c \text{ or } b+d) \end{bmatrix} / \text{Overall total } (a+b+c+d)$$

If there is a large difference between observed and expected values, then that would suggest that the two groups differ in respect to the characteristic under consideration (e.g. regular smoking).

For a 2 × 2 table the formula for χ^2 is:

$$\chi^2 = \sum \frac{\left(|O - E| - \frac{1}{2}\right)^2}{E}$$

where O = observed value, E = expected value, Σ means 'sum' or add up and the 'l' means make the answer positive. This is known as a χ^2 with Yates correction, which allows for the fact that the distribution is continuous, but the numbers in the cells are discrete (whole numbers). This can be translated into a formula that is easier to calculate if doing it by hand:

$$\chi^2 = \frac{N(|ad - bc| - N/2)^2}{r_1 \times r_2 \times c_2} = 1.53$$

Assuming 1 degree of freedom the p value given in a statistical table can be seen to lie between 0.1 and 0.25. Results from a statistical package, however, gives the p value more accurately at 0.22, which is clearly not significant as it is >0.05.

Table 7.15 Distribution of smoking habits in two populations

Characteristic	Group 1: White European	Group 2: Asian	Total
Present: regular smoker	42 (37.9)	13 (17.5)	55
	a	b	$a+b$ (r_1)
Absent: non-smoker or occasional smoker	c	d	$c+d$ (r_2)
	302 (310.1)	148 (143.5)	450
Total	344	161	505
	$a+c$ (c_1)	$b+d$ (c_2)	$a+b+c+d=n$

Data from Croghan E et al. 2003 The importance of social sources of cigarettes to school students. Tobacco Control 12: 67–73.

area of London and shows that particle emission increases as the average car speed increases. From the graph it is possible to read off an average speed and predict what the environmental pollution is likely to be. This estimate is likely to be useful in health outcome planning in the future.

Statistical packages will give confidence intervals for b and its associated p value. The null hypothesis is that y does not change with x and hence $b=0$ (the best fit line will be horizontal, or not significantly different from the horizontal). In the case of Figure 7.23C we can see that y does change with x and $p<0.05$.

Logistic regression is a useful method of statistical analysis used widely for studies. It is used where the outcome is binary, e.g. dead or alive, or got the disease or not. The results are given as **odds ratios** and the predictors can be binary or numeric. In the former case the odds ratio could be of death if male rather than female, and in the latter the odds ratio would be of death given a unit change in, for example, a biochemical test result. **Conditional logistic regression analysis** is similar but takes account of paired data, and is therefore commonly used in case–control studies. It also adjusts for the situation where there is more than one control for a case, but not every case has the same number of controls.

Multivariate analysis

When investigating observational data, we are often interested in more than one predictor of outcome. Usually it is already known that one or more factors may be associated with the outcome (age and sex are obvious examples), and if they are also associated with the predictor as well then they could confound the results by either masking or exaggerating them.

If we use only **univariate** analysis, for example for investigating whether alcohol (the independent or explanatory variable) might have a causal association with lung cancer (the dependent or response variable), the positive and statistically significant association that we are likely to find, while being correct, will probably be inaccurate in terms of predicting the effect of changing the prevalence of alcohol use on the risk of contracting lung cancer. In other words, only reducing alcohol consumption in the population is unlikely to reduce, or significantly reduce, the risk of getting lung cancer. This is because alcohol use and lung cancer are each **independently** associated with smoking (the definition of a **confounding factor**). Including both alcohol use and smoking in a **multivariate** analysis will give us the effect of alcohol after adjustment for smoking (the alcohol effect will probably be

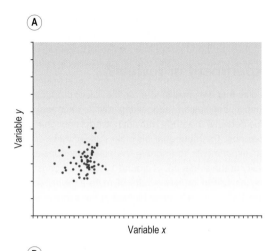

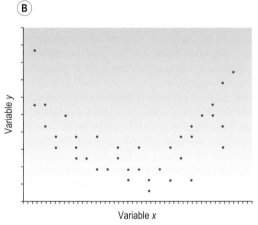

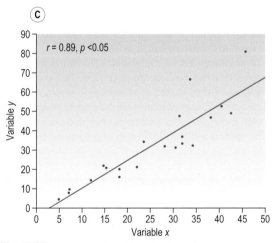

$r = 0.89, p < 0.05$

Fig. 7.23 Various scattergrams. (A) No linear relationship. (B) Curvilinear relationship. (C) Linear relationship. The direction of the slope indicated by the *red line* of best fit through the data shows a strong positive relationship, where as one variable increases, so does the other. In contrast, the slope for deaths from lung cancer in Figure 7.13 shows a negative relationship depending on the year of the study. The later the study, the lower the rate of death from lung cancer.

weak or non-existent and not significant), and this will reflect better the (limited) causal effect of alcohol on lung cancer.

■ In cohort studies, age and gender are usually adjusted for as they both are generally associated with risk of death or with being diagnosed with a specific disease and they may also be associated with potential risk factors.

■ In case–control studies, where cases and controls are often matched according to age and gender, any factors that are matched for will not be considered in the analysis. Thought has to be given to what factors may need to be included and therefore measured in the studies.

INVESTIGATION BY REVIEW

A review of a series of experiments is productive, not only because it gives credence to a single, apparently beneficial, treatment, but also because it can be a device for accumulating evidence over time and revealing effective treatments where individual studies had not been so convincing. In order to be sure that the review is free from bias it must be systematic in nature, the principle being to have a systematic and unbiased methodology to collect and evaluate all the available evidence, both published and unpublished.

The Cochrane Collaboration consists of a network of interested parties with a commitment to prepare systematic reviews of the evidence produced by RCTs. The collaboration is named in memory of the epidemiologist Archie Cochrane, whose forward-thinking idea it was in the 1970s. In 1979 he stated 'It is surely a great criticism of our profession that we have not organised a critical summary, by specialty or subspecialty, adapted periodically, of all relevant randomised controlled trials.' The collaboration began publication in 1993, forming the *Cochrane Library,* which includes the *Cochrane Database of Systematic Reviews.*

META-ANALYSIS

The Cochrane logo was developed from a systematic review, published in 1989, of trials of corticosteroids given to women at risk of giving birth prematurely (Fig. 7.24). Between 1972 and 1982, seven RCTs had been published. Figure 7.24 shows the results obtained in each study. Only two show a statistically significant effect (because the confidence interval does not cross the no effect line, where the odds are equal to 1), but combining information from all the studies increased the power and provided a significant effect estimate, the uncertainty of the combined measure being shown by the diamond at the base of the graph. The statistical method used to produce the combined effect is called a **meta-analysis**.

Cumulative meta-analysis

The review of treatment over time can be followed by constructing a cumulative meta-analysis, and can help avoid the continuation of RCTs where there is sufficient evidence of an effect. An early example, published by Antman and colleagues, examined 33 trials of the effect of intravenous streptokinase on death of people in hospital after a heart attack. These trials had been carried out over a period of time from 1959 to 1988, during which about 37 000 individuals had been randomised to receive streptokinase or a placebo (or no treatment).

Only six of the 33 trials reached statistical significance in favour of streptokinase but the meta-analysis (Fig. 7.25) revealed a highly significant odds ratio that was less than 1, reflecting an approximate 20% reduction in risk of death for those on treatment in comparison with those not given

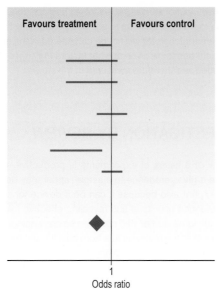

Fig. 7.24 Systematic review of the first seven trials investigating the use of corticosteroids to reduce risk of infant death from complications of giving birth too early. The horizontal line at the base shows the odds ratio scale with a vertical line being where the odds are equal to one (1:1, or no difference between treatment and control). The individual horizontal lines depict the 95% confidence intervals for the treatment effect for each of the seven published studies. Data from Crowley P et al. 1990 The effects of corticosteroid administration before preterm delivery: an overview of the evidence from controlled trials. British Journal of Obstetrics and Gynaecology 97:11–25.

streptokinase. Had a cumulative analysis been done as each study was published, the meta-analysis would have revealed a statistically significant difference ($p < 0.05$) as early as 1971 when around only 1000 individuals had been randomised, and would have reached $p < 0.01$ two years later after a total of only 2500 individuals had been randomised. This has major ethical implications since about 35 000 patients had been unnecessarily randomised, of whom about half would not have had a treatment that would have reduced their risk of death by about 20%. Possibly an additional 3500 individuals died as a result of this lack of a cumulative review. Even

after the meta-analysis was published, randomised trials of thrombolytic therapy continued for some time.

Experiment or review?

Studies that are small in size run the risk of producing a false negative conclusion, suggesting that a treatment is of no value because the study was not powerful enough to detect a difference. The meta-analysis makes use of these underpowered experiments to improve the power by considering the totality of the evidence. In around 10% of comparisons, conclusions based on the results of meta-analysis sometimes appear at odds with those looking at the same question but undertaken in large, sufficiently powered, clinical trials.

Differences between reviews and RCTs

There are several possible reasons for conflicting findings from systematic reviews and randomised clinical trials, some real and some spurious. One difficulty is **publication bias**, where published trials may not truly be representative of the truth since journals are more likely to publish those with statistically significant results and pharmaceutical industry-funded positive research findings are also more likely to be published in comparison with non-industry funded research. In addition, leading journals may be more likely to publish those where the results differ from before. On the other hand, single large clinical trials are probably not as representative of the whole population as a large collection of small clinical trials which provide information on more heterogeneous patient groups and hence are more likely to be representative of the population. Sometimes the criticism that the two methods are producing different results has been simply based on the fact that one method detects a statistical difference, while the other does not, when in fact the point estimates of effect measured in the two methods are very similar.

Other differences may be related to differences in the populations in the two methodological groups. Der Simonian and colleagues in 1999 looked at differences in recommendation for calcium supplementation in pre-eclampsia (characterised by high blood pressure, protein in urine and oedema, seen in the second and third trimesters of pregnancy) between a meta-analysis and a subsequent large clinical trial, the latter suggesting that there was no benefit to treatment. The clinical trial was undertaken in healthy women and when the

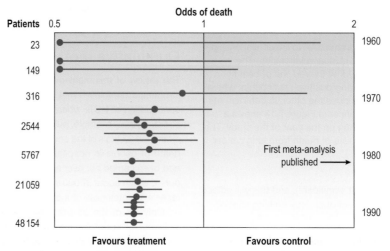

Fig. 7.25 Cumulative meta-analysis of thrombolytic therapy. Data from Lau J et al. 1992 Cumulative meta-analysis of therapeutic trials for myocardial infarction. New England Journal of Medicine 327:248–254.

trials involved in the meta-analysis were stratified according to risk, those at low risk also showed no treatment benefit, like the clinical trial, but a definite benefit was observed among the high-risk groups. Thus, what appeared to be a contradiction at first was due to a difference in the populations being studied.

Definition of best evidence

While both the clinical trial and meta-analysis are perceived as being the best forms of evidence, because of their methodological design focusing on the intervention of interest and avoidance of biases, it is important to remember that, in the best of all possible worlds, a clinical trial is always likely to be more convincing than the truth. People who consent to take part in a clinical trial are likely to be different from those who do not, and because this is an experiment, they are more likely to be compliant in undertaking their assigned treatment.

HEALTH EDUCATION AND PROMOTION

As well as doing the best for patients with disease (effective interventions), medical students and doctors in the 21st century need to understand the principles of disease prevention and the natural history of diseases to effectively practise the art of clinical medicine. An important role for doctors (and all health professionals) is in providing patients with information and support that enables them to make appropriate choices for either staying healthy or to be restored to an approximation of their previous state of health. Choices for making changes in behaviour and lifestyle may be necessary. It must, however, be remembered that the decision to make changes is for the patient to make, and their ability to change depends not only on their motivation and their individual skills, but also on their environment. However well motivated an individual is, it is more difficult to follow a healthy lifestyle if they have an inadequate income, poor housing and work in a dangerous environment. The aim in providing health education is to help people to understand what is at stake and take control over decisions that affect their health, not simply providing information and expecting a change in behaviour.

Clinical medicine concerns the understanding of how a disease progresses and how best to treat a person who has already developed the disease, whereas epidemiology tries to identify the factors that contribute to the development of the disease, its causes, and how to prevent it. Epidemiology also addresses the likely consequences of a disease process, the complications, in order to understand how these may be avoided or minimised for people who have developed the condition. Thus, prevention is about reducing the risk of disease, illness, injury or disability. Services include immunisation and screening, preventive health education, such as advice about sensible drinking, and preventive health protection, such as legislation for compulsory car seat belts, taxing tobacco and fluoridating water.

HEALTH EDUCATION

Agencies involved in health education include government, schools, local health promotion units and the media. For the doctor, the areas in which health education is most likely to be relevant are where there is evidence from epidemiological studies that particular diseases can be avoided, that the risk of developing a condition in a particular individual may be reduced, or that the risk of complications in a particular disease can be reduced by a particular action.

Approaches to health education

Three approaches to health education are often described:

- Disease orientated
- Risk-factor orientated
- Health orientated.

In disease-orientated health education there is a focus on a particular disease, e.g. cardiovascular disease, and the action is focused on the risk factors, e.g. providing dietary advice. There is often an overlap in risk factors for many types of disease (e.g. smoking for coronary heart disease and lung cancer) in this approach, and it reflects the perspective of the healthcare provider. The expert (the doctor) focuses on an area of expertise (disease) and imparts information to the patient. This focus also emphasises the prevention of disease rather than promotion of health. An alternative approach is to focus attention and action on risk factors rather than on the associated disease; for example, focusing on smoking as a risk factor for carcinoma of the lung and coronary heart disease. This process recognises that single risk factors can be linked to more than one disease and therefore there is less duplication. But the approach is still from the expert's perspective and the emphasis is again on disease prevention rather than health promotion.

The health-orientated approach focuses attention and action on behaviours that contribute to positive health and prevent ill-health. For example, it can be pointed out that a healthy diet can be enjoyable, contributing to well-being in a positive way rather than just being a way of preventing diseases. On any occasion when there is interaction and communication with patients, some, or all, of the above approaches may be called into play.

Strategies for disease prevention and health promotion

There are two possible strategies for disease prevention and health promotion. The population strategy aims to reduce the risk of the whole population, usually by public health measures. The high-risk strategy focuses on the individual who is considered to be at high risk.

Population strategies

The rationale behind the population strategy is that the bulk of the morbidity and mortality of a disease in a population is contributed by those who have a moderate degree of risk. For example, the British Regional Heart Study about 'Who dies in a heart attack?' published in 1995 found that 60% of middle-aged British men have elevated total cholesterol levels, which carries at least a two-fold risk of major coronary heart disease. Only one-third of all the heart attacks, however, occur in the 20% of men with the highest level of cholesterol. The most effective way, therefore, of reducing morbidity and mortality from heart disease would be to lower the population mean cholesterol level, thus reducing the risk of the majority. In the case of cholesterol this would be mainly by dietary means, by reducing the proportion of calories from saturated fat. This is most likely to be achieved by public health measures such as general health education, food and pricing policy, labelling of foods and so on.

Another example of a population strategy is the reduction of alcohol-related morbidity and mortality. Reducing the number of people drinking at moderate risk levels (14–35 units/week in women and 21–50 units/week in men) would have a greater effect than identifying and offering treatment to those drinking at harmful levels (>35 units/week for women; >50 units/week for men).

High-risk strategy

While public health measures – dietary recommendations, raising the taxes on cigarettes and alcohol – are the most effective population strategies at a national level, the high-risk individual approach comes more naturally to the clinician. This approach aims to identify and treat individuals with a high risk of developing a disease (e.g. those with familial hypercholesterolaemia, individuals with high alcohol consumption). A combination of these two approaches is often the case, so that 'healthy eating' advice is given to everybody (through the media, schools and in primary care) together with screening and, when indicated, specific treatment (e.g. with lipid-lowering drugs) of those at particularly high risk. Statins, for example, have been estimated to save about 7000 lives annually in the UK.

Two concepts of 'risk'

A risk factor may be thought of as a factor that has been shown to have a **causal** association with a disease. For example:

- Cigarette smoking has a strong causal association with lung cancer (see above). Reducing this risk, by quitting smoking, reduces the 'risk 'of this individual developing lung cancer.

Alternatively, characteristics of an individual that may be **prognostic** markers for an increased likelihood to develop a disease are 'risk' factors that identify a person as being at high 'risk' for a disease.

- A middle-aged man who leads a sedentary life, is overweight, has a family history of coronary heart disease and smokes 30 cigarettes a day has a higher risk of coronary heart disease than a woman of similar age, but with none of the other characteristics. These factors, or a combination of factors, could be used for screening to identify individuals who would or would not have a coronary event within the next 5 years.

These two concepts of 'risk' should not be confused, nor are they interchangeable. Some risks, e.g. tobacco smoking, alcohol consumption, are modifiable, whereas others, e.g. genetic makeup, age, sex, are not modifiable.

Essentials for effective health education

Health education involves exchanging (not just giving) information between patient and doctor. This means that there must be good and effective communication between the patient and the person involved in providing health education. Effective communication – using the skills of active listening, open questioning and picking up verbal and non-verbal cues – is essential. Tuckett in 1985 provided evidence that patients' recall of information given during a consultation is significantly improved if some simple rules are followed. When talking to

patients about health education information and giving advice on healthcare, the following checklist could be helpful:

- Find out what the patient already knows (may be inaccurate)
- Use short words and short sentences
- Organise the information into clear categories
- Give instructions and advice early in the interview
- Stress the importance of the advice and the instructions you give
- Check patient understanding
- Repeat the advice during the course of the interview
- Give specific advice.

Besides using good communication skills, it is essential when giving information to ensure that there is an exchange of information and ideas between patient and educator. A **health education interview** can be conveniently divided into four phases:

- **Elicit** the person's health beliefs.
- **Information phase**: this is a two-way process with the educator seeking information from the patient and at the same time providing information.
- **Negotiating phase**: if the patient decides to make a change, an achievable and realistic target must be discussed, choices offered and action agreed. The desirability for continued support is then discussed.
- **Promote change**: ways of promoting change include support from family and friends, ways in which the individual recognises the achievement by rewarding him/herself, and perhaps general changes in lifestyle.

Studies have shown that reinforcing the verbal advice with appropriate written material helps the patient to retain information and make choices. Health education resources, such as leaflets and DVDs, are usually available from local health promotion units.

Ethical considerations in prevention and health promotion

A detailed discussion of the ethics of prevention is beyond the scope of this chapter. Remember that in prevention, just as in the treatment of disease, we have a duty to:

- Ensure that the benefit of any procedure outweighs any possible harm to the patient
- Respect the patient's autonomy
- Distribute our resources fairly.

Furthermore, as will be seen from the section on screening, identifying people as being 'at risk' of a condition when there is no effective treatment for the condition is unethical. It is extremely important to follow these basic ethical principles in preventive activities when it is usually the health professional, rather than the patient, who initiates the activity.

Case scenario: a new diagnosis of diabetes

Mr Tate comes to see you, highly embarrassed because of an itchy rash around his genitalia, which turns out to be *Candida* infection. He is aged 51, married, with a daughter at university and a son in his final year at secondary school. He has worked in a warehouse since his early 20s. You find that he has developed type 2 diabetes with no detectable complications; he is moderately obese with a body mass index (BMI) of 32 (see Ch. 16), although his blood pressure is normal. His fasting cholesterol is raised at 6.8 mmol/L (desirable <5.2 mmol/L) with triglycerides of 2.8 mmol/L (desirable <2.3 mmol/L). He does not smoke, and only drinks moderately on social occasions. You decide to try him on diet alone for glycaemic control.

Elicit the person's health beliefs

You discover that Mr Tate's mother died of a heart attack when she was 64 years old, and she was diabetic. On enquiry, he tells you that he thinks diabetes is something to do with sugar in the blood. His mother had taken tablets for her sugar for many years, but from about her mid-50s she had high blood pressure and trouble with her eyesight. You find that he is very anxious and upset about the diagnosis of diabetes, afraid that he might also have a heart attack or lose his eyesight.

Information phase

You ask if Mr Tate knows how his mother managed her medication and if he understands how they worked. He tells you that he had no idea of how she really managed her condition other than having to take different sorts of tablets, and he is worried that the tablets may not be effective.

Explanation of the diagnosis

You explain to Mr Tate that he is correct to think that diabetes is to do with sugar in the blood. It is characterised by persistently high levels, which can lead to complications by damaging other organs in the body. This is caused by a relative deficiency of, or resistance to, insulin, the hormone that regulates sugar metabolism. Diabetes also runs in families. Much of the longer-term complications of diabetes is related to the increased risk of atherosclerosis leading to hardening and narrowing of relatively large (macrovascular disease) and very small (microvascular disease) arteries. These in turn could result in coronary heart disease (macrovascular) and damage to the vessels in the eye (diabetic retinopathy, microvascular) as may have happened to Mr Tate's mother. There is also a risk of damage to kidney tissues, which could lead to high blood pressure. Mr Tate has normal blood pressure, which is very good news.

Information

It is, however, important to remember that these complications can be avoided, or at least minimised, by keeping the blood sugar levels within normal limits and keeping a very close eye on Mr Tate's blood pressure. The type of diabetes that Mr Tate has is known as non-insulin dependent and can be treated with diet alone, or medication to lower his sugar levels. He does not smoke, which is another risk factor for heart disease and high blood pressure, and only drinks alcohol (a risk factor for hypertension) occasionally in moderation, although his cholesterol is a little high. It may only be necessary, therefore, to use dietary control to get his weight down, to keep his blood sugar within normal limits and to bring his cholesterol down to desirable levels.

Negotiating phase

You ask Mr Tate to describe the meals that he takes on an average day. He has always had a good cooked breakfast as his work is physically quite hard. His wife usually cooks bacon and two eggs, sometimes with a sausage or two, and of course toast and marmalade. She also does a packed lunch of three rounds of sandwiches, usually with cold meat of some sort and a large flask of sweet tea to keep his energy up. The evening meal is usually meat with two vegetables, although lately she has taken to grilling the meat and using 'oven chips' instead of frying, which is supposed to be less fattening. She makes a dessert only for lunch on Sundays since the children have grown up, and she is trying to lose a bit of weight herself. He tells you that they have only full cream milk in the house as he dislikes semi-skimmed milk.

Information

You tell Mr Tate that the main principles of healthy diet for diabetes include:

- Low sugar intake (although not sugar free), sugar-free drinks.
- High intake of starchy carbohydrates (up to 50% of total energy) which are slowly absorbed, e.g. pasta, long-grain rice, wholemeal bread, cereals such as oats, pulses, fruit.
- High intake of dietary fibre, to include five portions of fruit and vegetables per day. This helps to smooth the post-prandial peaks in blood glucose.
- Low intake of dietary fat, particularly saturated fat.

Mr Tate should try to reduce salt intake and avoid special 'diabetic' food, which may be expensive and is not of any real benefit. You also refer him to a specialist dietitian for further advice, and draw his attention to the website for Diabetes UK, advising him that they have excellent information on diabetes. He should also see the nurse for monitoring his blood glucose and weight, and be taught how to monitor his sugar himself. You suggest that Mr Tate should try to lose 0.5 kg per week until you see him again.

You understand that there is a great deal to take in, and think about. Mr Tate wants to discuss all this with his wife, and also talk to his daughter, who is studying nutrition at university. You arrange to see him again in 4 weeks.

Promoting change

Mr Tate comes with his wife on the next appointment. You are very interested in how he is getting on. He tells you that the nurse has weighed him, he has lost 3 kg, his sugar is normal and so is his blood pressure. He is learning to keep a diary for self-monitoring. You congratulate him, and enquire how he is getting on, and is his wife also coping. Mrs Tate had been to see the dietitian with her husband, and they later talked over the difficulties of changing their eating habits with their daughter. Breakfast now consists of porridge (oats) and fruit, and only skimmed milk is used in the house. Lunch is two sandwiches, but made with wholemeal bread and a low-fat spread, and tea with no sugar, and also an apple and a banana. They have reduced their intake of red meat to twice per week, with more fish and chicken. Although they are finding it very hard to give up butter, most of the cooking is done with oil. It is taking a little time to get used to this, but they are getting there. The most difficult part has been with shopping, as the labels on the supermarket shelves are confusing about food values. Mrs Tate produced some food labels and asks your advice. You are very pleased to advise her (see Ch. 16).

PREVENTION

Preventive measures can be taken at different stages of a disease, often classified as **primary**, **secondary** or **tertiary**. This classification has been criticised on the grounds that it focuses on disease and includes a consideration of treatment, and also that there is no standard definition of the terms primary, secondary and tertiary. For example, the term secondary prevention is sometimes used to describe interventions that aim to prevent re-occurrence of an illness, such as the use of aspirin after myocardial infarction. All classifications draw boundaries that at times seem artificial, but they are useful as long as the reservations are borne in mind; the classification of prevention is no exception to this. Other terms that have been used with reference to prevention are health promotion, health education, health protection, emphasising the dual role of preventing ill health and promoting positive health.

Primary prevention

Primary prevention includes all activities aiming to remove the cause of disease in individuals, or to reduce the susceptibility of the individual to the causative agent. Some are general social or economic measures that may be part of national strategy. The example of the Broad Street pump led to the national public health policy of clean water, thereby removing a major cause for the transmission of infectious diseases. Although a direct link between environmental, social and economic determinants of health and specific diseases is difficult to demonstrate, and may not be amenable to medical intervention, government policies to reduce poverty, improve housing conditions, living standards and nutrition are important strategies for reducing the risk of mortality and morbidity in vulnerable population groups. Current examples of primary prevention are:

- Immunisation programmes
- Legislation by Parliament (e.g. car seat belts) and fiscal policies (e.g. increased taxation of tobacco and alcohol)
- Helping patients to avoid coronary heart disease and to promote their well-being, e.g. providing dietary advice, sensible drinking, how to stop smoking
- Promoting information to patients about the appropriate use of health service resources; for example, giving advice about childhood immunisation, or about influenza vaccination for older people during the winter months.

Immunisation

The discovery of the cowpox vaccine by Edward Jenner in the early 1800s led to the widespread use of vaccination to prevent and eradicate infectious diseases by reducing individuals' susceptibility to the infecting agent. Compulsory vaccination against smallpox was introduced by British governments from the mid-19th century onwards through Acts of Parliament. Although immunisation programmes are taken for granted in developed and developing countries, the original laws were seen as a violation of civil liberty and later changed to voluntary immunisation.

The World Health Organization (WHO) used a strategy of surveillance and containment to control smallpox. Reporting of cases elicited a reward and suspected cases were isolated while known contacts in the previous 2 weeks were traced and vaccinated. WHO declared the world free of smallpox in 1980.

Immunisation is an example of primary prevention where the aim is to eliminate the risk of the infectious disease in the individual occurring through reducing the susceptibility of the whole population. The WHO set out the aims of eliminating polio, diphtheria, tetanus in the newborn, measles and congenital rubella by the year 2000. To achieve this, all children (at least 95%) needed to receive the appropriate vaccine before the age of 2. The European Region was certified free of poliomyelitis in 2002, at which time it had been free of indigenous poliomyelitis for over 3 years. Since then there have been a few minor outbreaks – one in eastern Turkey in 1998, when a 2-year-old unvaccinated boy was paralysed by the virus, and another outbreak of virus imported from India into Tajikstan in 2010, associated with a number of deaths. To sustain Europe's status of being free of indigenous infection, maintenance of immunisation, surveillance and the ability to respond to imported virus are essential. The most recent outbreak was supported with national immunisation days in Tajikstan and neighbouring countries. The best way of ensuring a polio-free Europe would be to reduce the susceptibility of children to poliomyelitis worldwide.

The efficacy of vaccination is shown in Table 7.16, which illustrates the reduction in mortality and incidence of infectious diseases after the introduction of immunisation.

Public perception and immunisation coverage

A combined vaccination for measles, mumps and rubella (MMR) was introduced in 1988, resulting in significant reduction in the incidence of these diseases. Table 7.17 shows the rate of serious complications of these diseases.

In the 1970s, there was a loss of confidence in the whooping cough vaccine, when it was suggested that the vaccine was a significant cause of brain damage. As a result there were three major whooping cough epidemics; there were over 300000 disease notifications, a large number of children were admitted to hospital and an estimated 100 died unnecessarily. More recently, there were concerns over a possible association between the MMR vaccine, autism and bowel

Table 7.16	Mortality and incidence of infectious diseases in the UK before and after introduction of an immunisation policy					
	Last year of no immunisation			**After immunisation**		
Disease	**Year**	**Deaths (all ages)**	**No. of cases**	**Year**	**Deaths (all ages)**	**No. of cases**
Diphtheria	1939	2133	47061	1996	0	12
Tuberculosis	1952	10590	48093	1996	420	5859
Whooping cough	1956	92	92410	1996	2	2387
Tetanus (not notifiable until 1968)	1960	32	?	1996	0	8
Measles	1967	99	460407	1996	0	5613
Congenital rubella syndrome	1971	–	162	1996	–	21
Haemophilus influenzae meningitis	1991	22	417	1996	0	38

Data from Salisbury D, et al. Joint Committee on Vaccination and Immunisation, D Salisbury, M Ramsay, Great Britain: Department of Health, K Noakes. 2006 Immunisation against infectious disease. The Stationery Office, London.

Table 7.17	Serious complications of measles, mumps and rubella	
Disease	**Complication**	**Incidence**
Measles	Ear infection	1 in 20
	Pneumonia/bronchitis	1 in 25
	Convulsion	1 in 200
	Diarrhoea	1 in 6
	Hospital admission	1 in 100
	Meningitis/encephalitis	1 in 1000
	SSPE	1 in 8000 under 2 years
	Death	1 in 2500–5000
Mumps	Painful testicles in older males	1 in 5
	CNS symptoms:	
	• Meningitis/encephalitis	1 in 200
	Pancreatitis	1 in 5000
	Deafness (with full or partial recovery)	1 in 30
	Spontaneous abortion	1 in 25
Rubella	Encephalitis	1 in 6
	Bleeding disorders	1 in 3
	Joint symptoms	
	Spontaneous abortion	
	Congenital rubella syndrome resulting in babies born with:	
	• Deafness	
	• Blindness	
	• Heart problems	
	• Brain damage	
	• Other serious problems	

SSPE, sub-acute sclerosing pan encephalitis (a rare degenerative neurological disorder developing some years after measles infection, causing brain damage and resultant death).
Data from Department of Health 2002 MMR fact sheets 1–4. Crown Copyright.

problems. MMR is given routinely to babies aged between 12 and 15 months, with a pre-school booster to increase coverage and protection. Reports of an association between the measles virus and Crohn disease (a chronic inflammatory bowel disease), and between MMR and autism (associated with intestinal symptoms), has led to widespread public concern over the vaccination policy. While the bulk of the reported evidence is against a causal association in either case, this has not prevented the decision by some parents not to vaccinate their children with MMR, or choosing to have the vaccines given separately, spaced over 1 year.

There is considerable public health concern over the reluctance of parents to allow their children to be vaccinated, or vaccinated on time, because, once immunisation rates fall below 75%, community outbreaks of MMR will occur, along with the serious complications reported in Table 7.17. Across the UK vaccination rates vary from about 90% to below 50% and a rate of over 95% is needed to provide full community immunisation and prevent outbreaks. Rising from a level of a few cases per year, 2012 saw nearly 2000 cases of measles in UK, placing it second in Europe and early in 2013 there was a major outbreak in Wales, the majority in non-immunised children.

Primary prevention of coronary heart disease

The Joint British Societies' evidence-based guideline (JBS 2) on the prevention of cardiovascular disease was published in 2005 and updated guidelines were published through NICE (the National Institute for Health and Care Excellence) in conjunction with the British Hypertension Society (http://guidance.nice.org.uk/CG127) and offers the current best advice on coronary heart disease prevention. Their priorities are to focus on healthy individuals who are at high risk of developing coronary heart disease or other major atherosclerotic disease and they have produced 'Coronary Risk Charts' that can assess the risk of developing coronary heart disease over the next 10 years using information about an individual's gender, age, smoking status, systolic blood pressure and total cholesterol, although these charts are not appropriate for patients with pre-existing major atherosclerotic disease, inherited dyslipidaemia, chronic renal dysfunction or diabetes mellitus, have a first degree relative with middle age coronary vascular disease (CVD) onset, or are of South Asian heritage, who are all at a higher risk of CVD.

High risk strategy for the prevention of coronary heart disease

At every level of risk the total coronary heart disease risk of a diabetic patient is much higher than that of a comparable non-diabetic and separate risk calculators are available for these patients. Where the absolute risk for an individual is judged to be more than 20% over the next 10 years then intensive risk factor modification is recommended including, where appropriate, proven drug therapies. Lifestyle interventions, such as stopping smoking, making healthier food choices and becoming physically active, are particularly important in this context (Table 7.18).

Secondary prevention

Secondary prevention concerns the detection and treatment of disease before symptoms or disordered function develop, or before irreversible organ damage occurs as the consequence of the disease process. The possibility of being able to detect and treat pre-symptomatic disease and thus prevent or at least reduce morbidity and mortality has, in the past, generated considerable enthusiasm.

The finding of hidden morbidity among the people screened at the Peckham (London, UK) pioneer health centre, and the description by Last in 1963, provided the impetus to expand screening activities. Last used epidemiological methods to estimate the expected numbers of individuals with particular conditions within an average general practice and compared these numbers with actual numbers known to the practitioners. Last referred to the diseases being picked up by general practitioners as being only the 'tip of the iceberg'. Screening is perhaps the best example of secondary prevention, with different programmes for detecting disease before symptoms develop, as in population screening strategies in a healthy population, or more targeted screening of populations with a known high risk of disease.

Screening or diagnosis

Screening could be defined as the systematic application of a test (or enquiry) to identify individuals at risk of a specific disorder, who would benefit from further investigation or preventive treatment, among people who have not sought medical advice on account of symptoms of that disorder.

The main difference between screening and diagnosis is that the former is used to assess risk in the healthy population while the latter is normally done for the purpose of establishing

Table 7.18   **Lifestyle and therapy goals for healthy individuals at high risk of coronary heart disease (CHD)**

Definition of a healthy person at high risk of CHD	Absolute risk of 20% or more over 10 years, or over 20% risk if projected to age 60
Lifestyle change goals	Stop smoking; healthy food choices; increased physical activity; achieve ideal weight
Other desirable risk factor changes. If these are not achieved by the lifestyle changes then blood pressure and cholesterol lowering drug therapies should be used	Blood pressure <140/90 mmHg; total cholesterol <5.0 mmol/L; low-density lipoprotein (LDL)-cholesterol <3.0 mmol/L
Other prophylactic drug therapies	Aspirin (75 mg) in treated hypertensive patients and in men at particularly high risk of CHD (in the top 20% of a risk score, or living in the top 25% of regions with the highest CHD mortality rate)
Other actions	Screen close relatives if familial hypercholesterolaemia or other inherited dyslipidaemia is suspected

an actual diagnosis. It follows, therefore, that when a diagnostic test is inexpensive and without risk, it can be offered to everyone, thus screening to select those at high risk is pointless. For example, the 'Guthrie' test is a routine screening test of newborn babies done in the UK on a blood spot card. The test detects high levels of thyroid-stimulating hormone (TSH), an indication of primary hypothyroidism and, if the replacement thyroid hormone T_4 is given within the first few months of life, it will prevent the development of cretinism in those infants.

Clinical versus laboratory diagnosis or screening

In many ways, the 'medical interview' is an enquiry, clinical 'screening' by the doctor, into the likelihood of an individual having a particular condition. The suspicion that there may be a condition is normally prompted by the presence of symptoms and/or signs of disease, which is then confirmed (or refuted) by further investigation with screening or diagnostic tests (Information box 7.27).

Screening strategies

Various screening strategies have been described using confusing definitions such as:

- **Population or mass screening**: this applies to a screening procedure which is offered to a whole population (Information box 7.28).
- **Multiple or multiphasic screening**: this means a variety of screening tests are carried out simultaneously, often adopted by private healthcare organisations offering

Information box 7.27   **Diagnosis of pleural effusion**

A clinical diagnosis of a **pleural effusion** (an excessive amount of fluid in the space between the two connective tissue layers that cover the lungs, the pleura) can be made simply and reliably by being able to distinguish, through clinical examination, a characteristic loud, sharp sound from a soft dull sound when tapping the chest wall and listening through a stethoscope (**auscultatory percussion**).

To confirm the diagnosis of pleural effusion and ascertain its precise cause, a chest radiograph is first performed, which may be considered a **screening** test, to confirm (or refute) the presence, and site, of fluid in the pleural cavity. If the presence of pleural effusion is confirmed, a pleural biopsy, an invasive and technically demanding diagnostic procedure to obtain a sample of fluid and pleural tissue, will be needed for laboratory examination to determine the cause of the effusion, i.e. what type of cells (blood, cancer, bacteria) the fluid might contain, and if there is disease of the pleura.

When a diagnostic procedure is hazardous or expensive, it would be appropriate to limit access to this procedure by identifying, through screening, those at high enough risk of the disorder to justify the hazard and expense of diagnosis.

Information box 7.28   **Examples of 'mass' screening**

Table 7.19 sets out the purpose of population screening.

Ideally, the person or team responsible for the care of the individual should carry out the screening procedure. Any intervention or treatment which is required is then an integral part of the individual's overall care. Screening carried out by a group or organisation which does not have responsibility for the overall care of the individual is an example of the separation of prevention from care and cure.

Table 7.19   **Reasons for mass screening**

	Description	Who benefits
Determining the prevalence of a disorder	Surveillance	Community at large
Keeping an eye on a situation, ready to act if necessary	Monitoring	Community at large
Identifying high risk people early enough to help them	Screening	Individuals
Testing employees' fitness for work (e.g. food handlers)	Occupational testing	Customers/ employers

screening packages. Some national health services have also adopted this policy from time to time.

- **Selective screening** (or targeted screening): this is the offering of a screening procedure to selected groups in a population that are considered to have an increased risk of having the condition, e.g. mammography for women aged over 50 years.
- **Surveillance**: this is the long-term observation of individuals or populations, e.g. developmental screening for pre-school children.
- **Case finding** is the screening of patients already in contact with the health services and is the same as opportunistic screening such as the 'new patient check' in UK general practice. The contact, but not always the screening activity, is usually patient initiated.

Important characteristics of all types of screening are that the person being screened is asymptomatic for the condition being sought and that the procedure is usually initiated by the medical authorities.

Criteria for population screening strategies

Criteria that should be fulfilled before screening for a particular condition is adopted were defined by Wilson and Jungner in 1968, and adopted by the WHO as **principles for screening**. These principles are still applicable today.

- The condition should be an *important health problem*
- The *natural history* of the disease should be adequately understood
- There should be a *recognisable latent* or *early symptomatic stage*
- There should be a *suitable test or examination,* i.e. simple to perform and interpret, acceptable to those taking part, accurate and repeatable, and *sensitive and specific* (see below)
- Treatment started at an early stage should be of more benefit than treatment started at a later stage
- There should be *accepted treatment* for patients with recognised disease. This principle is extremely important, but not always adhered to
- There should be an agreed *policy* on who should receive treatment
- Diagnosis and treatment should be cost-effective
- Case finding should be a continuing process.

Ethical considerations about screening

It behoves all planning and policy-makers to consider each and every one of the Wilson–Jungner criteria for ethical implications before implementing screening programmes. 'Do no harm' is the ethical principle that applies. Some of these will be discussed here.

Screening or early diagnosis resulting in the 'labelling' of a person as being at high risk of developing a disease, or indeed having the disease, can hurt people, especially if there is no known effective intervention to ameliorate the condition. Often only a small proportion of those people screened as being at high risk will go on to develop the disease and so it is important to consider if there is a benefit to early labelling. If an early diagnosis is made, is there available a treatment that will benefit the individual if started early and which will outweigh the negative effects of loss of 'healthy time'?

Research published in 2010 of the UK mammography screening programme suggested that between 2 and 2.5 lives were saved for every over-diagnosed case and it is this study that supports the NHS breast screening programme. A 2013 Cochrane review of breast mammography screening has, however, reported no benefit in lives saved. This latter review suggested that of every 2000 women invited for screening over 10 years, one will avoid dying from breast cancer and 10 healthy women will be treated unnecessarily. The discrepancy between this and previous reported outcomes is explained by the authors by the poorer methodology in studies that show benefit. While it is difficult for clinicians not to be able to give clear messages to their patients it does highlight the importance of having a frank discussion about benefits, harms and uncertainties. False positive (see below) screening tests can only harm, even if further tests prove negative. Macdonald and colleagues in 1984, in a review of the consequences of disease 'labelling', reported a series of studies showing that individuals who were told they had high blood pressure (were hypertensive), and who were not subsequently treated, had higher levels of absenteeism from work. Psychological well-being was also shown to be lower in those with high blood pressure and in those with normal blood pressure (were normotensive) but who had been wrongly labelled, compared with unaware normotensives. The adverse impact of screening on vocational and economic opportunities (e.g. life insurance, mortgages) have also been cited as 'doing harm'.

Screening and diagnostic test characteristics

Ideally, a screening test should select only those people who, on further (diagnostic) testing, are found to have the disease (the diagnostic test should ideally be 100% **sensitive**, with no false positives). All people without the disease should produce a negative screening test (the screening test should be 100% **specific**, with no false negatives). In reality such an ideal test does not exist but sensitivity and specificity (see below) should both be as high as possible for a test to be useful (Table 7.20).

Given that there is no perfect screening test, false positives will inevitably arise. Apart from the psychological harm discussed in the ethical considerations above, the WHO principle that there should be an agreed policy on who should receive treatment is an important one for those who screen false positive. An example of what can go wrong if no agreed policy for people that screen positive is the over-diagnosis of breast cancer in the population screening programme in the UK. Some women had unnecessary mastectomies as the result of false positive findings.

In some cases it may be important to trade sensitivity in favour of specificity (for example, if it is more important to detect as many people as possible who truly do not have the disease (true negatives)) because the available treatment for the disease is particularly toxic, or to trade specificity in favour of sensitivity (for example, if it is more important to detect as many people as possible with the disease (true positives)) because, when treatment is available, lives will be saved.

Screening and diagnostic tests use these factors, in addition to the feasibility, cost and invasiveness of a particular

Table 7.20	Characteristics of screening and diagnostic tests		
Test	**Ideal**	**Purpose**	**Problem**
Screening	High sensitivity (ability to detect true positives). They will, therefore, have a low false-negative error rate (low type II error)	To detect as many people as possible who definitely have the disease (true positives). Ensures that not many true cases are missed. Those screening as negative are very likely not to have the disease. If the test is highly sensitive, it can be used to 'rule out' the diagnosis	Will also include people who do not have the disease (false positives). Further (diagnostic) tests may be needed to deal with a high number of false positives
Diagnosis	High specificity (ability to detect true negatives). They will, therefore, have a low false-positive error rate (low type I error)	To detect as many people as possible who definitely do not have the disease (true negatives). Ensures that not many cases are misdiagnosed, and inappropriately treated. Those screening positive are very likely to have the disease. If the test is highly specific it can be used to 'rule in' the diagnosis	Will also exclude people who do have the disease (false negatives). Prior (screening) tests may be needed to deal with a high number of false negatives

test, to determine the actual test to be used in each particular circumstance. Often they will be used sequentially, screening tests being designed to work best in the asymptomatic population, with diagnostic tests working better in a situation where the disease is more prevalent (in the screen-positive population).

Diagnostic tests and non-dichotomous values

In many branches of medicine, a diagnostic test will often be something that gives a range of values (e.g. biochemical tests, haemoglobin estimates, blood pressure) rather than a dichotomous answer (yes/no). For tests of sensitivity and specificity, a dichotomous (or binary) concept, such as 'true' or 'false' is used. In such cases we need to convert the range into a binary answer by deciding on a **cut-point**. A cut-point is the limits of the range within which normal values lie. Outside of these limits, the value would be deemed 'abnormal', and thus the values can be dichotomised into normal/abnormal. In psychological tests for intelligence, for example, the range of intelligence quotients (IQ) follows a normal distribution curve. The 'cut-point' for normality is 2 standard deviations below the mean, below which the IQ is impaired. As these limits can vary, thus varying the cut-point, what might have been a positive test indicating an actual abnormality may become a false positive (a type I error).

Receiver operating characteristic (ROC) curves were first used during World War I for testing the sensitivity of radar receivers to detect objects such as aircraft. ROC curves are used to plot different levels of sensitivity (to detect something) against the false-positive error rate (1 − specificity) produced by different cut-points in order to decide on the optimum cut-point (Fig. 7.26). The curves can also be used to compare the usefulness of a test between different subgroups, or to compare different tests. The closer the curve approaches the top left-hand corner of the graph the better the test.

Sensitivity and specificity

The **sensitivity** of a screening test (e.g. the cervical screening test) is the ability of a test to identify correctly those individuals who have the disease, as determined by a reference diagnostic test (e.g. cone biopsy), also known as the **gold standard**. It is a measure of the true positive rate, and is also referred

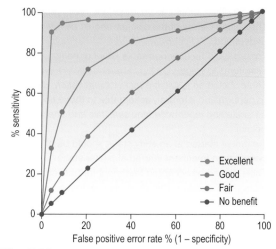

Fig. 7.26 Receiver operating characteristic (ROC) curves.

to as the **detection rate**. A highly sensitive test will have a low false-negative rate (see Information box 7.29). Therefore, a screening test with high sensitivity would suggest that those testing positive are extremely likely to have the condition and should progress to having a diagnostic test.

It is important to understand that the predictive value of a test depends on the prevalence of the disease (i.e. the total number of cases in a population) that is being screened for, unlike sensitivity and specificity. If a disease is common in the population that is being screened, then the proportion of true positives and thus the positive predictive value is greater than when the prevalence is low (see below).

The **specificity** of a screening test is the ability of the test to identify correctly those who do not have the disease. It is a measure of the true-negative rate. A highly specific test will have a low false-positive rate (see Information box 7.29). A screening test with low specificity would give rise to a high rate of false positives, causing alarm and anxiety among those testing positive, and necessitating a great number of additional diagnostic tests on patients without disease. Table 7.21 shows how the results of screening and diagnostic tests can be set out in order to assess their usefulness.

| Information box 7.29 | True and false in screening and diagnostic tests |

When evaluating the characteristics of screening and diagnostic tests, the concepts of 'true' and 'false' refer to whether or not the outcome of the test indicates the presence or absence of the condition or disease that is being tested for:

- True positive: positive test when the disease or condition is present.

- True negative: negative test when the disease or condition is absent.
- False positive: positive test when the disease or condition is absent. Also known in statistics as a type I error.
- False negative: negative test when disease or condition is present. Also known as a type II error.

| Table 7.21 | How to calculate important statistics in screening and diagnosis |

		Condition screened for (as determined by a reference, diagnostic test, the 'Gold standard')		
		Present	**Absent**	
Test result	Positive	True positive	False positive	Positive predictive value
		a	b	a/(a + b)
	Negative	c	d	d/(c + d)
		False negative	True negative	Negative predictive value
		a/(a + c)	d/(b + d)	
		Sensitivity	Specificity	

The other important characteristics of a test are its positive and negative predictive values (Table 7.22). The values are not the same as sensitivity and specificity, although related, because a positive screening test identifies the risk of developing disease, when the disease may not actually be present. It is relevant when you have a test result from your patient and want to determine from that the chance that your patient has, or has not, the disease in question.

- The **positive predictive value** (**PPV**) is the proportion of people with a positive screening test who actually have the disease. Another way that this can be expressed is by the odds of being affected given a positive result (OAPR).
- The **negative predictive value** (**NPV**) is the proportion of people who screen negative and who do not have the disease.

Calculations for evaluating screening and diagnostic tests

Screening and diagnostics tests both identify the likelihood that a condition is present or absent. A diagnostic test, however, must give much more certainty so that a positive test has to identify the presence of a condition with close to 100% certainty, i.e. a sensitivity of 100%, and, equally, if the test were negative, then the specificity should be as close to 100% as possible. In contrast, the performance of screening tests is likely to be less sensitive and less specific, because they can be backed up by diagnostic tests. Because, as outlined above, the predictive value of these tests depends on the prevalence of a condition, the concept of pre-test probability comes into play. **Pre-test probability** is the judgement of the clinician about whether, based on symptoms, signs and personal characteristics such as age, sex, occupation etc., the patient is likely to have a particular disease. If nothing is known about the patient then disease prevalence might be the only clue.

Calculating and evaluating the functions of diagnostic and screening tests follow similar procedures. The following example illustrates how this is done.

Diagnosis of pulmonary embolism

This example for evaluating a diagnostic test for pulmonary embolism (PE, where a thrombus has broken away from its source and lodges in the pulmonary arteries) is taken from an article by Qanadli SD et al., published in the journal *Radiology* in 2000. The authors wanted to see if dual-section helical computed tomography (CT; involves an X-ray tube rotating round the patient to provide a series of cross-sectional images) functioned as well as pulmonary arteriography, the 'gold standard' diagnostic test that diagnosed pulmonary embolism with certainty. PE is a life-threatening condition needing a reliable diagnostic test, but pulmonary arteriography is highly invasive, technically difficult and expensive to perform. The alternative tests were chest radiographs, which are usually normal in PE, or lung scans that are sensitive (high proportion of true positives) but not specific (high proportions of false negatives).

The study was carried out with 157 patients admitted as emergencies with suspected pulmonary embolism. Table 7.22 shows the results of pulmonary arteriography and dual CT scans. Of the 157 patients, 65 tested positive for PE on dual CT scan, of which 59 were positive on pulmonary arteriography ('gold standard'). The disease prevalence in this population was calculated as the proportion of 'disease positives' in the sample (39.5%). Of the 92 patients who were negative on dual CT scanning, 3 were positive on arteriography. The sensitivity, specificity and predictive values can now be calculated to show that the dual CT scan has a:

- Sensitivity of 0.952: the dual CT scan can pick up 95.2% of patients that have PE
- Specificity of 0.937: of the patients who do not have PE, 93.7% will test negative
- Positive predictive value of 0.908, meaning that 90.8% of patients who test positive on dual CT scanning actually have PE
- Negative predictive value of 0.967, meaning that 96.7% of patients testing negative on dual CT scanning do not have PE.

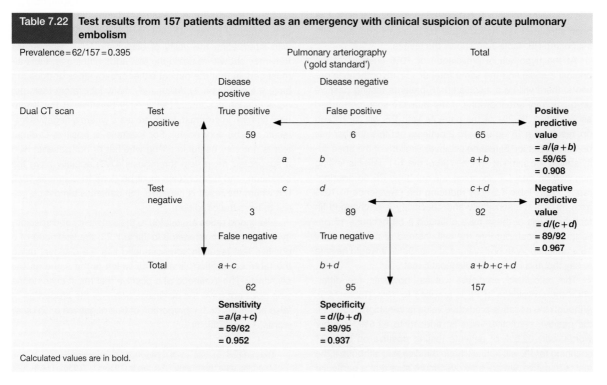

| Table 7.22 | **Test results from 157 patients admitted as an emergency with clinical suspicion of acute pulmonary embolism** |

Prevalence = 62/157 = 0.395

		Pulmonary arteriography ('gold standard')		Total	
		Disease positive	Disease negative		
Dual CT scan	Test positive	True positive	False positive		**Positive predictive value** = a/(a + b) = 59/65 = **0.908**
		59	6	65	
		a	b	a + b	
	Test negative	c	d	c + d	**Negative predictive value** = d/(c + d) = 89/92 = **0.967**
		3	89	92	
		False negative	True negative		
	Total	a + c	b + d	a + b + c + d	
		62	95	157	
		Sensitivity = a/(a + c) = 59/62 = **0.952**	**Specificity** = d/(b + d) = 89/95 = **0.937**		

Calculated values are in bold.

Table 7.23   **Test results from 157 hypothetical patients among whom the prevalence of the condition is only around 10%, instead of about 40% in the previous example (Table 7.22)**

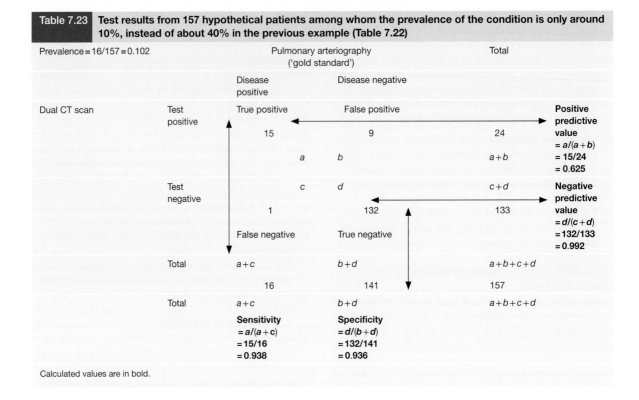

Prevalence = 16/157 = 0.102

		Pulmonary arteriography ('gold standard')		Total
		Disease positive	Disease negative	
Dual CT scan	Test positive	True positive	False positive	**Positive predictive value**
		15	9	24 **= a/(a + b)**
		a	b	a + b **= 15/24**
				= 0.625
	Test negative	c	d	c + d	**Negative predictive value**
		1	132	133 **= d/(c + d)**
		False negative	True negative	**= 132/133**
				= 0.992
Total		a + c	b + d	a + b + c + d
		16	141	157
Total		a + c	b + d	a + b + c + d
		Sensitivity	**Specificity**	
		= a/(a + c)	**= d/(b + d)**	
		= 15/16	**= 132/141**	
		= 0.938	**= 0.936**	

Calculated values are in bold.

The dual helical CT scan can therefore be reliably used to diagnose pulmonary embolism accurately for *patients suspected of PE on clinical grounds,* as examined in this study. The dual CT scan, however, is expensive, and needs an experienced radiologist for interpretation. There are now quicker and cheaper tests, and quicker biochemical tests may be preferred, but will need assessment in an analogous fashion.

The effect of prevalence on sensitivity and predictive values

To show how prevalence affects the functions of diagnostic and screening tests, a hypothetical prevalence of 10% has been attributed to a hypothetical 157 patients admitted with suspected PE. Table 7.23 shows the results.

At the hypothetical prevalence of 10% (instead of the original 39.5%) and the same total of 157 (hypothetical) patients, there will be a calculated 16 patients testing positive on pulmonary arteriography. If the dual CT scan performed as expected, 95.2% of the patients with PE will be picked up, resulting in 15 (actually 15.2 patients but this number has been reduced to 15) testing positive. Similarly, if the specificity stayed the same at 93.7%, 132 of the 141 patients testing negative on dual CT scanning will not have PE on arteriography. From Table 7.23, by reducing the prevalence to 10% from 39.5%, the sensitivity and specificity is unchanged (in fact the levels of these have changed a bit because 15 patients have been put into the cell, instead of an impractical 15.2 patients). With both values at over 90%, it would be safe to say that this is a 'good' diagnostic test.

The calculated predictive values, however, are different if the prevalence of PE is reduced to 10% (Table 7.23). Although the negative predictive value is very high at 99.2%, the positive predictive value is reduced to 62.5%. In other words, only 62.5% of patients testing positive on dual CT scanning for PE will actually have the disease, although if the test is negative, we are now even more sure that a particular patient would not have PE in these particular circumstances of low prevalence.

Likelihood ratios

In relation to screening and diagnostic tests, likelihood ratios (LR) refer to the likelihood of a positive test from a patient with the condition of interest (LRpos), or the likelihood of a negative test from a patient without the condition (LRneg), and obtaining the same result from a patient without, or conversely with, the condition.

Although likelihood ratios are not commonly used, they offer a very simple way of evaluating a test result in the context of a particular patient. Understanding these concepts helps with interpreting the utility of diagnostic tests. Sometimes they may show that doing the test adds nothing and it is almost certain that the patient either already does or does not have the condition. Unfortunately many laboratory tests are done in such circumstances, simply because of the 'litigation' culture. In contrast, there are tests where a negative test result can be very useful. For example, a positive D-dimer test is not very useful in telling whether or not patients with a suspected deep vein thrombosis (DVT) actually have the condition, and further tests must be done to diagnose DVT, but where the result is negative, the patient is almost certain *not* to have the condition.

Likelihood ratios are related to the sensitivity and specificity of a test. With reference to Table 7.23, the likelihood of a positive test result in someone who has the disease, using the table convention, is $a/(a + c)$, which is the same as the sensitivity. The likelihood of a positive test result in someone who does not have the disease is $b/(b + d)$, the proportion of false positives, or 1 − proportion of true negatives or, in other words, 1 − specificity.

Thus LR positive test result = sensitivity/1 − specificity
Using the data from Table 7.23, this is 0.938/(1 − 0.936) = 14.6

We can interpret this by saying that a positive test result is about 14–15 times more likely to be seen in someone with the disease than in one without.

> The LR negative test result = 1 – sensitivity / specificity
> Using the data from Table 7.23, this is $(1 - 0.938) / 0.936 = 0.066$

We can interpret this by saying that a negative test result is 0.066 times more likely to be seen in someone with the disease, than in one without or, in other words, is less likely. As we discussed before when talking about risk and benefit, it might be simpler to invert this figure for easier interpretation: $1/0.066 = 15.2$ can be interpreted as a negative result being about 15 times more likely to be seen in someone *without* the disease, than in someone with.

In addition to the diagnostic test that has been performed, the clinical examination of the patient, or simply knowledge of the prevalence of the condition in your setting, will provide an idea of how likely it is that the patient has the condition (the pre-test odds) before you do any diagnostic tests. Putting these two pieces of information together – the usefulness of the diagnostic test and your best clinical assessment – produces a better estimate of whether or not your patient has the condition (the post-test odds). The calculation is simple:

> Post-test odds (of having the condition) = Pre-test odds
> (clinical odds of having the condition) × LRpos (likelihood
> ratio of a positive test)

Many people prefer to think in terms of 'probability' of a condition, instead of 'odds'. Although they are mathematically linked it is easier to use a nomogram (Fig. 7.27) to determine the post-test probability after seeing your patient and doing a test.

Evaluating a diagnostic test

If a diagnostic test is to prove itself, it must be assessed against the 'truth', and undertaken without knowledge of that truth, avoiding the problems of conscious and unconscious bias. Knowing the truth is, of course, problematic, but we aim in clinical diagnosis to get as close as possible to the truth by direct examination of the gross and cellular pathology with the use of autopsy or biopsy. The former can only be done after the patient has died and so evaluation in this way can be severely delayed. Biopsy, where tissues are taken for microscopic examination by a pathologist, is inevitably an invasive process and its use in the evaluation of screening tests (see below, breast cancer screening example) can be problematic. Sometimes a 'reference' standard may be developed. We call these various standards 'gold' standards. Whatever method is used to provide the truth, we must be sure of its validity, as this is the measure against which we will assess the diagnostic test – how gold is gold?

The 'truth' derived from any gold standard can only be as good as the reference standard, or those individuals who may interpret the results of any autopsy or biopsy. Two individuals may agree in their interpretation and be correct (reliable), or both be incorrect (unreliable), or differ from each other (inter-observer variation). A single individual who repeats the examination, without knowledge of the repetition, may disagree with the original interpretation (intra-observer variation). For example, in a study of interpretation of chest radiographs for progression of tuberculosis, Yerushalmy and colleagues in 1950 showed that pairs of individuals

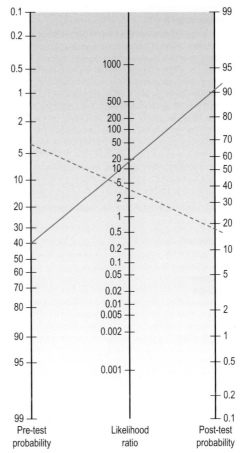

Fig. 7.27 **Updating a diagnostic test result with clinical information.** Using this diagram we can draw a straight line between the pre-test probability (clinical assessment or prevalence) of a condition, through the LRpos point, in order to assess the post-test probability. Using the example in the text, which had a LRpos of about 15 for the computed tomography (CT) scan test and considering that the patients being admitted had a pre-test probability (prevalence in this example) of PE of 40%, the fact that this patient had a positive test result would result in a post-test probability of PE of over 90%, converting doubt into almost certainty, shown by the *solid line*. It will be clear from this diagram that, depending on the LRpos value of the test, and the prevalence of the condition (the pre-test probability), finding a positive test result may not result in any significant change in opinion. A hypothetical example is shown by the *dashed line* where doing the test and getting a positive result has increased the chance that the patient has the condition by less than 5%. In these circumstances doing a test is often a waste of resources.

frequently disagreed, and individuals disagreed with their own interpretation almost as frequently.

Measuring clinical agreement

It is possible for two examinations to be interpreted in the same way just by chance alone and so we need to know how good the agreement is beyond chance. This is measured by 'kappa' (see Information box 7.30). Kappa levels are often disappointingly low. For example, an article published in 2002 by Speciale et al. on the assessment of lumbar spine stenosis into categories of normal, mild, moderate or severe stenosis, reported an average inter-observer kappa of only

---

Information box 7.30 **The kappa statistic**

Suppose two radiologists are asked to review radiographs from 100 patients and decide whether there were degenerative changes in the lower spine. In 60 patients, they agreed that there were no changes, and in another 20 they agreed that degenerative changes were present. They disagreed about the changes in the other 20 and their observations (fictitious data) are recorded in Table 7.24.

The radiologists agreed about 80% $(20 + 60)/100$ of their patients, as shown in cells 'a' and 'd'. But some of this agreement could just be due to chance. What would happen if the radiologists were to each toss a coin and record that outcome instead? If we applied the χ^2 test, we can calculate what each cell would be expected to contain by chance alone, assuming the totals were to remain the same (which they would because the average totals reflect the prevalence of the condition in the population).

Expected value = row total × column total / overall total

These expected values are shown in parentheses in the table. The agreement by chance is:

$(8.91 + 48.91)/100 = 57.82\%$

The actual agreement beyond chance is:

80 − 57.82 = 22.18%

The potential further agreement beyond chance is:

100 − 57.82 = 42.18%

Kappa is the ratio of the actual agreement beyond chance and potential further agreement beyond chance:

22.18/42.18 = 53%

Kappa values have been given qualitative labels according to the ranges:
- 0–20% – slight agreement
- 20–40% – fair agreement
- 40–60% – moderate agreement
- 60–80% – substantial agreement
- 80–100% – almost perfect agreement.

Table 7.24 **Observations of lower spine degenerative changes by two radiologists**

		Radiologist 1 (first observation)		Total
		Present	**Absent**	
Radiologist 2 (second observation)	Present	20 (8.91)	13 (24.09)	33
		a	*b*	*a+b*
	Absent	*c*	*d*	*c+d*
		7 (18.09)	60 (48.91)	67
	Total	*a+c*	*b+d*	*a+b+c+d*
		27	73	100

Expected values in brackets.

26%, and intra-observer kappa of 11%, although they were increased when the scales were combined to produce just two categories (to 33% and 43%, respectively), or when the observers were particularly experienced (to 32%), or in particular occupational groups (radiologists to 40%).

The surgical management of lumbar spine stenosis, by decompression, can produce excellent results in many patients, but a substantial number of those who seem to be good candidates do not benefit. Magnetic resonance imaging (MRI) has become the gold standard for evaluating lumbar spine stenosis, but, with poor agreement between observers about the extent of the problem, it may be that there is significant misdiagnosis and inadequate surgical decompression, resulting in a poorer than expected prognosis. Information box 7.31 provides a summary of strategies, suggested by Sackett et al. in *Clinical Epidemiology*, to reduce clinical disagreement.

Consider the prevalence of disease

A second important consideration when evaluating a diagnostic test is to make sure it has been used in a patient sample that contains the same spectrum of disease that would be found within the population of interest. The population of interest will, for example, be different between primary care and secondary care because the prevalence of the condition will be different. For example, a particular test for myocardial infarction that works well in patients admitted to hospital with chest pain, e.g. electrocardiogram (ECG) (where

---

Information box 7.31 **Six strategies for preventing or minimising clinical disagreement**

- Match the diagnostic environment to the diagnostic task.
- Seek collaboration of key findings:
  - Repeat key elements of your examination
  - Corroborate important findings with documents and witnesses
  - Confirm key clinical findings with appropriate tests
  - Ask 'blinded' colleagues to examine your patients.
- Report evidence as well as inference, making a clear distinction between the two.
- Use appropriate technical aids.
- 'Blind' your assessments of raw diagnostic test data.
- Apply the social sciences, as well as the biological sciences, of medicine.

---

the proportion of patients experiencing chest pain due to a myocardial infarction is likely to be high), may be completely useless within the setting of general practice (where the proportion of patients experiencing chest pain due to a myocardial infarction is likely to be very low). Prevalence affects the predictive value of the diagnostic test (see above).

Clinical suspicion: pre-test probability

A diagnostic test may readily distinguish between people that definitely do, or do not have, the disease, and may in fact be a biochemical test that does no better than consideration of a patient's signs and symptoms. A test will only be useful if it can discriminate in cases where there is some doubt about the clinical diagnosis, in the spectrum between these two extremes. For example, many conditions may exhibit symptoms of irritability, anxiety, trembling and sweating. These are also symptoms of mild hyperthyroidism (thyroid overactivity, also called thyrotoxicosis). In hyperthyroidism, measurement of the level of thyroid-stimulating hormone (TSH) can be a very useful diagnostic test as it is normally low in this condition (see Ch. 10).

Harming the patient

If the gold standard test is invasive, involving a risky clinical procedure, there may be some reluctance on the part of the evaluators of the test to submit all their patients to both tests. Nevertheless, the evaluation depends on both assessments being made in every case. An alternative has been proposed in order to rule out the disease that involves the absence of any adverse health outcome in a patient after long-term follow-up without that patient being treated for the condition.

Consistency of findings

Finally, as in all situations, a finding may be due to chance alone and it is important always to be able to evaluate the performance of a test in a second, independent, group of patients.

Screening for breast cancer

In the UK, there is a free, 3-yearly national breast screening programme for women aged between 50 and 64. Policies for the secondary prevention of breast cancer vary in developed countries, depending mainly on the way that health services are funded.

Case scenario: how effective is breast screening?

You are a general practitioner in the UK. Mrs A has just passed her fiftieth birthday, and was invited to attend the local unit for mammography screening. She comes to see you because although she has a general idea of what mammography is for (the letter inviting her to attend explained the procedures (the test involves a small dose of X-rays) and the reasons for screening), she is undecided about whether or not to attend. She is perfectly well in herself, has no history of breast cancer, and is not aware that anyone in her family has suffered from breast cancer. She wants to know what benefits and harms there are of having a mammogram in order to balance these against the inconvenience and discomfort.

There are several questions and other matters that both the patient and clinician might want to consider in this context (Wilson–Jungner criteria, see above). An example is discussed below that uses some historic data for illustration of how the consultation might proceed.

How effective is breast cancer screening for preventing death from breast cancer?

Breast cancer is the leading cause of death from malignant neoplasm for women in England. The national screening programme aims to reduce deaths from breast cancer. Mammography screening is the most effective tool for the early detection of cancer at a stage when effective treatment is possible. Combined mortality data from various developed countries worldwide, from randomised controlled and case–control studies over 7–12 years, published by Blamey et al. in 2000, showed that breast screening reduced deaths

from cancer, and was most effective in the over-50 age group, suggesting that the reduction in the screened population could be up to 29%.

Will the X-rays be harmful, as the screening test has to be repeated every 3 years?

There is a minute possibility (if 2 million women aged over 50 were screened, there might be one extra cancer after 10 years) of the radiation causing cancer, which is far outweighed by the incidence of 2000 cases per million women aged 60.

Is the test acceptable?

There is evidence to show that psychological problems such as anxiety are not associated with invitation and attendance for mammography, but awaiting the results could be anxiety provoking.

What happens after the mammogram? How accurate is mammography at early diagnosis of cancer?

Mammography is a screening test which detects abnormalities including cancer. However, the sensitivity and specificity of the test is not known, because they are not directly measured. The gold standard for mammography is breast biopsy, a painful, hazardous procedure. It would be ethically unacceptable to subject women with normal mammograms to breast biopsy.

From data from all the basic or first screening tests (**prevalent screening**) performed in the UK in 1997–8, 8.3% (23 637/286 184) were reported as abnormal in a publication in 2000 (Table 7.25). Those women with abnormal mammograms are recalled for repeat screening (**incident screening**), and about two-thirds will be shown to be negative after further mammography or ultrasound scan. The remaining third who are still positive on the retest will then be referred for clinical assessment and fine needle aspiration or core needle biopsy.

In 1997–8, a total of 1800 (1800/23 637 testing positive on the first test = 7.6%) were diagnosed with breast cancer (Table 7.25). We refer to the 7.6% as the positive predictive value (PPV). About 8 (7.6) women in 100 with an initial positive mammogram will end up being diagnosed with breast cancer. Thus the PPV is also referred to as the 'odds of being affected given a positive result, OAPR'. Even if the repeat screening is positive (one-third of 23 637 = 7879) of which 1800 will be diagnosed with breast cancer, the positive predictive value is still below 50% (1800/7879 = 22.8%), meaning that even if a woman has two positive screening tests it is still more likely that she does *not* have breast cancer.

Table 7.25	Results from a UK breast screening programme in women aged 50–64 (1998–9), first screening
No. of women screened	286 184
No. of women referred	23 637 (8.3%)
No. of cancers detected	1800
Cancer detection rate	6.29 per 1000
Positive predictive value (%)	7.6

Data from Blanks RG, Moss SM, Patnick J 2000 Results from the UK NHS breast screening programme 1994–1999. Journal of Medical Screening 7:195–198.

Tertiary prevention

Tertiary prevention is the monitoring and management of established disease in order to prevent disability or handicap. In many ways, the practice of medicine, whether managing chronic or acute episodic conditions, could be thought of as tertiary prevention. In a person who presents with symptoms of coronary heart disease – stable angina (chest pain ranging from a central mild ache to a severe pain that may radiate to the jaw and/or arms and may cause sweating and breathlessness, often provoked by exertion), unstable angina (recent onset severe angina, worsening angina or angina at rest), or acute myocardial infarction (a thrombotic occlusion of one of the heart blood vessels resulting in loss of blood and therefore of oxygen delivery to a significant area of heart muscle) – the aim of treatment would be to slow the progression of coronary artery disease, if possible, to induce disease regression, and to reduce the risk of thrombotic complications. As a result it is hoped that, not only will the risk of a further non-fatal or fatal event be reduced, but the patient will also have a better quality of life and longer life expectancy. Here, knowledge of the effectiveness of diagnosis and treatment discussed above is essential for good clinical practice.

Components for tertiary healthcare delivery

Components for effective tertiary healthcare delivery have been formulated. For example, cardiac rehabilitation programmes are evolving to include a wide range of activities, therapies, lifestyle changes, psychologies and networks supported by a multidisciplinary team of healthcare professionals, integrated between hospitals and the community (Table 7.26). The WHO has defined such a programme (Needs and priorities in cardiac rehabilitation and secondary prevention in patients with coronary heart disease. WHO Technical Report Series 831, Geneva, 1993) as:

The rehabilitation of cardiac patients is the sum of activities required to influence favourably the underlying cause of the disease, as well as the best possible physical, mental and social conditions, so that they may, by their own efforts, preserve or resume when lost, as normal a place as possible in the community. Rehabilitation cannot be regarded as an isolated form of therapy but must be integrated with the whole treatment of which it forms only one facet.

These components are essential for delivering the best care for any patient after any acute, major event.

Evidence-based medicine

Central to the practice of medicine as an art based in science is the integration of individual clinical expertise and the best external evidence. Clinical expertise is built on basic clinical skills, then derived from experience, and expressed as judgement (**clinical acumen**). Making clinical judgements is about the skill to make the best clinical decision for the patient, and to help the patient to make choices about their treatment. There are many components to the process of making clinical decisions. Some have good external scientific evidence in support. Of importance to how we present choices to the individual patient are her/his personal circumstances, social, psychological and educational background and, to some extent, public policy.

The best available external evidence is clinically relevant research. This covers the accuracy of diagnostic and screening tests, identifying risk factors and prognostic markers, and evaluating the efficacy and safety of therapeutic, preventative and rehabilitative interventions. The 'evidence' in support of evidence-based medicine is mostly

Table 7.26	Main components of a cardiac prevention and rehabilitation programme*	
Component	**Activity**
Lifestyle and cardiovascular risk assessment	Assessment of: smoking, diet, physical activity, blood pressure and lipid levels. Integration of all these factors is needed to shape a programme according to the particular needs of the individual
Educational	Education about: the disease, its causes, how causes can be modified, medical and surgical treatments and resuscitation. Education is provided to patients and their families
Behavioural	Behavioural 'stages of change': preparation – preparing and advising change; action – assisting change; maintenance – providing follow-up. Done in partnership with patient and doctor and tailored to the needs and level of understanding of the patient
Health promotion	Promoting a healthy lifestyle: avoiding tobacco, making healthy food choices, becoming physically active
Family-based intervention	Assisting the patient by the family or partner: being tobacco free, participating in healthy diet changes, supporting leisure time exercise in the household, participating in programmes that address psychosocial and sexual problems
Risk factor management	Monitoring: weight, blood pressure, lipids, blood glucose. The monitoring is used to set goals, suggest lifestyle changes and introduce drug therapies as necessary
Drug therapies and compliance	Ensuring that: treatment and dose are the most appropriate, according to the best available evidence. The importance of sustained therapies should be emphasised with the patient
Psychology	Emotional response to development of disease by: stress management and relaxation
Screening of first degree blood relatives	In patients with premature disease (men under 55 and women under 65) screening of: parents, siblings and offspring (over 13) for blood pressure, lipids and glucose
Vocational	Advice on: preparations for return to work, seeking alternative work, driving licence considerations
Quality assurance	Audit of, for example: which patients take up and adhere to the programme, the quality and accessibility of information provided to the patients, the ability of the programme to make changes in factors such as blood pressure and cholesterol. Audit of a programme is necessary for any programme to evolve and improve in order to achieve the stated objectives

* Information taken from 1998 Prevention of coronary heart disease in clinical practice. Recommendations of the Second Joint Task Force of European and other Societies on Coronary Prevention. European Heart Journal 19:1434–1503.

quantitative, in the form of RCTs, emphasising the quantifiable and measurable aspects of medical practice. In the real-life situation, there may be areas of clinical uncertainty. The less easily measured factors that influence clinical decisions, such as the psychological and social condition of the patient, and the patient's own concerns and expectations are equally, or more, important and only to be ignored at the doctor's peril. It would be worthwhile to reflect upon these aspects and their relevance to the preferences of the patient sitting in front of you.

The epidemiologist, David Sackett, has described the discipline of evidence-based medicine as 'the integration of best research evidence with clinical expertise and patient values'. While much epidemiological research may relate more to an overall strategy for managing a population of patients, for example all people with diabetes, the practice of evidence-based medicine encourages individual learning and fosters important research by the health professional in order to offer the best possible care to the individual patient.

8 The nervous system

Brian Pentland

Introduction	**337**
Embryology	**337**
Gross anatomy	**339**
Central nervous system	339
Peripheral nervous system	345
Meninges	349
The ventricular system	**351**
Cells of the nervous system	**352**
Blood supply to the brain and brain metabolism	**353**
Arterial blood supply	353
Blood–brain barrier	355
Metabolic requirements of the brain	356
Transmission of neural signals	**356**
Action potentials	356
Synapses	358
Neurotransmission	359
Motor control and pathways	**364**
Motor cortex	365
Brainstem	365
Spinal cord	367
Cranial nerve reflexes	369
Cerebellum	369

Basal ganglia	372
Eye movements	373
Sensory systems	**375**
Special senses	**381**
Vision	381
Vestibular system	386
Auditory system	388
Smell	392
Taste	392
Central autonomic networks	**392**
Examples of central autonomic control	394
Consciousness	**395**
Sleep and wakefulness	**395**
Emotion	**396**
Motivation and goal-directed behaviours	**398**
Higher cortical functions	**399**
Cognition	399
Memory	399
Attention	401
Agnosias	401
Apraxias	401
Language	401
Brain death	**402**

INTRODUCTION

The nervous system detects details about the external and internal environments, processes them and determines behaviour and controls body activities. Sensory information is carried to the brain from specialised receptors in the skin, muscles and joints; from special sense organs (for vision, hearing, smell and taste); and from visceral receptors in internal organs (e.g. gut and bladder). The incoming data are integrated with or modified by other information from related areas and, after processing, the brain then sends signals to excitable cells in skeletal muscles, internal organs (e.g. heart and lungs) and glands.

The nervous system is anatomically divided into:

- **Central nervous system**: consisting of the brain and spinal cord
- **Peripheral nervous system**: this is further divided into:
  - **Somatic nervous system**: sensory and motor supply to skin, muscles and joints
  - **Autonomic nervous system**: supplies smooth muscles, glands and specialised effector cells (e.g. pacemaker cells in the heart).

EMBRYOLOGY

Embryologically, the nervous system develops from the ectoderm (which also forms the skin). It is an extremely complex system originating from stem cell precursors that differentiate into nerve cells (neurons) and glia. The immature neurons then migrate to their eventual destinations whether in the brain or spinal cord, and form outgrowths of axons. These are then guided towards their postsynaptic partners. Neural development, however, continues after birth and into adulthood, where the nature/nurture mechanisms become important.

Neurodevelopmental mechanisms are either activity (neuronal activity) independent or activity dependent.

- Activity independent mechanisms are thought to be genetically determined (hard wired) and include the differentiation of neurons, neuron migration to target areas, axon growth and guidance toward postsynaptic partners.
- Activity dependent mechanisms occur once the neurons are in place, when neural activity and sensory stimuli mediate the formation of new synapses, synapse plasticity and the development of neural circuits. These activities come into play once the axons reach their postsynaptic targets.

Neurulation

At about the third week of gestation, signals from the mesoderm activate the part of the ectoderm destined for the nervous system to differentiate into neuro-ectoderm, which thickens to form the neural plate. The neural plate develops into the brain and spinal cord (see Fig. 8.1). The neural plate forms a groove, which elongates and grows outwards, then folds and curls into the neural tube, a process known as **neurulation**. The neural tube continues to elongate and has a central neural canal. The folds fuse from about where the embryonic neck would be and proceeds rostrally (forwards towards the head), and caudally (backwards, towards the tail). The ends close off at about the end of the 4th week of gestation. Defects in neurulation can occur at this stage, which could have serious or even fatal consequences (see Clinical box 8.1).

The anterior, or ventral, part of the neural tube is known as the **basal plate**, the posterior or dorsal part the **alar plate** (Fig. 8.2). Cells of the alar and basal plates differentiate into neurons with different functions. In the caudal part of the neural tube designated to become the spinal cord, the alar plates give rise to sensory areas while the basal plates become motor areas. Neurons of the autonomic nervous system originate in the intermediate area between the alar and basal plates. Cell differentiation in the parts designated for the brain is more complex.

Brain development

The neural tube continues to enlarge by elongation and thickening, through proliferation of neurons and connecting structures. The rostral end enlarges to form three primary brain vesicles or swellings:

- The **prosencephalon** which later becomes the forebrain
- The **mesencephalon** becomes midbrain
- The **rhombencephalon** destined for hindbrain.

At about the end of 3 weeks, it flexes at the level of the mesencephalon in the **cephalic flexure** (see Fig. 8.3) and at the end of the 4th week the **cervical flexure** develops between the rhombencephalon and spinal cord.

The optic vesicle (future optic nerve, retina and iris) develops in the basal plate of the prosencephalon.

By the end of 5 weeks of gestation the prosencephalon enlarges to form the **telencephalon** (the future cerebral hemispheres) and the **diencephalon** (see below). The third vesicle, the rhombencephalon, also divides into the **metencephalon**, which becomes the pons and cerebellum, and the **myelencephalon**, which is the future medulla oblongata.

Ventricles

The neural canal develops into the ventricular system of the brain, containing cerebrospinal fluid (CSF). Within the cerebral hemispheres, the neural canal dilates to form the lateral ventricles. The third ventricle forms in the diencephalon, and the fourth ventricle in the rhombencephalon. The ventricles communicate with each other: the pair of lateral ventricles communicate with the third, and the third and fourth ventricles communicate via the cerebral aqueduct (of Sylvius) in the midbrain. CSF leaves the fourth ventricle to enter the spinal canal in the spinal cord.

CSF is secreted by the choroid plexuses formed by invagination of capillaries in the ventricles. Obstruction at any point in the communicating channels between ventricles and the spinal cord would lead to accumulation of CSF within the ventricle increasing CSF pressure, and eventual dilatation of the ventricles: hydrocephalus (see Ventricular system, below).

Spinal cord development

The caudal part of the neural tube becomes the spinal cord. Neuroepithelial cells in the walls differentiate into neuroblasts that form the grey matter, with nerve fibres emerging from them (Fig. 8.4). Cells in the alar plates differentiate into sensory neurons, receiving dorsal nerve roots growing in from the spinal ganglia, while the basal plate cells differentiate into motor neurons that give off the ventral nerve root. The nerve roots also carry autonomic fibres from autonomic neurons that lie in between the alar and basal plates. The dorsal and

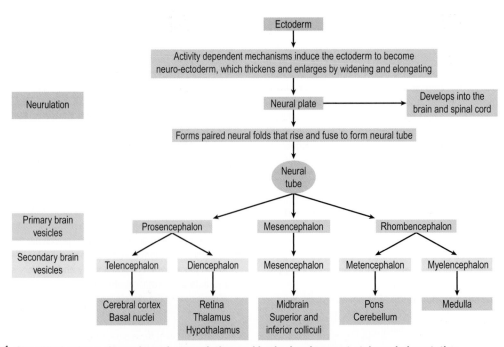

Fig. 8.1 Simplified scheme for embryonic neurulation and brain development at 4 weeks' gestation.

Clinical box 8.1   Open neural tube defects

Congenital abnormalities arise as the result of failure of the neural tube to close properly. Possible causes include folic acid deficiency and the administration of anti-epileptic medication, e.g. sodium valproate, during pregnancy. Folic acid supplementation is recommended before conception and during early pregnancy. Conditions include:

- Anencephaly: absence of a brain, which is invariably fatal.
- Meningoencephalocoele: where part of the brain and meninges protrude through a midline defect in the skull, which may be small or massive.
- Meningomyelocoele: where parts of the spinal cord, nerve roots and meninges protrude through a defect in the spinal column. If severe, the lower limbs and sphincters may be paralysed. Infections, e.g. meningitis, may ensue if left uncorrected.
- Spina bifida: where the lumbosacral neural tube fails to close. This is often associated with meningomyelocoele, hydrocephalus and intellectual impairment.
- Spina bifida occulta: failure of lumbosacral arch fusion, Often only seen on X-ray, and may be associated with a sacrococcygeal dimple with an overlying tuft of hair. Usually not associated with clinical abnormalities.

ventral nerve roots join to form the spinal nerves that are segmental, emerging from the bony vertebral canal. The spinal cord is the pathway for information transmission between the external environment, musculoskeletal system and internal organs of the body and the brain. Development of the motor and sensory pathways is activity dependent on neuronal activity from the various segments and organs that they serve.

Information from the head is routed via the cranial nerves which develop from various nuclei within the brain substance, and are described in detail later in this chapter.

Developmental disorders of the nervous system

Developmental disorders of the nervous system leading to congenital abnormalities may be genetic. They also occur due to metabolic disorders, infection, malnutrition, exposure to toxins, including drugs, or hypoxia during pregnancy. Most are associated with intellectual impairment from damage to the developing brain, so clearly, the earlier the insult occurs, the greater the effects will be on the unborn child (Clinical box 8.2).

GROSS ANATOMY

CENTRAL NERVOUS SYSTEM

The central nervous system (CNS) consists of the **brain** and **spinal cord** (Fig. 8.5). The brain has a **forebrain**, a **midbrain** and a **hindbrain**. The forebrain consists of the **cerebrum** (**telencephalon**) and a central core, the **diencephalon**. The midbrain is the smallest part of the brain and the hindbrain is composed of the pons and medulla anteriorly and the cerebellum posteriorly. The midbrain, pons and medulla make up the **brainstem**.

Brain

Cerebrum (telencephalon)

The cerebrum is made up of two **cerebral hemispheres** connected to each other by bundles of axons which cross the midline in tracts called **commissures**, the largest of which

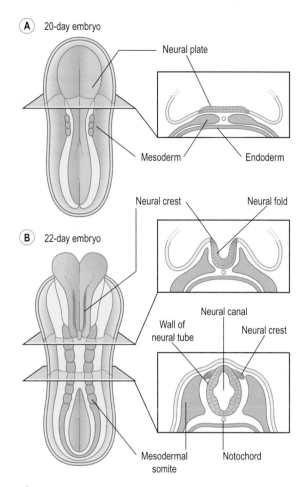

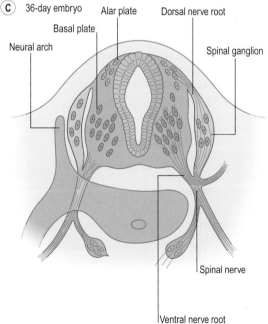

Fig. 8.2 **Alar and basal plates.** (A) Development within a 3-somite (20-day) embryo. (B) Development within an 8-somite (22-day) embryo. (C) Neural tube and spinal nerve of a 6-week embryo.

is the **corpus callosum**. Each cerebral hemisphere has four lobes: frontal, parietal, temporal and occipital (Fig. 8.6). Within the hemispheres lie groups of cell bodies, components of the **basal ganglia** and **limbic system**.

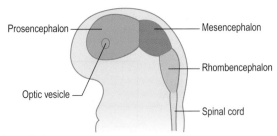

Fig. 8.3 Primary brain vesicles at 4 weeks' gestation.

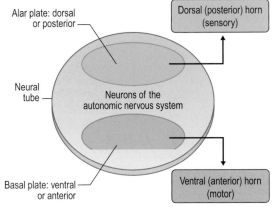

Fig. 8.4 Spinal cord development at 4 weeks' gestation.

Cerebral cortex

The **cerebral cortex** covers the surface of the brain and is made up of grey matter, varying in thickness from 1.5 to 4.5 mm. It is wrinkled in appearance with folds (**gyri**) and furrows (**sulci** or **fissures** if they are deep) (see Fig. 8.6). The cortex has two distinct structures:

- **Neocortex**, which accounts for about 95% of the cortex, has six layers with varying histology and connections (Fig. 8.7 and Table 8.1).
- **Archicortex** is older and has three layers. The main area with archicortex is the hippocampus.

Clinical box 8.2	Developmental disorders of the nervous system

Some of the more common congenital disorders of the nervous system are:

- **Genetic**: the best known neurodevelopmental disorder is Down syndrome or trisomy 21 (see also Clinical box 5.1). Clinically it is characterised by short stature, epicanthic folds, an extra palmar crease, congenital heart defects, immunodeficiency, hypothyroidism and widely varying degrees of intellectual impairment. Another example is Fragile X syndrome, an X-linked disorder with severe intellectual disability.
- **Infections**: rubella infection in early pregnancy (before 18 weeks) affects the developing foetus causing multiple defects including brain damage (with associated severe visual and auditory defects) and valvular heart disease. If the infection is severe in very early pregnancy foetal death and spontaneous abortion occurs. Rubella immunisation in early childhood has almost eliminated the occurrence of rubella embryopathy. Other infections in pregnancy causing a variety of congenital neurological impairments include toxoplasmosis and syphilis.
- **Malnutrition**: folate deficiency during pregnancy typically causes open neural tube defects.
- **Metabolic**: type 2 diabetes mellitus in the mother is associated with developmental delay in the baby, thought to be due to exposure of the foetus to either too much or too little blood glucose, if the mother's blood glucose levels are not tightly controlled. Thyrotoxicosis in the pregnant mother can lead to hypothyroidism in the baby. The excessive circulating thyroid hormone in the foetus suppresses thyroid gland development, and the lack of thyroxin could result in impairment of foetal brain development.
- **Drugs and alcohol**: a variety of drugs can lead to congenital brain damage, of which anti-epileptic medication is the best documented but antibiotics (e.g. nitrofurantoin and sulfonamides) have also been implicated. Excessive maternal alcohol intake during pregnancy as the cause of foetal alcohol syndrome is increasingly recognised as associated with stunted growth and intellectual impairment in the child.
- **Toxins**: exposure to heavy metals, such as mercury, lead and cadmium, and to pesticides in pregnancy, especially early pregnancy, can lead to neurodevelopmental disorders in the baby.

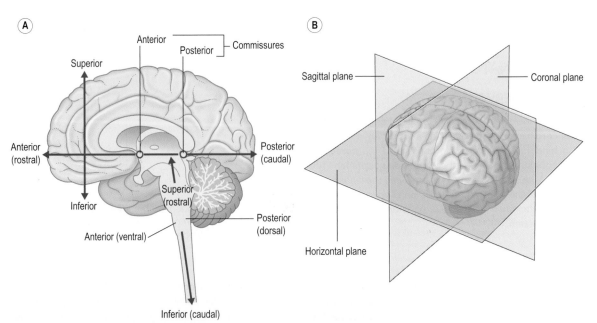

Fig. 8.5 Anatomical axes (A) and principal planes (B) of the human nervous system.

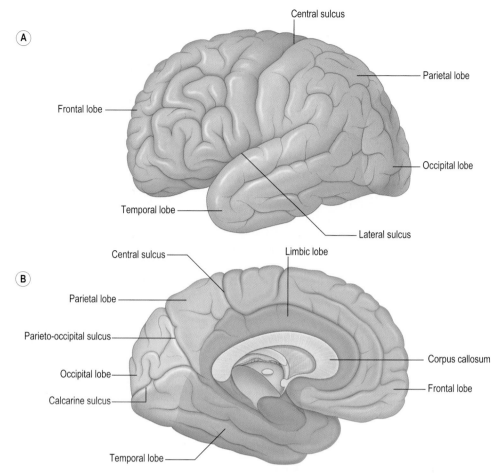

Fig. 8.6 **Left cerebral hemisphere.** (A) Lateral surface, (B) medial surface, showing lobes, principal gyri and sulci.

While specific functions (e.g. motor, sensory, language) are located in particular areas, most of the cortex is designated as **association cortex**. Cortical maps are composed and used to signify different areas of function (Fig. 8.8). The best known example is **Brodmann's** in which the cortex is divided into 52 areas.

Basal ganglia

The basal ganglia (Fig. 8.9) comprises:

- Caudate nucleus
- Lentiform nucleus consisting of the putamen and globus pallidus
- Subthalamus (in the diencephalon)
- Substantia nigra (in the midbrain).

The caudate and lentiform nuclei are situated deep in the white matter of the cerebrum and are separated by the internal capsule. Functionally, however, the caudate and putamen are homologous and so are together referred to as the **dorsal striatum**.

There are extensive interconnections between the basal ganglia and with the thalamus and parts of the cortex. These connections constitute the **extrapyramidal system** involved in motor control.

Limbic system

There is no universally accepted anatomical definition of the **limbic system** but most of the structures involved are located on the medial aspect of the temporal lobe, forming a rim around the corpus callosum (Figs 8.9 and 8.10). It includes:

- Areas of cerebral cortex: orbital prefrontal cortex, cingulate and parahippocampal gyri and the hippocampus
- Nuclei: the mammillary bodies, amygdala, ventral striatum and medial dorsal thalamus.

These structures are heavily interconnected and involved in functions such as learning, memory and emotion.

Diencephalon

This central core of the forebrain is continuous with the midbrain and contains four major parts:

- The **thalamus**: the largest part of the diencephalon consists of five groups of nuclei (Table 8.2). All sensory input to the brain, with the exception of smell, relays via the thalamus. In addition it connects to parts of the cerebrum concerned with movement, emotion and cognition.
- The **hypothalamus** is part of the **limbic system**. It is involved in thermoregulation, in triggering sleep, and in the regulation of the endocrine system by connections to the **pituitary gland** (see Ch. 10).
- The **epithalamus** contains the **pineal gland**.
- The **subthalamus** at the junction of the diencephalon and midbrain is part of the **basal ganglia**.

Brainstem

The **brainstem** consists of midbrain, pons and medulla. Apart from the nuclei of the olfactory (I) and optic (II) cranial nerves, the nuclei of the other 10 cranial nerves lie in the brainstem

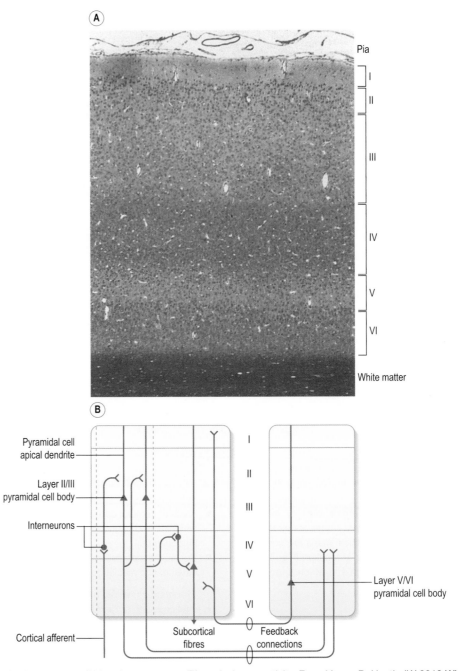

Fig. 8.7 **Cerebral neocortex.** (A) Laminar structure; (B) cortical connectivity. From Young B, Heath JW 2013 Wheater's functional histology, 6th edn. Churchill Livingstone, Edinburgh, with permission.

Table 8.1	Features of the neocortical layers			
No.	**Layer**	**Principal cell type**	**Input from**	**Output to**
I	Molecular layer	Apical dendrites of pyramidal cells	Cortex	
II	Outer granular layer	Small pyramidal cells		Ipsilateral cortex
III	Outer pyramidal cell layer	Medium-sized pyramidal cells		Contralateral cortex
IV	Inner granular layer	Spiny stellate cells (many interneurons)	Thalamus	
V	Inner pyramidal cell layer	Large pyramidal cells		Striatum, brainstem, spinal cord
VI	Fusiform layer	Modified pyramidal cells	Cortex	Thalamus

(Figs 8.11 and 8.12) where numerous other discrete nuclei are embedded. The latter include the **reticular formation** which extends throughout the brainstem and is involved with various networks including arousal, autonomic reflexes and posture control (see below). Most of the rest of the brainstem is the white matter of the ascending and descending fibre tracts to and from higher levels of the CNS along its long axis (the **neuraxis**).

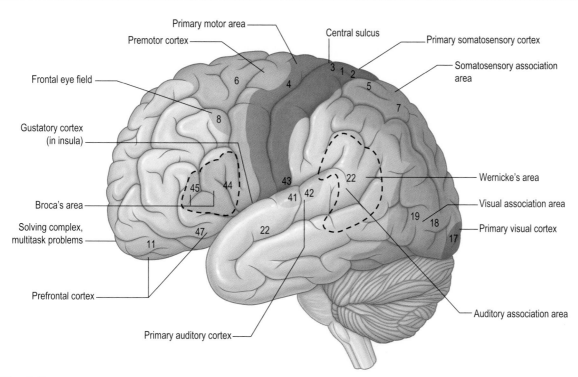

Fig. 8.8 Functional areas of the cerebral cortex, including Brodmann's areas (numbered). Red: motor cortex; blue: sensory cortex; pale blue and pale red: association cortex.

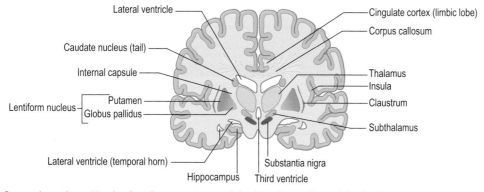

Fig. 8.9 Coronal section of brain showing structures of the basal ganglia and the limbic system.

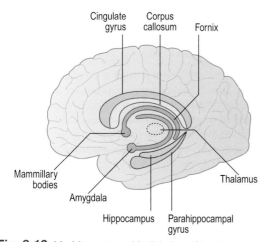

Fig. 8.10 Limbic system. Medial view of hemisphere showing main structures.

Midbrain

The midbrain consists of the **tegmentum** ventrally and the **tectum** dorsally with the cerebral aqueduct running through it.

- The **tegmentum** has the nuclei of cranial nerves III (oculomotor) and IV (trochlear) concerned with eye movements embedded within it. It also contains the substantia nigra (see Basal ganglia, above) and the red nucleus. Both are concerned with the modulation of motor function.

- The **tectum** consists of two pairs of colliculi (singular: colliculus). The **superior colliculi** receive input from optic nerves, while vestibulocochlear nerves send signals to the **inferior colliculi**. Thus they are involved with visual and auditory reflexes.

- The **periaqueductal grey (PAG) matter**, as its name implies, surrounds the cerebral aqueduct and is thought to modulate pain sensation and defensive behaviour.

Table 8.2	**Thalamic nuclei**		
	Nuclei	**Connections**	**Function**
Anterior group	Anterior nucleus	Limbic system	Emotion
Medial group	Mediodorsal nucleus	Basal ganglia and amygdala Frontal cortex	Memory
Ventral group	Ventrobasal nuclei	Basal ganglia Cerebellum Motor cortex Somatosensory systems	Sensory and motor
Posterior group	Medial and lateral geniculate nuclei Posterior nucleus Pulvinar	Auditory and visual input	Pain perception Visual attention
Non-specific	Intralaminar nuclei Midline nuclei Reticular nuclei	Widespread and diffuse	Sleep/wakefulness and arousal

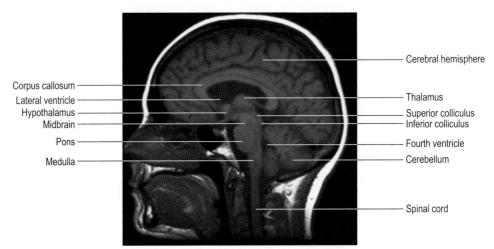

Fig. 8.11 Magnetic resonance (MR) image of the midsagittal section of the brain and spinal cord.

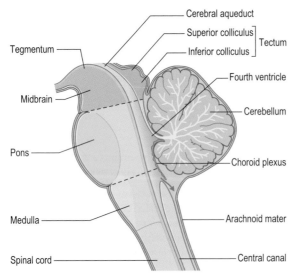

Fig. 8.12 Brainstem anatomy. Sagittal section through the brainstem.

Pons and medulla

The pons and medulla contain the nuclei for cranial nerves V–XII and have neural networks that play a central role in the autonomic control of the cardiovascular, respiratory and alimentary systems.

Cerebellum

The cerebellum (little brain) lies posterior to the pons and inferior to the cerebral hemispheres in the posterior fossa of the cranium. It essentially consists of two **hemispheres** and a central **vermis** (see Fig. 8.37, below). Packed with neurons, the cerebellum has a major role in motor control, contributing to coordination, precision and timing of voluntary movement and motor learning. It may also have a role in higher level functions, such as cognition and emotional responses.

Spinal cord

The **spinal cord** is a long, thin tube made up of columns of nervous tissue, with a **central canal**. It is enclosed by the bony vertebral column, and begins at the medulla, emerging from the skull at the foramen magnum (an opening in the occiput) and extending to the level of the second lumbar vertebra (L2). There are 31 segments to the spinal cord, corresponding to the vertebrae in the bony spine (see Ch. 9). These give rise to 31 pairs of spinal nerves. There are two bulges in the spinal cord:

- The **cervical enlargement** receives sensory input and sends motor output to the arms, and is located between C3 and T2 spinal segments
- The **lumbar enlargement** deals with sensory input and motor output from and to the legs, and is found between L1 and S3 spinal segments.

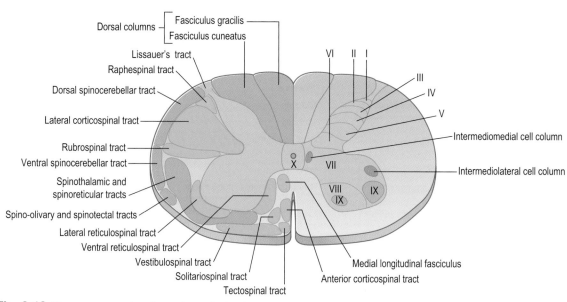

Fig. 8.13 Transverse section through cervical spinal cord. White matter pathways are shown on the left, descending in green, ascending in brown; Rexed's laminae are depicted on the right.

At its lower end, the adult spinal cord tapers into the **conus medullaris**. Whilst the spinal nerves (see below) from the upper segments exit directly from the cord, those from the lower segments have to travel obliquely down a distance within the vertebral column before emerging, and those emerging below the conus medullaris form the **cauda equina** (horse's tail).

In transverse section (Fig. 8.13), the cord shows the central butterfly-shaped region of grey matter surrounded by white matter, and encloses the central canal. The central canal is a continuation of the ventricular system, but closed to CSF in most adults. Transverse sections of the spinal cord at all levels show similar structures, but the ratio of grey to white matter is greatest at the lowest segments, with the highest segments containing the most white matter.

Grey matter

The different columns of grey matter in the spinal cord are characterised by their neuron populations and their connections. In transverse section the columns form the wings of a 'butterfly', each wing consisting of a **dorsal**, a **lateral** and a **ventral horn** whose principal functions are sensory, autonomic and motor, respectively. The columns form layers known as **Rexed's laminae** in transverse sections.

- Neurons in the **dorsal horns (Rexed's laminae I–VI)** are the targets of primary afferent sensory neurons. Lamina VI is confined to spinal segments C5–T1 and L2–S3 receiving sensory information from muscles and joints in the upper and lower limbs, respectively.
- Neurons in the **lateral horns (Rexed's lamina VII)** are the cell bodies of preganglionic **sympathetic** fibres in T1–L2 and of preganglionic **parasympathetic** fibres in the sacral region.
- Neurons in the **ventral (or anterior) horns (Rexed's laminae VIII and IX)** are motor cell bodies that send their axons to skeletal muscles.

White matter

The white matter consists of nerve fibres running in ascending tracts towards the brain or descending tracts from the brain. The terminology used to identify these usually refers to their origin and destination (e.g. the spinothalamic tract conveys sensory information from the spinal cord to the thalamus and the corticospinal tract relays motor signals from the cortex to the motor neurons in the ventral horn of the spinal cord). Some tracts carry information between segments within the spinal cord, and are known as **propriospinal fibres**.

Because of its compact nature damage to the spinal cord results in a constellation of symptoms and signs (Information box 8.1).

PERIPHERAL NERVOUS SYSTEM

The network of nerves that transmit information to and from the central nervous system is known as the **peripheral nervous system**, and is subdivided into:

- **Somatic** nervous system (see below)
- **Autonomic** nervous system (see Ch. 4) which includes the **enteric** nervous system (see Chs 15 and 16).

Information box 8.1	Localisation of spinal cord lesions

When considering the anatomical basis of spinal cord disease, the segmental properties and internal structure of the spinal cord must be taken into account. Although many conditions affect all components, some damage specific areas such as the white or grey matter, or the spinal nerve roots. Damage to a spinal nerve root leads to symptoms confined to the specific dermatome or muscles supplied by it. Causes of spinal root compression include tumours, haematoma and intervertebral disc disease and infection.

These same pathologies may occur within the spinal cord (intramedullary lesions) and also result in compression as the spinal canal is a rigidly exposed space. These result in segmental signs.

White matter damage can result in a combination of sensory, motor and autonomic symptoms and signs. An example is multiple sclerosis where patches of demyelination may occur at different sites in the cord.

Other conditions affect the neurons of the grey matter. For example, in motor neuron disease the α motor neurons in the ventral horns may be affected with lower motor neuron signs in the muscles supplied (Clinical box 8.16). Damage to the dorsal horns leads to sensory and reflex changes (Clinical box 8.26).

Table 8.3	Cranial nerves		
Nerve	**Type (motor/sensory/both, parasympathetic)**	**CNS origin/destination**	**Function**
I Olfactory	Sensory	Olfactory bulb	Smell
II Optic	Sensory	Thalamus	Vision
III Oculomotor	Motor, parasympathetic	Midbrain	Eye movements, pupil constriction
IV Trochlear	Motor	Midbrain	Eye movements
V Trigeminal	Both	Pons and medulla	Sensory from head and face, motor to jaw
VI Abducens	Motor	Pons	Eye movements
VII Facial	Both, parasympathetic	Thalamus (sensory), pons (motor)	Motor to face, taste, sensory from palate, secretomotor to salivary and lachrymal glands
VIII Vestibulocochlear	Sensory	Thalamus (auditory division), medulla (vestibular division)	Hearing and balance
IX Glossopharyngeal	Both, parasympathetic	Thalamus (sensory), medulla (motor)	Taste, motor to pharynx, secretomotor to salivary glands
X Vagus	Both, parasympathetic	Thalamus (sensory), medulla (motor)	Taste, sensory from viscera, motor to pharynx and larynx, visceral motor
XI Accessory	Motor	Medulla, spinal cord C1-C5	Motor to palate and some neck muscles
XII Hypoglossal	Motor	Medulla	Motor to tongue

Somatic nervous system

The **somatic nervous system** shows bilateral symmetry with 12 pairs of **cranial nerves** and 31 pairs of **spinal nerves**.

Cranial nerves

The cranial nerves provide all the sensory input from the special senses, general sensory input from and motor output to the head and neck, and most of the parasympathetic (visceral efferent) output to the head. They are given Roman numerals according to the order in which they emerge from the brain. The main function and nuclei for each are outlined below and in Table 8.3, but more detail of their function is discussed in the relevant sensory and motor sections below. (The relationship between the cranial nerves and the brainstem is shown in Fig. 8.14.)

Olfactory (I) nerve

The olfactory nerve carries special sensory afferents for **smell**; its connections and central pathways are described below.

Optic (II) nerve

The optic nerve is also purely sensory responsible for transmitting the special sense of **vision** from the retina to the brain. By development criteria the retina and optic nerve could be regarded as part of the CNS.

Oculomotor (III) nerve

This nerve sends motor fibres to four of the six extraocular muscles responsible for **eye movements** (see below) and the muscle of the upper eyelid (levator palpebrae superioris). It also carries proprioceptive afferents from these muscles to the brain. The **motor nucleus of III** lies in the periaqueductal grey matter of the midbrain at the level of the superior colliculus.

In addition the oculomotor nerve has preganglionic parasympathetic fibres that arise in the **Edinger Westphal nucleus**, just dorsal to the motor nucleus, and end in the ciliary ganglion. These fibres are involved in the pupillary light reflex (see Clinical box 8.34, below).

Trochlear (IV) nerve

The trochlear nerve innervates the superior oblique muscle which moves the eye inferomedially (see Eye movements) and carries proprioceptive information from the muscle. The **motor nucleus of IV** is situated in the periaqueductal grey matter at the level of the inferior colliculus. The trochlear nerve is the only nerve to emerge from the dorsum of the brainstem but it passes around the midbrain to its ventral surface.

Trigeminal (V) nerve

The trigeminal nerve is so named because it divides into three major peripheral nerves (**ophthalmic**, **maxillary** and **mandibular**). It is a mixed nerve with both sensory and motor divisions.

Sensory division

Sensation from the head is carried in afferent fibres whose cell bodies are contained in the trigeminal ganglion, with the exception of proprioceptive fibres.

- Pain and temperature axons leave the trigeminal ganglion enter the pons and run caudally to form the **spinal tract of V** terminating in the **nucleus of the spinal tract of V** as they pass through the pons, medulla and upper cervical spinal cord
- The centrally directed axons for touch and pressure end in the **principal (or chief) nucleus of V** in the pons
- Proprioceptive fibres have their cell bodies in the **mesencephalic nucleus**.

Motor division

The **motor nucleus of V** lies laterally in the upper pons and sends motor fibres to the muscles of mastication (chewing).

Abducens (VI) nerve

The abducens nerve innervates the lateral rectus muscle responsible for abducting the eye (see Eye movements) and carries proprioceptive afferents from the muscle.

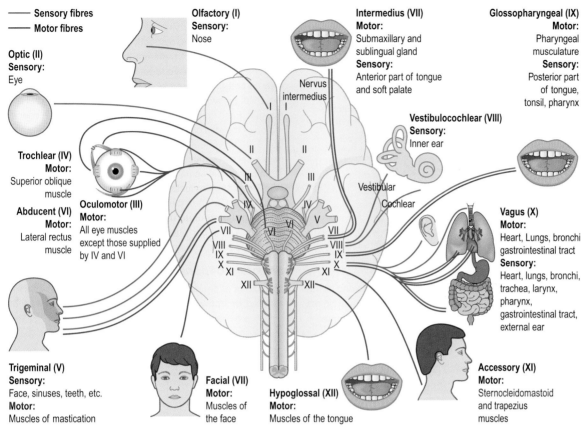

Fig. 8.14 Emergence of cranial nerves from the brain and brainstem.

Facial (VII) nerve

The facial nerve is a mixed nerve with motor, sensory and parasympathetic components (see Clinical box 8.3).

- Motor fibres from the **motor nucleus of VII** in the pons supply the muscles of facial expression, muscles in the throat and the stapedius muscle.
- Somatic sensory information from the external ear runs to **the spinal tract and nucleus of V**.
- Special sensory afferents for **taste** from the soft palate and anterior two thirds of the tongue end in the **nucleus of the solitary tract (NST)**.
- Preganglionic parasympathetic fibres arise in the superior salivatory nucleus and pass via the **nervus intermedius** to the **pterygopalatine** and **submandibular ganglia**. Postganglionic fibres from these ganglia terminate in the lacrimal gland and submandibular salivary gland respectively.

Vestibulocochlear (VIII) nerve

The vestibulocochlear nerve carries special sensory information and is essentially two nerves: the vestibular concerned with **balance** and the cochlear with **hearing** (see below).

Clinical box 8.3 **Bell's palsy**

Bell's palsy results from a facial nerve lesion of unknown cause, although it may be associated with a viral infection (e.g. herpes simplex). The patient experiences unilateral facial palsy with loss of the sense of taste in the anterior two-thirds of the tongue and increased sensitivity to sound (hyperacusis) on the same side. Most patients (80%) recover in 4–8 weeks.

Glossopharyngeal (IX) nerve

Another mixed nerve, the glossopharyngeal has motor, general and special sensory and parasympathetic fibres. It is functionally closely related to the vagus (X) nerve.

- Motor fibres from the **nucleus ambiguus** supply the stylopharyngeus muscle.
- Fibres carrying general sensory information from the mucosa of the pharynx, Eustachian tube, middle ear and from the posterior third of the tongue have cell bodies in the petrosal ganglion and send axons to the **NST**. Special sensory taste fibres from the posterior third of the tongue also terminate in the **NST**.
- Preganglionic parasympathetic fibres from the **inferior salivary nucleus** end in the **otic ganglion** and postganglionic fibres supply the parotid gland.

Vagus (X) nerve

The vagus nerve has motor sensory and parasympathetic fibres:

- The **nucleus ambiguus** gives rise to fibres supplying muscles of the soft palate, pharynx and larynx.
- General sensory information from the pharynx, larynx and organs of the thorax and abdomen is sent to the **NST**.
- Preganglionic parasympathetics from the **dorsal nucleus of the vagus** send their axons to parasympathetic terminal ganglia located near or within the viscera they innervate. The effects of stimulation of vagal parasympathetics include slowing the heart, constricting smooth muscle of the bronchial tree, promoting peristalsis in the gut and secretion of gastric and pancreatic juices (see Ch.4).

Accessory (XI) nerve

This nerve has two roots:

- The **cranial root** originates in the caudal end of the **nucleus ambiguus** and innervates muscles of the soft palate and pharynx.
- The **spinal root** arises from the **spinal accessory nucleus** in the ventral horn of C2–C5 and supplies the sternocleidomastoid and trapezius muscles.

Hypoglossal (XII) nerve

The muscles of the tongue get their motor supply from the hypoglossal nerve, the nucleus of which is a column of cells extending nearly the entire length of the medulla.

Spinal nerves

The 31 pairs of **spinal nerves** (Fig. 8.15) each arise from a single segment of the spinal cord and leave the vertebral column via an intervertebral foramina. The first seven spinal nerves (C1–C7) emerge above the corresponding vertebrae C1–C7 but the eighth (C8) emerges below the C7 vertebra and all the others emerge below their numbered vertebra. Each spinal nerve is formed by the union of two nerve branches, a dorsal and a ventral root carrying sensory and motor (both somatic and autonomic) fibres, respectively. Thus, they are all mixed nerves containing both afferent and efferent fibres. Primary afferent fibres are pseudo-unipolar (having a single axon with central and peripheral branches and no dendrites (see Fig. 8.20, below) and have their cell bodies in the **dorsal root ganglia**. Each spinal nerve carries information from a specific region of the skin called a **dermatome** (Fig. 8.16, Information box 8.2).The ventral roots contains α **motor neurons** that innervate skeletal muscles.

In places the spinal nerves join together to form plexuses (see Fig. 8.15). For instance the **brachial plexus** arises from spinal roots C5–T1. It then gives rise to a network of branches including the **median**, **ulnar** and **radial nerves** to the hand and arm. These **peripheral nerves** represent the most distal part of the peripheral nervous system.

Structure of peripheral nerves

The axons of neurons within peripheral nerves may be myelinated or unmyelinated. Unlike myelinated fibres in the

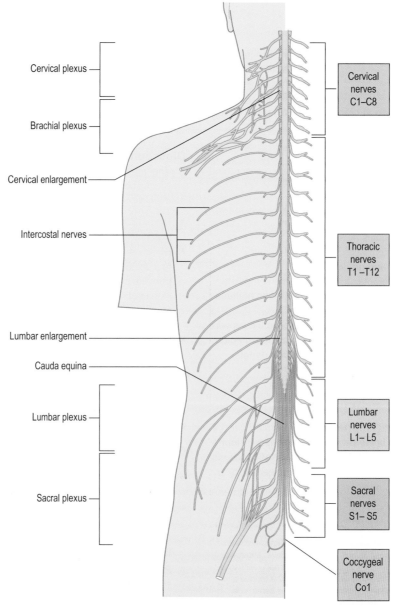

Fig. 8.15 **Spinal nerves.**

Information box 8.2   Dermatomes

The region of skin innervated by a spinal nerve is called a **dermatome** (Fig. 8.16). By mapping which dermatomes have normal sensation and which do not, it is possible to estimate at which level the spinal cord is injured. However, the following provisos should be noted:

- Dermatomes vary from one person to another
- Dermatomes overlap, and the overlap is more extensive for touch, pressure and vibration than it is for pain and

temperature, so pain sensation is the best guide to the level of cord injury

- Proprioceptor fibres follow the distribution of muscle innervation rather than dermatomes.

Because in **herpes zoster** (shingles) specific dorsal roots are infected with the virus, the resulting skin lesions and pain follow dermatomes.

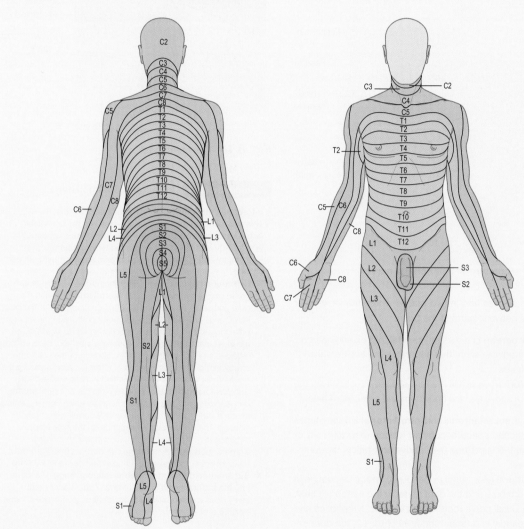

Fig. 8.16 **The dermatomes.**

CNS those in peripheral nerves have, in addition, a **neurolemma** (or **sheath of Schwann**) outside the myelin. The nerve fibres are held together by connective tissue, the **endoneurium**, and are gathered into bundles called **fascicles** surrounded by more connective tissue, the **perineurium**. A peripheral nerve contains one or more fascicles along with blood vessels ensheathed in an **epineurium** (Fig. 8.17).

Nerve fibre classification

Nerve fibres in the peripheral nervous system are classified according to their diameter (Table 8.4). This is closely linked to the speed with which impulses spread along them, i.e. their conduction velocity, and allows fibres to be crudely characterised as to function. The fastest fibres

are the myelinated large diameter motor neurons (Aα) and the slowest unmyelinated small (C) fibres which transmit pain impulses.

MENINGES

The **meninges** are three connective tissue membranes that ensheath the CNS: the **dura**, **arachnoid** and **pia maters** (Fig. 8.18).

Dura mater

The **dura mater** is a dense structure with an outer periosteal layer attached firmly to the inner surfaces of the cranial bones and an inner meningeal layer. These layers are generally fused except where they separate to provide space for

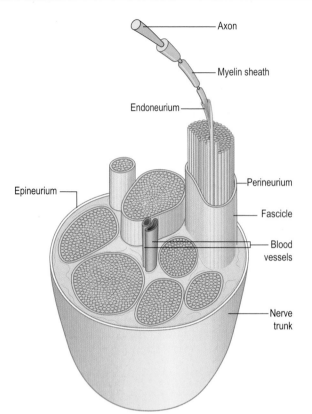

Fig. 8.17 Structure of a peripheral nerve.

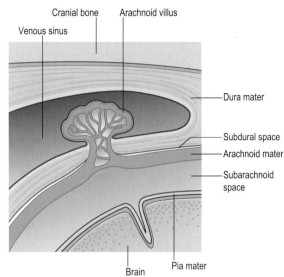

Fig. 8.18 The meninges.

the venous sinuses and in two places where the inner layer forms folds between parts of the brain:

- The **falx cerebri** is a midline, sagittal fold extending into the longitudinal fissure that separates the two cerebral hemispheres
- The **tentorium cerebelli** is a tent-shaped structure with the cerebrum above and the brainstem and cerebellum below.

The terms **supratentorial** and **infratentorial** are sometimes used to describe space-occupying lesions (e.g. tumours or haemorrhage, Clinical box 8.4), above and below the tentorium cerebelli.

The **epidural** (extradural or peridural) **space** lies between the bony vertebrae and the dura mater in the vertebral canal. It contains spinal nerve roots, blood vessels, lymphatics and fat. At the caudal end (about the level of L1–L2) the dura extends as a blind-ending sac (see Clinical box 8.5).

Arachnoid mater

Lying close to the dura is the **arachnoid mater** which is separated from the dura by the narrow **subdural space** and from the underlying pia mater by the **subarachnoid space** which is filled with **cerebrospinal fluid (CSF)**. Larger spaces within the subarachnoid space are known as **cisterns**

Clinical box 8.4   Intracranial haemorrhage

Intracranial haemorrhage refers to bleeding within the skull. This may occur at the brain surface or within the brain itself (**intracerebral haemorrhage**). When the haemorrhage results in a collection of blood this is referred to as a **haematoma**. Head injury and cardiovascular disorders are the most common causes.

- **Extradural haemorrhage**. Bleeding from the meningeal arteries results in an extradural haematoma, between the dura and skull. This can cause brain compression and raised intracranial pressure (ICP). Vasomotor neurons in the medulla drive increased sympathetic vasoconstriction, which raises mean arterial blood pressure (**Cushing's reflex**). Baroreceptor reflexes (see Ch. 11) then cause a slowing of the heart rate (bradycardia). The combination of a rise in blood pressure and bradycardia in a head-injured patient indicates raised ICP.
- **Subdural haemorrhage**. Bleeding into the subdural space between the dura and the arachnoid is usually from superficial cerebral veins going from the cerebral cortex to the venous sinuses. The clinical picture depends on the time elapsing between the injury and presentation (hours to months). Chronic subdural haemorrhage can occur in the elderly as a result of brain shrinkage rupturing superficial cerebral veins.
- **Subarachnoid** and **intracerebral haemorrhage**. Bleeding into the subarachnoid space or brain occurs after head injury or as a cerebrovascular accident or stroke (see Clinical box 8.8 and Information box 8.7).

(e.g. the cisterna magna is where the arachnoid bridges over the space between the medulla and the cerebellum). The arachnoid mater is a delicate fibrocellular layer and it forms **arachnoid villi** which protrude through the dura into the venous sinuses of the brain, allowing CSF to enter the bloodstream. **Trabeculae** extend across the subarachnoid space to provide support for superficial cerebral vessels.

Table 8.4	Erlanger–Gasser classification of nerve fibres		
Fibre type	**Diameter (mm)**	**Conduction velocity (m/s)**	**Functions (example)**
Aα	12–20	72–120	Motor neurons
Aβ	6–12	36–72	Skin touch afferents
Aγ	2–8	12–48	Motor to muscle spindles
Aδ	1–6	4–36	Myelinated skin temperature and pain afferents
C	0.2–1.5	0.4–2.0	Unmyelinated skin pain afferents

Epidural anaesthesia

The epidural space is distinct from the subarachnoid space which contains CSF. It can be accessed easily via a catheter inserted between L2 and L3 vertebrae with low risk of spinal cord injury. The technique of epidural anaesthesia involves the introduction of local anaesthetic by this route and is often used in surgical procedures, particularly in obstetrics (e.g. caesarean section) and the catheter can be left in situ to provide postoperative analgesia. Opiates may also be given by this method to control intractable pain in patients with terminal malignancy.

Pia mater

This is the innermost layer of the meninges investing the brain and spinal cord. Water and small molecules can pass through the pia allowing metabolites to diffuse from the extracellular fluid of the brain into the CSF.

THE VENTRICULAR SYSTEM

The brain and spinal cord are suspended in CSF, a clear liquid that fills the subarachnoid space and a series of cavities within the brain called the **ventricles**. The four ventricles (two lateral, a third and a fourth) are connected to each other, the central canal of the spinal cord and the subarachnoid space (Fig. 8.19).

Secretion and circulation of CSF

CSF is formed principally by the **choroid plexuses**. There are large plexuses in the floors of each lateral ventricle and smaller ones in the roofs of the third and fourth ventricles. The choroid plexuses are capillary networks surrounded by cuboidal epithelium of ependymal origin and produce 500 mL of CSF daily. The vessels are quite permeable, so

CSF secretion starts with the formation of an ultrafiltrate of plasma. However, the ependymal cells are coupled by tight junctions and so act as a **blood–CSF barrier**, selectively absorbing some substances while secreting others, so that CSF has a different composition from blood (Table 8.5).

The fluid leaves the lateral ventricles via the **interventricular foramina** into the third ventricle then passes through the cerebral aqueduct to the fourth ventricle. Two **lateral** and one **medial foramina** in the roof of the fourth ventricle connect to the subarachnoid space. CSF flows continuously from the ventricles to the spinal cord in the subarachnoid space (Clinical box 8.6).

Table 8.5   Composition of CSF compared with blood plasma

	CSF	Plasma
Protein (mg/dL)	35	7000
Glucose (mmol/L)	3.3	5
Na$^+$ (mmol/L)	138	138
K$^+$ (mmol/L)	2.8	4.5
Ca^{2+} (mmol/L)	2.1	4.8
pH	7.33	7.41

Lumbar puncture

Although the spinal cord ends around the level of L1/L2, the subarachnoid space continues until vertebra S2. Thus the space below L2 forms a large lumbar cistern containing CSF. By introducing a needle, usually at the L3/4 intervertebral space CSF can be sampled by lumbar puncture. The freely floating spinal nerves are not at risk of damage as they will drift away from the point of the needle. However, lumbar puncture should not be performed under circumstances of raised intracranial pressure as this can cause herniation of the brain.

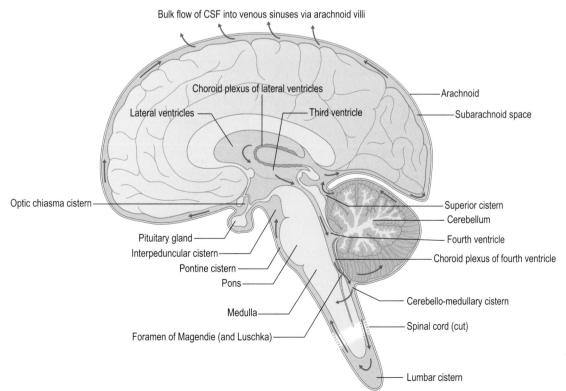

Bulk flow of CSF into venous sinuses via arachnoid villi

Choroid plexus of lateral ventricles

Lateral ventricles

Third ventricle

Arachnoid

Subarachnoid space

Optic chiasma cistern

Pituitary gland

Interpeduncular cistern

Pontine cistern

Pons

Medulla

Foramen of Magendie (and Luschka)

Superior cistern

Cerebellum

Fourth ventricle

Choroid plexus of fourth ventricle

Cerebello-medullary cistern

Spinal cord (cut)

Lumbar cistern

Fig. 8.19 **The ventricular system of the brain and circulation of the cerebrospinal fluid (CSF).**

Absorption of CSF

The **arachnoid villi** (see Fig. 8.18) allow CSF to flow into the blood whenever the pressure in the subarachnoid space exceeds the pressure in the venous sinus (Clinical box 8.7).

Functions of CSF

CSF has two major functions.

Metabolic functions

The constituents of CSF are in equilibrium with brain extracellular fluid and so maintain a constant environment for brain cells. CSF drains unwanted metabolites into the venous blood via arachnoid villi, acting as a lymphatic system for the brain. It may also provide some nutrients to cells and act as an intracerebral transporter carrying hormones from one part of the brain to another.

Clinical box 8.7 | **Hydrocephalus**

An obstruction to the circulation of CSF, due to a developmental abnormality, a tumour or in meningitis, causes fluid to accumulate in the space between cells (**interstitial cerebral oedema**); ventricles become progressively dilated, leading to brain compression and cerebral ischaemia.

In infants in whom the cranial sutures are unfused, increased volume is partly accommodated by enlargement of the head; however, neural damage may happen very early in development in congenital hydrocephalus.

Some types of hydrocephalus can be treated by the insertion of a shunt which can divert the flow of excess CSF into a neck vein.

Mechanical functions

- The weight of the brain is effectively reduced from about 1350 g to 50 g because it floats buoyantly in a 'pool' of CSF.
- The CSF and meninges dampen forces produced by head movement.
- The volume of the CSF compartment can undergo minor adjustments to resist the changes in intracranial pressure (ICP) that occur due to alterations in cerebral blood flow (CBF). When CBF rises, the subarachnoid space around the spinal cord can expand to accommodate CSF displaced by the increase in intracranial blood volume.

CELLS OF THE NERVOUS SYSTEM

Neurons (nerve cells) and glial cells are the main types of cells in the nervous system, as described in Chapter 2. Neurons can be classified according to their size, shape (morphology), their connections, and their chemistry.

Size

The cell bodies of neurons vary in diameter from about 6 to 8 μm for the granule cells of the cerebellum to 50 μm or more for α-motor neurons of the spinal cord. The most common type of nerve cells in the cerebral cortex, the pyramidal cells, have cell bodies 12–20 μm across.

Morphology

Different types of neuron can be distinguished by the number of neurites (see Fig. 8.20).

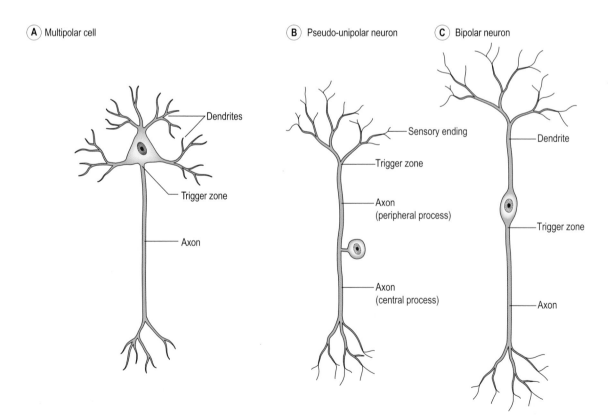

(A) Multipolar cell — Dendrites, Trigger zone, Axon

(B) Pseudo-unipolar neuron — Sensory ending, Trigger zone, Axon (peripheral process), Axon (central process)

(C) Bipolar neuron — Dendrite, Trigger zone, Axon

Fig. 8.20 **Three common neuron types.** (A) Multipolar neuron. (B) Pseudo-unipolar neuron. (C) Bipolar neuron. Redrawn from Michael-Titus A, Revest P, Shortland P 2006 The nervous system. Churchill Livingstone, Edinburgh, with permission.

- **Multipolar** neurons are the most common and have an axon and multiple dendrites.
- **Pseudo-unipolar** neurons have a single axon that bifurcates within a short distance of the cell body but no dendrites. In somatic sensory neurons one branch of the axon goes to a sense organ, the other to the CNS.
- **Bipolar** neurons have an axon at one pole of the cell body and a single dendrite at the opposite pole. These are located in the retina, and cochlear and vestibular ganglia.

Connectivity

Classifying nerve cells by how they are connected is useful because it says something about their functions.

- **Afferent neurons** transmit signals towards the CNS, so providing input.
- **Efferent neurons** transmit signals away from the CNS towards the periphery and thus serve as the route for nervous system output. **Motor neurons** signal to muscles and **secretomotor neurons** stimulate glandular secretion.
- Networks of **interneurons** connect afferent and efferent neurons and transform input to output. They make up most of the nerve cell population.

Chemistry

Different nerve cells release different chemical transmitters; for example, cholinergic neurons release acetylcholine, dopaminergic neurons release dopamine and glutaminergic neurons release glutamate.

BLOOD SUPPLY TO THE BRAIN AND BRAIN METABOLISM

The brain has a rich blood supply because of its high oxygen requirements. It consumes 20% of total body oxygen despite accounting for only 2% of the body mass.

ARTERIAL BLOOD SUPPLY

The major blood supply to the brain comes from two pairs of arteries:

- The **internal carotid arteries** anteriorly. The internal carotid arteries are branches of the common carotid arteries.
- The **vertebral arteries** which fuse together to form the **basilar artery** posteriorly. The vertebral arteries arise from the subclavian arteries.

The **circle of Willis** is an arterial loop lying at the base of the brain formed by the junction of the two internal carotid arteries and the basilar artery by an **anterior communicating artery** and a pair of **posterior communicating arteries** (Fig. 8.21). This ensures that, should flow be obstructed to any one vessel, blood can still be delivered to all regions of the brain (Information box 8.3). The anatomy of this arterial circle varies greatly between individuals.

The principal arteries arising from the circle of Willis are the **anterior**, **middle** and **posterior cerebral** arteries.

The circulation can be divided into the:

- **Anterior cerebral circulation** that supplies most of the cerebral hemispheres and forebrain with the exception of the occipital lobe and medial and inferior temporal lobe
- **Posterior cerebral circulation** supplying the occipital lobe and medial and inferior temporal lobe and the brainstem.

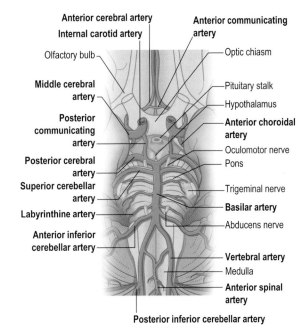

Fig. 8.21 Circle of Willis and principal arterial blood supply to the brain.

Information box 8.3   Loss of brain blood supply

Depriving a brain region of its blood supply for longer than a few minutes results in a region of damaged tissue called an **infarct**. This consists of **core**, in which hypoxia is so profound that cells undergo **necrotic cell death** surrounded by a **penumbra** in which hypoxia causes excessive release of the excitatory transmitter glutamate and cell death occurs partly by apoptosis (see Ch. 2). Because death of cells in the penumbra is not inevitable, treatment is aimed at salvaging them.

Neurological consequences depend on infarct size and location.

- Even small infarcts in the **brainstem** can be devastating because here neural structures are densely packed
- Blockages (occlusions) in the **circle of Willis** or the principal cerebral vessels are often **circumvented** by flow through alternative routes so infarction is avoided
- Because distal deep **end arteries** in the brain lack anastomoses, the deep brain regions they supply (**end zones**) are almost completely deprived of their blood supply by a bleed from, or occlusion of, these vessels.

Occlusion of an artery with the loss of blood supply to the territory it supplies results in a cerebrovascular accident (CVA, stroke) and 75% of CVAs occur in the anterior circulation (see Clinical box 8.8).

Anterior cerebral circulation

The anterior circulation comprises the **anterior cerebral arteries** and anterior communicating artery; the **middle cerebral arteries** and some direct branches from the internal carotid arteries.

Anterior cerebral arteries arch over the corpus callosum to supply the medial and superior parts of the frontal and parietal lobes (Fig. 8.22). A CVA in this territory can lead to paresis and sensory loss in the opposite lower limb.

Middle cerebral arteries give off deep branches (**lenticulostriate arteries**) which supply the anterior limb of the internal capsule and part of the basal ganglia. They then pass out to the lateral surface of the cerebral hemisphere with branches to the frontal, parietal and superior temporal lobes (Fig. 8.22). The clinical effects of occlusion depends on the

Clinical box 8.8 | **Cerebrovascular accidents (strokes)**

Definition: Any focal neurological deficit of vascular origin which is either fatal or lasts longer than 24 hours.

There are two types of stroke:

- **Occlusive strokes** (84% of all strokes) are typically the result of:
  - Atherosclerosis within cerebral vessels leading to thrombosis (see Ch. 11)
  - Migration of thrombo-emboli into cerebral vasculature from other sites (usually left side of a heart afflicted by atherosclerosis or valvular disease, or neck vessels)
- **Haemorrhagic strokes** are due to rupture of blood vessels and result in subarachnoid or intracerebral haemorrhage and are typically the result of:
  - Hypertension
  - Aneurysms (see Ch. 11).

It is important to determine which type, usually by neuroimaging, as thrombolytic agents (that dissolve clots) are appropriate for occlusive strokes but contraindicated in haemorrhagic strokes.

site and whether the dominant or non-dominant hemisphere is affected but severe cases lead to contralateral hemiplegia, sensory loss and hemianopia (i.e. paralysis, sensory and visual field loss on opposite side).

Posterior cerebral circulation

Arterial branches of the **posterior cerebral, basilar and vertebral arteries** make up the posterior cerebral circulation.

Posterior cerebral arteries supply the occipital lobe, medial and inferior parts of the temporal lobes, and the midbrain (Fig. 8.22).

Basilar artery gives rise to the **superior** and **anterior inferior cerebellar arteries** that supply the lateral pons and cerebellum; and to small **pontine arteries** to the medial pons.

Vertebral arteries give off the **posterior inferior cerebellar arteries** supplying the cerebellum and lateral medulla. The medial medulla is supplied by branches of the **anterior spinal artery**.

Strokes in the posterior circulation, particularly those involving the basilar and vertebral arteries, are often fatal or lead to profound consequences due to the loss of blood supply to the brainstem. For example, complete occlusion of the basilar artery can result in loss of consciousness, bilateral motor and sensory dysfunction, cerebellar signs and cranial nerve signs.

Arterial blood supply to the spinal cord

There are three principal arteries that supply the spinal cord:

- A single **anterior spinal artery** formed by two branches of the vertebral artery that join at the level of the foramen magnum. The anterior spinal artery supplies the anterior two thirds of the cord, which is mainly a motor area.
- Two **posterior spinal arteries** each arising from the posterior inferior cerebellar artery at the foramen magnum. The posterior spinal artery supplies the posterior one third of the cord – a predominantly sensory area.

This central supply is supplemented by a peripheral system of **radicular arteries** (21 pairs) arising from segmental spinal arteries that contribute to the spinal arteries and supply the nerve roots. Segmental spinal arteries enter the intervertebral foramina at every level arising from the vertebral and deep cervical arteries in the neck, the posterior intercostal arteries in the thorax, and the lumbar arteries in the abdomen.

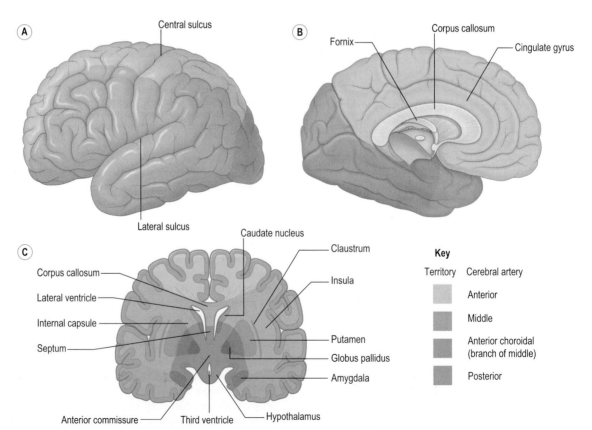

Fig. 8.22 **Territories of the cerebral arteries.** (A) Lateral view; (B) medial view; (C) coronal section through the brain at the level of the anterior commissure.

Venous drainage

Deoxygenated blood from the brain is carried to the superior vena cava via the internal jugular veins through a complex arrangement of superficial and deep venous systems:

- The superficial (or external) veins drain the superficial surfaces of both hemispheres
- The deep (or internal) cerebral veins drain blood from the deep white matter of the cerebral hemispheres and the basal ganglia.

Blood from the cerebral veins then connect to **venous sinuses** which are venous channels made of rigid layers of dura mater lined with endothelium. Unlike veins, dural sinuses lack tunica muscularis so that they do not collapse with raised intracranial pressure; they also lack valves so that blood can flow in any direction. The sinuses also receive CSF from the subarachnoid space through the arachnoid granulations. The major sinuses and veins are shown in Figure 8.23.

The superficial cerebral veins lie in the subarachnoid space, and blood is drained into the nearest venous sinus:

- The **superior sagittal sinus** runs at the site of the attachment of the falx cerebri. A mediolateral group of superficial veins drain blood from the upper part of both cerebral hemispheres into it. The **inferior sagittal sinus** receives blood from the falx and small veins from medial cerebral hemispheres and joins the great cerebral vein to form the **straight sinus**.
- Superficial veins from ventrolateral areas of each hemisphere drain to a **transverse sinus**.
- An anterior group of veins from the orbits and inferior frontal and parietal lobes go to the **cavernous sinus**. The cavernous sinus is a network of dural venous channels between the sphenoid and temporal bones lateral to the sella turcica, which contains the pituitary gland. It is also traversed by the IIIrd, IVth and VIth cranial nerves associated with eye movements and the ophthalmic and mandibular divisions of the trigeminal (V) nerve.

Deep veins receive blood from the deep white matter of the brain, the basal ganglia and thalamus and drain into two **internal cerebral veins**.

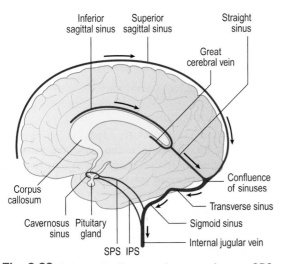

Fig. 8.23 **Schematic diagram of venous sinuses.** SPS, superior petrosal sinus; IPS, inferior petrosal sinus.

Labels: Inferior sagittal sinus; Superior sagittal sinus; Straight sinus; Great cerebral vein; Corpus callosum; Cavernosus sinus; Pituitary gland; SPS IPS; Confluence of sinuses; Transverse sinus; Sigmoid sinus; Internal jugular vein

- The two internal cerebral veins join under the corpus callosum to form the **great cerebral vein** (of Galen). This unites with the inferior sagittal sinus to form the straight sinus.

The superior sagittal and straight sinuses meet at the *confluence of sinuses* where blood then proceeds to drain into the transverse sinuses and on to the **sigmoid sinus** and **internal jugular vein**. The cavernous sinus drains via the superior and inferior petrosal sinuses to the sigmoid sinus and internal jugular vein, respectively (see Fig. 8.23).

Damage to the superficial cerebral veins, usually from trauma, can result in subdural haemorrhage (see Clinical box 8.4). Thrombotic occlusion of the venous system although rare is an important form of stroke (Clinical box 8.9).

BLOOD–BRAIN BARRIER

The blood–brain barrier separates blood in the systemic circulation from the extracellular fluid of the brain. It has a metabolic function supplying the brain with nutrients and removing waste products. It is also protective, preventing bacteria and large molecules from entering the brain. Drugs targeted at the brain need to 'breach' or bypass the barrier. Inflammation can disrupt the blood–brain barrier increasing its permeability so allowing antibiotics to pass. However, this increased permeability also allows proteins to enter the extracellular space leading to cerebral oedema (Information box 8.4).

The blood–brain barrier is formed by brain capillary endothelial cells that are held together by **tight junctions** (Fig. 8.24). Astrocyte projections, known as end feet, surround the endothelial cells and provide metabolic and mechanical support.

Water and some water- or lipid-soluble substances can traverse the blood–brain barrier by **passive diffusion** across the plasma membranes of endothelial cells. Other water-soluble substances require **facilitated diffusion**, e.g. glucose using GLUT 1 transporters (see Ch. 2). Amino acids produced by the brain are removed by **carrier-mediated active transport**: one each for basic (e.g. arginine), neutral (e.g. phenylalanine) and acidic (e.g. glutamate) amino acids. Some large molecules (e.g. insulin, leptin) cross the blood–brain barrier by receptor-mediated endocytosis.

Some areas of the brain are not on the brain side of the blood–brain barrier. These are the **circumventricular organs**, e.g. the pineal and posterior pituitary glands. The capillaries

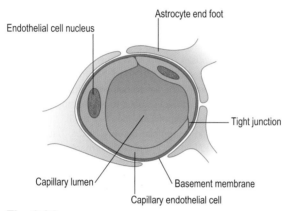

Fig. 8.24 **Blood–brain barrier.** Endothelial cells line the lumen and are joined by tight junctions. These are surrounded by a basement membrane and astrocytic end feet.

of circumventricular organs are fenestrated allowing them to secrete large molecules into the circulation (e.g. the pineal gland releases melatonin directly into the systemic circulation). Also by being in direct contact with the blood these organs can monitor the levels of hormones in peripheral blood. For example, the posterior pituitary gland monitors endocrine hormone levels (see Ch. 10).

METABOLIC REQUIREMENTS OF THE BRAIN

The preferred energy substrate for brain is glucose which is transported into the brain mostly via glucose transporters on capillary endothelial cells, neurons and astrocytes. Some glucose is transformed to lactate by astrocytes which supply the lactate to neurons described as the astrocyte–neuron **lactate shuttle** (see Ch. 3).

The brain consumes about 60% of the body's glucose, most of which is used to maintain the ion transport processes needed for neural signalling. Under conditions of starvation for several days, ketones (acetoacetate and D-3-hydroxybutyrate) can substitute for glucose as the main energy source. This occurs naturally in breastfed infants in whom lipids provide over half of the brain's total calories. Ketones can be used by both neurons and astrocytes, but

the β-oxidation of fatty acids (see Chs 2 and 3) which generates them occurs only in astrocytes.

Functional brain imaging (Information box 8.5) is based on detecting metabolism in different brain regions.

TRANSMISSION OF NEURAL SIGNALS

Stimulation of **excitable cells** (neurons, muscle cells, and some endocrine and exocrine cells) reverses the **resting membrane potential** producing an **action potential** which spreads at high speed over the surface of the cell. Action potentials in neurons are often called **nerve impulses** and are responsible for signalling between neurons at junctions, known as **synapses**, and triggering contraction in muscle cells and secretion in glands. The transmission and processing of information by neurons is referred to as **neural signalling**.

ACTION POTENTIALS

Equilibrium potentials

Ions are distributed asymmetrically across the plasma membrane of cells resulting in the **resting membrane potential** (see Ch. 2, Table 2.4). This net charge across the membrane means the cell is **polarised** with the inside negative. In most cells the resting potential is of the order of −60 mV but is usually higher in excitable cells ranging to as high as −90 mV in some muscle cells.

The origin of the resting potential can be explained using a model cell. The membrane is quite permeable to potassium cations (K⁺) but not to protein anions inside the cell where the K⁺ cations are balanced by an equal number of anions (Fig. 8.25A).

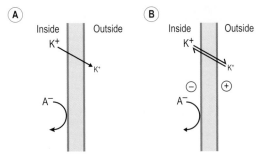

Fig. 8.25 The origin of the resting potential. (A) Initially K$^+$ ions leak down their concentration gradient; the membrane is impermeable to large anions (A$^-$). (B) At equilibrium a small potential difference is established by the separation of charges.

This results in a high concentration of K$^+$ inside and a low concentration of K$^+$ outside. This leads to a **diffusion force** acting to drive K$^+$ ions down this concentration gradient and out of the cell. However, if K$^+$ ions leave the cell an equivalent number of negative charges on intracellular anions are unmasked creating an **electrical force** acting in the opposite direction to the diffusion force. With time, the diffusion and electrical forces equal each other and a state of equilibrium exists.

At equilibrium there remains a very low concentration of K$^+$ outside and a small deficit of K$^+$ inside creating a potential difference across the membrane (Fig. 8.25B). This potential, the **potassium equilibrium potential** (E_K), is when the number of K$^+$ ions leaving and entering the cell is exactly balanced.

The resting potential in neurons is not as large as the E_K because Na$^+$ ions also contribute. The actual potential lies between the E_K which is −94mV and the E_{Na} of +62mV but is much closer to E_K because the resting membrane has a much lower permeability for Na$^+$ than for K$^+$ and typically is between −60mV and −85mV.

Depolarisation and hyperpolarisation

Neurons are constantly bombarded with stimuli that alter membrane permeability and change the membrane potential. If the changed permeability allows more cations (e.g. Na$^+$) to enter a neuron its membrane potential decreases (becomes less negative), and the cell is said to be **depolarised**. Conversely, if the change leads to either the efflux of positive charges (e.g. K$^+$) or entry of negative charges (e.g. Cl$^-$) the potential increases (becomes more negative), and the cell is **hyperpolarised**. The ions then redistribute across the membrane depending on their equilibrium potentials and permeabilities. The flow of charges stops and the membrane potential rapidly returns to the resting value.

Generation of action potentials

An action potential is a rapid depolarisation of the cell membrane potential which travels along the length of the cell without a decrease in amplitude. It is caused by the opening of voltage-gated ion channels (see Ch. 4) specifically for Na$^+$ and K$^+$. The opening of these channels change the conductance (Information box 8.6) of Na$^+$ and K$^+$ with resulting changes in the membrane potential.

The action potential can be divided into four phases (Fig. 8.26):

1. **Initiation**: A stimulus results in depolarisation of the membrane potential to a **threshold voltage**.
2. **Upstroke**: There is a rapid increase in the membrane potential which includes an **overshoot** to a positive value (e.g. +30 to +50mV).

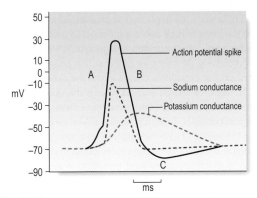

Fig. 8.26 Potential and conductance changes during a neural action potential.

3. **Repolarisation**: The membrane potential returns to a negative value and in fact falls transiently to below the normal resting potential – described as **after-hyperpolarisation**.
4. **Refractory period**: After repolarisation triggering of a further action potential is impossible or requires a much stronger stimulus.

Initiation

Typically, neurons must be depolarised to between about −60 and −50mV (the threshold voltage) before they fire an action potential. The stimulus that makes a cell fire on 50% of the occasions on which it is applied is the **threshold stimulus**. Action potentials obey an **all-or-nothing** rule in that they either do or do not fire.

Upstroke

When the depolarising stimulus reaches threshold voltage, **voltage-gated sodium channels** open resulting in a marked rise in **Na$^+$ conductance**. Na$^+$ ions flood into the cell. These channels stay open for only about a millisecond and then go into an **inactivated state** in which they are 'locked shut'. Thus the increased Na$^+$ conductance is switched off. Also the electrochemical gradient driving sodium inwards reduces as the membrane potential approaches the sodium equilibrium potential (E_{Na}).

Repolarisation

The same depolarisation stimulus that opens the sodium channels also triggers the opening of **voltage-gated potassium channels**. They take longer to respond and their opening is delayed and occurs about the same time as the sodium channels are inactivated. The opening of the potassium channels results in a rise in **K$^+$ conductance** causing an outward flow of K$^+$ ions that quickly drives the membrane potential towards the potassium equilibrium potential (E_K). This is slightly more negative than the resting potential, hence the **after-hyperpolarisation**.

Refractory period

The refractory period can be divided into two phases. When the voltage-gated sodium channels are inactivated a further action potential cannot pass. This is called the **absolute refractory period**.

Shortly after this sodium channels gradually recover. Around the same time the after-hyperpolarisation briefly makes the membrane potential more negative. This is the **relative refractory period** during which a greater than normal stimulus is needed to fire another action potential.

Conduction of action potentials

Action potentials are generated at an area within the neuron called the **axon hillock** and are propagated along the axons because local circuit currents are generated in front of the action potential. At the spike of the action potential there is a slight excess of positive charge inside the axon and an excess of negative charge outside. This is the opposite of the normal resting potential of the axon membrane just ahead of the action potential. Thus, a potential difference builds up between the region of axon undergoing an action potential and the region ahead. This causes local circuit currents to flow from A to B intracellularly (and from B to A extracellularly), which depolarises the membrane just ahead of the action potential, opening sodium channels so that the action potential advances (Fig. 8.27A). Current does not pass backwards as the membrane region behind the action potential is in a refractory state.

The **speed** of conduction depends on the diameter of the axon: the larger the diameter, the higher the conduction velocity (see Table 8.4). It also depends on whether or not an axon is **myelinated**. Because the myelin sheath has a high electrical resistance, local circuit currents can flow only between adjacent, low resistance, nodes of Ranvier. Action potentials jump between successive nodes, a process known as **saltatory conduction** (Fig. 8.27B). Saltatory conduction in myelinated fibres is faster than conduction in non-myelinated fibres. Demyelination of axons in the CNS occurs in multiple sclerosis (Clinical box 8.10). In the peripheral nervous system one way of classifying the many forms of peripheral neuropathy is into either demyelinating (Clinical box 8.11) or axonal neuropathies.

SYNAPSES

The specialised structure that allows a neuron to pass a signal to another cell, which may be another neuron, a muscle or gland cell, is known as a **synapse**. There are two types of synapse: **electrical** and **chemical**.

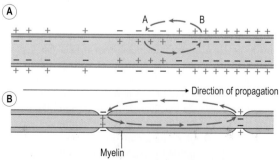

Fig. 8.27 **Propagation of the action potential in (A) unmyelinated and (B) myelinated axons.**

Clinical box 8.10　**Multiple sclerosis**

Multiple sclerosis is a disease of unknown cause but involves a disorder of immunity in which T cells (see Ch. 6) inappropriately target CNS myelin proteins, producing demyelination of axons.

In myelinated axons, although the Na$^+$ channels are confined to the nodes of Ranvier, the K$^+$ channels are expressed all along the axon. Demyelination uncovers these K$^+$ channels which can then be inappropriately activated by local circuit currents. Increased K$^+$ efflux hyperpolarises the axon, rendering it less excitable. This causes **conduction block**, which accounts for the paralysis and sensory losses. Demyelination also results in the expression of a type of voltage-dependent Na$^+$ channel that does not inactivate readily in the exposed and previously internodal membrane. If these channels are activated, bursts of improperly conducted action potentials are generated; these cause **paraesthesias** ('pins and needles').

Treatment for multiple sclerosis is aimed at curtailing the immune disturbance. For example, a number of cytokines which curb T cells are currently being evaluated, including β-interferon.

Clinical box 8.11　**Guillain–Barré syndrome**

Guillain–Barré syndrome (GBS; or acute idiopathic polyneuropathy) is the most common acquired demyelinating polyneuropathy.

Over half of those affected suffer symptoms of a respiratory or gastrointestinal infection 1–3 weeks prior to developing GBS. Both antibody and cell-mediated reactions to peripheral nerve myelin appear involved. There is segmental demyelination and, in severe cases, secondary axonal damage occurs.

The first symptoms are usually paraesthesia (pins and needles) in feet, then hands, but are followed by weakness which may be generalised, proximal or start distally in the feet and ascend. Tendon reflexes are lost. In severe cases the weakness may affect respiration and the patient requires ventilation.

Intravenous immune globulin speeds recovery and improves outcome. The overall prognosis is favourable but mortality is around 2% and about 25% of patients are left with some disability.

Electrical synapses

Electrical synapses are formed by **gap junctions**, where the plasma membranes of adjacent cells are only 2–3.5 nm apart. A gap junction is made up of one **connexon** from each connecting cell, forming a channel with a diameter of 1.5 nm. Each connexon is composed of six protein subunits called **connexins**.

The gap junction allows the flow of ions (e.g. Na$^+$, K$^+$, Ca^{2+}) and small molecules (e.g. ATP) between the cytoplasm of the connecting cells. Electrical synapses allow the rapid (0.1 ms) and bi-directional flow of currents between adjacent neurons (e.g. retinal interneurons) but these synapses are predominantly found in cardiac and smooth muscle.

Chemical synapses

Most synapses in the nervous system are chemical and, unlike electrical synapses, are unidirectional. The neuromuscular junction between a motor neuron and skeletal muscle is a chemical synapse (see Ch. 9) and is not discussed further here.

Between neurons the synapse is a junction between the **terminal bouton** of the axon of one neuron and the target cell. A **synaptic cleft**, a gap 30 nm wide, separates the **presynaptic membrane** of the terminal bouton and **postsynaptic membrane** of the target cell (Fig. 8.28). The presynaptic terminal has **synaptic vesicles** which contain the chemical neurotransmitter and its membrane has an **active zone** where synaptic vesicles can dock and release transmitter. The postsynaptic membrane opposite the active zone has a **postsynaptic density** packed with receptors capable of binding transmitter.

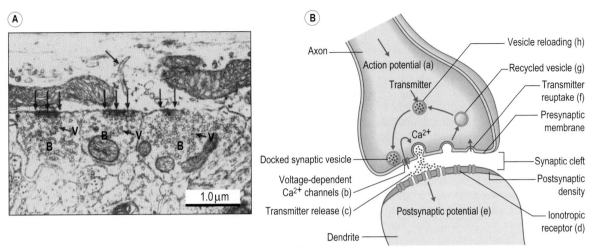

Fig. 8.28 (A) Electron micrograph of a central synapse. Arrows indicate active zones with postsynaptic densities; B, bouton; V, vesicle. From Young B, et al. (eds) 2012 Wheater's functional histology, 6th edn. Churchill Livingstone, Edinburgh. (B) Diagrammatic illustration of events in chemical transmission at central synapses. For explanation of the steps please see the text.

NEUROTRANSMISSION

Neurotransmission is an example of **excitation-secretion coupling**. A summary of the sequence of events during neurotransmission at a synapse (see Fig. 8.28B) is:

a. An action potential arrives at the presynaptic terminal
b. Depolarisation opens voltage-gated calcium channels in the presynaptic membrane allowing Ca^{2+} to enter the terminal
c. The rise in Ca^{2+} concentration triggers the release of transmitter from a synaptic vesicle into the synaptic cleft
d. The transmitter diffuses across the cleft, and binds to its receptors on the postsynaptic membrane
e. Binding of transmitter and receptor alters the conductance of the postsynaptic cell to ions, producing a postsynaptic potential – precisely which ions depends on the nature of the transmitter and on which of its receptors is involved
f. Transmitter is transported back into the neuron (but see neurotransmitter inactivation below)
g. The synaptic vesicle is recycled and reloaded with transmitter (h).

The outcome is either to increase or decrease the probability that the postsynaptic cell will fire action potentials. A transmitter acting to increase the chance of firing is described as **excitatory** whereas if it decreases the firing probability it is **inhibitory**. A given transmitter might be excitatory at one synapse but inhibitory at another, depending on which of its receptors is present.

Neurotransmitters

There are two broad categories of neurotransmitters (see Table 8.6):

- **Classical transmitters**: small molecules such as amino acids and monoamines. These are stored in **small synaptic vesicles** which are clear, spherical, membrane-bound organelles about 50 nm across.
- **Peptide neurotransmitters (or neuropeptides)**: these are synthesised on ribosomes, secreted into the rough endoplasmic reticulum and packaged into **large (dense core) vesicles** (120–200 nm) by the Golgi apparatus.

The release of neuropeptides is typically slower than that of the classic transmitters and their effects are much more prolonged.

Neurotransmitter release

Classical neurotransmitter secretion occurs by vesicle exocytosis triggered by the sudden rise in intracellular calcium brought about by action potential depolarisation. The vesicle membrane fuses with the presynaptic membrane to open a pore through which transmitter is discharged, after which the pore closes and the vesicle disengages. This is **fast release** (as opposed to slow release which occurs at the neuromuscular junction) and is able to support long periods of high synaptic activity.

Exocytosis of transmitter from **small synaptic vesicles** has several steps. Vesicles are normally anchored to the cytoskeleton by **synapsin I**. Calcium-dependent phosphorylation of this protein frees vesicles into a releasable pool. These vesicles dock with specific sites at the **active zone** by interactions of proteins termed **SNARES**. Hydrolysis of ATP now causes partial fusion of vesicle and presynaptic membranes so that the vesicle is now ready to release its contents. Botulinum and tetanus toxins disrupt SNARES, interfering with neurotransmitter docking.

Dense core vesicles can liberate their **neuropeptide transmitters** from anywhere in the terminal membrane, not only from the active zone. Higher concentrations of calcium are required to trigger exocytosis of large dense core vesicles, hence higher firing frequencies are needed to liberate neuropeptides.

Many synapses can release more than one transmitter. This is termed **co-transmission** and often involves the secretion of a classic transmitter in response to a modest firing frequency, supplemented by release of a neuropeptide at higher frequencies.

Neurotransmitter receptors

Generally neurotransmitters attach to two types of cell surface receptors (see Chs 2 and 4):

- Ligand-gated ion channels (**ionotropic receptors**): membrane receptors coupled directly to an ion channel. Transmission is fast occurring in a few milliseconds.

- G-protein-coupled (**metabotropic**) receptors: the neurotransmitter modulates the activity of ion channels indirectly and so transmission is slower (>100 ms).

Many classic transmitters have both ionotropic and metabotropic receptors and hence are both fast and slow transmitters.

When a neurotransmitter binds to an ionotropic receptor ion channels open permitting ions to flow in. This produces a **postsynaptic current** which changes the membrane potential, generating a **postsynaptic potential**, which is either excitatory or inhibitory.

If activation of a receptor causes a net inward current, the postsynaptic membrane depolarises. This is an **excitatory postsynaptic potential** (**EPSP**) as it brings the cell closer to the threshold for firing action potentials. Glutamate and acetylcholine produce EPSPs via non-selective cation channels (Fig. 8.29A).

Conversely receptor activation that results in a net outward current makes the membrane potential become more negative and produces an **inhibitory postsynaptic potential** (**IPSP**), so reducing the probability of the postsynaptic neuron firing. **GABA** (γ-aminobutyrate) and glycine are the principal inhibitory neurotransmitters and act on ion channels selective for chloride or potassium (Fig. 8.29B).

Summation

In contrast to action potentials which maintain their amplitude as they pass along the axon, postsynaptic potentials get smaller, or decay, both with time and distance. At any given instant one neuron may receive EPSPs and IPSPs from hundreds or thousands of neurons. However, postsynaptic potentials can combine together to form a larger potential. This is referred to as summation.

Whether or not the postsynaptic neuron fires is dependent on the summed potential (i.e. the combined effects of EPSPs and IPSPs) arriving at its axon hillock.

There are two types of summation, temporal and spatial (see Fig. 8.30). If for simplicity we imagine only EPSPs:

- Temporal summation occurs when EPSPs arrive rapidly one after the other at the same target cell, without the time to decay, bringing the membrane potential to threshold
- Spatial summation is when EPSPs from different sites on the neuron combine at the same time.

If only IPSPs were summed the membrane potential would move away from threshold.

Neurotransmitter inactivation

The effect of the neurotransmitter is terminated in three main ways:

- **Reuptake** of the transmitter by the presynaptic neuron or by glial cells.
- **Enzymatic destruction** for example of acetylcholine which is broken down into acetate and choline by the enzyme **acetylcholinesterase**. Several drugs act on acetylcholinesterase (see Ch. 4).
- **Diffusion** away from the synaptic cleft. This occurs slowly with peptide transmitters explaining their long duration of action.

Presynaptic receptors

Presynaptic receptors can regulate neurotransmitter synthesis and release in the CNS and peripheral nervous system. A presynaptic receptor that is stimulated by the same transmitter

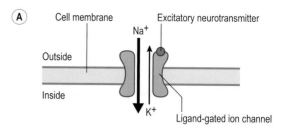
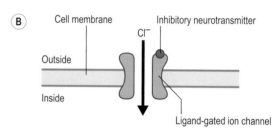
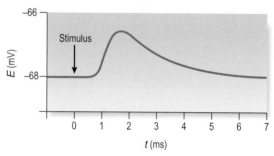
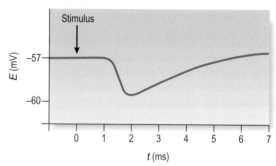

Fig. 8.29 **Ligand-gated ion channels and synaptic potentials.** (A) Glutamate and acetylcholine produce excitatory postsynaptic potentials (EPSPs); (B) γ-aminobutyrate (GABA) and glycine produce inhibitory postsynaptic potentials (IPSPs). Redrawn from Longstaff A 2005 Instant notes in neuroscience, 2nd edn. Taylor & Francis, Abingdon, with permission.

released by the neuron is known as an **autoreceptor**. These can be inhibitory or excitatory. When a transmitter different to that released by the neuron acts on the presynaptic receptor it is termed a **heteroceptor**.

Types of neurotransmitters

There are five main types of neurotransmitter: amino acids, acetylcholine, monoamines, purines and peptides (Table 8.6) (see also Ch. 4).

Amino acids

Excitatory amino acids

The principal excitatory amino acid transmitter is **glutamate**. It is widespread throughout the CNS and most cells in the cerebral cortex respond to glutamate.

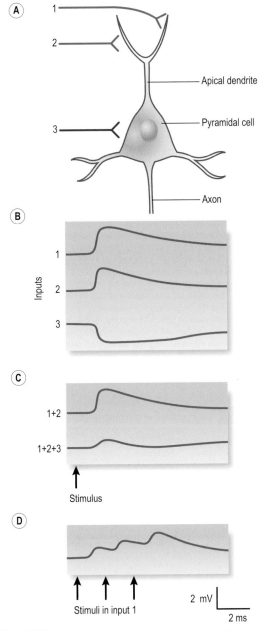

Fig. 8.30 Summation. (A) Three inputs onto different regions of a cortical pyramidal cell. 1 and 2 are excitatory, 3 is inhibitory. (B) Postsynaptic potentials recorded from the cell body after stimulating each of the inputs individually. (C) Spatial summation: postsynaptic potentials caused by stimulating pairs of inputs at the same time. (D) Temporal summation: the postsynaptic potential generated by repeated stimulation of an excitatory input.

Glutamate is synthesised in neurons from glutamine and is then pumped into vesicles. After release it is removed from the synaptic cleft by glutamate transporters in neurons and glia (Fig. 8.31A). In neurons the glutamate is probably metabolised although some may be re-used as a transmitter but in glial cells it is converted to glutamine which is taken up by neurons.

Glutamate acts at both ionotropic and metabotropic receptors responsible for fast and slow transmission respectively. Two populations of ionotropic receptors mediate glutamate fast transmission:

- **AMPA** receptors: when glutamate binds a conformation shift allows an influx of Na^+ ions. A less common subtype, **AMPA**-kainate receptors, are also permeable to Ca^{2+}.

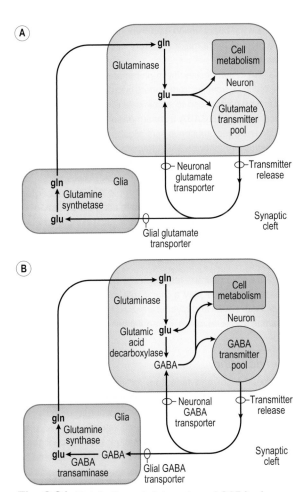

Fig. 8.31 Metabolism of glutamate and GABA. gln, glutamine; glu, glutamate.

Table 8.6	Major neurotransmitters			
	Classical transmitters			**Peptide transmitters**
Amino acids	**Monoamines**	**Purines**		
Glutamate	Acetylcholine	Adenosine		Substance P
GABA	Epinephrine (adrenaline)	ATP		Met-enkephalin
Glycine	Norepinephrine (noradrenaline)			β-Endorphin
	Dopamine			Dynorphins
	Serotonin			Somatostatin
	Histamine			Cholecystokinin

- **NMDA** receptors: these are ion channels particularly permeable to Ca^{2+}. These channels need to bind not only to glutamate but also to glycine, as a **co-agonist**, to open. In addition, at normal resting membrane potentials the ion channel is blocked by Mg^{2+} ions, which must be removed by depolarisation to allow Ca^{2+} to enter. NMDA receptors have a role in the rewiring of neural circuits during development and are involved in learning.

In high concentration glutamate is toxic to the brain. It may be responsible for cell death in stroke (Information box 8.7) and in status epilepticus. Reduced reuptake by glial glutamate transporter may underlie the excitotoxicity seen in motor neuron disease, a condition characterised by loss of motor neurons.

Inhibitory amino acids

The main inhibitory amino acid throughout the CNS is GABA while **glycine** has a major inhibitory role in the brainstem and spinal cord.

GABA is synthesised from glutamate; after release GABA is taken up by specific transporters into both neurons and glia, and is then catabolised to succinic semialdehyde by the mitochondrial enzyme **GABA transaminase** (see Fig. 8.31B). The GABA analogue anticonvulsant vigabatrin is an irreversible competitive inhibitor of GABA transaminase and is thought to act by increasing the neurotransmitter pool of GABA.

There are both ionotropic ($GABA_A$) receptors (see Information box 8.8) and metabotropic ($GABA_B$) receptors. Binding of GABA to $GABA_A$ receptors allows the influx of Cl^- ions causing hyperpolarisation of cells and taking the neuron further from its threshold potential.

Glycine receptors have a similar mode of action to $GABA_A$ receptors.

GABAergic neurons represent the sole output of the cerebellar cortex and play a major role in basal ganglia pathways. Both GABA and glycine are used by many interneurons including those involved in regulation of muscle tone (see below).

Acetylcholine

The metabolism and receptors for acetylcholine (ACh) are described in Chapter 4 and at the neuromuscular junction in Chapter 9. There are four major cholinergic pathways in the CNS (Table 8.7). In the brain, cholinergic pathways are thought important in memory formation. Loss of cholinergic neurons occurs in Alzheimer disease, in which symptoms are aggravated by anticholinergic drugs.

Information box 8.7   **Excitotoxicity and strokes**

Cell death that occurs in the penumbra of a stroke infarct are caused by the excessive release of glutamate from neurons. This phenomenon is termed **excitotoxicity**. The sequence of events is as follows:

1. Hypoxia from the lack of blood flow causes failure of the Na^+/K^+-ATPase leading to **cytotoxic oedema** and a fall in the extracellular fluid (ECF) volume
2. K^+ ions accumulate in the ECF, depolarising neurons, opening voltage-gated Ca^{2+} channels driving the release of glutamate
3. Large scale activation of AMPA receptors lifts the Mg^{2+} block on NMDA receptors, allowing more Ca^{2+} influx
4. In the absence of energy to power them, transport mechanisms that keep cytoplasmic concentrations low are overloaded
5. High intracellular Ca^{2+} triggers apoptosis or cell death.

Information box 8.8   **Drugs acting at $GABA_A$ receptors**

Several drugs act at $GABA_A$ receptors, particularly barbiturates and benzodiazepines.

The **barbiturates** (e.g. phenobarbital) and **benzodiazepines** (e.g. diazepam) both bind to separate sites which allosterically alter the affinity for GABA binding. Binding of the drug and GABA produces a greater flux of Cl^- through the $GABA_A$ receptor than does GABA alone, thereby enhancing inhibition.

Both these drug groups cause sedation. Highly lipophilic barbiturates (e.g. thiopental) cross the blood–brain barrier very easily and are used intravenously for rapid induction of anaesthesia. Benzodiazepines can be used intravenously to provide sedation for minor procedures and are used to terminate seizures in status epilepticus. Some are used orally in epilepsy treatment (e.g. clonazepam) but sedation limits their usefulness. Some barbiturates (e.g. phenobarbital) have a specific anticonvulsant action and are used in the long-term management of epilepsy. Oral benzodiazepines are sometimes used short-term as anxiolytics (i.e. anxiety reducing agents).

Ethanol acts on $GABA_A$ receptors and this contributes to the intoxication and ataxia of drunkenness.

Flumazenil, an antagonist of the benzodiazepine binding site on the $GABA_A$ receptor, reverses the effects of benzodiazepine overdose and the CNS effects of acute ethanol intoxication. There are compounds which bind to the $GABA_A$ benzodiazepine site which reduce the GABA-evoked chloride flux. These **inverse agonists** have the opposite pharmacological profile to the usual agonist benzodiazepines; they are proconvulsants and anxiety-producing.

Table 8.7   **Major cholinergic pathways**

Origin	Destination	Role
Pontine reticular formation	Forebrain (thalamus) and spinal cord	Sleep and wakefulness
Forebrain	Cerebral cortex	Cortical arousal
Septum	Hippocampus	Learning and memory
Ventral horn of spinal grey matter	Skeletal muscle	Movement

Monoamines

The major brain monoamines are:

- The catecholamines: norepinephrine (noradrenaline) and epinephrine (adrenaline), dopamine
- Serotonin (5-hydroxytryptamine, 5-HT)
- Histamine.

The metabolism and receptors for norepinephrine and epinephrine and the metabolism of dopamine are dealt with in Chapter 4. Dopamine receptors are G-protein-coupled receptors and fall into two families: D_1 family (D_1 and D_5) act through G_s, increasing cAMP levels causing excitation; and D_2 family (D_2, D_3 and D_4) which are G_i linked, reduce cAMP and are inhibitory.

Serotonin is synthesised from **tryptophan** first by hydroxylation then decarboxylation. Serotonin is removed from the synaptic cleft by a specific transport system. The synthesis and release of transmitter from many catecholaminergic neurons and serotonergic neurons is regulated by autoreceptors. Histamine receptors are discussed in Chapter 6.

The cell bodies of neurons containing monoaminergic transmitters are mainly found in the brainstem but their axons

Table 8.8	Noradrenergic and adrenergic pathways	
Origin	**Destination**	**Role**
Locus coeruleus (dorsal pons)	Widely throughout brain but especially cerebral cortex	Sleep and arousal
Nucleus ambiguus (ventral medulla)	Hypothalamus	Endocrine and cardiovascular functions
Nucleus of the solitary tract	Hypothalamus Parabrachial nucleus	Effects on visceral and ventilatory networks
Motor nucleus of vagus nerve (dorsal medulla)		
Pons	Spinal cord	Pain perception (AD) Tonic vasoconstriction (NA)

Table 8.9	Major dopaminergic pathways	
Origin	**Destination**	**Role**
Substantia nigra (nigrostriatal)	Striatum	Intentional movement
Tegmentum (mesolimbic)	Limbic system	Reward, motivation
Tegmentum (mesocortical)	Prefrontal cortex	Working memory Cognitive tasks
Hypothalamus (tuberoinfundibular)	Median eminence	Pituitary secretion of prolactin
Hypothalamus	Spinal grey matter	Sympathetic

Table 8.10	Major serotonergic pathways	
Origin	**Destination**	**Role**
Medulla and ventral pons	Spinal cord	Pain perception Autonomic modulation Modulation of motor output
Dorsal pons and midbrain	Medial forebrain bundle, especially hypothalamus	Cardiovascular and thermoregulatory homeostasis
Dorsal pons and midbrain	Cerebral cortex	Cortical modulation
Dorsal pons	Pons (cholinergic neurons)	Termination of rapid eye movement (REM) sleep
Several raphe nuclei	Cerebral blood vessels	Regulation of cerebral blood flow
	Choroid plexus	Secretion of cerebrospinal fluid

are widely distributed throughout the CNS. Tables 8.8–8.10 summarise the main pathways; brief notes on each follow:

- **Norepinephrine and epinephrine**: noradrenergic neurons in the **locus coeruleus** are important in sleep and brain arousal systems (see Fig. 8.67). Others are involved via the hypothalamus with endocrine and autonomic function, and those to the spinal cord modulate pain transmission.

- **Dopamine**: the largest concentration of dopaminergic neurons is in the nigrostriatal pathway in the basal ganglia system. Loss of these neurons occurs in Parkinson disease. The mesolimbic and mesocortical pathways are involved in reward, motivation and cognitive pathways. D_1 agonists are used in Parkinson disease and in some endocrine disorders (see Ch. 10). D_2 antagonists are used in schizophrenia, which is associated with defects in dopamine neurotransmission in the mesolimbic and mesocortical systems.

- **Serotonin**: there are multiple serotonergic pathways; ascending pathways participate in regulation of temperature, sleep, eating, and in emotional responses. The latter explains the probable relation between reduced serotonergic transmission and depression and the use of **selective serotonin reuptake inhibitors** (**SSRIs**) in its treatment. The recreational drug 'Ecstasy' (3,4-methylene-dioxymethamphetamine, MDMA) reduces anxiety and produces euphoria by competing with serotonin for the reuptake system, thus increasing cytoplasmic serotonin levels (see also Information box 8.9).

- **Histamine**: concentrated in the tuberomamillary nucleus, histaminergic neurons project widely in the CNS. They are involved in sleep and arousal system. Antihistamines (H_2 antagonists) that cross the blood–brain barrier may cause drowsiness as a side effect.

Purines

The purine neurotransmitters are **ATP** and **adenosine**. A number of receptors have been identified (Table 8.11) at sites in both the CNS and PNS. Their function is not fully understood.

ATP is co-released with classical transmitters from post-ganglionic autonomic fibres and some central synapses. Thus it acts as a co-transmitter with norepinephrine in some sympathetic pathways and with acetylcholine in certain post-ganglionic parasympathetic synapses. There is also evidence of its release from sensory afferents in the spinal cord.

Adenosine acts at A_1 presynaptic receptors reducing the release of a number of transmitters in the peripheral

Information box 8.9	Serotonin, GABA and anxiety

Serotonin neurotransmission is implicated in anxiety:
- In animal experiments, destruction of serotonergic neurons reduces behaviours associated with anxiety.
- There is an association between anxiety and a long version of the gene for the serotonin transporter that clears serotonin from the synaptic cleft faster than the short version.
- Serotonin 5-HT$_{1A}$ receptors are inhibitory metabotropic autoreceptors of serotonergic nerve terminals which decrease serotonin secretion. Partial agonists of 5-HT$_{1A}$ receptors (e.g. buspirone) – which reduce serotonin release – have proved to be clinically potent **anxiolytic** (anxiety-reducing) agents.

GABA transmission is implicated in anxiety because high numbers of GABA$_A$ receptors are found in the limbic system, particularly in the amygdala, and benzodiazepines (Information box 8.8) are anxiolytic. Benzodiazepine inverse agonists are actually **anxiogenic** (anxiety-generating) agents. It is possible that there are endogenous inverse agonists which are mediators of anxiety.

Serotonergic neurons are inhibited by GABAergic neurons so indirect actions on serotonin transmission may contribute to the anxiolytic actions of benzodiazepines.

Table 8.11	Receptors for purine neurotransmitters		
Receptor	**Transduction**	**Endogenous agonists**	**Antagonists**
A_1	G-protein-coupled receptor, increases cAMP	Adenosine	Caffeine, theophylline
A_2	G-protein-coupled receptor, decreases cAMP	Adenosine	
P_{2X}	Ligand-gated cation channel	ATP	
P_{2Y}	G-protein-coupled receptor	ATP, ADP	

Table 8.12	Opioid receptors		
Receptor	**Location**	**Endogenous ligand**	**Preferential agonists***
μ	Ubiquitous	β-Endorphin, dynorphin	Morphine and analogues (e.g. fentanyl)
δ	Spinal cord	β-Endorphin, enkephalins	
κ	Peripheral nervous system	β-Endorphin, dynorphin	Benzomorphans (e.g. pentazocine)

*All receptors are blocked by opioid antagonists (e.g. naloxone).

and CNS, particularly excitatory glutamate. Adenosine levels rise when brain metabolism is very high (e.g. during an epileptic seizure), or during ischaemia. By inhibiting glutamate release, adenosine may naturally curtail seizure activity and be neuroprotective in ischaemia. A_2 receptors are located in nociceptors in the heart. Adenosine levels rise in cardiac ischaemia and these receptors may help mediate the pain of angina.

Peptides

There are a large number of neuropeptides. They include some originally identified in the gastrointestinal tract and so are sometimes termed gut-brain peptides. These include cholecystokinin, vasoactive intestinal peptide, somatostatin and substance P. Substance P belongs to a family of peptides called **tachykinins**. The other major family is the **opioids**.

- Tachykinins: substance P is an excitatory transmitter in several brain regions including the cerebral cortex, striatum and substantia nigra. It is released by both central and peripheral terminals of C fibre primary afferents. The central terminals carry pain and temperature information to dorsal horn cells while release from peripheral terminals causes neurogenic inflammation (see below). Other members of the tachykinin family include substance K and neurokinins A and B.
- Opioids: act on opioid receptors, the targets for opiate drugs such as morphine. Opioids make up an entire class of transmitters. They include enkephalin, met-enkephalin and leu-enkephalin, β-endorphin and dynorphin. They are generally inhibitory and co-released with classical transmitters, e.g. GABA and serotonin. They are widely distributed including in the basal ganglia, limbic system and hypothalamus. Opioid transmission is thought to be important in analgesia pathways in the CNS and is also implicated in emotion and behavioural pathways.

The properties of **opioid receptors** are summarised in Table 8.12. There are three populations – all are G-protein-coupled receptors. The euphoria, dependence and respiratory depression of opiate drugs relate to the μ opioid receptors. The symptoms of opiate drug overdose may be treated with **opiate antagonists** (e.g. naloxone).

MOTOR CONTROL AND PATHWAYS

The control of motor activities involves a multiplicity of systems and pathways. It is useful to consider a **hierarchy** of motor systems which are interconnected with sensory input at all levels. Beginning at the highest level of motor function the hierarchy is as follows:

- The **motor cortex** in the frontal lobe is where voluntary movements are planned and executed from. Signals are sent from here by descending pathways to motor nuclei in the brainstem and spinal cord.
- The **basal ganglia** are also involved in the initiation and scaling of motor actions through connections with the motor cortex.
- The **cerebellum** also influences activity in the motor cortex and is important in the timing, coordination and accuracy of movements.
- At an intermediate level a number of **nuclei in the brainstem** (e.g. reticular, vestibular and red nuclei) provide descending tracts that influence lower motor neurons particularly involved in postural mechanisms.
- The lowest level of the hierarchy is represented by the **motor neurons of cranial nerves** in the brainstem and the α **motor neurons** in the spinal cord which are the targets of the descending motor pathways. These neurons and their axons to muscles are described as the final common pathway for motor action.

Voluntary, goal-directed motor sequences require the involvement of the highest levels while some coordinated, largely automatic movements, such as walking or the maintence of posture, rely on intermediate levels of function. Many reflexes, however, occur at the lowest level only involving sensory input and the action of cranial nerve and spinal cord motor neurons.

Sensory input is important at all levels of the hierarchy and plays an important role in feedback and feedforward controls of voluntary movements:

- **Feedback control**: when a voluntary movement is made, sensory signals in the form of proprioception (which provides information about the position of joints and muscles and muscle movement) are sent to the cerebrum and cerebellum. If there is a difference between the desired position and actual position it is termed an **error signal**. This allows a correction to be made to the movement.
- **Feedforward control**: sensory information gives advance information so the required movement can be anticipated and directed to the target (e.g. picking up a pencil).

MOTOR CORTEX

The motor cortex is the part of the cerebral cortex where voluntary movements are planned, controlled and executed. It is composed of the primary motor cortex and the premotor and supplementary motor cortices. Its principal output is by the lateral motor pathways.

Primary motor cortex

Immediately anterior to the central sulcus is the precentral gyrus of the frontal lobe (see Fig. 8.8). This is the site of the **primary motor cortex** (**M1** or **motor strip**), Brodmann's area 4. Each motor strip controls movement of the opposite (contralateral) side of the body. It has a somatotopic map of body movements in which areas such as those controlling hand, tongue and larynx are disproportionately large reflecting the complexity of movement associated with these structures. The map is termed the motor **homunculus** (Fig. 8.32). Lesions, particularly tumours, affecting particular parts of the primary motor cortex can lead to disturbance of function in individual parts of the head or body (Clinical box 8.12). The map also helps explain the way in which partial motor seizures (Jacksonian epilepsy) start with clonic movements in one area which may spread (e.g. begins in fingers and can spread to arms and then becomes more generalised).

The motor cortex controls movements rather than the activation of single muscles. Populations of cortical neurons act together to determine the direction and force of movements. The main function of the primary motor cortex is the **execution of movements** with projections to brainstem and spinal motor neurons principally in the **corticospinal tract**.

Premotor and supplementary motor cortices

Immediately anterior to the primary motor cortex is the **premotor cortex** (Brodmann's area 6) and anterior to it is the **supplementary motor cortex**. These are thought to **plan movements** because functional imaging shows increased activity in these areas when subjects are asked to think about a motor activity without actually doing it.

The premotor cortex receives input from sensory and visual cortices and from the basal ganglia and cerebellum via the thalamus. It projects to the reticulospinal and corticospinal tracts.

The supplementary motor area also receives input from the basal ganglia and from the contralateral motor cortex. It appears to have a role in integrating movements performed simultaneously by both sides of the body.

Lateral motor pathways

There are two lateral motor pathways. The major tract and principal controller of muscle activity is the **corticospinal tract**. The other, the **rubrospinal tract**, originates in the same motor cortex areas as the corticospinal tract and runs in the corticorubral tract to the red nucleus in the midbrain. The rubrospinal tract is functionally similar to the corticospinal tract and is not discussed further in this chapter.

The **corticospinal (or pyramidal) tract** (Fig. 8.33) arises from neurons in the motor cortex, and fibres descend as the **corona radiata** and **internal capsule** (Clinical box 8.13) to enter the brainstem. Here it gives off fibres, the **corticobulbar tract**, to supply motor nuclei of the cranial nerves supplying face, jaw and tongue muscles.

In the medulla the corticospinal tract bunches up to form a discrete bundle, known as the **pyramid**. At the lower end of the medulla, 80–90% of the fibres cross to the other side in the **pyramidal decussation**. These crossed fibres descend in the spinal cord as the **lateral corticospinal tract**, while the remaining uncrossed fibres run down the anterior column of cervical and upper thoracic segments as the **anterior corticospinal tract**.

The final destination of the corticospinal tract is the α motor neurons in the spinal cord.

BRAINSTEM

Medial motor pathways

The other descending motor pathways arise from nuclei in the brainstem and are located in ventromedial positions in the spinal cord. They are principally involved in control of the anti-gravity muscles, the axial and proximal muscles controlling posture (Fig. 8.34 and Table 8.13).

- **Tectospinal tract**: begins in cells in the superior colliculus whose axons cross the midline and descend only as far as cervical cord neurons.
- **Vestibulospinal tracts**: vestibular nuclei in the medulla give rise to medial and lateral vestibulospinal tracts. The former descends as the **medial longitudinal fasciculus** to the cervical spinal cord and helps control head and neck posture. It also mediates vestibulocollic reflexes (see below). The **lateral vestibulospinal tracts** supply proximal limb extensors.
- **Reticulospinal tracts**: the diffuse network of nuclei throughout the brainstem known as the reticular formation is responsible for two main tracts: the **pontine**

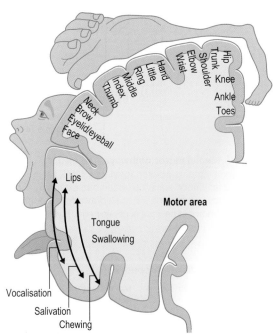

Fig. 8.32 Somatotopic map of the primary motor cortex. Compare it with the somatosensory map in Figure 8.43. Redrawn from Penfield W, Rasmussen T 1952 The Cerebral Cortex of Man. New York, Macmillan Press, with permission.

Clinical box 8.12 **Parasagittal meningioma**

Meningiomas are slow growing tumours that arise from arachnoid granulations. When they develop in the midline near the vertex they can extend through the falx and by causing pressure on both motor homunculi lead to bilateral leg weakness, which might be misinterpreted as arising from a spinal cord lesion.

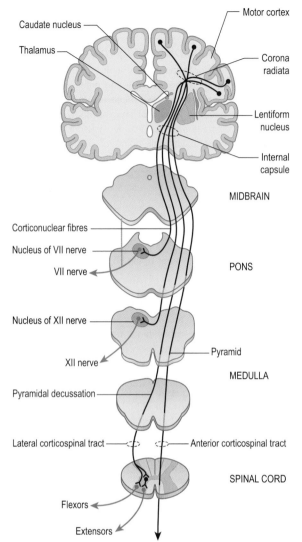

Fig. 8.33 **Lateral motor pathways: the corticospinal and corticobulbar pathways.** The rubrospinal tract is not shown. Only two cranial nerve motor nuclei, facial (VII) and hypoglossal (XII), with their corresponding corticonuclear fibres are depicted.

> **Clinical box 8.13** **Internal capsule**
>
> All the corticospinal tract fibres are packed close together in the internal capsule which receives its blood supply from the lenticulostriate branches of the middle cerebral artery. When these branches, or the middle cerebral artery itself, are occluded in a stroke the result is paralysis of the lower part of the face and of the arm and leg on the opposite side of the body (i.e. a contralateral hemiplegia).

reticulospinal tract which projects uncrossed to supply extensor motor neurons and the **medullary reticulospinal tract** which is partly crossed and is excitatory to flexor motor neurons. Both these tracts synapse with interneurons shared with the corticospinal tract. Damage to reticulospinal pathways can lead to spasticity (Clinical box 8.14).

Upper and lower motor neurons

All movement of skeletal muscles is dependent on signals from the α **motor neurons** in the ventral (anterior) horn of the spinal cord (and the **motor cranial nerves** in the brainstem). These are referred to as **lower motor neurons**.

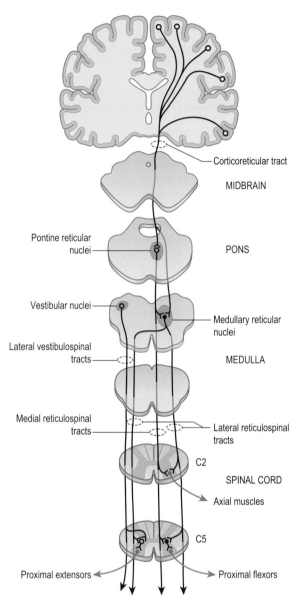

Fig. 8.34 **Medial motor pathways.** The medial vestibulospinal tract is omitted for clarity. Black filled neurons are inhibitory, black open neurons excitatory. Red neurons are lower motor neurons. Redrawn from Longstaff A 2005 Instant notes in neuroscience, 2nd edn. Taylor & Francis, Abingdon, with permission.

Table 8.13 **Medial motor pathways**

Tract	Distribution	Main effect* on α motor neurons	
		Excitatory to:	Inhibitory to:
Lateral vestibulospinal	Ipsilateral	Axial and proximal limb extensors	Axial and proximal limb flexors
Medial vestibulospinal	Bilateral	Ipsilateral axial muscles	Contralateral axial muscles
Pontine (medial) reticulospinal	Ipsilateral	Axial and proximal limb extensors	Proximal limb flexors
Medullary (lateral) reticulospinal	Bilateral	Proximal limb flexors	Axial and proximal limb extensors

*Both direct and indirect (i.e. via interneurons).

Spasticity is one of the consequences of damage to cortical motor neurons that regulate **muscle tone**, the background level of activity in skeletal muscles. Muscle tone depends on discharge of α motor neurons, but this is established by firing of the γ efferents to muscle spindles.

Normally a rise in muscle tone is brought about by increasing the gain of the muscle spindle reflex, i.e. increasing γ efferent firing rate. However, in spasticity the enhanced muscle tone (**hypertonus**) is not the result of enhanced γ efferent activity but exaggerated drive on α motor neurons from Ia primary afferents. This is due to the loss of presynaptic inhibition on the Ia terminals.

Normally, reticulospinal neurons synapse with presynaptic inhibitory interneurons that release GABA. This acts on both GABA$_A$ and GABA$_B$ receptors to reduce glutamate release from the Ia terminal. The reticulospinal neurons in the brainstem are in turn driven by **corticoreticular axons** that descend with the corticospinal tract (see also Clinical box 8.15).

Pure lesions of the motor cortex, or of corticospinal fibres above the medulla, initially cause a contralateral flaccid paralysis that is most severe in the limbs. Axial muscles are relatively spared because they are controlled by medial motor pathways. Subsequently there is some return of muscle tone but the ability to make fine movements with distal muscles is lost. There is no spasticity.

However, generally, lesions (most commonly the result of strokes) damage corticoreticular fibres that descend along with corticospinal fibres so the final clinical picture is of an **upper motor neuron** (**UMN**) **syndrome** characterised by:
- Paralysis of movements rather than individual muscles.
- **Spasticity**; increased muscle tone (**hypertonus**)
- **Hyperactive stretch reflexes and clonus** (rhythmic, 3–7 Hz contractions of muscle triggered by muscle spindles)
- **Loss** of superficial reflexes (e.g. abdominal reflex)
- **Extensor plantar reflex** (**Babinski's sign**), which is extension of the toes on hard stroking of the sole of the foot.

Loss of lower motor neuron function results in:
- **Paralysis** (lack of movement) or **paresis** (weakness) of muscles
- **Hypotonia** (flaccidity) of affected muscles
- **Disuse atrophy** (wasting) of the affected muscles
- Loss of stretch reflexes (**areflexia**)
- **Fasciculations**, contractions of all the muscle fibres in a motor unit caused by spontaneous firing (injury potentials) of damaged α motor neurons
- **Fibrillation**, the spontaneous contractions of individual muscle fibres. Fibrillation is due to **denervation supersensitivity**; the massive upregulation of nicotinic receptors in denervated skeletal muscle is enough to make the muscle responsive to circulating acetylcholine.

As explained above many descending motor pathways influence lower motor neuron activity, but clinicians usually use the term **upper motor neuron** to refer to the corticospinal tract and associate specific patterns of clinical features with damage to each (see Clinical boxes 8.15 and 8.16).

SPINAL CORD

Motor reflexes

Motor reflexes are characterised by lower motor neurons causing contraction or relaxation of muscles in response to sensory input. In addition to the sensory and motor neurons there is often one or more interneurons involved in the reflex circuit. Reflexes may be classified according to the number of interneurons and synapses they contain:

- **Monosynaptic**: no interneurons and only one synapse (i.e. the sensory neurons synapse directly with the motor neurons)
- **Disynaptic**: one set of interneurons and two synapses
- **Polysynaptic**: many interneurons and synapses.

Stretch reflex

The **muscle stretch** (**myotactic** or **spindle**) **reflexes** prevent overstretching of a muscle by opposing an increase in muscle length. It is, therefore, a negative feedback mechanism. Clinicians examine these reflexes which they refer to as **tendon reflexes**. Using a hammer a sharp tap to a tendon stretches the attached muscle and elicits a contraction that restores the muscle to its original length (Clinical box 8.17).

Muscle spindles

Muscle stretch is detected by muscle spindles. A **muscle spindle** (Fig. 8.35A) consists of a connective tissue capsule containing about seven modified muscle fibres called **intrafusal fibres**. The spindles lie in parallel to the ordinary muscle fibres outside the spindle (**extrafusal fibres**) and experience the same forces as the muscle. Essentially muscle spindles are proprioceptors measuring the length and rate of change of length (velocity) of the muscle.

The intrafusal fibres have contractile ends (poles), but non-contracting middle regions; there are two principal types of intrafusal fibre:

- **Nuclear chain fibres** which are short and thin are the most numerous and are innervated by two types of myelinated sensory fibre: large diameter **Ia afferents** and smaller diameter **II afferents**.
- **Nuclear bag fibres** are longer and larger and most are innervated by **Ia afferents** only, although a few smaller types, called B2 fibres, have type II afferents.

When a muscle is stretched, so is the spindle and its afferent sensory neurons fire, synapsing directly with a pool of motor neurons which supply extrafusal muscle fibres in both the same (**homonymous**) muscle and synergist (**heteronymous**) muscles (Fig. 8.35B). As there are no interneurons involved it is an example of a monosynaptic reflex. When a muscle shortens the spindle relaxes and the afferent firing rate drops.

In testing tendon reflexes (or jerks) the patient should be relaxed and the examiner uses a tendon hammer to make a sharp tap on the muscle tendon. The principal reflexes and their innervations routinely tested clinically are:
- Upper limb: biceps (C5–C6), triceps (C7) and brachoradialis (C5–C6)
- Lower limb: knee (L3) and ankle (S1).
  If initially absent **reinforcement** of tendon reflexes is achieved by simultaneous voluntary contraction of muscles elsewhere (e.g. clenching teeth or pulling the flexed fingers of the two hands against each other – Jendrassik's manoeuvre). This acts by increasing activity in the γ efferent system.

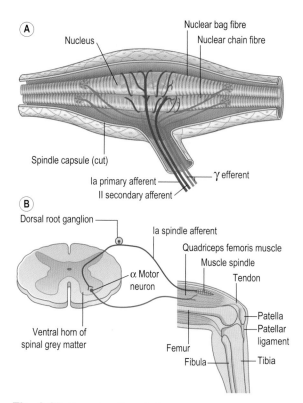

Fig. 8.35 Stretch reflex. (A) Structure and innervation of a muscle spindle; (B) myotatic reflex circuitry. Redrawn from Longstaff A 2005 Instant notes in neuroscience, 2nd edn. Taylor & Francis, Abingdon, with permission.

The sensitivity of the intrafusal fibres is increased by the action of small diameter myelinated γ **efferents** which innervate their contractile poles. Firing of the γ efferents causes the poles to contract keeping their central regions taut and sensitive to stretch even as the muscle contracts. This means that the stretch reflex can work over a wide range of muscle lengths.

Golgi tendon organ reflex

Golgi tendon organs are proprioceptors arranged in series with the collagen fibres connecting a muscle to a tendon. They consist of an encapsulated network of collagen fibres with a **Ib sensory afferent** winding around the collagen fibres. When the Golgi tendon organ is stretched the firing rate of the Ib afferent increases. The afferent synapses with an inhibitory interneuron which, in turn, synapses with the α motor neuron in the spinal cord innervating the same muscle. It is, therefore, a di-synaptic reflex. The **Golgi tendon organ reflex** is an example of negative feedback that maintains a set point in muscle tension. By inhibiting muscle contraction they protect the muscle from excessive tension and so may prevent injury.

Cutaneous reflexes

An example of a polysynaptic reflex in the spinal cord is the **flexion withdrawal reflex** that protects a limb from potential injury. If one accidentally touches a hot stove or stands on a tack the flexors of the affected limb contract and the extensors relax so the limb is withdrawn. The sensory fibres are referred to as flexor reflex afferents and they synapse with interneurons that excite the α motor neurons of the flexors and inhibit the α motor neurons of the extensors.

An even more complicated polysynaptic reflex specific to the lower limbs is the **crossed extensor reflex**. When one steps on the tack the flexion withdrawal reflex occurs in the ipsilateral limb but simultaneously the contralateral limb extends to support the body's weight.

Locomotion

Normal gait involves alternate flexion and extension of opposite legs (see Ch. 9). This is dependent on central pattern generators (CPGs). These are clusters of interneurons in the spinal cord that can generate coordinated rhythmical movements autonomously, although initiation of locomotion comes from higher centres. Each limb has a CPG consisting of two half-centres: a flexor half-centre and an extensor half-centre. These are mutually inhibitory. The output of the half-centres is modulated by proprioceptor input.

Muscle tone

Muscle tone is essentially a clinical concept, describing the resistance to the passive manipulation of the limbs by an examiner. Tonic firing of spinal motor neurons (α and γ) is the final pathway but the firing frequency is set by various inputs including from stretch receptors and from higher centres through corticospinal, reticulospinal and vestibulospinal tracts which are influenced by connections with the basal ganglia and cerebellum. There are two key abnormalities of tone:

- Hypotonia: decrease in resistance to passive manipulation of the limb
- Hypertonia: an increase in resistance.

If either the ventral root carrying motor fibres or the dorsal root containing sensory fibres from muscles is cut hypotonia results. Hypotonia can also result from disease affecting higher centres, particularly the cerebellum.

There are two main forms of hypertonia: spasticity and rigidity. In spasticity the examiner detects an initial increased resistance sometimes followed by a sudden decrease, referred to as the clasp-knife phenomenon. Rigidity usually results from basal ganglia disorders (e.g. Parkinson disease). The resistance is uniform in degree throughout the full range of movement and is described as plastic or lead-pipe. When tremor is superimposed it is called cog-wheel rigidity.

Spinal cord injury

The spinal cord can be damaged by trauma and a wide range of diseases (Clinical box 8.18) and by disease or trauma to the bony canal. These result in combinations of sensory, motor and autonomic dysfunction. Trauma causing bilateral damage at the thoracic or lumbar spinal levels results in paralysis of the lower limbs (**paraplegia**) while cervical lesions can cause paralysis of all four limbs (**quadriplegia** or **tetraplegia**).

Complete transection of the spinal cord results initially in **spinal shock** – a general hyperpolarisation of neurons below the lesion, possibly due to disinhibition of glycinergic interneurons. There is:

- A flaccid paralysis of denervated skeletal muscles
- Hypotonia
- Areflexia

Clinical box 8.18   **Some diseases of the spinal cord**

Disease of the spinal cord affects mobility, sensation and autonomic function, particularly bladder and bowels. There are diverse conditions, too numerous to discuss here. Some examples are cited here to illustrate their possible underlying scientific basis. Trauma is discussed in the text and not covered further here.

An inflammatory condition of the cord is termed a **myelitis**, and non-inflammatory disorders **myelopathies**.

- **Hereditary**: examples are the hereditary ataxias (e.g. **Friedreich's ataxia**) and hereditary spastic paraplegia. Among other features these conditions lead to disturbances of gait.
- **Nutritional**: vitamin B_{12} deficiency (e.g. in pernicious anaemia) is associated with **subacute combined degeneration of the spinal cord**. Demyelination affects the dorsal column causing sensory impairment and lateral columns affecting the corticospinal and spinocerebellar tracts causing spasticity and ataxia. Folic acid deficiency can also cause a myelopathy.
- **Vascular**: atherosclerosis of the spinal arteries themselves is rare but spinal cord infarction can result from diseases in vessels supplying them (e.g. atheroma or dissection of the aorta). Arteriovenous malformations can cause subarachnoid haemorrhage in the cord and haematomas result in compression.
- **Infection**: although **poliomyelitis** has been largely eradicated by the WHO campaign it is still endemic in four countries: Nigeria, India, Pakistan and Afghanistan. It is an acute viral infection in which α motor neurons and cranial nerve motor neurons are selectively involved. Acute viral myelitis is rare but causes include measles, mumps, herpes and HIV.
- **Inflammation**: **transverse myelitis** is usually preceded by an infectious illness 1–3 weeks earlier and is thought likely to have an immunological basis. As its name implies, its effects are across the whole spinal cord. There is in some cases demyelination. Weakness and paraesthesia develop in the lower limbs with urinary retention or incontinence common. A more common inflammatory condition is **multiple sclerosis** (see Clinical box 8.10).
- **Tumours**: these may be arise outside the cord, **extramedullary** (e.g. meningiomas, neurofibromas), or inside, **intramedullary** (e.g. gliomas, ependymomas). Their effects are often due to compression or to occlusion of arteries and veins to the spinal cord.

- Loss of all sensation
- Paralysis of bladder and rectum (loss of drive to the preganglionic autonomic neurons).

After a few weeks, reflexes return with appearance of signs of an **upper motor neuron** syndrome (see Clinical box 8.15).

A lesion of one side of the spinal cord (hemisection) results in the Brown-Séquard syndrome (Fig. 8.36, Clinical box 8.19).

Damage to the **cauda equina** below the conus medullaris results in a lower motor neuron weakness of muscles supplied by sacral roots (i.e. the plantar flexors and evertors of the foot), loss of ankle jerks and a sensory deficit over the saddle area of the perineum and buttocks. In addition overflow incontinence and impotence occurs.

CRANIAL NERVE REFLEXES

Several reflexes involve the cranial nerves such as postural reflexes and pupillary light and autonomic reflexes (see below). There are two other important reflexes used in clinical practice.

- **Corneal (blink) reflex**: when a foreign body touches the cornea of one eye both eyes close briskly. Sensory fibres

Clinical box 8.19   **Brown-Séquard syndrome**

Lesions confined largely to one side of the spinal cord give rise to a characteristic pattern of sensorimotor loss, the **Brown-Séquard syndrome**. There is ipsilateral paralysis, loss of touch and position sense, but contralateral loss of pain and temperature sense because the anterolateral pathway decussates within a couple of segments of the primary afferents (Fig. 8.36).

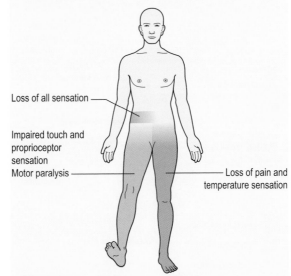

Loss of all sensation

Impaired touch and proprioceptor sensation

Motor paralysis

Loss of pain and temperature sensation

Fig. 8.36 **Brown-Séquard syndrome.** Cord hemisection on right side at level of T10. The ipsilateral motor deficit is largely an upper motor neuron syndrome.

in the **trigeminal (V)** nerve send impulses to the **spinal tract** and **nucleus of V** which connect to the **motor nucleus of the facial (VII) nerve**. This sends motor signals to the orbicularis oculi which closes the eye on the side touched (**direct corneal reflex**) but, because interneurons from the spinal nucleus connect with the opposite VIIth nerve nucleus, the opposite eye also closes (**consensual corneal reflex**).

- **Gag reflex**: touching the posterior wall of the pharynx results in contraction of the muscles of the soft palate and pharynx. The afferent arm of this reflex is provided by sensory fibres of the **glossopharyngeal (IX) nerve** which enter the **solitary tract**. Interneurons connect to the **nucleus ambiguus** which sends motor impulses via the **IXth** and **vagus (X) nerve** to the muscles.

CEREBELLUM

Anatomy

The cerebellum, part of the hindbrain, sits in the posterior fossa behind the pons and below the cerebrum. It consists of a midline vermis and two hemispheres and is divided into three lobes (anterior, posterior and flocculonodular) by the primary and posterolateral fissures (Fig. 8.37). The surface is tightly folded grey matter which forms transverse ridges called **folia**, similar to the gyri in the cerebrum.

Within the white matter of each hemisphere are the deep cerebellar nuclei: **dentate**, **interposed** (globose and emboliform) and **fastigial nuclei**.

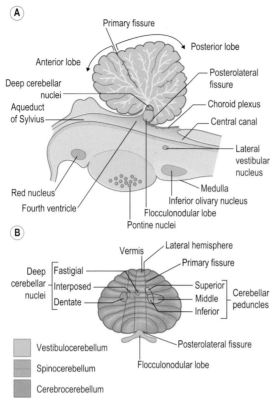

Fig. 8.37 Anatomy of the cerebellum. (A) Midsagittal section; (B) flattened view of the cerebellar surface with location of intracerebellar nuclei.

Three pairs of cerebellar peduncles connect the cerebellum to the brainstem:

- Superior cerebellar peduncle is the main output route from the cerebellar nuclei to the cerebral cortex via the thalamus and red nucleus

- Middle cerebellar peduncle takes signals from motor and sensory cerebral cortex that relay via pontine nuclei to the cerebellum
- Inferior cerebellar peduncle receives input from the lateral vestibular nucleus and inferior olive in the brainstem and from ascending tracts from the spinal cord.

Functional subdivisions

On the basis of function and their inputs and outputs, the cerebellum is divided into three functional units (Fig. 8.37B and Table 8.14):

- The **vestibulocerebellum** comprises the flocculonodular lobe and receives its input from the vestibulocochlear (VIII) nerve and sends output to vestibular nuclei. It is important to maintenance of posture and eye movements in the vestibulo-ocular reflex (see below).
- The **spinocerebellum** consists of the vermis and paravermis, a medial strip of hemisphere (Clinical box 8.20). It receives proprioceptive information from the spinal cord via **spinocerebellar and cuneocerebellar tracts**. In addition it gets visual, vestibular and auditory input.

Output is through the **fastigial nucleus** which projects to the motor cortex and reticular formation controlling trunk and proximal extensor muscles; and through the **interposed nuclei** which project via the thalamus and red nucleus to motor cortex for control of distal muscles. Thus the spinocerebellum's principal functions relate to posture and locomotion.

- The **cerebrocerebellum** is the lateral part of the hemisphere and receives motor and sensory information from the cerebral cortex relayed via pontine nuclei in the corticopontine cerebellar tract.

Its output is from the dentate nuclei to contralateral ventrolateral thalamus and red nucleus to motor cortex. It controls rapid and complex movements (Information box 8.10).

Table 8.14	Input–output relations of the cerebellum				
Input	**Origin**	**Tract**	**Subdivision**	**Output nucleus**	**Destination**
Balance	Inner ear	Cranial nerve VIII	Vestibulocerebellum	Vestibular nuclei	Vestibulospinal tracts
Proprioceptive from face and jaw	Cranial nerve V	Trigeminocerebellar	Spinocerebellum	Globose and emboliform nuclei	Ventral lateral thalamus → cerebral cortex red nucleus (hence lateral motor pathways)
Proprioceptive from neck and arm	Accessory cuneate nucleus	Cuneocerebellar			
Proprioceptive from trunk and leg	Clarke's column	Dorsal spinocerebellar			
Proprioceptive	Ventral horn	Ventral spinocerebellar			
Vision, hearing	Tectum	Tectocerebellar		Fastigial nucleus	Reticulospinal tracts
Sensorimotor	Cerebral cortex → pontine nuclei	Pontocerebellar	Cerebrocerebellum	Dentate nucleus	Ventral lateral thalamus
Motor error signal	Inferior olivary nucleus	Olivocerebellar*	All		

*Climbing fibres; all other inputs are mossy fibres.

Cerebellar cortex and circuitry

There are three layers to the cerebellar cortex: granule cell, Purkinje cell (or piriform) and molecular layers. These contain five cell types arranged in a circuit (Fig. 8.38).

- **Purkinje cells**: constitute the sole cerebellar output neurons. They send inhibitory (GABAergic) output to deep cerebellar nuclei which project to other parts of the CNS. They receive input from two sources: **climbing fibres** arising from the inferior olivary nucleus and **parallel fibres** from **granule cells**.
- **Granule cells**: these small, excitatory (glutamatergic) interneurons are estimated to account for about half the cells in the CNS. They give rise to parallel fibres supplying many Purkinje cells. Their input is from **mossy**

fibres which come from the corticopontine cerebellar and spinocerebellar tracts.
- **Basket cells** and **stellate cells** are inhibitory interneurons which get input from parallel fibres and inhibit adjacent rows of Purkinje cells.
- **Golgi cells** receive input from parallel fibres but also send inhibitory output back to the granule cells in a feedback loop.

The cerebellum receives a large amount of motor and sensory information via afferents from the cerebral cortex, brainstem and spinal cord. The output from the Purkinje cells in the cerebellar cortex is inhibitory to the deep cerebellar nuclei which project via the thalamus to the cerebral cortex. Through the information received and interactions through the deep nuclei the cerebellum is able to monitor ongoing movements and trigger new movements. It makes sure that the speed and accuracy of movement are appropriate and adequate for the motor task being undertaken. These involve feedforward and feedback mechanisms.

Mossy fibre circuits are the key to **feedforward** commands. Mossy fibres excite deep nuclei on their way to the cerebellar cortex but also inhibit the deep nuclei via the mossy fibre–granule cell–parallel fibre–Purkinje cell circuit (see Fig. 8.38). At rest the low tonic firing rate of mossy fibres means that excitation of deep nuclei predominates. During a voluntary movement mossy fibre firing increases and Purkinje cell inhibition of the deep nuclei cells dominates, which reduces the activity in corresponding cells in the thalamus and motor cortex (Information box 8.11).

Feedback error correction is dependent on climbing fibre circuitry. Climbing fibres convey information from the **inferior**

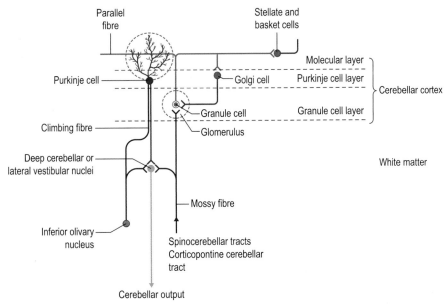

Fig. 8.38 **Cerebellar cortical circuitry.**

olivary nucleus. Sensory and motor information from the cerebral cortex is sent to the inferior olivary nucleus which also gets input from the spinal cord via the spino-olivary tract. The inferior olivary nucleus transforms the sensory information about the movement to be executed into the necessary motor signals. It also detects any mismatch between the actual movement and the intended movement. This error signal allows correction to be made. Climbing fibre activity is also thought to influence motor learning by inducing changes to synaptic activity of Purkinje cells when a new motor skill is acquired.

Damage to the cerebellum may result from trauma, tumours, haemorrhage or ischaemia and cerebellar pathways are disrupted in inherited disorders such as Friedreich's ataxia and other spinocerebellar ataxias or in acquired conditions such as multiple sclerosis and alcoholic cerebellar degeneration. In these circumstances a variety of motor problems may occur (Clinical box 8.21). These can interfere with many activities of daily living such as eating, dressing, writing and locomotion.

In addition to its role in movement, evidence is growing to indicate that the cerebellum participates in certain cognitive functions (Information box 8.12).

Clinical box 8.21   **Motor signs in cerebellar disorders**

Lesions of the cerebellum or its pathways can result in several motor signs:
- **Decomposition of movement**: a motor action is performed in a jerky, irregular manner.
- **Dysmetria**: a disturbance in the trajectory of a movement (e.g. when asked to touch an examiner's finger in the 'finger-nose test' the patient's finger overshoots).
- **Intention tremor**: as the patient's finger approaches the examiner's a tremor develops which gets worse the nearer the finger is to the target.
- **Dysdiadochokinesis**: a difficulty performing rapid, alternating movements (e.g. patting the palm of one hand with the palm and back of the other hand).
- **Rebound phenomenon**: when the outstretched arm is displaced by the examiner, on return it flies past the original position.
- **Hypotonia**: there is decreased resistance to passive movements of the limbs. This may be associated with pendular tendon reflexes.
- **Ataxia**: this term is sometimes used to describe disturbances of stance and gait where the patient stands on a broad base and walks unsteadily but is also used more generally to include the effects of decomposition of movement of the limbs.
- **Dysarthria**: speech is slow and slurred.

Information box 8.12   **Cerebellar cognitive deficits**

Cerebellar lesions such as infarcts, olivopontinecerebellar atrophy and trauma, as well as surgery, can cause:
- Impaired estimation of elapsed time and poor judgement of the relative speeds of moving objects or relative lengths of tones
- Degraded frontal cortex functions such as abstract reasoning, planning and working memory
- Loss of visuospatial skills, particularly with left-sided damage
- Defects in language, especially with right-sided lesions
- Flattening of affect, particularly associated with vermis lesions.

A constellation of the last four items on this list is called the **cerebellar cognitive-affective syndrome.**

BASAL GANGLIA

The anatomy of the basal ganglia is outlined above (see Fig. 8.9). The five nuclei that comprise the basal ganglia form a closed loop with each other and with the motor cortex via the thalamus.

They account for the major part of the extrapyramidal system which modulates motor activity.

The motor cortex sends excitatory (glutamatergic) signals to the dorsal striatum (caudate and putamen) via the corticostriatal tract (Fig. 8.39). The great majority of cells in the striatum are medium spiny neurons, all of which have an inhibitory (GABAergic) output. There are two subgroups of these neurons distinguished according to their dopamine receptors and co-transmitters:

- **D_1 receptors** have substance P and dynorphin as co-transmitters and send their axons to the **globus pallidus pars interna** (**GPi**) and the **substantia nigra pars reticulata** (**SNpr**) which in turn project to the thalamus and thence to the motor cortex in the **thalamocortical tract**. This is referred to as the **direct pathway** (Fig. 8.39, *black arrow*). When the striatum inhibits the GPi/SNpr it reduces the inhibitory effect of the GPi/SNpr on the thalamus, effectively encouraging the thalamus to fire and stimulate the cortex.
- **D_2 receptors** use enkephalin as co-transmitter and project to the **globus pallidus pars externa** (**GPe**) which has its output to the **subthalamic nucleus** (**STN**). The STN relays to the GPi/SNpr and so to the thalamus and cortex. This is the **indirect pathway** (Fig. 8.39, *red*). The STN's output to the GPi/SNpr is excitatory. Thus, when the striatum inhibits the GPe, this reduces the GPe's inhibition of the STN. The STN then excites the GPi/SNpr which inhibits the thalamus and so reduces the stimulation of the cortex.

However, the medium spiny neurons also receive projections from the largest dopaminergic pathway in the brain, the **nigrostriatal pathway**. These fibres originate in the **substantia nigra pars compacta** (**SNpc**) (Fig. 8.39, *blue*). This enhances cortical activation of D_1 medium spiny neurons but suppresses activation of D_2 neurons.

Much of our understanding of basal ganglia function comes from study of disorders affecting them such as **Huntington disease** (Clinical box 8.22) and, especially, **Parkinson disease** (PD).

The three cardinal clinical features of PD are **bradykinesis, rigidity and tremor**. Bradykinesis (slowness of movement) includes delay in initiation of and poverty of movement (hypokinesis) and difficulty stopping one motor action and starting another. Rigidity is an increase in muscle tone (see above). The tremor of PD is maximal at rest and reduced by voluntary movement.

Although the actual cause of PD remains unknown, pathologically it is characterised by loss of the dopaminergic neurons of the nigrostriatal pathway. This results in excessive inhibition of the GPe by the striatum and disinhibition of the STN (Fig. 8.40B). The increased excitatory drive from the STN to its targets (GPi/SNpr) reduces the activity of the thalamocortical neurons and this is assumed to account for the bradykinesis in PD.

The treatment of PD is summarised in Clinical box 8.23. The mainstay of treatment is **L-dopa** which readily crosses the blood–brain barrier and is decarboxylated to dopamine,

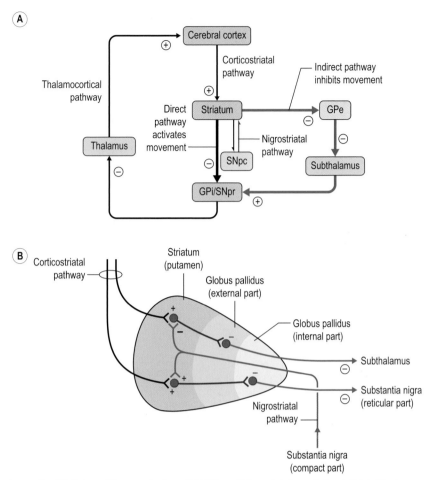

Fig. 8.39 **Basal ganglia.** (A) Schematic organisation. (B) Differential modulation of direct (thick black arrow) and indirect (red) pathways by dopaminergic neurons from the compact part of the substantia nigra (blue). Excitatory connections, +; inhibitory connections, −. GPi, globus pallidus (internal part); GPe, global pallidus (external part); SNpc, substantia nigra (compact part); SNpr, substantia nigra (reticular part).

Clinical box 8.22 **Huntington disease**

Huntington disease (HD) is an inherited (autosomal dominant) progressive neurodegenerative disorder (see Ch. 5) with a mean onset of motor and cognitive symptoms at age 40 years.

The mutation in HD is an excessive number of trinucleotide (CAG) repeats on the huntingtin gene which codes for the **huntingtin (Htt)** protein. Htt accumulates around the nuclei of and kills preferentially striatal medium spiny neurons of the indirect pathway. So HD can be viewed as a failure of the indirect pathway to suppress unwanted motor sequences (Fig. 8.40A) and is a **hyperkinetic** condition, characterised by random twitching or writhing movements (choreoathetosis).

---

which is released in a physiologically appropriate manner provides good control of the symptoms of PD initially but within 2 years of starting treatment most patients develop **dyskinesia** (involuntary movements of face and limbs). The precise cause of dyskinesia is uncertain but probably results from long-lasting synaptic changes that alter the balance of activity in direct and indirect pathways in the basal ganglia. Dopamine agonists do not cause dyskinesia but tend to lose effectiveness over time.

In addition to the role in motor function in the motor loop described above, there are a number of non-motor **basal ganglia circuits** or loops. One is involved in emotional expression (**limbic loop**), another in the control of saccadic (fast) eye movements (**oculomotor loop**). In PD, there is oculomotor hypokinesia where some saccades are slow or inadequate and loss of facial expression is common. Another of these so-called **parallel circuits** is involved in executive motor planning (**cognitive loop**). Damage to these non-motor areas of the basal ganglia have been hypothesised in disorders such as Tourette syndrome, obsessive compulsive disorders and schizophrenia.

EYE MOVEMENTS

Each eye is moved by three pairs of **extraocular muscles**:

- Medial and lateral rectus
- Superior and inferior rectus
- Superior and inferior oblique.

The muscles originate from the rear of the orbit and insert into the sclera. Rectus muscles are inserted in front and oblique muscles behind the equator of the eyeball (Fig. 8.41).

The muscles act in complementary pairs to move both eyes in the same direction (e.g. looking to the left, the left lateral rectus abducts the left eye and the right medial rectus adducts the right eye). They are innervated by motor neurons of the oculomotor (III), trochlear (IV) and abducens (VI) cranial nerves (Table 8.15). Damage to these nerves causes typical changes in gaze and/or double vision (Clinical box 8.24).

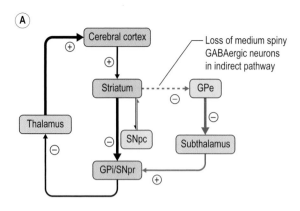

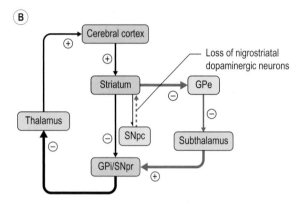

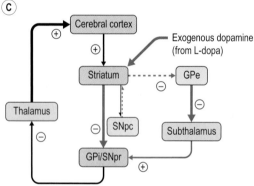

Fig. 8.40 Functional derangements of basal ganglia circuitry. (A) Huntington disease; (B) Parkinson disease; (C) L-dopa-induced dyskinesia. Compare with the normal state shown in Figure 8.39. GPi, globus pallidus (internal part); GPe, global pallidus (external part); SNpc, substantia nigra (compact part); SNpr, substantia nigra (reticular part).

Control of eye movements

Eye movements direct the fovea (the point of highest visual acuity) onto points of interest in the visual scene, either **stabilising** gaze during head rotation or **shifting** gaze to track a moving object or jump to a different part of the visual scene.

Gaze stabilisation

- **Vestibulo-ocular reflexes** move the eyes in the opposite direction when the head is rotated (see vestibular pathways, below)
- **Opticokinetic reflexes** use visual input to hold the retinal image stable during slow head movements. The magnitude of the eye movement is equal and opposite to that of the head.

Drug treatment
The principal approaches to treatment are:
- Provision of the dopamine precursor **L-dopa** (L-3,4-dihydroxyphenylalanine)
- Inhibiting dopamine catabolism by blocking **monoamine oxidase B** (e.g. selegiline) or **catechol-*O*-methyl transferase** (e.g. entacapone)
- Activating dopamine D_2 receptors by **dopamine agonists** (e.g. ropinirole).

Surgical treatment
Hyperactivity of the STN is an essential feature of PD. This drives GPi and SNpr cells to excessive inhibition of their thalamic and cortical targets. These observations form the basis for surgical treatment which involves making selective lesions of the STN (subthalamotomy) or GPi (pallidotomy). Alternatively functional blockade of these structures is achieved by delivering an electrical current through implanted electrodes (**deep brain stimulation**).
   A further approach is the injection of dopaminergic cells (e.g. produced from neural stem cells) into the striatum; these survive to form synapses with striatal neurons and secrete dopamine.

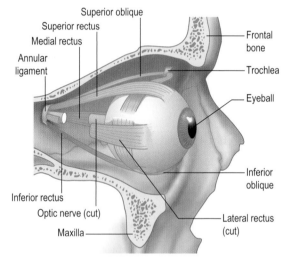

Fig. 8.41 Extraocular muscles of the right orbit.
Redrawn from Longstaff A 2005 Instant notes in neuroscience, 2nd edn. Taylor & Francis, Abingdon, with permission.

Gaze shift

- **Saccades** are extremely rapid eye movements, which occur every 300 ms, bringing new targets onto the fovea. Saccadic eye movements are generated in the brainstem reticular formation under the influence of a circuit that involves the frontal eye fields, pulvinar nucleus, superior colliculus and basal ganglia.
- **Smooth pursuit** describes voluntary movements that allow tracking a moving target and are much slower than saccades.
- **Vergence** changes the gaze of both eyes to allow refocusing as an object moves closer (convergence) or further away (divergence).

In saccades and smooth pursuit both eyes move in the same direction (**conjugate gaze**), whereas in vergence they move in opposite directions (**disconjugate**).

Table 8.15		Innervation and actions of extraocular muscles				
Muscle	**Nerve**	**Movement**	**Direction of weakness after nerve injury**	**Direction of gaze causing double vision**	**Complementary muscle in contralateral eye**
Lateral rectus	VI	Abduction (out)	In (convergent squint)	Out	Medial rectus
Medial rectus	III	Adduction (in)	Out (divergent squint)	In	Lateral rectus
Superior rectus	III	Elevation after abduction (up and out)	Down and in	Up and out	Inferior oblique
Inferior oblique	III	Elevation after adduction (up and in)	Down and out	Up and in	Superior rectus
Superior oblique	IV	Depression after adduction (down and in)	Up and out	Down and in	Inferior rectus
Inferior rectus	III	Depression after abduction (down and out)	Up and in	Down and out	Superior oblique

Clinical box 8.24 Oculomotor disorders

Squint (**strabismus**) is convergent if the visual axes cross or divergent if the visual axes diverge.
- **Paralytic squint** is an acquired defect in an extraocular muscle or its innervation and causes double vision.
- **Non-paralytic squint** is a developmental defect, manifesting early in childhood, in which the deviating eye moves so that the squint is the same for all directions of gaze, and there is no double vision.

If non-paralytic squint is not corrected very early – usually surgically by functionally shortening the appropriate muscle – the visual system wires itself to ignore the signals from the affected eye (unless the normal eye is closed) resulting in a functional blindness in the squinting eye termed **amblyopia**, in which stereopsis is permanently impaired.

Double vision (**diplopia**) generally accompanies paralysis of a cranial nerve controlling eye movements and is caused by the inability of the visual system to implement stereopsis when the visual axes of the two eyes are misaligned. Diplopia occurs when attempting to look in the direction that compensates for the eyeball deviation caused by the damage (see Table 8.15).

SENSORY SYSTEMS

Sensory systems carry information about the external and internal environments of the body to the brain and can be divided into:

- **Cutaneous senses**: receptors in the skin detect pain, thermal, touch and pressure sensations
- **Position senses (proprioception)**: mechanical changes in the muscles and joints provide information on the position of the body and limbs in space both when static and in movement
- **Visceral senses**: these receptors respond to distension and contraction of internal organs
- **Special senses**: include sight, hearing, balance, smell and taste.

Specific sensory entities are termed the **sensory modalities** and include the special senses, pain, temperature, touch and proprioception. Within the latter four senses there are individual receptors for **submodalities** (e.g. hot and cold; light touch and deep pressure) (Table 8.16).

Modality is conferred by whichever neurons are being stimulated (Clinical box 8.25).

Table 8.16	Stimulus modalities		
Modality	**Stimulus**	**Physiological receptor**
Somatosensory: touch, pressure, vibration	Mechanical forces acting on skin	Skin mechanoreceptors
Proprioception	Mechanical forces acting on joints and muscles	Muscle and joint mechanoreceptors
Temperature	Heat	Cold and warm thermoreceptors
Pain	Mechanical force on skin and viscera, heat on skin, chemical on skin, mucous membranes and viscera	Mechanical, thermal and polymodal nociceptors
Itch	Chemical on skin and mucous membranes	Itch receptors
Vision	Light	Retinal photoreceptors
Hearing	Sound	Cochlear hair cells
Balance	Head acceleration and velocity	Vestibular hair cells
Smell	Chemical	Olfactory sensory neurons
Taste	Chemical	Taste cells

Clinical box 8.25 Synaesthesia

Synaesthesia, a condition in which people have perceptions that are out of step with their sensory experience (e.g. 'seeing' colours in response to sounds), presumably occurs via neural circuitry which allows crosstalk between different sensory modalities.

Sensory receptor transduction

Sensory receptors convert (**transduce**) the energy of the stimulus into a change in membrane potential termed a **receptor (or generator) potential**. Like synaptic potentials (see above), but unlike action potentials, these potentials get smaller with both the duration and distance they are conducted and they summate. Sensory receptors have the following properties:

- Each type of receptor responds to a **specific** stimulus. Thus mechanoreceptors respond to mechanical forces by opening ion channels whereas in vision (phototransduction) light triggers a G-coupled, secondary cascade (see below).
- The **receptive field** describes the area over which the receptor responds to the stimulus. Receptive fields vary in size. For example, in the skin, the palmar aspect of the fingers has many sensory neurons each with a small receptive field. A healthy subject can distinguish two touch stimuli 2–5 mm apart on the fingertips but only 20–30 mm on the dorsum of the hand which has fewer neurons each with a larger receptive field. This is tested clinically by the **two-point discrimination test** which uses an instrument like a pair of blunt-tipped school dividers to provide the stimuli at various degrees of separation.
- Different receptors detect different aspects of a stimulus changing their firing rate in relation to the constancy or intensity of the stimulus – a process termed **adaptation**. **Rapidly adapting receptors** respond to changes in the intensity of the stimulus but fire only transiently to a constant stimulus. **Slowly adapting receptors** remain responsive for the duration of a constant stimulus.

Receptive field structure

Within one receptive field, there may be two or more regions that determine the response of a neuron:

- **On-centre cells**: where stimulation of the inner zone increases neuronal firing, and stimulation of the outer zone decreases firing
- **Off-centre cells**: where the regions are reversed.

Surround (lateral) inhibition occurs when an excited neuron suppresses activity in neighbouring neurons. This is achieved by GABAergic interneurons and enables more accurate spatial location of a stimulus. A simple example is a bee sting; sensory neurons at the point of contact would fire, while those in the surrounding area would be suppressed, allowing the bee sting to be located. Neurons that exhibit surround inhibition are found in visual, auditory and touch pathways. This phenomenon also contributes to **selective attention**.

Touch and proprioception

The receptors in the skin responsible for detecting tactile sensations are the **skin mechanoreceptors**. These react to the stimulus of deformation of the skin when an object exerts pressure on it. Lying in the superficial layers of non-hairy skin are **Meissner's corpuscles** and **Merkel's discs**. These have small receptive fields and detect light touch and are important in tactile discrimination. **Pacinian** and **Ruffini corpuscles** are located in the deeper layers, have large receptor fields and are responsive to vibration and stretch (Table 8.17). Hairy skin does not have Meissner's corpuscles but has **hair follicle receptors** that react to hair displacement.

Other mechanoreceptors, including muscle spindles and Golgi tendon organs, are found in muscles and joints. These are involved in spinal cord reflexes (see above) and

Table 8.17	**Properties of non-hairy skin mechanoreceptors**		
Receptor	**Location**	**Adaptation***	**Sensation**
Meissner's corpuscle	Superficial	RAI	Touch, stroking, flutter
Pacinian corpuscle	Deep	RAII	Vibration
Merkel's disc	Superficial	SAI	Light pressure
Ruffini's corpuscles	Deep	SAII	Stretch

*RA, rapidly adapting; SA slowly adapting; type I, high resolution; type II, low resolution.

in proprioception. Proprioceptive information is conveyed to conscious awareness along the same pathways as touch and by other pathways principally to the cerebellum.

Touch and conscious proprioception pathway

Touch is a complex phenomenon and does not run in a single pathway. The following pathway describes the route for light touch and proprioception. Some mechanoreceptors, described as detecting crude touch, run with the pain and temperature pathways (see below).

Primary afferents from mechanoreceptors have their cell bodies in dorsal root ganglia. They synapse with interneurons which send their axons ascending in the **dorsal columns** of the spinal cord (Clinical box 8.26). Fibres from the legs make up the medial part of the dorsal column as the **gracile tract** (or fasciculus gracilis), while those from the arms comprise the lateral part, the **cuneate tract** (or fasciculus cuneatus). These fibres end in the **dorsal column nuclei**, the gracile and cuneate nuclei, in the lower medulla. Second order neurons from these dorsal column nuclei cross (decussate) to the opposite side of the medulla in the **decussation of the medial lemniscus** and ascend as the **medial lemniscus** to the **ventroposterior thalamus**. The pathway is termed the dorsal column–medial lemniscus pathway (Fig. 8.42).

The equivalent mechanoreceptor fibres from the face and head have their cell bodies in the **trigeminal ganglion**. The fibres travel in the **trigeminal nerve** to the **principal nucleus of V** in the pons. Second order neurons from this nucleus cross the midline in the **trigeminal lemniscus** and end in the ventroposterior thalamus.

Thus, the ventroposterior thalamus receives information from both face and body and its third order neurons project to the **somatosensory cortex**.

Clinical box 8.26 **Dorsal column lesions**

Compression of the spinal cord on one side will compress the dorsal columns within the cord. This will result in the patient experiencing a loss of feeling and a disturbance of position sense on the ipsilateral (same) side below the level of the injury.

One variant of CNS involvement in tertiary syphilis is **tabes dorsalis**. In this condition loss of dorsal column function causes postural instability and an unsteady gait hence its synonym of locomotor ataxia. These features are particularly prominent in the dark when visual cues are lost

Vitamin B$_{12}$ deficiency can lead to **subacute combined degeneration** of the spinal cord in which loss of dorsal column functions is accompanied by peripheral neuropathy, with associated loss of sensation, pain and poor muscle control.

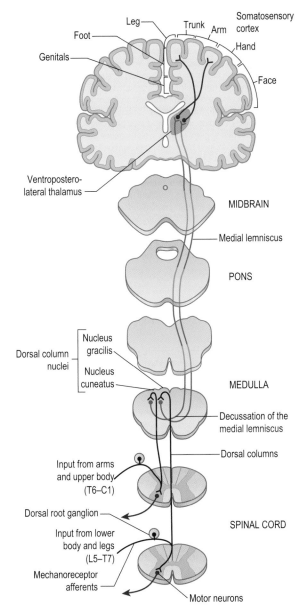

Fig. 8.42 Dorsal column–medial lemniscal pathways for transmitting skin mechanoreceptor sensations.

Table 8.18	Functions of the primary somatosensory cortex	
Brodmann area	**Submodality**	**Input from**
1	Perception of surface texture	Cutaneous mechanoreceptors
2	Shape and size of a grasped object	Joint proprioceptors
3a	Position and direction of movement	Muscle proprioceptors
3b	Perception of surface texture and shape discrimination	Cutaneous mechanoreceptors

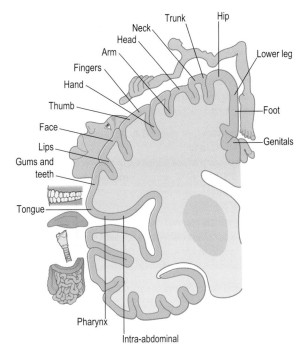

Fig. 8.43 Somatotopic map of the primary somatosensory (SI) cortex. Compare it with the somatosensory map in Figure 8.32. Redrawn from Penfield W, Rasmussen T 1952 The Cerebral Cortex of Man. New York, Macmillan Press, with permission.

Somatosensory cortex

The **primary somatosensory cortex (SI)** lies in the **post-central gyrus** of the parietal lobe (Brodmann's areas 1, 2, 3a and 3b) (see Fig. 8.8). Each of these four areas is dominated by a particular submodality (Table 8.18).

The information from the medial and trigeminal lemniscus is in the form of a topographic map which is passed from the thalamus to the somatosensory cortex. This **somatotopic map** is represented by a **sensory homunculus** in which areas of high sensitivity or complexity (e.g. the fingers and face) are disproportionately large (Fig. 8.43). On the other side of the central sulcus is the pre-central gyrus which contains the motor homunculus.

Four other maps of the body surface lie in the **secondary somatosensory cortex (SII)** and the **somatosensory association area** in the posterior parietal cortex. There are extensive interconnections between SI, SII and the posterior parietal lobe. The posterior parietal area has important functions in integrating sensory, including visual, and motor information (Clinical box 8.27).

Clinical box 8.27	Posterior parietal cortex lesions

Lesions of the posterior parietal cortex occur most commonly as a result of a stroke. These do not affect the ability to detect a stimulus but affect the ability to know what the stimulus means. This can result in:

- **Astereognosis**, the inability to recognise the shape of objects by touch.
- **Sensory neglect syndrome**, in which sensory information from a part (usually half) of sensory space is not perceived. This can manifest itself as a failure of the patient to recognise one half of their own body. It can also include visual neglect of half of the visual field.

Sensory neglect syndrome implies that the posterior parietal cortex has two **cognitive maps** (representations of where things are in space): one for body self-image and a second for extrapersonal space.

These problems are more likely to occur if the injury is on the right side as this part of the cortex is larger on the right.

Other proprioception pathways

There are two other important pathways that do not involve conscious awareness. The first is that involved in stretch and Golgi tendon organ reflexes. Skin, muscle and joint mechanoreceptors also send axons to the nucleus dorsalis (Clarke's nucleus) in the dorsal horn of the spinal cord and the accessory cuneate nucleus in the lower medulla. These provide second order neurons that form the dorsal (posterior) spinocerebellar and cuneocerebellar tracts which pass via the inferior cerebellar peduncle to the cerebellum (see above).

Pain and temperature

The sensations of pain and temperature share the same pathway. It is convenient to describe the receptors for temperature (thermoreceptors) first.

Thermoreceptors

The detection of the sensations of cold and warmth, rather that the pain of extreme cold or heat, is by **thermoreceptors** which consist of naked nerve endings which have small diameter, thinly myelinated (Aδ and some C) afferent fibres. There are two populations of thermoreceptors:

- **warm receptors** that respond to temperatures in the range 29–48°C, and
- **cold receptors** that are sensitive to skin temperatures between 5°C and 40°C with maximal activity at 25°C.

Nociceptors

The naked terminals of small diameter (Aδ and C) nerve fibres constitute the peripheral receptors for pain, termed **nociceptors**. Pain refers to noxious stimuli. Different nociceptor types respond to different forms of noxious stimuli:

- **Mechanical nociceptors** are stimulated by intense pressure and have fast conducting myelinated Aδ afferents. These give rise to a sharp **fast (first) pain** which is localised.
- **Polymodal nociceptors** respond to multiple stimuli including molecules released from tissue damage. Their afferents are C fibres which are slower than Aδ afferents and result in **slow (second) pain** of an aching or burning nature. **Itch receptors** that respond to histamine released from mast cells also have C fibre afferents.
- **Thermal nociceptors**, with C fibre afferents, respond to extremes of hot and cold.

In response to injury a number of chemicals, including inflammatory mediators, are released from leaky blood vessels and damaged tissue. These include a long list of substances including ATP, prostaglandins, histamine, serotonin, bradykinin and substance P (Information box 8.13). These agents directly excite nociceptors or make them more sensitive to other agents.

Pain and temperature pathways

The primary nociceptor sensory afferents have their cell bodies in the dorsal root ganglion and enter the dorsal horn. Here they bifurcate into ascending and descending branches, forming the **dorsolateral tract** (of Lissauer). These axons terminate on the cell bodies of the second order **projection neurons** in Rexed's laminae I, II and V within one or two spinal segments.

Information box 8.13 **Neurogenic inflammation**

Action potentials triggered by exciting polymodal nociceptor terminals are not only conducted centrally but, in what is termed an **axon reflex**, can also travel the 'wrong way' alongside branches of the axons (axon collaterals) to stimulate secretion of **substance P** from their peripheral terminals. This contributes to the classic signs of inflammation at an injury site in what is termed **neurogenic inflammation**. Substance P vasodilates post-capillary venules, which produces heat and redness. It increases capillary permeability, which causes swelling and pain and can cause itching by liberating histamine from mast cells, which excites itch C fibres.

Capsaicin, the active compound responsible for the hot taste of chilli peppers, acts on **vanilloid receptors** in thermal and polymodal nociceptors. Vanilloid receptors transduce noxious heat stimuli (burning sensations). Capsaicin causes pain by releasing substance P from nociceptors, but repeated application causes depletion of the transmitter and hence a reduced sensitivity to nociceptor stimuli. Recovery takes days to weeks. Vanilloid receptor ligands are being explored as potential novel analgesics.

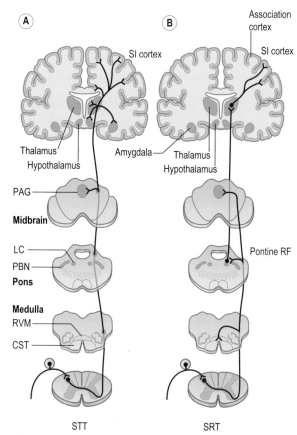

Fig. 8.44 Pathways for transmission of pain, temperature and crude touch sensations. (A) Spinothalamic tract. (B) Spinoreticular tract. CST, corticospinal tract; LC, locus coeruleus; PAG, periaqueductal grey; PBN, parabrachial nucleus; RF, reticular formation. Redrawn from Michael-Titus A, Revest P, Shortland P 2006 The nervous system. Churchill Livingstone, Edinburgh, with permission.

Axons from these projection neurons cross over within one or two segments to ascend in the **anterolateral pathway**. This term is used as it is located in the anterolateral column of the spinal cord. The main components are the **spinothalamic and spinoreticular tracts** (Fig. 8.44).

Projection neurons from lamina I, conveying fast fibre (Aδ) pain, go via the lateral **spinothalamic tract** (STT) and terminate in the **posterior nucleus** of the thalamus. Axons from lamina V account for the majority of STT fibres. These neurons receive input from both Aδ and C fibres but also from large diameter (Aβ) mechanoreceptor afferents. They are termed **wide dynamic range (WDR) cells** and their axons terminate in the **posterior** and **ventral posterior lateral (VPL)** nuclei of the thalamus. Lamina I cells have large receptive fields, relay to thalamic nuclei but do not have topographic projections to the cortex whereas lamina V do have somatotopic projections to the thalamus. Thus, localisation of painful stimuli relies on simultaneous firing of both types of cell.

The **spinoreticular pathway** principally transmits slow (C fibre) pain and makes extensive connections in the reticular nuclei in the brainstem as well as with the thalamus. The reticular nuclei throughout the brainstem contribute to autonomic responses to pain and the increased arousal associated with pain. Midbrain reticular nuclei include the **periaqueductal grey (PAG)** matter which modulates nociceptor input and the parabrachial nucleus which projects to the amygdala and is thought to be involved in emotional responses and learning to fear painful situations. Many spinoreticular axons do not cross the midline but ascend ipsilaterally.

Crude touch sensation is conveyed to the ventral lateral nuclei of the thalamus from mechanoreceptor stimulation of lamina V cells.

The **trigeminal pathway** is the route for pain, temperature and crude touch sensation of the face. The primary afferents responsible have their cell bodies in the **trigeminal ganglion** and their centrally directed axons run in the **trigeminal (V) nerve** to the **spinal nucleus of V**. Second order neurons then go to the **posterior** and **ventral posterior medial (VPM)** nuclei of the thalamus (see Clinical box 8.28).

The anterolateral and trigeminal pathways relay in the thalamus which makes connections with the cerebral cortex, basal ganglia and limbic systems. Connections with the hypothalamus activate the hypothalamic–pituitary–adrenal axis stress response.

Summary of the ascending sensory pathways

As explained above, but worthy of repetition, both the main ascending sensory pathways cross before reaching the thalamus but at different positions. The touch and conscious proprioception pathway crosses in the lower medulla but the anterolateral pathway fibres cross soon after the primary afferents have entered the spinal cord. This explains the pattern of sensory loss in the Brown-Séquard syndrome (see above).

Clinical testing of these two pathways is summarised in Clinical box 8.29.

Clinical box 8.28 **Trigeminal neuralgia**

Trigeminal neuralgia (or tic douloureux) is characterised by attacks of excruciating pain in the face lasting for only a few seconds at a time. Often there is an area of the face, known as a **trigger zone**, which when stimulated by light touch, a change of temperature or facial movement sets off a paroxysm of pain. The cause is unknown but is thought to be caused by an aberrant artery in some cases.

Clinical box 8.29 **Clinical examination of ascending sensory pathways**

With the patient's eyes closed or averted the examiner tests the **mechanoreceptor pathways** by the following:

- **Light touch:** a wisp of cotton wool is dabbed on the skin and the patient reports when it is felt
- **Vibration:** a 128 Hz tuning fork is first placed over the tip of the big toe then moved proximally over joints to see if a 'buzzing' sensation is experienced
- **Joint position sense:** conscious proprioception is examined by holding the distal phalanx of the patient's big toe and is asked to report when they sense it being moved up or down.

  The anterolateral pathway is tested similarly:
- **Pain:** a pin is used to determine areas of loss of superficial pain. (NB: pin is disposed of after use.) Deep pain is tested by squeezing muscle bellies (e.g. calf muscles).
- **Temperature:** the patient is touched with a cold metal object (e.g. tuning fork) and asked if it feels cold. More accurate testing requires tubes of hot and cold water at controlled temperatures but is seldom performed.

Pain regulation

Mechanisms to reduce nociceptor input operate at both the spinal and supraspinal level. These are exploited in treating pain in clinical practice.

The **gate control theory** is thought to explain why rubbing the site of a painful stimulus helps alleviate the pain. This occurs at the level of the spinal cord (Fig. 8.45). According to the gate control theory concurrent activity in large diameter (Aβ) primary afferents reduces the transmission of pain signals in small (Aδ and C) diameter afferents. The WDR projection neurons in lamina V transmit excitatory pain signals to the thalamus. These neurons receive input from both large mechanoreceptor and small nociceptor afferents. However, they also receive inhibitory input from interneurons in lamina II. Collaterals of the large afferent stimulate these interneurons while small afferent collaterals inhibit them.

In response to a painful stimulus the small afferents stimulate the lamina V neurons directly and their collaterals by inhibiting the inhibitory neuron stimulate them indirectly. This opens the gate. If large mechanoreceptors are excited at the same time, their collaterals stimulate the inhibitory interneuron, countering the effect of the small afferent. Thus the gate is closed.

The gate control theory is the basis for transcutaneous electrical nerve stimulation (TENS), used to relieve pain (Clinical box 8.30).

Pain can also be modulated by supraspinal pathways. Brainstem nuclei such as the raphe nucleus and **locus coeruleus** send descending fibres to dorsal horn cells reducing nociceptor transmission. The PAG has fibres that release the opioid peptide, enkephalin which binds to the presynaptic membrane of nociceptor fibres inhibiting pain signals (Information box 8.14).

The PAG is considered important in **emergency analgesia**. This refers to the lack of pain at the site of a painful injury described by those in high arousal states such as warfare or sport. Rapid in onset this effect can last a few hours. Also thought to involve the PAG is the more generalised reduction in pain awareness that occurs in those recovering from a stressful event, termed stress analgesia.

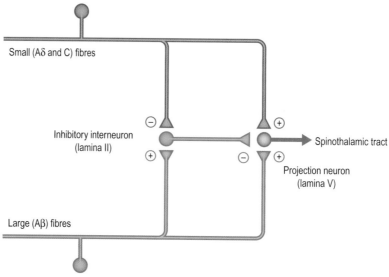

Fig. 8.45 **Gate control theory of pain.** The neurons which transmit pain signals are stimulated by both small (Aδ and C) fibres and large (Aβ) fibres. Collaterals from both of these inhibit and stimulate, respectively, lamina II interneurons.

Clinical box 8.30   **Therapeutic application of pain modulation mechanisms**

Transcutaneous electrical nerve stimulation (TENS) delivers high-frequency, low-intensity currents sufficient to stimulate Aβ and Aδ fibres and hence close the pain gate. However, it may work by stimulating the production of endorphins (endogenous opioids) as the analgesia produced by TENS can be blocked by opioid receptor antagonists.

Although TENS is widely used in the treatment of acute and chronic pain and in labour, evidence-based reviews have failed to show benefit over placebo (sham TENS).

Stimulus-induced analgesia in rats involves stimulation of the PAG by implantation of electrodes.

Information box 8.14   **Opioid analgesics**

Opioids are ligands of opioid receptors. Analgesia is attributed to agonist or partial agonist activity at opioid receptors, mimicking the actions of the endogenous opioids in the pain-modulating pathways. The effects of opioid analgesics can be rapidly reversed by their competitive antagonists. There are a number of unwanted side effects of opioid analgesics:

- Respiratory depression (which occurs at therapeutic doses) and vomiting are due to activation of opioid receptors in the medulla
- Constipation from an increase in tone but reduced motility in the gastrointestinal tract due to the stimulation of peripheral opioid receptors in visceral smooth muscle
- Morphine and some other opioids may cause tolerance and dependence.

Analgesic agents

The most common analgesics used clinically are:

- **Opioid analgesics**: act on opioid receptors and are usually reserved for moderate to severe pain (Information box 8.15). These include morphine and structurally related drugs (e.g. diamorphine, codeine) and synthetic agents (e.g. fentanyl, pethidine).
- **Non-steroidal anti-inflammatory drugs** (**NSAIDs**): inhibit cyclo-oxygenase which acts on arachidonic acid to produce prostaglandins which sensitise nociceptors to inflammatory mediators (e.g. serotonin, bradykinin). They also inhibit leukotrienes which prolong inflammation

---

Information box 8.15   **Acupuncture**

Effective **acupuncture** relies on stimulation of small diameter (group II and III) afferents from skeletal muscle and joints. This is thought to activate a descending endorphinergic pathway from the arcuate nucleus of the hypothalamus to the ventrolateral periaqueductal grey matter (PAG), the midbrain region that is thought to be responsible for stress analgesia. Acupuncture produces a state similar to stress analgesia, and both can be reversed by the opioid receptor antagonist naloxone.

(see Ch. 6). NSAIDs include aspirin, paracetamol, ibuprofen, mefenamic acid etc.

- **Local anaesthetics**: reversibly block the conduction of action potentials by blocking Na^+ channels in the axonal membrane. Local anaesthetics are weak bases which are mainly in the form of positively charged cations that cannot enter the Na^+ channel until it is open. This occurs when the axon membrane is inactivated (see Action potentials above). At low concentration local anaesthetics affect only small diameter (Aδ and C) myelinated and unmyelinated fibres, reducing pain and temperature signals but sparing proprioceptive and motor fibres.

In addition to these agents a number of drugs are used to relieve pain in specific situations (e.g. carbamazepine in trigeminal neuralgia; almotriptan and sumatriptan for migraine).

Placebo effect

In medical research, a placebo is an inert substance or sham procedure used as a control when comparing the effectiveness of a therapeutic intervention with no treatment. A placebo should have no physiological or pharmacological effects, so that any demonstrable change is known as the **placebo effect**. This effect varies widely between individuals, and as much as a difference of 30% in the measurements used has been demonstrated. In patients, the effect is most marked in subjective symptoms which are difficult to measure such as pain, and weak in more objective measures such as clearance of bacteria in patients with septicaemia.

Whilst poorly understood, there is some research evidence to suggest the mechanism behind placebo analgesia. fMRI studies have demonstrated increased activity in the brain concerned with cognition, the dorsal lateral prefrontal cortex, instead of pain sensitive regions (e.g. thalamus), where activity decreased. This suggests that the expectation of pain relief may trigger activity in the sensory, supraspinal opioid pathways to block the transmission of pain sensation.

Visceral sensation

Pain from viscera often comes from nociceptors in covering tissues, such as peritoneum, pleura and dura mater, rather than the parenchyma of internal organs. In addition, however, mechanoreceptors respond to excessive distention or contraction of hollow organs (e.g. bladder and bowel).

Visceral afferents from nociceptors follow sympathetic pathways, have cell bodies in dorsal root ganglia and their axons terminate in the dorsal horn and intermediate grey matter of the spinal cord. These second order neurons project to the anterolateral system. Fibres conveying non-painful sensation from viscera travel primarily in the vagus nerve to the nucleus of the tractus solitarius.

Referred pain

Visceral pain tends to be poorly localised. Nociceptors from viscera and skin converge on the same spinothalamic neurons and the brain interprets the visceral pain as coming from an area of skin that may be quite far from the internal organ (see Fig. 8.46). This is called **referred pain**. Pain from the heart in myocardial ischaemia may be felt in the left axilla or down the inside of the left arm. Other examples include inflammation of the peritoneum covering the diaphragm, which is referred to the shoulder, and pain from an inflamed appendix, which is felt around the umbilicus.

Phantom pain

Phantom pain is the perception of pain in a body part that is absent. For example, most patients experience sensation, including pain, in a limb that has been amputated. These phantom pains can sometimes be attributed to abnormal

growth of injured nerve fibres forming neuromas at stump sites. However, children born with congenital limb deficiencies can also experience phantom pain, suggesting other mechanisms. Theories include alteration of pain pathways and reorganisation of the cerebral cortex. Phantom sensations can also result from loss of other body parts such as a breast (mastectomy), penis, eye, tongue or even internal organs.

SPECIAL SENSES

VISION

Vision, or seeing, is a complex set of processes in which light rays reflected from objects pass through the cornea and lens of the eye to reach photoreceptors of the retina which send signals via the visual pathways principally to the visual cortex in the occipital lobe.

The anatomy of the eyeball

The structure of the eyeball is shown in Figure 8.47. It has three concentric layers:

- An outer fibrous layer that consists anteriorly of the transparent **cornea** covered by a thin epithelium, the **conjunctiva**, and the posterior five-sixths is the opaque **sclera**
- A middle vascular layer that includes the **iris**, **ciliary body** and **choroid**
- The innermost nervous layer is the **retina**, consisting of the light-sensitive **neural retina** and the single layer of **retinal pigmented epithelium** (**RPE**).

The **iris** is a circular structure with a central opening, the pupil. As well as collagen fibres and the pigment cells, responsible for its colour, it contains two sets of smooth muscle fibres: the **pupillary sphincter** and the **pupillary dilator**. The iris divides the internal space into an **anterior chamber** in front of the iris and **a posterior chamber** between the iris and the lens. Both chambers contain **aqueous humour** which is secreted by the ciliary body in the posterior chamber and drains through a trabecular meshwork into the **canal of Schlemm** at the **iridocorneal angle** of the anterior chamber (Clinical box 8.31). A transparent gel, the **vitreous humour**, fills the main cavity of the eye behind the lens and helps maintain the shape of the eyeball.

Optics of the eye

To reach the retina the light rays have to pass through the conjunctiva, cornea, aqueous humour, lens (Clinical box 8.32) and vitreous humour. Smooth **ciliary muscles** in the ciliary body are attached to the lens by a suspensory ligament and can alter its shape. When the ciliary muscles are relaxed the lens is relatively flat and parallel rays of light from distant objects are brought to focus on the central part of the retina, but when the muscles contract the lens becomes more spherical and light rays from near objects, which are diverging as they enter the eye, are focused onto the retina. A number of conditions are associated with **refractive errors** (Clinical box 8.33) that interfere with the ability of the eye to focus light rays onto the retina.

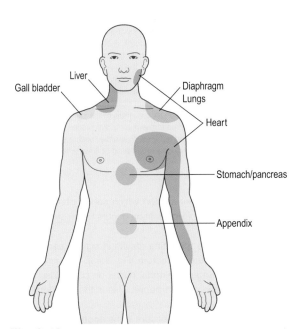

Fig. 8.46 **Referred pain.** Sites at which visceral pain from internal organs can be felt.

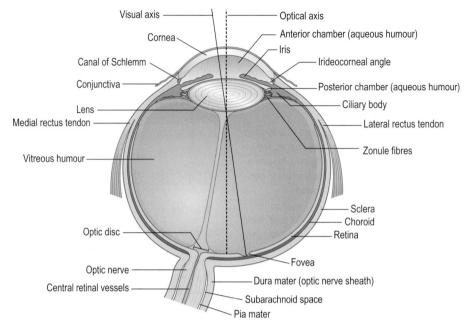

Fig. 8.47 **Horizontal section through a human eye.**

Labels (clockwise from top):
Visual axis — Optical axis — Anterior chamber (aqueous humour) — Iris — Irideocorneal angle — Posterior chamber (aqueous humour) — Ciliary body — Lateral rectus tendon — Zonule fibres — Sclera — Choroid — Retina — Fovea — Dura mater (optic nerve sheath) — Subarachnoid space — Pia mater — Central retinal vessels — Optic nerve — Optic disc — Vitreous humour — Medial rectus tendon — Lens — Conjunctiva — Canal of Schlemm — Cornea

---

Clinical box 8.31 Glaucoma

In glaucoma the drainage of aqueous humour into the trabecular meshwork is impaired, resulting in an increase in intraocular pressure. This can lead to damage to the nerve fibres in the retina and to the optic nerve. There are four main types of glaucoma:

- **Chronic open-angle glaucoma**: this is the most common and develops slowly. It is more common in short-sighted people and its incidence rises with age
- **Angle-closure glaucoma**: this is uncommon and is associated with a narrow iridiocorneal angle
- **Secondary glaucoma**: results from eye injury or inflammation (e.g. uveitis)
- **Developmental** (congenital) **glaucoma**: present at birth or shortly thereafter.

Clinical box 8.32 Cataract

The lens of the eye consists of a capsule, epithelium and lens fibres. The lens fibres are elongated cells that lose their nuclei and mitochondria and are packed with proteins, called **crystallins**, which are normally transparent. An opacity of the lens is termed a **cataract**. Various changes to the lens fibres and capsule occur with ageing resulting in senile cataract. Other causes include:

- Hyperglycaemia that attends poorly controlled diabetes mellitus. The lens contains **aldose reductase** which catalyses the synthesis of sorbitol from glucose. The osmotic action of excess sorbitol causes fluid to accumulate in the lens.
- Infection, inflammation, trauma including eye surgery can result in cataract.
- UV-B radiation destroys proper crystallin folding causing opacity.
- **Congenital cataract** can occur with maternal rubella infection or with inherited disorders such as Down syndrome, dystrophia myotonica and galactosaemia.

Pupillary reflexes

Stimulation of the pupillary sphincter produces constriction of the pupil (**miosis**) while the dilator muscle increases pupil size (**mydriasis**). The sphincter receives parasympathetic fibres that run in the oculomotor (III) nerve. These fibres originate in the **Edinger–Westphal nucleus** in the midbrain

Clinical box 8.33 Refractive errors

Refractive errors can result in a failure to bring light from distant objects to focus at the retina. They may be due to a defect in the lens or in the shape of the eyeball or both.

Myopia (nearsightedness): light is focused in front of the retina so distant objects are blurred. Because of the greater refractive power the eye can view close objects with less accommodation. Correction is with a concave lens of appropriate power. Myopia is extremely common and may be a modern disease. It is thought that an eye mechanism which regulates eyeball growth to ensure light is focused on the retina is disrupted by the large amount of near vision children engage in when they read, write and use computers.

Hyperopia (farsightedness): light is focused behind the retina. The accommodation reflex is in play continuously to bring distant objects to focus, but the lower refractive power of the hyperopic eye is unable to focus nearby objects. It is corrected with convex lenses.

Presbyopia: with age the lens becomes less elastic and less able to relax into the high-refractive-power spherical shape needed to focus close objects. Hence the closest point that can be clearly focused, the **near point**, recedes with age. The increased stiffness of the lens, and its tendency to become more convex with time because of the continual activity of the proliferative epithelium, also means it may not be so effectively flattened by tension in the suspensory ligaments. The result is a loss in the ability to focus on distant objects with age.

Astigmatism: the radius of curvature of the surface of the cornea or the lens is not the same in all radial planes, so that points of light are focused as lines. Presented with a starburst of lines the patient sees only one orientation of lines in focus.

and end in the ciliary ganglion which sends postganglionic fibres to the muscle. Pupil dilation occurs under sympathetic stimulation.

Light shining on the retina results in signals sent via the optic (II) nerve to the pretectum (Fig. 8.48). Pretectal axons stimulate the Edinger–Westphal nuclei on both sides which cause constriction of both pupils. This is the **pupillary light reflex** (Clinical box 8.34).

Pupil constriction also occurs in the **accommodation reflex** when both eyes are adducted to focus on a near object. At the same time the ciliary muscles make the lens bulge.

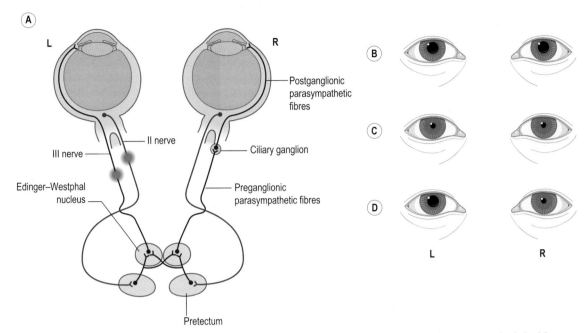

Fig. 8.48 **Pupillary light reflexes following damage to either optic (II) or oculomotor (III) nerves on the left side.** (A) Reflex pathway; (B) optic nerve damage, left eye stimulated; (C) optic nerve damage, right eye stimulated; (D) oculomotor nerve damage, either eye stimulated.

Clinical box 8.34   **Clinical utility of pupillary reflexes**

Pupillary light reflexes can be used to diagnose visual system lesions. Normally, light shone into one eye causes constriction of the pupil of the same eye (direct reflex) and of the other eye (consensual reflex). **Optic nerve lesions** abolish the direct, but not the consensual, reflex (see Fig. 8.48B, C). **Oculomotor nerve lesions** result in a **fixed dilated pupil** on the afflicted side (i.e. loss of direct and consensual reflexes so no reaction on that side to light shone in either eye, Fig. 8.48D). Third nerve palsy also causes a **divergent squint** (the eye deviates laterally) and **ptosis** (drooping of the eyelid).

Retina

The neural retina contains five basic types of neuron (Fig. 8.49): **photoreceptors** (**cones** and **rods**) lying in close contact with the RPE; three populations of interneurons (**bipolar cells**, **horizontal cells** and **amacrine cells**); and the **ganglion cells** of the optic nerve.

Optic nerve fibres from throughout the retina converge and leave at one area known as the **optic disc** (Figs 8.47, 8.50, Clinical box 8.35). There are no photoreceptors at the optic disc and testing of the central visual field shows this as a blind spot but it is not noticeable in normal vision. Rods are fairly evenly distributed throughout the retina but cones are clustered mainly in an area called the **macula lutea** lateral to the optic disc. Within the macula is a conical pit, the **fovea centralis**, that contains only cones. The macula and fovea are the areas of highest visual acuity (Information box 8.16).

Photoreceptors

Rods are very sensitive and respond to dim light (scotopic vision) and cones operate in bright light (photopic vision). Rods and cones have different structures but share certain features. Both have an **outer segment** packed with highly folded plasma membrane containing visual pigment; an **inner segment** housing the nucleus and mitochondria; and a **synaptic terminal**.

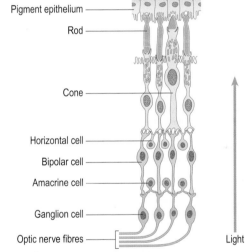

Fig. 8.49 **The cellular organisation of the retina.** From Douglas et al. (eds) 2013 Macleod's Clinical examination, 13th edn. Elsevier, Edinburgh, with permission.

- Rod cells have **rhodopsin** as visual pigment. This consists of the protein **opsin** and a prosthetic group, **11-*cis* retinal**, derived from vitamin A in the diet.
- Cones have three different types of opsin (or **iodopsin**), each absorbing light maximally at a different part of the visible light spectrum (Fig. 8.51): **short** (**S, blue**), **medium** (**M, green**) and **long** (**L, red**) **wavelength**. Colour blindness results from defects in cone opsins (Clinical box 8.36).

Phototransduction is similar in rods and cones in that the absorption of light energy isomerises pigment molecules which starts a cascade of chemical reactions. Here the process in rods is described in a little more detail. In the dark Na^+ (and Ca^{2+}) ion influx occurs through cGMP-controlled cation channels which **depolarises** the rod cells to about $-40\,mV$. When a photon is absorbed by 11-*cis* retinal it is isomerised

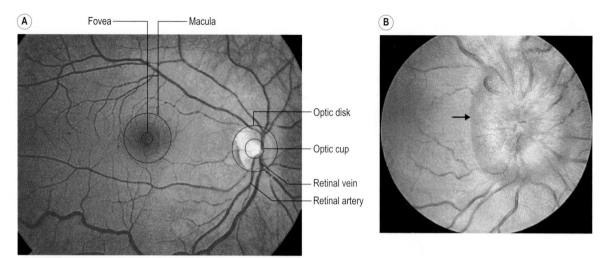

Fovea — Macula
Optic disk
Optic cup
Retinal vein
Retinal artery

Fig. 8.50 **Funduscopy.** (A) Normal eye showing optic disc and retinal arteries. From Kumar P, Clark M. Clinical medicine, 8th edn. Elsevier, Edinburgh, 2012, with permission. (B) Papilloedema with bulging of the optic disc. From Colledge NR, et al. (eds) 2010 Davidson's principles and practice of medicine, 22nd edn. Churchill Livingstone, Edinburgh, with permission.

| Clinical box 8.35 | Funduscopy and retinal disorders |

The examination of the retina with an ophthalmoscope, called **funduscopy** (Fig. 8.50), is an important part of the neurological examination, for example:

- Because the optic nerve lies within the meninges, a rise in intracerebral pressure is transmitted through to the optic disc and can be diagnosed by **papilloedema**, a swelling of the disc
- Characteristic alterations of retinal blood vessels (e.g. retinal haemorrhages) allow the diagnosis of a number of conditions, e.g. hypertensive and diabetic retinopathy.

Trauma can cause a **detached retina** where the neural retina peels away from the retinal pigmented epithelium. The loss of contact causes the death of the photoreceptors because they rely on the epithelium for metabolic support.

Macular degeneration is a failure of central vision that accounts for almost half of visual impairment in patients over 65. There are two types, both resulting from the functional disconnection of photoreceptors from the pigment epithelium.

| Information box 8.16 | High acuity vision |

High acuity vision is achieved by the fovea centralis because it:
- Has the highest density of cones
- Lies at the optical axis where light comes through the optically best central parts of the cornea and lens
- Has all retinal layers above the cones displaced laterally so light does not have to pass through them
- Has a low number of blood vessels, thus minimising diffraction.

Only about 1/1000 of the visual field is seen by the fovea centralis at any instant and it is the only part in sharp focus, hence gaze must be frequently and rapidly shifted to view a significant portion of the visual field clearly. This is the purpose of **saccades**. These are rapid movements of both eyes simultaneously which jump around the visual field allowing the gaze to be fixed on one point after another.

---

to **all-*trans* retinal** (photoisomerisation), rhodopsin is activated and binds to a GTP-bound protein called **transducin**. The GTP-bound α subunit of transducin dissociates and activates a phosphodiesterase which hydrolyses cGMP to 5′-GMP which closes the cation channels reversing the depolarisation and causing hyperpolarization (Fig. 8.52).

Exposure to bright light desensitises rod cells as all-*trans* retinal dissociates from rhodopsin which is said to be

---

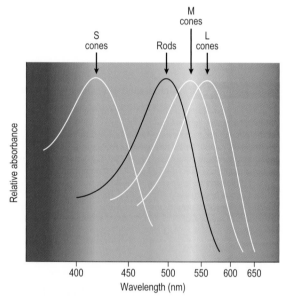

S cones   M cones   L cones   Rods

Fig. 8.51 **Absorption curves for photoreceptors.**

| Clinical box 8.36 | Photoreceptor dysfunction |

Abnormalities of cone opsins
Inherited defects in colour vision occur mostly as a result of abnormalities in one or more cone opsins. By far the commonest is **red–green colour blindness**, an X-linked recessive trait that afflicts up to 8% of European males and 0.4% of females. It arises because of mutations in M or L cone opsins which renders red and green indistinguishable from each other (and from grey). **Blue colour blindness** is a rare autosomal dominant trait due to a defect in the S opsin gene.

Lack of cones
More rarely defects in colour vision occur because of the lack of one, two or all three populations of cone. Patients missing two types of cone have no colour vision and those completely without cones are completely blind in daylight when their rods are saturated, but have scotopic vision at night.

Loss of both rods and cones
Retinitis pigmentosa is a blanket term for a set of heritable disorders characterised by progressive loss of both rods and cones, accompanied by disruption of the pigment epithelium and abnormal migration of pigment into the neural retina where it forms clumps. Most retinitis pigmentosa involves mutations of the various photoreceptor-specific proteins.

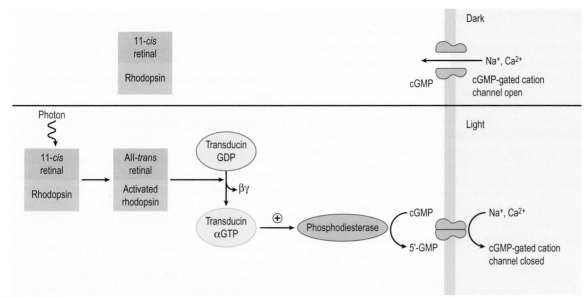

Fig. 8.52 Rod cell phototransduction. In the dark cGMP-controlled cation channels are open. Light stimulates a cascade of events which results in the breakdown of cGMP which closes the channels and hyperpolarises the rod.

bleached. Retinal isomerase must convert all-*trans* retinal to 11-*cis* retinal for rods to regain function and explains the delay in adjustment to dim light.

Retinal processing

All photoreceptors synapse with bipolar cells which then signal to ganglion cells of the optic nerve. The photoreceptors synapse with two types of bipolar cells which have different glutamate receptors. In the dark there is a constant release of glutamate which is reduced in response to light. One type of bipolar cell (**on-centre** cells) is hyperpolarised in the dark and depolarise in the light; and **off-centre** cells are depolarised in the dark and hyperpolarise in light. Each population of bipolar cells is connected to the equivalent population of ganglion cells. Thus, for example, on-centre ganglion cells get their input exclusively from on-centre bipolar cells and so in response to light the bipolar cell depolarises and the ganglion cell is excited and increases its firing frequency.

The receptive fields of the bipolar and the ganglion cells are circular with opposite responses between the central zone and the peripheral zone, a phenomenon known as centre-surround inhibition (see above) (Fig. 8.53).

- **On-centre** (or on-centre/off-surround) **cells:** the bipolar cell centre depolarises to light while the surrounding area is hyperpolarised; the ganglion cell centre is excited and its surround inhibited
- **Off-centre** (or off-centre/on-surround) **cells:** the bipolar cell centre is hyperpolarised in response to light, the surround depolarised; ganglion cell centre is inhibited and surround excited.

Direct photoreceptor-bipolar-ganglion cell connections are responsible for the central zone response while connections via interneurons produce the opposite response from the periphery. For cone cells this mechanism is mediated by horizontal cells and for rod cells the interneurons are amacrine cells. The effect of these two antagonistic actions enhances contrast.

Retinal output, transmitted by axons of ganglion cells, essentially consists of information about small

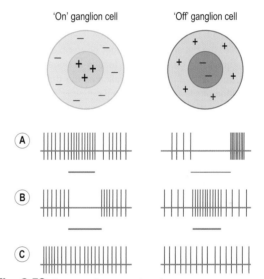

Fig. 8.53 Surround antagonism in an on-centre ganglion cell. Top: receptive fields. Responses to: (A) central illumination; (B) surround illumination; and (C) overall illumination. From Michael-Titus A, Revest P, Shortland P 2006 The nervous system. Churchill Livingstone, Edinburgh, with permission.

differences in light intensity and colour. Centre-surround antagonism, which acts particularly to produce contrasts of colour and at dark/light boundaries, signals differences in space, giving rise to the perception of form, while the parallel on- and off-channels signal changes in time. Correlating the differences in space and time gives movement perception.

The retina processes information about form and colour and movement separately. **P (parvocellular)** ganglion cells transmit information about form and colour, and **M (magnocellular)** ganglion cells process information about movement. These cells connect to visual pathways that are anatomically separate; the P and M pathways. This is known as **parallel processing**, where separate streams of information are simultaneously processed, but separately.

Central visual pathways

Axons of the ganglion cells leave the eye in **optic (II) nerves**. The majority (>90%) synapse with cells in the **lateral geniculate nuclei (LGN)** of the thalamus that project to visual cortex and the remainder end in midbrain structures involved in visual reflexes and eye movements.

The optic nerves from each eye combine to form the **optic chiasma** in front of the pituitary gland stalk. Nerve fibres from the nasal half of the retina (i.e. the temporal half of the visual field) cross over in the optic chiasma to join the optic tract (Fig. 8.54). Thus the right optic tract contains information from the left half of the visual field from both eyes. Each **LGN** has six layers and each layer receives input from only one eye. Thus the right LGN receives input from the right eye to layers 2, 3 and 5 and from the left eye to layers 1, 4 and 6. Layers 1 and 2 are supplied by M ganglion cells (one from each eye) while layers 4–6 get input from P ganglion cells.

Axons leave the LGN in the optic radiation by two slightly different routes to the **primary visual cortex** (V1). One route carries information from the fovea and the lower part of the visual field and passes directly through the parietal lobe, while the other fibres travel more laterally through the temporal lobe.

Visual fields are examined clinically by the **confrontation method** where the examiner compares their own visual field with that of the patient using a finger or an object such as a white-headed pin. More detailed testing is done instrumentally by **perimetry**. Figure 8.54 indicates the defects occurring at different sites along the visual pathway.

In addition to the primary visual cortex (V1), in the occipital lobe around the calcarine sulcus visual information is processed by **secondary** and **association visual cortex** (V2–5) (see Fig. 8.55).

Visual perception

Perception of depth in the visual field is computed in V1 by a number of mechanisms. For objects further than about 30 m away, binocular vision is not required and information from individual eyes (**monocular clues**) is involved, including:

- **Parallax**: near objects appear to move more than more distant ones
- **Perspective**: distant objects appear smaller than near ones
- **Occultation**: near objects obscure distant ones
- **Chiaroscuro**: near objects cast shadows over more distant ones.

Nearer than 30 m these monocular clues are supplemented by comparison of images from both eyes, **stereopsis**, or binocular vision. Both eyes turn inwards to focus the image of an object on the fovea of both eyes, known as the **vergence reflex**. Because the eyes are about 6.3 cm apart images of objects closer to, or further from, the fixation point will fall onto slightly different positions on the two retinas, known as **retinal disparity**.

The **magnocellular (M) pathway** from the LGN is the principal route for information required for **movement perception** and relays via V5 in the middle temporal area (Fig. 8.56). This pathway is closely related to eye movement pathways.

Colour perception goes by the **parvocellular (P) pathway** from the LGN and these neurons relay in V4 (Fig. 8.56).

VESTIBULAR SYSTEM

The vestibular system helps maintain balance, contributes to posture mechanisms and keeps the eyes fixed on an image as the head moves. Its sensory receptors are located in the inner ear and are sent to the CNS alongside hearing fibres in the vestibulocochlear (VIII) nerve.

Anatomy

The inner ear consists of the **bony labyrinth**, a series of interconnected cavities in the petrous part of the temporal bone, inside of which is the **membranous labyrinth**, a system of

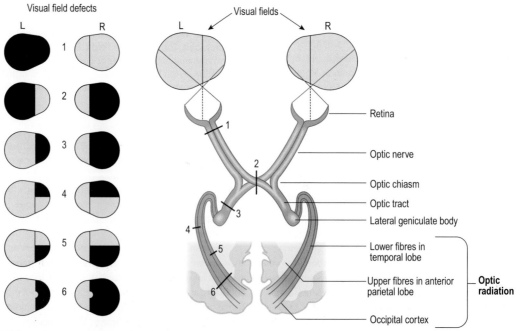

Fig. 8.54 **Visual pathways and field defects.** From Douglas G, et al (eds) 2013 Macleod's Clinical examination, 12th edn. Churchill Livingston, Edinburgh, with permission.

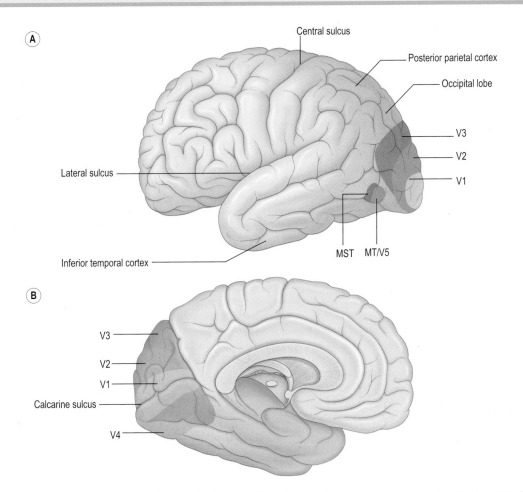

Fig. 8.55 **Visual cortex.** Location of visual cortical areas in the left hemisphere: (A) lateral aspect; (B) medial aspect. MT, middle temporal area; MST, medial superior temporal area.

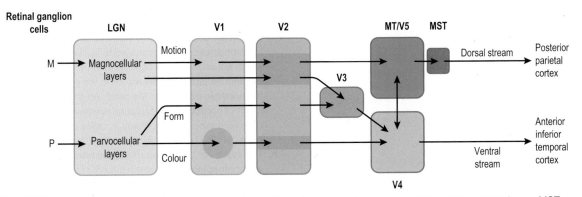

Fig. 8.56 **Processing pathways in the visual system.** LGN, lateral geniculate nucleus; MT, middle temporal area; MST, medial superior temporal area.

tubes and sacs. Fluid called perilymph fills the space between the bony and membranous labyrinths. It is secreted by the periosteum and has a similar composition to CSF. The membranous labyrinth contains a different fluid, **endolymph**, which has a higher specific gravity and viscosity than perilymph and its composition is similar to intracellular fluid. It drains into the **endolymphatic sac** and is absorbed into the CSF (Clinical box 8.37). There are small connections between both endolymph and perilymph in the vestibular system and the cochlea. The vestibular apparatus consists of two **otolith organs**, the **utricle** and **saccule**, and three **semicircular canals**: lateral, posterior and anterior (Fig. 8.57). In all five **hair cells** are the sensory receptors.

Clinical box 8.37   **Ménierè disease**

In Ménierè disease endolymph reabsorption is impaired and the increase in endolymph volume damages the membranous labyrinth and hair cells in the vestibular inner ear and the cochlea. The result is:

- Intermittent, relapsing **vertigo** (the illusion of rotatory movement) and loss of balance often accompanied by nausea and vomiting
- **Tinnitus** (ringing in the ears)
- Progressive **hearing loss**.

The disorder is usually unilateral and what triggers it is unknown. In severe cases surgical destruction of the afflicted labyrinth alleviates the vertigo. The vestibular system adapts to receiving unilateral input, so normal vestibulo-ocular reflexes and sense of balance are restored.

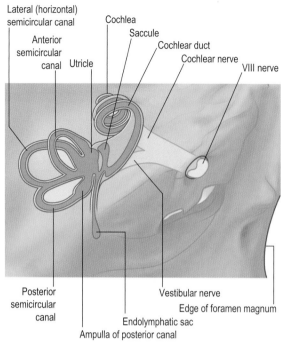

Fig. 8.57 **The left vestibular apparatus and cochlea viewed from above.** The membranous labyrinth is shaded. Redrawn with permission from Longstaff A 2005 Instant notes in neuroscience, 2nd edn. Taylor & Francis, Abingdon.

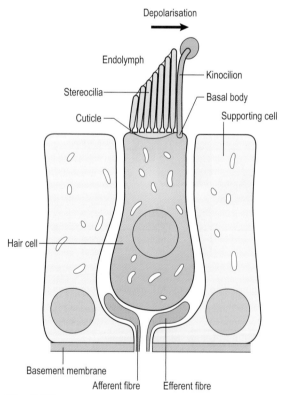

Fig. 8.58 **Vestibular hair cell.**

Hair cells (Fig. 8.58) are arranged in bunches of **stereocilia**, graduated in height becoming taller until the tallest, the **kinocilium**. **Transduction** occurs when the tips of the stereocilia are bent towards the kinocilium. The tips of the stereocilia contain transmembrane ion channels and when a mechanical force deflects the stereocilia the ion channels

open and depolarisation occurs. Movement in the opposite direction closes the channel resulting in hyperpolarisation.

- In otolith organs hair cells are in the **macula** with the tips of the hair bundles embedded in a gelatinous **tectorial membrane** which is studded with calcium carbonate crystals called **otoconia**. Linear acceleration displaces the tectorial membrane relative to the hair cells due to the inertia of the otoconia. This deflects the hair cell one way and the opposite way when head movement stops. The utricle and saccule detect linear acceleration in the horizontal and vertical axes, respectively.
- The hair cells in the semicircular canals are located in a small hillock, the **crista**, in a small swelling, the **ampulla**, at the base of each canal. The tips of these hair cells extend into the gelatinous **cupula**. The three semicircular canals lie at right angles to each other and detect rotation, or angular acceleration, in all three planes of three-dimensional space. Transduction is similar to that of the otolith organs with the inertia of the cupula bending the hair cells.

Central vestibular pathways

The afferents from the vestibular hair cell have their cell bodies in the **vestibular (Scarpa's) ganglion**. These are bipolar cells and their central processes run in the vestibular division of the **vestibulocochlear (VIII) nerve** to the **vestibular nuclei** in the medulla. These nuclei have various outputs including:

- The **medial vestibular nuclei** project to the motor nuclei of the IIIrd, IVth and VIth cranial nerves which control eye movements. The **vestibulo-ocular reflexes (VOR)** keep gaze steady when the head rotates. Rotation of the head stimulates the semicircular canals which work in pairs so that hair cells on the side towards which the head is turning are depolarised and those on the opposite side hyperpolarised. This is signalled to the vestibular nuclei which act on the nuclei controlling opposing pairs of extraocular muscles. This results in the eyes moving in the opposite direction to the head. An example of the effect of horizontal head rotation is shown in Figure 8.59. Clinicians assess this pathway in cases of suspected brainstem injury using caloric testing (Clinical box 8.38).
- The vestibular nuclei give rise to the **lateral** and **medial vestibulospinal tracts** which strongly facilitate motor neurons to antigravity muscles involved in posture control.
- Axons from vestibular nuclei cross to the contralateral ventroposterior lateral nucleus of the thalamus which sends information to the cerebral cortex providing conscious awareness of posture and balance.

AUDITORY SYSTEM

Sound

Sound consists of pressure waves transmitted through a medium (e.g. air or fluid). The **frequency** of the wave is the number of oscillations, expressed in hertz (Hz) which is perceived as the **pitch**. Pure tones at frequencies of between 20 Hz and 20 kHz are heard by young people but there is a loss of high frequencies in older people (**presbycusis**).

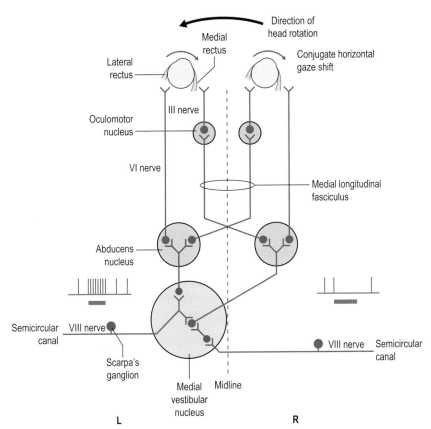

Fig. 8.59 The circuitry of the rotational vestibulo-ocular reflex. Stimulation of the horizontal semicircular canals by leftward head rotation (red bars) excites motor neurons to ipsilateral medial rectus and contralateral lateral rectus muscles. Motor neurons to the antagonists are silenced by inhibitory (red) neurons.

Clinical box 8.38   **Vestibular testing of brainstem function**

Brainstem lesions can often be assessed by examining the performance of the vestibular system because its circuitry lies in the medulla, pons and cerebellum. Hence, unilateral damage to the vestibular system can result in pathological nystagmus in the absence of head rotation.

Damage to the brainstem can be tested by examining the vestibulo-ocular reflex (VOR) in response to stimulating the semicircular canals using the **caloric test**. With the head at an angle of 30° the horizontal canals lie vertically, and irrigating one ear with cold water causes convection currents in the endolymph which mimic head rotation. In a normal subject this causes a nystagmus with a slow component towards the irrigated ear and a fast saccade away from it. Unconscious patients cannot make saccades, so only the slow component is normally visible. A low brainstem lesion abolishes the slow component in both eyes while a lesion to the medial longitudinal fasciculus abolishes the slow component in the eye on the non-irrigated side.

The **amplitude** of the wave is the difference in pressure during the passage of the waveform. Pressure is expressed on a logarithmic scale as the **sound pressure level** which is measured in **decibels** (dB). Amplitude is perceived as **loudness**, although loudness also depends on frequency, since sensitivity is maximal around 3 kHz and falls away at higher and lower frequencies. Speech is usually about 65 dB but exposure to sounds greater than 120 dB can cause pain and damage to hearing.

External and middle ear

Hearing occurs through a series of transformations of sound waves. The ear is anatomically divided into the external, middle and inner ear. Sound waves are funnelled from the **pinna** of the external ear into the **external auditory meatus**, which acts as a resonating tunnel, to impinge on the eardrum, or **tympanic membrane**, that sits at the entrance to the air-filled middle ear.

Vibration of the tympanic membrane is transmitted to a relay of tiny bones, the **ossicles** (**malleus**, **incus** and **stapes**) which act as a lever system amplifying the pressure changes that impinge on the **oval window** (Fig. 8.60). Here the pressure waves in air are converted to oscillations in the fluid of the inner ear. As the area of the oval window is about 20 times smaller than that of the tympanic membrane the pressure of the sound wave is greatly increased when it arrives at the entrance to the inner ear (Clinical box 8.39).

Two muscles, the **tensor tympanum** attached to the malleus and **stapedius** to the stapes, dampen down extreme vibrations of the ossicles. As the mucosa of the middle ear absorbs air the pharyngotympanic (or Eustachian) tube allows air from the pharynx into the middle ear to equilibrate air pressure on either side of the tympanic membrane.

Inner ear (cochlea)

The **cochlea** is the structure in the inner ear that converts sound waves into nerve impulses (Fig. 8.61). Shaped like a snail shell it is a bony canal with 2.25–2.5 turns spiralling around a central pillar (the modiolus). There are three compartments that run the whole length from its wide **base** to its pointed **apex**:

■ The **scala vestibuli**, adjacent to the oval window is the upper compartment filled with perilymph.

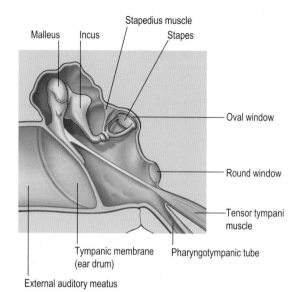

Malleus Incus Stapedius muscle Stapes
Oval window
Round window
Tensor tympani muscle
Tympanic membrane (ear drum) Pharyngotympanic tube
External auditory meatus

Fig. 8.60 **The anatomy of the middle ear.**

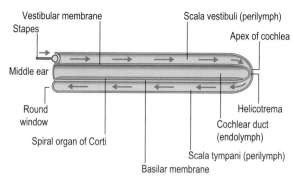

Vestibular membrane Scala vestibuli (perilymph)
Stapes Apex of cochlea
Middle ear
Round window Helicotrema
Spiral organ of Corti Cochlear duct (endolymph)
Basilar membrane Scala tympani (perilymph)

Fig. 8.61 **The propagation of sound through the cochlea (depicted uncurled).** The base is tuned to high frequencies while the apex is more sensitive to low frequencies.

Clinical box 8.39 **Clinical investigation of deafness**

There are simple tests for the two forms of hearing loss:
- **Conduction deafness** – a middle ear defect prevents sound reaching the inner ear
- **Sensorineural deafness** – the defect is cochlear or more central.

Rinne's test and Weber's test exploit the fact that sound is conducted by bone, albeit less well than by air. In **Rinne's test**, the base of a ringing tuning fork (frequency 256 Hz) is applied to the mastoid bone:
- If the sound can be heard, even though it cannot be heard when simply held close to the ear, this demonstrates that sensory transduction in the inner ear has been activated, bypassing a defect in the middle ear, i.e. it implies **conductive deafness**
- If the patient is unable to hear a tuning fork normally, or by bone conduction, this implies **sensorineural deafness** in which the inner ear is defective.

The most common cause of conduction deafness is **otosclerosis**, a disorder in which the ossicles fuse so that energy transfer from eardrum to oval window is compromised.

Weber's test investigates sensorineural deficit. The base of a tuning fork is placed on the middle of the patient's forehead:
- If the sound is located more on one side, then either conduction deafness exists on that side, or sensorineural deafness exists in the other. The test is repeated by covering the ear in which the sound was faintest. Normally the closed ear hears best by bone conduction.
- If no sound is heard in the covered ear sensorineural deafness is confirmed.

The frequency response and dynamic range of hearing can be tested by **audiometry**. Tones with different SPL and frequency are transmitted to one or other ear through headphones, and the patient says when they can hear them.

- The **scala tympani** is the lowest compartment, also filled with perilymph, and is connected to the scala vestibuli at the apex of the cochlea.
- Lying between the two is the **scala media (cochlear duct)** filled with endolymph. The roof of the scala media is the **vestibular membrane** while its floor, which lies above the scala tympanum, consists of the **basilar membrane** on which sits the **organ of Corti**.

The sound waves on the oval window cause a pressure wave through the scala vestibuli to the scala tympani after

which it is dissipated at the **round window**. The pressure wave in the perilymph is transmitted to the basilar membrane of the scala media resulting in a travelling wave which moves along the basilar membrane from its basal to its apical end. The basilar membrane is narrow and stiff at the base of the cochlea and wider and less stiff at the apex. These shorter, stiffer fibres at the base have a higher resonant frequency than the longer ones at the apex (i.e. the basal end is tuned to high frequencies and the apex to low frequencies, Fig. 8.61).

The **organ of Corti** (Fig. 8.62) on the basement membrane of the cochlear duct contains hair cells from which **stereocilia** extend in ascending order of height. The tips of the stereocilia are close to, or inserted into, the **tectorial membrane**, a mucopolysaccharide gel. Vibrations of the basilar membrane cause the stereocilia to bend to and fro, swaying at the same frequency as the part of the basilar membrane that the hair cell sits on. These movements result in alternate depolarisation and hyperpolarisation of the hair cells.

Hair cells are arranged in rows on either side of pillar cells in the organ of Corti:

- **Inner hair cells** are in a single row. They are responsible for the main afferent output from the hair cells to the vestibulocochlear (VIIIth cranial) nerve and so they transmit sound information.
- **Outer hair cells** (OHCs) are in rows of three. The OHCs are contractile getting shorter with depolarisation and longer with hyperpolarisation. This increases the amplitude of basilar membrane vibrations and raises the sensitivity of inner hair cells. This is described as a cochlear amplifier. Efferents from the superior olivary nucleus supply the OHCs via the VIIIth nerve and release ACh which hyperpolarises the OHCs dampening their amplifier effect. Excessive exposure to aminoglycoside antibiotics (e.g. streptomycin, kanamycin) causes selective loss of OHCs resulting in hearing loss (Information box 8.17).

Central auditory pathways

The hair cells form synapses with axons of the **cochlear division** (auditory part) of the VIIIth nerve, the cell bodies of which lie in the **spiral ganglion**, and the central processes of which end in the **cochlear nuclei** which lie in the rostral

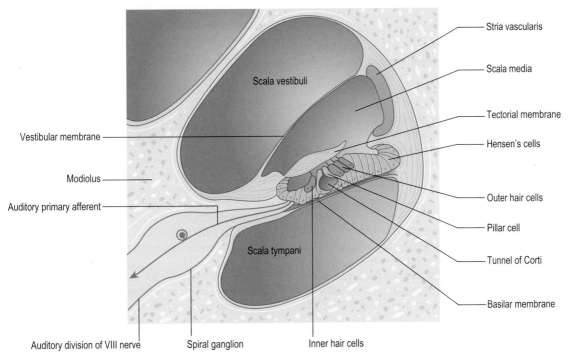

Fig. 8.62 Transverse section through the cochlea to show the organ of Corti.

Labels on Fig. 8.62:
Scala vestibuli
Stria vascularis
Scala media
Tectorial membrane
Hensen's cells
Vestibular membrane
Modiolus
Auditory primary afferent
Scala tympani
Outer hair cells
Pillar cell
Tunnel of Corti
Basilar membrane
Auditory division of VIII nerve
Spiral ganglion
Inner hair cells

Information box 8.17   Cochlear implants

A cochlear implant is able to restore limited but useful sound sensation in patients with deafness due to cochlear damage, provided that there is still a functioning auditory nerve. The implant itself is a linear array of 22 electrodes, inserted through the mastoid bone and round window into the scala tympanum at the basal end of the cochlea, so that it follows the first 1.5 turns towards the apex. At its distal end is a radio receiver, and externally there is a microphone, speech processor and radio transmitter.

Sounds picked up by the microphone are analysed by the speech processor – a computer that filters sounds into frequency bands optimal for understanding speech – and the processed signal is transmitted to the implant. This crosstalk between the electrodes, which are spread along the cochlear implant, degrades the quality of the perceived sound, but with experience patients can follow a conversation.

As well as being used for acquired deafness, cochlear implants are useful in congenital deafness. Because maximum plasticity of the auditory system occurs in the first 2 years of life, the implants are given as early as 12 months, optimising the conditions for language acquisition.

---

medulla (Fig. 8.63). These nuclei have three projections (dorsal, intermediate and ventral acoustic striae). Fibres in the ventral stria terminate in **nuclei of the trapezoid body** and **superior olivary nuclei** (not shown in Fig. 8.61) on both sides. These then send fibres via the lateral lemniscus to the **nuclei of the lateral meniscus** and the **inferior colliculi** of the midbrain. Dorsal and intermediate striae fibres cross, to end in the lateral lemniscus and inferior colliculi nuclei. Put simply, there are extensive reciprocal connections across the midline between nuclei within auditory pathways which explains the fact that unilateral damage to central auditory pathways does not result in deafness in one ear.

Neurons in the inferior colliculus project to the **medial geniculate nuclei (MGN)** of the thalamus. Fibres from the MGN go in the **acoustic radiation** to the **primary auditory cortex (A1)**, Brodmann's areas 41 and 42, on the superior medial aspect

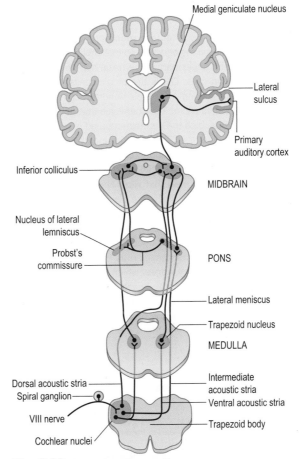

Fig. 8.63 Central auditory pathways.

Labels on Fig. 8.63:
Medial geniculate nucleus
Lateral sulcus
Primary auditory cortex
Inferior colliculus
MIDBRAIN
Nucleus of lateral lemniscus
Probst's commissure
PONS
Lateral meniscus
Trapezoid nucleus
MEDULLA
Dorsal acoustic stria
Spiral ganglion
VIII nerve
Cochlear nuclei
Intermediate acoustic stria
Ventral acoustic stria
Trapezoid body

of the temporal lobe. Next to this and extending to cover the lateral surface of the superior temporal gyrus is the **secondary auditory cortex (SAC)**, Brodmann's area 22. This area is important in sound localisation and is involved in aspects of language and music perception (see Language, below).

Sound frequency coding

As explained above, the basal end of the cochlea is sensitive to higher frequencies and the apical end to lower frequencies. This is termed **place coding**, the hair cell's position along the membrane specifies the frequency. However, for lower frequency sounds (<1–3 kHz) groups of different afferent neurons have a greater probability of firing at different phases of the waveform. This **phase locking** results in a complete representation of the waveform when the signals from the different groups are integrated. Throughout the entire auditory pathway from cochlea to cortex information is held in **tonotopic** (frequency) **maps**.

Sound localisation

Sound waves reach the tympanic membrane through the external auditory meatus directly but also indirectly after being reflected off the irregular surface of the pinna. The time delay in those arriving by the indirect route enables detection of the origin of the sound in the vertical plane, i.e. the **elevation** of a sound. Determining the angle from which direction the sound comes, the **azimuth**, is dependent on the differences in sound levels and arrival time of sounds to the two ears. Sound localisation enables brainstem reflexes to alter gaze and head orientation in response to a noise.

SMELL

Smell is detected by **olfactory receptor neurons (ORNs)** which are located in the olfactory epithelium in the roof of the nasal cavity and upper part of the nasal septum, alongside mucus-secreting cells. ORNs are bipolar cells which have **olfactory cilia** coming from their dendritic endings at the surface of the epithelium. The chemicals that act as stimuli, termed **odorants**, bind to G-protein-coupled receptors in the plasma membrane of cilia altering the membrane potential. For example odorants binding to G_{olf} receptors that activate adenylate cyclase (see Chs 2 and 4) result in a rise of cAMP which opens ion channels that allow Na^+ and Ca^{2+} to enter and depolarise the cilia. There are over a thousand different odorant receptor proteins on olfactory cilia.

The central processes of ORNs are small diameter, unmyelinated axons that pass through the cribriform plate of the ethmoid bone, forming numerous bundles that together constitute the **olfactory nerve**, which enters the **olfactory bulb** (see Clinical box 8.40). These axons in the olfactory nerve synapse with **mitral** and **tufted cells** in **glomeruli** in the olfactory bulb. The axons of the mitral and tufted cells project in the olfactory tract to a number of destinations in the cerebrum.

Clinical box 8.40   **Anosmia**

The small axons of the olfactory receptor neurons can become torn by acceleration-deceleration forces in high speed road accidents and trauma can lead to fracture of the cribriform plate and damage to the olfactory bulbs or tracts. These injuries can result in loss of the sense of smell (**anosmia**).

The most common causes of anosmia are upper respiratory tract and nasal sinus infections. Other causes include tumours of the frontal lobe, drug use (e.g. cocaine, amphetamines), pernicious anaemia and Parkinson disease.

Complete anosmia results in the inability to recognise flavours as the olfactory and gustatory systems operate together in the perception of flavours.

These destinations include the piriform cortex, which receives mainly mitral cell axons, and may be involved in odour discrimination, and the amygdala and hippocampus responsible for emotional and behavioural responses to smell. Projections to the hippocampus are thought to be responsible for the olfactory component of episodic memory (see Memory, below).

TASTE

Taste receptor cells are clustered together in **taste buds** which are present on the tongue, oral mucosa, pharynx and oesophagus. On the dorsum of the tongue they form small protuberances called **papillae**. Taste cells have microvilli on their apical border that have specific receptors for taste stimulating ions and molecules called **tastants**. Tastants get to the microvilli through taste pores on the top of the taste buds.

There are five principal taste stimuli: salt, sweet, sour (acid), bitter and umami (savoury flavour) although other less defined submodalities exist. The manner in which each causes depolarisation of the taste receptor membrane (i.e. how it effects transduction of the taste signal) varies:

- **Salty** tastes are detected by Na^+ ions passing through amiloride-sensitive channels.
- **Sourness** is the result of H^+ ions binding to and blocking voltage-gated K^+ channels.
- **Sweet**, **bitter** and **umami** (L-glutamate) activate G-protein-coupled receptors (GPCR). A taste-specific G protein, **gustducin**, is linked to many of the GPCRs. Some bitter tastes (e.g. quinine) block K^+ channels.

In all cases the effect of depolarisation is to trigger a rise in intracellular Ca^{2+} and the release of serotonin.

Central pathways of taste

Primary taste afferents have their cell bodies in the ganglia of the facial (VII), glossopharyngeal (IX) and vagus (X) cranial nerves. Input from the anterior two-thirds of the tongue run in the chorda tympani of the VIIth nerve while afferents from the posterior third of the tongue are relayed in the IXth. Those from the epiglottis and oesophagus are conveyed in the Xth nerve.

The afferents terminate in part of the **nucleus of the solitary tract (NST)** in the medulla termed the **gustatory nucleus** (Fig. 8.64). Neurons from the gustatory nucleus project via the ventroposterior medial nucleus of the thalamus to an area of cortex next to that which maps somatosensation from the tongue. The latter receives information from non-taste receptors which detect texture, temperature and irritants in the mouth. The NST is also thought to send projections to the amygdala and hippocampus involved in behavioural responses to taste.

CENTRAL AUTONOMIC NETWORKS

The cell bodies of preganglionic autonomic fibres are located in the CNS: sympathetic fibres arise in the lateral grey matter of the spinal cord in segments T1–L2; cranial parasympathetics from the brainstem and sacral parasympathetics from S2–S4 segments (Ch. 4 and Fig. 4.22). The output pathways of the autonomic nervous system are modulated by **central autonomic networks** in the brainstem and forebrain (Fig. 8.65).

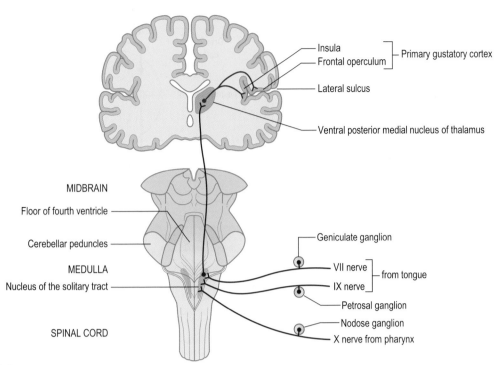

Fig. 8.64 **Central taste pathways.**

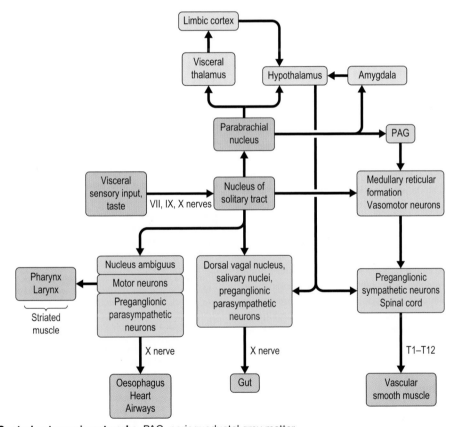

Fig. 8.65 **Central autonomic networks.** PAG, periaqueductal grey matter.

Visceral sensory input (e.g. chemoreceptor, baroreceptor and taste afferents) goes principally to the **nucleus of the solitary track** (NST). The NST sends fibres to:

- Medullary reticular formation vasomotor and cardio-accelerator neurons that project to preganglionic sympathetic neurons

- Dorsal vagal nucleus and salivatory nuclei which send parasympathetic output to the salivary glands and gut
- Nucleus ambiguus which sends parasympathetic output to the oesophagus, heart and airways and special visceral motor neurons to striated muscle in the pharynx and larynx for controlling swallowing.

In addition, the NST projects to the **parabrachial nucleus** (in the pons) and a network of structures including the periaqueductal grey matter, the thalamus, hypothalamus, amygdala and limbic cortex. This network integrates visceral and somatic motor responses in various emotional and social behaviours.

EXAMPLES OF CENTRAL AUTONOMIC CONTROL

Thermoregulation

Control of body temperature is an example of a physiological homeostatic negative feedback system (see Ch.1). The central control involves integration of signals in the hypothalamus. Nuclei in the preoptic region and anterior hypothalamus contain **internal warm thermoreceptors**. These are receptors for core body temperature, i.e. the temperature of the blood supplied to the hypothalamus. The hypothalamus also receives information about the body surface temperature from **cutaneous thermoreceptors** (see above) and integrates this with core temperature signals.

The posterior hypothalamus acts as a thermostat as it has temperature-insensitive interneurons, the signal from which is a **set point**. This is the core temperature which the thermoregulatory mechanisms attempt to maintain. The set point is altered by circadian rhythms (with lowest core temperature at night) and hormones (e.g. rise in progesterone during the menstrual cycle; see Ch. 10).

The fever that can accompany infections is caused by resetting of the set point by cytokines; for example, macrophages challenged by bacterial endotoxins secrete interleukin 1 and virus-infected cells release interferons (see Ch. 6). The rise in core temperature – if not excessive – is adaptive as it raises metabolic rate, increasing the rate of immune responses such as antibody synthesis and may compromise the growth of microorganisms. Damage to the areas of the hypothalamus containing the internal warm receptors interferes with heat dissipation mechanisms such as peripheral vasodilation, sweating and moving to somewhere cooler resulting in hyperthermia. Lesions to the posterior hypothalamus are associated with hypothermia as they interfere with the generation of heat through peripheral vasoconstriction, shivering and seeking a warmer environment.

Regulation of feeding and satiety

The control of food intake is described in Ch. 16. Central regulation is by two parallel brain pathways which originate in the **arcuate nucleus** of the **hypothalamus**. An **orexigenic** (anabolic) **pathway** promotes feeding while an **anorexigenic** (catabolic) **pathway** reduces feeding (Fig. 8.66). Leptin reduces food intake by inhibiting the orexigenic and stimulating the anorexigenic pathways.

Orexigenic pathway

The first order neurons from the arcuate nucleus use **neuropeptide Y** as a transmitter in the orexigenic pathway and project to the **lateral hypothalamus**, synapsing with second order neurons that secrete peptide transmitters termed **orexins (hypocretins)** which act on neurons in the **nucleus of the solitary track (NST)** decreasing their sensitivity to satiety factors (e.g. glucose).

Anorexigenic pathway

First order cells in the anorexigenic pathway contain **pro-opiomelanocortin (POMC)**, the precursor protein for the neurotransmitter **melanocortin**. The axons from these arcuate

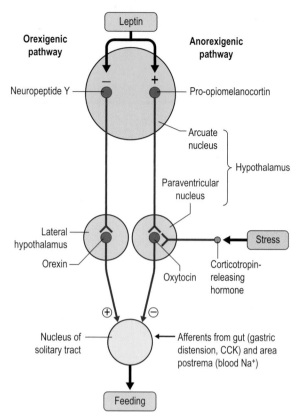

Fig. 8.66 Central pathways involved in feeding. CCK, cholecystokinin.

nuclei cells project to the **paraventricular nucleus (PVN)** of the hypothalamus, which contains neurons that use oxytocin, thyrotropin-releasing hormone or corticotropin-releasing hormone (CRH) as transmitters. These molecules suppress feeding by increasing the sensitivity of neurons in the NST to satiety factors. Stress probably reduces appetite by exciting the CRH neurons in the anorexigenic pathway. This may be a factor in the eating disorder, **anorexia nervosa** (Clinical box 8.41).

Clinical box 8.41   **Anorexia nervosa**

In anorexia nervosa, the patient deliberately opts to maintain extremely low food intake, often accompanied by very high levels of physical activity. Socio-cultural factors are very important, though there is evidence for a genetic predisposition, and there may be an underlying brain deficit, as evinced by evidence for reduced cerebral blood flow localised to specific limbic structures.

Anorexia is probably a constellation of related disorders and is often associated with depression or obsessive compulsive disorder. There are numerous psychological theories for the origin of the disease, all hard to test. Neurobiology-based ideas must distinguish cause from the effect of starvation, which is also difficult to do.

Anorexics have heightened secretion of corticotropin-releasing hormone (CRH) and glucocorticoids, a stress response perhaps caused initially by anxiety about eating, and subsequently reinforced by the normal stress response to starvation. Whatever the reason, raised CRH secretion in the anorexigenic pathway could lead to suppression of appetite, though it is not clear why this is not overridden by the low leptin concentrations that are seen in untreated anorexics. The orexigenic pathway also appears to be defective in anorexia nervosa because the low leptin concentrations do not result in increases in neuropeptide Y. Leptin concentrations rise in weight-recovering anorexics in an apparently physiological fashion, but are higher than in normal women with the same body mass index (BMI).

Regulation of thirst and drinking

The main stimuli for thirst are increase in tissue osmolality and decrease in blood volume (see Ch.1). Osmotic pressure-sensitive neurons in the hypothalamus, called osmoreceptors, shrink or swell in response to changes in plasma osmolality. If osmolality rises above 280 mOsmol/kg, the osmoreceptors stimulate other neurons in the supraoptic and paraventricular nuclei of the hypothalamus which have their axon terminals in the posterior pituitary from where they release vasopressin (antidiuretic hormone, ADH).

ADH-secreting neurons also receive afferents via the glossopharyngeal and vagus nerves from two sets of baroreceptors. Low blood volume acts on the low pressure baroreceptors in the great veins and right atrium of the heart while low blood pressure acts on high-pressure arterial baroreceptors in the carotid sinus and aorta (see Ch. 11).

Decrease in ECF also leads to renal hypotension which results in release of **angiotensin II** (see Ch. 14). Angiotensin II is a potent **dipsogen** (thirst provoker) and stimulates neurons in the **subfornical organ** (**SFO**), which is a circumventricular organ (i.e. lies outside the blood–brain barrier). The SFO connects to the preoptic nucleus of the hypothalamus, which itself uses angiotensin II as a neurotransmitter, and connects to the nucleus of the solitary tract to enable drinking behaviour.

Thirst is temporarily sated by the activity of afferents in the mouth, pharynx, oesophagus and stomach long before deficits in blood osmolality and volume are corrected. This means that several small drinks are taken at intervals until the loss is made up. This pattern of drinking is thought to prevent dilution of extracellular fluid and hypotonicity (**water intoxication**).

Regulation of sexual function

Sexual arousal is brought about by psychological inputs and physiological control is by the sacral parasympathetic neurons. Activation of the parasympathetic neurons leads to engorgement of the penis or clitoris, when acetylcholine (ACh) stimulates nitric oxide (NO) synthesis. NO is a vasodilator, causing relaxation of vascular smooth muscle thus increasing blood flow to the corpora cavernosa. Activation of the sympathetic neurons in the thoracic and lumbar regions then stimulates smooth muscle contraction leading to ejaculation in men and orgasm in women. Depending on the level, lesions of the spinal cord affect sexual function, but do not necessarily abolish it.

CONSCIOUSNESS

One of the greatest challenges to neuroscience is providing a clear and agreed definition of **consciousness**. Two components are generally accepted: **wakefulness** and **awareness** of self. Wakefulness refers to how alert an individual is, while awareness includes various aspects of knowledge of the internal and external environment and includes aspects of cognition, often referred to by clinicians as **higher cortical functions** (see below).

Common terms for altered states of consciousness are:

- **Confusional state**: minor disorientation, faulty memory, short attention span and some difficulty following commands
- **Delirium**: disorientation, irritability, motor restlessness and hallucinations

---

Information box 8.18 **Disorders of consciousness**

Cerebral cortical arousal can be impaired by metabolic disturbance, drugs and traumatic or non-traumatic injury to either the cortex itself or the ascending arousal system for generating consciousness. The most extreme case is **coma** which refers to a state of unrousable unconsciousness without any response to external stimuli or internal need. Clinicians use the **Glasgow Coma Scale** to determine a patient's conscious level by measuring their response to graded stimuli in terms of eye opening, motor response and verbal response. Stimuli include speaking or shouting commands and applying pain as supraorbital or nail-bed pressure to the patient.

Loss of large numbers of cortical neurons, with an intact arousal system, can result in **persistent vegetative state**. These patients breathe spontaneously, have a stable circulation and exhibit eye opening and closure that simulates sleep–wake cycles but show no evidence of self-awareness.

This contrasts with the rare condition of **locked-in syndrome** resulting from damage (usually infarction) to the ventral pons. This spares the ascending arousal system and the cortex is unaffected. The patient is fully aware but has total paralysis of the limbs and cranial nerves (V–XII). As cranial nerves III and IV are functioning they can move the eyes up and down but not laterally because of involvement of cranial nerve VI.

- **Stupor**: unresponsive and only aroused by vigorous stimulation
- **Coma**: unresponsive and unrousable.

As the definition of these terms is often imprecise, in clinical practice standardised scales such as the Glasgow Coma Scale are used to describe different levels of reduced consciousness (Information box 8.18).

SLEEP AND WAKEFULNESS

Sleep is a state of reduced responsiveness to, and interaction with, the environment which is readily reversible. Its exact function remains unclear but theories include homeostatic mechanisms such as replenishment of glycogen stores and consolidation of memory.

There are two types of sleep which can be characterised by electroencephalogram (EEG) (Information box 8.19) and other features.

Information box 8.19 **Electroencephalography**

EEG is a non-invasive method for measuring the surface electrical activity of the brain. Large numbers of cerebral cortical cells fire in synchrony and consequently their summed activity produces field potentials large enough to be recorded with electrodes attached to the scalp. An array of electrodes allows activity of different brain areas to be examined.

The EEG shows characteristic patterns when a person is alert, drowsy or asleep. It is possible to analyse the patterns of activity to assess changes in amplitude and frequency of the waveforms. A frequency that is too fast or too slow can indicate impaired cortical function. In addition, the presence of unusual waveforms such as sharp spikes, spike-and-wave potentials or unusually slow waves indicates a brain lesion or seizure disorder.

The EEG waveform ranges in frequency from 1 Hz to 30 Hz and frequency ranges are conventionally grouped:

- Alpha (8–13 Hz) – typically seen in relaxed wakefulness
- Beta (13–30 Hz) – seen when an individual is alert or engaged in intense mental activity
- Delta (0.4–4 Hz) and theta (4–7 Hz) – seen during drowsiness and NREM sleep.

- **Rapid eye movement (REM)** is characterised by low voltage, high frequency waveforms similar to the awake state (this is why REM sleep is sometimes called **paradoxical sleep**). There is loss of muscle tone, muscle twitches and rapid eye movements. Dreams occur during this phase.
- **Non-rapid eye movement (NREM)** has high voltage, low frequency waveforms. It is divided into stages 1–4. As a person falls asleep they drop progressively through these stages from β to α waves in stage 2 and δ waves in stages 3 and 4 (**delta** or **slow wave sleep**) and the arousal threshold increases.

During a normal night the amount of time in deep, slow wave NREM becomes less and NREM sleep is interrupted by progressively longer intervals of REM sleep. In adults about 25% of total sleep is REM.

Arousal system

The **arousal system** consists of monoaminergic neurons in the brainstem called the **ascending reticular formation** (or reticular activating system) (Fig. 8.67). This generates the awake state and has two branches:

- **Wake-on/REM-off cells** are noradrenergic and serotonergic neurons that project via the hypothalamus to the cerebral cortex. These fire at the highest rate in wakefulness, have low firing rates during NREM sleep and go silent during REM sleep.
- **Wake-on/REM-on cells** are cholinergic neurons in the pons that project to the thalamus. These are active during wakefulness and REM sleep but go quiet during NREM sleep.

The two groups of cells in the ascending reticular formation are connected and reciprocally inhibit neuron firing when regulating sleep–wake and arousal transitions. This inhibition is abolished during waking when both groups of cells are excited. Disruption of the ascending reticular formation can lead to loss of consciousness. The thalamus has a major role in the regulation of sleep and wakefulness. **Thalamic relay cells** innervate areas of the cortex via thalamo-cortical nerve fibres. They are activated by sensory stimuli and transmit excitatory signals to the cerebral cortex.

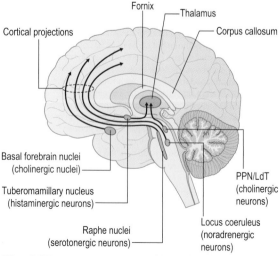

Fig. 8.67 Brain arousal systems. PPN/LdT, pedunculopontine nucleus/lateral dorsal tegmental nucleus.

Labels in figure:
- Fornix
- Thalamus
- Cortical projections
- Corpus callosum
- Basal forebrain nuclei (cholinergic nuclei)
- Tuberomamillary nucleus (histaminergic neurons)
- PPN/LdT (cholinergic neurons)
- Locus coeruleus (noradrenergic neurons)
- Raphe nuclei (serotonergic neurons)

NREM sleep

Sensory information is no longer transmitted from the thalamus to cortex during NREM sleep and the EEG shows regular repeating wave patterns (i.e. it becomes synchronised).

Antihistamines that cross the blood–brain barrier reduce the excitation of thalamic relay neurons, causing drowsiness. Bursting, periods of rapid neuron firing followed by quiet periods, of thalamic neurons is associated with absence seizures (petit mal).

Although poorly understood, the timing of sleep is related to the circadian clock in the **suprachiasmatic nucleus (SCN)**, and a rise in core temperature detected by hypothalamic warm receptors. The thalamus stops sending signals to the cortex during NREM sleep. Melatonin (*N*-acetyl-5-methoxytryptamine) is a hormone secreted by the pineal body directly into the bloodstream. Blood levels vary in a daily cycle, which enables the entrainment of a circadian, light/dark rhythm to the sleep–wakefulness cycle.

REM sleep

During REM sleep sensory input is relayed to the cortex and the EEG is desynchronised, i.e. the wave pattern is irregular.

Despite the sensory input there is no movement as inhibition of motor neurons results in an almost complete motor paralysis (REM atonia). Some sleep behaviour disorders, such as sleep walking, are thought to be due to lack of REM atonia. Neurons known as REM-on cells, located in the tegmentum of the pons, are very active during REM sleep, and thought to be the cause of rapid eye movements.

EMOTION

Emotions arise in response to changes in the external or internal environment. The primary emotions are fear, anger, disgust, pleasure or happiness, and sadness. **Feelings** can be considered to be the conscious experience of the emotion.

Emotions involve multiple pathways in the brain and nervous system, including cognitive components and autonomic, hormonal and motor responses. Although functional imaging techniques in humans are rapidly increasing our understanding from previous knowledge based on animal experiments and injuries in humans, many of the networks involved remain unclear.

Limbic system

The part of the brain most involved with emotion is the limbic system. As explained above, it includes areas of the cerebral cortex (orbitofrontal cortex, cingulate gyrus and hippocampus), the amygdala, mamillary bodies, and the ventral striatum (nucleus accumbens) of the basal ganglia.

The **amygdala** is concerned with inborn and learned fear responses, avoidance behaviour, and recognition of emotions in facial expressions. It consists of a cluster of nuclei in the white matter of the temporal lobe, lying anterior to the tail of the caudate nucleus. Afferents carry sensory information (visual, auditory and somatosensory) from the thalamus to the **lateral nucleus** of the amygdala which also receives input from the hippocampus. Output from the **central nucleus** of the amygdala to the hypothalamus and brainstem is via

Table 8.19 Functions of amygdala outputs

Output target/pathway	Effect
Periaqueductal grey/raphe spinal tract	Decreased pain transmission
Periaqueductal grey/ reticulospinal tract	Fear responses
Nucleus coeruleus	Arousal
Noradrenergic cells in medulla/ preganglionic sympathetic neurons	Cardiovascular fear responses (e.g. tachycardia)
Hypothalamus/dorsal vagal nucleus	Bradycardia (vasovagal syncope)
Hypothalamus (arcuate nucleus)	Release of corticotropin-releasing hormone
Parabrachial nucleus/medulla respiratory neurons	Hyperventilation

stria terminalis, while the **ventral amygdalofugal pathway** conveys connections to the nucleus accumbens. The functions of these outputs are summarised in Table 8.19.

The pathways of fear

When the brain receives a sensory stimulus indicating a danger (e.g. the sight of a snake; the sound of an explosion), it is routed via the thalamus to the amygdala by two parallel pathways (see Fig. 8.68):

- The thalamo-amygdala pathway (or short route).
- The thalamo-cortico-amygdala pathway (or long route).

The short route is subcortical (i.e. no cognition is involved) and conveys a fast impression to the lateral nucleus and the central nucleus generates an emotional response. Thus the amygdala can trigger immediate flight and fight responses to a threatening situation before there is conscious recognition of the situation.

Subsequently the information travelling by the long route is processed and informs the amygdala as to whether or not the stimulus represents a real threat. This is achieved by different levels of cortical processing. First the various modalities of the perceived object are processed in the primary sensory cortex and this provides the amygdala with a representation of the object. At a higher level the polymodal association cortex conceptualises the object and informs the amygdala. This detailed representation of the object is then compared with the contents of explicit memory (see below) in the hippocampus which gives it context (i.e. is this a threat or not). Armed with this information the amygdala can adjust its output from the central nucleus to increase or decrease the emotional response.

In infancy and early childhood the amygdala develops more rapidly than the hippocampus. It is suggested that fearful memories may be acquired during this time which cannot later be consciously accounted for and so could underlie some specific phobias (Clinical box 8.42).

Emotion recognition

Activity is increased in the amygdala in subjects shown fearful faces, and in the left amygdala the extent of the response increases the more fearful the expression. Patients with damage to the amygdala lose the ability to recognise fearful expressions but they are still able to identify a familiar face. The amygdala has a role also in recognising other expressions such as disgust and anger.

Emotional expression

Facial expressions engendered by emotions (e.g. smiling, frowning etc.) are brought about by extrapyramidal pathways that run in the brainstem reticular formation (see Clinical box 8.43). In response to fear the amygdala sends output to the brainstem resulting in altered expression.

Clinical box 8.42 **Anxiety disorders**

While anxiety in a threatening situation is adaptive, it is debilitating when it occurs excessively or unnecessarily. **Anxiety disorders**, which occur when fears or phobias impair normal daily activities, are the commonest psychiatric disorder.

Altered **serotonin** transmission may underlie some anxiety states, and limbic structures implicated in fear learning, such as the amygdala, septum and hippocampus, receive projections from raphe nuclei serotonergic neurons.

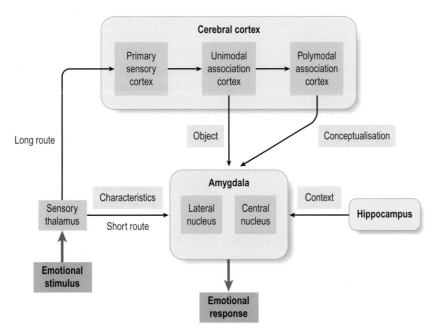

Fig. 8.68 **Circuitry involved in emotions.**

Patients with unilateral damage to corticobulbar fibres descending from the motor cortex have voluntary motor paresis on the opposite side. When asked to smile on demand their smile is lopsided. However, when genuinely amused their smile is natural and bilateral (**Duchenne smile**) because different emotion-driven motor pathways are engaged.

There is no coherent science model for depression but there are a number of observations that must be accounted for in any theory.

All antidepressants increase serotonin neurotransmission. However, in no case is this directly brought about by their immediate action. Instead, delayed adaptive changes are thought to be responsible because therapeutic effects are not seen for several weeks. In the case of **monoamine oxidase inhibitors (MAOIs)**, **selective serotonin reuptake inhibitors (SSRIs)** and **5-HT$_{1A}$ receptor agonists**, the mechanism appears to be a decrease in the sensitivity of 5-HT$_{1A}$ and 5-HT$_{1B}$ inhibitory autoreceptors, so serotonin release is enhanced.

Tricyclic antidepressants (which block the reuptake of serotonin and norepinephrine from the synaptic cleft) increase the sensitivity of postsynaptic serotonin receptors. Long-term antidepressant therapy also results in changes in noradrenergic transmission, e.g. the downregulation of β-adrenoceptors. However, this requires intact serotonergic transmission, which shows that interactions between neurotransmitter systems are likely to be important in depression (see also Ch. 4).

There is excessive secretion of corticotropin-releasing hormone and hence of adrenocorticotropic hormone and cortisol, coupled with a loss of circadian variation in cortisol secretion and blunting of negative feedback mechanisms that control cortisol secretion (see Ch. 10). The significance of these neuroendocrine changes is unclear – they are not exclusive to depression – but they are probably associated with the disturbed sleep patterns experienced by depressed patients.

Prefrontal cortex and emotion

The **prefrontal cortex** is all of the frontal lobe cortex other than premotor and motor cortices and has extensive connections with brain structures implicated in emotion, including the amygdala, nucleus accumbens and hypothalamus. PET scans of depressed patients show decreased activity in the prefrontal cortex (Information box 8.20). Functional images also suggest that separate sectors of the prefrontal area mediate positive and negative emotional states with evidence of lateralisation. Thus, activity in the dorsolateral left prefrontal cortex generates positive affect or happiness while the ventromedial orbital area on the right leads to sadness or disgust. Bilateral lesions of the prefrontal cortex can lead to the individual appearing depressed and apathetic or inappropriately cheerful and disinhibited. They tend to lack social graces and show little concern for others. Such bilateral frontal damage is common in severe head injury and survivors are often described as having undergone a personality change with many of the above features evident.

MOTIVATION AND GOAL-DIRECTED BEHAVIOURS

Volition refers to the complex process of determining what one needs or wants and deciding how to realise the need or want. **Goal-directed behaviours** are purposeful actions aimed at achieving this. **Motivation**, including the ability to initiate activity, is a prequisite to such behaviour. These behaviours may be to meet basic physiological needs (e.g. drinking and feeding) and are homeostatic, and normally self-limiting in that the internal cues that drive them, thirst and hunger, are sated by consumption (see above). Others may encompass more abstract and long-term goals (e.g. buying a home, promotion at work etc.).

The brain reward system

The motivation of behaviour is thought to come about by activity in the brain reward system. The key pathways at the basis of this system are thought to consist of **dopaminergic neurons** in the **ventral tegmental area (VTA)** of the midbrain. These neurons project their axons to the nucleus accumbens, striatum, amygdala and other limbic structures as the **mesolimbic system**, then to the frontal cortex as the **mesocortical system**. There are also connections to the hippocampus as memory can inform motivational behaviour by providing details of past behaviour when goals were obtained.

The brain reward system is responsible for the positive reinforcing properties of natural rewards (such as food, drink and sex). Natural rewards, self-stimulation (through implanted electrodes) and addictive drugs all increase dopamine release from mesolimbic terminals in the nucleus accumbens, and the reinforcing properties of these stimuli are blocked by dopamine receptor antagonists.

The predictability of a natural reward determines the firing of mesolimbic neurons; expected rewards elicit small effects, whereas novel rewards bring about a strong response that reduces on repetition.

Drugs and the brain reward system

Recent research on addiction suggests that some addictive drugs act on the brain reward system to enhance dopamine transmission, perhaps mimicking the effect of natural rewards (Information box 8.21). A well-known example is cocaine (see Information box 8.22). Other addictive drugs (e.g. **barbiturates** and **benzodiazepines**) do *not* activate dopamine transmission, so the brain reward system does not fully explain all addictive behaviour.

Addiction is a goal directed behaviour, where satisfying the addiction brings its own reward; known as **positive reinforcement**. Characteristics of addiction to drugs are:

■ **Tolerance** – where the substance becomes less effective on repeated administration, and increasing doses are needed to achieve the desired effect.
■ **Dependence** – when normal function is only possible in the presence of the substance.

● **Cocaine** – see Information box 8.22.
● **Nicotine** acts on cholinergic receptors on the dopamine cell bodies in the VTA enhancing dopamine synthesis and release.
● **Cannabis** acts on excitatory cannabinoid receptors on dopamine terminals to increase dopamine release.
● **Opioids** (e.g. **morphine** and **heroin**) act on δ and μ opioid receptors to hyperpolarise GABAergic interneurons in the VTA that normally tonically inhibit the dopaminergic cells, so disinhibiting the mesolimbic system.
● **Alcohol** reduces activity in most neuronal pathways but increases activity in inhibitory interneurons in the VTA.

Cocaine blocks the **dopamine transporter** in the presynaptic terminals of mesolimbic neurons, limiting dopamine reuptake so that the concentration of transmitter in the synaptic cleft is raised. Cocaine administration in addicts causes transient activity in the VTA and nucleus accumbens (nAc) as recorded by brain imaging. However, a stronger nAc signal is seen in addicts who are craving the drug. This implies that the nAc is more important for learning contextual cues associated with drug taking than with the reinforcement and euphoria.

A single dose of cocaine can make the neurons of the VTA more sensitive to the drug by inducing long-term potentiation. This may be important in the early stages of addiction by enhancing the learning that leads to craving.

Tolerance develops later because the increase in synaptic dopamine concentration causes downregulation of postsynaptic dopamine receptors. Higher amounts of transmitter, and hence drug, are needed to achieve the same level of dopamine transmission.

During **withdrawal**, dopamine concentrations drop back to baseline, but because there are fewer postsynaptic receptors, dopamine transmission in the mesolimbic system is decreased. This rebound drop in the effectiveness of the brain reward system is probably responsible for the **anhedonia** (lack of pleasure), reduced activity, depression and anxiety seen with drug withdrawal.

Brain imaging shows that cocaine causes an enduring reduction of dopamine synthesis in mesolimbic neuron terminals that gets worse the longer the period of abstinence. These long-term alterations seem to underlie persistent craving and provide a serious challenge to the treatment of drug addiction.

- **Withdrawal (abstinence) symptoms** – once dependence occurs, withdrawal of the substance can lead to symptoms such as anxiety, cold sweats, hallucinations, delirium, tremor and ataxia among others. The symptoms can be very unpleasant, and may even be long lasting.
- **Craving** – after withdrawal of the substance, the addict experiences the intense need for it. Craving involves neural pathways that are different from other pathways in addiction. Neuroimaging has shown increased activity in the dorsolateral prefrontal cortex (cognitive pathway), medial temporal cortex (explicit learning) and the nucleus accumbens (brain reward system).

Other forms of addiction including alcohol, tobacco, gambling, sex and even exercise, can show similar patterns of behaviour.

HIGHER CORTICAL FUNCTIONS

There are a number of complex processes referred to as **higher cortical functions** that form part of the clinical examination. These include assessment of the state of arousal and emotional state (or **affect**), discussed above, but also cognition, memory, attention and language.

COGNITION

Cognition is behaviour based on **knowledge** which is stored in the brain as **semantic networks** that allow associations to be forged between all the disparate elements that make up the mental image of an object or abstract concept. Cognitive function is a mental process that includes memory, attention,

language and decision making. It is a process of organising information and applying knowledge to solving problems, which requires **thinking**, i.e. arranging ideas represented by words and numbers, organising mental images of objects and past actions, planning, reasoning and generating new ideas. Cognitive tasks include:

- Language that is a function of the left cerebral hemisphere
- Visual spatial tasks (e.g. catching a ball, driving a car) involve the right hemisphere.

Studies suggest that men and women use different parts of the brain for visual-spatial tasks. There is also some evidence to suggest that women are better at language tasks, and, on average, men have better visual-spatial skills than women.

MEMORY

Memory is the ability to recall knowledge and skills **learned** in the past. This is how information is *encoded*, *stored* and *retrieved*, and two categories are described:

- **Declarative (explicit) memory** is the recall of new facts (**semantic memory**), such as the capital of France is Paris, and events (**episodic memory**), which relate to personal experience of specific occasions or episodes (e.g. seeing a play). Semantic memories include facts such as being able to identify a small red-breasted bird as a robin, and knowing the meaning of words – essential for verbal reasoning.
- **Procedural (implicit or motor) memory** applies to memory of motor skills. Learning a motor skill (e.g. riding a bike) is a relatively slow process requiring repetition. However, performance does not need conscious recall (hence implicit) and, once learned, is rarely forgotten. The cerebellum has an important role in procedural memories and motor learning (see under Cerebellum, above).

Declarative memory

There are at least two phases to declarative memory:

- **Short-term (recent) memory (STM)**: can only be retained for a few seconds to a minute without rehearsal; is limited in capacity, i.e. only 4–5 items can be stored at one time, and requires continuous rehearsal to retain. Irrelevant or distracting information interferes with encoding.
- **Long-term (remote) memory (LTM)**: in contrast, long-term memory can store much larger quantities of information that can be retained almost indefinitely, and does not need rehearsal.

STM and LTM appear to be separate, but parallel processes. Not all items in STM are stored as LTM. Only selected items are retained through a process known as **consolidation**. Some forms of memory loss, known as **amnesias**, affect LTM only, and not STM. The reverse occurs in other forms of amnesia. Loss of STM is a prominent feature in dementias, e.g. Alzheimer disease (see Clinical box 8.44).

A further elaboration to STM is the concept of **working memory** which is a form of temporary storage of several types of information from multiple areas of the brain all held simultaneously. It briefly stores and processes information

---

Clinical box 8.44   **Alzheimer disease**

Alzheimer disease (AD) is the commonest dementia and memory impairment is a central feature. Inability to retrieve semantic memories occurs early and manifests as difficulty in finding the words to formulate or follow speech, failure to recognise or identify people or objects and being unable to navigate through once familiar surroundings. The ability to make new declarative memories and retrieve motor skills (e.g. dressing) is subsequently eroded.

AD is characterised pathologically by death of pyramidal cells, neuritic plaques and neurofibrillary tangles, particularly in the hippocampus, locus coeruleus and temporoparietal and frontal cortices. Plaques are extracellular deposits of amyloid surrounded by glial processes, abnormal nerve endings and dendrites. Tangles are intraneuronal, located in the cytoplasm and consisting of bundles of filaments made of highly phosphorylated tau, a protein which normally regulates the polymerisation of microtubules in the cytoskeleton (see Ch. 2).

CT and MRI scans show cortical and subcortical atrophy with enlargement of the ventricles. Brain mass may be reduced by 30–40%. Functional imaging reveals hypometabolism in posterior temporal and parietal areas.

Information box 8.23   **Hippocampal cognitive maps**

PET scans of London taxi drivers show increased activity in the right hippocampus while they are recalling familiar routes. This, and considerable work with rats, suggests that the hippocampus houses a **cognitive map** which facilitates navigation through the environment. However, it is likely that the hippocampus is not restricted to the consolidation of spatial memories, but involved in an eclectic range of episodic memories, at least in humans.

---

needed in planning and problem solving. Functional imaging indicates that various regions of the left hemisphere contribute to **verbal working memory tasks** while areas of the right hemisphere are involved in **spatial** (**non-verbal**) **tasks**.

Anatomical structures and declarative (explicit) memory

The **limbic system** (see above) has a major role in declarative memory. The **hippocampus** appears essential for the consolidation of LTM (Information box 8.23). When the hippocampus is damaged in diseases, such as herpes simplex encephalitis, patients suffer severe **anterograde amnesia** and cannot store information in LTM (although STM and procedural learning are unaffected). This is very disabling as the individual has difficulty remembering appointments or recalling seeing a friend or conversations on the telephone.

Limbic structures are also damaged in **Korsakoff syndrome**, a condition associated with thiamine deficiency seen most commonly in chronic alcoholics. There is **mammillary body** atrophy and neuronal loss in the **medial dorsal thalamus**. These patients suffer **retrograde amnesia**, i.e. loss of LTM and anterograde amnesia. They often exhibit **confabulation** in that they can tell a coherent, and sometimes convincing, account of recent experience which is false.

Long-term potentiation and depression

At the cellular level, **learning** requires the strengthening or weakening of synapses. This can involve de novo synthesis of proteins, with changes to the shape and form of synapses. Some neurites are lost, and new ones may develop. These cellular events are called **long-term potentiation** and **long-term depression**, respectively. Epilepsies are thought to involve the same synaptic mechanisms (Clinical box 8.45).

Clinical box 8.45   **Epilepsies**

Epileptic seizures are self-limiting episodes of abnormal, synchronised firing of large populations of neurons. The cause of the hyperexcitable state that predisposes to seizures is unclear but, in some cases, it seems to involve synaptic changes similar to those that underlie learning.

Animal models which are thought to emulate temporal lobe epilepsy (TLE or complex partial seizures) in humans help our understanding of epilepsy. Susceptibility to seizure activity is thought to be due to a hyperexcitable state of synapses between mossy fibres and CA3 pyramidal cells in the hippocampus. CA3 cells have three features that contribute to their ability for prolonged synchronised firing:

- They fire bursts of action potentials spontaneously, like pacemakers.
- They are heavily interconnected by recurrent axon collaterals by which each cell excites its neighbours and re-excites itself.
- There are gap junctions which allow adjacent CA3 cells to be electrically coupled for rapid spread of activity throughout the entire hippocampus. These electrical synapses are opened by a rise in pH. This is interesting because:
  - Hyperventilation, which produces a respiratory alkalosis, is used in EEG recording to induce seizure activity
  - Ketogenic diets, which produce metabolic acidosis, reduce seizure frequency
  - The local fall in pH produced by high neural activity during a seizure may limit it.

In contrast, CA1 cells in the hippocampus are only sparsely interconnected with each other and normally cannot be driven to burst fire by CA3 cells because they are inhibited by GABAergic interneurons. However, in epilepsy CA1 cells do burst fire, which implies a weakening of the GABAergic inhibition, and this allows the seizure to spread out of the hippocampus into the cortex of the temporal lobe.

Neural activity is very high during a seizure and intracellular adenosine concentration rises in consequence and adenosine may terminate individual seizures. It is transported out of the cell where it increases local blood flow and it binds to adenosine receptors in neurons causing hyperpolarisation, which curtails firing.

Causes of epileptogenesis

Inherited epilepsies have been linked to mutations in voltage-gated sodium or potassium channels or in ionotropic receptors (nicotinic receptor α subunits) that increase neural excitability.

Epileptogenesis in acquired epilepsies is far more difficult to account for. One thing is clear, however – seizure activity makes future seizures more likely, i.e. seizures are themselves epileptogenic. A possible mechanism for this is that seizures induce the expression of growth factors which enhance glutamate transmission but dampen GABA transmission (i.e. promoting excitatory transmission while suppressing inhibitory transmission) or trigger the formation of new synaptic connections between cells.

The pharmacological treatment of epilepsy is predicated on the notion that epilepsy is a matter of too much neural excitation or too little inhibition.

Principal modes of action of anti-epileptic drugs are:
- Blockade of voltage-dependent sodium channels (e.g. phenytoin, carbamazepine), or calcium channels (ethosuximide)
- Increasing GABAergic inhibition by blocking GABA reuptake (e.g. tiagabine) or inhibiting GABA transaminase, the enzyme responsible for inactivating GABA (e.g. vigabatrin)
- Mimicking GABA inhibition with GABA$_A$ receptor agonists (barbiturates and benzodiazepines).

Long-term potentiation (**LTP**) is an increase in the efficacy of synapses with repetitive stimulation. Repeated depolarisation of the postsynaptic membrane causes alteration in the NMDA glutamate receptors allowing calcium to enter the cell. A variety of biochemical processes that increase synaptic transmission are triggered. Both post- and presynaptic changes take place to maintain LTP, but it appears that new synapses are formed by splitting pre-existing ones. LTP was first discovered in the hippocampus but has subsequently been shown in the cortex, amygdala and other structures.

Long-term depression (**LTD**) is the reduction of synapse strength. It is dependent on strong synaptic stimulation with long periods of patterned, high activity (takes place in Purkinje cells), or persistent, weak synaptic stimulation (occurs in the hippocampus). L-Glutamate is the commonest neurotransmitter involved in LTD. The process is best characterised in the cerebellar Purkinje cells where LTD takes place at the synapse between Purkinje cells in response to high activity in parallel fibres representing error signals; the synapse becomes less responsive to the glutamate released by the parallel fibres.

It appears that LTD selectively weakens specific synapses to limit error, to increase the effectiveness of synaptic strengthening by LTP. It is proposed that cerebellar LTD is important for motor learning, and hippocampal LTD helps to clear redundant, old traces of memory.

ATTENTION

Attention may be described as a cognitive process of focusing on one aspect of the environment while ignoring everything else. Psychologists have defined an executive attention system that selects what is stored and organises and retrieves the relevant information in working memory (see above). Anatomically, the cognitive basal ganglia circuit in the dorsolateral prefrontal cortex has been identified for executive attention. The executive attention system searches for specific memories relevant to the task in hand. It also maintains a relevant cognitive set despite distracting stimuli and attempts to maintain a consistent behavioural response during repetitive activity by recalling past experience. It is also thought responsible for the ability to switch attention from one item or task to another.

AGNOSIAS

Comprehension or knowing (gnosis) involves a comparison of current sensory input with past experience. Agnosia is a failure to recognise stimuli when the appropriate sensory systems are functioning. Visual, auditory and tactile agnosias are associated with different cortical lesions.

In visual agnosia there is no defect in vision but the patient cannot recognise an object although they may be able to do so if they can touch and feel it. Bilateral lesions of the temporal aspect of the visual association area are usually responsible. Bilateral lesions to the posterior part of the superior temporal lobe (area 22) are responsible for auditory agnosia. Despite intact hearing, there is failure to recognise specific sounds, including speech and music. Lesions of the supramarginal gyrus (area 40) can cause tactile agnosia in which there is inability to identify objects by touch despite intact sensory pathways.

APRAXIAS

Apraxia can be defined as the loss of the ability to carry out a motor task, the nature of which the person understands, in the absence of weakness, ataxia or sensory loss. There is some debate as to the exact anatomical site of lesions responsible for different types of apraxia.

In **ideomotor apraxia** there is separation between the idea of a movement and its execution. Affected individuals cannot carry out a verbal command but can perform the movement under different circumstances (e.g. asked to protrude the tongue the person cannot do it, but may do so to lick his lips spontaneously moments later). This is usually associated with a lesion of the supramarginal gyrus of the dominant (left) parietal lobe.

Lesions of the frontal lobe can result in **ideational apraxia**, the inability to carry out a sequence of movements, each of which can be performed separately.

Non-dominant (right) parietal lobe damage is thought responsible for **constructional apraxia** which is apparent as the inability to copy a geometric pattern (e.g. an arrangement of matchsticks or the drawing of a cube).

LANGUAGE

Speech is the motor production of language. Language refers to the vocabulary and grammar (or syntactic rules) needed for verbal communication. In 90% of people the left hemisphere carries out language processing and is called the dominant hemisphere for both right-handed and left-handed individuals. A considerable volume of brain is involved in language (see Fig. 8.69).

- The superior temporal cortex is involved in the input of language information. It includes the auditory cortex and **Wernicke's area** (area 22). Lesions to Wernicke's area result in **sensory** (**receptive or posterior**) **aphasia** (Information box 8.24), which is a deficit in auditory comprehension. Speech, while fluent, becomes unintelligible because patients cannot understand what they are saying.

Bordering Wernicke's area lies the angular gyrus (area 39), which receives extensive visual input from the extrastriate cortex (area 19). Damage to the angular gyrus, such as infarction, can result in the loss of the ability to read (**alexia**) and write (**agraphia**).

- **Broca's area** (Brodmann's areas 44 and 45) lies in the inferior frontal gyrus, in the premotor area for speech, sending its output to the face and tongue areas of the motor cortex. Planning the articulatory movements needed for speech relies on input from verbal working memory input in the prefrontal cortex which projects to Broca's area and the **insula** (floor of the lateral sulcus) which directs motor control for articulation. Lesions that include Broca's area cause **motor** (**expressive or anterior**) **aphasia**, which ranges from difficulty finding words to the complete inability to speak.
- Wernicke's and Broca's areas are reciprocally interconnected. Lesions to these connections result in conduction aphasia. This usually causes a fluent aphasia with poor repetition of spoken language.

It is important to distinguish these disorders of language from disturbances to the motor actions responsible for speech. These can be divided into the production of sounds as air passes through the vocal cords (phonation) and the manipulation of sound as it passes through the upper airways by the palate, tongue, teeth and lips (articulation). Damage to the recurrent laryngeal nerve or respiratory muscle weakness can result in **dysphonia** in which speech volume is reduced and sounds are hoarse. Difficulties in the articulation are **dysarthrias** and occur with damage to articulatory structures themselves or to motor pathways.

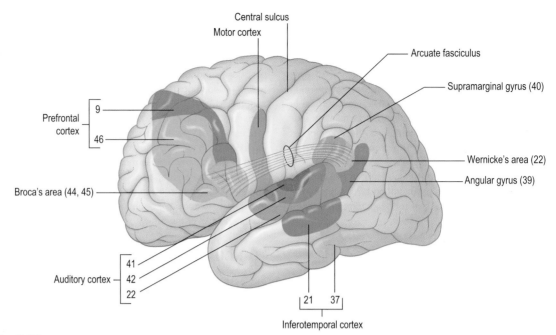

Fig. 8.69 **Cortical areas implicated in language by functional brain imaging studies.** Green regions show increased blood flow when listening to words (active listening). The auditory cortex (red), but not other regions, is also activated by tones (passive listening). Blue regions are, in addition, engaged during reading aloud.

Information box 8.24 **Prefixes a- and dys-**

The prefixes a- (or an- before a vowel) and dys- are often used interchangeably although, strictly speaking, a- refers to loss of or inability to perform a function, while dys- indicates difficulty in or abnormal performance of an activity. Thus alexia is the loss of the ability to read and dyslexia is difficulty in reading. However, clinicians use terms like apraxia and dyspraxia, and aphasia and dysphasia as if they were synonyms, as do some textbooks.

BRAIN DEATH

In most cases death is diagnosed by the absence of pulse and heart sounds and fixed pupils. However, when a patient is on life support different criteria are required. Death is then defined as the irreversible loss of both the capacity for consciousness and the capacity to breathe. There are three prerequisites for the diagnosis:

- There is no doubt that irremediable brain damage of known cause has occurred
- There is deep coma in the absence of the effects of drugs, hypothermia, and potentially reversible metabolic or endocrine disturbances
- Spontaneous respiration is inadequate or has ceased.

Tests are done repeatedly to confirm the diagnosis and are essentially aimed at brainstem reflexes (see above) and function. Hence it is more accurate to refer to brainstem death. These tests include:

- Loss of pupillary light reflexes
- Loss of corneal reflex
- Loss of gag reflex
- Loss of vestibulo-ocular reflex
- No spontaneous respiration after turning off the mechanical ventilator even when extreme levels of hypercapnia are reached.

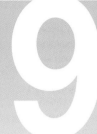

Bone, muscle, skin and connective tissue

Lesley Robson and Denise Syndercombe Court

Introduction	**403**	**Skeletal muscle**	**432**
Imaging in medicine	403	The neuromuscular junction and	
The skeletal system	**404**	muscle innervation	432
Cartilage	404	Isotonic versus isometric contraction	435
Bone microanatomy	405	The skeletal muscle fibre	435
Bone formation	406	The contractile process	438
Skeletal components	406	Muscle metabolism	440
Structure of bone	406	Types of muscle fibres	441
Bone development	411	The connective tissue of muscle	441
Bone growth	412	Muscle growth and repair	442
Bone's role in calcium		Muscle nomenclature	442
homeostasis	415	**Posture and locomotion**	**443**
Bone healing	417	Standing	444
Joints	**418**	Walking	444
Bony joints	418	**Specialised connective tissues: skin,**	
Fibrous joints	418	**hair and nails**	**444**
Cartilaginous joints	419	Structure of skin	444
Synovial joints	419	Hair	447
Tendons and ligaments	428	Nails	448
Anatomical relationships	432	**Generalised connective tissue**	**448**

INTRODUCTION

The **musculoskeletal system** is composed of the skeleton, the muscles and accessory tissues, which together allow movement of the body.

The bones of the **skeleton** are living tissue, and they can be found in a variety of shapes and sizes depending on their function. The skeleton is composed of approximately 206 individual bones that articulate with each other via a network of joints. **Joints** vary in their structure and function, with some joints allowing a wide range of movements while other joints are virtually fixed and are designed for stability.

The **skeletal muscles** provide power to move and support the skeleton, often linking two bones across a joint. Most of them are attached to the skeleton via **tendons** which transmit the muscular contraction to the bones which move at the joints. The skeletal muscles of the face attach not only to the skull but also to other facial muscles and the skin, and contraction of these muscles changes the facial expression. The muscles that act on the skeleton are all under voluntary control and contain the contractile proteins, actin and myosin.

Knowledge of the musculoskeletal system is vital for medical practitioners as a third of general practitioner (GP) consultations involve the musculoskeletal system in some way. Conditions that affect the musculoskeletal system include osteoarthritis, which affects two-thirds of individuals over 75 years of age and 20% of the total population, and back pain, which affects 2.5 million people every day in Britain and accounts for 6% of all GP consultations. Around

400 thousand of us take time off work because of back pain. Musculoskeletal disorders therefore cost the UK economy considerable sums each year.

The **integumentary system** (integument means covering) is formed by the skin plus associated glands, hair and nails. It covers the entire body and has four main roles:

- Protection: it protects the body from the external environment
- Homeostasis: it controls body temperature (see also Ch. 1)
- Perception: the skin contains receptors for pain, temperature and touch (see Ch. 8)
- Metabolism: synthesis of vitamin D (see Ch. 10).

Generalised **connective tissue** forms an extracellular matrix inside the body, separating and supporting the organs and is composed predominantly of collagen and elastin.

IMAGING IN MEDICINE

Different imaging techniques form an important part of being able to visualise what is in the body.

- **Radiographs** are the earliest form of imaging techniques and are produced by **X-rays**. Standard radiographs will normally involve two views: anteroposterior (AP) and lateral. Higher energy X-rays are used in medical imaging as they can easily pass through soft tissue, but are stopped by hard tissue. X-rays interact with tissue in different ways but visualisation is possible through photoabsorption.

- **Photoabsorption** takes place when the X-rays meet high density material, particularly where high atomic number elements are involved. Bones have a high calcium content and calcium also has a high atomic number, facilitating absorption of the X-rays.
  - Photographic film is coated with a light sensitive silver halide emulsion. Light (and X-rays) interact with the emulsion, releasing silver which appears black when the film is developed. Because bone absorbs the X-rays then these are visualized as white 'shadows' on a film placed on the far side of the body from the X-ray source. Gas, such as air within the lungs, shows up clearly as a dark image as there is little attenuation.
- **Dual-energy X-ray absorptiometry (DXA scanning)** uses two X-ray beams with different energies to measure bone density. This technique is particularly useful in the diagnosis of osteoporosis.
- **Computed tomography (CT)** or **computed axial tomography (CAT)** scans are computer generated images from a large number of two-dimensional X-rays, producing a three-dimensional image which can then be examined in a series of cross-sectional images through the body. This technique is particularly useful as a transverse plane image (horizontal section across the body) is almost impossible to produce using standard X-rays. CT scans also provide a greater grey scale separation which allows soft tissue types to be more easily differentiated.
- **Magnetic resonance imaging (MRI)** uses nuclear magnetic imaging. The human body contains a large amount of water that contains two hydrogen nuclei (protons) which are magnetised and aligned when the human body is located within a large magnetic scanner. Varying the magnetic field leads the nuclei to spin at a particular frequency (resonance), which then stops when the magnetic field is switched off. The rate at which the protons return to their original relaxed state varies according to the tissue and the spatial organisation of the nuclei and this is used to inform the final image. Fourier transformation is a mathematical technique used to produce the image. Because of their high water content, MRI scans are very useful in examining soft tissues such as nervous tissue, muscles, ligaments and also in the detection of tumours.
- **Ultrasound** waves are particularly useful for imaging soft tissue. Different frequencies facilitate different penetration into tissue, the tissue reflecting the sound waves in ways that provide fine differentiation within variable tissue types. The technique has high utility across much of medicine, including in foetal medicine enabling examination of the developing foetus, in echocardiography to examine the heart structure, and being able to detect fluid.
- **Bone scans.** The radio-isotope technetium (^{99m}Tc) is bound to bisphosphonates which are taken up by osteoblasts on injection. The technique is very sensitive in the detection of bone rebuilding activity and is therefore useful in the examination of fractures and tumours that invade bone. Detection is with a gamma camera.
- **Positron emission tomography (PET)** scans. This technique uses molecules such as glucose analogues that are labelled with a short life radionuclide, as a radiotracer, and injected into the body. The radionuclides emit positrons, releasing gamma rays as they decay and their distribution within body tissue can be examined. This technique is particularly useful to diagnose and monitor cancer as rapidly growing cells utilise the sugar, phosphorylating it by the action of hexokinase, which effectively then traps the labelled compound within the cell, producing an intense signal. It is also used to examine the activity of different areas of the brain.

THE SKELETAL SYSTEM

Skeletal tissues are modified connective tissues in which the fibres are often organised and condensed to produce strong or rigid tissues. The skeleton is mainly composed of bones which form a framework for the rest of the body tissues. Bone is a complex and dynamic living tissue. It is continually being broken down and replaced by new bone. The adult skeleton also contains cartilage, which is more elastic than bone and forms a semi-rigid part of the skeleton and a protective layer at many joint surfaces. Other fibrous connective tissues form tendons and ligaments which provide strength, without being rigid or elastic.

CARTILAGE

Cartilage, which consists largely of water, contains two cell types:

- Immature **chondroblasts** which secrete the extracellular matrix of cartilage, composed of collagen fibres, elastin fibres and other proteinaceous components, such as proteoglycans (heavily glycosylated proteins), glycoproteins and water.
- **Chondrocytes**, which are mature cartilage cells, derived from chondroblasts that are trapped within spaces called **lacunae**, surrounded by the extracellular matrix.

Cartilage does not contain blood vessels so all metabolites are exchanged by diffusion. Although cartilage has a low metabolic rate, diffusion limits its potential thickness and prevents rapid repair following injury. The high water content of cartilage ensures that it is resilient and retains its shape under pressure, as water is virtually incompressible.

Three types of cartilage are found in the adult body:

- **Hyaline (glassy) cartilage**: covers the ends of synovial joints (**articular cartilage**, see below), connects the ribs to the sternum (**costal cartilage**), forms the larynx and part of the nose and reinforces the trachea and bronchi. **Osteoarthritis** is caused by degeneration of cartilage at the joints.
- **White fibro-cartilage**: has less matrix and more collagen than other cartilage, which makes it more compressible and able to resist high pressures. It is found in discs in areas of high stress such as between the vertebrae (**intervertebral disc**) and in the knee joint (**meniscus**).
- **Elastic (yellow) cartilage**: is found in only two places: the external ear, where it forms the **pinna** and the external auditory canal, the **Eustachian tube**, and in the throat where it forms the **epiglottis**. Elastic cartilage contains high levels of elastic fibres, which gives these tissues a large degree of flexibility.

Hyaline and elastic cartilage, but not the articular cartilage within synovial joints, are surrounded by a fibrous layer, the **perichondrium**, containing fibroblasts along with type

I collagen in the outer layer and chondroblasts in the inner layer. It is continuous with the periosteal bone and the surface of surrounding connective tissue and forms the **periosteum** as it becomes vascularised, lining the outside surface of all bones. In the embryo (at 6 weeks) the skeleton is composed of hyaline cartilage and fibrous tissue formed by mesenchymal cells. These are then converted to bone by endochondral ossification and intramembranous ossification, respectively (see below).

BONE MICROANATOMY

Bone is classified as a connective tissue, as it shows the characteristics of all connective tissues: relatively acellular, with osteogenic (bone generating) cells widely separated within an abundant matrix.

Bone matrix

In bone, the matrix is composed of approximately:

- 25% water
- 25% organic protein fibres
- 50% crystallised mineral salts.

Most (90–95%) of the organic component of bone consists of **collagen fibres**, 90% of which are type I.

About 50% of the bone is composed of **inorganic crystals** made up of the mineral **hydroxyapatite**, which itself is composed of calcium phosphate, calcium carbonate, calcium fluoride, calcium hydroxide and citrate.

Cellular content of bone

There are four types of cells in bone (Fig. 9.1):

- Osteogenic progenitor cells
- Osteoblasts
- Osteocytes
- Osteoclasts.

The **osteogenic progenitor cells** are the precursors of the osteoblasts and are derived from mesenchymal cells. The osteogenic progenitor cells are found in the periosteum and endosteum (lining the medullary cavity) of the bone and also in the canals within the bone that contain blood vessels (see below) and differentiate into osteoblasts.

Osteoblasts are the cells that make new bone matrix. They synthesise and secrete collagen fibres and other organic components, in particular alkaline phosphatase (ALP) which dephosphorylates many molecules, initiating the calcification of the matrix by laying down deposits of calcium phosphate.

In the presence of normal liver function, increased serum ALP is a strong indicator of increased osteoblast activity and is useful in the diagnosis of **Paget disease**, in which increased bone resorption is compensated for by increased osteoblast activity.

Osteocytes are found in the more mature bone and were once osteoblasts, but have now become surrounded and entrapped in their own matrix. They no longer secrete matrix, and their role is to maintain the daily cellular activities of the bone tissue. These activities include the exchange of nutrients and waste products with the blood.

The final type of cell found in bone is the **osteoclast** whose role is the removal of old bone. Historically it was

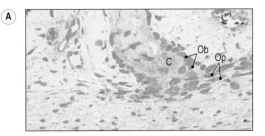

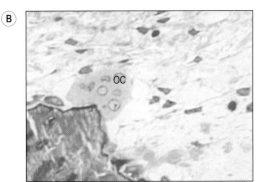

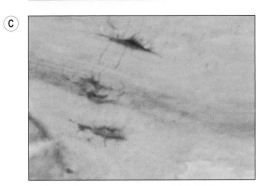

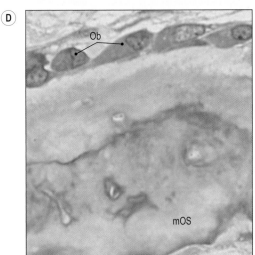

Fig. 9.1 **Bone cell types.** (A) Osteogenic progenitor cells; (B) osteoclasts; (C) osteocytes; (D) osteoblasts. C, osteoid collagen (unmineralised osteoid); mOS, mineralised osteoid; Ob, osteoblast; OC, osteoclast. From Stevens A, Lowe J 2004 Human histology, 3rd edn. Mosby, Edinburgh, with permission.

believed that osteoclasts were formed from osteoblasts but they have been shown to have different lineages, osteoclasts originating from monocyte-macrophage precursors. They are very large and concentrated in the **endosteum** (the layer of connective tissue lining the bone medullary cavity).

The plasma membrane of the osteoclast facing the bone surface has a deep ruffled border and releases powerful lysosomal enzymes and acids that digest and dissolve the protein and mineral matrix. The removal of old bone matrix is usually balanced with the osteoblasts' production of new bone (see below).

BONE FORMATION

The bone matrix is unlike other connective tissues because it contains lots of inorganic salts, the main one being **hydroxyapatite**, which is mainly calcium phosphate, but there is also some calcium carbonate and small amounts of other calcium salts along with magnesium hydroxide, fluoride and sulphate. These are all deposited on the framework of collagen fibres secreted by the osteoblasts. As the minerals crystallise they harden the tissue, in a process called **ossification**.

The hardness of the bone depends on the amount and type of the crystallised salts. Bone must remain slightly flexible to be able to withstand the forces it is subjected to daily and this is dependent on the presence of collagen fibres which provide the bone with tensile strength. Calcification only takes place in the presence of the collagen fibres, with mineral salts first crystallising in the microscopic spaces between the collagen fibres (see Clinical box 9.1). Once these spaces have been filled, more mineral crystals accumulate around the collagen fibres.

While the presence of calcium salts gives bone its great compressional strength, collagen increases its tensile strength (the ability to endure a stretching force). Bone does not, however, have great torsional strength and many

---

Clinical box 9.1   Osteogenesis imperfecta

Osteogenesis imperfecta, or brittle bone disease, is a genetic disease that affects the production of collagen type I. Collagen has a triple helix formation and in type I forms tightly packed microfibrils. This collagen is important in forming the organic scaffold of bone. The inheritance pattern is autosomal dominant and osteogenesis imperfecta is the result of a genetic mutation that results in either less collagen type I being produced (due to a premature stop codon or mutant mRNA) or an abnormal collagen type I protein to be made (usually when the mutation substitutes a glycine amino acid with cysteine or alanine. The former glycine is a very small molecule and facilitates the super helix formation of collagen type I which gives it its strength; larger molecules produce abnormal chains which are much weaker). New spontaneous mutations account for 25% of cases.

At least seven types of osteogenesis imperfecta have been identified: type 1 is the most common form of the disease and also the mildest, whereas type 2 is the most severe (often leading to perinatal death), and those with type 3 are often wheel-chair bound. Other types are milder. The main symptom is that the bones fracture easily so that X-rays of an affected person usually show evidence of multiple fractures that have healed or are in the process of healing. As collagen type I is found elsewhere in the body besides bone, osteogenesis imperfecta also affects other tissues and organs. For example, in the eyes, the sclera (the whites of the eye) have a tendency to be blue rather than white, joints tend to be loose or lax as tendons and ligaments are partly composed of collagen type I, and patients often have low muscle tone, brittle teeth and may suffer from hearing loss. Other features include increased perspiration and easy bruising, as the skin tends to be thin and smooth, as collagen type I is also found in the dermis of the skin.

Osteogenesis imperfecta is usually diagnosed during infancy, as babies with the more severe types are often born with fractures and babies with type 1 often have their first fracture in the first year of life; some milder forms are not diagnosed until teenage or even into adulthood.

---

fractures result from excessive twisting forces applied to long bones.

Bone is not completely solid and contains many small spaces, some of which provide space for blood vessels to supply the bone cells with nutrients and remove waste products. Other spaces are filled with bone marrow (haemopoietic cells). Bone can be divided into two categories, compact and spongy, depending on the distribution of the spaces. Overall 80% of the total skeleton is **compact bone** and 20% is **spongy** (**cancellous**) **bone**, although bones in the axial skeleton are 70% spongy bone.

SKELETAL COMPONENTS

The skeleton can be divided into two parts:

- **Axial skeleton**, which forms the long axis of the body and contains the skull, vertebral column (Anatomy box 9.1) and ribs
- **Appendicular skeleton**, which consists of the limb bones and their attachments or **girdles**, the pelvis and scapula and clavicle.

There are many different types of bone and they can be classified according to their shape (Fig. 9.2):

- **Long bones** are longer than their width and are the most common. They are mainly formed from compact bone with spongy bone in their centres and at their ends (see below). Examples include the long bones of the arms (humerus, radius and ulna) and legs (femur, tibia and fibula) as well as the small bones of the fingers and toes. The tibia is a particularly important bone as pain in the lower leg is a common complaint (Clinical box 9.4).
- **Short bones**: these are cuboidal and contain mainly spongy bone with a surface layer of compact bone. Examples of these are the bones of the wrist and ankles, as well as the **sesamoid** bones such as the patella (kneecap), which are found within some tendons.
- **Flat bones**: these are flat, thin and usually slightly curved. They consist of two thin layers of compact bone, surrounding a thin layer of spongy bone. The skull, ribs, sternum (breast bone) and scapula (shoulder blade) are all flat bones.
- **Irregular bones**: these are bones that do not fit the other categories. They are made from spongy bone covered with compact bone. The bones of the vertebrae (Anatomy box 9.2) and pelvis are irregular bones.

STRUCTURE OF BONE

A typical long bone (Fig. 9.3) consists of the following regions:

- The **diaphysis**, which is the shaft of the long bone and is the main portion of the bone
- The **epiphyses**, which are the distal and proximal ends of the bone
- The **metaphyses**, which are the regions in a mature bone where the diaphysis joins the epiphysis. In a growing bone the metaphysis is the region occupied by the **epiphyseal growth plate**.

Articular cartilage is a thin layer of hyaline cartilage that covers the epiphyses. The articular cartilage reduces the friction at the joints and acts as a shock absorber at freely moveable joints.

Anatomy box 9.1 The vertebral column

The **vertebral column** is a rigid yet flexible structure that extends from the base of the skull to the tip of the coccyx (Fig. AB1). The vertebral column allows trunk movement, helps to maintain an upright posture, supports the weight of the body and head and allows the head to turn. It also protects the spinal cord, which runs down through a canal formed by the vertebrae.

The vertebral column is composed of 24 moveable **vertebrae**:

- 7 in the **cervical** (neck) region (C1–C7) (Clinical box 9.2)
- 12 in the **thoracic** region (T1–T12)
- 5 in the **lumbar** region (L1–L5).

There are also two immobile composite vertebrae, the **sacrum** which is composed of five fused segments (S1–S5) and the **coccyx**, which is composed of three to five fused vertebrae. This gives a total of 33 ± 1 vertebrae. The number of vertebrae is fairly constant, with an estimated 5% of the population having a slight variation.

The movements that the vertebral column can perform are:

- Anterior, posterior and lateral flexion
- Extension
- Rotation.

The movement between any two vertebral segments is relatively small, but added together there is a considerable range of movement possible.

The length of the vertebral column is 72–75 cm in adults; with three-quarters of the length made up by the **vertebral bodies**, and the rest of the length made up by the **intervertebral discs** that lie between the vertebrae.

Curvatures (see Clinical box 9.3)

In the adult there are four curves in the vertebral column (Fig. AB1).

- Two primary curvatures: the **thoracic** and **sacral** curves. These curves develop in utero and give the newborn a single concave 'C' shaped curve to their backs.
- Two secondary curves: the convex **cervical** and **lumbar** curves. The cervical curve develops when the baby starts to hold up its head, and the lumbar curve develops when the infant starts to stand up and begins to walk.

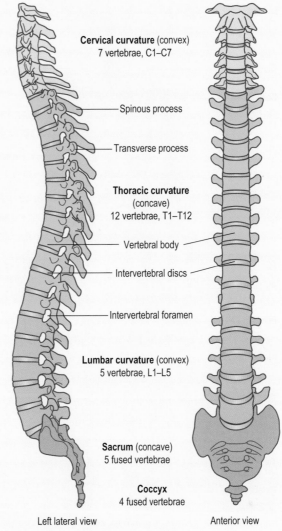

Cervical curvature (convex)
7 vertebrae, C1–C7

Spinous process

Transverse process

Thoracic curvature
(concave)
12 vertebrae, T1–T12

Vertebral body

Intervertebral discs

Intervertebral foramen

Lumbar curvature (convex)
5 vertebrae, L1–L5

Sacrum (concave)
5 fused vertebrae

Coccyx
4 fused vertebrae

Left lateral view   Anterior view

Fig. AB1 **The vertebral column.**

Clinical box 9.2 Neck pain

Neck pain is a common complaint. Chronic pain, often extending to the shoulders, is commonly associated with sedentary occupations that lead to poor neck posture over prolonged periods (such as computer usage). **Cervical spondylosis** is the most common degenerative condition affecting the neck, especially at C5–C6. Narrowing of the cervical canal from various causes can lead to cord compression and affect upper limb movement. **Whiplash injury** is a common cause of persistent neck pain. Classically the injury occurs as the result of a rear impact into a stationary or slow moving car, which then is propelled into another object in front. The resultant force on the mass of the car occupant's head leads to a rapid extension, followed by flexion of the cervical spine.

Clinical box 9.3 Abnormal curves

Scoliosis is a lateral curvature of the vertebral column. Most cases are idiopathic but some are due to a developmental defect. The lateral curvature of the spine often results in one shoulder and possibly one side of the pelvis being higher than the other. If the curvature is slight there may not be any significant defect when standing but the abnormal curve becomes more noticeable on bending over. Severe curves may restrict the lungs and the other internal organs, leading to the need for surgery to fuse the curve, preventing further deterioration.

Kyphosis, also known as 'dowager's hump', is an increased thoracic curvature; although more commonly postural, it can also form because of osteoporosis, where the thoracic vertebral bodies collapse. The progressive erosion and collapse of the vertebral bodies can result in an overall loss of height. In severe cases it may restrict breathing by reducing the capacity for the lungs to expand within the thoracic cage.

An increase in the lumbar curvature is called **lordosis** and is often associated with weakened trunk muscles. Lordosis can also result from obesity or during the latter stages of pregnancy, where the increase in weight anterior to the vertebral column pulls the lumbar vertebrae forwards. This abnormal curvature tends to be temporary and the vertebral column will revert to its normal curves after the baby is born or if the individual loses weight. If the abnormal curvature is severe enough then it can cause problems, again by restricting the internal organs, or by impinging on the nerve roots as they leave the spinal cord.

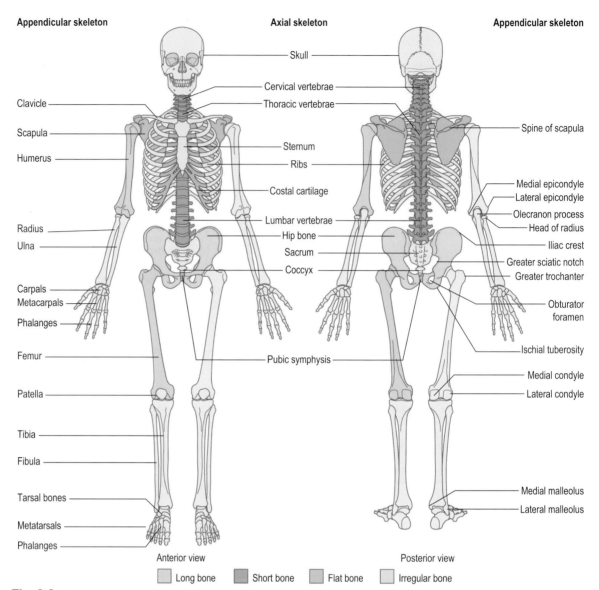

Fig. 9.2 The adult skeleton showing the types of bone.

Pain originating in the anterior or posterior aspect of the tibia is a common bone pain complaint and can be the result of various causes.

In the anterior aspect:

- **Osteitis** – inflammation of the bone in the metaphyseal areas – seen mainly in children
- **Bone tumour** – a common site for primary bone tumours
- **Anterior tibial compartment syndrome** – a common complication of tibial fractures producing inflammation and ischaemia of the tibialis anterior and extensor hallucis longus muscles, leading to an inability to extend the ankle and big toe. There may be an absent dorsalis pedis pulse and sensory loss due to ischaemia of the deep peroneal nerve. Relief of pressure in the area to prevent muscle necrosis can be a surgical emergency
- **Stress fracture** – also more common in **Paget disease** (localized bone remodelling).

In the posterior aspect:

- **Ruptured plantaris tendon** – more probably due to tearing of muscle fibres of the gastrocnemius or soleus muscles, rather than the plantaris muscle, causing sudden activity-related pain in the calf
- **Thrombophlebitis** – thrombosis in the superficial calf veins leading to inflammation and pain in the calf is a common sign. Deep vein thrombosis, a common postoperative complication, is often silent.

The **periosteum** is a tough layer of dense irregular connective tissue surrounding the bone surface where it is not covered by the articular cartilage. It contains the osteogenic progenitor cells and as these differentiate into osteoblasts they allow the bone to grow in thickness. The periosteum also helps to protect the bone, assists in fracture repair, helps nourish the bone tissue and serves as an attachment point for tendons and ligaments.

The **medullary cavity** in the centre of the bones is sometimes called the **marrow cavity** and is the space within the diaphysis that contains the bone marrow. Two types of bone marrow are found in the medullary cavity:

- **Red marrow**, which produces red and white blood cells and platelets (haemopoietic tissue)
- **Yellow marrow**, which contains fat and connective tissue and produces some white blood cells.

The two types of bone marrow are interconvertible. At birth there is only red bone marrow present and as the person grows the red marrow in many of the bones is replaced by yellow marrow. By adulthood, only about half of the bone marrow is red. The change from red to yellow is due to a decrease in the level of the haemopoietic stimulant,

Anatomy box 9.2   The 'typical' vertebra

The **vertebral body** is the weight-bearing part of the vertebra; it is a solid block of bone that is the anterior part of the vertebra (Fig. AB2). Inferiorly the vertebral bodies become progressively greater in size, especially from T4, reflecting the increased weight that the vertebrae have to carry; the largest vertebral body is that of L5. In the sacrum and coccyx, the size of the vertebral body decreases.

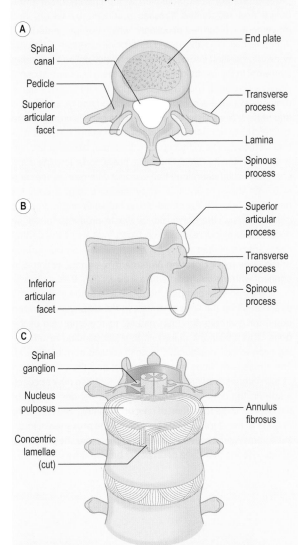

Fig. AB2   A typical vertebra. (A) Cross-sectional view; (B) lateral view (showing vertebral body, pedicles, laminae, spinal cord, processes, intravertebral disc and ligaments); (C) section showing intervertebral discs.

The **vertebral arch**, or **neural arch**, is composed of the **pedicles** and **laminae**, which form a ring through which the spinal cord passes called the **vertebral foramen** (spinal canal) (Fig. AB2). There are notches in the superior and inferior borders of the pedicles called the **vertebral notches**. These form an **intervertebral foramen**, through which the nerve roots exit and enter the spinal cord.

Each vertebral arch has seven processes which are attachment sites for muscles and ligaments:
- Four articular processes
- Two transverse processes
- One spinous process.

The vertebrae from different regions show a number of modifications, especially the atlas (C1) and axis (C2) vertebrae of the neck which form a specialised pivot joint (see below).

Joints and ligaments of the vertebral column
Between C2 to S1 adjacent vertebrae articulate at three joints:
- Two synovial (zygapophyses) between the vertebral arches
- One symphysis between the vertebral body and the intervertebral disc.

The **zygapophyses** are synovial joints of the planar kind and allow limited gliding movements between the vertebrae. Osteoarthritis may attack these joints, and the bony growths that form in this condition may reduce the size of the intervertebral foramen, leading to pressure on the spinal nerves.

The pivot joint between C1 and C2 allows the head to tip forward (the 'no' joint), and the atlanto-occipital joint between C1 and the base of the skull is the flexion/extension joint and therefore is the 'yes' joint.

Ligaments strengthen and stabilise the vertebral column and stop any excessive movements. The **anterior and posterior longitudinal ligaments** prevent hyperextension and hyperflexion, respectively. There are also short ligaments joining adjacent vertebrae: the **ligamentum flavum**. There are also **interspinous** and **supraspinous** ligaments and some specialised ligaments around the atlanto-axial joint.

Intervertebral discs
The joints between the vertebral bodies are secondary cartilaginous joints or symphyses designed for weight bearing and strength. The articulating surfaces of the adjacent vertebrae are connected by an **intervertebral disc**.

The intervertebral disc is composed of two parts: the **annulus fibrosus** is a fibrous ring consisting of alternating layers of obliquely orientated collagen fibres surrounding the central gelatinous **nucleus pulposus**, which is a turgid gel composed of 70–90% water, proteoglycans and some collagen fibres which allows compression between adjacent vertebrae. When weight is applied to the disc the nucleus becomes flattened and the annulus fibrosus bulges between the vertebrae.

The water content of the intervertebral discs declines with age so the intervertebral discs are better shock absorbers in the young than in the elderly and this also accounts for some of the loss of height that is experienced with age. If the intervertebral discs reduce in height, the intervertebral foramen also reduces in size, which may lead to entrapment of the spinal nerves (Clinical box 9.5).

Clinical box 9.5   Slipped disc (herniation or prolapse of the intervertebral disc)

A **slipped disc** is a protrusion of the nucleus pulposus through the annulus fibrosus. The protrusion can press on the spinal nerve roots, causing referred pain. This commonly takes place in the lumbar region, leading to **sciatica**, where the pain is felt in the lower back, posterior thigh and leg, which is the course of the sciatic nerve. Neurological disturbances can also occur which are segmental and dependent on the level and side of the prolapse. Where the prolapse is large and central and below L1/L2 this can also affect the **cauda equina**, so called because of the 'horse tail' appearance of the nerves at the base of the spinal cord. Bladder incontinence is a common symptom and the condition may become a surgical emergency as it can lead to paraplegia. Approximately 95% of herniations of the nucleus pulposus in the lumbar region take place most commonly at the L5/S1, then L4/L5 levels.

Muscles of the vertebral column
There are superficial, intermediate and deep muscles around the vertebral column. The superficial muscles are located around the back of the neck and shoulders and act to help move the shoulders. The intermediate group of muscles is located in the lower neck and thoracic level and may be related to inspiration. The deep back muscles maintain posture and move the vertebral column.

Extreme movements of the vertebral column may lead to back strain. The term 'strain' is used to indicate some degree of stretching of the muscles and or ligaments of the back.

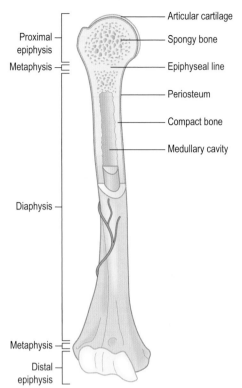

Articular cartilage
Spongy bone
Proximal epiphysis
Metaphysis
Epiphyseal line
Periosteum
Compact bone
Medullary cavity
Diaphysis
Metaphysis
Distal epiphysis

Fig. 9.3 **Structure of a typical long bone.**

erythropoietin, the hormone that regulates red cell mitosis and differentiation, which reduces with age such that in the elderly only about 30% of the bone marrow is red bone marrow. Red bone marrow is found mostly in the ribs, sternum (breastbone), scapulae (shoulder blades), clavicles (collarbones), pelvis (hip bones), skull and vertebrae.

The **endosteum** is a membrane that lines the medullary cavity and contains bone-forming cells; it is the equivalent of the periosteum surrounding the outside of the bone. It serves as the site of formation for new bone and contains the osteogenic precursor cells.

Compact bone

Compact bone forms the outer layer of all bones, where it provides support and protection to the spongy bone in the centre and resists the stresses produced by weight and movement. It is formed of collagen which is impregnated with inorganic calcium salts, giving its exterior hardness. Compact bone is organised into **osteons**, sometimes called **Haversian systems**. In the centre of each osteon there is a **central canal (Haversian canal)** which runs longitudinally through the bone; running through this central canal are blood and lymph vessels and nerves. Around the central canal the bone is arranged into concentric layers (**lamellae**) which are rings of calcified matrix. Osteocytes lie within spaces (**lacunae**) between the layers. Lacunae join in small finger-like projections, forming small channels called **canaliculi** that connect with one another and also with the central canal. They therefore form a complex branching network for blood-borne nutrients and oxygen to diffuse through the bone and for waste products to diffuse back to the blood vessels. The blood vessels of the central canal are connected to the periosteal vessels on the surface of the bone by **perforating (Volkmann's) canals**, which also connect with the internal medullary cavity (Fig. 9.4).

The osteons in compact bone are all aligned in the same direction along the lines of stress. In the diaphysis of a long bone, for example, they run parallel to the long axis of the bone. This allows the diaphysis to resist bending or fracturing even when considerable force is applied from either end. The stresses on bone are not constant and the organisation of the osteons is dynamic in response to these new stresses made on the bone, and is part of the normal destruction of old bone and the formation of new bone matrix. The response of bone to new stresses can be seen by the presence of interstitial lamellae between the osteons; these are the remnants of old osteons that have been partly broken down.

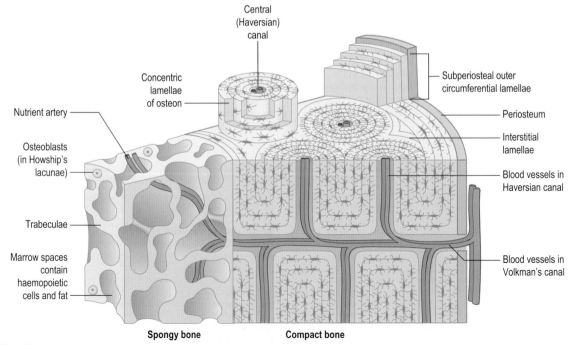

Central (Haversian) canal
Concentric lamellae of osteon
Subperiosteal outer circumferential lamellae
Periosteum
Interstitial lamellae
Nutrient artery
Osteoblasts (in Howship's lacunae)
Blood vessels in Haversian canal
Trabeculae
Marrow spaces contain haemopoietic cells and fat
Blood vessels in Volkman's canal
Spongy bone
Compact bone

Fig. 9.4 **Compact and spongy bone.**

Spongy bone

Spongy bone does not contain true osteons and consists of lamellae arranged into an irregular lattice of thin interconnecting partitions (**trabeculae**). The spaces between the trabeculae are filled with red or yellow bone marrow, which is responsible for the production of blood cells. Within each trabecula osteocytes lie in lacunae with radiating canaliculi, much like in the osteons of the compact bone. The osteocytes in the spongy bone trabeculae receive their nutrients directly from the blood circulating through the medullary cavity (Fig. 9.4).

Spongy bone makes up the majority of bony tissue in the short, flat and irregularly shaped bones and the epiphyses of the long bones, and lines the medullary cavity of the diaphysis of the long bones.

The orientation of the trabeculae in spongy bone is along the lines of stress, like the osteons in compact bone. This characteristic helps bone resist stresses and the transfer of force without breaking. Spongy bone is located where bones are not heavily stressed or where the stresses are applied from many directions, as this type of bone has both flexibility and strength. Spongy bone has a higher rate of turnover than compact bone, and so responds to the changing stresses placed on it faster than compact bone does. For this reason osteoporosis is more evident in the spongy bone compartments than in compact bone.

Spongy bone reduces the weight of the skeleton, so that the muscles acting on the skeleton do not have to work as hard. In the adult the spongy bone and its red bone marrow is the only site of haemopoiesis, especially the spongy bone of the pelvis (hip), ribs, sternum (breast bone), vertebrae and the ends of the long bones.

Blood and nerve supply to bone

Certain regions of bone contain large quantities of red bone marrow and these regions have a very good blood supply that passes from the periosteum into the interior of the bone. The **periosteal arteries** are accompanied by nerves and they enter the diaphysis through the perforating Volkmann's canals. They supply the periosteum and the compact bone. Near the centre of the diaphysis there is a large **nutrient artery** that passes obliquely through the compact bone through a hole – the nutrient foramen. When the nutrient artery reaches the medullary cavity it divides into proximal and distal branches, which supply both the inner layers of compact bone and spongy bone of the diaphysis and the red marrow as far as the epiphyseal growth plates (or lines). The number of nutrient foramina varies from bone to bone – the tibia has only one nutrient artery while the femur has many; this variation is due to the size of the bone and the relative amounts of red bone marrow that the bone has. The ends of the bone are supplied by the **metaphyseal and epiphyseal arteries**. These arteries arise from those that supply the joint. Both the metaphyseal and epiphyseal arteries also enter the bone and supply the red bone marrow in their respective regions.

There are usually one or two nutrient veins that accompany the artery in the diaphysis, and there are many epiphyseal and metaphyseal veins which also exit with the respective arteries. Finally, there are also periosteal veins that drain blood from the periosteum.

Nerves accompany the blood vessels of bone. The periosteum has a rich supply of sensory nerves, some of which transmit pain sensations. These nerves are sensitive to tearing or tension and explain the severe pain from a fracture or a bone tumour.

BONE DEVELOPMENT

Bony tissue is formed by one of two processes during embryonic development:

- Endochondral ossification: the **replacement** of hyaline cartilage with bone tissue
- Intramembranous ossification: the **direct ossification** of the mesenchymal cells.

Ossification begins during the sixth or seventh week of human development; once they are fully formed the bones produced by these two processes are indistinguishable in structure.

Endochondral ossification

The majority of the bones in the body are formed from cartilage by endochondral ossification. Hyaline cartilage forms an initial model of the future bone from mesenchymal cells that differentiate into chondroblasts. Once the hyaline model of the bone has formed, osteoblasts gradually replace the cartilage with bone matrix, which is then ossified. The process is most clearly seen in the long bones of the arms and legs (Fig. 9.5).

The process begins with mesenchymal cells at the site of the future bone condensing into a rough approximation of the bones. These mesenchymal cells differentiate into chondroblasts (precursors of cartilage) under the influence of various factors in the environment. The chondroblasts then begin to secrete a cartilage matrix around themselves, with a membrane (the **perichondrium**) forming around the cartilage model containing the chondroblast precursors. As more cartilage matrix is produced the chondroblasts become buried in the matrix, and they mature into **chondrocytes**.

As the foetus grows so does the cartilage model. The chondrocytes can divide and the new chondrocytes produce more cartilage matrix, causing an increase in the *length* of the cartilage bone model. This is called **interstitial** growth. The increase in the *thickness* of the bone **appositional** growth) comes from new chondroblasts differentiating from the precursors in the perichondrium and becoming incorporated into the cartilage bone model.

As the cartilage model grows, the chondrocytes in the centre of the model hypertrophy. Some of the hypertrophied cells burst and release their contents into the cartilage matrix around them. This changes the pH of the matrix and it is this change in pH that triggers the calcification of the cartilage matrix. As the cartilage begins to calcify, chondrocytes begin to die as their nutrients can no longer diffuse through the calcifying matrix. Where the chondrocytes had been, spaces called **lacunae** form and these eventually merge together forming small cavities within the calcifying matrix.

For bone formation or ossification to begin a nutrient artery must pierce the perichondrium and the calcifying matrix in the mid region of the cartilage model. This stimulates the osteogenic precursor cells in the perichondrium to become osteoblasts. Initially these remain just under the perichondrium and secrete a thin shell of compact bone called the **periosteal bone collar**. Once the perichondrium starts to produce bone rather than cartilage it becomes the **periosteum**. Osteoblasts are carried into the disintegrating calcified

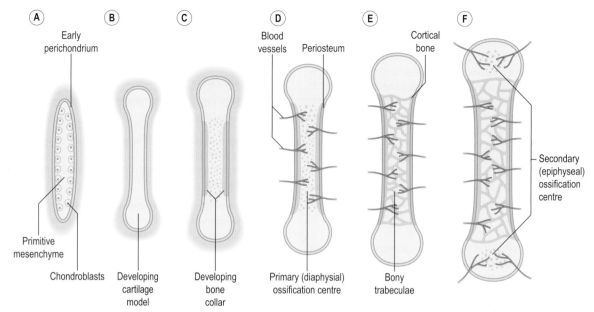

Fig. 9.5 **Endochondral ossification.**

matrix by the nutrient artery and its capillaries. Once these are within the cartilage model they begin to form bone and the **primary ossification centre** is formed. **Spongy** bone is formed as osteoblasts deposit bone matrix on the remains of the calcified cartilage. As the ossification centre enlarges towards the ends of the bone, osteoclasts start to break down the new spongy bone to form the **medullary cavity** in the centre of the bone, where the bone marrow will be located. Primary ossification therefore proceeds inwards from the external surface to the centre of the bone.

Primary ossification forms the diaphysis or shaft of the long bones, composed of an outer core of compact bone, lined with spongy bone surrounding a medullary cavity which is filled with red bone marrow. **Secondary ossification centres** form the epiphyses at the ends of the long bones and these usually develop at around the time of birth. The formation of bone in the secondary ossification centres is much the same as for that in the primary ossification centres. However, there is one difference in that spongy bone remains in the interior of the epiphyses. Secondary ossification also proceeds in an outward direction from the centre of the epiphysis towards the outer surface of the bone.

The still-growing bone has two regions composed of hyaline cartilage: the first is the cap of **articular cartilage** that covers the epiphyses at both ends of the bone, and the second is the **epiphyseal growth plate** located between the epiphysis and the diaphysis, which is responsible for the growth in length of the bones during childhood. The articular cartilage cap at the end of the bone is retained throughout life and helps to reduce the friction between the articulating bones.

Intramembranous ossification

The second process by which bone is formed is **intramembranous ossification**, where bone forms directly in the condensed mesenchymal cells without first going through a cartilage step (Fig. 9.6). This type of ossification tends to be found in the flat bones of the skull, the lower jaw, and the scapula of the pectoral girdle. At the site of future bone the mesenchymal cells condense as for endochondral

ossification, but they differentiate into osteogenic cells rather than chondroblasts. The osteoblasts cluster together forming a centre of ossification and secrete the organic bone matrix around themselves. Once surrounded, the osteoblasts become osteocytes located in lacunae and they extend fine cytoplasmic processes into canaliculi in all directions. Calcium and other mineral salts are deposited in the matrix within a few days and this hardens and calcifies forming **bony spicules**. The matrix develops into spongy bone with **trabeculae** (small pieces of bone) separated by spaces. The connective tissue associated with the blood vessels in the trabeculae differentiates into red bone marrow that fills the spaces. On the outside of the bone the mesenchyme condenses and develops into the periosteum. Finally, the most superficial layers of spongy bone are remodelled into compact bone with spongy bone remaining in the centre.

BONE GROWTH

During childhood the bones grow both in thickness and in length. The bones continue to grow in length until about 25 years of age, although they may still increase in thickness after this time.

Bone growth in length

Bone growth in length, especially the long bones, is by the addition of new bone on the diaphyseal side of the epiphyseal growth plates. The epiphyseal growth plate is composed of hyaline cartilage and separates the epiphyses from the diaphysis of the growing bones. It can be divided into four zones (Fig. 9.7).

■ Zone 1 is the zone of **resting cartilage**. It is closest to the epiphysis and is made up of small, scattered chondrocytes that have a low rate of proliferation. These cells do not have a function in the growth of the bone; their role is to anchor the epiphyseal growth plate to the bone of the epiphysis and to provide the supplies for the developing cartilage cells and to store the necessary materials (lipids, glycogen, proteoglycan aggregates) for growth.

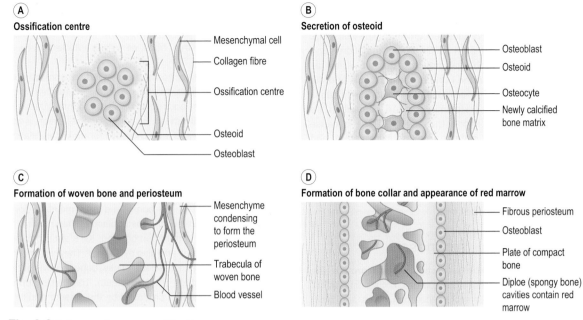

A

Ossification centre

- Mesenchymal cell
- Collagen fibre
- Ossification centre
- Osteoid
- Osteoblast

B

Secretion of osteoid

- Osteoblast
- Osteoid
- Osteocyte
- Newly calcified bone matrix

C

Formation of woven bone and periosteum

- Mesenchyme condensing to form the periosteum
- Trabecula of woven bone
- Blood vessel

D

Formation of bone collar and appearance of red marrow

- Fibrous periosteum
- Osteoblast
- Plate of compact bone
- Diploe (spongy bone) cavities contain red marrow

Fig. 9.6 **Intramembranous ossification.**

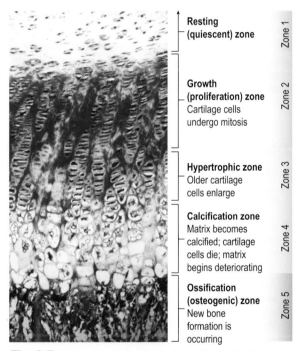

- Resting (quiescent) zone — Zone 1
- Growth (proliferation) zone — Cartilage cells undergo mitosis — Zone 2
- Hypertrophic zone — Older cartilage cells enlarge — Zone 3
- Calcification zone — Matrix becomes calcified; cartilage cells die; matrix begins deteriorating — Zone 4
- Ossification (osteogenic) zone — New bone formation is occurring — Zone 5

Fig. 9.7 **Bone growth in length.** From Young B, Heath JW 2014 Wheater's functional histology, 6th edn. Edinburgh, Churchill Livingstone, with permission.

- Zone 2 is the zone of **proliferating cartilage**. The chondrocytes are slightly larger and are stacked like coins. The chondrocytes are dividing and replacing the ones that are dying at the diaphyseal side of the epiphyseal growth plate. These chondrocytes produce the necessary matrix and are responsible for longitudinal growth of the bone via active cell division.
- Zone 3 is the zone of **hypertrophic cartilage**. This zone can be further subdivided into maturation, degeneration and provisional calcification zones. The chondrocytes increase in size, still in their columns, and they accumulate calcium within their mitochondria;

this causes them to deteriorate, and ultimately leads to their cell death. Upon their death, calcium is released from matrix vesicles, impregnating the matrix with calcium salt. The calcification of the matrix is necessary for invasion of metaphyseal blood vessels, destruction of cartilage cells, and the formation of bone along the walls of the calcified cartilage matrix. No active growth occurs in this layer; columns of cells extending toward the metaphysis are at various stages of maturation. This is the weakest portion of the physis and is commonly a site of fracture or alteration (e.g. widening, as in rickets).

- Zone 4 is the zone of **calcified cartilage**. This layer is only a few cells thick and is composed of mainly dead or dying chondrocytes, because they have become surrounded by a calcified matrix. The calcified matrix is removed by the action of osteoclasts and invaded by osteoblasts. The osteoblasts lay down new bone matrix and therefore result in the diaphyseal border being firmly attached to the epiphyseal growth plate. It is only by the action of the epiphyseal growth plate that the diaphysis can increase in length. Cartilage is replaced by bone at the diaphyseal end of the growth plate and new chondrocytes are added to the epiphyseal growth plate to maintain its size. Thus the thickness of the epiphyseal growth plate is maintained.

Between the ages of 18 and 25 the epiphyseal growth plates begin to close. The main stimulus for growth by the epiphyseal growth plate is **human growth hormone (hGH)**, which is secreted by the pituitary gland and promotes growth during childhood and adolescence. Growth hormone acts on the liver and other tissues to stimulate production of **insulin-like growth factor 1 (IGF-1)**, which is responsible for the growth-promoting effects of growth hormone and also reflects the amount produced. The amount of hGH, and so IGF-1, declines with age.

As the levels of hGH and IGF-1 begin to decline the chondrocytes in zone 2 stop dividing and so the thickness of the epiphyseal growth plate gets thinner as bone gradually replaces the cartilage. Eventually only the epiphyseal line remains as a bony feature on the bones, indicating that the bones have stopped growing. The last bone to finish growing is the clavicle. On X-rays of children and young adults, the epiphyseal growth plates are visible as a black region between the bone of the epiphysis and the diaphysis, as cartilage is radiolucent. If a fracture damages the epiphyseal growth plate while it is still open, then the fractured bone may be shorter than normal. This is because the epiphyseal growth plate is an avascular structure and damage to it accelerates the closure of the plate and so growth of the bone is reduced. If the rate of bone formation is reduced then the affected bone will be shorter and may cause misalignment of joint surfaces, and in severe cases shorter stature (Clinical box 9.6).

Growth in bone thickness

Bone can increase in thickness by **appositional growth**. The periosteal cells at the bone surface differentiate into osteoblasts and components secrete collagen fibres and other organic and inorganic matter forming the bone matrix. The osteoblasts become surrounded by the matrix and develop into osteocytes. This forms bone ridges along the bone on either side of a periosteal blood vessel. As more bone matrix is produced, the ridges grow and form a groove for the blood vessel, eventually fusing into a tunnel for the vessel. The former periosteum now becomes endosteum that lines the tunnel.

Bone deposition continues from the osteoblasts in the endosteum forming concentric lamellae that proceed towards the centre of the tunnel. Once the tunnel is filled in with bone it is a new osteon. As an osteon is forming, osteoblasts under the periosteum deposit a new circumferential lamella, which further increases the thickness of the bone. This process continues as new periosteal blood vessels become enclosed.

As new bone is being added on the outer surface of the bone, the bone lining the medullary cavity is being destroyed by osteoclasts in the endosteum. Therefore, the medullary cavity gets larger as the bone increases in diameter.

Clinical box 9.6	Achondroplasia (without cartilage formation)

Achondroplasia is the commonest cause of short stature, with an average adult height of about 1.2 m (4 ft) for affected men and women, and it occurs in around 1:22 000 live births. Achondroplasia is an autosomal dominant disorder, but approximately 80% of cases represent new dominant mutations. Achondroplasia is due to a mutation in the **fibroblast growth factor** receptor 3 (*FGFR3*) gene on chromosome 4, 99% of them being due to an A to C point mutation leading to an amino acid substitution.

The mutation affects endochondral ossification through inhibition of chondrocyte proliferation in the growth plate cartilage, affecting the growth of the limbs in particular and leading to short bones and reduced height. The diagnosis of achondroplasia is based on a number of very specific features that can be seen in X-rays, such as frontal skull 'bossing' and a 'champagne glass' pelvis, and 'trident' hands, in which the fingers are of similar length.

Children affected with achondroplasia frequently have delayed motor milestones, otitis media and bowing of the knees. Although infants with the condition are at an increased risk of death, most thereafter lead independent and productive lives and are of normal intelligence.

Factors affecting bone growth

Adequate dietary intake of minerals and vitamins is essential to maintain the growth of bone, as well as sufficient levels of several hormones.

Calcium and phosphorus are needed in considerable quantities during bone growth. Fluoride, magnesium, iron and manganese are required in smaller amounts. Vitamin C is required for the synthesis of the collagen – which is the main bone protein – and is also needed for the differentiation of osteoblasts into osteocytes. The vitamins K and B_{12} are required for protein synthesis, and vitamin A stimulates the activity of osteoblasts.

IGFs are the most important hormones during childhood to stimulate growth of the bones and help maintain bone mass in the adult, stimulating osteoblastic differentiation of mesenchymal cells in bone remodelling. IGFs are produced by the bone tissue itself and also by the liver. They act by promoting cell division and synthesis of new bone proteins at the epiphyseal growth plate and periosteum. The production of IGF is stimulated by hGH produced by the anterior pituitary. The thyroid hormones T_3 and T_4 and insulin are also required for normal bone growth.

At puberty the ovaries and testes secrete sex steroids which stimulate IGF-1. Initially the sex steroids cause a sudden growth spurt and the oestrogens in the female start to cause changes in the female skeleton, such as a wider pelvis. The sex steroids, especially oestrogens, contribute to the shutting down of the epiphyseal growth plate. Females have more circulating oestrogens than males, who have higher androgens; therefore, the lengthwise growth of bones stops earlier in females than in males.

Bone remodelling

In normal life there is constant bone remodelling, where the resorption of bone by osteoclasts matches the formation of new bone by the osteoblast cells.

- **Resorption.** Osteoclasts attach to the surface of old bone that is about to be resorbed. The ruffled border of the osteoclast faces the bone surface; they seal themselves onto the bone surface when activated. They secrete enzymes such as **collagenases** and **lysosomal enzymes** that attack the organic portion of the bone under the leak-proof seal beneath their ruffled border. They also secrete acid to dissolve the inorganic salts of the bone matrix. Both bone proteins and minerals – mainly calcium salts – enter the osteoclasts and pass through to be excreted into the extracellular space (Fig. 9.8).
- **Formation.** The next step is that osteoblasts migrate into the hollowed out space prepared by the osteoclasts. They synthesise **type I collagen**, **osteocalcin** (also known as **bone Gla protein**), and the other organic components of bone such as proteoglycans and growth factors that together form osteoid. The osteoblasts also control the mineralisation of the bone. The osteoid matrix is gradually coated in calcium salts and hardens.
- **Quiescence.** As the osteoblasts become embedded in the mineralising matrix, they slow down their production of matrix protein and become osteocytes. The bone is now in a resting phase of the remodelling cycle.

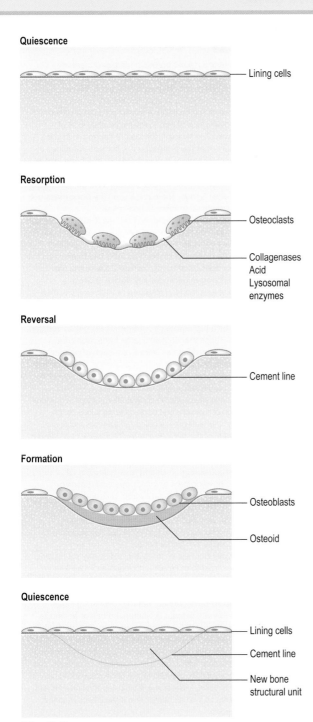

Quiescence

— Lining cells

Resorption

— Osteoclasts

— Collagenases
Acid
Lysosomal
enzymes

Reversal

— Cement line

Formation

— Osteoblasts

— Osteoid

Quiescence

— Lining cells

— Cement line

— New bone
structural unit

Fig. 9.8 **Bone remodelling.**

Resorption and new formation are normally well balanced but where resorption is increased a basophilic lesion occurs (the **cement line**) where remodeling is obvious histologically as new bone fills a resorbed cavity.

This remodelling cycle is the same for both compact cortical bone and the trabecular network of the internal spongy bone. This constant remodelling means that old bone is removed before it can deteriorate, and also redistributes the bone matrix along lines of mechanical stress. Uncoupling bone resorption from bone formation leads to the bone conditions with a loss or increase in the body's bone mass, as seen in osteoporosis, osteomalacia or Paget disease (Clinical box 9.7)

The whole process of bone remodelling takes between 160 and 200 days from when the osteoclasts begin to remove the old bone and when the osteoblasts have become

---

Clinical box 9.7   **Paget disease (osteitis deformans)**

In **Paget disease** there is accelerated bone turnover, which is indicated by an increased osteoclast-mediated bone resorption. The osteoclasts seen in Paget disease patients are numerous and large, with up to 100 nuclei in them. The alkaline phosphatase levels are very high as well indicating increased osteoblast activity. The increase in bone turnover leads to thicker but softer bones and is frequently associated with fractures.

Paradoxically there is also **bone thickening**, but the new bone is new woven bone as there is no remodelling to stronger compact and trabecular bone. This thickening of the bone may trap nerves, resulting in severe bone pain. Untreated, the disease progresses and the legs may bow, the spine develops a curvature and the skull may increase in size with the person's hat size going up several sizes. If there is severe skull enlargement there can be problems with the patient's vision and hearing as the nerves become trapped. Treatment includes the administration of drugs that reduce bone turnover, such as bisphosphonates and analgesics.

Paget disease increases in prevalence with age and is more common in those with northern European ancestry. The cause is unknown although both genetic and environmental factors are thought to play a part.

---

embedded in the mineralised bone matrix. The final stage of bone healing after a fracture occurs by the same process as happens in bone remodelling (see below).

BONE'S ROLE IN CALCIUM HOMEOSTASIS

The main calcium store for the body is the bone, with 99% of the total body calcium stored in the skeleton; serum calcium represents less than 1% of the body's total calcium. The serum calcium level is extremely important for many vital bodily functions, such as blood clotting, nerve cell activity and many other cellular activities. The concentration of calcium ions in the blood plasma must be maintained within a narrow range (9–10.5 mg/dL, 2.2–2.6 mmol/L), as even small changes outside of this window can be fatal, from heart or respiratory arrest due to either calcium concentrations that are too high or low, respectively. The level of calcium in the blood must therefore be very tightly regulated by controlling the rate of calcium resorption from bone into the blood, and calcium deposition into the bones. There are two major hormones and one minor hormone that control calcium homeostasis.

Parathyroid hormone

Parathyroid hormone (**PTH**) is an 84-amino acid peptide which is secreted by **chief cells** within the four parathyroid glands, located on the back of the thyroid gland in the neck. PTH is the most important regulatory hormone of calcium concentration in the bone and blood and is linked to several negative feedback systems that adjust blood calcium ion concentration. A fall in blood calcium ions is detected by the PTH receptors, and PTH synthesis is increased and is released into the blood. PTH affects the activity of osteoclasts indirectly through its binding to osteoblasts, which increase the resorption of bone, thus resulting in the release of calcium from the bone into the blood. PTH also acts on the kidneys to increase calcium reabsorption, phosphate excretion and 1,25-dihydroxyvitamin D synthesis. Normally 95% of the calcium filtered by the kidney is reabsorbed, PTH actually decreases calcium reabsorption from the proximal tubule but increases the reabsorption from the distal nephron. There is also decreased phosphate reabsorption from the proximal tubule, which results in its increased excretion.

Vitamin D

1,25-Dihydroxyvitamin D (dihydroxycholecalciferol) is the second factor that controls serum calcium levels. Vitamin D is derived from two sources: the diet (D3) or by synthesis in the skin (D2). This is then converted to **25-dihydroxyvitamin D** in the liver, and then to the active 1,25-dihydroxyvitamin D in the kidneys. 1,25-Dihydroxyvitamin D is a very potent stimulator of intestinal calcium and phosphate absorption, and is also a stimulator of bone resorption, although only at high concentrations. At normal physiological levels 1,25-dihydroxyvitamin D is necessary for proper bone mineralisation, and the lack of vitamin D either due to dietary deficiencies or lack of sunlight exposure leads to osteomalacia (Clinical box 9.8).

The principal role of 1,25-dihydroxyvitamin D is the increased mineralisation of the bone matrix, a part of this is due to the raised plasma Ca^{2+} levels from the action of 1,25-dihydroxyvitamin D on the gut. 1,25-Dihydroxyvitamin D can also stimulate the proliferation and activity of the osteoblasts, which are producing the new bone matrix.

Calcitonin

Calcitonin (thyrocalcitonin) also contributes to the control of blood plasma calcium. It is released from the parafollicular cells of the thyroid gland in response to rising serum Ca^{2+} concentration (e.g. after a meal) and directly inhibits osteoclast activity, inhibits Ca^{2+} absorption by the intestines and inhibits renal tubular Ca^{2+} reabsorption, thus reducing plasma Ca^{2+} (and phosphate) concentrations. Therefore, calcitonin leads to less calcium resorption from the bones and more calcium is incorporated into the bone tissue. Under normal physiological conditions calcitonin has only minor effects, which, as outlined above, are the opposite of PTH.

Other factors affecting bone mass

Oestrogen

Oestrogen increases the activity of osteoblasts and decreases the activity of the osteoclasts that resorb bone. It therefore has a protective effect in women. Loss of oestrogen at the menopause removes this protective effect and there is

---

Clinical box 9.8 **Osteomalacia**

Osteomalacia is a softening of the bones and the childhood variety of this condition is **rickets**. There is no loss in the mass of the bones, but the ratio of matrix to mineral changes so that there is more bone matrix and less bone mineral than in the normal bones. It can produce similar symptoms to osteoporosis but they have different causes. Osteomalacia is due to the inadequate mineralisation of newly formed bone matrix. In contrast, in osteoporosis, mineralisation is normal. Rickets is only seen before the epiphyseal growth plate has closed, and causes a bowing of the legs as the bones are softer and bend. This may be due insufficient calcium absorption because of a lack of dietary calcium, or a lack of activated vitamin D, or phosphate deficiency from increased renal loss. In children, the bones are soft anyway because they are growing, so the deformities produced by osteomalacia may be severe, with curvature of the spine in addition to the bowed legs. In children the epiphyseal growth plate is widened and may be cup or trumpet shaped, and the line of ossification is less distinct. In adults, because the bones have stopped growing, the deformities are less severe, and the symptoms are more like osteoporosis. On an X-ray of an adult with osteomalacia, there may be pseudofractures visible on regions of bones that have muscle attachments. These radiolucent lines on the bones are called '**Looser's zones**' (Looser's lines).

Clinical box 9.9 **Osteoporosis**

Osteoporosis literally means porous bones, and there is a generalised loss of bone mass making the bones more insubstantial and brittle. In both men and women, bones reach their maximum density in early adulthood. By the age of 20 years, 90–95% of the peak bone mass has been attained and from around 40 years of age there is a gradual loss of bone mass. However, in women, the loss of oestrogen at the menopause means that the protection the hormone provides in preventing osteoclast activity is now removed, and bone loss is increased. As women's skeletons tend to be lighter to begin with, a relatively small loss of bone mass can have severe implications on the health of their bones. There is a loss in the bone mass but the ratio of bone matrix to mineral is unchanged.

The condition is usually diagnosed from the X-ray appearance of the bones where they appear more radiolucent and less dense than normal. However, normal X-rays are relatively insensitive to the loss of bone mass and as much as 50% has to be lost for it to be clearly seen on an X-ray. Instead **DXA scans** are used to measure **bone mineral density** (**BMD**) in which a density **T-score** of less than 2.5 standard deviations away from normal is considered to indicate osteoporosis. In most cases of osteoporosis the loss of bone is not evenly distributed; trabecular (spongy) bone has a higher rate of bone remodelling than cortical (compact) bone. Those that contain a large trabecular bone framework are particularly at risk, with a reduction of between 2% and 3% per year, in comparison with cortical bone where the loss averages 1–2% per year. Bones forming the hip, spine, shoulder and forearm are particularly at risk.

The loss of bone mass has no clinical effect unless a fracture occurs. Fractures of the vertebral bodies create a loss in the anterior height of the vertebrae, leading to kyphosis (excessive posterior curvature) of the back. Fracture of the neck of the femur increases with age until by the age of 75 it is the most common type of fracture, due to the osteoporosis seen in the elderly.

Genetic, hormonal, nutritional and activity factors all play a role in the development of osteoporosis. Excessive glucocorticoid activity, either naturally from an adrenal tumour or from artificial sources such as the prolonged use of corticosteroids, also lead to the loss of bone mass and osteoporosis. Excessive alcohol and smoking can also lead to the loss of bone mass and brittle bone.

To prevent osteoporosis, children and especially young girls should be encouraged to maintain an adequate dietary intake of calcium, and to exercise, both of which will build up the strength of the bones. Throughout life adequate dietary calcium and exercise should be continued, not to prevent bone loss but to minimise the rate of loss. In women the use of **hormone replacement therapy** (**HRT**) has been shown to slow down the development of osteoporosis in postmenopausal women.

Apart from HRT another treatment available for osteoporosis are **bisphosphonates**. These are pyrophosphate analogues that bind to the hydroxyapatite crystals of the bone matrix and so inhibit bone breakdown. They also inhibit osteoclast attachment to the bone matrix, as well as stimulating osteoblasts to inhibit osteoclast formation.

---

a rapid loss of bone mass in the 5 years around the time of the menopause (Clinical box 9.9).

Exercise

As bone is continually being formed and broken down it has the ability to alter its strength in response to **mechanical stress**. More new bone is deposited along the lines of stress, and calcitonin production is increased to inhibit bone resorption. With no mechanical stress, bone does not undergo normal remodelling and bone resorption outweighs bone formation. The main mechanical stress that bone encounters is from the contraction of skeletal muscles and the pull of gravity. If a person is bedridden or has a fractured bone that is placed in a cast, the strength of the unstressed bones reduces. Astronauts who live in a low gravity environment for even a short length of time lose bone mass dramatically – as much as 1% a week. The bone of athletes on the other hand, whose bones are continually under repetitive stress, become thicker. Any weight-bearing activity helps to maintain bone mass and this is especially vital just prior to the closure of the epiphyseal growth plate, as it helps to build up bone mass prior to the inevitable loss with age. Even in the elderly, weight-bearing activities can help to slow the loss of bone mass.

Diet and bone mass

A calcium intake of between 800 mg and 1500 mg per day is considered to be adequate for most adults; children and teenagers require higher levels of calcium in their diet as their bones are actively growing. However, the amount of calcium required to be taken in from dietary sources must be considered alongside those of the other dietary components that affect absorption of calcium from the gut, and also those factors that influence calcium losses.

Calcium is lost from the body in urine, gut secretions and sweat. To avoid a net loss of calcium from the bones the calcium absorbed from food in the gut must balance the losses. Otherwise, the body will take calcium from bone to maintain the required level of calcium in the blood. The body contains about 1 kg of calcium in the bones. Even a small excess in the loss of calcium compared with absorption of just 30 mg per day, will after a year result in a 1% loss of calcium from the bones.

The typical diet of North Americans and Europeans contains four dietary components with equal importance that also lead to a net calcium *loss*: high sodium, high protein, low potassium and low bicarbonate intakes.

- Increasing the sodium intake from 1000 mg to 4000 mg per day causes an additional 52 mg of calcium loss per day.
- Increasing the protein intake from 40 g to 100 g per day will cause an additional calcium loss of 66 mg per day.
- Decreasing the potassium intake from 8000 mg to 2000 mg per day will increase calcium losses by 31 mg per day.
- Decreasing the bicarbonate intake from 100 mmol to 20 mmol per day will increase calcium losses by 32 mg per day.

In children, adolescents and younger adults, calcium absorption is more efficient and adapts better to increased losses with better production of 1,25-dihydroxyvitamin D. Older individuals of both sexes show a decline in calcium absorption of about 30–40% less at 80 years than at 30 years of age, and so they are affected more by these dietary factors.

The best foods for increasing calcium absorption without effecting calcium loss are the green leafy vegetables, such as kale and spring greens. There is no evidence that high dairy food consumption increases calcium levels and these foods are also usually associated with high saturated fat intake, and the high calcium content of many of these foods is often offset by their high sodium and protein content. Foods such as meat, fish and eggs, which are low in calcium, but which also drive high calcium losses should be eaten in moderation, while some low-calcium foods, such as bananas and oranges stimulate calcium absorption, providing a boost.

The Asian diet is also not without problems for calcium absorption. Phytic acid is found in high quantities in *chapatti* flour and combines with calcium in the gut to make it unabsorbable. The pH of the blood also plays a significant factor in osteoblast and osteoclast activity. As the blood pH drops, the balance is shifted in favour of osteoclasts and therefore bone density declines. The pH of the blood decreases with age, as kidney efficiency declines, and it is also more sensitive to the balance between acid and bicarbonate from the diet. Consuming alkaline foods, which are typically high in potassium relative to protein, will increase the pH of the blood, thereby shifting the balance in favour of the osteoblast activity. However, a low protein diet causes a decline in the production of growth hormones and even of bone proteins such as collagen. It is therefore very important to maintain adequate protein intake while eating plenty of alkaline foods such as fruits and vegetables to balance the acid from the protein. It should be noted that proteins that come from vegetable sources (other than grains and some nuts) are usually alkaline, whereas proteins from animal sources are usually acidic.

BONE HEALING

A **fracture** is any break in the bone; the process of bone healing is an ordered progression of steps. Bone is about the only tissue in the body that when it heals it is stronger than before the fracture. Usually scar tissue is weaker than the original, but with bone the healing process leads to new bone tissue which is as strong if not stronger than the old bone that broke.

There are three phases in the healing process: reactive, reparative and remodelling.

- **Reactive phase**. The first step in the repair process is the formation of a **fracture haematoma**. There are numerous blood vessels throughout the bone. As a result of the fracture the blood vessels that cross the fracture line are damaged and blood leaks out into the fracture site. A blood clot forms 6–8 hours after the fracture. The blood supply to the bone cells that lie on either side of the fracture is disrupted, and they begin to die. The dead cells induce macrophages and osteoclasts to start removing the dead bone and other cells from the fracture site and these cause a localised swelling and inflammation. The haematoma serves as a focus for the healing process.

  The next step in the healing process is to re-establish the blood supply to the area, so that new cells can begin to heal the fracture. Blood capillaries grow into the haematoma. This stage may last several weeks but it is during this process that the presence of nicotine in the system can inhibit this capillary ingrowth, and for smokers there is an increased length of fracture healing compared with non-smokers.

- **Reparative phase**. The next step is the formation of a **fibrocartilaginous callus**; the new blood vessels that grow into the haematoma begin to organise it into a granulation tissue, called initially a **procallus**. Fibroblasts from the periosteum, and osteogenic progenitor cells from the periosteum, endosteum and the red bone marrow start to invade the procallus. Collagen is produced by the fibroblasts, which become chondroblasts, and these connect the two ends of the fracture together. The osteogenic progenitor cells enter the bordering regions of healthy bone on the edges of the dead bone, ready to start making new bone matrix. As more chondroblasts form they begin to make fibrocartilage which replaces the procallus. This stage lasts about 3 weeks. The procallus and the fibrocartilaginous callus that replaces it are very soft in the first 4–6 weeks of fracture healing, so there is need for adequate support and bracing until the callus begins to ossify.

The next step in the healing process is the formation of the **bony callus**. The osteogenic progenitor cells that invaded the procallus and migrated to the borders of the dead/healthy bone region form into osteoblasts and begin to secrete bone matrix. They form spongy bone trabeculae which at this stage are not arranged in an ordered way and so the new bone is called **woven bone**. The trabeculae join the living bone tissue on either side of the fracture. Depending on the size of the bone and the severity of the injury, it may take up to 3 months for the whole of the fibrocartilaginous callus to be transformed into bone of adequate strength.

- **Remodelling**. The final step in the healing process is bone remodelling. The woven bone lattice is rearranged into the normal cortical and spongy bone arrangement. The woven bone is removed gradually by the action of the osteoclasts and replaced by other osteoblasts. Sometimes the repair is so good that the fracture line is undetectable even on an X-ray.

JOINTS

Joints occur at the joins between two or more bones and can be classified according to the type of connecting material into four types:

- Bony joints
- Fibrous joints
- Cartilaginous joints
- Synovial joints.

They can also be classified according to the amount of movement that is possible at the joint:

- Synostoses and synarthroses – fixed, unmovable joints
- Amphiarthroses – where some movement is possible
- Diarthroses – which are freely movable.

BONY JOINTS

Bony joints are formed where a previous gap between two bones ossifies, effectively forming a single bone – a synostosis. For example the right and left frontal and mandibular bones in infants fuse, and in the elderly some of the cranial bones may fuse. The first rib and the sternum can also fuse with age, as do the epiphyses and diaphysis of the long bones.

FIBROUS JOINTS

Fibrous joints are connected via fibrous tissue, with no cavity between them. These are **synarthroses**, as there is usually very little movement at the joint because the bones are held together very closely via fibrous tissue crossing the joint. There are four types of fibrous joint:

- Suture
- Syndesmosis
- Gomphosis
- Schindylesis.

Suture

A type of fibrous joint called a **suture** is found between the bones of the skull where dense connective tissue is found

between the closely interlocked bones. They may be **serrate**, as seen in the parietal bones, **bevelled**, as seen associated with the temporal, sphenoid and occipital bones, or **butt**, seen in the roof of the mouth where the palantine and maxilla bones meet.

At birth the bones of the skull vault are separated via broad fibrous bands of tissue called **fontanelles**. These allow an easier passage of the baby's head through the birth canal (pelvic outlet) during labour, by letting the skull mould, with the parietal bones over-riding each other. This makes the baby's head temporarily smaller and a few days after birth the head returns to its normal shape. The fontanelles are also vital *after* birth as they also allow the brain to grow.

The anterior fontanelle is the largest and generally closes by 18–24 months after birth. While it is open it can be used to help in the diagnosis of raised intracranial pressure. As the fontanelle is composed of fibrous tissue rather than bone it can be gently palpated; a fontanelle that is dome-shaped and does not depress when gently pressed indicates a raised intracranial pressure.

The fontanelles remain open until at least 18 months after birth; however, the sutures are still separated by fibrous tissue. The sutures can still be seen on the adult skull, as most never fully close (Clinical box 9.10).

Syndesmosis

Another type of fibrous joint is a **syndesmosis**. These are formed by either a bundle or sheet of fibrous tissue between the bones. The bundles are **ligaments** while the sheets are called **interosseous membranes**. Syndesmoses are found in the lower legs between the distal tibia and fibula, forming the **distal tibiofibular joints**. These joints have a short ligament between the bones so they are very rigid. Another syndesmosis is found in each lower arm between the radius and ulna, forming the **radioulnar interosseous joints**. These bones are connected by an interosseous membrane so these joints do allow a little movement between the bones, especially in the radius and ulna, allowing pronation and supination, and so functionally are **amphiarthroses**.

Clinical box 9.10   **Craniosynostosis syndromes**

Clinically there are a number of conditions where the fontanelles and the sutures close prematurely; these are all classified as **craniosynostosis syndromes**. The sutures may close before birth, making labour difficult and life-threatening for both the baby and the mother, and such babies are often delivered by caesarean section. Children born with one of these conditions may have to undergo extensive and repeated surgery to open the sutures to allow the brain to develop and grow; without this the intracranial pressure rises, which can cause brain damage. The sutures and fontanelles also allow the face to grow after birth, and if they close prematurely then the skull is attached to the base of the skull earlier than normal and the face tends to appear flat with bulging eyes as the orbit fails to grow to accommodate the eyes, and the mandible protrudes giving malocclusion of the teeth. The genetic basis of many of the craniosynostosis syndromes have been linked to mutations in the fibroblast growth factor receptor genes or in the TWIST genes. These mutations result in an activated receptor even in the absence of the ligand, which seem to cause premature ossification of the skull bones. In a few conditions other regions of the skeleton are also affected, mainly the hands and feet, with fused digits (**syndactyly**).

Gomphosis

Each tooth is connected to the bone of the upper or lower jaw via a fibrous joint called a **gomphosis**. The dense fibrous connective tissue between the tooth and its socket in the alveolar bone is called the **periodontal ligament**. In most healthy cases there should be no or only very limited movement between the elements of the joint; only in dental gum disease does the gomphosis become weakened and the tooth loosen in its socket.

Schindylesis

The last type of fibrous joint is the **schindylesis**; this is an articulation where a thin plate of bone is received into a cleft or fissure formed by the separation of two laminae in another bone. An example of a schindylesis is the articulation of the rostrum of the sphenoid and perpendicular plate of the ethmoid with the vomer (all found in the upper facial part of the skull), or in the reception of the latter in the fissure between the maxillae and between the palatine bones.

CARTILAGINOUS JOINTS

Cartilaginous joints are generally classified as amphiarthroses in that they allow slight movement. In this class of joints, the bones are connected via cartilaginous connecting material and there is no synovial cavity between the bones. There are two types of cartilaginous joints:

- Primary
- Secondary.

Primary cartilaginous joints called **synchondroses**, where the joint is bridged by hyaline cartilage, tend to be temporary and are associated with the growth of the bones (especially the long bones). The epiphyseal growth plates are examples of a primary cartilaginous joint. They are temporary in that the epiphyseal growth plate will close and become bone when bone growth stops (becoming bony joints). There is little or no movement possible at these growth plates although the hyaline cartilage that joins the two parts of the bone can slip and cause problems (Clinical box 9.11).

A persistent synchondrosis is the joint between the first rib and the manubrium of the sternum, which usually remains cartilaginous throughout life but may ossify in later life as a bony joint.

Secondary cartilaginous joints are the **symphyses**, which are permanent joints that are designed for strength, resilience and limited mobility. In a symphysis the ends

of the bone are covered by hyaline cartilage, with fibrocartilage connecting the bones together. An example of this type of joint is the pubic symphysis, where the two coaxial bones of the pelvis are joined at the front; other examples are the anterior intervertebral joints between the vertebrae, and the manubriosternal and xiphisternal joints, which join the manubrium (superior) and xiphoid process (inferior) to the body of the sternum. Although the movement between the joints is limited, between the vertebrae the collective effect of all of the intervertebral discs allows significant spinal flexibility. All symphyses are located in the midline of the body.

SYNOVIAL JOINTS

Synovial joints are the largest and most important class of joints. They are all diarthroses, in that they allow free movement of the joint, although movement is more limited in the joints within the wrist and ankle. Most of the joints in the body are of this type and all the limb joints are synovial.

The normal synovial joint is highly effective at allowing low friction movement between the articular surfaces of the opposing bones. To achieve this low friction the articular cartilage is elastic and the joint is filled with fluid, which is kept in place by a relatively impervious layer of calcified cartilage and bone. Load-induced compression of the articular cartilage forces the interstitial fluid to flow laterally within the tissues through adjacent cartilage, which assists in protecting the cartilage from mechanical injury.

Synovial joint structure

Synovial joints all have the same characteristic features (Fig. 9.9). These are:

- **Articular cartilage** covering the ends of the bones
- An **articular capsule** consisting of a **fibrous capsule** surrounding the joint and a **synovial membrane** lining the cavity
- A **joint cavity** filled with **synovial fluid**.

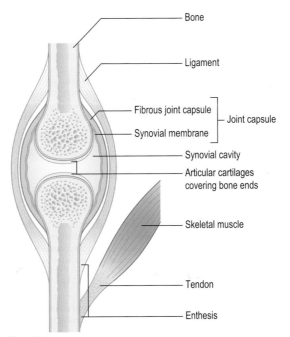

Fig. 9.9 Structure of a synovial joint.

The joint is usually reinforced by ligaments, external and/ or internal. Besides these features, which are present in all these joints, several other structures can be found in some synovial joints such as articular discs (menisci), labrum, ligaments and fat pads.

Articular cartilage

The ends of the bones are covered by a layer of articular cartilage, around 2–3 mm thick, separated by a narrow space, the joint (synovial) cavity. The cartilage is normally hyaline cartilage, except for in a few cases where coverage is with fibrocartilage. Hyaline cartilage provides the joint with a very smooth and slippery surface, which reduces the friction between the articulating bones and helps to absorb shock through its content of water and extracellular matrix proteoglycans. Although avascular, it readily absorbs synovial fluid which delivers both nutrients and oxygen to the chondrocytes within it. Loss and damage of the articular cartilage can lead to osteoarthritis (Clinical box 9.12).

Clinical box 9.12 | Osteoarthritis

Osteoarthritis is a degenerative condition which primarily affects the articular cartilage. Previously thought to be a 'wear and tear' condition, it is now considered to be due to abnormal mechanics and inflammation from cytokines and metalloproteinases released into the joint. It mainly affects the main weight-bearing joints of the body such as the hip and knee.

Early in the process the cartilage swells as the chondrocytes increase the synthesis of proteoglycans in a hypertrophic repair process. Later the amount of proteoglycans decreases and the cartilage loses its elasticity, which compromises the articular surface integrity, leading to bone being exposed. The protective effect offered by the articular cartilage is reduced, leading to pain and limits joint movement. On an X-ray you can see a loss of joint space as the articular cartilage is lost from the ends of the bones: as cartilage is radiolucent and does not show up on the X-ray, most of the gap normally seen between the adjacent bones is the articular cartilage. The joints can also become noisy (**crepitus**) as the rough surfaces move against each other.

The bone tries to compensate for the loss of the articular cartilage by producing new bone, leading to the growth of bony spurs (**osteophytes**) at the joint margins, which may reduce the movement at the joint even further. They can grow quite extensive, and may eventually break off, leading to loose bodies in the synovial fluid that may cause the joint to seize up completely. The production of osteophytes also leads to the presence of calcium pyrophosphate crystals in the synovial fluid; this is known as pseudo-gout. In the knee these calcium phosphate crystals may become embedded in the menisci and lead to their calcification, which is visible in X-rays as a white line in the middle of the joint.

As the articular cartilage is lost over the articular surface and bone is exposed, the underlying bone responds by making new bone subchondrally. This leads to a thickening of the bone or **bone sclerosis**, immediately under the remaining articular cartilage of the joint. However, the new bone produced is disorganised and weaker than normal bone, and may not withstand the normal stresses, leading to trabecular fractures. These are small fractures in the underlying bone, due to the new compression forces on the bone from being exposed to the synovial fluid directly, which can cause subchondral **cysts** to form. These may be the result of a group of trabecular fractures collapsing to form a cavity in the bone.

The end point of untreated osteoarthritis is that the head region of the bone may collapse completely and the complete loss of the articular cartilage may produce an **arthrodesis** of the joint. This is the fusion of the bone on each side of the joint, leading to the joint becoming immovable.

Articular capsule

The **articular** or **joint capsule** is a sleeve-like structure that surrounds and encloses the synovial cavity; it also acts to join the articulating bones together. It is composed of two layers.

- There is an outer **fibrous capsule**, which is composed of dense irregular connective tissue attached to the periosteum of the articulating bones. The fibrous capsule allows considerable movement while still maintaining great tensile strength. These features give synovial joints a great degree of movement with stability. Often there are fibres arranged into parallel bundles incorporated into the fibrous capsule, **ligaments**, often with individual names. Ligaments give added strength to the joint and help to prevent dislocations of the articulating bones.
- The inner layer of the articular capsule is the **synovial membrane** or **synovium**. This is composed of areolar connective tissue with elastic fibres. These allow the capsule to stretch during movement and to return to the resting position after the movement has stopped.

In many joints, the synovial membrane has accumulations of adipose tissue, which are called **articular fat pads**. The knee has several of these fat pads.

The synovium

The **synovium** is the inner lining layer of the joint cavity. It is composed of a layer of specialised cells, between one to three cells thick, called **synoviocytes**, and a **subintima** (Fig. 9.10). The synoviocytes line the inner surface of the synovium, which is composed of at least two types of synoviocytes, designated type A and type B, also called the intima. There are also some other immediate cells (type C) which may be precursors.

Type A synoviocytes are derived from the bone marrow macrophage lineage. These synoviocytes mediate cytokine release in response to small immune complexes. There are also dendritic cells, which are antigen-processing cells that are involved in the generation of an immune response.

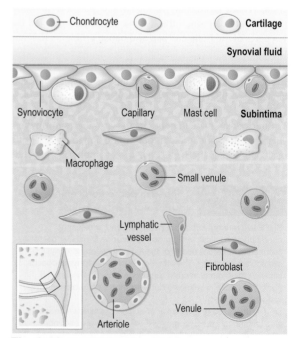

Fig. 9.10 **Structure of the synovium.**

Type B synoviocytes are of the fibroblast-like mesenchymal cell lineage. These synoviocytes keep the surface intact, smooth and non-adherent. The type B synoviocytes synthesise large amounts of the proteoglycan, hyaluronic acid, which then passes into the synovial fluid (see below). The synovium is permeable to water, small molecules and small proteins, but not to hyaluronic acid. This allows the synovium to trap the synovial fluid within the cavity.

The synoviocytes lie in a matrix of collagen fibrils and proteoglycans; no basement membrane separates this from the subintima, so forming one continuous layer. The subintima is made from loose connective tissue and contains a dense network of fenestrated capillaries, which allow the diffusion of nutrients and metabolic waste between the synovium and the blood. Lymphatic capillaries remove large molecules from the synovium. The synovium contains nerve endings that produce pain, particularly during inflammation (Clinical box 9.13). Tendon sheaths and bursae are also lined with similar synovium (see below).

The synovial fluid

The **synovial fluid** is present in relatively small quantities in normal synovial joints; even the largest joints such as the knee and the hip may only have a few millilitres of fluid. Normal synovial spaces contain only a microscopic film of fluid (about 50 μm thick) at sub-atmospheric pressure. In the healthy joint, the synovial fluid should be clear and a very pale straw colour, or colourless; it is a relatively acellular liquid and has high viscosity. Synovial fluid is an ultrafiltrate of blood plasma and contains **hyaluronic acid**, secreted by the synovial membrane. Hyaluronic acid (hyaluronan) is a long-chain glycosaminoglycan with a molecular mass of about 1 million. The hyaluronic acid gives the synovial fluid its high viscosity so it acts as a lubricant for the movement of the articular cartilage against each other. A non-Newtonian fluid (as is paint and blood), the viscosity of synovial fluid increases as the shear rate decreases. Not only does the synovial fluid have lubricant abilities but it also allows the exchange of metabolites between the plasma and the surrounding synovial membrane and articular cartilage. The half-life of hyaluronan in the joint cavity is about 24 hours. It eventually seeps out by a process of 'reptate diffusion', which can be considered as molecular 'snaking' through the tissue surface associated with the untangling and movement of long polymeric chains. Normal synovial fluid contains 3–4 mg/mL hyaluronic acid.

Lubricin, also known as proteoglycan 4, is a specialised glycoprotein which plays an important role in lubricating synovial joints at the boundary interface between opposing articular cartilage surfaces. The hyaluronic acid as well as helping to lubricate the joint also helps to maintain the thickness of the lubricating fluid film.

Water is able to enter the joint very quickly during inflammation, but once it mixes with the hyaluronan it cannot leave as quickly, and so a joint may swell within a few hours although the resultant inflammation may take several days to reduce. The synovial fluid also provides a cushion for the synovial lining by filling the crevices, which the synovial tissue cannot reach. The synovial lining cannot fill the space between the cartilage surfaces perfectly in all positions. If it did the joint would be like a vacuum pack and the synovium would probably be caught between the articular cartilages and damaged. If the joints are stretched suddenly, even the fluid does not fill all the space (synovial cavitation) and the

---

Clinical box 9.13 | **Rheumatoid arthritis**

Rheumatoid arthritis (RA) is the classic inflammatory arthropathy (joint disease) affecting about 1% of all populations and more common in females. The synovium undergoes characteristic changes histologically, although these are not specific for the disease. Eventually the changes in the synovium may lead to the destruction of the articular cartilage and result in the destruction of the joint.

The cause of RA is unknown but there are a variety of factors that are considered significant:

- Genetic factors account for 50% of the risk of developing RA and many share a particular epitope (antibody binding region) of the **human leucocyte antigen (HLA)-DR4** cluster. Other non-MHC (major histocompatibility complex) are also involved. The prevalence of this disease in the female is thought to be linked to **epigenetic factors** inherited from the parents. Epigenetic factors are differential methylation patterns within the DNA resulting in different expression derived from maternal and paternal genes.
- Infectious factors – various infectious agents have been linked to RA: *Mycoplasma* organisms, periodontopathic bacteria, Epstein-Bass virus (EBV) and rubella.
- Hormonal factors may be involved as pregnancy often results in quietening of the disease which emerges again post-partum, and a reduced prevalence has been reported in women taking oral contraceptives. Increased serum prolactin may be a risk factor for RA.
- Immunological factors. T cells are thought to be pivotal in the initiation of RA, leading to the activation of macrophages and fibroblasts within the synovium. Antigen-presenting B cells secrete cytokines and also produce autoantibodies which serve as diagnostic indicators of RA:
  - **Rheumatoid factor (RF)** is an IgM antibody often seen in RA although levels fluctuate and RF can be detected in a small number of individuals without RA
  - **Anti-nuclear antibody (ANA)** are seen in about 40% of individuals with RA

- **Anti-cyclic citrullinated protein antibody (ACPA)**, or **anti-CCP**, positivity is considered to offer high sensitivity and specificity in the diagnosis of RA, at least equaling that of RF.

In the early stages of rheumatoid arthritis, the synovium becomes swollen with excess fluid, thickened and hyperplastic with the synovial cells multiplying to such an extent that the synovium develops villi. There is endothelial cell activation which leads to the abnormal production of various cytokines and other inflammatory mediators (such as interleukin (IL)-1, IL-6, IL-8, tumour necrosis factor (TNF)-α, transforming growth factor (TGF)-β, fibroblast growth factor (FGF) and platelet-derived growth factor (PDGF) and involvement of B-cells, CD4 T cells, neutrophils, mononuclear phagocytes, fibroblasts and osteoclasts).

In the later stages of the disease, the inflamed synovium develops a layer of inflamed fibrous tissue known as **pannus**. In the pannus, new blood vessels form and allow more pannus formation. The pannus may spread over and even invade the articular cartilage, depriving the cartilage of its nutrients and leading to the death of the cartilage, and erosion of the bone underneath.

The synovial fluid often appears cloudy owing to the increased number of white blood cells, mainly neutrophils, which it now contains. It tends to have a lower viscosity than normal synovial fluid because of the biochemical breakdown of hyaluronic acid.

Unlike osteoarthritis, rheumatoid arthritis often involves periarticular structures as well as the joints, with any structure that has a synovial membrane affected; this includes tendon sheaths and bursae.

Juvenile RA (**juvenile idiopathic arthritis**) is a common arthritis in children and is also associated with a life-threatening complication (**macrophage activation syndrome**) due to the uncontrolled T lymphocyte and macrophage proliferation with consequential cytokine over-production and increased phagocytosis producing a pancytopenia.

lining may jump into the vacuum formed producing a noise (such as when finger joints are 'cracked').

Accessory ligaments

Many of the synovial joints have accessory ligaments, which are also called **extracapsular** and **intracapsular** ligaments, depending on whether they lie outside or inside the articular capsule. Examples of the extracapsular ligaments are the medial and lateral collateral ligaments of the knee. The intracapsular ligaments lie within the articular capsule but are excluded from the synovial cavity by folds in the synovial membrane. Examples of this type of accessory ligament are the anterior and posterior cruciate ligaments of the knee.

Articular discs

In some joints there are pads of fibrocartilage inside the synovial cavity, which are attached to the fibrous outer capsule and lie between the articular surfaces. These pads are called **articular discs** or **menisci**. The knee joint has lateral and medial menisci; they modify the shape of the articular surfaces of the bones so that they fit together better. They also direct the synovial fluid to the areas of greatest friction, thus giving added stability to joints and protecting the joint from damage during heavy work.

Blood and nerve supply to the joint

The nerves that supply the joint are the same that supply the skeletal muscles around the joint. The nerve endings are distributed around the articular capsule and associated ligaments. Some of the nerves convey pain from the joint to the brain. Others convey the degree of stretch that the joint is undergoing (see below).

The arteries around the synovial joint send out many branches that supply the ligaments and articular capsule with oxygen and nutrients. The veins remove the waste products of metabolism from the joints. However, as mentioned above, the articular cartilage gets its nutrition from the synovial fluid and not directly from the blood.

Types of synovial joints

There are six subtypes of the synovial joint, classified according to the shapes of the articular surfaces (Fig. 9.11):

- Planar
- Hinge
- Pivot
- Condyloid or ellipsoid
- Saddle
- Ball and socket.

The synovial joints can also be classified according to the type of movement that is performed at the joint. Movement can occur in a variety of axes.

- Non-axial: gliding movement only in a single plane
- Uniaxial/monoaxial: in a single axis
- Biaxial: in two axes
- Multiaxial: in many axes.

Planar or gliding synovial joint

The **planar** or **gliding joints** are non-axial joints which have the form of two flat plates which slide against each other. The articulating surfaces of these joints are usually flat or only slightly curved; there is only a limited range of movement

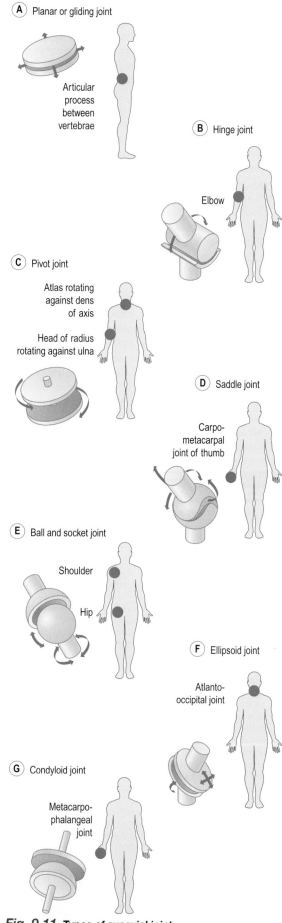

Fig. 9.11 Types of synovial joint.

possible at these joints, but the combined action of several allows for a significant range of movement. They allow a side-to-side, back and forth movement. Examples of planar joints are the intercarpal and intertarsal joints in the hands and feet (see Anatomy box 9.4, below) and between the vertebrae.

Hinge joint

The **hinge joint** consists of a convex part of one bone which fits into the concave part of another to allow uniaxial movement, as in a door hinge. Examples include the humeroulnar joint of the elbow (Anatomy box 9.3), the ankle joint and

---

Anatomy box 9.3   A simple hinge joint – the elbow

The elbow is possibly the most important joint of the upper limb as it brings the hands towards the head and the body. The elbow flexors are the 'hand to mouth' muscles producing movements which are vital in everyday life, such as in eating, washing and dressing.

The elbow extensors allow the upper limb to form a firm brace that can be used to push objects away from the body. People who have lost the use of their lower limbs rely on the elbow extensors to lift their body so that they can use crutches and to rise from a chair. The elbow is a hinge joint, but the forearm can rotate so that the lower end of the radius rotates around the ulna, carrying the hand with it (pronation or supination).

The elbow joint is a complex of three joints functionally, with all three joints within the same synovial cavity (Fig. AB3). The three joints are the:

- Humeroradial

- Humeroulnar
- Superior (proximal) radioulnar.

The humeroradial and humeroulnar joints allow flexion and extension of the elbow. The superior (proximal) radioulnar joint allows the pronation and supination of the forearm and hand.

The hinge joint between the humerus and ulna has bony surfaces that are interlocked in such a way as to constrain the flexion and extension movements of the elbow, preventing hyperextension and flexion of the joint. The flexion of the joint is not restricted by the ligaments that surround the elbow joint, but extension is limited by the contact of the olecranon process of the ulna with the floor of the olecranon fossa of the humerus. Adduction and abduction on the other hand are limited by the ligaments that surround the joint.

Acute and chronic conditions include dislocation (see Clinical box 9.14) and tennis elbow (see Clinical box 9.15).

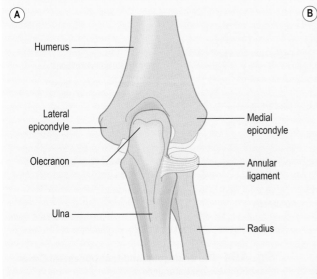

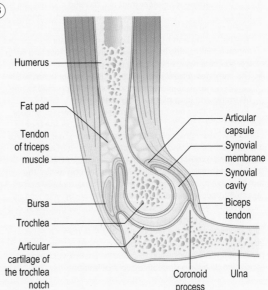

Fig. AB3 **The elbow joint.** (A) External view. (B) Cross-sectional view.

Clinical box 9.14   Elbow dislocation

The elbow may dislocate, normally posteriorly, in children who fall on their hands with their elbows flexed. The distal end of the humerus is driven through the weak anterior part of the elbow joint's fibrous capsule as the radius and ulna are displaced posteriorly. There is often an associated fracture of the head of the radius, coronoid process or olecranon processes of the ulna. Because of the posterior displacement of the radius and ulna, the ulnar nerve may be stretched or torn and results in numbness of the little finger and weakness in flexion and adduction of the wrist.

Clinical box 9.15   Tennis elbow

Pain around the lateral epicondyle of the humerus may be due to **tennis elbow**, also known as **lateral epicondylitis**. It is an overuse injury, causing inflammation of the common extensor tendon insertion although muscle fibrosis or a nerve entrapment syndrome are alternative causes of the pain. The main muscle that is affected is the extensor carpi radialis brevis, although the other extensor muscles may also be involved. The clinical signs of tennis elbow include a localised tenderness over the lateral epicondyle. Pain occurs when trying to extend the elbow with a pronated flexed hand, and is also experienced when pronating the arm when the elbow is fully extended. Attempts to lift a chair with fully extended elbows will also result in pain in this condition (the **chair test**), and pain on resisted extension of the wrist or middle finger (**Thomsen's test**). A similar condition can occur over the medial epicondyle, **golfer's elbow**, and is an inflammation of the flexor tendons. Both of these conditions can occur in individuals who do not play tennis or golf and are caused by repetitive elbow activity.

Anatomy box 9.4   **A modified simple hinge joint – the ankle and phalanges of the foot**

At the ankle (Fig. AB4A), a hinge joint is present between the inferior surface of the **tibia**, the medial surface of the lower **fibula** and the trochlear surface of the **talus**. Movement at the joint enables plantarflexion by **gastrocnemius** and **soleus** muscles, and dorsiflexion by **tibialis** and other extensor muscles with tendons within synovial sheaths that extend down the front of the leg and ankle joint into the foot. These tendons are prevented from 'bowstringing' by a thick fascia (**superior and inferior extensor, and superior and inferior peroneal retinaculum**) that form 'straps' across the front of the foot. The ankle joint is reinforced by three ligaments:

- **Medial (deltoid) ligament** attached to the medial malleolus of the tibia and to the navicular, talus and calcaneus bones
- **Lateral ligaments – anterior and posterior talofibular and calcaneofibular –** attached to fibula, talus and calcaneus
- **Inferior tibiofibular ligaments** (anterior and posterior) binding the medial condyles of the tibia and fibula and the talus.

While the ankle joint and its supporting ligaments provides great strength, excessive force that might be encountered in several sports, for example, can result in injury (Clinical box 9.16).

The **tarsal** bones illustrate different types of joints. The most important are:

- Between the talus and the posterior facet on the calcaneus is the planar **subtalar joint**, supported by the **interosseous talocalcaneal ligament**.
- The **talocalcaneonavicular joint** is a ball and socket joint formed by the hemispherical head of the talus and concave facets on the calcaneus and navicular bones, supported by the **medial, spring and bifurcate ligaments**. The spring ligament is important in maintaining the medial arch of the foot and laxity in this ligament results in **flat feet (pes planus)**.
- The **calcaneocuboid joint** is a concavo-convex condylar joint between the calcaneus and cuboid bones, supported by the **bifurcate and long plantar ligaments**.

In the foot the **metatarsophalangeal** and **interphalangeal** planar joints, forming the bones of the toes, enable the foot to plantarflex (through action of **flexor hallucis** (big toe) and **flexor digitorum** muscles) and dorsiflex (through action of **extensor hallucis** and **extensor digitorum** muscles) (Fig. AB4B). The digits are normally maintained parallel to the long axis of the foot by these muscles and their tendons. Hypermobility of the first metatarsophalangeal joint, that might develop with loss of muscle tone, leads to excessive pronation forces that result in the metatarsal moving medially and the toe laterally. The more the joint is displaced, so the tendons on one side gain a mechanical advantage and the pull on the metatarsal head causes bone proliferation and remodelling to produce a **hallux valgus** which might also develop a protective bursa or **bunion**.

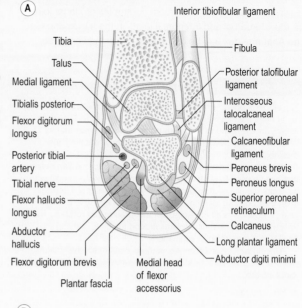

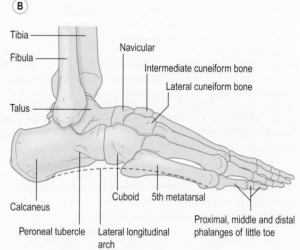

Fig. AB4 **The ankle joint and foot bones.** (A) Cross-sectional view. (B) Lateral view.

Clinical box 9.16   **Ankle fractures**

Previously also called **Pott's fracture**, this describes a range of ankle fractures caused by a combination of forced eversion or inversion to the extent that, for example, forced inversion causes the medial ligament to tear, fracturing the medial malleolus of the tibia. The talus moves laterally and shears off the lateral malleolus of the fibula and the tibia moves to the anterior and its posterior margin is sheared off by the tallus.

the interphalangeal joints (Anatomy box 9.4). The movement possible at a hinge joint is a simple opening and closing movement – **flexion** and **extension** at the elbow, **dorsiflexion** and **plantarflexion** at the ankle (Information box 9.1).

Pivot joints

The **pivot joint** allows uniaxial movement and in this type of joint there is usually a peg of bone that fits into another bone or ligament. An example of this type of joint is the atlanto-axial joint (between the C1 (atlas) and C2 (axis) vertebrae) in the neck. The movement is a rotational movement, thus the atlantoaxial joint allows one to say 'no' by turning the head from side to side. Another pivot joint is the superior (proximal) radioulnar joint, where the head of the radius fits into the annular ligament of the ulna. This joint allows one to **pronate** and **supinate** the forearm and hand. A third pivot joint is the inferior (distal) radioulnar joint at the wrist, where the lower end of the radius and the fibrocartilaginous disc over the head of the ulna articulate.

Condyloid or ellipsoidal joint

Condyloid or ellipsoidal joints allow biaxial movement; the articulation at the wrist between the radius and carpal bones and the metacarpophalangeal joints are examples of this type of joint (Anatomy box 9.5). One of the articular surfaces has a convex oval shape while the other has a concave depression into which the convex surface fits. The movements possible at these types of joints are **extension, flexion, abduction** and **adduction**, a mixture of all these movements producing **circumduction**.

Information box 9.1   Movements at joints

The different movements at the joints have specific names (Fig. 9.12). These are particularly useful in describing the available movement during a clinical examination.

- **Flexion** – decreasing the angle of the joint. For example, moving the head forwards at the neck or raising the arm above the head.
- **Extension** – increasing the angle of the joint. For example, moving the arm behind the body line.
- **Dorsiflexion** – upward movement of the foot, lifting the toes towards the front of the leg.
- **Plantarflexion** – lowering the toes away from the ankle (pointing the toes).
- **Abduction** – away from the midline of the body. For example, raising the arm to the side or spreading of the fingers.
- **Adduction** – towards the midline of the body. For example, moving the arm towards the body or closing the fingers.
- **Circumduction** – this is a combination of extension, flexion, abduction and adduction which allows a limb to draw a cone in space in a sort of stirring motion.

Special movements at particular joints

- **Supination and pronation** – this refers to a rotation of the hand involving the radius and ulna. Supination rotates the palm upwards and pronation rotates the arm to face the palm downwards.
- **Inversion and eversion** – this turns the sole of the foot. Inversion turns the sole inwards, facing the other leg, and eversion turns it outwards.
- **Protraction and retraction** – these movements move the body part forwards and backwards in the transverse plane. Jutting out the jaw is protraction and holding the shoulders back is an example of retraction.
- **Elevation and depression** – this is moving the body part upwards (elevation) or downwards (depression) in the frontal plane. An example of this is chewing where the lower jaw (mandible) is alternately elevated and depressed.

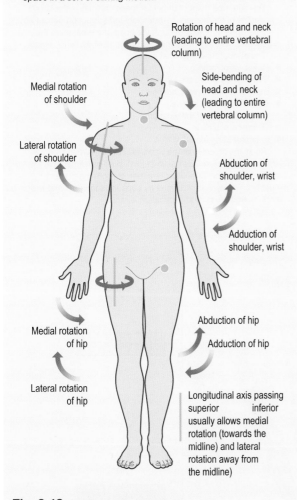

Fig. 9.12 **Anatomical movements.**

The stability of the wrist depends on capsular ligaments crossed by long tendons, which means that dislocations are rare. This region is called the **carpal tunnel** which connects the forearm to the palm (Anatomy box 9.5)

Saddle joint

Saddle joints can be considered a modified condyloid joint; they allow multi-axial movement, compared with the bi-axial movement of the condyloid joint, so the movement is freer. In the saddle joint, one bone is the rider and the other bone the saddle; one example is the carpometacarpal joint of

the thumb. At these types of joints a slightly larger range of movement is possible than at the condylar joints.

Ball and socket joint

The most versatile type of synovial joint is the **ball and socket joint**. There are only four ball and socket joints in the body, the two shoulder (glenohumeral) joints and the two hip (femoral-acetabular) joints (Anatomy boxes 9.6 and 9.7). These joints allow multi-axial movement and have the greatest range of movement among the joints, allowing extension, flexion, abduction, adduction, medial and lateral rotation and circumduction.

Anatomy box 9.5   Pivot, condylar and saddle joints – the wrist

The different joints within the wrist ensure the manual dexterity which is essential for both work and leisure activities.

The distal radioulnar joint forms a **pivot type synovial joint**. The rounded head of the ulna articulates with the ulnar notch on the medial side of the radius, so that during pronation and supination of the forearm, the head of the ulna rotates within the ulnar notch of the radius.

Condylar joints connect the radius to the proximal carpal bones, and form most of the metacarpophalangeal joints, apart from the articulation between the trapezium and the first metacarpal bone of the thumb, which is a **saddle joint**, enabling movement in two direction: **circumduction** (movement in a circle) and **opposition** (allowing the thumb to oppose the remainder of the digits in order to facilitate gripping of objects).

The eight carpal bones are arranged in two rows, the **scaphoid** and **lunate** bones articulate with the radius with the **pisiform** and **triquetrum** bones situated more medial to the lunate bone. The four distal bones (the **hamate, capitate, trapezoid** and **trapezium**) articulate with the metacarpals of the fingers (Fig. AB5A).

Fractures to the wrist are one of the most common fractures seen in the emergency department (Clinical box 9.17).

Two sets of movements are possible at the wrist joint, caused by radial and ulnar deviation, respectively:
- Flexion/extension
- Abduction and adduction.

Flexion-extension takes place about a mediolateral axis through the lunate and, due to the mobility of the carpal bones, also about the mediolateral axis of the capitate bone. Muscles passing anterior to these axes will act as flexors, while the muscles that pass posterior to these axes will act as the extensors.

The flexors of the wrist are the:
- Flexor carpi radialis
- Palmaris longus
- Flexor carpi ulnaris.

These muscles all have a common point of origin on the medial epicondyle of the humerus. The tendons of these three muscles can be seen on the anterior surface of the wrist when the hand is made into a fist and the wrist is flexed.

The palmaris longus is the central tendon, with flexor carpi radialis lying next to it on the radial (thumb) side. The tendon of flexor carpi ulnaris is harder to see but runs along the ulnar (little finger) side of the wrist. It is estimated that in 13% of the population, palmaris longus is missing. It is a weak wrist flexor and its main action is to tense the palmar fascia but the absence of the muscle has no significant effect on the flexion of the wrist. Because of this, it is a prime candidate for surgical removal for use as a tendon for the repair of damaged ligaments or tendons elsewhere in the body, such as for anterior cruciate knee ligament replacement.

The extensor muscles of the wrist are the:
- Extensor carpi radialis longus
- Extensor carpi radialis brevis
- Extensor carpi ulnaris.

The common point of origin for these muscles is the lateral epicondyle of the humerus. Abduction and adduction occurs about the anteroposterior axis through the head of the capitate, the largest and centrally positioned carpal bone of the wrist region.

The abductors of the wrist are:
- Flexor carpi radialis
- Extensor carpi radialis longus
- Extensor carpi radialis brevis
- Abductor pollicis longus.

The adductors of the wrist are:
- Flexor carpi ulnaris
- Extensor carpi ulnaris.

As all the muscles of the wrist, except for palmaris longus, have two actions across the wrist joint, pure movements at the wrist require simultaneous contraction of more than one of the muscles. The wrist is stabilised by capsular ligaments and the tendons that cross, and dislocation is rare.

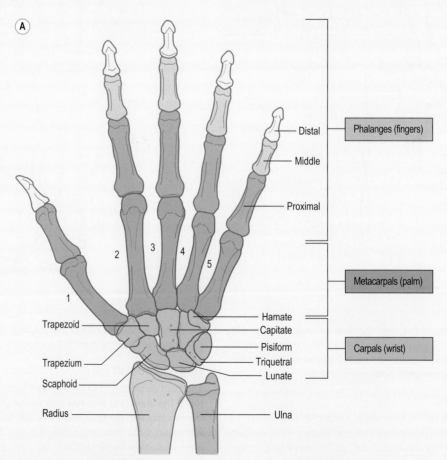

Fig. AB5 **The wrist.** (A) Bones of the hand.

Anatomy box 9.5 | Pivot, condylar and saddle joints – the wrist—cont'd

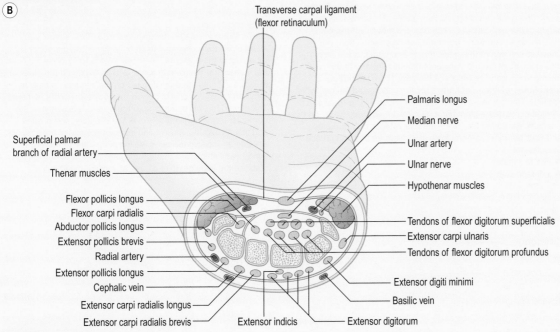

Transverse carpal ligament (flexor retinaculum)

Palmaris longus

Median nerve

Ulnar artery

Ulnar nerve

Hypothenar muscles

Tendons of flexor digitorum superficialis

Extensor carpi ulnaris

Tendons of flexor digitorum profundus

Extensor digiti minimi

Basilic vein

Extensor digitorum

Extensor indicis

Extensor carpi radialis brevis

Extensor carpi radialis longus

Cephalic vein

Extensor pollicis longus

Radial artery

Extensor pollicis brevis

Abductor pollicis longus

Flexor carpi radialis

Flexor pollicis longus

Thenar muscles

Superficial palmar branch of radial artery

Fig. AB5 cont'd – (B) Carpal tunnel.

The relationship between structures in the wrist is important but complex. The carpal tunnel is an area within the wrist on the palmar aspect bound by:

- The transverse carpal ligament (flexor retinaculum), on the volar (palmate) aspect
- The scaphoid tuberosity and trapezium, radially
- The pisiform and hook of the hamate, ulnarly
- The carpal bones and the deep volar radiocarpal and volar interosseous ligaments.

Running through the carpal tunnel is the median nerve, four flexor digitorum superficialis tendons, four flexor digitorum profundus tendons and the flexor pollicis longus muscle where it forms a flattened tendon at its distal end in the wrist (Fig. AB5B). **Carpal tunnel syndrome** occurs when the median nerve becomes trapped (Clinical box 9.18).

Clinical box 9.17 | **Wrist fractures – fracture of the distal radius (Colles and Smith)**

Colles' fractures are very common, and distal wrist injuries such as these account for 17% of fractures treated in the emergency department. A Colles' fracture occurs when a person falls onto their outstretched hand in the pronated position. The fracture site is usually 2–3 cm up the radius and the fragment is displaced proximally, causing a shortening of the radius, and dorsally, giving the broken wrist the resemblance of a dinner-fork.

Smith fractures are the reverse of a Colles' fracture and much less common. They are caused by falling backwards onto the palm of an outstretched hand, which leads to pronation of the upper extremity while the hand is fixed in supination by contact with the ground.

Clinical box 9.18 | **Carpal tunnel syndrome**

Carpal tunnel syndrome is the result of compression of the median nerve within the carpal tunnel leading to paraesthesia (pins and needles sensation) in the hand, sometimes accompanied by numbness, weakness and pain in some areas. Damage to the nerve leads to its demyelination and axonal degeneration as a result of increased pressure causing venous blockage, oedema and ischaemia. It is seen more commonly in women in middle age. Surgery, in which the transverse carpal ligament is divided, relieves the pressure and is highly successful, although long-term success is reduced.

Anatomy box 9.6 | **Ball and socket joints – the shoulder** (Clinical boxes 9.19 and 9.20)

Both the shoulder and the hip joints are ball and socket joints. However, there are significant differences between these joints which relate to their flexibility and the load bearing capacity of the different joints.

Shoulder joint

The shoulder joint itself is the joint between the head of the **humerus** and the **glenoid cavity** of the scapula: the **glenohumeral joint**. This is the most mobile joint in the body (Fig. AB6); the joint is so mobile because it is held away from the trunk by the **pectoral girdle**, which itself is largely suspended from the trunk via muscles rather than through joints.

The **clavicle** (collar bone) and the **scapula** (shoulder blade) form the **pectoral girdle**, which links the upper limb and the trunk. There is a large range of movements possible for the scapula and

a large part of the overall mobility of the shoulder is due to the mobility of the scapula. This is in contrast to the lower limb where the pelvis (the equivalent of the pectoral girdle) is firmly fixed to the axial skeleton, and so sacrifices mobility for increased stability and better load bearing capacity.

The head of the humerus lies in a rather flat **glenoid fossa**, and so its movements are not constrained by bony boundaries. The humeral head is four times larger than the glenoid cavity; this allows the head of the humerus a great range of movement around the glenoid cavity. The glenoid fossa is deepened a little by a ring of fibrocartilage called the **glenoid labrum**, and this does give the joint a small degree of stability. The joint capsule for the glenohumeral joint is also rather 'baggy', especially inferiorly, which allows the arm to be raised above the head. As well as being lax

Continued

Anatomy box 9.6   **Ball and socket joints – the shoulder—cont'd**

and loose, the articular capsule of the shoulder is also relatively weak, giving the glenohumeral joint plenty of 'give' before the extent of the joint capsule is reached and movement restricted.

The **coracohumeral ligament**, which extends from the coracoid process of the scapula to the humerus, is the only strong ligament around the glenohumeral joint and this serves mainly to support the weight of the arm. There are three **glenohumeral ligaments**, the superior, middle and inferior, which are only simple thickenings of the joint capsule. This means that the ligaments of the glenohumeral joint are relatively weak, and the muscles around the joint – the four **rotator cuff muscles** and their tendons – are the main stabilisers for the joint. These muscles are:

- Supraspinatus
- Infraspinatus

- Teres minor
- Subscapularis.

All four originate on the posterior side of the scapula and insert close to the humeral head on to either the greater or lesser tubercles of the humerus. Their main role is to stabilise the head of the humerus in the glenoid fossa, and to work with the other larger muscles such as the deltoid to act on the shoulder, mainly to rotate the humerus and to help in the abduction of the humerus. The deltoid muscle extends from the deltoid tuberosity on the humerus, forming the muscle over the shoulder, and divides and inserts into the clavicle and different regions of the scapula. Another stronger stabiliser is the **intracapsular tendon of biceps** (long head) which runs through the joint capsule and helps to stabilise the shoulder joint as well as moving the shoulder.

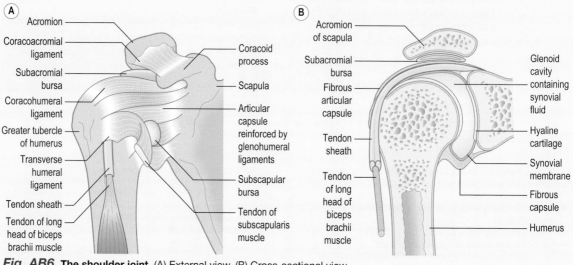

Fig. AB6 **The shoulder joint.** (A) External view. (B) Cross-sectional view.

Clinical box 9.19   **Shoulder dislocations**

As a consequence of the freedom of movement of the glenohumeral joint, it is likely to be dislocated by either a direct or an indirect injury. Because of the positions of the reinforcing elements and the position of the acromion and coracoid processes of the scapula, most dislocations are forwards (anterior). Posterior dislocations are the next most common; inferior dislocations are rare.

Two types of movement commonly produce dislocation of the shoulder:

- Excessive extension and lateral rotation of the humerus can drive the head of the humerus inferoanteriorly, which may tear the inferior part of the glenoid labrum as it is forced out of the joint. This is known as **Bankart lesion**.
- A hard blow to the humerus when the glenohumeral joint is fully abducted tilts the head of the humerus inferiorly onto the weaker part of the joint capsule. This may result in tearing the capsule and dislocates the shoulder so that the head of the humerus now lies inferior and anterior to the glenoid cavity.

After dislocation the strong flexor and abductor muscles around the joint pull the head of the humerus into a subcoracoid

position. The patient is unable to use the arm and commonly will support it with the other hand.

Two consequences of a shoulder dislocation are clinically relevant:

- The **axillary nerve** may be damaged by the displaced humeral head. This denervates the deltoid muscle and gives cutaneous denervation to a small area of skin covering the central part of the deltoid. Testing for the loss of sensation over the deltoid muscle is a sign of axillary nerve damage. If the axillary nerve is damaged then the deltoid muscle may waste and the rounded profile of the shoulder will be lost.
- The glenoid labrum may be torn. This forms a weak spot so that in the future the shoulder is easier to dislocate again and requires less force to do so.

Almost all the muscles that move the shoulder are innervated by the branches of the **brachial plexus** so damage to the brachial plexus, which can occur when the limb is pulled hard or by a severe blow to the top of the shoulder, can cause weakness and/or paralysis to the whole upper arm.

Clinical box 9.20   **Frozen shoulder**

Frozen shoulder or **idiopathic adhesive capsulitis** defines the syndrome in which both passive and active movement of the glenohumeral joint are severely restricted and extremely painful over a prolonged period of time. The cause is unclear but subacromial bursitis, calcifying tendinitis and partial rotator cuff tears have all been described as producing this clinical condition.

A complex joint

The knee is also considered to be a hinge joint although it is more complex as it has both condylar and planar joint elements (Anatomy box 9.8).

TENDONS AND LIGAMENTS

Tendons and ligaments are important tissues that normally serve to bind structures, such as joints, together and keep

The hip joint, where the **head of the femur** articulates with the **acetabulum** of the pelvis, is a strong weight-bearing joint but it has much less flexibility than the shoulder. Like the shoulder, the hip joint is another ball and socket synovial joint, but the acetabulum into which the head of the femur fits is already deep and is deepened even further by the presence of a ring of fibrocartilage, the **acetabular labrum** (Fig. AB7).

The joint has a strong fibrous **joint capsule** that is attached to the acetabular margin and to the pelvis and anterior femur. Inferiorly the capsule extends some way down the medial border of the femur; this gives the capsule enough slack to allow abduction of the hip joint. The fibres of the capsule form three strong ligaments that help to stabilise the joint. The **iliofemoral ligament** strengthens the front of the joint capsule, and the **pubofemoral** and **ischiofemoral ligaments** reinforce the back of the joint capsule.

The large muscles and tendons which cross the joint increase the stability of the joint but this is insignificant compared with the stability produced by the deep acetabulum and strong ligaments.

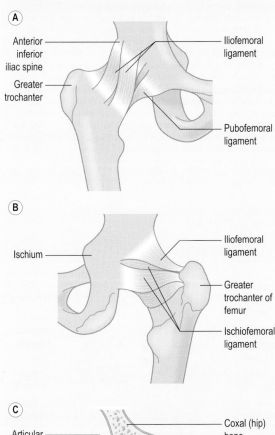

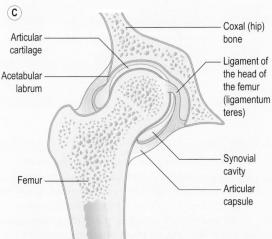

Fig. AB7 **The hip joint.** (A) Anterior external view. (B) Posterior external view. (C) Cross-sectional view.

Due to its stability, dislocations of the hip joint are rare, but **fractures of the femoral neck** are fairly common, especially in elderly women or any person with **osteoporosis**. The head and neck of the femur are mainly supplied with blood from the gluteal and obturator arteries (branches of the internal iliac artery). Following a fracture of the femoral neck, if the gluteal artery is damaged **avascular necrosis** of the femoral head may occur as the obturator artery is not sufficient to maintain the bone of the head of the femur. Avascular necrosis of the femoral head may occur in children spontaneously and is called **Perthe** or **Legg–Calves–Perthe disease**.

The nerve supply to the hip joint is via branches of the femoral, obturator, sciatic and gluteal nerves. Some of these nerves also give off branches that supply the knee joint as well as the hip. Therefore, pain originating in the hip may be referred to the knee.

Developmental dislocation of the hip (DDH), in which the femoral head is displaced relative to the acetabulum of the pelvis, is seen in about one in 60 newborns and is more common in girls, and in the first born. If it is untreated it disrupts the normal development of the hip and results in significant morbidity. The cause is unknown, although there are several risk factors.

A screening test (**Ortolani**) was devised for all newborns in which the knees are flexed and encircled with fingers lying over the trochanter. The hips are then flexed to a right angle and abducted. If the femoral head slips from the acetabulum this will be felt and a 'clunk' may be heard on subluxation and on reduction of the joint as the bone slips out and back in. Ortolani screening did not pick up all children at risk, however, and now a series of tests are used:

- All children are examined by experienced screeners twice, before 3 months of age.
- High risk children (breech presentation, family history of DDH, clicking hips) should also have ultrasound screening and rechecked when the child begins to stand.
- **Barlow's test** is also used to see if dislocation can be forced. The pelvis and sacrum are fixed with one hand and the other hand attempts to dislocate the hip with firm backward pressure. If the femur head is felt to sublux backwards then a wider abduction will reduce it and be felt by the screener.

them stable. They also have elastic properties that allow them to store energy and release it to muscle with no additional work.

Tendons and ligaments are soft collagenous tissues made of parallel rows of fibroblasts organised in microfibrils and 'wavy' fibrils which contribute to their non-linear strength. These are organised in separate fascicles within a single tendon, which can glide across each other within a sheath, independently.

- Tendons connect muscles to bones
- Ligaments connect bones to bones

Age and immobilisation change the structure of the collagen matrix, affecting its mechanical strength (Clinical box 9.23).

Injuries to these structures often produce severe pain and reduced mobility over a considerable time while the tissue repairs itself (Clinical box 9.24). The joint, or articular, capsule surrounds synovial joints and is usually composed of a network of independently moving ligaments and tendons associated with sheets of coarse fibrous connective tissue called **fascia**. Some joints, such as the sacroiliac joint, are surrounded almost exclusively by ligaments while

Anatomy box 9.8   A complex joint – the knee

Perhaps the most complex joint in the body is the **knee joint**. It is partly a hinge joint, allowing flexion and extension, but it also has **condylar joint** characteristics, which adds rotational movements to the list of movements possible at the knee. Standing in the anatomical position the knee is in extension in a stable configuration.

The knee is a compromise between mobility and stability. It is most stable when fully extended as it 'locks', making the lower limb a solid column and well adapted for weight-bearing. However, for locomotion the knee must unlock, and for this to happen the **popliteus muscle** contracts, causing the femur to rotate laterally so that flexion (unlocking) of the knee can occur. The knee joint is one of the most frequently used joints and as a result one of the most frequently injured joints.

The knee joint is surrounded by strong muscles and by ligaments that are arranged both inside and outside the fibrous joint capsule, which help to maintain the stability of the knee joint when it is straightened.

The knee is composed of articulations between three bones:
- Femur
- Tibia
- Patella.

The knee consists of three joints that are combined together (Fig. AB8). At the centre of the knee is the **femoropatellar joint**, a plane joint between the patella and the distal femur. The patella is a sesamoid bone (one that protects a tendon that crosses a joint) that is held at the front of the knee between the tendon of the quadriceps muscle and the **patellar ligament**. The other two joints are between the medial and lateral condyles of the femur and tibia, the **tibiofemoral joints**. Unusually the joint cavity is only covered by the capsule on the lateral and posterior sides. On the anterior surface the joint is covered by ligaments.

The menisci and the ligaments of the knee joint
The condyles of the femur and tibia do not fit very closely so to help with the stability of the joint there are two semicircular rings of fibrocartilage called the **menisci**. The **lateral and medial menisci** help to pack the joint so that the femur and tibia fit together better. They also help to distribute the load and direct the synovial fluid to the most stressed part of the joint.

The medial meniscus is partly attached to the **medial (tibial) collateral ligament**. This ligament is a broad band that partly blends with the joint capsule and so is partly attached to the medial meniscus. Often when one is injured the other is also damaged due to this connection. The lateral meniscus is completely separate from the lateral collateral ligament. The **lateral (fibular) collateral ligament** is a rope-like structure that is also separated from the joint capsule. These collateral ligaments prevent the knee joint from opening medially and laterally. They help to supply stability when the knee moves from side to side or when you make sharp twisting movements. Other ligaments outside the joint capsule are the **oblique and arcuate popliteal ligaments**, which reinforce the posterior of the knee. The front of the knee is stabilised in the middle by the patellar ligament and by the **lateral and medial patellar retinacula** ligaments, which extend from the quadriceps femoris muscle to the articular capsule on either side of the knee.

Inside the joint are two more ligaments that prevent the tibia from moving too far forwards or backwards on the femur. These are the cruciate ligaments, as they cross each other. The **anterior cruciate ligament** originates near the back of the femur and runs downwards to attach to the anterior of the tibia, while the **posterior cruciate ligament** runs from the anterior of the femur to the posterior of the tibia. On the tibia they attach to the tibial spines while on the femur they attach to the intercondylar notch.

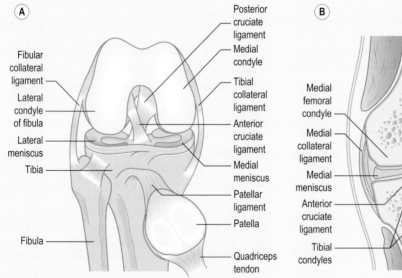
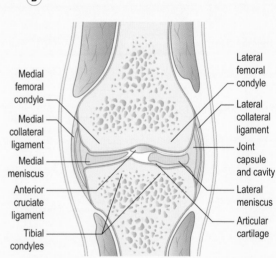

Fig. AB8   **The knee joint.** (A) External view. (B) Cross-sectional view.

Clinical box 9.23   Ageing and the changes in the joints

Production of synovial fluid decreases with age, while the articular cartilage loses water and so becomes thinner. The ligaments lose some of their flexibility. Therefore, by the age of 80, everyone will have degenerative changes in the major joints of the body such as the shoulder, elbow, hip and knee. Some of these degenerative changes can be seen in X-rays as early as 20 years of age.

others are surrounded by tendons, such as the rotator cuff muscle tendons around the shoulder. Tendons can pass through joint cavities, such as in the shoulder where the tendon of the long head of the biceps muscle enters the joint cavity and helps to stabilise the joint. **Aponeuroses** are flat, sheet-like tendons which attach muscles to bones or to other muscles.

The point on a bone where a ligament, tendon or apo-neurosis attaches is called an **enthesis**. The entheses are

Clinical box 9.24 | **Sprains and tears**

A sprain occurs when some of the fibres of a ligament are torn, often when a joint is over-extended. Sometimes there can be a complete tear, or rupture. Excessive repetitive overload can also produce a tendinopathy, with associated inflammatory processes. Although any joint can be affected common injuries are seen to the knee and ankle.

- The knee is stabilised by a series of ligaments: cruciate, posterior and capsular, which, along with collagenous pads (menisci), can become injured. Tears to the medial meniscus are commonly seen in association with injury to the anterior cruciate ligament

  The **anterior cruciate ligament** (**ACL**) is easily injured and accounts for 70% of cruciate ligament injuries. This high proportion of injuries is in part due to the close association it has with the **medial meniscus**, so that damage to the medial meniscus can cause tears not only in the medial collateral ligament but also in the anterior cruciate. Likewise, damage to the anterior cruciate can lead to damage to the medial meniscus and collateral ligament – an injury **triad**.

  Several provocative exercises are useful in the diagnosis of these injuries:

- The **anterior drawer test** attempts to jerk the lower leg forward when the knee is flexed to 90°, holding the thumbs over the tibia tubercle. If there is a differential displacement in the two legs and if the displacement is more than 1.5 cm then this suggests damage to the ACL. Variations to this test with the foot rotated externally or internally can also reveal involvement of the medial ligament, posterior and posterior cruciate ligaments, but all these tests will also produce a false positive if the posterior cruciate ligament is torn.
- The **posterior drawer test** is the opposite of the above, forcing the tibia backwards to detect posterior cruciate ligament injury
- The **Lachman test** is also used to detect ACL instability. With the knee in slight flexion one hand fixes the femur laterally and the other hand holds the tibia medially placing the thumb on the joint. An attempt is made to pull the tibia forwards and the end-points compared between the legs. A positive test is when the end-point is 'spongy' – normally there should be a firm stop.

  Injuries to the ankle are extremely common, especially to the lateral ligament – the **sprained ankle**.

  Injuries to the **Achilles tendon** are common in athletes, ranging from a tendinitis through to a traumatic rupture. Degenerative ageing changes to the collagen matrix (tendinosis) will also weaken this tendon in particular.

  Tendon and ligament injuries are extremely painful. Initial treatment involves: rest (to facilitate early cellular repair mechanisms); ice, to reduce pain and swelling; compression, to provide stability to the joint; and elevation, to minimise swelling (**r**est, **i**ce, **c**ompression, **e**levate – **RICE**).

Clinical box 9.25 | **Seronegative spondyloarthropathies**

Diseases that fall into this class of inflammatory conditions (associated with the human leucocyte antigen (HLA)-B27 class I allotype) are **ankylosing spondylitis** (**AS**), **psoriatic arthritis** and **reactive arthritis**. Typically, there is inflammation in the synovium and bony enthuses including CD4+ and CD8+ T lymphocytes and macrophages and secretion of various cytokines, such as TNF-α and TGF-β. In AS the sacroiliac joints are always involved.

The synovium in these conditions may be difficult to distinguish from rheumatoid arthritis microscopically but the synovium does not develop extensive pannus formation and consequently there is less invasion of the bone and articular cartilage than in rheumatoid arthritis.

The enthesis becomes infiltrated by non-specific granulation tissue. In more severe forms of the disease, enthesopathy is followed by calcification and ossification of the enthesis, thus reducing the movement possible at the joints affected. Because there are many entheses around the spine, due to the large number of joints and muscle/tendon insertions, the spine is often affected by such conditions and has a bamboo-like appearance radiologically.

The characteristic history is of insidious onset of low back pain associated with marked stiffness lasting for an hour or more after waking in the morning. The pain and stiffness is usually relieved by exercise and begins again when resting.

Clinical box 9.26 | **Inflammation of the bursae**

Diseases that affect the synovial joints usually also affect all types of synovial cavity, which include bursae and tendon sheaths. The overuse of muscles or tendons in regions where bursae are found, as well as continuous external compression or trauma, can cause **bursitis** (inflammation of the bursae). The symptoms of bursitis include swelling, pain and often a loss of muscular strength and range of motion in the joint. Repeated cumulative trauma may eventually lead to the formation of calcium deposits and to degeneration of the internal lining of the bursa.

Bursitis of the shoulder is often seen in athletes who participate in sports that require repetitive throwing and swinging motions and who use the shoulder joint throughout its entire range of motion, such as in swimming, gymnastics and tennis to name a few.

The knee joint contains a number of bursae, and bursitis of the prepatellar bursa is colloquially known as '**housemaid's knee**'. Tendon sheaths are elongated bursae which surround the tendon where it could be subjected to friction. The synovial tendon sheaths line the tendons only where they pass through narrow passages or **retinacula** such as in the palm of the hand, the wrist and around the ankles. Elsewhere the tendon lies in a bed of loose fibrous tissue.

Clinical box 9.27 | **Ganglion cysts**

If there is a small hole in the tendon sheath specifically, the synovial fluid may leak out and expand the tough fibrous outer connective tissue layer. Water and small molecules are able to diffuse away leaving the hyaluronan behind. This forms a very thick hyaluronan-rich fluid sac called a ganglion. These often form at the wrist where there are many long tendon sheaths passing over the wrist into the hand. A ganglion can be excised if it causes pain by pressing on nerves. Historically known as 'bible cysts', because a bible provided a suitably heavy object with which to try and burst the membrane and disperse the fluid through the surrounding tissue; treatment nowadays more normally includes needle fluid aspiration.

important because they are the main target in a group of inflammatory disorders known collectively as the **seronegative spondyloarthropathies** (Clinical box 9.25).

Bursae and tendon sheaths

Bursae and **tendon sheaths** are flattened sacs made of fibrous material containing synovial fluid. The synovial lining of these structures is similar to that found within the joints, with a slippery non-adherent surface that allows movement between the planes of the tissues. The sacs lie under and around structures in the joint to reduce friction.

Bursae are located at sites where the muscle or fascia may experience shearing forces due to being close to the surface or being embedded in the subcutaneous tissues. For example, in the shoulder there is a bursa which lies between the outside of the joint capsule and the overlying ligament (Clinical Box 9.26). Many bursae form during development but new or adventitious bursae can occur at sites of occupational friction. Bursae are located predominantly between bony prominences, muscles or tendons, and their main function is to provide cushioning and support in areas where repetitive motion occurs. Cysts (**ganglion cysts**) sometimes develop over joints and are more commonly seen at the wrist (see Clinical box 9.27).

ANATOMICAL RELATIONSHIPS

The skeleton cannot always be considered in isolation from other important tissues which are in close association with the bone. In addition to the wrist (Clinical box 9.18), important examples are:

- The spinal canal, which passes through the vertebral column. The position of a spinal fracture will influence the amount of cord damage and subsequent paralysis of affected muscles (see Ch. 8).
- The nerves, muscles and arteries that are associated with the elbow (cubital fossa) (Anatomy box 9.9)
- The nerves and blood vessels that run at the back of the knee (popliteal fossa) (Anatomy box 9.10)

SKELETAL MUSCLE

Skeletal muscle is the most abundant of the three types of muscle found in the body. Its main function is to provide the force for locomotion; to do this it converts chemical energy in to mechanical energy. Skeletal muscle is under the voluntary control of the nervous system. Besides its role in locomotion, it has other functions as well, such as acting as a reservoir for 80% of the body's water and as a pool for the storage of intracellular ions such as potassium. Its conversion of chemical energy to mechanical work generates heat and contributes to the maintenance of the body's temperature.

THE NEUROMUSCULAR JUNCTION AND MUSCLE INNERVATION

Skeletal muscle is under voluntary control and the axons of the motor neurons extend to the muscles and form synapses at the neuromuscular junctions. The neuromuscular junction is located at the centre of the muscle fibre rather than at the ends. As muscle fibres can be up to 10 cm in length, the neuromuscular junction is located near the mid-point and the action potential is then propagated towards both ends of the fibre. This allows a near simultaneous activation and contraction of the fibre.

Anatomy box 9.9   **Muscles of the arm and the cubital fossa**

Muscles of the arm

The three flexors lie in the anterior compartment of the upper arm. The main flexors are the **biceps** (**biceps brachii**) and the **brachialis**, which insert into the radius and ulna, respectively. The third flexor, **brachioradialis**, is only really effective when the forearm is partially flexed as it originates on the distal humerus and inserts into the distal radius (Fig. AB9).

There are two muscles that bring about extension of the forearm, the large **triceps brachii** and the much smaller **anconeus**, which are both contained in the posterior compartment.

The biceps muscle is also the main supinator and this action prevents it being an effective flexor of the pronated forearm. The **supinator** and **pronator quadratus** muscles, lying down the forearm, are roughly equal in strength but the great size of the biceps relative to the **pronator teres** muscle enables a person to supinate the forearm with much greater force than he or she can pronate. The strength of this action has led to screws being designed so that they can be tightened by this action.

The brachial arteries

The **brachial artery** is a continuation of the axillary artery and begins at the lower border of teres major where it inserts into the humerus. The brachial artery descends through the arm in the flexor compartment of the arm and is crossed by the median nerve half way down the upper arm,. The **deep brachial artery** is given off from the brachial artery soon after its origin. It descends deep through the arm following the spiral groove on the posterior side of the humerus, along with the radial nerve.

- The deep brachial artery is, therefore, vulnerable to damage by a mid-shaft fracture of the humerus.

The brachial pulse may be palpated by pressing the artery from the medial aspect against the humerus. The brachial artery passes anterior to the elbow joint; it then bifurcates in the cubital fossa into the **radial** and **ulnar arteries**.

The cubital fossa

The triangular area in front of and slightly distal to the elbow is the **cubital fossa**, or antecubital fossa. The fossa is bounded proximally by an imaginary line joining the two humeral epicondyles and distally by the pronator teres muscle on the ulnar side and the brachioradialis on the radial side. The floor of the fossa is formed by the brachialis and supinator muscles. The roof of the fossa is formed by the deep fascia and the bicipital aponeurosis.

The cubital fossa usually contains the terminal part of the brachial artery before it divides into the ulnar and radial arteries. The brachial artery lies between the biceps tendon, which has to be pushed aside to feel the brachial pulse, and the median nerve.

Accompanying the arteries are the deep veins so the brachial vein or veins are located in the fossa. The tendon of biceps brachii and the median nerve all pass through the fossa. Superficial to the fossa are the superficial veins, such as the median cubital vein, which makes the fossa a good site for venepuncture.

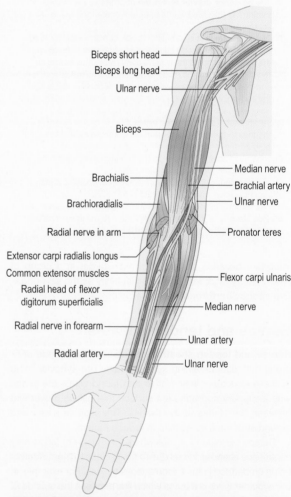

Fig. AB9 **Muscles, nerves and arteries running either side of the elbow.**

Anatomy box 9.10   **The popliteal fossa**

The **popliteal fossa** (Fig. AB10) is a diamond-shaped fossa located at the back of the knee joint. Its boundaries are the hamstring muscles (**semitendinosus**, **semimembranosus and biceps femoris**) superiorly and the two heads of the **gastrocnemius** muscle inferiorly. The fossa is important as all the important blood vessels and nerves from the thigh pass through the popliteal fossa to reach the leg.

The **popliteal artery** is a continuation of the **femoral artery**; it runs immediately next to the posterior surface of the femur and is thus the deepest structure in the fossa.

- The popliteal artery can be vulnerable to a fracture of the supracondylar femur when the pull of the gastrocnemius on the distal fragments can cause the artery to be severed by the sharp bone.

The **popliteal pulse** can be difficult to locate because of its deep location and because of the overlying leg fascia. It is felt by pressing from behind against the back of the femur, but to feel the pulse the leg muscles must be relaxed and the knee flexed, which helps to relax the popliteal fascia.

At the lower border of the popliteal fossa the popliteal artery bifurcates to give rise to the **posterior tibial artery**, which travels

down through the posterior compartment of the leg, and the **anterior tibial artery**, which descends in the anterior compartment of the leg. The posterior tibial artery usually gives off the **fibular artery**, which runs close to the fibula in the posterior compartment of the leg.

The **sciatic nerve** is the largest nerve in the body, originating in the lumbosacral plexus. passing through the greater sciatic foramen in the pelvis into the posterior compartment of the thigh, dividing into the **tibial and common fibular nerves** at the upper border of the popliteal fossa. The tibial nerve descends vertically down the leg, while the common fibular passes laterally around the neck of the fibula.

- Both tibial and common fibular nerves are vulnerable to trauma in the fossa.

The **sural nerve**, the sensory branch of the sciatic nerve in the posterior calf, is composed from nerve fibres from both the tibial and the fibular nerves.

- As the common fibular nerve winds round the neck of the fibula it is vulnerable to damage from strikes to the lateral leg. Unfortunately, the neck of the fibula is the right height for impacts from car bumpers. Damage to the common fibular nerve causes foot drop.

Anterior

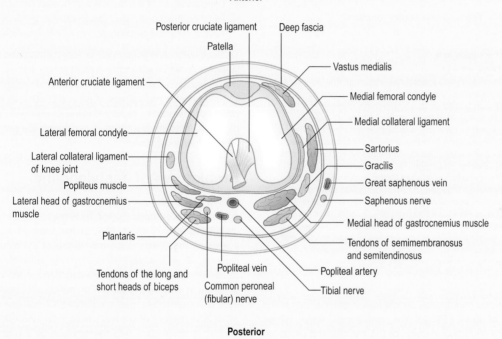

Fig. AB10 **The popliteal fossa.**

Acetylcholine receptors

Following release ACh diffuses across the synaptic cleft to the ruffled sarcolemma of the muscle fibre where ACh receptors (AChRs) are located (see Fig. 9.13). There are 30–40 million AChRs embedded into the muscle fibre membrane at each synapse and the postsynaptic membrane is thickened with cytoskeletal proteins that hold the receptors in place. All of the AChRs on skeletal muscle are nicotinic acetylcholine receptors (nAChR). These are ligand-gated ion channels that open an integral ion channel permeable to Na^+ and K^+ in response to the binding of two molecules of ACh. The rapid movement of sodium ions changes the membrane voltage leading to an electrochemical gradient. Once the resting potential voltage of around $-70\,mV$ reaches a threshold (around $-55\,mV$) an action potential results as the ion channels open

At the neuromuscular junction the motor neuron axon branches into a number of endings (Fig. 9.13). Each of the axon branches ends with an elongated terminal bouton, which contains thousands of synaptic vesicles loaded with the neurotransmitter **acetylcholine** (ACh). The sarcolemma of the muscle fibre under these endings is thrown into ruffles or 'junctional folds'.

Neurotransmitter release

An action potential in the motor neuron causes the exocytosis of several hundred vesicles into the synaptic cleft. Each synaptic vesicle contains approximately 10^4 ACh molecules so the simultaneous release of so many vesicles results in large amounts of ACh being released (Information box 9.2).

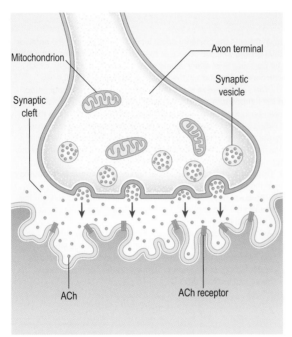

Fig. 9.13 **The neuromuscular junction.**

Labels in figure: Mitochondrion, Axon terminal, Synaptic vesicle, Synaptic cleft, ACh, ACh receptor

---

Information box 9.2   **Botulinum toxin**

There are several plant substances and drugs that selectively block the neuromuscular junction. The toxin produced by *Clostridium botulinum* (botulinum toxin) prevents the exocytosis of ACh from the synaptic vesicles. Therefore, no ACh is released and the muscle does not contract. The bacteria can be found in improperly canned foods, and the toxin is one of the most lethal chemicals known, causing death by paralysis of the diaphragm.

The toxin is also marketed as Botox. In clinical use Botox injections into the muscle can help patients with strabismus, blepharospasm or cerebral palsy, by relaxing the muscles. The effects of Botox last from 2 to 6 months. Its other uses have been cosmetic, with injections into the facial muscles, reducing the appearance of fine lines and wrinkles by again relaxing the muscles attached to the skin of the face. The long-term risks of Botox injections have not been assessed.

---

more and the membrane 'depolarises' reaching membrane voltages of up to +100 mV. The membrane voltage change caused by this depolarisation of the sarcolemma produces an electric current, which is propagated across and into the inside of the muscle fibre by **transverse tubules (T tubules)**. The depolarisation then rapidly reverses as the polarity of the membrane changes and the sodium channels close. Potassium channels are then activated and potassium ions flow out, returning the electrochemical gradient to its resting level. In fact there is a slight hyperpolarisation, to below the normal resting level, preventing the current from returning to its source.

Neuromuscular blockade

Several drugs produce muscle paralysis by affecting AChRs. They are used during surgery to produce relaxation of skeletal muscle. Much surgery requires the separation of muscle layers, and this requires these layers to be relaxed. The use of muscle relaxants requires the patient to be artificially ventilated via an endotracheal tube (intubation), which also cannot be inserted without relaxation of the muscles of the larynx.

Information box 9.3   **Curare**

Curare is derived from a South American plant, and is used by the local Indians to tip their arrows and darts. It causes muscle paralysis, by binding to the AChR and blocking normal activation of the receptor. Curare-like drugs, such as cisatracurium, are often used as muscle relaxants before surgery. **Neostigmine** (an anticholinesterase) is used as an antidote for curare poisoning and terminates its effect after surgery. Neostigmine is usually administered with atropine to block the muscarinic effects of increasing the amount of circulating ACh.

The two types of muscle relaxant are:

- Non-depolarising drugs such as **tubocurarine** and its safer synthetic alternatives are competitive antagonists of nAChRs. These drugs bind to AChRs but do not cause depolarisation. They are fairly long-lasting (up to 60 min) and can be reversed by drugs, such as neostigmine, which increase the local concentration of ACh (Information box 9.3).
- Depolarising drugs such as **succinylcholine** are ACh agonists. They bind to AChRs and cause a long-lasting depolarisation of the muscle which, after disorganised initial contractions called fasciculations, produces a flaccid paralysis possibly due to AChR desensitisation.

Succinylcholine is normally rapidly metabolised by circulating cholinesterases and so is short acting. It is usually used only to provide relaxation during intubation. However, about 1 in 3000 patients have a type of plasma cholinesterase which does not metabolise succinylcholine so the neuromuscular blockade lasts several hours during which the patient must be continually ventilated.

Breakdown of acetylcholine

ACh is broken down in the synaptic cleft by cholinesterase enzymes concentrated on the basement membrane, which hydrolyses approximately 30% of the released ACh before it reaches the postsynaptic membrane of the muscle fibre. However, as ACh is released in such large quantities, with up to 10 times more ACh being produced than is needed, muscle contraction is usually assured. For muscle contraction to fail, 90% of the receptors must be blocked (Clinical box 9.28).

ACh is broken down into acetic acid and choline. The choline is taken back into the synapse by the action of a specific Na⁺-dependent choline transporter. This is a rate-limiting step for the synthesis of ACh and this transporter can be blocked by the drug **hemicholinium**. This results in a depletion of ACh in the synapse and a reduction in ACh release. Another drug, **vesamicol**, prevents the transport of synthesised ACh into vesicles.

Motor units

Each muscle is innervated by at least one motor neuron which branches to supply a number of muscle fibres within the muscle. The motor neuron and all the muscle fibres it supplies are called a **motor unit**. The average number of fibres in a motor unit is about 150 but the number varies according to the degree of fine movement or force required from that muscle. The number of fibres innervated by a single neuron varies enormously, from hundreds in large, weight-bearing muscles such as those around the hip to as few as four in the tiny ocular muscles which control eye movements.

The ACh receptors (AChRs) on skeletal muscle normally turn over with a half-life of 10 days, with new receptors constantly being made and incorporated into the postsynaptic junctional folds, and the old receptors removed and degraded by lysosomes.

In myasthenia gravis the immune system makes antibodies to the AChR. The antigen-antibody complex has a half-life of only 2 days, leading to a progressive loss of AChRs. Certain muscles are affected more than others; those innervated by the cranial nerves, for example, are affected more than the somatic muscles of the body. For this reason myasthenia gravis clinically is characterised by muscle weakness of the muscles in the face and this is especially noticeable in the muscles around the eyes and mouth. The limb muscles are usually less affected but in severe cases these will be weakened as well. In the most severe cases, the muscles of swallowing and respiration are affected and this can be life-threatening.

Treatment for myasthenia gravis involves the administration of an anticholinesterase drug such as pyridostigmine or neostigmine. This prevents the breakdown of ACh as it is released from the motor axon and allows it to bind to the remaining AChRs, thus improving the contractile power of the muscles.

The antibodies that are produced originate in the thymus gland which in affected individuals is hyperplastic, and in 10% of cases there is a lymphoid tumour in the thymus gland. The removal of the thymus may therefore be beneficial in individuals with severe symptoms that are not controlled by the usual drug regimen.

The fibres innervated by a single motor unit are distributed through a muscle so activation of a single motor unit causes a weak contraction of the whole muscle. As more motor units are activated, fibres throughout the muscle are activated until maximum tension is reached with the activation of all the motor units supplying a given muscle.

Development of sustained tension

A single action potential in a motor neuron will cause a small twitch in a muscle, and repeated low frequency stimulation will produce a series of twitches which match the frequency of stimulation.

When a skeletal muscle is stimulated at 20–30 times a second, it is only partly able to relax between the stimuli. This results in a sustained but wavering contraction called **unfused tetanus**. Stimulating the muscle at 80–100 times a second results in no relaxation between repeated stimuli and a **fused tetanus** occurs with a sustained constant tension.

In both unfused and fused tetanus the level of Ca^{2+} builds up inside the muscle and the peak tension that can be generated is 5–10 times greater than for a single contraction.

Muscle tone

In skeletal muscle, a muscle is never totally inactive; a few motor units are always being activated to produce a sustained contraction of their muscle fibres. The proportion of the motor units that are active is only very small and so the muscle is relaxed but has 'tone'. The motor units that are active constantly shift so that fatigue does not set in. Muscle tone keeps the muscle firm but is not strong enough to cause movement. For example, when standing the muscles of the leg and back help to maintain an upright posture but are mainly relaxed with only a few motor units active to stop us from falling down.

Sensory innervation of muscle

Apart from the motor neuron innervation of muscle there is also sensory innervation of skeletal muscle. Sensory nerves convey information about muscle length and tension in order to coordinate muscle contraction. The main sensory organ in muscle, the muscle spindles, which are embedded between the contractile fibres, are up to 1 cm in length and can vary in number from a dozen to several hundred in different muscles. They are more numerous in the antigravity muscles such as the muscles along the vertebral column and in the legs, and in the intrinsic muscles of the hand. All these muscles tend to have more type 1 fibres while the muscles rich in type 2 fibres tend to have fewer muscle spindles (see Ch. 8).

ISOTONIC VERSUS ISOMETRIC CONTRACTION

Not all muscle contraction results in the shortening of a muscle:

- **Isotonic** contractions result in muscle shortening and move the body and external objects
- **Isometric** contractions stabilise joints and are vital in maintaining posture; they do not produce movement but still use energy as the muscle tension increases.

An example of an isometric contraction is when you are holding a book in an outstretched arm. Considerable tension is generated by the muscles in the arm – as the book drags the arm down, the shoulder and arm muscles must compensate by contracting. Therefore, the stretching and contraction of the muscle in opposite directions keeps the arm level.

Isotonic contractions can be subdivided into concentric and eccentric contractions:

- **Concentric contractions** cause a muscle to shorten and produce a movement that reduces the angle at a joint (flexion). Picking up a book from a table is a result of a concentric contraction of the biceps brachii muscle in the front of the upper arm.
- **Eccentric contractions** are where a muscle contracts but the length of the muscle gets longer. As you lower the book gradually to the table the biceps brachii still contracts to prevent the book from dropping, yet the actual length of the muscle increases.

Repeated eccentric contractions produce more damage to the muscle fibres as it is thought that the myosin heads are pulled off the actin filaments by the stretching of the muscle that takes place. In most daily activities there is a mixture of isotonic and isometric contractions.

THE SKELETAL MUSCLE FIBRE

Each muscle is composed of a collection of muscle fibres, which are bound together by connective tissue (Fig. 9.14). Each fibre within the muscle is itself formed by the fusion of many myogenic cells into a single multinucleated cell. Individual muscle fibres can measure up to 10 cm in length with a diameter ranging from 10 μm to 100 μm. In the mature muscle fibre the nuclei are arranged around the periphery, as the fibre is packed with contractile proteins, but during development or repair after damage the nuclei of the newly added myogenic cells appear in the centre of the muscle fibre.

Muscle
(organ)

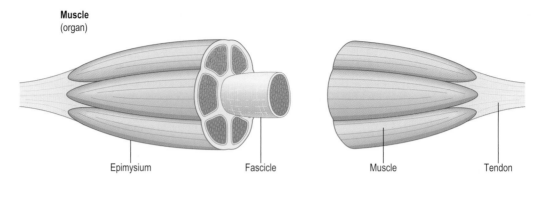

Epimysium Fascicle   Muscle Tendon

Fascicle
(a portion of the muscle)

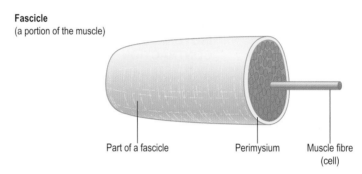

Part of a fascicle   Perimysium   Muscle fibre
(cell)

Muscle fibre
(cell)

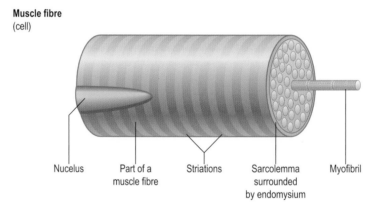

Nucelus   Part of a   Striations   Sarcolemma   Myofibril
           muscle fibre   surrounded
                                         by endomysium

Myofibril or fibril
(complex organelle composed of bundles of myofilaments))

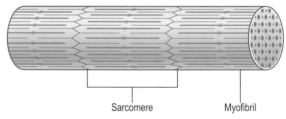

Sarcomere   Myofibril

Fig. 9.14 **Macroscopic structure of skeletal muscle.**

Each muscle fibre contains many **myofibrils**. These long rod-like structures run the entire length of the cell and contain the contractile proteins. Each fibre contains between hundreds and thousands of myofibrils depending on its size. The myofibrils take up more than 80% of the cell volume, with the **sarcoplasm** (muscle cell cytoplasm), mitochondria and the other cellular components packed in between. The sarcoplasm contains relatively high levels of glycogen and the red, oxygen-carrying molecule, **myoglobin**.

The contractile proteins

As in all types of muscle, the contractile proteins of skeletal muscle are **actin** and **myosin**, plus a number of accessory muscle proteins (see Ch. 2, Table 2.14). Actin and myosin form the **thin** and **thick** filaments, respectively, which are arranged in a very ordered lattice arrangement (Fig. 9.15), giving skeletal muscle its other name of 'striated muscle'. The interactions between the thick and thin filaments form the basis of muscle contraction by the

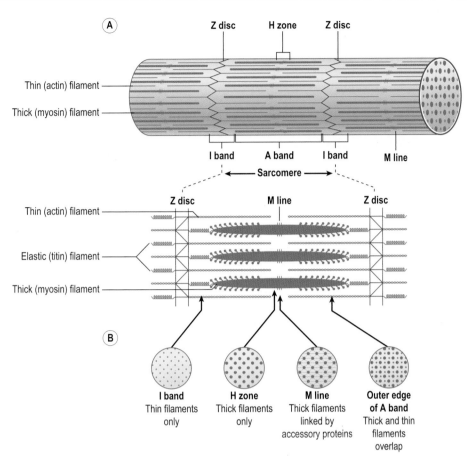

Fig. 9.15 **The sarcomere.** (A) Longitudinal view showing A and I bands, M and Z lines and H zone. (B) Cross-sectional view showing geometrical arrangement of thick and thin filaments.

binding of myosin and actin in the presence of calcium and ATP (adenosine triphosphate).

The thin and thick filaments are attached at regular intervals to accessory proteins, which are visible as lines that divide the myofibril into its functional unit, the **sarcomere**. The actin filaments insert into the **Z disc**, while the myosin filaments insert into the **M line** (Fig. 9.15A). Each sarcomere extends from one Z disk to the next and is composed of alternating light and dark bands. These are formed depending on the overlap between the thin and thick filaments. The length of the thick filaments is shown by the **A band**, whose length remains constant even during muscle contraction. The light band called the **H zone** is the region that contains just myosin filaments whereas the light **I band** is where there are only actin filaments (Fig. 9.15B).

Thin filaments

The thin filaments, anchored to the Z disc, extend across the I and A bands where they interdigitate with the thick filaments, but don't extend into the H zone. They are made from actin plus two regulatory proteins, troponin and tropomyosin.

Long flat strands of actin, **F-actin** (fibrous actin), are formed by the polymerisation of the **G-actin** (globular actin) subunits, consuming ATP. Two F-actin strands coil around each other in a helix forming the thin filaments. The thin filaments extend into the sarcomere from the Z disc, partly overlapping with the myosin chains that extend from the M line. In a muscle fibre there are approximately twice as many actin filaments as myosin filaments, leading to an array where each myosin filament is associated with six actin filaments, and each actin filament with three myosin filaments (Figs 9.15 and 9.16).

Two other proteins, **tropomyosin** and **troponin**, are associated with the actin filament. Tropomyosin is a filamentous protein that lies in the groove of the coiled F-actin filaments. It strengthens and stiffens the F-actin, and at rest, in the absence of Ca^{2+}, covers the myosin-binding site on the actin filament, inhibiting muscle contraction.

Troponin, found in skeletal and cardiac muscle, but not smooth muscle, consists of three proteins:

- Troponin T which binds to tropomyosin, forming the troponin-tropomyosin complex
- Troponin I which is an inhibitory subunit, stabilising the complex
- Troponin C which binds calcium causing a conformational change leading to disclocation of troponin I and then tropomyosin, enabling myosin to bind to actin, initiating contraction.

Thick filaments

The thick filaments are made up mainly of myosin. Myosin II is a multimeric elongated protein with two long tail regions each with a globular head. It is made up of two heavy and four light chains. The two heavy chains form an extended α helix, while at each end a light chain binds to form a globular domain, the 'head' region. A flexible hinge region (the 'neck') near the globular head divides the protein into light meromyosin (LMM, helical region) and heavy meromyosin (HMM, the short helical region and the globular domains). The thick filaments of muscle are formed by the self-association of LMM helices, with up to 400 myosin 'tail' molecules in each thick filament. The thick filaments extend outward from the M line

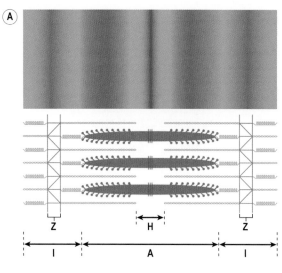

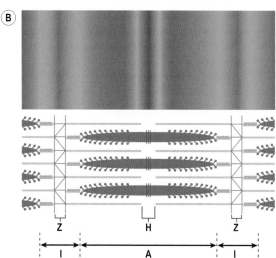

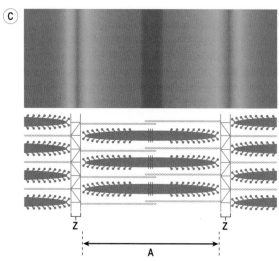

Fig. 9.16 **Sliding filament model of muscle contraction:** (A) at rest, (B) during contraction and (C) fully contracted.

towards the Z disc of each myofibril, with the globular heads protruding from the bundles of myosin molecules. A second hinge region is defined between the globular domains (S1) which bind to actin and ATP, and the short helical region (S2) of the HMM.

Each of the globular domains contains a calcium-dependent ATPase. Binding of ATP to ATPase reduces the affinity of binding between actin and myosin, and hydrolysis of ATP by ATPase provides the energy required to shorten the muscle.

The sliding filament model of muscle contraction

During muscle contraction it can be seen that while each sarcomere shortens, the length of the separate thin and thick filaments does not change. This is because during contraction the thin and thick filaments slide along one another with increasing degrees of overlap.

1. At rest, when the muscle is at its maximum length, there is only a small amount of overlap between the thin and thick filaments, as shown by the wide H zone and I band (Fig. 9.16A).
2. As the muscle shortens the H zone gradually disappears as the ends of the thin filaments get closer. The I band also narrows as the ends of the thick filaments get closer to the Z disc (Fig. 9.16B).
3. At maximum contraction the thin filaments from the opposing ends of the sarcomere overlap where the H zone was and the thick filaments reach the Z disc, thus abolishing the I band. The A band is the same length as at rest with the thick filaments now filling the space between the two Z discs (Fig. 9.16C).

The method by which the muscle shortens is due to a cycle of making and breaking of **cross-bridges** between the thick and thin filaments. At each cycle the energy from the hydrolysis of ATP causes the myosin head region to move backwards (towards the tail region) pulling the thin filament along the thick filament (see below).

THE CONTRACTILE PROCESS

Muscle contraction is triggered by the activity in the motor neuron supplying the muscle. The process by which the electrical signal produces contraction is called **excitation–contraction coupling**.

Excitation–contraction coupling

Intracellular calcium release (Fig. 9.17A)

The **sarcolemma** (muscle fibre plasma membrane) has invaginations that penetrate deep into the muscle fibre, called **T tubules** (transverse tubules). These occur at the Z discs where, along with the terminal cisternae of the **sarcoplasmic reticulum** (SR, the endoplasmic reticulum of the muscle), they form a structure called a **triad** where the T tubules and the SR are linked by structures called **end feet**. The SR stores high concentrations of calcium whereas free calcium levels in the sarcoplasm at rest are very low (about 10^{-8} M) (Clinical box 9.29).

When the sarcolemma is depolarised by the motor neuron at the neuromuscular junction, the electrical impulses are propagated across the surface of the muscle and deep into the T tubules by the activation of voltage-dependent sodium channels. The T tubule system allows the simultaneous contraction of all the muscle fibres in the muscle, thereby avoiding damage from parts of the muscle contracting while other parts are inactive.

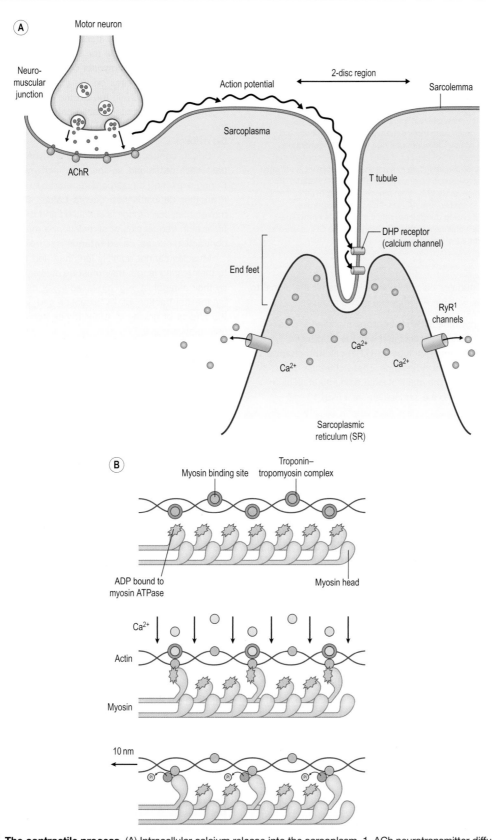

Fig. 9.17 **The contractile process.** (A) Intracellular calcium release into the sarcoplasm. 1. ACh neurotransmitter diffuses across the junction. 2. Binds to AChR receptors in sarcolemma and ion channels open. 3. Na^+ influx changes membrane voltage producing a current (action potential) that propagates across membrane. 4. Action potential transmitted to sarcoplasmic reticulum end feet through dihydropyridine (DHP) receptor calcium channels. 5. Ca^{2+} stores in sarcoplasmic reticulum released into sarcoplasma as RyR_1 channels open. (B) Cross-bridge formation and muscle contraction. 1. Resting. 2. Cross-bridge formation, Ca^{2+} binds to troponin–tropomysin complex, myosin head binds to myosin binding site on actin filament. 3. Movement of actin strand across myosin in 'ratchet' mechanism, cross-bridge causes conformation change (ATP > ADP + Pi) releasing stored energy, actin filament moves across myosin filament and muscle contracts. 4. Relaxation, Ca^{2+} removed by active transport into SR, troponin–tropomyosin blockage restored, myosin heads released from actin and muscle relaxes.

Malignant hyperthermia is a rare genetic defect which is caused by a defect in the control of calcium release from sarcoplasmic reticulum (SR). It is only manifested when the susceptible individual is given halothane anaesthesia or a muscle relaxant. Muscle spasms result due to excessive calcium release from mutant RYR1 channels that trigger massive cross-bridge cycling and adenosine triphosphate (ATP) consumption, and a rapid rise of body temperature, due to the heat generated by the regeneration of large quantities of ATP. Metabolism can become anaerobic, resulting in the generation of lactic acid with subsequent metabolic acidosis. Depletion of ATP leads to the release of high levels of K^+ from muscle, causing hyperkalaemia with a risk of cardiac arrhythmias. As well as supportive treatment, the drug dantrolene, which inhibits the ryanodine-sensitive Ca^{2+} channels in the membranes of the SR, is used to prevent further Ca^{2+} release.

In the T tubules calcium channels transmit the signal to the end feet, which are composed of two proteins:

- **Dihydropyridine (DHP) receptors**, modified L-type calcium channels, associated with the T tubules
- **Ryanodine-sensitive type 1 (RYR1) calcium channels** with a very high conductance. These channels open rapidly to allow the efflux of large amounts of calcium from the SR into the sarcoplasm, reaching 10^{-5} M.

Cross-bridge formation and muscle contraction (Fig. 9.17B)

Prior to contraction, the binding of ATP to the myosin ATPase and its subsequent hydrolysis to adenosine diphosphate (ADP) and Pi move the myosin head to point forwards along the axis of the myosin filament in a high energy conformation. ADP and Pi remain bound to the myosin head and this complex has a high affinity for the binding site on the actin filaments. However, this is inhibited by tropomyosin which blocks the binding site.

When Ca^{2+} is released from the SR it binds to troponin C, which undergoes a conformational change allowing the myosin binding sites to become available. The myosin heads now bind to the thin filaments forming **cross-bridges**. This binding triggers a conformation change in the myosin head, releasing the stored energy, which moves the head region backwards, pulling the thin filament about 10 nm along the thick filament. This also releases the ADP and Pi from the ATPase.

The myosin ATPase now binds ATP, which causes the release of the cross-bridge, followed by hydrolysis of the ATP and movement of the myosin head back to the forward-pointing position. This high-energy conformation is then ready to reattach to the thin filament and repeat the stroke 10 nm further along, rachet-like.

This cycle of cross-bridge formation, movement and release is repeated over and over again by all the myosin heads until the Ca^{2+} is removed or ATP is depleted. Because, at any given time, about half of the cross-bridges will be attached, this prevents the filaments sliding apart.

Calcium removal and muscle relaxation

During a muscle contraction the muscle will typically shorten by about 30% although it can reduce its length by up to 70%, which requires many cross-bridge cycles. The contraction is terminated by the removal of Ca^{2+} from the sarcoplasm by the action of Ca^{2+}-ATPase pumps present on the SR membrane which actively transport Ca^{2+} back into the SR. As the Ca^{2+} levels drop in the sarcoplasm of the muscle fibre, the troponin–tropomyosin complex once again covers the myosin-binding sites on the actin filament, and so the cross-bridges detach. In the SR the Ca^{2+} is sequestered by a calcium-binding protein called **calsequestrin**. This allows the concentration of Ca^{2+} to be 10 000 times greater than in the cytosol.

During contraction the actin and myosin filaments slide past each other and so the sarcomere reduces in length. During relaxation the sarcomere returns to its resting length. If another depolarisation occurs before all the Ca^{2+} is removed then contraction is sustained and is strengthened until, at high frequencies of stimulation, a maximum sustained contraction occurs, called **tetanus** (see below).

Muscles cannot actively lengthen and in order to return to their resting length they must be actively stretched, either by their antagonist, e.g. a relaxed flexor muscle is stretched by the contraction of its extensor and vice versa, or by the effects of gravity or other forces acting on the muscle (Information box 9.4).

Muscle length and tension

The optimal overlap between the actin and myosin filaments is at a sarcomere length of 2.0–2.4 μm, and at this length the muscle fibre is able to develop its maximum tension. If the muscle fibre is stretched so that overlap between the actin and myosin is reduced, fewer myosin cross-bridges are able to make contact with the actin filament, and thus the muscle cannot generate the same degree of tension. At 170% of its optimal length there is no overlap between the actin and myosin, and the muscle will not generate any tension. If the sarcomere length becomes shorter the tension that can be generated by the muscle again is reduced. This is because the myosin filaments are compressed and crumple against the Z disc, and consequently fewer myosin heads are able to make contact with the actin filament. The resting length of muscle is held very close to the optimal length by the firm attachments of the skeletal muscle to the bones via their tendons.

MUSCLE METABOLISM

Muscle goes from times when it is virtually inactive and using only small amounts of ATP, to contracting continually, when ATP is being used at a rapid rate. The ATP stored in muscle is only enough to power contraction for a few seconds, so additional ATP must be continually synthesised if contraction of the muscle is to continue without fatigue. Muscle has three sources of ATP synthesis:

ATP is required by the muscle both to release the myosin heads from the actin and to remove Ca^{2+} from the sarcoplasm. After death **rigor mortis** occurs as a result of the inability to regenerate ATP. The hydrolysis of any remaining ATP to ADP and the maintenance of a high sarcoplasmic Ca^{2+} concentration mean that the myosin heads remain bound to the actin filament forming a rigid muscle tissue. Rigor mortis sets in 3–4 hours after death and lasts for approximately 24 hours. Then it disappears gradually due to the release of proteolytic enzymes that digest the myosin cross-bridges from the myosin filaments.

- Creatine phosphate
- Anaerobic cellular respiration
- Aerobic cellular respiration.

The first of these is unique to muscle fibres, while all cells utilise the other two sources of ATP and are considered elsewhere (see Ch. 2).

Creatine phosphate

When the muscle is relaxed and at rest, excess ATP is being produced and some of this excess ATP is diverted to the synthesis of **creatine phosphate**. This is an energy-rich molecule produced by the enzyme creatine kinase. The enzyme catalyses the transfer of one high energy phosphate group from ATP to creatine, forming creatine phosphate and ADP. In the sarcoplasm of the muscle fibre, creatine phosphate is three to six times more abundant than ATP. As contraction of the muscle begins, the ADP levels begin to rise and creatine kinase catalyses the return of the high energy phosphate group from creatine phosphate back to ADP, forming ATP. The creatine phosphate and ATP stores in muscle can fuel muscle contractions for about 15 seconds, which is sufficient for short bursts of activity.

Creatine supplementation

Creatine is a small amino acid-like molecule, which the body can synthesise, as well as it being derived from the diet. Adults need to synthesise and ingest around 2 g of creatine daily to replace the loss of creatine as its breakdown product **creatinine**, which is expelled in the urine. During intense exercise improved performance has been shown in subjects who had taken creatine supplements of up to 15 g per day for 28 days prior to the exercise. The subjects also gained muscle mass and were able to lift greater weights. However, such a large intake of creatine causes the body's own production of creatine to stop, and research on the consequence of long-term use has not provided sufficient data to check whether, after cessation of supplementation, the body's own synthesis of creatine is restored to normal levels.

Muscle fatigue

After a prolonged period of muscle contraction the muscle becomes fatigued. However, this is not due to a lack of ATP in the muscle, as the levels of ATP in fatigued muscle are often not much lower than in resting muscle. The depletion of creatine phosphate may trigger muscle fatigue as can insufficient oxygen, depletion of glycogen and other nutrients, the build-up of lactic acid and ADP, and the failure of the motor neuron to release sufficient acetylcholine (ACh). Certain muscle fibres are more resistant to fatigue such as the type 1 slow fibres, while the type 2b fast glycolytic fibres are more susceptible to fatigue.

TYPES OF MUSCLE FIBRES

Muscle fibres can be divided on the basis of their morphology and physiochemical characteristics into one of two main groups which have different functions.

- **Type 1 muscle fibres** are slow in their speed of contraction and have high resistance to fatigue. The metabolism of type 1 fibres is oxidative and they have an increased concentration of myoglobin, which gives them their red appearance and an increased capacity to hold oxygen. The type 1 fibres tend to have more mitochondria and generally a larger capillary blood supply than type 2 fibres.
- **Type 2 muscle fibres** use glycogen as their energy source and an anaerobic metabolism. The fibres contract at a faster rate and have a lower resistance to fatigue. Type 2 fibres may be further subdivided into **type 2a** and **type 2b** fibres. Type 2a have a mixed metabolism, which is oxidative and glycolytic, and therefore have a mixed phenotype with some features of a type 1 fibre.

During development the pattern of fibre types is established before innervation, but in the adult, fibre types are maintained by the innervation to that fibre, although circulating hormones such as thyroid hormone can also influence the fibre types in muscle. All the muscle fibres supplied by a single neuron are of the same histological type. The proportions of different fibre types within a muscle can vary because of exercise or inactivity.

The distribution of type 1 and type 2 fibres depends on their function, so that more type 1 fibres are located in the deeper muscles and are involved in the maintenance of posture, while the type 2 fibres are located more superficially and are mainly associated with movement.

THE CONNECTIVE TISSUE OF MUSCLE

Surrounding each muscle is the **fascia** (bandage); it lies deep to the skin and is a sheet of fibrous connective tissue. Several layers of the fascia can be identified.

- The **superficial fascia** separates the muscles from the skin. It allows a route for nerves and blood vessels to both enter and exit the muscle, and therefore it is composed of a loose areolar connective tissue. There is also a layer of adipose tissue, which helps to protect the underlying muscle from everyday traumas, as well as acting as an insulator that prevents too much loss of the heat generated by the muscles.
- The **deep fascia** is composed of dense irregular connective tissue. It separates functionally similar muscles together. The nerves and blood vessels travel between the sheets of the deep fascia.

Around each individual muscle is the **epimysium**. The **perimysium** separates the muscle fibres into **fascicles** of around 10–100 muscle fibres. Finally, around each individual muscle fibre is the **endomysium**. Both the epimysium and the perimysium are made up of dense, irregular connective tissue, while the endomysium is composed of an areolar connective tissue.

The deep fascia, epimysium, perimysium and the endomysium are continuous with and contribute collagen fibres to the tendons (see above). The tendons are dense regular connective tissue cords and bands that connect muscle to the bone's periosteum. The tendon that attaches the muscle to the stationary part of the body is known as the **origin**, while the tendon that connects the muscle to the more mobile part of the body is known as the **insertion**. These terms are not precise as in some cases the muscle will act over several joints and both ends of the muscle are therefore mobile, but usually the distal end of the muscle has the 'insertion' tendon attachment.

MUSCLE GROWTH AND REPAIR

Skeletal muscle is able to repair itself by the activation of a population of resident muscle precursors that lie under the basal lamina of the muscle fibres, called **satellite cells**. These satellite cells remain quiescent until the muscle fibre is damaged, when they become activated to re-enter the cell cycle. They initially undergo symmetrical division (producing two identical daughter cells) like any stem cell population and then a proportion will undergo asymmetric division and one of the daughter cells will drop out of division and will fuse with the damaged muscle fibres and differentiate. The muscle contractile proteins of the differentiated cell will span the damaged region, repairing the defect.

The activated satellite cells that do not differentiate and help repair the damaged region will become quiescent again and remain dormant until needed. In this way, there is always a population of repair cells available to the muscle, although with age the ability of the satellite cells to re-enter the cell cycle declines and thus repair in the elderly is reduced. This may be related to the number of cell divisions that the satellite cells have had to undergo in a lifetime, reducing their ability to replicate. This has implications for muscle diseases such as muscular dystrophy as the satellite cells normally constantly repair damaged muscle. It is thought that one of the reasons for the reduced lifespan of these patients is that their satellite cells reach their maximum number of divisions earlier in life than in normal individuals and are thus unable to repair the muscle after the early to mid-twenties (see Clinical box 9.30).

After growth has stopped no new muscle fibres are formed and any increase in muscle bulk is due to the incorporation of more myogenic cells into pre-existing fibres (**hyperplasia**). This also means that if a muscle fibre is extensively damaged,

---

Clinical box 9.30 | Duchenne muscular dystrophy

Duchenne muscular dystrophy (DMD) is a genetic disorder caused by a defect in the muscle protein **dystrophin**. Dystrophin is an accessory muscle protein that helps to reinforce the muscle fibres' plasma membrane; in its absence the plasma membrane can be damaged more easily, leading to muscle fibre degeneration and even muscle fibre death. This results in a loss of muscle bulk and replacement with fibrous scar tissue in affected individuals. The gene for dystrophin is located on the X chromosome and so the disease is more commonly found in males. The gene is very long (nearly 2.5×10^{6} base pairs) and mutations in the gene are relatively common. DMD has an occurrence of 1 in 3500 male births and is therefore one of the most common genetic disorders. DMD presents with progressive muscle weakness, which results in affected individuals being wheelchair-bound by puberty and dying, usually in their early to mid-twenties, from respiratory and cardiac failure.

---

the satellite cells cannot repair the damage, and the fibre is lost and replaced by fibrocollagenous scar tissue.

Recently, evidence has emerged of a circulating population of stem cells derived from bone marrow, which can also contribute to the repair of muscle. However, satellite cells still make up the majority of the repair cells in muscle and are responsible for replacing cells lost in the day-to-day microtrauma that muscle has to withstand. The newly identified stem cells form only a very small proportion of the muscle repair mechanism and are only activated after extensive muscle fibre damage.

MUSCLE NOMENCLATURE

Muscle shape

The arrangement of the fascicles in each muscle can vary and is used to describe the shape of the muscle (Fig. 9.18).

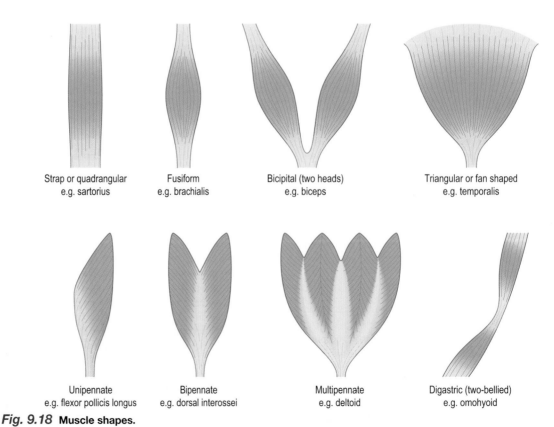

Strap or quadrangular
e.g. sartorius

Fusiform
e.g. brachialis

Bicipital (two heads)
e.g. biceps

Triangular or fan shaped
e.g. temporalis

Unipennate
e.g. flexor pollicis longus

Bipennate
e.g. dorsal interossei

Multipennate
e.g. deltoid

Digastric (two-bellied)
e.g. omohyoid

Fig. 9.18 **Muscle shapes.**

The deltoid muscle is a **pennate** muscle which has its fascicles arranged in a feather-like arrangement. Pennate muscles may be uni-, bi- or multi-pennate muscles, examples of each being the extensor digitorum longus, rectus femoris and the deltoid, respectively.

The biceps brachii muscle is an example of a **fusiform** muscle, which is spindle shaped, with tapered ends and a fatter belly. The biceps brachii is also a **bicipital** muscle that has two heads which are separate proximally, but which at the distal end merge into one tendon. A **quadrate** muscle has four equal sides; an example is the pronator quadratus muscle.

When the muscle fibres surround an opening, and contraction of the muscle causes a constriction of the opening, these are called **circular** or **sphincter** muscles, such as the orbicularis oculi and oris muscles in the face.

Muscle names

Muscles are named according to several factors, including their **location** and **function**. Some are named according to the bones they are attached to. For example:

- The cricothyroid muscle in the neck attaches to the cricoid cartilage inferiorly, and to the thyroid cartilage superiorly.
- The abductor digiti minimi abducts the little finger.

Muscle names may also be derived from their **position** (e.g. the flexor digitorum superficialis is the superficial flexor of the digits) or **length** or **size** (the extensor pollicis longus and extensor pollicis brevis are the long and short extensor muscles of the thumb, respectively).

Some muscles are named according to the **shape** and **direction** of their fascicles. For example, the deltoid muscle is roughly triangular (deltoid means triangle) whereas the rectus abdominis has its fascicles running straight (rectus) with respect to the midline.

Figures 9.19 and 9.20 illustrate the major muscles in the body (Information box 9.5).

POSTURE AND LOCOMOTION

Posture refers to the arrangement of the limbs, trunk and head in relation to the centre of gravity. It is controlled by

---

Information box 9.5   **Major skeletal muscles of the body**

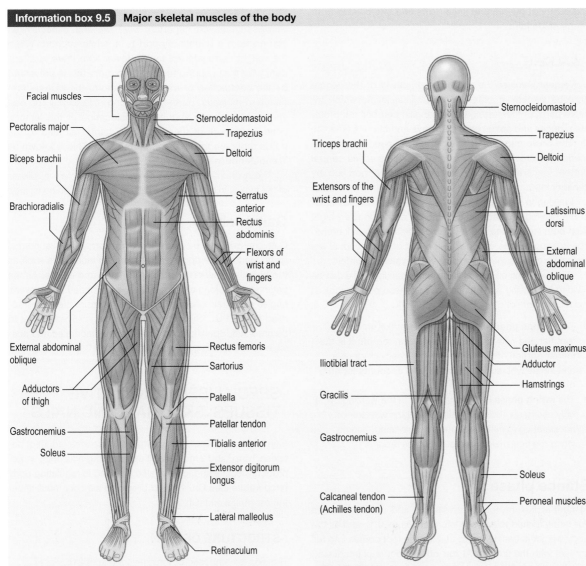

Fig. 9.19 **Superficial muscles of the body: anterior view.**

Fig. 9.20 **Superficial muscles of the body: posterior view.**

reflexes which enable the body position to remain stable, especially during movement which moves the centre of gravity. Postural reflexes which automatically adjust the body position in response to sensory input are organised by the brainstem (see Ch. 8). The main muscles involved in posture are the axial trunk extensors and the proximal limb muscles.

STANDING

When standing normally the feet are slightly apart and laterally rotated with the toes pointing outwards. Because of the arrangement of the joints in the lower limb, they tend to be in their most stable position when standing, with the hip and knee extended. This means that when standing there is little muscular activity needed to maintain the upright position.

The ankle is the most unstable joint of the lower limb so there is some muscular activity in the muscles of the leg to prevent falling. The centre of gravity when standing passes down through the mastoid process, located on the base of the skull just behind the ear. It continues down through the vertebral column, to pass just behind the centre of the hip and knee joints and ends just in front of the ankle joint.

WALKING

Movement involves the coordinated activity of the central nervous system at different hierarchical levels which involve parts of the cortex, basal ganglia, cerebellum, brainstem nuclei and spinal cord pathways and circuits (see Ch. 8). The basic patterns of muscle activity needed for locomotion are provided by spinal cord networks called central pattern generators which are subsequently modified by sensory input.

Walking is a complex process that requires coordination of the two legs; it also requires transfer of the body's weight from both legs to one leg. A basic understanding of locomotion is important as changes in the gait of an individual are indicative of joint, muscle and nervous system disorders.

When walking on a level surface the walking cycle can be divided into swing and stance phases; these phases look at the movements of a single leg as you walk.

- The **stance phase** begins with heel-strike, through to foot flat and mid-stance and ends with toe-off; it is the longer portion of the walking cycle, has both double and single limb support phases, and accounts for 60% of the cycle
- The **swing phase** is the smaller part of the walking cycle, only taking up 40% of the time; it begins with toe-off, accelerating to mid-swing then decelerating, ending when the heel makes contact with the ground.

Stance phase

At **heel-strike** the foot is dorsiflexed and usually inverted (for terms related to gait see Information box 9.1), and as the body weight is transferred to that leg the foot comes into full contact with the ground. At **toe-off** the foot is plantarflexed and slightly everted.

If the triceps surae (gastrocnemius and soleus) is paralysed or the calcaneus tendon is ruptured, toe-off is less

---

Disorders of gait can be caused by both mechanical and neurological problems. Mechanical causes include osteoarthritis, muscle strains and blisters, while neurological problems include deficits in perception and damage to nerves.

A commonly seen abnormal gait is seen in Parkinson disease, with short shuffling steps and rigidity in the knee and hip extensors.

---

effective; the gluteus maximus and hamstrings can lift the leg off the ground by extending the thigh at the hip joint but the movement is not as efficient.

Swing phase

During the swing phase the toes are prevented from dragging on the ground by the simultaneous flexion of the hip and knee joints. The foot is also dorsiflexed by the action of the muscles in the anterior compartment of the leg.

During normal walking the quadriceps and gluteus maximus contribute little but become more active when walking up and down hills or when climbing stairs.

Stabilisation

Stabilisation is very important when walking, especially as you go from a double support to a single support. When the weight is transferred to one lower limb there is a tendency for the unsupported pelvis to drop; this is prevented by the contraction of the hip abductors, the gluteus medius and minimus, on the supporting side to pull the pelvis level. Weak hip abductors, dislocation of the femoral head or fracture of the greater trochanter all lead to the pelvis dropping to the unsupported side. This is known as **Trendelenburg's sign**.

The invertors and evertors of the foot are the main stabilisers of the foot, with movements adjusting to the ground constantly.

Gait analysis

Gait analysis can be used for both normal and abnormal gaits. Markers are applied to anatomical landmarks such as the bony landmarks on the pelvis, knee and ankles. As the patient walks along a walkway they are videoed from several angles and strain gauges in the floor measure the forces applied by the feet. This allows the movement of each joint to be analysed. Specific conditions can be diagnosed and possible treatments suggested (Clinical box 9.31).

SPECIALISED CONNECTIVE TISSUES: SKIN, HAIR AND NAILS

Skin covers the whole body with a surface area (adult) of between $1.5\,m^2$ and $2\,m^2$. As well as providing a flexible, waterproof protective surface it is also involved in regulating body temperature (see Ch. 11) and providing sensory input about the external world (Ch. 8).

STRUCTURE OF SKIN

The skin is composed of three layers (Fig. 9.21):

- Epidermis, the most superficial layer of the skin, formed mainly of keratinocytes

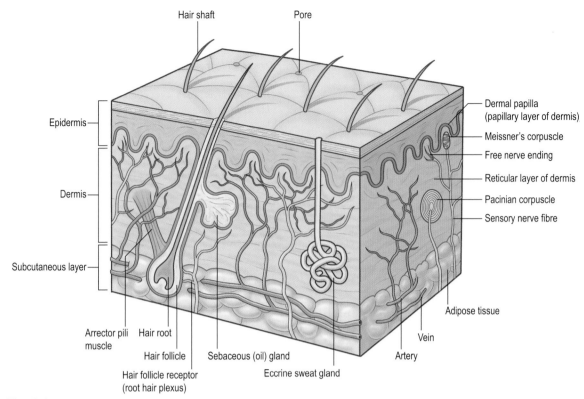

Fig. 9.21 **Structure of skin.**

- Dermis, the middle layer containing large quantities of connective tissue and the dermal capillaries which provide nutrients to the skin
- Subcutaneous layer, the deepest layer, formed from loose connective tissue and fat cells (adipose tissue).

Epidermis

The **epidermis** is a stratified squamous epithelium containing mainly **keratinocytes** with some **melanocytes**. The epidermis sits on a basement membrane composed mainly of type IV and VII collagens. Defects in these collagens result in skin fragility.

The epidermis is composed of four to five layers which represent different stages in the maturation of **keratin**, a fibrous protein which is secreted by the keratinocytes. The surface layers of the epidermis consist of toughened dead cells which are continually being shed. They are replaced from below by new cells produced at the base of the epidermis, the entire epidermis being replaced about every 40 days.

- **Stratum basale** (basal layer) is the layer closest to the basement membrane and contains the youngest keratinocytes which are rapidly dividing forms of epidermal stem cells. These columnar keratinocytes are anchored to the basement membrane by **hemidesmosomes** (small rivet-like structures).
- **Stratum spinosum** (spiny layer) consists of several layers of polyhedral keratinocytes linked by **desmosomes** (a complex of transmembrane proteins, specialised for cell to cell adhesion). These cells contain bundles of **prekeratin** which form **tonofilaments** which confer strength and distribute stress horizontally. The 'spines' are artefacts of tissue fixation but the name remains.
- **Stratum granulosum** (granular layer) consists of three to five layers of flattened keratinocytes. These cells have thickened membranes and, as well as tonofilaments,

contain two types of granule: **keratohyalin granules** (see below) and **lamellar granules** containing waterproofing glycolipids which are secreted into the extracellular space. This waterproofing slows water loss across the skin. Above this layer the cells are dead as they are too far away from the dermis to receive adequate nutrition.
- **Stratum lucidum** (clear layer) is only present in thick skin (palms, fingertips and soles of the feet) and consists of a few layers of dead keratinocytes with the keratin fibrils formed from the association of keratohyalin and tonofilaments.
- **Stratum corneum** (horny layer) is the thickest layer, 20–30 cells thick, and consists of dead cells called **corneocytes** filled with keratin fibrils. Their thick membranes and their waterproof coating produce a strong impermeable layer which protects the body from damage and dehydration. Cells from this layer are continually being shed, and can been seen as skin flakes and dandruff.

Melanocytes

Melanocytes are found in the stratum basale where they synthesise **melanins**, stimulated by the tyrosinase enzyme, which give the skin its characteristic colour (Information box 9.6). Melanin accumulates in melanocytes as membrane-bound melanosomes which move along the arm-like processes of the melanocytes, where they are then taken up by the nearby keratinocytes. The melanin granules take up position above the keratinocyte nucleus. As melanin absorbs ultraviolet radiation by scavenging for free radicals, they protect the skin from the damaging effects of exposure to sunlight (Clinical box 9.32).

The epidermis also contains **Langerhans' cells** (**epidermal dendritic cells**), a type of macrophage, mainly in the stratum spinosum. They not only ingest foreign material but also activate the immune system as they present antigens to lymphocytes. **Merkel's cells** are found in the stratum basale and consist of sensory receptors which respond to touch (see Ch. 8).

Information box 9.6 Skin colour

The relative number of melanocytes is the same in all humans; therefore an individual's skin colouration is dependent on the kind and amount of melanin that is made. Melanin is manufactured from tyrosine and is produced in two forms:
- Eumelanin, which is more abundant in people with dark skin
- Phaeomelanin, which has a pinkish colour and is more prominent in red hair and areas of the skin that have a pink/red tinge – the lips, nipples, penis glans and vagina.

Skin colour depends on the type and quantity of melanin present in the skin. Darker-skinned individuals produce more of the darker form of melanin and it is retained for longer.

Variation in skin colour is mainly under genetic control and the main gene responsible for determining the different melanin proportions is the melanocortin 1 receptor (*MC1R*) gene. Although it is thought that the lighter skin of individuals living at more northerly or southerly latitudes, where the incident radiation is less, has evolved in response to the need to produce sufficient vitamin D in the skin, the lighter skin colours seen in European and East Asian populations, while having some similarities in the genes that are involved, appear to have different genetic roots that have resulted in the lighter coloured skin of these populations.

Melanin production is stimulated by exposure to the sun to give a 'tan'; however, this also increases cross-linking of collagen fibres in the skin which produces wrinkles and there is an increased risk of skin cancer. The low incidence of skin cancer in dark-skinned individuals, especially in countries with a high incident solar radiation, shows how effective melanin is as a sun shield.

Albinos, who lack all melanin, are at grave risk of skin cancer unless they avoid going in the sun and use high strength UV-protective creams.

Clinical box 9.32 Skin cancer

While there are many types of benign tumours of the skin, exposure to UV radiation, especially in light-skinned individuals, is one of the major causes of malignant skin cancer. This is thought to be due to the inhibition of the tumour suppressor gene, *p53*. There are three main types:
- **Malignant melanoma** – this tumour, derived from melanocytes, is the most dangerous with 5-year survival rates for the severe forms being less than 40%. The CDKN2A cyclin-dependent kinase inhibitor has been implicated in the cause of this disease. Treatment involves surgical removal of the cancer plus a wide surrounding region with subsequent chemotherapy.
- **Basal cell carcinoma** – this tumour is derived from basal keratinocytes; it is the most common type of skin cancer and the least dangerous. Also known as rodent ulcers, these cancers are slow growing and can usually be cured by simple excision. Defects have been observed in the transmembrane receptor protein genes – PTCH.
- **Squamous cell carcinoma** – this tumour is derived from mature differentiated keratinocytes, and can metastasise to local lymph nodes. A genetic link has not been discovered but many genetic disorders have an increased risk of skin cancer and the aetiology is likely to be complex.

Public awareness campaigns aim to encourage the use of powerful sunscreens, limiting sun exposure times and periodic examination of any new lesions as a way of preventing and limiting skin cancer.

Dermis

The dermis consists of connective tissue containing cells such as fibroblasts and macrophages in a matrix of collagen and elastin. The dermis has large numbers of capillaries, nerve endings and lymphatics.

The dermis consists of two layers:
- Papillary layer – this thin uppermost layer has numerous raised projections which interdigitate with the epidermis. These either contain loops of capillaries or sensory nerve endings.
- Reticular layer – this layer contains bundles of collagen fibres which give strength and flexibility to the skin. This layer contains the sweat and sebaceous glands and the hair follicles.

Damage to the dermis can occur when the skin is burnt (Clinical box 9.33). Different types of burn affect different layers.

Clinical box 9.33

Blisters

Acute trauma such as digging the garden with a spade can cause shearing forces between the epidermis and the dermis of the hands, producing a friction blister. The separation between the epidermal and dermal layers of the skin is filled with fluid that leaks from the capillaries in the dermis.

Burns

When the skin is exposed to high temperatures (around 45°C or higher), proteins begin to break down and the cell membrane is disrupted with loss of potassium and gain of sodium and water. If sufficiently extensive, this can be life-threatening, so initial treatment is concentrated on maintaining fluid balance. If the patient survives this, then the major problem is infection due to the loss of the protective barrier. The extent of burns (in adults) is estimated by the **rule of nines** which divides the body into 11 regions (Table 9.1), each of which represents 9% of the surface area (total 99%) plus the perineum (1%).

Burns are classified according to the thickness of the burnt layer.
- **First-degree (superficial) burns** only involve damage to the epidermis. There is swelling, pain and localised redness, but the epidermis heals in 2–3 days without specialist treatment. Unless severe, sunburn is usually a first-degree burn.
- **Second-degree (superficial partial thickness) burns** involve the epidermis and the upper dermis. They produce blistering but if infection is avoided there are enough remaining live cells to produce regeneration within about 4 weeks.
- **Third-degree burns** involve the destruction of the entire epidermis and dermis and so are called **full-thickness burns**. These burns are not painful as the nerve endings are also destroyed but due to the complete loss of tissue they can only regenerate round the edge, which is very slow, so treatment usually involves skin grafting. New techniques involving growing the patient's own epidermal cells in culture to provide unlimited sheets of tissue with no rejection problems may eliminate many of the problems associated with traditional methods.

Table 9.1 Rule of nines – body surface area percentages

Area	%
Head and neck	9
Anterior upper trunk	9
Posterior upper trunk	9
Anterior lower trunk	9
Posterior lower trunk	9
Anterior arms	9
Posterior arms	9
Anterior leg (×2)	18
Posterior leg (×2)	18
Perineum	1
Total	100

Sweat glands

Sweat glands, which are found over most of the body, secrete water with varying amounts of sodium chloride and other metabolic compounds.

There are two types of sweat glands:

- **Eccrine glands** – these are found everywhere on the body except mucous membranes, and they secrete a watery hypotonic fluid which produces cooling of the skin as it evaporates. This varies from a minimum of 0.5 L/day to a maximum of 2 L/hour. This is a major mechanism in the control of body temperature, although it is much less effective when the external humidity is high. The fluid is slightly acidic (pH 4–6), which reduces fungal growth and also lubricates the skin surface. The glands consist of a simple secretory coil in the epidermis with a duct that opens onto the skin surface with a pore.
- **Apocrine glands** are found mainly in the axillae (armpits) and anogenital area. Their secretions are more viscous as they contain more fats and proteins than eccrine secretions and are not secreted onto the skin but into hair follicles. Although the secretions are initially odourless, bacteria on the skin break them down to give a musky smell which is the basis of body odour. They only become active after puberty and there are suggestions that they may be involved in sexual signalling.

Sebaceous glands

These glands secrete an oily substance called **sebum**, usually into the hair follicles or occasionally onto the skin. This softens the hair and skin and helps to reduce water loss from the skin surface. Sebum is also strongly bactericidal. The glands are especially numerous on the face and scalp. They are activated by androgens and become particularly active during puberty when they may cause acne (Clinical box 9.34).

Subcutaneous layer

This layer, which is also called the **hypodermis**, consists of areolar connective tissue and adipose tissue. As well as providing an energy store, the fat layer also acts as a shock absorber and insulator. The hypodermis allows the skin to slide over the underlying structures, reducing the severity of trauma.

HAIR

Structure of hair

Although humans are relatively hairless compared with most other mammals, most of the body is covered with hairs of some kind. Hair consists of the hair shaft, which is the external hair, and the root, which lies in the dermis and epidermis.

Clinical box 9.34   Acne

Excessive production of sebum along with infection by *Propionibacterium acnes* and a blockage of the sebaceous duct by hyperplasia lead to the release of cytokines and inflammation. Skin lesions can cause varying degrees of both temporary and permanent disfigurement. There are a number of treatments but the condition tends to improve over time, although it can sometimes be persistent.

The hair shaft consists of three concentric rings of keratinocytes, which contain hard keratin:

- Medulla – an inner core of large cells
- Cortex – several layers of flattened cells
- Cuticle – a single layer of overlapping highly keratinised cells.

Structure of hair follicle

In the dermis the **hair follicle** is where the hair shaft is produced. The developing shaft is surrounded by the **root sheath** which consists of two layers: the **inner** and **outer** root sheath. At the base of the follicle is the **hair bulb**. This consists of a loop of capillaries which project into a dermal papilla, which is covered by a single layer of cells from the stratum basale. Growth signals from the papilla reach a group of stem cells situated just above the hair bulb, called the **hair matrix,** and cause the cells to divide. This pushes the older cells upwards towards the skin surface. Just as in the different layers of the epidermis, the cells become more keratinised until they die and form the hair shaft.

Hair growth is not continuous, otherwise all our hair would keep growing until it broke. There are three phases of hair growth:

- **Anagen** – the active growth phase
- **Catagen** – the resting phase during which no growth occurs, the hair bulb partially atrophies and the hair shaft is released from the matrix with a short club root
- **Telogen** – during this phase the hair is shed and a new hair shaft develops at the matrix. The old hair is either pushed out by new hair or it falls out.

Most (80–90%) of the scalp hair is in anagen and about 10–20% in catagen. Fewer than 1% of scalp hair is in telogen, with the loss of about 90 hairs per day.

Hair growth is usually out of phase so there is no detectable reduction in hair volume, but a number of factors, such as stress, fever, surgery and childbirth, can cause synchronisation during anagen and so large numbers of hairs are lost at the same time leading to hair thinning (Clinical box 9.35). A common cause of hair thinning in women is iron-deficiency anaemia and this is reversed after treatment of the anaemia. However, other types of hair loss may be permanent. Women

---

Clinical box 9.35   Baldness and hirsutism

Alopecia

Both sexes can suffer varying degrees of baldness (or alopecia) and this can be linked to illness, stress, diet or other factors. However, the commonest type of baldness is **male pattern baldness**. This is androgen dependent and results from the shortening of the cycle of hair growth so that the hair shaft is so short that it does not emerge from the skin before shedding. Any hairs that do emerge are vellus rather that terminal hairs, leading to a fuzzy appearance. Although 80% of 70-year-old men show some baldness, the pattern of baldness (timing and shape) is often inherited. A common pattern starts with bi-temporal recession followed by crown thinning. Treatment with minoxidil, which increases blood flow, is effective in a third of cases but the drug has to be taken continually.

Hirsutism

Excessive hairiness or hirsutism can result in women from abnormally high levels of androgens. There are normally small amounts of androgens produced by the ovaries and adrenal glands, but tumours in these glands can lead to the formation of facial and chest hair as well as other masculinisation effects.

may also have excessive hairiness due to high levels of androgen hormones (Clinical box 9.35).

Each hair follicle is connected to a smooth muscle called the **arrector pili**, which can pull the hair into a more vertical position in response to cold or fear. In humans this gives the skin a dimpled appearance known as 'goose bumps' but in more hairy mammals this can either increase heat retention by trapping more air between the hairs or give the impression that the animal is larger (and possibly fiercer).

Hair density (number of hair follicles within a fixed area) also varies from person to person, fine hair being more dense.

Types of hair

There are three types of hair, of different length and thickness:

- **Lanugo** are fine, long hairs which are produced in utero and are shed before birth, hence they are usually only seen in premature babies.
- **Vellus** hairs are the short, fine hairs which cover most of the body, particularly in women and children.
- **Terminal** hairs are the thicker, longer hairs which cover the scalp and eyebrows. They grow in the axillae and pubic regions of both sexes after puberty and also form the beard and chest hairs in males.

The rate of hair growth is dependent on many factors including nutritional and hormonal status and normally is about 0.4 mm per day. The length of hairs in the different areas of the body is dependent on the length of time the hair follicles are in their active phase. Scalp hair is in the anagen phase for between 3 and 7 years but for eyebrow hair this is less than 4 months.

The hair shaft which projects from the skin varies in its cross-section. Evolutionary influences, possibly related to comfort, have led to differences in the shape of the follicles that lead to curly (oval or flat section) or straight (round section) hairs being produced. Hair colour is dependent on melanocytes in the hair follicle, which transfer melanins to the cortex of the growing hair and the balance of the different melanin types. Grey or white hair is due to reduced quantities of melanin being produced.

NAILS

Nails are derived from the epidermis and consist of hardened keratin which forms the hard **nail plate**. Nails grow from the proximal end, which consists of a **nail matrix** that produces the keratinocytes. These become heavily keratinised as they emerge to form the nail plate. The area of the nail matrix can be seen as a white crescent called the **lunula**, at the base of the nail. Under the nail plate lies the nail bed, which is pink due to the presence of dermal capillaries. Skin lies over the nail plate on each side, forming the **lateral nail folds**, and over part of the matrix, the **cuticle**.

Finger nails grow faster than toe nails; it takes 6 months to replace a finger nail and 12 months for a toe nail. The reason is unclear but is likely to be related to environmental exposure (with faster growth on exposure to sunlight) and usage (friction). However, there are many disease processes which can affect nail growth and distinctive patterns in nail growth can reflect current or previous medical history:

- **Nail pitting**. Small depressions in the surface, often seen in association with psoriasis, but can also be related to other connective tissue disorders.
- **Nail clubbing**. This is seen when the ends of the fingers enlarge and the nails curve around the tips. This development is often linked to reduced oxygen availability and is associated with a large number of lung and cardiovascular diseases, but is also seen with other conditions.
- **Koilonychia**. In this the nails appear spoon shaped. Seen in association with iron deficiency anaemia and **haemochromatosis** (excess iron) and hypothyroidism.
- **Terry's nails**. The nails have a white 'ground glass' appearance with dark bands near the tips. This condition can be seen in the aged or in association with liver disease, heart failure and diabetes.
- **Beau's lines** are ridges in the nail caused by a temporary halt in nail growth which might be the result of trauma, infections associated with high temperatures, uncontrolled diabetes and zinc deficiency.
- **Oncholysis**. Separation of the nail and the nail bed is normally associated with fungal disease, but can also result from trauma, thyroid disease, psoriasis and some drug interactions. Oncholysis of a single digit is likely to be the result of tumour.
- **Yellow nail syndrome**. Seen in chronic bronchitis and other respiratory disease conditions.
- **Oil spots** are darkish brown discolourations often associated with psoriasis.

GENERALISED CONNECTIVE TISSUE

Connective tissue is mainly composed of **collagen** and **elastin** which together form matrices that protect organs within the body.

Elastin, so called because of its stretching ability, is the major component of ligaments and skin.

Collagen is found in many different forms, and abnormalities are seen in autoimmune and vascular conditions and in inflammatory processes. It is a widely dispersed connective tissue organised into fibrils. Types I–V are the most abundant:

- **Type I**: about 90% of the collagen in the body is type I; it is the main component of bone and is utilised in repair. It is not found in cartilage.
- **Type II**, formed of copolymers, is the main component of cartilage and is also found in the cornea and vitreous humour.
- **Type III** is found in arteries and hollow organs, often in combination with type I.
- **Type IV** forms the basement membrane.
- **Type V** is found in cell surfaces, placenta and hair, often in combination with types I and II.

There are many different diseases associated with abnormalities in collagen production, many of them from genetic causes (see Clinical box 9.36). The main collagen diseases include:

- **Rheumatoid arthritis** where there is immune inflammation, mainly of the joint membrane.
- **Scleroderma** in which immune cell activation produces scar tissues in skin, blood vessels and organs.

Clinical box 9.36   Collagen diseases

Type I collagen is the most abundant in the body and is also the collagen used in tissue repair. It is present in cartilage, tendons, skin, artery walls and in the endomysium of myofibrils. Defects in the *COL1A1* and *COL1A2* genes have been reported in diseases such as:

- **Osteogenesis imperfecta** (Brittle bone disease, see Clinical box 9.1).
- **Ehlers–Danlos syndrome** which shows wide heterogeneity affecting a range of tissues but thin stretchy skin, joint hypermobility and fragile blood vessels are all common observations in this condition.
- **Type II** collagen is found in hyaline cartilage and in the vitreous humour of the eye. The *COL2A1* gene is responsible for its production and chondrodysplasia is one condition that is seen in association with mutations producing various skeletal abnormalities and an increased risk of developing osteoarthritis. In **Stickler syndrome** individuals typically have a very flat face.
- **Type III** collagen is a rapidly produced type of collagen from young fibroblasts and is found in granulation tissues, artery walls, skin and internal organs, developing before, and in association with, type I collagen. Defects in *COL3A1* genes are also associated with Ehlers–Danlos syndrome.
- **Type IV** collagen is found in the basement membrane and in the lens of the eye. It also forms an important component of capillaries and the kidney glomerulus. There is a family of genes, *COL4A1–6*, which are involved in producing this form of collagen. Alport syndrome is associated with mutations in types 3–5 and the resultant defects in the basement membrane in the kidney leads to kidney failure. Goodpasture syndrome is an auto-immune condition which also results in kidney disease, but there are also lung manifestations and haemorrhage is a common observation, along with antibodies to glomerular basement membrane (anti-GBM).
- **Type V** collagen is found in most interstitial tissue and forms fibrillar collagen. Defects in the *COL5A1* gene are also associated with Ehlers–Danlos syndrome.

- **Sjögren syndrome** in which the inability to secrete saliva and tears occurs. This sign may also be associated with other collagen diseases.
- **Systemic lupus erythematus** (**SLE**) which is a widespread inflammation of connective tissues in all organs and is aggravated by sunlight.
- **Wegener's granulomatosis** which mainly causes inflammation in the upper respiratory tract.
- **Mixed connective tissue disorders** combining many of the above conditions.

Many of these disorders show a 3:1 female to male ratio.

10

Endocrinology

Joy Hinson and Peter Raven

Introduction	451
The endocrine system	451
Neuroendocrinology	455
Important concepts in endocrinology	455
Endocrine regulation – the role of the hypothalamus and pituitary	458
Growth hormone	461
ENDOCRINE HOMEOSTASIS	464
Thyroid gland and the regulation of metabolism	464
The structure and location of the thyroid	464
Hormone synthesis in the thyroid gland	465
Control of thyroid function	466
Hormones and 'stress'	467
Adrenal cortex and medulla	468
Endocrine control of glucose metabolism	471
Regulation of plasma glucose concentration	471
Endocrine pancreas	471

Endocrine control of blood calcium	475
Calcium homeostasis	475
Control of blood calcium and phosphate concentrations	475
REPRODUCTIVE PHYSIOLOGY	478
Male reproductive endocrinology	478
Hypothalamic–pituitary–testicular axis	479
Female reproductive endocrinology	481
Hormonal control of the ovary and menstrual cycle	481
Puberty	484
Pregnancy	486
Fertilisation	486
Foetal development	488
Parturition – labour	488
Infertility (subfertility)	491
The endocrinology of ageing (including menopause)	491

INTRODUCTION

The human body is an astonishingly well-coordinated organism. Made up of several billion cells, the body depends on communication systems which are precisely regulated and which reach every one of those cells. There are two main communication systems in the human body, the **nervous system** and the **endocrine system**. In Chapter 8 we saw how the nervous system is constructed and how it processes information and controls a range of processes from regulation of blood pressure to movement of our limbs. In this chapter we shall look at the endocrine system and how it interacts with the nervous system to control the body's homeostatic and reproductive systems (see Information box 10.1).

Information box 10.1 Comparison of nervous and endocrine systems

Both systems use chemical signals (**hormones and neurotransmitters**). The nervous system is hard-wired with the signalling molecule delivered precisely to the point where it is needed. This means that only a very few different signalling molecules are required as they do not affect any cells except at their site of delivery. The endocrine system is not hard-wired. All the cells in the body are exposed to hormones so there is a wide range of signalling molecules needed.

Both systems need receptors for their chemical signals. In the nervous system specificity is conferred by hard-wiring: the neurotransmitter is delivered directly and specifically to the cell which has the receptor and responds to the transmitter. In the endocrine system, where hormones are delivered to all cells, specificity comes only from expression of the receptor for the hormone. Only cells with receptors for a hormone can respond to that particular hormonal signal.

The endocrine, or hormonal, system is responsible for regulating most of the systems of the body. You will find descriptions of hormones and their effects throughout this book: on energy metabolism (Ch. 3), bone (Ch. 9), the cardiovascular system (Ch. 11), bone marrow and haemopoiesis (Ch.12), the renal system (Ch. 14), the gastrointestinal system (Ch. 15) and the regulation of food intake (Ch. 16). It is also responsible for regulating reproductive processes.

THE ENDOCRINE SYSTEM

The endocrine system is made up of a number of hormone-producing glands. These are called **endocrine glands** (Fig. 10.1). Examples of endocrine glands include the pituitary and the thyroid glands. These glands do not have secretory ducts like the **exocrine glands** (e.g. salivary glands), but instead they release **hormones** directly into the bloodstream. In addition to these discrete endocrine glands, there are various different endocrine cells found in other tissues of the body, such as the G cells, located in the antrum of the stomach, which secrete gastrin. Isolated endocrine cells such as the G cells are often collectively referred to as the 'diffuse endocrine system'.

Hormones released by endocrine glands and cells circulate in the blood and so all cells in the body, by virtue of having a blood supply, are exposed to all hormones. But only the cells which have a specific receptor for a hormone are able to 'see' the hormone and respond to the hormonal signal. These cells are called '**target cells**' for the hormone.

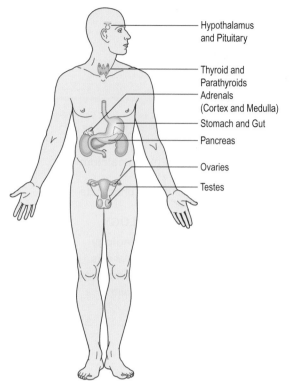

Fig. 10.1 **The location of the human endocrine glands.** The skin and vascular systems also have endocrine functions.

The labels in Fig. 10.1 point to:
- Hypothalamus and Pituitary
- Thyroid and Parathyroids
- Adrenals (Cortex and Medulla)
- Stomach and Gut
- Pancreas
- Ovaries
- Testes

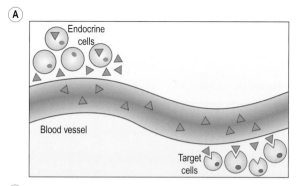

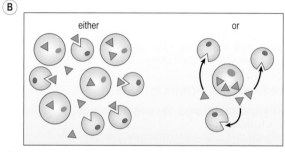

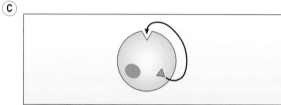

Fig. 10.2 Comparison of (A) endocrine, (B) paracrine and (C) autocrine regulation.

Hormone receptors have a very high affinity for their hormones, which means that even very low circulating concentrations of hormones are biologically effective. Most hormones circulate in picomolar or nanomolar concentrations (10^{-15} to 10^{-12} moles per litre).

Classically, hormones are released into the bloodstream and act on tissues which are distant from the site of hormone production, an endocrine effect. However, some hormones act locally within the tissue where they are produced. These are called 'local hormones' or '**paracrine**' effects. Some hormones have both local and systemic effects and so act in a paracrine and endocrine manner (Fig. 10.2). An example is testosterone, which has local actions in the testes and hormonal effects on muscle. Some hormones, particularly growth factors, exert their actions on the cells which secrete them. These are called '**autocrine** effects' (see Ch. 2).

There are three broad groups of hormones: **peptides**, **steroids** and **amino acid derivatives** (Table 10.1).

Peptide hormones: secretion and mechanisms of action

The largest group of hormones, and the most diverse, is the peptide hormones. These vary in size from just three amino acids, such as **thyrotropin-releasing hormone** (**TRH**), to 30 kDa glycosylated proteins, such as **thyroid-stimulating hormone** (**TSH**, also called **thyrotropin**). Peptide hormones are made in a similar way to all secreted proteins. Most peptide hormones are the product of a single gene which encodes a larger protein, called a **pre-prohormone**. After production of the protein in the rough endoplasmic reticulum of the endocrine cell, the protein is processed in the Golgi apparatus and the secretory granules. The initial N-terminal

Table 10.1	The chemical nature of some key hormones (closely related peptides/proteins are grouped together)
Chemical class	**Hormone**
Amino acid derivative	Epinephrine (adrenaline)
	Thyroid hormones (T_3, T_4)
Steroid	Oestrogens (e.g. oestradiol)
	Androgens (e.g. testosterone)
	Progesterone
	Cortisol
	Aldosterone
Peptides	Thyrotropin-releasing hormone (TRH)
	Gonadotropin-releasing hormone (GnRH)
	Vasopressin
	Oxytocin (OT)
	Vasoactive intestinal peptide (VIP)
	Glucagon
	Adrenocorticotropic hormone (ACTH)
	Somatostatin
Proteins	Insulin
	Insulin-like growth factors (IGFs)
	Growth hormone (GH)
	Prolactin (PRL)
	Placental lactogen (PL)
	Parathyroid hormone (PTH)
Glycoproteins	Thyroid-stimulating hormone (TSH)
	Follicle-stimulating hormone (FSH)
	Luteinising hormone (LH)
	Chorionic gonadotropin (CG)

signal sequence is cleaved, leaving the **prohormone**. The action of other proteolytic enzymes produces the mature hormone with associated peptide fragments which are secreted together with the hormone. Peptide hormones are usually stored in secretory granules within the cell until they are released in response to an appropriate signal. Secretion is by non-constitutive exocytosis which depends upon increases in intracellular calcium acting as a second messenger (see Ch. 2).

There are several distinct 'families' of peptide hormones. These are groups of structurally similar hormones which may have arisen through duplication of an ancestral gene. However, not all peptide hormones are members of a family.

Peptide hormones are water soluble and so are readily transported in blood without needing specific carrier proteins. The half-life in blood of most peptide hormones is short, a matter of a few minutes only, and they are inactivated and degraded by proteolysis.

Peptide hormones all bind to receptors located on the plasma membrane of their target cells and exert their effects on the cell by either the direct activation of a protein kinase or by the generation of a second messenger and the indirect activation of a protein kinase (see Ch. 2 for more details). In either case, the net result is phosphorylation of target proteins within the cell and altered cell function.

Steroid hormones: synthesis, actions and metabolism

There are five major classes of steroid hormone (Fig. 10.3) although **calcitriol**, the active form of vitamin D3 is often counted as a sixth class. The steroid hormones are all synthesised from **cholesterol**, which is either taken up by the cell from circulating lipoproteins by receptor-mediated endocytosis, or is made de novo, from acetate, within the cell. In contrast to the peptide-secreting cells, those that secrete steroids do not store the final hormonal product, but instead store cholesterol, the precursor for steroid synthesis. The cholesterol is stored in an esterified form in lipid droplets within the cell. Steroid synthesis takes place in the mitochondria and smooth endoplasmic reticulum, and the abundance of these organelles, together with the lipid droplets, gives steroid-secreting cells a characteristic appearance under electron microscopy.

The pathway of steroid synthesis is shown in Figure 10.4. Most of the enzymes involved belong to the **CYP** gene family, encoding the **cytochrome P450 steroid hydroxylases**. The initial step, the conversion of cholesterol to **pregnenolone**, is common to the synthesis of all the steroid hormones and is the rate limiting step of steroidogenesis. Unusually, it is not the activity of the enzyme cytochrome $P450_{scc}$, which cleaves the side chain from cholesterol to form pregnenolone, which limits the rate of steroidogenesis (see Information box 10.2), but rather the rate of delivery of cholesterol into the mitochondrion.

Steroid synthesis is a multi-step process which involves the movement of steroid hormone precursors between the mitochondria and the smooth endoplasmic reticulum. This process is not well understood but it is clear that there is a mechanism for holding the steroid within the cell until the final hormonal steroid has been made. Unlike peptide hormones there is no specific secretory mechanism for steroids; they are thought to simply diffuse out of the cell down a concentration gradient. What prevents the intermediate products from escaping the cell is, as yet, unknown.

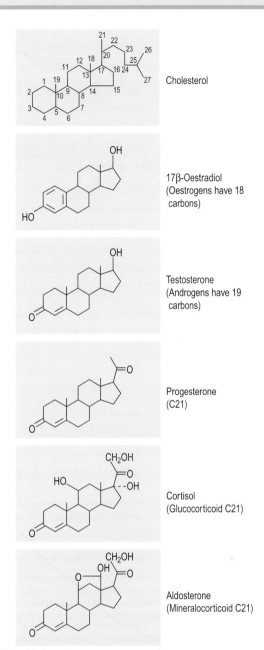

Fig. 10.3 Major classes of steroid hormone and the structure of cholesterol showing numbering of carbon atoms.

The steroid hormones are lipophilic and do not readily dissolve in blood. They mostly rely on specific transport proteins, a group of steroid binding globulins, to carry them in blood. As a result, steroid hormones have a half-life in plasma of an hour or longer. They are metabolised in the liver into less active compounds. The liver enzymes which metabolise steroids belong to the same two families as the main enzymes of steroid synthesis: the **hydroxysteroid dehydrogenases** and the CYP family of hydroxylases. In addition, steroids are conjugated in the liver to produce glucuronides and sulphates which increases their solubility and allows them to be excreted in bile or urine. Not all steroid metabolism results in deactivation, however. For some hormones, such as testosterone, peripheral metabolism in adipose tissue or muscle produces either the more potent androgen, **dihydrotestosterone**, or **oestradiol**, the main female sex steroid. In the case of **vitamin D3**, metabolism in the liver and kidney is essential to produce the active hormone.

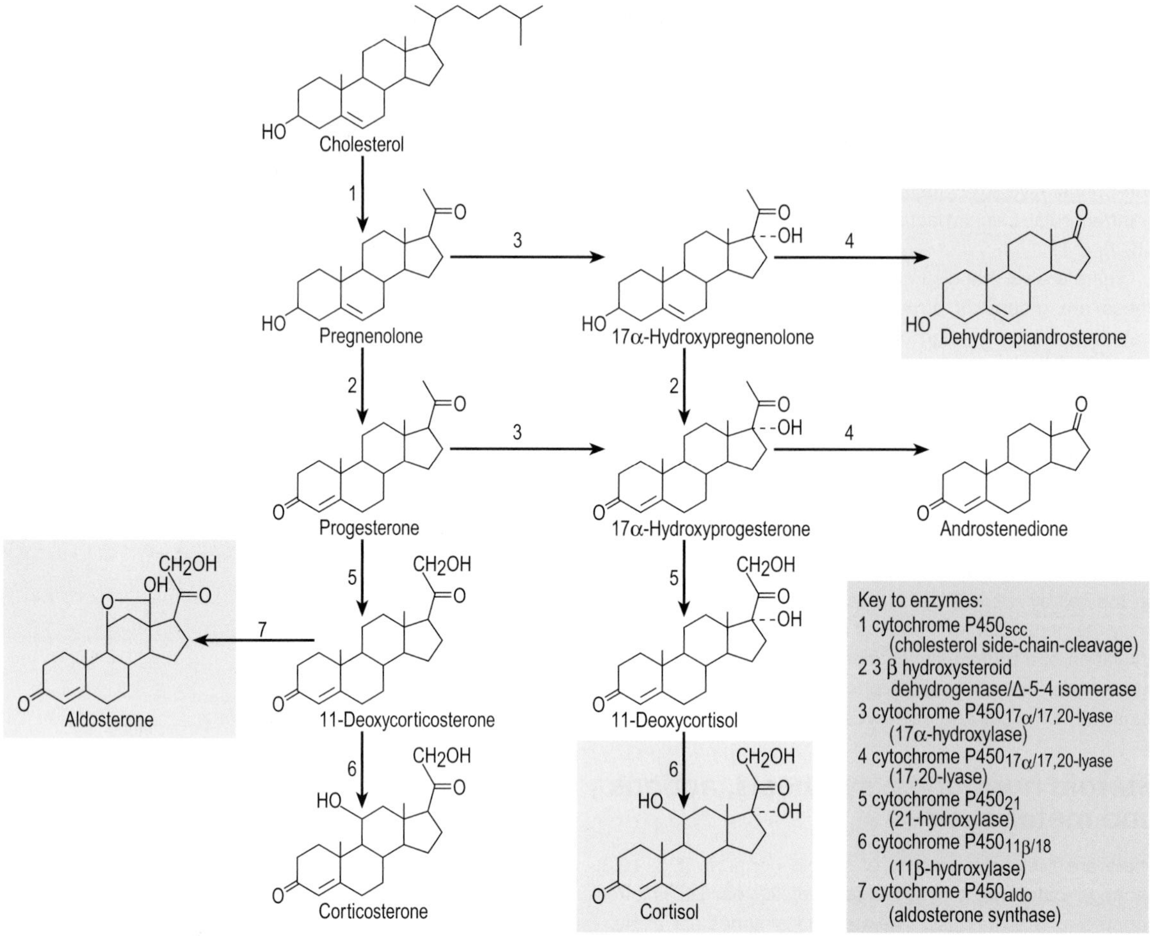

Fig. 10.4 **Outline of steroid synthesis from cholesterol.** There is no single tissue in which all these pathways occur. The CYP genes are expressed in a highly tissue-specific manner.

Information box 10.2	The rate limiting step of steroidogenesis

In order to reach the enzyme which catalyses the first reaction of steroid biosynthesis, cholesterol has to travel from its storage site in lipid droplets to the inner mitochondrial membrane. The protein which facilitates this transfer is called **StAR, steroidogenesis acute regulatory protein**, and is found in all the cells of steroid synthesis in the adrenal glands and the gonads. Only very low levels of steroid synthesis can occur in the absence of functional StAR protein. Mutations in the gene encoding StAR result in a disorder termed '**lipoid congenital adrenal hyperplasia**' which is characterised by a failure of appropriate sexual differentiation during foetal development, and by severe glucocorticoid deficiency early in life. The affected adrenal cells have a characteristic lipid-rich appearance under microscopy.

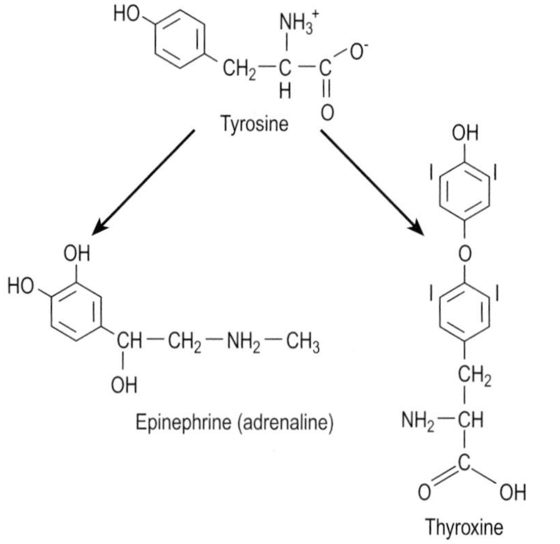

Steroid hormones are small and lipophilic and readily cross the plasma membrane of cells. They act by binding to intracellular receptors which function as transcription factors, in turn binding to response elements in the promoter regions of certain genes and so modifying gene transcription (see Ch. 2). In some tissues steroids also appear to act by binding to cell-surface receptors, but this mode of action is unusual.

Modified amino acids: thyroid hormones and catecholamines

The final group of hormones comprises those derived from the amino acid **tyrosine** (Table 10.1). These are the adrenal catecholamines, **epinephrine (adrenaline)** and **norepinephrine**

Fig. 10.5 **Thyroid hormones and catecholamines are produced by the metabolism of tyrosine.**

(**noradrenaline**), and the **thyroid** hormones (Fig. 10.5). Despite their common precursor these are very different hormones. The catecholamines are synthesised by step-wise modification of free tyrosine residues, then stored in secretory vesicles and released in response to an action potential. The thyroid hormones, **thyroxine (T_4)** and **tri-iodothyronine (T_3)**, on the other hand, are formed by the iodination of pairs of tyrosine residues, held within a large precursor molecule called **thyroglobulin**. The thyroid hormones generally behave like steroid hormones, binding to intracellular receptors and altering gene transcription, while the catecholamines bind to cell surface receptors and act by the generation of second messengers. One difference between the thyroid hormones and steroids is the requirement for thyroid hormones to have a specific mechanism for crossing the plasma membrane. They also have very different half-lives in blood. Thyroid hormones have the longest half-life of hormones, circulating in blood for days before being de-iodinated and conjugated in the liver. Catecholamines have the shortest half-life of all hormones, lasting only a few seconds before they are degraded by **monoamine oxidase**, an enzyme found in most tissues.

NEUROENDOCRINOLOGY

There is a degree of interaction between the nervous system and the endocrine system. Several hormones are released from neurons, in response to an action potential, in exactly the same way that neurotransmitters are released. These are called **neurohormones**. However, instead of being released into a synaptic cleft, neurohormones are released into the blood, where they circulate and exert their effects on target tissues (Information box 10.3). The major neuroendocrine tissues are the hypothalamus, the posterior pituitary and the adrenal medulla.

IMPORTANT CONCEPTS IN ENDOCRINOLOGY

Patterns of hormone secretion

Most hormones are secreted in response to a specific stimulus. In some cases this means that their secretion is episodic. **Insulin**, for example, is secreted in response to high blood glucose and so it is secreted in an episodic manner,

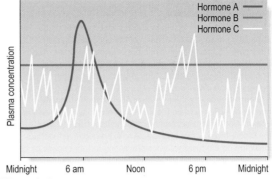

Fig. 10.6 **Patterns of hormone secretion.** Some hormones, such as hormone A, have a pronounced diurnal variation in their secretion. An example would be cortisol. Other hormones, such as hormone B, are maintained at constant levels throughout the day, e.g. thyroxine. Hormone C shows episodic secretion. This pattern of secretion is common to many hormones.

whenever blood glucose reaches the appropriate threshold (Fig. 10.6, see also Fig.1.2). At some times the plasma level of insulin may be very high, while at other times it is undetectable. Other hormones, such as thyroxine, which is needed to maintain physiological functions all the time, is secreted in a manner that allows a constant plasma concentration of the hormone over a period of days or weeks. This is a form of 'set point' regulation of a hormone: levels fluctuate only slightly around a constant set point. In other cases, particularly the adrenal corticosteroid, cortisol, secretion is subject to diurnal variation which means that there is a fairly predictable pattern of hormone secretion over a 24-hour period. The diurnal variation in hormone secretion is controlled by the **suprachiasmatic nucleus** (**SCN**) in the hypothalamus. Most hormones that are subject to diurnal variation also have some episodic secretion superimposed on this daily variation so that there is some response to immediate physiological demand as well as the underlying pattern (see Information box 10.4).

Negative feedback

The concept of negative feedback regulation is fundamental in understanding homeostatic mechanisms including the endocrine system (see Fig. 1.1). The body has some fairly basic mechanisms to protect it from excess of any kind, and this includes protection against hormonal excesses. The simplest form of negative feedback regulation is illustrated by the control of parathyroid hormone (PTH) secretion (see later). The main action of PTH is to increase plasma calcium and when this rises above a set point further production of PTH is inhibited. In an endocrine axis the final hormonal product of the axis exerts feedback inhibition on the other elements higher up the axis. An example of negative feedback is seen in the **hypothalamic–pituitary–thyroid axis** (see Fig. 10.7).

Endocrine disease

The endocrine system involves finely controlled patterns of hormone secretion. When these patterns are disrupted then disease occurs. In terms of clinical medicine, endocrinology is very simple: there can either be too much or too little of a hormone. An imbalance either way causes disease. Most endocrine disease is caused by autoimmune disorders. These usually result in loss of endocrine function, such as

---

| **Information box 10.3** | **Hormone transport in blood** |

In general, peptide hormones are hydrophilic and readily soluble in blood and so circulate in blood in a free, unbound form. Plasma albumin does bind small peptide hormones but this is a loose association and does not have a regulatory function. One peptide hormone, **insulin-like growth factor 1** (**IGF-1**), does have a specific plasma binding protein, but this is unusual.

Steroid and thyroid hormones, however, are lipophilic and poorly soluble in blood. These are usually transported bound to a specific binding globulin:

- **Thyroid hormone binding globulin** (**THBG**), binds thyroxine
- **Sex hormone binding globulin** (**SHBG**), binds oestradiol and testosterone
- **Cortisol binding globulin** (**CBG**), is also called **transcortin**
- **Vitamin D** binding protein.
   Aldosterone is usually transported like small peptides, loosely bound to plasma albumin.
   These hormone binding globulins have several functions:
1. They increase the solubility of steroid hormone and thyroxine.
2. They increase the plasma half-life of these hormones by protecting them from renal filtration and peripheral metabolism. Cortisol, bound to CBG, has a half-life in plasma of around 90 minutes, while aldosterone, which does not have a specific binding protein, has a half-life of about 15 minutes.
3. They may act as an accessible store of hormone in blood.
4. They may serve to deliver hormones to specific target tissues.

The hypothalamus and pituitary gland have a role in orchestrating the activity of several other parts of the endocrine system. They achieve this through a number of endocrine axes. The hypothalamic–pituitary–thyroid axis is illustrated here (Fig. 10.7). The hypothalamus releases TRH (thyrotropin releasing hormone) in response to a stimulus such as cold. TRH acts on the anterior pituitary to stimulate the release of TSH (thyroid stimulating hormone), which acts on the thyroid gland to increase release of thyroxine. Thyroxine, being small and lipophilic, crosses the blood–brain barrier and is able to exert negative feedback inhibition on the hypothalamus preventing further release of TRH. Thyroxine also acts on the anterior pituitary inhibiting further TSH release.

There is also a **hypothalamic–pituitary–adrenal axis**, a **hypothalamic–pituitary–gonadal axis** and a **hypothalamic–pituitary–IGF axis**.

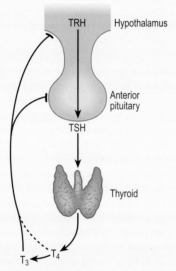

Fig. 10.7   The hypothalamic–pituitary–thyroid axis. Thyrotropin releasing hormone (TRH), from the hypothalamus, stimulates the release of thyroid stimulating hormone (TSH) from the anterior pituitary. The TSH stimulates the thyroid gland to release T_3 and T_4, which exert a negative feedback inhibitory effect on the hypothalamus and pituitary gland.

Primary adrenocortical insufficiency – Addison disease
Failure of the adrenal cortex to secrete aldosterone and cortisol is most commonly due to autoimmune disorder or tuberculosis. Other autoimmune disorders (e.g. type 1 diabetes mellitus, Hashimoto's thyroiditis, Graves disease, vitiligo) are commonly seen in patients with autoimmune Addison disease. The signs and symptoms are predictable from the actions of the missing hormones (Table 10.2). Pigmentation of the skin, due to the excess ACTH secretion from the anterior pituitary released from its glucocorticoid negative feedback, is often the first manifestation and distinguishes it from secondary adrenocortical insufficiency.

Secondary adrenocortical insufficiency
Loss of ACTH secretion from the anterior pituitary, either because of hypopituitarism or because of atrophy of corticotropes induced by long-term glucocorticoid treatment, results in a failure of the zona fasciculata and zona reticularis to secrete glucocorticoids and androgens. However, the output of aldosterone by the zona glomerulosa is normal. Secondary adrenal insufficiency is easily distinguished from primary:

- There is no pigmentation
- ACTH concentrations are low
- ACTH injection will stimulate cortisol secretion (note that in very long-standing cases of secondary adrenocortical insufficiency the response will be slow, so that a 3-day test, at the least, will be needed)
- No effects attributable to lack of aldosterone are seen
- Other evidence of pituitary failure (hypogonadism, hypothyroidism) except when the insufficiency follows withdrawal of long-term glucocorticoid therapy.

Table 10.2   Clinical features of primary adrenal insufficiency (Addison disease)

Loss of aldosterone	Loss of cortisol
Na⁺ loss: hyponatremia hypovolemic shock raised plasma renin	*reduced gluconeogenesis, increased glucose transport and utilization by muscle and fat:* hypoglycemia
impaired excretion of K^+ and H^+: hyperkalemia metabolic acidosis	*loss of enhanced catecholamine actions:* postural hypotension, hypotension
	loss of appetite stimulation and GI trophic effects: anorexia, weakness, fatigue, nausea, vomiting
	increased ACTH from loss of negative feedback: hyperpigmentation
	decreased secretion of adrenal androgens: loss of pubic and axillary hair in women

the autoimmune destruction of the endocrine pancreas which results in **type 1 diabetes**, or autoimmune loss of adrenal function causing **Addison disease** (Clinical box 10.1). However, in some cases, autoantibodies cause stimulation of an endocrine gland with an increase in hormone secretion. The commonest example of this is **Graves disease** of the thyroid (Clinical box 10.2).

Hormone-secreting tumours, called **adenomas**, are relatively uncommon but result in significant disease. Adenomas have usually lost the normal endocrine regulation and so the tumour produces hormone in an uncontrolled manner. The commonest endocrine tumour is a **prolactinoma**, a tumour of the posterior pituitary which secretes **prolactin** (Clinical box 10.3). The hormone secreted by the tumour presents one set of problems, but in the pituitary gland where space is limited, the presence of a tumour displaces other endocrine cells resulting in loss of other hormones and the symptoms of hormone deficiencies.

Chromosomal abnormalities are responsible for most of the disorders of sexual differentiation, but endocrine disorders can also result from defects of the hormone receptor,

such as **androgen insensitivity syndrome** and, of course, the insulin resistance seen in **type 2 diabetes**. Finally, it is important to be aware that some endocrine disease is iatrogenic, for example the **Cushing syndrome** commonly caused by prolonged therapeutic use of high levels of glucocorticoids (Clinical box 10.4).

Endocrine testing

When endocrine disorders are suspected it is usual to carry out a range of clinical tests. In most cases hormone concentrations are measured directly in blood samples. However, there are many factors which need to be taken into consideration when endocrine tests are carried out. A key factor is the pattern of hormone secretion. It is obviously easiest to take a blood sample and measure hormone levels at a time

Clinical box 10.2 Hyperthyroidism

Hyperthyroidism is overactivity of the thyroid gland. Many of the consequences of exposure to excess thyroid hormone – **thyrotoxicosis** – are related to the physiological effects of the hormones.

Graves disease

The commonest form of hyperthyroidism is **Graves disease**, an autoimmune disorder in which naïve T helper lymphocytes (Th2 cells) are inappropriately primed to recognise TSH receptors on thyroid follicle cells. The activated Th2 cells stimulate cognate B lymphocytes to produce antibodies to the TSH receptors. These are termed **thyroid-stimulating immunoglobulins** because in effect they act as agonists of the TSH receptor and the consequence is unregulated thyroid hormone production. The high thyroid hormone concentration clamps TSH at low levels by intense negative feedback.

Thyroid eye disease in Graves disease (ophthalmopathy)

Retro-orbital connective tissues suffer autoimmune attack by activated Th2 cells because they express TSH receptors:

- Fibroblasts secrete glycosaminoglycans, generating oedema, which pushes the eyes forward **(proptosis)** and may produce visual impairment by compression of the optic nerve
- Cytokines from activated lymphocytes stimulate abnormal growth of the extraocular eye muscles causing disturbance to gaze and vision
- Overactivity of sympathetic transmission (an effect of elevated thyroid hormone levels) retracts the eyelids; inability to cover the eyes results in conjunctival oedema and corneal damage, with scarring.

Total thyroidectomy and treatment with radioactive iodine (^{131}I) are the most effective treatments for ophthalmopathy because they remove the source of self-antigens. Less drastic management includes corticosteroids to suppress the autoimmune inflammatory response.

Neonatal Graves disease

Graves disease can occur in neonates due to placental transfer of thyroid-stimulating immunoglobulins from an afflicted mother. The disorder resolves over 4–12 weeks as the infant clears the offending antibodies.

Management of hyperthyroidism

- Anti-thyroid drugs inhibit thyroid peroxidase, blocking iodide organification and coupling reactions. The main ones are the **thioamides (carbimazole** or its metabolite **methimazole**, and **propylthiouracil**). Because of the long half-life of T_4, it can take 3–4 weeks for clinical improvement.
- **Iodides** (e.g. potassium iodide) at high concentrations suppress organification and thyroid hormone synthesis via the Wolff–Chaikoff effect. Because iodide administration produces improvement within 2–7 days; it is used (along with β-blockers which antagonise the Th-mediated increase in β-adrenoceptors, and other measures) in **thyrotoxic crisis** (or **'thyroid storm'**), a rare but rapid, life-threatening, worsening of hyperthyroidism that is usually triggered by stress.
- **Iodine radioisotope**: ^{131}I is rapidly absorbed by the gut and concentrated in the thyroid by iodide trapping. It decays by emitting electrons (β$^-$ particles), and has a **biological** half-life of 5 days. The electrons have sufficient energy to penetrate 0.4–2.0 mm and kill large numbers of thyroid cells. Because ^{131}I crosses the placenta and is secreted into milk it is not used in pregnant or lactating women. Early fears that the radiation would lead to increased incidence of leukaemias or thyroid cancers have not been borne out. It restores normal thyroid hormone levels in most patients, but hyperthyroidism often re-occurs.
- **Subtotal thyroidectomy**: care must be taken not to remove all the parathyroid glands and to avoid damaging the recurrent laryngeal nerve.

Clinical box 10.3 Hyperprolactinaemia

Hyperprolactinaemia is the over-production of prolactin, and may be physiological, e.g. during pregnancy and lactation. Pathological causes include:

- Prolactin-secreting tumours, which account for over 70% of all anterior pituitary tumours (commonly a microadenoma)
- Lesions of the hypothalamus or pituitary stalk
- Dopamine (D$_2$) receptor antagonist drugs, which interfere with dopaminergic inhibition of prolactin secretion, e.g. metoclopramide, phenothiazines.

Hyperprolactinaemia causes infertility in both sexes by suppressing:

- The secretion of GnRH
- The gonadotrope response to GnRH
- The response of the gonads to LH.

Clinical box 10.4 Effect of excess glucocorticoids – Cushing syndrome

Long-term therapeutic use of pharmacological doses of synthetic glucocorticoids is the commonest cause of **Cushing syndrome**. The condition could also be secondary to an ACTH-secreting adenoma of the pituitary or ectopic ACTH sources (e.g. small cell carcinoma of the lung). Primary Cushing disease is uncommon and usually due to an adrenal tumour. Major features of Cushing syndrome are:

- Skin pigmentation, which is infrequent in the secondary syndrome, but is seen, particularly, in the case of ectopic ACTH-secreting tumours. It is not seen in the primary disease since here ACTH concentrations are low
- Hyperglycaemia – which results because of the **diabetogenic effect** of glucocorticoids, i.e. they raise blood glucose concentration
- Increased appetite, with truncal obesity adding to insulin resistance
- Increased proteolysis, which reduces muscle mass, with weakness and wasting, especially of the proximal limb muscles
- Enhanced actions of catecholamines resulting in hypertension
- Bone demineralisation and hence **osteoporosis**, which often leads to pathological fractures
- Decreased collagen synthesis, which increases wound healing time and is the cause of **abdominal striae**
- Immune suppression, which increases the risks of infection
- Increased **erythropoietin** production which increases red cell number.

when the patient happens to be in a clinic. This is entirely appropriate for some hormones, notably calcitriol and thyroid hormones. Both these hormones have fairly constant levels in plasma, as they are maintained at a set point. It therefore does not matter when the hormone is measured. For hormones with a pronounced diurnal rhythm this can be used to judge the most appropriate time for sampling. In the case of cortisol, which peaks in the morning and has a low point around midnight, then the morning peak can be used to determine whether there is sufficient cortisol secretion. Determining whether there is over-secretion of a hormone is more difficult. For growth hormone, which is often undetectable during the day but which exhibits episodic secretion, there is no good time to take a blood sample. One way of getting round these problems is to use dynamic testing of endocrine systems (Clinical box 10.5).

The principles of dynamic testing are very simple: a challenge is applied to the endocrine system, and the hormonal response is measured. If a clinician suspects that there is a hormone deficiency, then the challenge used is designed to stimulate hormone secretion. If there is a suspected hormone excess, then the challenge is designed to inhibit hormone secretion.

Growth hormone is secreted in an episodic manner. It is very often completely undetectable during the day, but there are peaks of secretion. A patient with excess growth hormone secretion has plasma growth hormone that is always detectable, but this is difficult to differentiate from a normal secretory peak.

In order to be certain of the diagnosis a dynamic test is performed. This uses the negative feedback effect of high blood glucose on growth hormone. One of the effects of GH is to increase blood glucose, so a rise in blood glucose concentration acts on the hypothalamus and pituitary to suppress further GH secretion. In a person with normal GH secretion a rise in blood glucose leads to a fall in blood GH to being undetectable within 60 minutes. In a patient with abnormal GH secretion (e.g. **acromegaly**), GH suppression by glucose will not occur. So a patient is fasted overnight then given 50 g glucose in a drink. GH is measured after 60 minutes. If GH is still detectable then this confirms GH excess (Fig. 10.8).

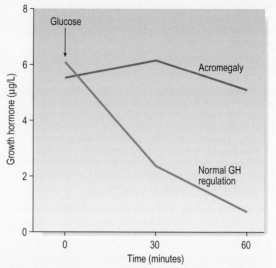

Fig. 10.8 Glucose suppression of GH secretion in a normal person and failure of suppression in a person with acromegaly.

Measuring hormones in blood

In order to investigate endocrine disease it is important to be able to measure circulating hormone levels. The fact that hormones circulate in such low concentrations makes this measurement more challenging than most clinical assays. In the early days of endocrinology, hormone assays relied on measuring responses of a biological system to different hormone concentrations. These bioassays were expensive, relatively insensitive and highly variable. Now it is possible to purchase kits to reliably and reproducibly measure every hormone. The modern kits use immunological methods to detect small concentrations of hormone (Information box 10.5).

ENDOCRINE REGULATION – THE ROLE OF THE HYPOTHALAMUS AND PITUITARY

The hypothalamus and pituitary are important coordinators of the endocrine system. The hypothalamus is part of the brain and integrates a variety of different internal and external inputs to produce a range of neural and hormonal outputs which control various homeostatic functions. The role of the hypothalamus in the regulation of appetite is covered in Chapter 16, while its role in the control of blood pressure and volume is covered in Chapter 11. The hypothalamic nuclei produce an array of regulatory hormones which control the hormonal output of the anterior pituitary gland. These pituitary hormones in turn regulate the activity of the thyroid gland, the adrenals and the gonads, as well as controlling growth.

Functional anatomy of the hypothalamus and pituitary

The hypothalamus is located at the base of the brain, adjacent to the third ventricle (Fig. 10.10). Like all brain areas it is composed of a collection of nuclei, several of which are neurosecretory. The hypothalamus is connected to the pituitary by the pituitary stalk which contains both neural and vascular

elements (Fig. 10.11). The pituitary gland is formed from two quite distinct tissues. The posterior pituitary is derived from neural ectoderm and is connected to the hypothalamus by the axons of secretory neurons. These neurons have their cell bodies in the hypothalamus but their nerve endings in the posterior pituitary. The anterior pituitary is derived from an outgrowth of the oral ectoderm, called Rathke's pouch, which grows to meet the neural ectoderm of the posterior pituitary and finally separates from the buccal cavity. The anterior pituitary is joined to the hypothalamus by a portal vascular system which has its primary capillary bed in the hypothalamus and the secondary capillary bed in the anterior pituitary. Hormones secreted by the hypothalamic neurons into the portal system act on the cells of the anterior pituitary (see Information box 10.6).

The pituitary gland is located in a hollow in the sphenoid bone and is almost completely surrounded by bone. A tumour or other increase in size of the pituitary results in pressure upwards, towards the hypothalamus. The proximity of the optic chiasma to the hypothalamus means that a pituitary tumour causes pressure on this structure, resulting in visual disturbances. These are important diagnostic features of a pituitary tumour. See Clinical box 10.6 for hypopituitary states.

The hypothalamus controls hormone secretion by the anterior pituitary

The hypothalamus secretes a range of 'releasing hormones' which bind to receptors on the anterior pituitary cells and modify their function. The main effect of these releasing hormones is to stimulate the release of hormones from the anterior pituitary. The anterior pituitary hormones then act on other endocrine tissues and so form the central part of an endocrine axis.

The anterior pituitary secretes six hormones which are all regulated by hypothalamic hormones. Five of these hormones are regulated by stimulatory hormones from the hypothalamus:

Information box 10.5   Techniques for measuring hormones

As hormones circulate in such low concentrations, usually in the nanomolar range, measuring hormones in blood presents a significant challenge. The earliest hormone measurements used a biological response to a hormone, i.e. bioassays. Pregnancy tests, for example, used an animal which would be injected with the urine from a patient. A positive test would be seen if the animal ovulated. This sort of test was unreliable and raised significant ethical issues. Modern testing uses immunological methods for measuring hormone concentrations, relying on specific anti-hormone antibodies. The most common methods are immunometric assays and immunoassays. Immunometric assays are more sensitive and more readily automated than immunoassays, and therefore more widely used. These tests are simple to perform, very reliable and rapid. It is now possible to buy assay kits which measure all the known hormones at the concentrations found in human blood.

Immunoassay (Fig. 10.9)

The principle of **immunoassay** (**RI**) is that an unknown amount of hormone and a known amount of labelled hormone compete for a limited number of binding sites on anti-hormone antibodies.

- Known amounts of labelled hormone and antibody are added to samples containing an unknown hormone concentration. The label may be a radioactive tracer (**radioimmunoassay**, **RIA**), a fluorescent molecule or some other marker.
- The lower the unknown concentration of hormone in the samples, the greater the amount of labelled hormone that binds the antibody.
- A variety of methods are then used to separate antibody-bound and free hormone and the ratio of bound to free labelled hormone (B/F) is measured.
- The B/F ratio is a measure of the competition between labelled and non-labelled hormone and the unknown hormone concentration is found by comparison with a standard curve prepared from a range of known concentrations of unlabelled hormone.

Immunometric (sandwich) assays (two site non-competitive assay)

- This method uses two antibodies that bind to different epitopes on the hormone.
- One antibody is adsorbed onto the surface of a multi-well plate. This serves to anchor the unknown amount of hormone present in the samples added to the wells. The antibody must be present in large excess to ensure all the hormone is captured.
- The second **reporter antibody** is now added and the amount of this antibody that binds is in direct proportion to the amount of anchored hormone. The reporter antibody is so

called because it bears an easily measured marker such as a fluorescent tag or an enzyme.

- When the marker is an enzyme the assay is called an **enzyme-linked immunosorbent assay** (**ELISA**) (see also Ch. 6).

A specific antibody is needed

The antibody is chemically bound to a solid surface

The sample containing the hormone is added to the surface

Two methods are used:

1. Single-site competitive assay (for small-sized hormones)

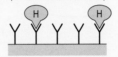

The antibody binds the hormone

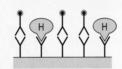

A competitor for the antibody is added and binds free sites. The competitor is labelled and emits a signal that can be measured

The amount of hormone is deduced from the total antibody sites minus free sites

2. Two-site non-competitive assay (for large-sized hormones)

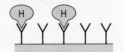

The antibody binds the hormone

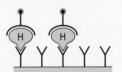

A different antibody binds the hormone at a second site. The second antibody is labelled and measured

Fig. 10.9 **Immunological methods for measuring hormone concentrations.**

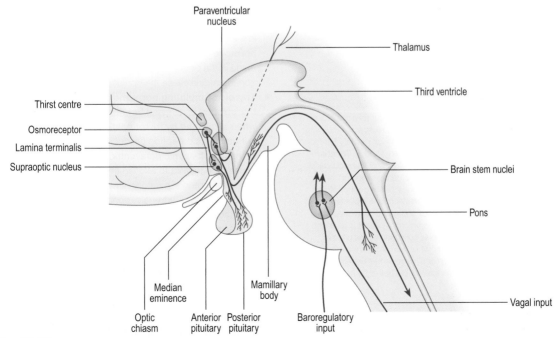

Fig. 10.10 Location of the hypothalamus and pituitary.

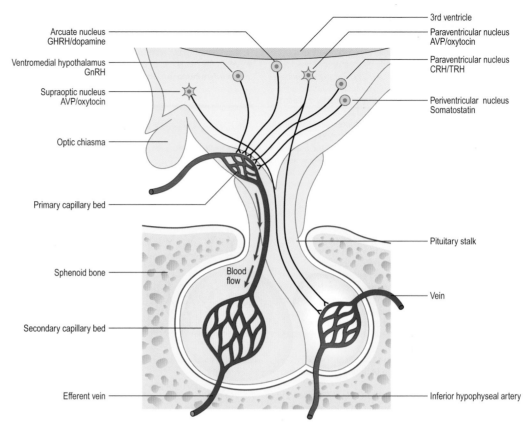

Fig. 10.11 Neural and vascular connections between the hypothalamus and pituitary. The hypothalamus and posterior pituitary have a direct neural link, whereas the anterior pituitary has a vascular connection to the hypothalamus. Note the separate blood supply to the two parts of the pituitary. Disruption of the portal system results in failure of anterior pituitary hormone secretion, but usually not of posterior pituitary hormones. The neurons with star-shaped cell bodies are magnocellular neurons; the round cell bodies indicate parvocellular neurons. AVP, arginine vasopressin; CRH, corticotropin-releasing hormone; GnRH, gonadotropin-releasing hormone; PVN, paraventricular nucleus; TRH, thyrotropin releasing hormone.

- **Adrenocorticotropin (ACTH)** is released by pituitary corticotrope cells in response to **corticotropin-releasing hormone (CRH)**, a 41-amino acid peptide from the hypothalamic paraventricular nucleus. ACTH acts on the adrenal to stimulate the release of cortisol.
- **Luteinising hormone (LH)** and **follicle stimulating hormone (FSH)** are collectively known as the gonadotropins. They are released from gonadotropic cells in the pituitary when stimulated by **gonadotropin-releasing hormone (GnRH)**, a 10-amino acid peptide which is mainly made in the pre-optic area of the hypothalamus. The gonadotropins cause the gonads to secrete sex steroids.
- **Thyroid stimulating hormone (TSH**, also called **thyrotropin**) is released from pituitary thyrotrope cells when stimulated by thyrotropin-releasing hormone (TRH), a 3-amino acid peptide produced in the medial neurons of the hypothalamic paraventricular nucleus. TSH causes the thyroid to release thyroxine. In each of these cases the anterior pituitary hormone causes the final endocrine gland, adrenals, gonads or thyroid, to produce a hormone which exerts a negative feedback inhibition of the hypothalamus, preventing further release of the 'releasing hormone' and shutting down the axis.
- The fifth pituitary hormone is **growth hormone (GH**, also known as **somatotropin**) which is partly regulated by **growth hormone-releasing hormone (GHRH)**, a 44-amino acid peptide produced by the arcuate nucleus of the hypothalamus. The other factors involved in the complex regulation of growth hormone secretion are discussed below.

The hypothalamic releasing hormones are all peptides. However, the hypothalamus also produces two release-inhibiting hormones: prolactin from the arcuate nucleus and **somatostatin** from the periventricular nucleus.

Prolactin secretion is under inhibitory regulation (Fig. 10.12)

Prolactin is unique in endocrinology. It is the only hormone whose secretion is under tonic inhibitory regulation. If the connection between the hypothalamus and pituitary is cut, then the secretion of all the other anterior pituitary hormones falls dramatically. The exception is prolactin which needs the influence of the hypothalamus to keep its secretion in check. Without the hypothalamus, prolactin secretion increases several-fold (see Clinical box 10.7). In order to achieve this effect the hypothalamus produces a release-inhibiting factor, **dopamine**, the only one of the hypothalamic hormones that is not a peptide. Dopamine is a catecholamine, derived from tyrosine and an intermediate in epinephrine production. It is normally considered to be a neurotransmitter, but in the control of prolactin secretion it is a neurohormone, like all the other hypothalamic hormones. Dopamine acts on the lactotrope cells of the anterior pituitary and inhibits prolactin secretion.

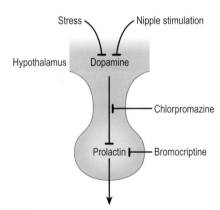

Fig. 10.12 Regulation of prolactin secretion. Prolactin is under tonic inhibitory control by dopamine. This means that prolactin is released only when dopamine secretion by the hypothalamus is inhibited. Drugs that mimic dopamine, such as bromocriptine, inhibit prolactin, but dopamine *antagonists,* such as chlorpromazine, stimulate prolactin release. There does not appear to be any negative feedback regulation in the control of prolactin secretion.

Clinical box 10.7 Hyperprolactinaemia

Hyperprolactinaemia is the over-production of prolactin. Pathological causes include:
- Prolactin-secreting tumours, which account for over 70% of all anterior pituitary tumours (commonly a microadenoma)
- Lesions of the hypothalamus or pituitary stalk
- Dopamine (D_2) receptor antagonist drugs, which interfere with dopaminergic inhibition of prolactin secretion, e.g. metoclopramide, phenothiazines.

Hyperprolactinaemia causes infertility in both sexes by suppressing:
- The secretion of GnRH
- The gonadotroph response to GnRH
- The response of the gonads to LH.

Treatment of hyperprolactinaemia with a D_2 receptor **agonist** (e.g. bromocriptine) is usually effective (see Fig. 10.12). Surgery may be required for pituitary tumours.

GROWTH HORMONE

Growth hormone is produced by the somatotrope cells of the anterior pituitary and is under dual regulation of a hypothalamic-releasing hormone, GHRH, and an inhibitory hormone, somatostatin. We shall go on to consider the regulation of growth hormone secretion and its role in the regulation of growth.

Growth

Between birth and adolescence children grow in a fairly predictable way. There are childhood growth charts which allow clinicians to compare the growth of their young patients with the published average, and so determine whether growth is progressing as it should. These charts are gender specific and are constructed using both height and weight measures (Fig. 10.13). **Body mass index** (**BMI**), weight in kg divided by the square of height in metres) is not used as a clinical measure in children as this varies greatly through childhood. At puberty there is a growth spurt which lasts around 4 years, during which a child can increase in height by around 10 cm each year.

Growth hormone is the main driver of growth in children: the level of circulating growth hormone increases throughout childhood, peaking at the age of about 15, and then gradually declines through the rest of life. However, in order for childhood growth to proceed normally, the entire endocrine system needs to be working properly. While appropriate growth hormone secretion is essential for normal growth, thyroid function is also important as thyroxine has a significant permissive effect. Cortisol and insulin secretion are also required, along with appropriate hormonal regulation of calcium metabolism. There are several factors which can adversely affect childhood growth. These include chronic illness and psychosocial deprivation, as well as endocrine disease.

The regulation of growth hormone

Growth hormone is a polypeptide hormone secreted by the anterior pituitary. It is a member of a family of hormones that includes prolactin and **human chorionic somatomammotropin** (**hCS**, also known as **human placental lactogen, hPL**). The gene encoding growth hormone (**GH1**) is located on the long arm of chromosome 17, as part of a cluster of five highly conserved genes. The other genes in this cluster encode three different versions of hCS and a second form of growth hormone. *GH1* encodes a 191-amino acid peptide (22 kDa), which is known as growth hormone (GH) and is mainly expressed in the pituitary somatotrope cells, while the other genes in this cluster are mainly expressed in the placenta.

The synthesis and secretion of growth hormone are regulated by the hypothalamus: a releasing hormone, GHRH, and an inhibitory hormone, **somatostatin**, act together to produce pulses of growth hormone secretion (Fig. 10.14). Somatostatin is also known as **growth hormone inhibitory hormone** (**GHIH**) and **somatotropin release inhibitory factor** (**SRIF**). These names all refer to the same 14-amino acid hormone and are used interchangeably. The major stimuli to GHRH secretion are sleep, exercise, hypoglycaemia and high circulating concentrations of certain amino acids, particularly arginine. The satiety hormone produced by the gastric mucosa, **ghrelin** (**Growth Hormone RELease INducer**), is also a potent stimulus to GHRH secretion. Secretion of GHRH and GH is subject to negative feedback inhibition by **insulin-like growth factor 1** (**IGF-1**) and glucose (see Clinical box 10.8).

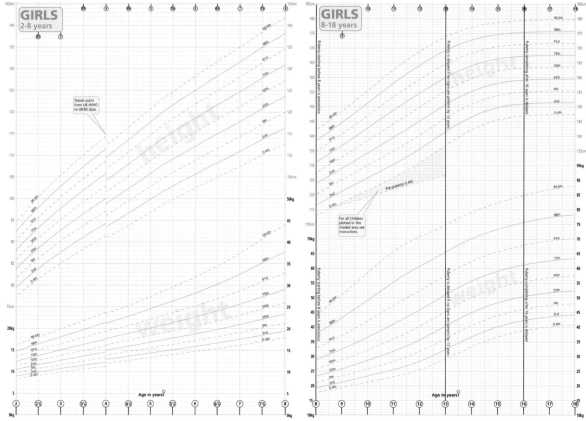

Fig. 10.13 **Growth chart for girls aged 2–18 years.** From the Royal College of Paediatrics and Child Health, with permission.

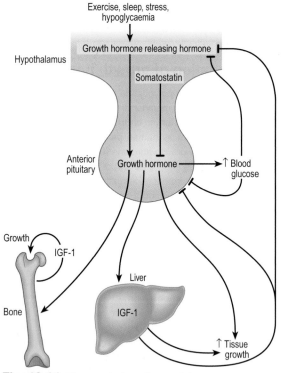

Fig. 10.14 **The regulation of growth hormone secretion.**

Actions of growth hormone

Growth hormone has some direct actions on metabolic processes, but most of its effects on growth are mediated by IGF-1. This growth factor is produced mainly by the liver,

Clinical box 10.8	Clinical tests for insufficient and excess growth hormone

If a clinician suspects insufficient GH secretion in a patient, tests which are designed to provoke GH secretion can be used. Potentially any of the known stimuli to GH secretion could be used: sleep, exercise, etc. Historically, hypoglycaemia induced by an injection of insulin was used as a clinical test. It was simple and gave reproducible standardised results. However, over time the dangers of insulin-induced hypoglycaemia became clearer and the current standard GH stimulation test involves an intravenous infusion of arginine.

If a clinician suspects over-secretion of growth hormone then the test is designed to suppress GH secretion. The simplest test is to administer a glucose drink to the patient, who has fasted overnight. In most people this will cause GH secretion to be suppressed and blood levels of GH to be undetectable after an hour. If the patient has a pituitary tumour secreting GH, the most likely cause of high GH levels, then it will not be suppressed by the glucose and after an hour blood GH levels will still be measurable.

but also by bone and other tissues in response to growth hormone stimulation. The IGF-1 produced by the liver has hormonal actions, including the feedback inhibition of hypothalamic GHRH secretion, while the IGF-1 produced by other tissues has mainly local, paracrine or autocrine effects. The effects of IGF-1 include the promotion of cell division in the growth plate and cellular maturation.

The metabolic effects of GH are wide ranging (Table 10.3). This hormone has a major effect on body composition and metabolism (see Information box 10.7 and Clinical boxes 10.9 and 10.10). It has profound effects on glucose metabolism, with some effects similar to those of insulin while also enhancing gluconeogenesis and glycolysis in the liver (see later section). During fasting, growth hormone increases lipolysis and promotes the oxidation of fatty acids, thus directing metabolic processes towards fat metabolism and away from protein. In general growth hormone has an anabolic effect on protein metabolism, reducing urea synthesis and excretion and promoting amino acid uptake into cells (see also Chs 3 and 16).

Table 10.3	Metabolic effects of growth hormone and IGF-1		
Metabolic measure		**GH**	**IGF-1**
Plasma glucose levels			↓
Hepatic gluconeogenesis			↓
Hepatic glycogenesis			↓
Insulin sensitivity		↓	
Glucose uptake (muscle, etc.)		↓	
Lipolysis			↓
Protein synthesis (muscle, etc.)			

The effects of IGF-1 are very similar to those of insulin as they are each able to bind to both receptors. In general, the effects of GH oppose those of insulin. However, both IGF-1 and GH act to increase protein synthesis in muscle.

Information box 10.7   Abuse of growth hormone

As growth hormone is anabolic and acts to increase lean body mass, it is perhaps an obvious drug of choice for athletes in power sports who wish to 'bulk-up'. It is on the list of 'banned substances' of the World Anti-Doping Agency, WADA. Because it is a polypeptide, growth hormone has to be administered by injection, with the risks inherent in injecting any illegal drugs. As GH is a naturally occurring substance in the body, with a short half-life in blood, it can be difficult to detect abuse. Indeed the only time when athletes have been banned for abusing GH is when vials of the hormone have been found in their kit. The most well-known occasion was when sufficient GH to supply the entire women's team was found during a customs search of the luggage of Chinese swimmer Yuan Yuan, at the World Aquatics Championship in Australia. Since 2004 it has been possible to detect artificial growth hormone and tests are now included in routine drug tests of athletes.

Growth hormone is also included in an array of hormones believed to have anti-ageing properties.

Clinical box 10.9   Excess growth hormone – gigantism and acromegaly

Excess growth hormone production is usually caused by a tumour in the pituitary gland which produces growth hormone in a largely unregulated manner. In children excess growth hormone causes an increase in linear growth, resulting in a condition called **gigantism**. In adults, after fusion of the epiphyseal plates so that linear growth has ceased, excess growth hormone causes a condition called **acromegaly**. The classical features of acromegaly are shown in Figure 10.15. Excess growth hormone secreted by a tumour does not respond to the normal negative feedback inhibition exerted by high plasma glucose. However, synthetic analogues of somatostatin such as octreotide are usually effective in both controlling the hormone secretion and shrinking the tumour in preparation for surgical removal.

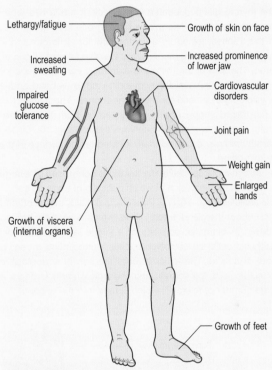

Fig. 10.15 Signs and symptoms of acromegaly (excess growth hormone in an adult).

Clinical box 10.10   Growth hormone insufficiency – dwarfism and growth hormone replacement

Insufficient growth hormone in children is one of the more unusual causes of short stature. The prevalence of idiopathic growth hormone deficiency in children has been reported to be between 1 in 3500 and 1 in 30 000. There is evidence to suggest that up to two-thirds of children diagnosed with growth hormone deficiency (see Table 10.4) later produce normal amounts of the hormone. The GH deficiency may be due to a mutation in any one of a number of genes, including the gene encoding the growth hormone receptor, which results in **Laron syndrome**. In adults growth hormone deficiency is usually the result of a pituitary tumour or other lesion which disrupts the pituitary architecture or blood supply. Until the mid-1990s adult growth hormone deficiency was not treated in Britain. It was believed that GH was necessary only for linear growth in childhood and was relatively unimportant to adults. It is now clear that appropriate GH secretion is important for the maintenance of body composition, particularly lean body mass

and bone density. It is also needed to maintain muscle strength and cardiac function as well as for a number of quality of life measures, including mood, motivation and fatigue levels.

Table 10.4	Causes of short stature

1. Genetic short stature
2. Constitutional growth delay
3. Short stature following intrauterine growth retardation (SGA)
4. Dysmorphic syndromes (including skeletal dysplasia)
5. Endocrine disorders
6. Chronic illness
7. Psychosocial deprivation

NB: Most children referred with short stature have a variant of normal growth.

ENDOCRINE HOMEOSTASIS

Hormones are involved in regulating several of the homeostatic processes in the body including water and electrolyte balance (see Ch. 1), digestion and appetite (see Chs 8 and 16), the basal metabolic rate and the metabolism of glucose and calcium.

THYROID GLAND AND THE REGULATION OF METABOLISM

THE STRUCTURE AND LOCATION OF THE THYROID

The thyroid gland is located in the neck. It has a two-lobed structure and looks like a bow tie with one lobe either side of the trachea, joined by a central isthmus. It is one of the largest endocrine organs, typically weighing about 20 g in an adult. The size of the thyroid is extremely variable, depending largely on the availability of iodine in the diet and on the physiological demand for thyroid hormones. The thyroid has a rich blood supply and is innervated by both the sympathetic and parasympathetic nervous system (Fig. 10.16). The parathyroid glands are normally located on the surface of the thyroid gland.

At a microscopic level the thyroid is composed of a large number of lobules, each of which consists of up to 40 spherical follicles (Fig. 10.17). Parafollicular cells are scattered throughout the gland. Each follicle, which is typically around 200 nm in diameter, consists of a single layer of cuboidal epithelial cells, called follicular cells, surrounding a central pool of colloid. The follicular cells are rich in endoplasmic reticulum and lysosomes, and the apical surface bears a large number of microvilli which extend into the colloid.

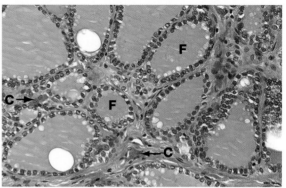

Fig. 10.17 **Histology of the thyroid gland (×150).** F, thyroid follicles containing thyroglobulin and surrounded by the purple follicular cells; C, capillaries. From Young B, Woodford P, O'Dowd G, et al. 2013 Wheater's functional histology: a text and colour atlas, 6th edn. Churchill Livingstone, Philadelphia.

Iodine – an important trace element

The thyroid gland requires a daily supply of at least 100 μg of the trace element **iodine** in the diet for normal hormone production. Sea fish, shell-fish, seaweed and sea salt are the main sources of dietary iodine, although in the UK iodine is also found in cow's milk, probably as a result of the use of iodine-based teat sterilants. In many countries iodine is added to table salts in order to ensure an adequate intake. Iodine deficiency (see Clinical box 10.11) results in inadequate production of thyroid hormones, which has serious consequences for foetal and childhood development. It has been estimated that iodine deficiency is the single commonest preventable cause of brain damage in the world, with around 43 million people affected worldwide.

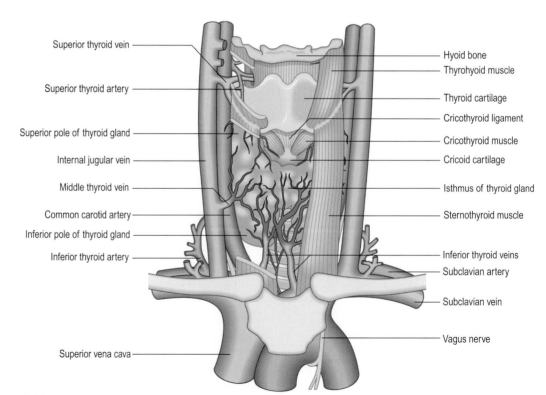

Fig. 10.16 **Anatomy of the thyroid gland.**

Clinical box 10.11   Goitre

When the thyroid gland grows beyond its usual size it forms a characteristic swelling in the neck, just above the sternal notch, called a **goitre**. A goitre may be diffuse, where the swelling is uniform throughout the gland, or nodular, where the swelling is patchy. The presence of a goitre is an important diagnostic sign in thyroid disease. However, it gives very little information other than the simple fact that the thyroid has become enlarged. There are different reasons why the thyroid might grow. For example, it could be a response to very low dietary iodine levels. If the thyroid is unable to obtain sufficient iodine to make enough thyroid hormone to meet the physiological demand, then the thyroid grows. This is in direct response to increased levels of thyroid stimulating hormone (TSH) from the anterior pituitary. In this case the goitre is a sign of hypothyroidism and is called a non-toxic goitre. Globally, a diffuse non-toxic goitre is commonly caused by iodine deficiency and is endemic in parts of the world. It may also be caused by ingestion of substances called **goitrogens**, which inhibit iodine trapping in the thyroid. Goitrogens are found in some vegetables such as brassicas and cassava. Some drugs are also goitrogenic, notably sulphonylureas and lithium.

Alternatively, goitre could be a response to the presence of antibodies which mimic the effects of TSH. These antibodies are produced in Graves disease and cause an over-stimulation of the thyroid gland with growth of the gland and excess hormone production. In this case the goitre is a sign of hyperthyroidism and is called a toxic goitre.

HORMONE SYNTHESIS IN THE THYROID GLAND

The thyroid makes three hormones: thyroxine (T_4) and tri-iodothyronine (T_3) are secreted by the follicular cells and calcitonin is secreted by the parafollicular cells. Calcitonin is involved in calcium metabolism (see p. 416 and below). Thyroxine and T_3 are both derived from modifications of the amino acid tyrosine (see Fig. 10.5). These hormones are synthesised by the cleavage of pairs of iodinated tyrosine residues from the pool of colloid in the thyroid follicle. This colloid is a glycoprotein called **thyroglobulin** which is synthesised by the epithelial cells. Thyroglobulin is particularly rich in tyrosine residues which are iodinated once the protein is transported to the lumen of the follicle.

The thyroid gland is extremely efficient at trapping circulating iodine, in the form of iodide. It does this through the action of an iodine pump which co-transports sodium and iodide together, utilising the sodium concentration gradient maintained by Na^+/K^+ - ATPase. In this way the concentration of iodine within the follicular cell can be many times higher than in blood. The iodide is not utilised within the follicular cell but passes through the cell into the lumen of the follicle. An enzyme called **thyroperoxidase** catalyses the iodination of tyrosine residues on the colloidal thyroglobulin (Fig. 10.18).

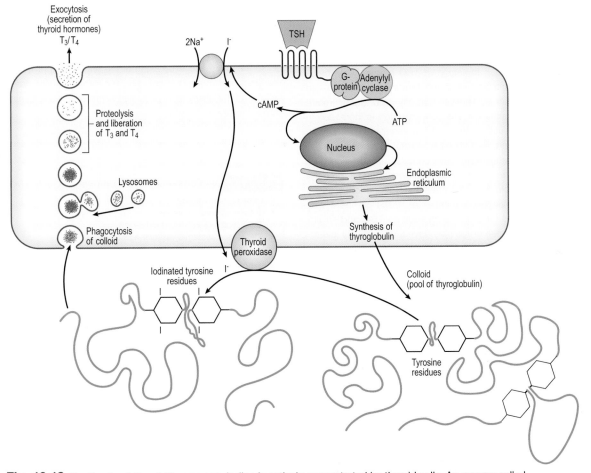

Fig. 10.18 Synthesis of thyroid hormones. Iodine is actively concentrated by thyroid cells. An enzyme called thyroperoxidase catalyses the addition of iodine to the tyrosine residues in thyroglobulin, a large protein, rich in tyrosine residues, which is synthesised in thyroid follicular cells. Iodinated thyroglobulin is stored in the thyroid follicles in the form of 'colloid'. In response to TSH stimulation, portions of colloid are taken back into the thyroid cell by phagocytosis and pairs of iodinated tyrosine residues (thyroxine) are released into the circulation. Anti-thyroid drugs, such as carbimazole, act by inhibiting thyroperoxidase activity. cAMP, cyclic adenosine monophosphate.

CONTROL OF THYROID FUNCTION

Thyroid function, including the synthesis and release of thyroxine, is regulated by the hypothalamic–pituitary–thyroid axis (see Fig. 10.7). Thyrotropin-releasing hormone (TRH) from the hypothalamus stimulates thyrotrope cells of the anterior pituitary to release TSH. This is a large glycopeptide hormone, in the same family as LH and FSH. TSH acts on thyroid follicular cells, binding to a G-protein coupled receptor. The actions of thyroid stimulating hormone include increasing the activity of the iodide pump and thyroperoxidase, stimulating synthesis of thyroglobulin and increasing thyroid blood flow.

Thyroid hormones in blood

Plasma thyroxine concentration is maintained at a set point with no diurnal variation. The half-life of thyroxine in the circulation is much longer than any other hormone and so there is very little variation in plasma concentration. The thyroid gland turns over only 1% of its iodide each day and so the gland contains a considerable reserve of hormone. The fact that so many factors all contribute to a very stable plasma concentration of thyroxine underlines the importance of maintaining appropriate thyroid hormone levels.

In blood thyroxine is bound to the proteins **thyroxine-binding globulin** (**TBG**) and **transthyretin** (**TTA**), with a small amount bound to albumin. Thyroid hormones are very poorly soluble and so almost all the thyroxine and T_3 in blood is bound to one of these proteins with about 75% bound to TBG. Each molecule of TBG has a single binding site for thyroid hormone and binds T_4 with a 10-fold higher affinity than T_3. There is typically around 270nmol/L TBG in plasma, although this concentration is increased in pregnancy, with use of the oral contraceptive pill, and in patients with acute liver disease. If total thyroxine is measured in these patients an elevated level may be recorded, although free thyroxine levels remain unchanged and so the patient is euthyroid (having normal thyroid function) (Clinical box 10.12). Conversely a number of drugs compete with thyroid hormones for the binding sites on TBG and so patients receiving these drugs may have a deceptively low total hormone level although free thyroxine is unchanged and the patient is euthyroid.

Clinical box 10.12 Tests of thyroid function

As thyroxine is maintained at a relatively unvarying level in plasma, thyroid function can be assessed using a single point hormone measurement. This is relatively unusual in endocrinology.

In neonates a heelprick blood test, the '**Guthrie test**' is carried out. This can detect a range of metabolic disorders, including hypothyroidism. This test measures thyroid stimulating hormone (TSH) rather than thyroxine as this is a better diagnostic indicator of thyroid function. An elevated TSH indicates hypothyroidism.

A standard thyroid function test involves measuring both T_4 and TSH. If both are within the normal range the person is said to be 'biochemically euthyroid'. In disease states, the body attempts to keep thyroxine within the normal range by increasing or decreasing TSH secretion. For example, a person who has thyroxine levels within the normal range may have a very high TSH. This demonstrates hypothyroidism as clearly the thyroid is relatively unresponsive to stimulation and, if left untreated, a goitre will develop.

Peripheral metabolism of thyroxine

Most of the thyroid hormone in the circulation is thyroxine (T_4). This needs to have one of its 5′ iodine atoms removed in order to form the more active T_3. This process of mono-deiodination takes place in peripheral tissues. It has been estimated that 80% of the T_3 in the circulation is derived from peripheral metabolism of T_4, with the rest produced directly in the thyroid gland. Removal of a different iodine from T_4 generates **reverse T_3**, or **rT_3**, which is inactive.

Functions of thyroxine (Table 10.5)

Thyroid hormones exert most of their effects by binding to intracellular receptors which act as transcription factors. It used to be believed that a small lipophilic hormone like thyroxine would simply diffuse into the cell, but it is now clear that specific thyroid hormone transporter proteins in the plasma membrane of target cells facilitate this process. The affinity of the thyroid hormone receptor for T_3 is about 15 times higher than for T_4 and so T_3 is generally considered to be the active thyroid hormone. There is now evidence that thyroid hormones also have non-genomic effects, acting through **mitogen-activated protein kinase** (**MAPK**) signalling.

Thyroid hormone receptors are found in most cells of the body and regulate large numbers of genes. Their actions are normally facilitatory and so it is difficult to list either key genes regulated by thyroid hormones or major physiological actions of thyroid hormones: their actions are mainly subtle and elusive. Their overall physiological effect is to increase the basal metabolic rate and raise the level of oxygen use by cells. They increase expression of the uncoupling protein in the electron transport chain, with the effect that increased cellular metabolism also produces more heat (see Clinical boxes 10.13 and 10.14).

Table 10.5 Actions of thyroid hormones

Cardiovascular effects
- Increased cardiac output
- Increased heart rate and stroke volume
- Decreased systemic vascular resistance
- Increased systolic pressure

Metabolic effects
- Increased basal metabolic rate
- Increased oxygen consumption
- Increased thermogenesis (increased expression of mitochondrial uncoupling proteins)
- Increased protein turnover (as a result of enhancing the actions of growth hormone, glucocorticoids, epinephrine, norepinephrine and glucagon)

Neurological effects
- Enhances
- Wakefulness
- Memory
- Alertness
- Reflexes
- Essential for maintenance of normal emotional tone

Growth and development
- Essential for normal foetal neural development
- Essential for normal bone growth after birth
- Required for normal tooth development

Reproduction
- Has a permissive role in both male and female reproduction: essential for normal reproductive function

Clinical box 10.13   **Disorders of thyroid function**

Over-secretion of thyroid hormones (hyperthyroidism, thyrotoxicosis)

The actions of thyroid hormones are best understood by looking at disorders of thyroid function. Broadly these are disorders in which either too much thyroid hormone is produced or too little is made. There is a strong link between disorders of the immune system and thyroid disease: autoimmune disorders are the commonest cause of thyroid dysfunction in the developed world where iodine supply is adequate.

Hyperthyroidism is a common endocrine disorder in women, with about 5% of all women having an overactive thyroid at some time in their life, but it is less common in men. The commonest causes of overproduction of thyroid hormones are Graves disease and toxic nodular goitre. Graves disease is an autoimmune disorder with antibodies directed against the thyroid stimulating hormone receptor on thyroid follicular cells. The antibodies

stimulate the receptor and increase thyroid hormone secretion. They also cause growth of the thyroid and so a goitre is formed.

People with excess thyroid hormone typically feel very warm, even on a cold day, and may dress inappropriately for the season. They often have weight loss, despite eating well, and may experience palpitations (Fig. 10.19). **Myxoedema** and **exophthalmos** are characteristic of Graves disease, but not other forms of hyperthyroidism.

Thyrotoxicosis can cause serious cardiac problems, usually tachycardia and arrhythmias, and so requires prompt treatment. Thyroxine has a very long half-life in blood and so in the short term β-blockers are used to prevent serious cardiac problems while thyroid hormone synthesis is blocked with a drug such as carbimazole. This acts by blocking the activity of thyroperoxidase and so preventing iodination of tyrosine residues. This treatment can take 4–6 weeks to be effective because the thyroid holds such a large store of thyroglobulin.

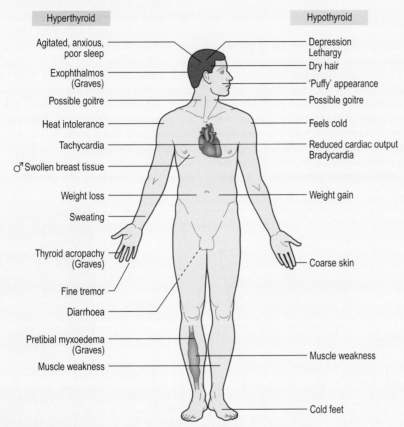

Fig. 10.19 Signs and symptoms of hyper- and hypo-thyroidism.

Clinical box 10.14   **Thyroid hormone deficiency (hypothyroidism)**

Like hyperthyroidism (Fig. 10.19), the commonest cause of hypothyroidism in the developed world is an autoimmune disorder, Hashimoto's thyroiditis, in which the body produces antibodies to thyroperoxidase. In the developing world, iodine deficiency is the major cause of hypothyroidism.

A deficiency in thyroid hormone causes a number of problems. In early childhood it results in neurological deficits, with severely reduced IQ (sometimes called **cretinism**), and so in many countries there is a standard check of thyroid function carried out on all newborn infants.

In adults thyroid hormone deficiency causes a general 'slowing down'. Patients may report tiredness and lethargy, lack of energy, constipation, and feeling cold all the time. They may report poor appetite but increased weight. Depression is a common feature of thyroid hormone deficiency. Physical signs include a slow pulse rate, 'puffy' appearance, coarse skin and thin hair.

Hypothyroidism is treated with thyroxine replacement therapy, which is given as a daily tablet.

HORMONES AND 'STRESS'

Stress is a difficult concept to understand. In its most basic form, anything which disturbs the homeostatic equilibrium can be defined as a 'stress' to the body. Medically a stress

includes infection, trauma, cold exposure, extreme exercise and anything that induces hypoglycaemia as well as psychological stress. Several hormones can be described as '**stress hormones**', as although the hormones of the adrenal glands are the most recognised stress hormones, other hormones also respond to stress. Growth hormone secretion is stimulated by stress, by hypoglycaemia and by exercise, as is prolactin; thyroid-stimulating hormone is increased by cold exposure. Therefore it is not only the adrenal gland that responds to 'stress'.

ADRENAL CORTEX AND MEDULLA

The adrenal gland produces the key hormones that enable the body to respond to 'stress', whether physiological or psychological. Although each adrenal is a single gland, there are two functionally distinct parts of the adrenal: the **cortex**, which produces steroid hormones such as cortisol and aldosterone; and the **medulla**, which produces the catecholamine norepinephrine (noradrenaline).

Structure of adrenals

The adrenals are paired glands, located on top of the kidneys. Their blood supply comes directly from the aorta, via the adrenal arteries. Their venous drainage is directly into the vena cava on the right and into the left renal vein on the left. The innervation to the adrenal glands is from the splanchnic nerve. Each adrenal is made up of two distinct tissues, the cortex and the medulla. The adrenal medulla is derived from the neural crest while the cortex is mesodermal in origin. During foetal life these tissues migrate together so that the adrenal medulla lies surrounded by cortical tissue. At birth

each adrenal gland weighs about 4 g, the same weight as in an adult. In the first year of life the foetal adrenal undergoes apoptosis and loses most of its cortical mass (the foetal zone), then grows proportionately throughout childhood.

The adrenal cortex comprises three distinct zones (Fig. 10.20): the **zona glomerulosa** lies immediately beneath the connective tissue capsule of the adrenal; the **zona fasciculata** lies beneath that; and the **zona reticularis** lies adjacent to the medullary tissue. The cells of the adrenal medulla, called chromaffin cells, retain their innervation and function like a modified sympathetic ganglion.

Stress: the adrenal medulla

Both parts of the adrenal are involved in the stress response. The medulla is the immediate response to threat, the 'fight or flight' reaction. When a threat is perceived, the sympathetic nervous system signals to the adrenal medulla to release norepinephrine, a catecholamine best known as a neurotransmitter, into the bloodstream. The catecholamines are modified amino acids, made from tyrosine (see Fig. 10.5). Norepinephrine binds to adrenergic receptors and causes an increase in heart rate and blood pressure, increased blood flow to skeletal muscle and increased respiratory rate: all parts of the classical fight or flight response. This reaction lasts usually only a few seconds. The half-life of catecholamines in blood is very short indeed. Surprisingly, if the adrenal glands are removed the response still remains as there is enough catecholamine released into

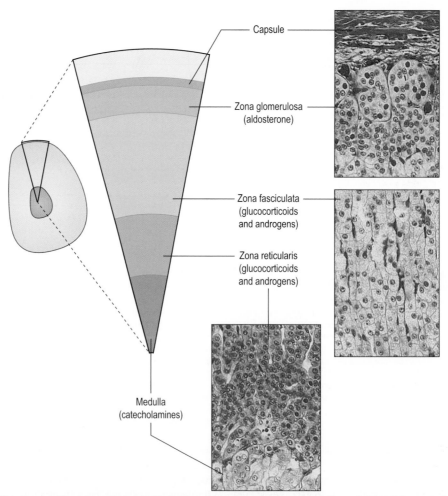

Fig. 10.20 **Structure of the adrenal glands.** From Young B, Woodford P, O'Dowd G, et al. 2013 Wheater's functional histology: a text and colour atlas, 6th edn. Churchill Livingstone, Philadelphia.

blood from the rest of the sympathetic nervous system even without the contribution of the adrenal medulla.

Stress: the adrenal cortex

The zones of the adrenal cortex each produce a characteristic set of hormones (Fig. 10.20). These are all steroid hormones, derived from cholesterol (see Fig. 10.4). Aldosterone, a mineralocorticoid produced by the zona glomerulosa is discussed in Chapter 14 as it has its major actions on the kidney. Cortisol is a glucocorticoid produced by the zona fasciculata and to a lesser extent the zona reticularis, while **dehydroepiandrosterone** is a weak androgen produced mainly by the zona reticularis. The classical hormone of the adrenal stress response is cortisol.

Regulation of cortisol secretion is through the hypothalamic–pituitary–adrenal axis (Fig. 10.21). 'Stress' of various sorts leads to secretion of CRH and **arginine vasopressin (AVP)** from the hypothalamus. Together these stimulate corticotrope cells of the anterior pituitary to release ACTH, which binds to melancortin receptors type 2 (MC2R, specific for ACTH) receptors on cells of the adrenal cortex and, acting via cAMP, stimulates cortisol secretion.

Cortisol in blood is mostly bound to a specific carrier protein, **cortisol binding globulin**, which serves to increase its solubility and extend its half-life in plasma. Cortisol is degraded by hepatic enzymes and excreted in bile salts and in the urine. (See Clinical box 10.15 and Information box 10.8.)

Actions of cortisol

Cortisol acts by binding to glucocorticoid receptors which are members of the family of steroid hormone receptors and which act as regulators of gene transcription. These receptors

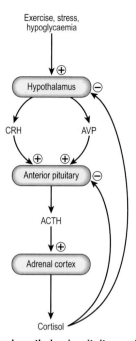

Fig. 10.21 **The hypothalamic–pituitary–adrenal axis.** Activity of this axis is stimulated by exercise, stress and hypoglycaemia. There is also a clear diurnal rhythm of activity of the axis with a peak at 6–8 a.m. and a nadir between midnight and 2 a.m. Corticotropin releasing hormone (CRH) and arginine vasopressin (AVP), from the hypothalamus, stimulate the anterior pituitary to release adrenocorticotropin (ACTH). ACTH acts on the adrenal cortex to stimulate the release of cortisol which, in addition to its other actions, exerts a negative feedback inhibitory effect on the hypothalamus and pituitary to decrease activity of the axis.

Clinical box 10.15   **Disorders of adrenal steroid synthesis – congenital adrenal hyperplasia**

Congenital adrenal hyperplasia (CAH) is the result of a deficiency in one of the enzymes of cortisol synthesis. The effect of decreased cortisol is that the usual negative feedback inhibition of the hypothalamic–pituitary–adrenal axis is removed and ACTH levels are increased. This is associated with growth of the adrenal gland, in a physiological attempt to correct the cortisol deficiency. CAH describes a spectrum of disorders from a mild cortisol deficiency to a complete absence of adrenal hormone synthesis although this is extremely rare. The commonest cause of CAH is a gene mutation causing reduced 21-hydroxylase activity (Fig. 10.22). This means that conversion of progesterone to aldosterone and

17α-hydroxyprogesterone to cortisol in the adrenal cortex is impaired. There is a build-up of progesterone and so the path of adrenal steroid biosynthesis is diverted towards androgen synthesis. This form of CAH is usually detected at birth. A baby girl whose adrenals have been producing large amounts of androgens often has 'ambiguous genitalia': an enlarged clitoris, partially fused labia and occasionally some pubic hair. In boys CAH is more difficult to detect and may be identified only when the child shows failure to thrive. Salt wasting may be a feature of CAH when insufficient mineralocorticoid is produced. The treatment of CAH is by replacement of adrenal steroids and surgical correction of the genitalia if necessary.

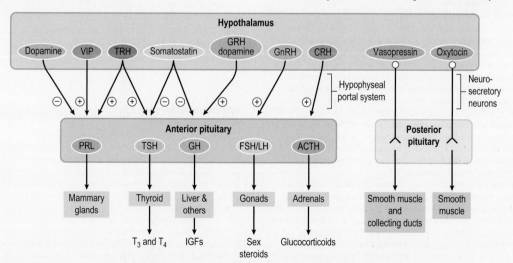

Fig. 10.22 **Pathway of steroid synthesis in CAH.** Loss of 21-hydroxylase activity results in an accumulation of the upstream steroids and so steroid synthesis is diverted towards androgen synthesis.

Information box 10.8 **Dehydroepiandrosterone**

DHEA is the major hormonal product of the adrenal cortex, circulating in far higher concentrations than either cortisol or aldosterone. Functionally, however, it is rather less important. DHEA is a weak androgen and is probably most important when metabolised to more potent androgens or oestrogens. It has an interesting age-related secretion pattern, with production increasing throughout childhood, peaking in early adulthood and then declining throughout the rest of life. It has been identified with youth and well-being and widely promoted as an anti-ageing hormone. There is no evidence to suggest that it delays the ageing process at all in humans, although it has some interesting effects in mice (which do not produce DHEA at all).

Table 10.6 **Effects of glucocorticoids**

Metabolic effects
- Stimulate mobilisation of glucose in liver (glycogenolysis and gluconeogenesis)
- Stimulate breakdown of fats and proteins
- Increase plasma concentrations of glucose, fatty acids and amino acids

Cardiovascular effects
- Maintain blood volume: increased glucose concentration draws water into blood compartment
- Maintain vascular responsiveness to catecholamines

Other effects
- Anti-inflammatory: inhibit prostaglandin synthesis
- Immunosuppressive

are located in most cells of the body and regulate a vast array of genes. There is no single target tissue for glucocorticoids and it is impossible to identify a key target gene. The actions of glucocorticoids are necessary for the expression of many genes, and without glucocorticoid action it is not possible to remain healthy for long. A summary of the major effects of glucocorticoids is shown in Table 10.6.

It is perhaps easiest to understand the actions of glucocorticoids by looking at the clinical conditions that arise from a deficiency and an excess of cortisol (see Clinical boxes 10.16, 10.17 and 10.18).

Clinical box 10.16 **Cortisol deficiency**

Cortisol deficiency may arise from a variety of causes. Primary adrenal insufficiency (Addison disease) is due to loss of adrenal function as a result of destruction of the adrenal tissue by autoimmune disease or infection (most commonly TB or HIV). Up to 90% of the total adrenal mass may be lost before symptoms are seen because the hypothalamic–pituitary–adrenal axis has a great amount of reserve which can be called upon to maintain levels of cortisol despite the loss of adrenal tissue. Cortisol deficiency may also arise when insufficient ACTH is produced by the anterior pituitary (secondary adrenal insufficiency). This may be the result of a tumour or trauma, or it may be the effect of suppression of pituitary function by the long-term therapeutic use of synthetic glucocorticoids.

It is possible for somebody with cortisol insufficiency to live for many months without adverse effect. However, as soon as they become exposed to 'stress', which might be as minor as the common cold, then they become very unwell: a condition termed an 'Addisonian crisis'. The typical symptoms are dizziness accompanied by nausea and vomiting. Blood pressure falls and the patient becomes very dehydrated. This results in coma and death if not treated promptly. Treatment is simply fluid and glucocorticoid replacement.

Clinical box 10.17 **Cortisol excess – Cushing syndrome**

There are several causes of cortisol excess: a cortisol secreting tumour in the adrenal glands, an ACTH secreting tumour either in the pituitary (Cushing disease) or from an ectopic source. By far the commonest cause of Cushing syndrome, however, is iatrogenic: from long-term use of prescribed glucocorticoids which switch off endogenous production of cortisol via negative feedback.

The signs and symptoms of Cushing syndrome are very characteristic (Fig. 10.23): moon face, truncal obesity with peripheral wasting (thin arms and legs), easy bruising, abdominal striae and plethoric cheeks as a result of skin thinning. These changes are accompanied by hypertension, osteoporosis, poor wound healing, impaired glucose tolerance and increased risk of infection.

The presence of hirsutism in women or baldness in men, and the nature of the mood change, is determined by the source of the excess cortisol. If the cause is iatrogenic then there is no excess androgen, only glucocorticoid, and these features are not seen.

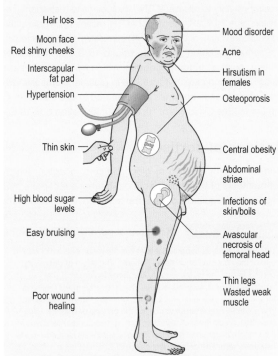

Fig. 10.23 **Major features of Cushing syndrome.** Acne, baldness and hirsutism are features of Cushing syndrome which is due to overactive adrenal glands as these symptoms result from excess production of adrenal androgens.

Clinical box 10.18 **Therapeutic use of glucocorticoids**

Glucocorticoids are powerful anti-inflammatory and immunosuppressive agents. A wide range of synthetic glucocorticoids is available for both topical and systemic use.

Glucocorticoid creams are used to treat skin conditions such as eczema and inhaled glucocorticoids are used for asthma. Topical use helps avoid the serious side effects that these drugs can cause.

Anybody who takes oral glucocorticoids for longer than 2 weeks should be given a steroid treatment card, warning of the dangers of stopping treatment suddenly. As oral glucocorticoid treatment 'switches off' the hypothalamic–pituitary–adrenal axis, the treatment needs to be tailed off gradually in order to allow the axis time to recover.

ENDOCRINE CONTROL OF GLUCOSE METABOLISM (details of biochemistry in Chs 2 and 3)

REGULATION OF PLASMA GLUCOSE CONCENTRATION

There are several hormones which influence plasma glucose concentrations and all but one of these hormones causes plasma glucose to increase. This reflects the physiological importance of maintaining blood glucose concentrations above a minimum level, usually considered to be around 3 mmol/L. As glucose concentrations fall below this level there is impaired cognition followed by loss of consciousness and death. It is therefore of great physiological importance that there should be a series of fail-safe mechanisms to prevent this. The hormones that act to increase plasma glucose concentrations are glucagon, growth hormone, cortisol and epinephrine. Any disorder resulting in an excess of any of these hormones (such as acromegaly or Cushing syndrome) is associated with impaired glucose tolerance, a pre-diabetic state in which the body is less able to handle a glucose load.

Plasma glucose concentrations are normally maintained at between 3 and 6 mmol/L. When concentrations increase above this level, insulin acts to bring glucose back within the optimal range (Fig. 10.24). Insulin is a peptide hormone secreted by the endocrine pancreas and is the only hormone that lowers blood glucose. A lack of effective insulin action results in the commonest of all endocrine disorders: diabetes mellitus.

ENDOCRINE PANCREAS

The pancreas is composed of two distinct parts: the bulk of the tissue comprises the exocrine pancreas, secreting enzymes into the duodenum via the pancreatic duct (see Ch. 15). Embedded within the exocrine tissues lie the islets of Langerhans, also called pancreatic islets (Fig. 10.25). These are clusters of endocrine cells, 50–500 μm in diameter, which secrete hormones directly into the bloodstream and make up only 1–2% of the pancreatic mass. There are several different cell types in the islets of Langerhans, each secreting a different hormone (Table 10.7). By far the most important, however, are the β cells which secrete insulin.

Insulin synthesis

Insulin is a two-stranded peptide hormone which is the product of a single gene (Fig. 10.26). The pro-insulin is processed in the Golgi apparatus of the β cell to form mature insulin

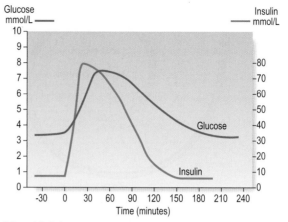

Fig. 10.24 **Plasma insulin and glucose levels following a meal.** Levels of both glucose and insulin increase rapidly after a meal (time 0). The time taken for values to return to fasting levels depends on both the size and composition of the meal. From Chew SL, Leslie D. 2006 Clinical endocrinology and diabetes: an illustrated colour text. Churchill Livingstone, Edinburgh.

and a non-functional peptide called **C-peptide**. Equimolar amounts of insulin and C-peptide are produced, and secreted, by the pancreas. The measurement of C-peptide is a useful proxy measure of endogenous insulin production in patients with type 1 diabetes who use injectable insulin, because it is not otherwise possible to differentiate between injected insulin and endogenous production.

Control of insulin secretion (Fig. 10.27)

When blood glucose rises above the normal fasting range, which typically happens after eating a meal, then insulin secretion is stimulated. The β cell effectively acts as a glucose sensor. Glucose binds to a GLUT2 receptor on the surface of the β cell, which allows the glucose to enter the cell. The glucose is then phosphorylated by glucokinase and enters the glycolytic pathway. This results in an increase

Table 10.7	Cell types in the islets of Langerhans		
Cell type	**Alternative name**	**Percentage of the islet**	**Hormone secreted**
A cell	α cell	10	Glucagon
B cell	β cell	60–80	Insulin
D cell	δ cell	~5	Somatostatin
F cell	PP cell	Varies	Pancreatic polypeptide

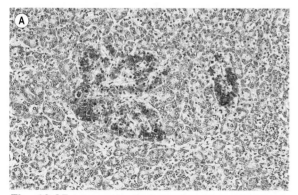

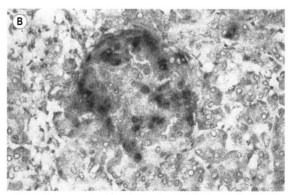

Fig. 10.25 **Islets of Langerhans.** From Young B, Woodford P, O'Dowd G, et al. 2013 Wheater's functional histology: a text and colour atlas, 6th edn. Churchill Livingstone, Philadelphia.

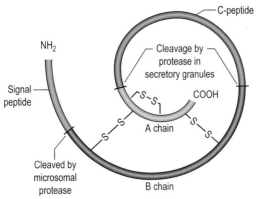

Fig. 10.26 Molecular components of preproinsulin. Mature insulin is formed by removal of the signal peptide and C-peptide in the endoplasmic reticulum and Golgi body of the β cells. Equimolar amounts of insulin and C-peptide are released.

in intracellular ATP which closes ATP-sensitive potassium channels, causing depolarisation of the cell, which in turn opens voltage-sensitive calcium channels, allowing an influx of extracellular calcium ions. The increase in intracellular calcium activates calcium-dependent protein kinase, which stimulates secretion of insulin by exocytosis of the insulin-containing secretory granules. Insulin secretion is also stimulated by the amino acids leucine, arginine and lysine, by parasympathetic nerve stimulation and by a number of hormones, including the gut hormones gastric inhibitory peptide (GIP), cholecystokinin and glucagon-like peptide-1 (GLP-1). Other hormones that stimulate insulin secretion include growth hormone, prolactin and cortisol.

Around half the total insulin secreted over a 24-hour period is produced under basal conditions, and the other half is secreted in response to meals.

Glucagon

The pancreatic islet α cells secrete **glucagon**, a 29-amino acid peptide hormone whose actions antagonise those of insulin.

Glucagon secretion is stimulated by low blood glucose, and inhibited by high blood glucose as well as by insulin itself. It appears to be the concentration of glucose within the α cell that regulates glucagon secretion and so concentrations of glucagon may be elevated in diabetes, even in the presence of high blood glucose. Glucagon mainly acts on the liver, stimulating glycogen breakdown and the conversion of amino acids to glucose. It also acts on adipose cells to stimulate lipolysis. Its overall effects are to increase plasma concentrations of glucose and free fatty acids. In diabetes the actions of glucagon contribute to both the hyperglycaemia and the ketosis.

Diabetes mellitus

Deficient secretion or action of insulin causes a condition known as diabetes mellitus, literally meaning 'sweet urine'. There are two types of diabetes mellitus: type 1, also known as **insulin-dependent diabetes**; and type 2, which is usually associated with a decreased effectiveness of insulin action. Over 85% of cases are of type 2 diabetes, the form of diabetes associated with obesity. In 2010 it was estimated that 170 million people worldwide had diabetes and this number is expected to increase to 365 million by 2030. Diabetes has been described as the greatest global health challenge of the twenty-first century.

Diabetes is a serious condition of chronic hyperglycaemia, which carries significant risk of cardiovascular disease, neuropathy and microvascular damage. If the disease is not adequately controlled this can result in blindness, renal failure, significant damage to the extremities, especially the feet, and increased risk of stroke and myocardial infarction. It is important that diabetes mellitus is diagnosed early and treated properly (see Clinical box 10.19).

Glycosuria

Glucose is not normally present in urine (see Ch. 14). Although glucose is a component of the renal filtrate, at concentrations lower than about 10 mmol/L all of the filtered glucose is reabsorbed and so none is lost in urine. If blood glucose

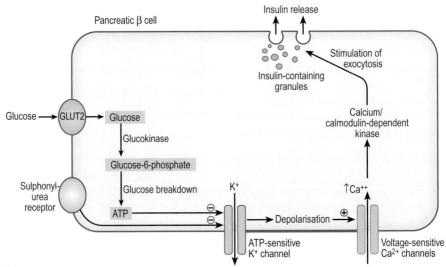

Fig. 10.27 Mechanism of glucose-stimulated insulin secretion. Glucose enters the pancreatic β cell through the GLUT2 transporter and is first converted to glucose-6-phosphate before undergoing glycolysis to generate ATP. This causes ATP-sensitive potassium channels to close, resulting in depolarisation of the cell which causes voltage sensitive calcium channels to open. The resulting increase in intracellular calcium activates calcium/calmodulin kinase, stimulating exocytosis of insulin-containing secretory granules and releasing insulin into the blood. One of the key treatments for type 2 diabetes is a class of drugs called sulphonylureas. These act on sulphonylurea receptors on the β cell causing the potassium channels to close and thus stimulating release of insulin.

A fasting blood glucose is the standard diagnostic test for diabetes. However, a very simple screening test can be carried out in a doctor's surgery by testing urine for the presence of glucose and ketones (see below).

In the past it was common to carry out an **oral glucose tolerance test**, although this is not often used now. The test is based on measuring how effectively a person can handle a glucose load. The person fasts overnight and in the morning is given a standard dose of glucose, usually in the form of a sweet drink. Blood samples are taken every 30 minutes for 2 hours and both glucose and insulin are measured (see Fig. 10.28).

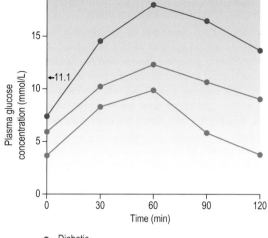

- ● Diabetic
- ● Impaired glucose tolerance
- ● Normal

Fig. 10.28 Typical oral glucose tolerance curves.

concentrations rise above this level, called the **renal threshold**, then the reabsorption mechanism in the kidney becomes saturated and so glucose is found in the urine. The sweet taste of urine from a person with uncontrolled diabetes used to be the basis of diagnosis and gives diabetes mellitus its name. The presence of glucose in urine causes an osmotic diuresis and so the patient needs to urinate frequently, causing an increase in thirst: polyuria and polydipsia are classical early symptoms of diabetes. The renal threshold is not an absolute constant. In older people, patients with renal disease and pregnant women the renal threshold is lower than 10 mmol/L and so it is more likely that glucose will be seen in the urine.

Type 1 diabetes

This form of diabetes results from loss of β cell function in the pancreatic islets. The reason why β cells are destroyed is complex and not fully understood. There is a genetic predisposition to developing diabetes, which may be linked to the **human leucocyte antigen (HLA)** genes. Current theories are that an environmental challenge is needed as a trigger for the β cells to become a target for autoimmune antibodies. The result is that pancreatic β cells are destroyed and the body is no longer able to produce insulin. This means that control of blood glucose has to be achieved by injecting insulin.

Type 1 diabetes usually starts in childhood or during adolescence. The diagnosis means that a young person has to learn to manage their blood glucose, taking regular measurements and injecting insulin. They also have to be careful about their diet.

Type 2 diabetes

Insulin resistance is strongly associated with the development of type 2 diabetes: the great majority of people with type 2 diabetes will have had a period of insulin resistance preceding the diabetes. This is most commonly seen in people who are overweight (Table 10.8). Insulin resistance means that the normal physiological response to insulin is impaired, so that blood glucose remains elevated for longer than normal after an oral dose of glucose or a meal. Insulin is also less effective at suppressing glucose output by the liver. The cellular mechanism of insulin resistance is poorly

understood: it does not appear to be a defect at the level of the receptor, but rather at some point downstream, in the complex insulin signalling pathway (see Ch. 3).

Impaired glucose tolerance may be assessed by an oral glucose tolerance test (see Fig. 10.28). Type 2 diabetes is treated principally through diet and exercise. In most cases, if the patient can reduce their BMI to the normal range of 20–25, their diabetes will resolve. However, this can be extremely difficult to achieve. Oral hypoglycaemic drugs such as **metformin** and **sulphonylureas** are used. These act in different ways. Metformin acts by inhibiting hepatic glucose synthesis and by stimulating cells to take up glucose. Sulphonylureas act by enhancing insulin release from pancreatic β cells (see Fig. 10.27).

Obesity

Obesity is associated with insulin resistance and impaired glucose tolerance. It is a major predisposing factor for the development of type 2 diabetes mellitus. In people with obesity there is a significantly higher rate of insulin secretion than in lean individuals and the pancreatic β cells appear to have a greater sensitivity to blood glucose levels (Clinical box 10.20). However, these individuals also have an impaired response to insulin and a higher fasting blood glucose level, so they are often in a state of **hyperinsulinaemia**.

Table 10.8   **Risk factors for developing type 2 diabetes:**

- Age (over 40)
- Obesity
- Ethnicity (Asian, especially South Indian, Maori, Polynesian. Black European/US populations have higher incidence than white European/US)
- Family history
- Western diet
- Physical inactivity
- City dwelling

Measurement of blood glucose is carried out by the patient themselves using a pocket-sized glucose meter. A finger prick blood sample is applied to a disposable stick which is inserted into the meter for an instant readout. People with type 1 diabetes need to check their blood glucose several times each day. For a newly-diagnosed patient frequent blood testing helps them learn to develop eating patterns and use of insulin to get the best control of their blood glucose.

Average blood glucose levels can be measured over a longer time period in the diabetic clinic. A blood sample is taken from the arm and the levels of **glycated haemoglobin (HbA₁c)** measured. As haemoglobin is found in red blood cells which have a life of about 120 days, the amount of glycated haemoglobin gives information about blood glucose over the previous 3 months. If the average blood glucose was 6 mmol/L (i.e. in the normal range) then the HbA₁c will be around 42 mmol/mol. An average blood glucose of 9 mmol/L results in an HbA₁c of 75 mmol/mol. Patients are usually monitored annually and aim for a target of lower than 48 mmol/mol (6.5 mmol/L glucose).

Complications of poorly controlled blood glucose 1: diabetic ketoacidosis

Diabetes is often described as 'starvation in the midst of plenty'. As insulin is either absent or ineffective, the body cannot handle glucose properly, with the result that blood concentrations of glucose may become very high. Without insulin this glucose cannot get into the cells to be used, and so the cells of the body are effectively in a starvation state despite the high blood levels of glucose. The body responds by trying to increase blood glucose, through increased release of glucagon and the stress hormones cortisol and epinephrine, which exacerbates the problem. As glucose cannot get into cells to be used as a metabolic fuel, the liver makes an alternative fuel by metabolising fatty acids to make ketones. An increase in ketone bodies causes metabolic acidosis or '**ketoacidosis**' (Fig. 10.29). This can cause nausea, dehydration and eventually lead to loss of consciousness and death. The physiological response to metabolic acidosis is hyperventilation as removal of carbon dioxide through respiration raises the pH of blood. This is seen as '**Kussmaul's respiration**'. Ketones in blood are excreted partly through the lungs: a person with ketoacidosis has characteristically sweet-smelling breath. Ketones are also excreted in urine and, together with the glucosuria, cause diuresis (see Ch. 3).

The treatment for diabetic ketoacidosis is fluid replacement followed by insulin treatment. Insulin action increases cellular uptake of potassium and so plasma potassium levels must be closely monitored to avoid hypokalaemia, which has dangerous effects on the heart.

Complications of poorly controlled blood glucose 2: HONK

Hyperosmolar non-ketotic states (**HONK**) is seen in some patients with type 2 diabetes and is commonly the first presentation. There is some insulin activity and so ketosis does not develop. Blood glucose may be extremely high and as a result there is osmotic diuresis and dehydration which may lead to coma. The blood becomes thicker and more likely to clot and so there is greatly increased risk of stroke, heart attack and deep vein thrombosis.

Complications of poorly controlled blood glucose 3: hypoglycaemia

In people with type 1 diabetes this is the result of taking their insulin but not eating enough to maintain blood glucose levels. It is a life-threatening condition which must be treated by prompt administration of glucose. Many diabetics learn to recognise 'early warning' signs of hypoglycaemia and carry glucose sweets to correct the hypoglycaemia.

In type 2 diabetes **hypoglycaemia** is unusual and occurs as a result of taking long-acting hypoglycaemic drugs or taking too much of their medication. Long-term consequences of poor glycaemic control are shown in Figure 10.30.

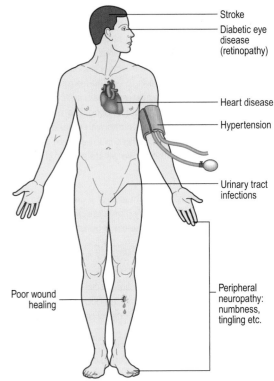

Fig. 10.30 **Long-term consequences of poor glycaemic control.**

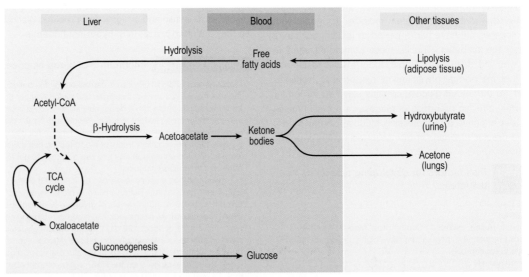

Fig. 10.29 **Pathways of ketone body formation in diabetes or starvation.** Entry of acetyl-CoA to the TCA cycle is impaired and so metabolism is diverted to acetoacetate and ketone body formation. Acetone is excreted via the lungs while hydroxybutyrate is excreted in urine. Oxaloacetate formed from the TCA cycle is diverted to a pathway of gluconeogenesis.

ENDOCRINE CONTROL OF BLOOD CALCIUM (details of bone in Ch. 9)

CALCIUM HOMEOSTASIS

Calcium is a metal ion: a divalent cation, with a very wide range of functions in the body. The vast majority of the total calcium in the body is in bones where it is an important structural component. This also acts as a reserve pool of calcium which can be mobilised if needed in order to maintain plasma calcium levels (Fig. 10.31). Plasma calcium concentrations are tightly regulated, normally between 2.2 and 2.5 mmol/L. If calcium concentrations fall below this level then neurotransmission at the neuromuscular junction is disrupted. This initially causes a 'pins and needles' sensation, followed by tetany, paralysis and convulsions. When the respiratory muscles become affected then low plasma calcium levels (**hypocalcaemia**) can be fatal. Higher calcium levels for any prolonged period lead to renal calculi (kidney stones), dehydration, renal failure, fatigue, constipation and depression.

CONTROL OF BLOOD CALCIUM AND PHOSPHATE CONCENTRATIONS

There are two hormones which play a major role in the regulation of plasma calcium levels: **parathyroid hormone (PTH)** and vitamin D. Parathyroid hormone is a peptide hormone secreted by the parathyroid glands. These glands are usually located on the under-surface of the thyroid gland and there are usually four parathyroid glands, but it is quite common to find more than this number and they may be distributed through the neck and upper thorax (see Fig. 10.16).

The secretion of parathyroid hormone is directly regulated by plasma calcium, detected by a calcium receptor on the surface of parathyroid cells. Low plasma calcium stimulates PTH release while high calcium inhibits it.

Parathyroid hormone has three main actions. It acts on the kidney to promote calcium reabsorption with the loss of phosphate and so prevents loss of calcium in urine. It also acts on bone to stimulate osteoclast activity, breaking down bone and so releasing calcium into the blood. The metabolic actions of PTH therefore result in increased plasma calcium concentrations by preventing urinary excretion and by sacrificing bone. Its third action is to increase the expression of the gene encoding a steroid hydroxylase enzyme in the kidney. This enzyme is needed for the activation of vitamin D. It is only through the actions of vitamin D that the body can increase the amount of calcium in the body by utilising dietary sources of calcium.

Vitamin D (also called **cholecalciferol**) is not a true vitamin as it is also made by the body and not, therefore, an absolute nutritional requirement. In fact, if we relied solely on dietary intake most people would be deficient in vitamin D. It is present in substantial amounts in oily fish and is also obtained from dairy products, but countries try to ensure an adequate intake of vitamin D in their populations by fortifying foods such as margarine (UK), milk and orange juice (USA). Breakfast cereals are also commonly fortified with vitamin D.

There are two forms of vitamin D: **D3** which is made in our skin by the action of ultraviolet light on **7-dehydrocholesterol** (Fig. 10.32); and vitamin **D2** which is made by plants and is the form most usually added to foods. Both forms of vitamin D undergo activation in the body and both act in the same manner to regulate plasma calcium.

Vitamin D (cholecalciferol) needs to be activated by two hydroxylation reactions in order to form the active hormone:

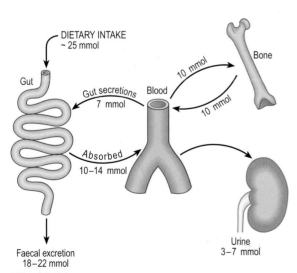

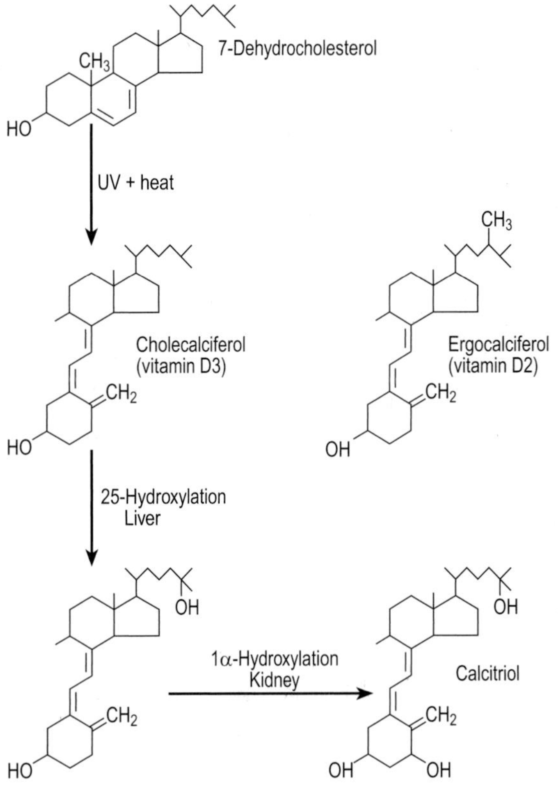

Fig. 10.31 Sources of plasma calcium. This shows the daily calcium turnover for an adult in calcium balance. It is important to recognise that calcium in bones is not all fixed, but can be mobilised to contribute to plasma calcium levels.

Fig. 10.32 Formation and structure of vitamin D3 (cholecalciferol) and D2 (ergocalciferol), and the formation of calcitriol. UV, ultraviolet light.

Information box 10.9 | **Metabolic effects of insulin**

Insulin binds to specific receptors in adipose tissue, muscle and the liver. It regulates a number of metabolic processes involving both glucose and other fuels. If insulin is absent or ineffective then these processes effectively go into reverse, an effect that is accelerated by the hormone glucagon.

Insulin stimulates uptake and storage of glucose
- In muscle and adipose tissue insulin increases glucose uptake via GLUT4 transporters, increases glycogen synthesis and inhibits glycogen breakdown.
- In the liver insulin acts to suppress gluconeogenesis. It also increases glycogen synthesis and inhibits glycogen breakdown.

Insulin promotes protein formation
- In muscle, adipose tissue and other tissues insulin increases uptake of amino acids, promoting protein synthesis and inhibiting protein breakdown.
- In the liver insulin inhibits conversion of amino acids into glucose and decreases urea formation.

Insulin promotes fat storage
- In adipose tissue insulin induces lipoprotein lipase and inhibits intracellular hormone-sensitive lipase so increases storage of triglycerides and esterification and storage of fatty acids.
- In liver insulin increases synthesis of triglycerides, cholesterol and very low density lipoproteins (VLDLs). It also inhibits the breakdown of fatty acids to ketones.

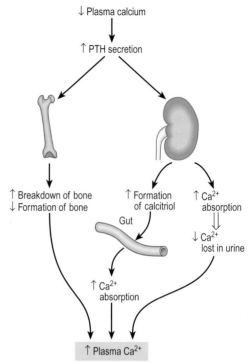

Fig. 10.33 Physiological response to hypocalcaemia.

Information box 10.10 | **Vitamin D**

Our understanding of the actions of calcitriol has increased greatly over the past two decades. It is now clear that bone disease represents only the most extreme effect of vitamin D deficiency. Sub-optimal levels of vitamin D have been associated with increased risk of a range of disorders with an autoimmune component, including type 1 diabetes and multiple sclerosis, as well as some forms of cancer. There is emerging evidence that supplementation with vitamin D can be a useful treatment for infective disorders such as tuberculosis. Each month it seems that vitamin D is implicated in yet another disease process. Vitamin D is a readily available dietary supplement with a wide therapeutic range. It is at worst harmless, within conventional dose ranges, and at best it may prove to be a significant health benefit.

1,2α-dihydroxyvitamin D or **1,25-dihydroxycholecalciferol**, more easily called calcitriol (see Information box 10.9). The first of these reactions is a **25-hydroxylation** and takes place in the liver. The second is a **1α-hydroxylation** and takes place in the kidney. It is this enzyme which is regulated by PTH.

The classical action of calcitriol is to increase the numbers of calcium channels in the gut, allowing for the effective utilisation of dietary calcium. This is the only way in which the body can increase its total calcium. When the body is able to use dietary calcium then bone health is preserved. In states of vitamin D deficiency the body effectively sacrifices bone minerals in order to maintain blood calcium (Figs 10.33 and 10.34; see also Information boxes 10.10, 10.11 and Clinical box 10.21).

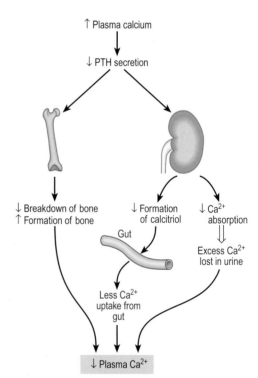

Fig. 10.34 Physiological response to hypercalcaemia.

Information box 10.11   The kidney as an endocrine tissue (details in Ch. 14)

The kidney has a range of important endocrine functions. Not surprisingly, it is the target tissue for the hormones involved in sodium and water balance. These hormones, aldosterone (sodium homeostasis) and vasopressin (also known as antidiuretic hormone, water homeostasis) are discussed in detail in Chapter 14.

The kidney is also, as we have just seen, critical in maintaining plasma calcium concentrations. It is the major target tissue for parathyroid hormone, which stimulates both an increase in calcium reabsorption and the excretion of phosphate into the urine. PTH also increases renal expression of the gene encoding the 1-α-hydroxylase enzyme responsible for the final step in the activation of vitamin D.

The kidney also produces a peptide hormone, **erythropoietin**, which stimulates bone marrow to produce more red blood cells, so increasing the oxygen-carrying capacity of blood. Finally, the kidney secretes **renin**, an enzyme which circulates in blood and acts to cleave angiotensinogen to produce **angiotensin II**, a potent vasoconstrictor and stimulant to aldosterone secretion.

Clinical box 10.21   Disorders of calcium metabolism

- **Hyperparathyroidism**: this is a disorder which is caused either by a tumour in parathyroid glands (primary hyperparathyroidism) or by chronic severe vitamin D deficiency (secondary hyperparathyroidism) which may result in the chronic high levels of PTH becoming autonomous. Hyperparathyroidism causes high plasma calcium levels and is associated with weak bones and renal calculi (kidney stones).
- **Hypercalcaemia** causes a number of clinical problems. Renal calculi are common. High plasma calcium causes osmotic diuresis and dehydration. Hypercalcaemia is also associated with peptic ulceration resulting from increased gastric acid secretion, severe constipation, cognitive impairment and depression.

- **Hypoparathyroidism**: a deficiency in PTH is a life-threatening disorder. Plasma calcium falls below the normal range which causes hyperexcitability of the neuromuscular junction. At first this causes paraesthesia, tingling of the fingers and toes and a pins and needles sensation. Ultimately PTH deficiency causes tetanic muscle contraction when is fatal when it reaches the respiratory muscles.
- **Vitamin D deficiency**. In children vitamin D deficiency causes a malformation of long bones called **rickets**. In adults the corresponding condition is called osteomalacia. Both conditions result in poor bone mineralisation with pain and weakness. In children the bones are deformed. This can be prevented very easily by giving vitamin D supplements.

REPRODUCTIVE PHYSIOLOGY

MALE REPRODUCTIVE ENDOCRINOLOGY

Male reproductive tract (Fig. 10.35)

The **testes** are the male gonads: paired glands located in the scrotum. They have a dual function, the production of male gametes, called sperm, and the production of male sex steroids, the androgens. The testes are located outside the abdomen and as a result are maintained at a lower temperature than normal body temperature as this is necessary for **spermatogenesis** to take place. The volume of each testis in an adult man is 20 to 25 mL. In a small number of baby boys one of the testes has not properly descended into the scrotum. This condition, known as **cryptorchidism**, is far more common in premature babies and is corrected by a surgical procedure to bring the testis into the scrotum where it is 'tethered'.

The testicular arteries, which provide the blood supply to the testis, arise from the abdominal aorta. Each artery arises independently so there is no connection between the blood supply to the left and right testis. This is significant. In late foetal life as the testes descend into the scrotum, or at any other stage in life, the testis can twist, causing a disruption of its blood supply, which is both painful and very disruptive to the function of the testis: this is treated as a surgical emergency. As each testis has an independent blood supply, such **testicular torsion** only disrupts the blood supply to one of the testes. Venous drainage on the right is into the vena cava and on the left into the renal vein.

There is both a sympathetic and a parasympathetic nerve supply which are important for sexual function. The parasympathetic innervation to the vas deferens controls ejaculation while the sympathetic supply controls erection.

Each testis consists of hundreds of tightly coiled **seminiferous tubules**. These tubules are connected to the **vas deferens** via the **rete testis** and the **epididymis** (Fig. 10.35). The seminiferous tubules are lined by **Sertoli** cells resting on a basement membrane (Fig. 10.36). Lying outside the basement membrane, scattered among the seminiferous tubules, are the **Leydig** cells. These are the site of steroid synthesis. The Sertoli cells are connected by tight junctions forming a blood–testis barrier. The blood–testis barrier is important for fertility. If it is breached then the immune system raises antibodies to spermatozoa which it recognises as foreign. In between the Sertoli cells are germ cells which undergo several divisions to form spermatozoa (Fig. 10.37). This process is controlled by hormones.

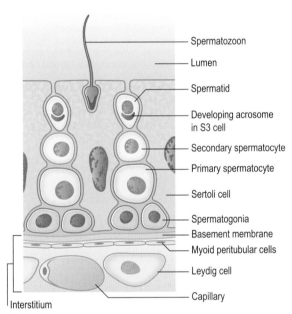

Fig. 10.36 **Seminiferous tubule – transverse section.**

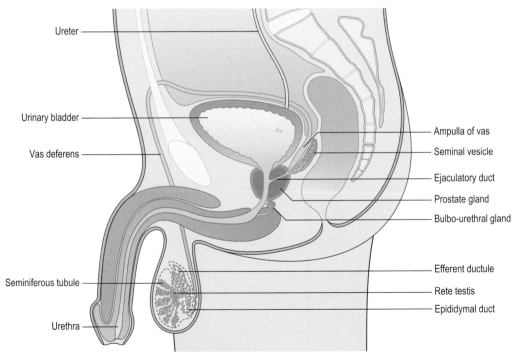

Fig. 10.35 **Mid-saggital section through the male pelvis.**

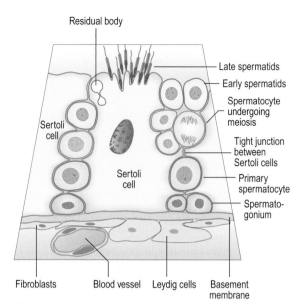

Fig. 10.37 Cells of the seminiferous tubule and the process of spermatogenesis. The germ cells originate next to the basement membrane, between the Sertoli cells. As these germ cells, known as spermatogonia, develop, they migrate towards the lumen of the seminiferous tubule, passing between the Sertoli cells. The immature spermatids are released from the secondary spermatogonia into the lumen of the seminiferous tubule leaving 'residual bodies' behind. The spermatids mature into spermatozoa as they pass along the tubules and through the epididymis.

HYPOTHALAMIC–PITUITARY–TESTICULAR AXIS

Testicular function is controlled by the hypothalamic–pituitary–testicular axis (Fig. 10.38). **Gonadotropin releasing hormone (GnRH)** from the hypothalamus stimulates the gonadotrope cells of the anterior pituitary to secrete the gonadotropins, luteinising hormone (LH) and follicle stimulating hormone (FSH).

LH acts on specific LH receptors on Leydig cells and stimulates steroidogenesis, in particular the production of testosterone (Fig. 10.39). Testosterone acts on the hypothalamus and pituitary to inhibit GnRH secretion as well as LH and FSH production.

FSH acts on Sertoli cells to stimulate the production of a specific high affinity androgen binding protein. This protein is responsible for maintaining the high intra-testicular concentration of testosterone necessary for spermatogenesis to take place. FSH also causes the Sertoli cells to produce **inhibin**, a peptide hormone which, together with testosterone, exerts a negative feedback effect on FSH secretion. Inhibin can be used as a marker of fertility as serum concentrations of inhibin are correlated with sperm count.

Androgens have a wide range of effects: sexual differentiation in foetal life; development and maintenance of male secondary sex characteristics; maintenance of libido; bone health; body composition; all in addition to the maintenance of spermatogenesis, the process of sperm formation (Table 10.9 and Fig. 10.40).

The effect of testosterone on spermatogenesis is a direct paracrine action, but most of the hormonal actions of testosterone are mediated by the active metabolite, **5-α-dihydrotestosterone (5αDHT)**. Testosterone also serves

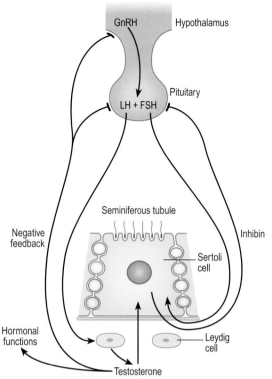

Fig. 10.38 Hypothalamic–pituitary–testicular axis. Gonadotropin releasing hormone (GnRH), released from the hypothalamus, stimulates the gonadotroph cells of the anterior pituitary to release luteinising hormone (LH) and follicle stimulating hormone (FSH). LH acts on Leydig cells to stimulate testosterone production, which acts with FSH on Sertoli cells to stimulate spermatogenesis. Testosterone and inhibin, a peptide secreted by Sertoli cells, exert negative feedback control of this axis.

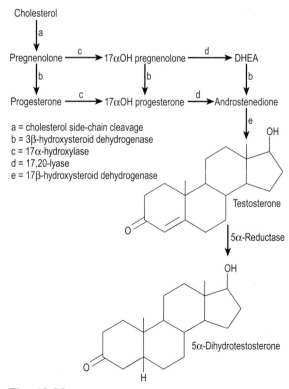

a = cholesterol side-chain cleavage
b = 3β-hydroxysteroid dehydrogenase
c = 17α-hydroxylase
d = 17,20-lyase
e = 17β-hydroxysteroid dehydrogenase

Fig. 10.39 Biosynthesis of testosterone in Leydig cells and its conversion to 5αDHT in peripheral tissues.

Table 10.9	Actions of androgens in man		
Intrauterine	**At puberty**		**In the adult man**
Development of male phenotype	Development of male secondary sex characteristics		Reproductive effects
Development of penis, scrotum, prostate, etc.	Hypertrophy of larynx (deepening of voice)		Maintenance of spermatogenesis
Testicular descent into scrotum	Development of seminal vesicles and prostate and initiation of sperm production		Maintenance of secondary sex characteristics including beard growth
Programming of male behaviour	Increased muscle mass		Maintenance of libido (sex drive)
Development of male phenotype	Increased skin thickness and sebum formation		Feedback inhibition of hypothalamic GnRH secretion
	Development of pubic and axillary hair		
	Fusion of epiphyseal plates in long bone		Metabolic effects
			Lipid metabolism, increasing circulating VLDL and LDL, decreasing HDL
			Increased metabolic rate
			Increased red blood cell number
			Maintenance of muscle mass
			Maintenance of bone density

as a precursor for oestrogen formation. Perhaps it would be more accurate to consider testosterone as a pro-hormone and a paracrine regulator.

Testosterone and 5αDHT act by binding to the androgen receptor. This is a member of the family of steroid hormone receptors which function as nuclear transcription factors. The androgen receptor is encoded by a gene on the X chromosome. So, paradoxically, men have only one copy of the gene for the androgen receptor while women have two copies. This means that any defect in the gene results in a condition of androgen insensitivity in men, while women are usually unaffected, acting only as carriers. Complete androgen insensitivity is unusual but there is a spectrum of disorders that arise from a defect in the androgen receptor gene, ranging from slightly impaired fertility to a full **androgen insensitivity syndrome** (Clinical boxes 10.22 and 10.23).

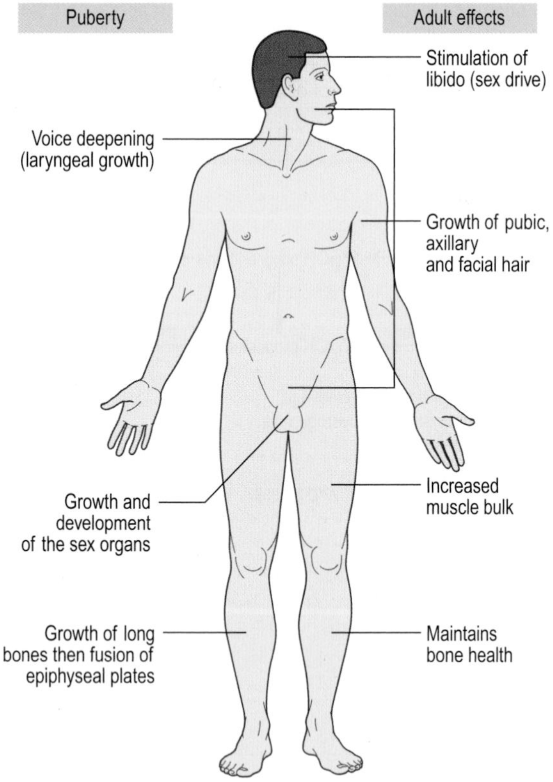

Spermatogenesis

The process by which sperm are formed is called spermatogenesis. This process is continuous from puberty until the end of a man's life. Men have testicular germ cells, **spermatogonia**, which constantly divide and renew, in marked contrast to a woman's ovaries which have a finite number of ova. Each spermatogonium first undergoes two divisions of

Fig. 10.40 **Actions of androgens.** The actions specific to puberty are shown on the left and the effects in adult men are shown on the right. The actions shown are mainly physiological effects on men. However, it should be noted that in women testosterone has an important role in stimulating libido, even though it circulates in only very low concentrations.

Puberty
Voice deepening (laryngeal growth)
Growth and development of the sex organs
Growth of long bones then fusion of epiphyseal plates

Adult effects
Stimulation of libido (sex drive)
Growth of pubic, axillary and facial hair
Increased muscle bulk
Maintains bone health

Clinical box 10.22 Androgen insensitivity syndrome

Testosterone is important in foetal development. In the absence of testosterone a male foetus (with an X and a Y chromosome) will develop female external genitalia and will be behaviourally programmed as a female. At birth it appears that the child is a normal baby girl and is raised as a girl. However, there is testicular tissue retained within the abdomen. At puberty there are very high levels of testosterone because there is no negative feedback inhibition of the hypothalamic–pituitary–testicular axis. Some of this testosterone is converted to oestradiol and so breasts develop. It is only when the girl does not start menstruation that she is referred to a doctor, to find that she is genetically male.

Clinical box 10.23 5α-Reductase deficiency

The enzyme 5α-reductase converts testosterone to the more active form, dihydrotestosterone (DHT) in peripheral tissues. Deficiency of 5α-reductase is an autosomal recessive condition that affects genetic males. Conversion of testosterone to DHT is important for development of normal male genitalia. In the absence of DHT in a male foetus varying degrees of feminisation of the genitalia occur and in some cases the child is raised as female. However, at puberty the greatly increased testosterone production causes testicular descent and growth of the penis. Gender identity is usually male, however severe the enzyme deficiency.

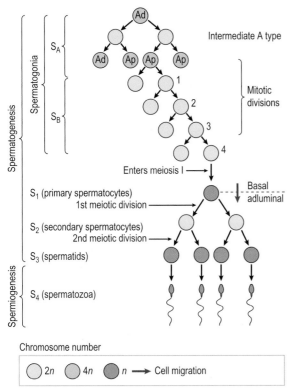

Fig. 10.41 Spermatogenesis.

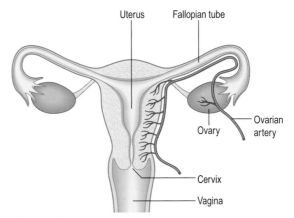

Fig. 10.42 The female reproductive system.

mitosis, resulting in four cells. One remains to continue dividing and giving rise to more spermatogonia while the other three undergo four more mitotic divisions followed by two meiotic divisions, giving rise to 64 **spermatids** (Fig. 10.41). A healthy man produces about 240 million sperm each day: or, looking at it another way, 2800 per second. It takes about 75 days to produce a mature sperm and up to 21 days to transport that sperm from the rete testis to the ejaculatory duct. The normal concentration of sperm in ejaculate is defined by the World Health Organization as greater than 15 million per mL. However, this is a threshold level used to define 'normal', and it is usual for each ejaculate to contain around 200 million sperm in a typical volume of 3 mL.

The testes require both testosterone and FSH for spermatogenesis, although in the absence of FSH low levels of sperm production can continue. The requirement for testosterone is absolute. The androgen binding protein produced by the Sertoli cells ensures that the concentration of testosterone in the testis is high enough to maintain spermatogenesis.

Clearly any agent which disrupts testicular testosterone production is a possible candidate for a male contraceptive. However, with about 96 days required for sperm production, it requires several months of treatment to reduce the numbers of sperm in ejaculate.

FEMALE REPRODUCTIVE ENDOCRINOLOGY

Female reproductive tract

The **ovaries** are the female gonads. Like the testes they have two functions: the production of gametes and the synthesis of sex hormones. The ovaries are each about 4 cm long and

lie within the abdominal cavity, connected to the **uterus** by structures called **fallopian tubes** (Fig. 10.42). The uterus is a muscular structure connected to the **vagina** via the **cervix**. The blood supply to the ovaries is directly from the aorta via ovarian arteries, while venous drainage on the right is into the vena cava and on the left into the renal vein: exactly the same arrangement as for the testes.

Each ovary contains a number of **primordial follicles** (Fig. 10.43), a pool of undeveloped **primary oocytes** with the capacity to develop into **ova**, the female gametes. At birth each ovary contains several million primordial follicles but this number declines over a woman's life; at puberty each ovary typically contains about 400 000 primary oocytes. During a woman's reproductive life an ovary will contain several oocytes at different stages of development and several **corpus albicans**, small white scar-like structures which are the remains of an ovulated follicle.

Gamete production in a woman is very different from a man. Men constantly produce sperm from puberty to the end of their life. Women have a narrow reproductive window, from puberty to menopause at around the age of 51 years, during which time they usually produce just one gamete each month.

Follicular development

Each primary oocyte consists of an ovum surrounded by a single layer of **granulosa cells**, all enclosed within a basement membrane (Fig. 10.43). The development of a follicle from selection to ovulation takes about 375 days. Several follicles are undergoing development at any one time, but the majority die by a process called **follicular atresia** and only one follicle usually enters the menstrual cycle each month.

HORMONAL CONTROL OF THE OVARY AND MENSTRUAL CYCLE

Ovarian function is controlled by the two gonadotropins secreted by the anterior pituitary, LH and FSH. The secretion of LH and FSH is controlled by GnRH secretion from the hypothalamus (Fig. 10.44).

Luteinising hormone acts on the developing follicle and then the corpus luteum to stimulate steroid hormone production while FSH stimulates follicular maturation. The **menstrual cycle** is the term given to the monthly cycle of gamete (ovum) production by the ovaries, and all the physical and hormonal changes which are associated with this process.

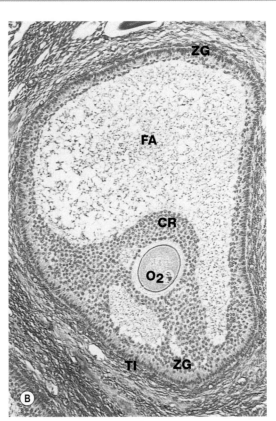

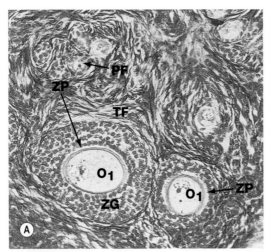

Fig. 10.43 **Follicular development.** (A) Primordial and primary follicles in the ovarian cortex. (B) Antral follicle. TA, tunica albuginea; O_1, primary oocyte; PF, primordial follicle; TF, thecal cells; ZG, granulosa cells; ZP, zona pellucida; CR, corona radiata (cumulus oophorus); FA, follicular antrum; O_2, secondary oocyte; TI, theca interna. From Young B, Woodford P, O'Dowd G, et al. 2013 Wheater's functional histology: a text and colour atlas, 6th edn. Churchill Livingstone, Philadelphia.

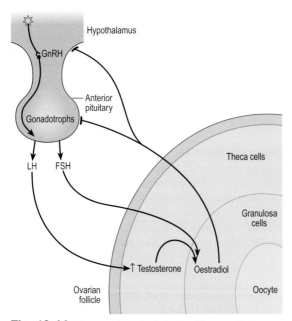

Fig. 10.44 **Hormonal control of steroidogenesis in the ovarian follicle.** The pulsatile release of gonadotropin releasing hormone (GnRH) from the hypothalamus stimulates release of luteinising hormone (LH) and follicle stimulating hormone (FSH) from the gonadotroph cells of the anterior pituitary. LH receptors are located on the theca cells and LH binds to these receptors, stimulating the secretion of androgens, particularly testosterone. The testosterone is converted to oestradiol in granulosa cells. Levels of the enzyme that catalyse this reaction, aromatase, are increased by the action of FSH on the granulosa cells. Oestradiol exerts a negative feedback effect on the hypothalamus and pituitary.

The menstrual and ovarian cycles

The typical menstrual cycle is 28 days long. The days of each cycle are numbered, starting with the first day of menstruation which is day 1 of the cycle. In this scheme, ovulation usually occurs on day 14. Although the interval between menstruation and ovulation may vary considerably, between 7 and 21 days, the interval between ovulation and the next menstruation is always 14 days, unless the ovum is fertilised and pregnancy results. At either end of her reproductive life, in puberty and when a woman is approaching menopause, the cycle length may be much longer.

The first phase of the menstrual cycle involves shedding the endometrial lining which grew and became vascularised during the previous cycle. This is seen as menstrual bleeding, a woman's 'monthly period', and usually lasts between 4 and 7 days. At this point the developing follicle is in the **pre-antral stage** (see Fig. 10.45) consisting of an ovum surrounded by four concentric layers of cells. The innermost layer is the granulosa which is surrounded by the **theca interna** and **theca externa**, all enclosed by the stromal layer.

During this time the developing follicle is secreting **oestrogens** under the influence of LH. This is a complex process. LH acts on the theca cells to stimulate hormone production, but these cells lack **aromatase**, the final enzyme required for oestrogen synthesis, and so produce only androgens. These androgens are converted by the adjacent granulosa cells into oestrogens, under the control of FSH, which regulates the expression of the gene encoding the aromatase enzyme (see Fig. 10.44).

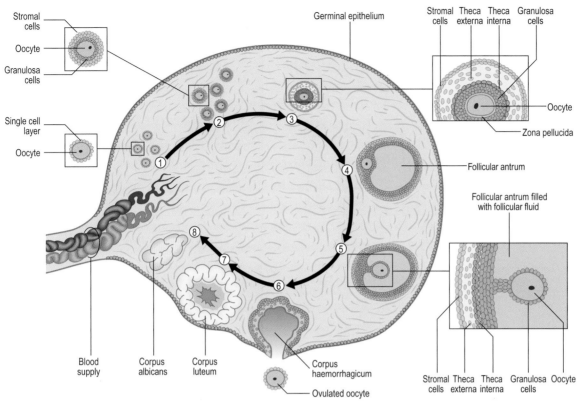

Fig. 10.45 **Stages of follicular development in the ovary.** (1) Primordial follicles consist of an oocyte surrounded by a single cell layer. (2) At the start of follicular development the cells divide to form a stromal layer and surround the granulosa cells. (3) Follicular development continues with the formation of the theca cells, which lie between the granulosa and stromal cells. The oocyte is surrounded by the zona pellucida. (4) The follicular antrum develops, filled with follicular fluid. (5) A mature oocyte: suspended in the follicular fluid, attached by a stalk to the granulosa cell layer. (6) As the follicle ruptures to release the oocyte (the point of ovulation), the antrum fills with blood to form a corpus haemorrhagicum, which develops into the corpus luteum. (7) Regression of the corpus luteum leads to formation of the scar-like corpus albicans. (8) The whole cycle shown here takes several months. The developing follicles are not drawn to scale; for comparison, the follicle at stage 2 is around 20 μm in diameter whereas the mature follicle at stage 5 is 250 times larger at 5 mm, easily visible by eye.

The second phase of the menstrual cycle is the **follicular phase** or **proliferative phase**. The oestrogens produced by the developing follicle act on the endometrium and stimulate its growth and vascularisation (Fig. 10.46). During this phase the follicle develops rapidly, forming a follicular antrum which is a fluid filled cavity in the follicle in which the mature oocyte is suspended.

Ovulation marks the end of this phase of the cycle. LH and FSH secretion has been rising through the follicular phase, increasing oestradiol production, with the usual negative feedback regulation of the hypothalamic–pituitary–ovarian axis. When oestradiol levels reach a certain point, the regulation switches from negative to positive feedback and the increasing oestradiol levels cause a further increase in LH. This is termed the LH surge and is the trigger for ovulation. Ovulation is the process by which the mature oocyte is released from the ovary and taken into the fallopian tube. It has some elements in common with an inflammatory process as it is dependent on cyclo-oxygenase inhibitors (e.g. COX2, see Ch. 4) and prostaglandins production. Local production of matrix metalloproteinases and other enzymes break down the stromal layer and basal lamina of the follicle and the germinal epithelium of the ovary, rupturing the follicle and allowing the oocyte to be released.

The LH surge also causes a switch in steroidogenesis in the ruptured follicle. The granulosa cells are triggered to become the major steroid secreting cells, effectively replacing the role of the theca cells. They begin to express the genes encoding steroidgenesis acute regulatory (**StAR**) protein (see Information box 10.2), **CYP11A1 (cholesterol side-chain cleavage)** and **3β-hydroxysteroid dehydrogenase**, allowing the granulosa cells to secrete **progesterone**.

The luteal phase, or secretory phase, is the final phase of the cycle. It always lasts for 14 days unless the oocyte is fertilised. This phase of the cycle is dominated by the corpus luteum and the actions of progesterone. The ruptured follicle fills with blood and forms a '**corpus haemorrhagicum**' within the ovary which matures into the corpus luteum. The corpus luteum consists mostly of granulosa cells which now secrete progesterone. Although LH and FSH levels decline dramatically following ovulation, progesterone secretion remains high. During this time the progesterone acts on the endometrium, maintaining the high degree of vascularity necessary for implantation and stimulating the production of a clear fluid from the endometrium, hence the term 'secretory phase' for this stage of the cycle. The life of the corpus luteum is 14 days in the absence of fertilisation of the oocyte. Towards the end of this period the corpus luteum begins to break down, a process termed **luteolysis**, and stops secreting progesterone. Without the high levels of progesterone to maintain the endometrial lining, it is shed; this is the start of menstruation and the next cycle.

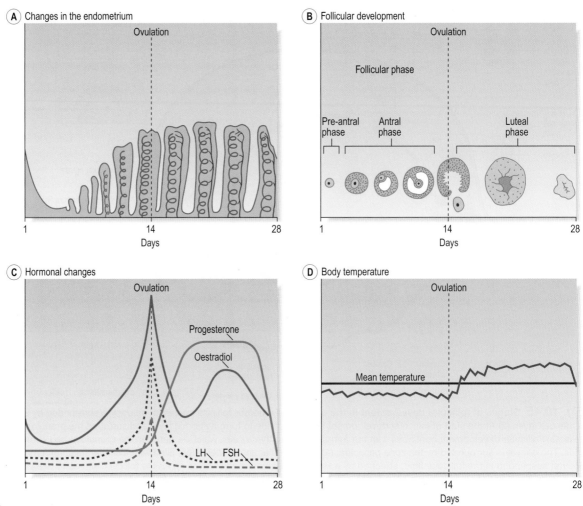

Fig. 10.46 **The menstrual cycle.** Conventionally, the days of the menstrual cycle are numbered from the onset of menstruation (day 1). Ovulation occurs on day 14 in the standard 28 day cycle. The duration of the proliferative phase (the interval from the onset of menstruation to ovulation) is variable and ovulation does not always occur on day 14. However, there is little variation in the length of the secretory phase. (A) Changes in the endometrium during the menstrual cycle. (B) Stages of follicular development during the menstrual cycle. (C) Hormonal changes during the menstrual cycle; the peak in oestradiol immediately precedes ovulation.

PUBERTY

The period of time that forms the transition between childhood and adulthood is called **puberty**. This is the time during which secondary sexual development takes place (Information box 10.12). There are characteristic physical changes which occur during puberty. In boys these changes include growth and development of the penis, testes and scrotum and the development of facial, axillary and pubic hair. In girls the changes include breast development, as well as growth of axillary and pubic hair. These particular changes in boys and girls have been used to classify the stages of pubertal development: the **Tanner** classification of puberty (Fig. 10.47). There are of course other physical changes. Boys and girls both undergo a change in body shape, boys have a lowering of the voice and girls begin to menstruate. There is also typically a growth spurt followed by the complete cessation of linear growth. All these changes are controlled by hormones (Information box 10.12).

Before puberty the hypothalamic–pituitary–gonadal axis is largely silent with very low levels of LH and FSH. As a child enters puberty the hypothalamus begins to produce GnRH, at first just during the night but later, as puberty progresses,

during the day as well. The GnRH is secreted in pulses, at first of low amplitude but increasing as puberty progresses. This change is paralleled by changes in LH and FSH secretion. The gonads produce sex hormones in response to the increased LH and FSH and it is these sex hormones which bring about most of the physical changes of puberty.

The timing of puberty is driven by the maturation of the hypothalamic neurons that control GnRH secretion. These neurons are sensitive to circulating oestrogens, particularly **oestrone**, and to **leptin**, the satiety hormone. In girls menstruation does not begin until they reach a weight of about 47 kg (Table 10.10). At this weight there is sufficient

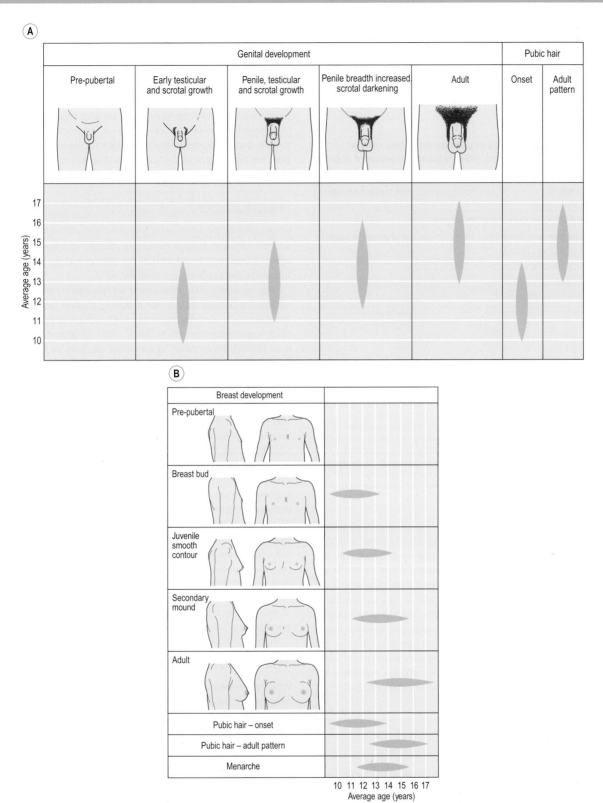

Fig. 10.47 **Tanner classification of pubertal development.** (A) Boys: stages of pubertal, genital and pubic hair development in boys, with the average age of each stage shown. (B) Stages of pubertal development in girls, with the average age of each stage shown.

body mass to produce leptin and sufficient adipose tissue to convert circulating androgens to oestrone. These hormones act on the hypothalamus, stimulating the maturation of a set of neurons which use **kisspeptin** as the transmitter. Increased release of kisspeptin allows GnRH secretion to develop its characteristic pulsatile pattern of secretion. If

GnRH is secreted constantly, rather than in pulses, then the anterior pituitary gonadotrope cells are no longer able to respond and the individual will have impaired fertility.

Puberty is associated with several other hormonal changes in addition to the activation of the hypothalamic–pituitary–gonadal axis. In late childhood there is an increase in adrenal

Table 10.10	Factors which influence the age of menarche

- Genetic component/ethnic variation
- Nutritional status
- Body mass index (body weight = 47 kg)
- Other factors

Table 10.11	Events of puberty (after Marshall & Tanner), fairly regular sequence of events between ages of 10 and 16 years in girls

Event	Age range (average)
Growth spurt (6–10 cm/year peak, 2.5 years' duration)	8–14 years (9 years)
Breast growth (thelarche)	8–13 years (11 years)
Pubic hair (pubarche) (first pubertal sign in 25%)	9–13 years
Axillary hair (adrenarche) (may follow menarche)	9.5–15 years
Menstruation (menarche)	10–16 years (13 years)

Clinical box 10.24   Failure of puberty

There are several reasons why somebody might not undergo the normal pubertal development, or where pubertal development is delayed (see Table 10.10). We have already looked at the androgen receptor defect which results in a genotypic male being phenotypically female and how this is not discovered until she is investigated for failure of menarche. There are several chromosomal abnormalities which cause a disorder of sexual differentiation which may not be detected until puberty. These include Klinefelter syndrome and Turner syndrome (see section on sexual differentiation).

size accompanied by a significant increase in adrenal androgen production, mainly dehydroepiandrosterone (DHEA) and its sulphate, DHEAS. This is called adrenarche (Table 10.11). These adrenal androgens are responsible for the development of axillary (armpit) hair during puberty. There is also an increase in growth hormone levels during puberty. This rise contributes to the growth spurt seen in both boys and girls, in which height increases by up to 10 cm per year. This growth spurt is brought to an end by the increase in circulating sex steroids which cause the epiphyseal plates in the long bones to close, preventing further growth (for failure of puberty, see Clinical Box 10.24).

PREGNANCY

In order for pregnancy to occur, an ovum needs to be fertilised by a single spermatozoon, an event which is sometimes called **conception**. Biologically, pregnancy begins with the **implantation** of the fertilised ovum in the wall of the uterus and ends with **parturition**, the process by which a baby is born. Medically, pregnancy is timed from the date of the last menstruation and not from conception, so is always about 2 weeks longer than the actual age of the foetus. The interval between the last menstruation and parturition (childbirth) is termed the **gestatory period**, and pregnancy is often referred to as **gestation**.

Conventionally, the duration of a pregnancy is divided into three time periods, called trimesters. So there is the first trimester, up to week 13 of a pregnancy, the second trimester, weeks

14–27, and the third trimester, which goes to the end of the pregnancy. A normal pregnancy, called 'full term', is about 40 weeks.

There are significant endocrine changes during pregnancy. This is partly because both the foetus and the placenta produce their own hormones, which can cross into the maternal circulation and so affect the mother's physiological processes, and partly because there are also some changes to maternal hormone production. The end of pregnancy, parturition, and the production of breast milk for the baby, **lactation**, are both regulated by hormones. The endocrinology of pregnancy begins with the process of fertilisation.

FERTILISATION

Fertilisation of the ovum usually occurs in the fallopian tube and the fertilised egg, or conceptus, travels into the uterus where it becomes embedded in the uterine wall and it is at this stage that pregnancy is established.

Approximately 100 million sperm are released in every ejaculation. The prostatic fluid, which makes up most of the volume of the ejaculate, contains prostaglandins which cause the sperm tail to move and the sperm to 'swim'. The vaginal environment is acidic and the entrance to the uterus can only be reached through a mucus plug. These two factors combine to the effect that only a small number of sperm reach the oocyte in the fallopian tube. Despite their slow rate of swimming, at around 1 mm per minute, sperm can be detected in the fallopian tube after only a few minutes. Their transport is aided by the contractile effects of prostaglandins on the uterine and fallopian tube smooth muscle. Before fertilising an oocyte a sperm has to undergo **capacitation** and the **acrosome reaction**. Capacitation occurs in the uterus where a range of enzymes produced by the endometrium act on the sperm, cleaving surface glycoproteins and increasing the membrane calcium permeability. This causes an increase in cAMP and results in hypermobility of the sperm, together with destabilisation of the membrane surrounding the acrosome at the head of the sperm, allowing it to fuse with the oocyte. When the sperm comes into contact with the cumulus layer surrounding the egg, the acrosome reaction is initiated. This allows the contents of the acrosome, including a number of enzymes, to be released. The enzymes allow the sperm to penetrate and fuse with the egg, and so fertilisation occurs.

The establishment of pregnancy

When the blastocyst becomes embedded in the endometrial lining of the uterus, it establishes a blood supply via the placenta. The placenta is an interesting tissue, forming the connection between the mother and the foetus, two genetically distinct individuals (see Information box 10.13). The outer layer of the blastocyst becomes the trophoblast and develops to form the outer layer of the placenta (Fig. 10.48). The placenta provides the blood supply to the foetus but also acts as a barrier between

Information box 10.13   The placenta

'Placenta' is derived from a Latin term meaning 'flat cake', which is approximately the appearance of the placenta. The placenta grows throughout pregnancy, reaching approximately 20 cm diameter and 2 cm thick at term. Typically a placenta weighs 500 g. It is the custom among some cultures, and normal behaviour for many mammalian species, to eat the placenta after childbirth. It has been suggested that the high levels of oestrogens in the placenta may be beneficial to the mother postpartum but there is no evidence to support this.

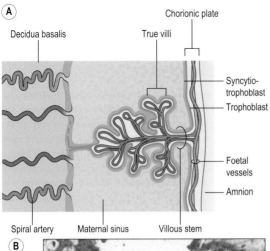

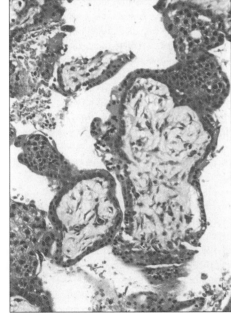

Fig. 10.48 Structure of the early placenta. (A) A chorionic villus; (B) histological section (×150). From Young B, Woodford P, O'Dowd G, et al. 2013 Wheater's functional histology: a text and colour atlas, 6th edn. Churchill Livingstone, Philadelphia.

Occasionally the conceptus does not reach the uterus but remains within the fallopian tube and begins to develop there. This is termed an 'ectopic pregnancy' and presents a serious health risk to the mother as the fallopian tube will rupture if the ectopic pregnancy is not detected at a very early stage. The risk of ectopic pregnancy is greatly increased by sexually transmitted infections which lead to pelvic inflammatory disease. Ectopic pregnancy can also occur if the conceptus remains within the ovary, in the abdominal cavity or in the cervix.

One explanation for the mistaken association of intrauterine contraceptive devices (IUCDs) with ectopic pregnancy is that IUCDs are very effective indeed at preventing uterine pregnancy, and so, if pregnancy does occur when using an IUCD, it is most likely to be ectopic.

---

the foetal and the maternal circulation. It is the placenta that is the key endocrine tissue of pregnancy, acting both to secrete and metabolise hormones, stimulating the corpus luteum to maintain pregnancy and regulating the endocrine environment in which the foetus develops. Clinical boxes 10.25 and 10.26 discuss clinical conditions that relate to failure of implantation.

Hormone production by the placenta

Within a few days of conception the placenta begins to produce hormones. The most important hormone in the early stages of pregnancy is **chorionic gonadotropin** (abbreviated to **hCG**), a hormone closely related to luteinising hormone.

The main action of hCG is to stimulate the corpus luteum to continue producing progesterone beyond the 14 days after ovulation when the corpus luteum would normally regress. Levels of hCG are highest in the first trimester of pregnancy, peaking around weeks 10–12, but hCG is produced throughout pregnancy. The placenta also produces a peptide hormone called **placental lactogen (hPL)**, which is also known as **chorionic somatomammotropin (hCS)**. This hormone is a member of the growth hormone family but is most closely related to prolactin. This is the hormone which causes maternal blood glucose levels to increase during pregnancy, which may contribute to the nutrition of the foetus. Its role in pregnancy is not really clear; despite its similarity to prolactin it does not appear to have a role in lactation. It is clearly not very important as levels of hPL may be undetectable in normal

---

Contraception is the practice of preventing pregnancy occurring following sexual intercourse. Globally a wide range of methods are used. These include the traditional low-tech forms which include avoiding sexual intercourse around the time of ovulation. Barrier methods of contraception such as condoms are widely used. These physically prevent the sperm from reaching the ovum. When used together with a spermicidal jelly, condoms are a very effective form of contraception.

Hormonal contraceptives such as the oral contraceptive 'pill' are the commonest form of contraception in the developed world. This pill is taken daily by women and usually consists of a combination of synthetic oestrogen and a progestogen, to counteract the hyperproliferative actions of oestrogen which increase the risk of endometrial cancer. Some oral contraceptives consist only of progesterone. The pill acts in two ways: first by negative feedback inhibition of the hypothalamus and pituitary, blocking LH and FSH secretion and so preventing ovulation; and secondly by increasing the viscosity of the mucus present in the cervix and so presenting a greater physical barrier to prevent sperm from entering the uterus. Sometimes the hormonal combination used in the oral contraceptive pill may be administered in the form of a slow release capsule injected under the skin, which may last for around 3 months.

The intrauterine contraceptive device (IUCD), also called the 'coil', is a small piece of plastic and copper that is inserted into the uterus. It is thought to act as a local irritant and prevent implantation of the fertilised ovum. A more modern method of contraception uses a small plastic device impregnated with the hormone progesterone. This is highly effective at preventing pregnancy for up to 5 years. It works through a combination of ways: the progesterone thickens the cervical mucus preventing the sperm from reaching the uterus; but it also thins the myometrium, so the environment of the uterus is not as suitable for implantation. It may also prevent ovulation.

Emergency hormonal contraception is sometimes called the 'morning after pill'. It consists of a single combined high dose of oestrogen and progestogen and is designed to prevent pregnancy following unprotected sexual intercourse. It appears to act by creating an intrauterine environment that is unfavourable for implantation.

Termination of pregnancy can be achieved hormonally, using the anti-progestin mifepristone. It is effective both as a morning after pill and for inducing termination of pregnancy once established. It is an effective alternative to the surgical termination of pregnancy which is more commonly practised.

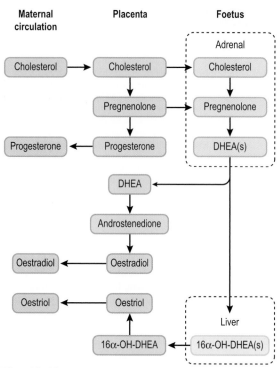

Maternal circulation	Placenta	Foetus

Fig. 10.49 Steroid biosynthesis by the placenta.

pregnancies which result in the delivery of normal infants. It has been used, however, as a marker of multiple births, as hPL levels are usually much higher than in a single pregnancy.

The placenta produces a range of steroids, taking over progesterone production from the corpus luteum in the 8th week of pregnancy (Fig. 10.49). Progesterone production continues through pregnancy and is important for the maintenance of the pregnancy. It prevents premature contractions of the uterine smooth muscle, the myometrium, partly by inhibiting oxytocin receptor expression but also by preventing the intrinsic contractile activity of the uterine muscle. The developing foetus also produces steroids, from the foetal adrenal gland, and these are metabolised by the placenta into oestrogens (Fig. 10.49). Placental oestrogens are important for stimulating uterine growth during pregnancy.

Pregnancy tests

Modern, commercially available, pregnancy tests detect the presence of hCG in the maternal urine. Although hCG is a large polypeptide hormone, consisting of two chains linked by disulphide bridges, sufficient quantities of the β chain are filtered unchanged in the urine to be detected. A standard pregnancy test uses plastic strips which support a sandwich ELISA: an antibody based test in which two different antibodies bind the hormone. One holds it in place while the second allows the hormone to be colour-tagged, and so the presence of hCG in the urine sample is indicated by a coloured strip appearing on the test stick. The urine tests are very sensitive indeed, detecting levels as low as 10 mIU/mL.

The placenta only produces hCG after implantation has occurred and it is detectable very soon after implantation. However, the time from ovulation to implantation can be up to 12 days and so tests carried out before a missed period (14 days after ovulation) can give a false negative result.

There is a new generation of pregnancy tests which measure **early pregnancy factor** (**EPF**). EPF is an immunosuppressant which appears in the maternal blood very soon after fertilisation. It can be detected 48 hours post-conception, but tests are currently very expensive and so not routinely available.

FOETAL DEVELOPMENT

The foetus develops rapidly; by 6 weeks a heartbeat may be detectable and by 8 weeks the different organ systems are in place. For an account of the development of the different organ systems see appropriate chapters. It is around this time that sexual differentiation takes place. The human foetus has 46 chromosomes: 22 pairs of chromosomes plus two sex chromosomes, designated X and Y. One X chromosome is essential for life but the second sex chromosome may be either X or Y. If there is a Y chromosome present the foetus is male; if not, it is female. The Y chromosome carries the **SRY** gene, sometimes called the 'testis determining factor'. The product of this gene is essential for normal male development to occur. The default state, in the absence of this gene, is the development of female genitalia.

At 7 weeks of gestation the foetus has a primitive gonad with the capacity to develop either male or female genitals (Fig. 10.50). Next to this gonad sit two pairs of ducts: the **Wolffian ducts** which form the male reproductive tract and the **Müllerian ducts** which form the female reproductive tract. At this stage both male and female foetuses look the same. In the absence of the SRY gene, the Müllerian ducts develop and form the fallopian tubes, uterus and vagina, while the Wolffian ducts gradually regress. This development takes place even if the foetal gonad is completely absent.

If the foetal gonad is a testis, however, the foetal Leydig cells begin to produce testosterone. This is converted to 5αDHT and the foetal Sertoli cells produce **anti-Müllerian hormone** (**AMH**). These two hormones together over-ride the default development of the female genitalia. The DHT works to stabilise the Wolffian ducts, preventing their regression and stimulating their development into the male reproductive tract, while the AMH causes the regression of the Müllerian ducts. This stage of development takes place within the first trimester of pregnancy and is complete by 12 weeks' gestation. (For screening for abnormalities, see Clinical boxes 10.27 and 10.28.)

PARTURITION – LABOUR

During pregnancy the high levels of progesterone maintain quiescence of the myometrium and it is thought to be a decrease in progesterone activity that initiates parturition. This is partly brought about by a decrease in circulating progesterone and partly by a decrease in progesterone receptors. There is also an increase in placental oestrogen production in the later stages of pregnancy which may be responsible for the increase in myometrial activity called **'Braxton-Hicks contractions'**. These appear almost like a rehearsal for the full contractions of parturition, and are irregular, weak contractions which occur in the last few weeks of pregnancy. The main hormone of parturition is the posterior pituitary peptide, **oxytocin**. Release of oxytocin is stimulated by activity of stretch receptors in the myometrium and oxytocin then acts on the myometrium causing contractions. There is only a small increase in oxytocin release at the time of parturition, but the fall in progesterone activity causes an increase in oxytocin receptor concentration in the myometrium and so oxytocin activity increases. Oxytocin stimulates the

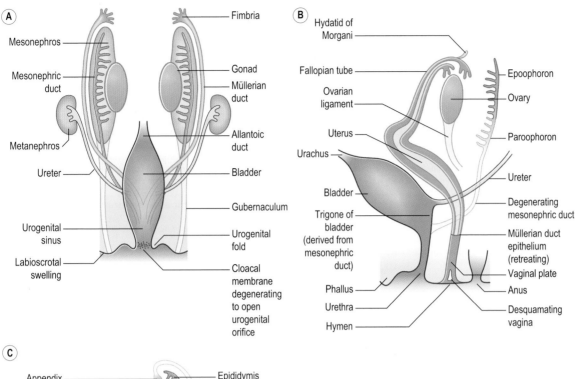

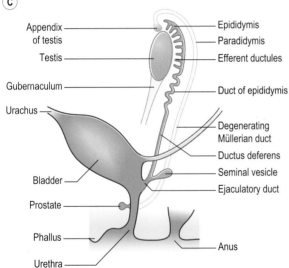

Fig. 10.50 **Sexual differentiation of the internal genitalia.**
(A) Primitive gonad at 7 weeks' gestation. (B, C) Differentiated
gonads (lateral view) at 12 weeks: (B) female; (C) male.

Clinical box 10.27   **Screening for foetal abnormalities**

During pregnancy various screening methods are used to
detect foetal abnormalities. These include ultrasound scans
to detect any gross abnormalities, and maternal blood tests.
One of the markers of foetal abnormality is α-fetoprotein
(**AFP**) which indicates the presence of a spinal tube defect. If
the maternal blood test indicates a high probability of a foetal
abnormality then amniocentesis may be performed. This is the
sampling of amniotic fluid surrounding the developing foetus,
by inserting a needle through the abdominal wall into the
uterus under ultrasound guidance. Foetal cells can be obtained
from the sample of amniotic fluid and these are screened
for the presence of abnormality. There is a significant risk
of miscarriage (unintentional termination of pregnancy) with
amniocentesis.

---

release of prostaglandins which act on the cervix, causing it
to become softer and thinner. This cervical 'ripening' is essential preparation for the cervix to dilate and allow the foetus
to pass through. The myometrial contractions stimulated by
oxytocin can then push the foetus through the cervix.

In many mammals the signal for parturition comes from
the foetal hypothalamic–pituitary–adrenal axis, but that is not
the case in humans. Corticotropin-releasing hormone (CRH)
does appear to have a role, however. This peptide hormone
is produced by the placenta in increasing concentrations
towards the end of pregnancy. It acts on the maternal and
foetal pituitary, increasing ACTH and so cortisol levels. In the
foetus this is important for lung maturation. In the uterus the
increased cortisol causes a further increase in CRH, which
stimulates prostaglandin synthesis.

Lactation

Breast development is stimulated during pregnancy by the actions of several hormones: progesterone, placental lactogen,
prolactin, insulin and cortisol (Fig. 10.53). Before parturition,
however, the high oestrogen levels effectively put a brake on
lactation. As soon as this brake is removed the breasts begin
to produce milk. The action of the baby suckling at the nipple
stimulates the release of two hormones: oxytocin from the

Clinical box 10.28 **Disorders of sexual differentiation: chromosomal abnormalities**

There are several disorders which are caused by abnormalities in the numbers of sex chromosomes. Two of these are relatively common. One copy of the X chromosome is essential for life, but the second sex chromosome may be missing, or there may be an additional copy of one of the sex chromosomes.

Klinefelter syndrome is the most common form of sex chromosome abnormality, affecting around one in a thousand men. It is classically associated with an additional copy of the X chromosome, so the karyotype is 47XXY. Boys with Klinefelter syndrome are obviously male and develop normally until puberty but then show symptoms of androgen insufficiency (Fig. 10.51): they don't undergo normal pubertal development, have symptoms of androgen insufficiency and are infertile. Men with Klinefelter syndrome are treated with androgens to stimulate development of secondary sex characteristics and to maintain musculoskeletal health.

Turner syndrome affects about one in 2500 women. Typically women with Turner syndrome have only one sex chromosome so the karyotype is 45X. These women often have a characteristic appearance (Fig. 10.52) and a range of associated health problems affecting the cardiovascular system, kidneys, thyroid etc. Women with Turner syndrome have undeveloped gonads called 'streak ovaries' and so have primary amenorrhoea and do not go through puberty. The treatment is with sex steroids to stimulate development of secondary sex characteristics and to maintain musculoskeletal health.

Other disorders of sex differentiation may be caused by defects in specific genes (Table 10.12). Earlier we saw how a defect in the androgen receptor gene can lead to a genetically male baby developing a female phenotype. This affects about 1 in 20 000 people who are genetically male.

Defects in the *SRY* gene can also result in genetically male babies developing a female appearance.

It is also the case that female babies exposed to high levels of androgens during foetal development may be born with a greatly enlarged clitoris and fused labia – 'ambiguous genitalia' – and may be assigned male gender.

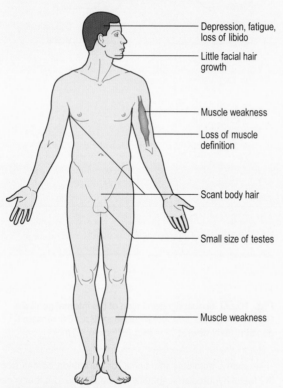

Depression, fatigue, loss of libido

Little facial hair growth

Muscle weakness

Loss of muscle definition

Scant body hair

Small size of testes

Muscle weakness

Fig. 10.51 **Features of androgen insufficiency as a result of hypogonadism.**

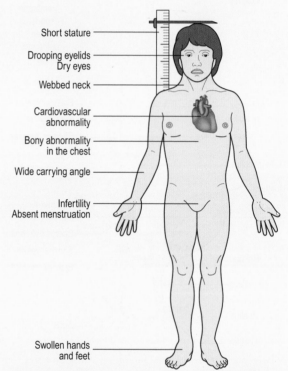

Short stature

Drooping eyelids
Dry eyes

Webbed neck

Cardiovascular abnormality

Bony abnormality in the chest

Wide carrying angle

Infertility
Absent menstruation

Swollen hands and feet

Fig. 10.52 **Features of Turner syndrome (karyotype 45X0).** In addition to the features shown, there is failure of normal pubertal development. The swelling of the hands and feet is due to lymphatic abnormalities.

Table 10.12 **Disorders of sexual differentiation**

Condition	Defect	Genotype	Phenotype
Turner syndrome	Lack of second sex chromosome	Female	Female
Klinefelter syndrome	Additional sex chromosome	Male	Male
Androgen receptor insensitivity	Mutation in the androgen receptor	Male	Variable, may be male or female
Congenital adrenal hyperplasia	Defect in adrenal cortisol biosynthesis	Male	Male
		Female	Ambiguous/male
5-α-Hydroxylase deficiency	Defect in enzyme converting testosterone to 5αDHT	Male	Variable, may be male or female
Kallman syndrome	Hypothalamic defect	Male	Male

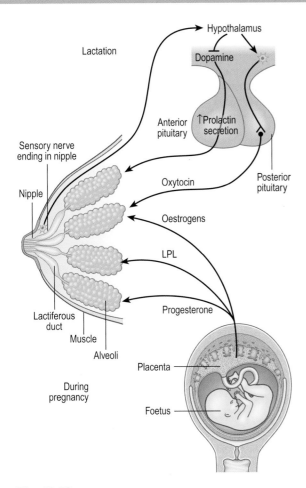

Fig. 10.53 Hormonal control of breast development during pregnancy and lactation. During pregnancy, hormones from the placenta, including human placental lactogen (hPL), progesterone and oestrogens, act on the breast and stimulate proliferation of the alveolar tissue in preparation for lactation. The oestrogens prevent lactation from occurring during pregnancy. After parturition, when the influence of the placenta is removed, suckling of the baby stimulates the release of prolactin from the anterior pituitary, thereby stimulating milk formation. Suckling also stimulates release of oxytocin from the posterior pituitary, causing contraction of the smooth muscle around the alveoli and expelling milk from the breast.

posterior pituitary and prolactin from the anterior pituitary. Prolactin stimulates lactogenesis, the formation of milk, while oxytocin causes contraction of the smooth muscle around the milk ducts, stimulating the 'let-down' reflex.

INFERTILITY (SUBFERTILITY)

In women, subfertility is often characterised by disorders of the menstrual cycle: absence of menstruation for three or more cycles is termed **amenorrhoea**. If this happens following the establishment of a normal cycle it is known as secondary amenorrhoea. If menarche is absent this is termed primary amenorrhoea and is usually investigated once a girl reaches the age of 16 years.

In men, subfertility is measured by semen quality. A normal sperm count is 20–40 million sperm per millilitre of semen. Subfertility is diagnosed with a sperm count of 15 million sperm per mL or lower, or when the sperm quality is poor; for example, if fewer than 50% of the sperm are motile or if there is a high percentage of abnormal sperm.

There are several causes of subfertility in men and women. In both genders these may be hypothalamic, pituitary or gonadal in origin: primary infertility (primary gonadal failure) is caused by a gonadal problem; secondary gonadal failure is caused by a pituitary defect; while tertiary gonadal failure is the result of a hypothalamic disorder.

Kallmann syndrome in men is an example of hypothalamic failure to produce GnRH. Women more commonly have hypothalamic GnRH failure in response to excessive dieting or exercise.

In some cases the gonadal failure may be secondary to a pituitary disorder, the commonest of which is a prolactinoma. Excessive prolactin secretion inhibits pulsatile GnRH secretion and leads to gonadal failure.

Primary hypogonadism in women may be due to a chromosomal disorder as in Turner syndrome. More common, however, are premature ovarian failure, also called premature menopause (defined as the cessation of menstruation before the age of 40), and polycystic ovarian syndrome (PCOS) (Clinical box 10.29).

Clinical box 10.29 Polycystic ovarian syndrome

This accounts for up to a quarter of cases of amenorrhoea. The ovaries develop a number of cysts which are 2–8 mm in diameter. The syndrome is associated with an increase in ovarian androgen production which causes acne, hirsutism and irregular monthly periods. Women with PCOS have a much higher incidence of type 2 diabetes than the general population. The degree of menstrual irregularity varies greatly between individuals with PCOS, and some women still ovulate, but most experience reduced fertility.

THE ENDOCRINOLOGY OF AGEING (INCLUDING MENOPAUSE)

Patterns of hormone secretion change as we get older. Growth hormone secretion declines with age, as does the adrenal androgen DHEA. There is an online market for hormone treatments to prevent ageing, as if taking GH or DHEA will somehow prevent the normal ageing process.

Perhaps the most significant endocrine ageing event, however, is the menopause. The menopause is the permanent cessation of menses as a result of loss of ovarian follicles. It requires an interval of 12 months since the last menses and so can only be classified retrospectively. Menopause usually occurs when a woman is 51 ±1 years of age, marking the end of her reproductive life just as menarche marks the start. Although the average life expectancy of women has increased significantly over the past 150 years, the average age of menopause has not changed at all. This means firstly that post-menopausal women were relatively less common 150 years ago, and now a woman can expect about 30 years of postmenopausal life. It is therefore important to understand the menopause and its consequences for women's health.

As the number of follicles in the ovaries declines, the plasma concentration of FSH increases. This is often used as a marker of the peri-menopausal period. As a woman approaches menopause, her monthly periods usually become more irregular and less frequent, and then cease completely.

The absence of responsive ovarian follicles means that oestrogen production falls and levels of FSH and LH remain very high, as there is no negative feedback inhibition. At the time of falling oestrogen levels many women experience a range of symptoms, including vasomotor symptoms such as hot flushes (called 'hot flashes' in the USA), night-time sweats, decreased libido and labile mood. Women's experience of menopausal symptoms is strongly culturally determined. In Western cultures around three-quarters of women report vasomotor symptoms, but this is much less common in other cultures. The longer term consequences of oestrogen deficiency include osteoporosis (see Ch. 9) and changes in the urinary and genital tracts, which may lead to vaginal prolapse and incontinence. Hormone replacement therapy (HRT) is used by many women to ameliorate the short term and longer term effects of menopause.

Introduction	493	The cardiac cycle	522
Clinical anatomy of the cardiovascular system	493	Cardiac output and heart failure	525
The heart	493	**Blood vessels**	**528**
The human circulation	497	The vessel wall	528
Embryology	**505**	Atherosclerosis	530
Development of the heart	506	Ischaemic heart disease	534
Development of the vasculature	508	Thromboembolism	539
Cellular structure and function of the heart	**510**	The microcirculation	541
		Mechanics of blood flow	546
Structure of heart muscle	510	**Systemic arterial blood pressure**	**554**
The contractile process	510	Regulation of arterial blood pressure	554
Electrical activation of the heart	512	Shock	556
		Hypertension	562

INTRODUCTION

The cardiovascular system is a network for blood distribution which functions to supply the cells of the body with oxygen and nutrients such as glucose and amino acids, to provide homeostatic control of acid–base balance, fluid balance and thermoregulation, and to transport hormones and immune cells to target tissues. It also transports CO_2 and other waste products of metabolism away from the tissues for excretion. The essential components of the cardiovascular system are the heart, blood vessels and blood. The lymphatic system also contributes to the cardiovascular system by returning blood plasma filtered from interstitial tissues as lymph to the circulation. Blood is discussed in detail in Chapter 12; this chapter will focus primarily on the heart and blood vessels.

CLINICAL ANATOMY OF THE CARDIOVASCULAR SYSTEM

The cardiovascular system consists of:

- The heart, which is the muscular pump that drives blood around the body
- Blood vessels, which are organised into two circuits which operate in series, the systemic circulation and the pulmonary circulation
- The blood and its constituents, the functions of which are discussed in detail in Chapter 12.

THE HEART

The heart is located in the middle mediastinum, between the lungs. It is protected by the sternum anteriorly, by the vertebral column posteriorly, and by the ribs. The heart's apex normally points leftwards; rarely (in about 1 in 12 000 people), it points to the right, a condition known as **dextrocardia**, which may be associated with other congenital abnormalities.

The adult heart weighs between 250 and 350 grams and is about the size of a fist. Its walls are composed of three layers of tissue (see Table 11.1):

- An outer layer of connective tissue known as the **epicardium** or **visceral pericardium** (see below).
- A middle layer known as the **myocardium**, which is composed of cardiac muscle and connective tissue. This is the contractile part of the heart.
- An inner layer, the **endocardium**, which is in contact with the blood, covers the heart valves and is continuous with the inner lining of the blood vessels, the vascular endothelium. It comprises a thin layer of connective tissue and endothelium.

The pericardium

The heart is covered by the **pericardium**. This is made up of three layers of connective tissue. The two layers closest to the heart are composed of a serous membrane which folds back on itself where the great vessels emerge from the heart. The inner-most layer is the visceral pericardium (or epicardium) and the second layer is called the parietal pericardium. The space enclosed between these two layers forms the pericardial cavity. This contains pericardial fluid which serves

Table 11.1	Tissue layers of the heart from the external surface of the heart working inwards
Fibrous pericardium	
Parietal pericardium	
Pericardial fluid (in **pericardial cavity**, between parietal and visceral pericardium)	
Visceral pericardium (epicardium)	
Cardiac muscle (myocardium)	
Connective tissue and endothelium (endocardium)	

as lubricant to allow the two layers to slide over each other as the heart contracts. The fibrous outer layer of the pericardium, the fibrous pericardium, anchors the heart in the mediastinum and protects the heart from trauma, the spread of infection from adjacent organs such as the lungs, and from over-expansion should intra-cardiac volume increase. The main pathology that affects the pericardium is called **pericarditis**, which is described in Clinical box 11.1.

The heart chambers

The heart consists of four chambers, two atria and two ventricles (Fig. 11.1). The atria are thin-walled structures which act as the initial collecting chambers for blood entering the heart. The right atrium forms part of the right heart border

Clinical box 11.1	Clinical features, causes and complications of pericarditis

Inflammation of the pericardium, or **pericarditis**, usually presents with sharp, pleuritic chest pain. The pain is classically exacerbated by lying flat and relieved by sitting forward. A pericardial friction rub may be heard and the electrocardiogram shows widespread 'saddle-shaped' ST elevation. The treatment is with non-steroidal anti-inflammatory agents.

There are many causes of pericarditis including:
- Idiopathic: the most common, where no identifiable cause is found
- Infective: viral (e.g. coxsackie virus, HIV, cytomegalovirus) or bacterial, including *Mycobacterium tuberculosis*
- Inflammatory: autoimmune conditions such as systemic lupus erythematosus
- Myocardial infarction: early, related to tissue necrosis, or occurring after 2–6 weeks due to an autoimmune phenomenon (Dressler syndrome)
- Postoperative: e.g. after coronary artery bypass graft (CABG)
- Metabolic: e.g. uraemia
- Malignancy
- Radiation
- Trauma: e.g. stab wound puncturing the pericardium
- Adverse effect of some drugs (e.g. warfarin, anti-tuberculosis medication).

Acute pericarditis usually resolves within 1–2 weeks but relapses may occur. The most common complication relates to the accumulation of fluid within the pericardial cavity called a pericardial effusion. The fibrous pericardium has a limited ability to stretch so large pericardial effusions or those which accumulate rapidly because an increase in the pressure in the pericardial cavity which restricts ventricular filling, lowers cardiac output, and causes shock. This condition is called **cardiac tamponade** and the pericardial fluid requires urgent needle aspiration or surgical drainage.

The second main complication of pericarditis is **constrictive pericarditis**. This occurs months to years after an episode of pericarditis (which may have been asymptomatic). Analogous to cardiac tamponade, the filling of the heart is restricted, in this case by a thickened, fibrotic, pericardium. Pericardectomy, surgical resection of the pericardium, may be required.

and receives the superior and inferior venae cavae while the left atrium lies posterior to the right atrium and receives the four pulmonary veins.

The ventricles have thick walls comprising mainly muscle and they make up the major bulk of the heart mass. The right ventricle lies anterior to the left ventricle and forms the mid-anterior surface of the heart. The left ventricle forms the posterolateral, lateral and anterolateral surface of the heart, and its apex. The left and right ventricles generate the force required to propel the blood round the systemic circulation and the pulmonary circulation, respectively, the left ventricle having a thicker myocardium because it is required to generate a much higher pressure than the right ventricle.

The apex of the heart

As the ventricles contract, they produce an impulse which can be palpated through the chest wall. The most inferior and lateral position at which the cardiac impulse can be palpated is called the **apex beat** (see Information box 11.1). The apex beat is best found by placing the right hand on the curve of the left lateral chest wall and drawing it medially. It is normally found in the fifth left intercostal space in the mid-clavicular line (Fig. 11.2). In males, this is inferior and medial to the nipple. Inferolateral displacement of the apex beat usually indicates left ventricular dilatation due, for example, to ischaemic heart disease, dilated cardiomyopathy, or a volume overloaded left ventricle due to aortic or mitral regurgitation.

The heart valves

There are four valves within the heart which, when functioning normally, ensure that the flow of blood through the heart is unidirectional. All of the valves have three cusps except the mitral valve which is a bicuspid valve. The valves, and the base of the aorta and pulmonary artery, are surrounded by four fibrous rings of dense collagenous connective tissue known as the **annulus fibrosus cordis**. These rings bolster the structure of the heart providing support to the heart valves; the muscle fibres of the atria and ventricles are attached to it as the fixed point about which muscular contraction takes place, and it provides electrical separation of the atria from the ventricles.

The **mitral valve** is located between the left atrium and the left ventricle and the **tricuspid valve** sits between the right atrium and the right ventricle (Figs 11.1B and 11.3A). Their positions denote these valves as the **atrioventricular (AV) valves**. The AV valves are attached to the **papillary muscles** on the inner wall of the ventricles via cord-like connective tissue and elastin tendons called **cordae tendineae**. The papillary muscles maintain closure of the AV valves and prevent regurgitation of blood back into the atria during ventricular contraction. When the ventricles relax and atrial pressures exceed ventricular pressures, the AV valves open allowing blood to flow from the atria into the ventricles.

The **aortic** and **pulmonary (semilunar) valves** sit between the left ventricular outflow tract and the aorta, and the right ventricular outflow tract and the pulmonary artery, respectively. When the ventricles contract and ventricular pressures exceed the pressures in the great arteries, the valve cusps open flat against the artery walls and blood flows out of the ventricles (Fig. 11.3B). Conversely, when the ventricles relax and the pressure in the great arteries exceeds that in the ventricles, the valve cusps come together in apposition and prevent the back flow of blood into the heart.

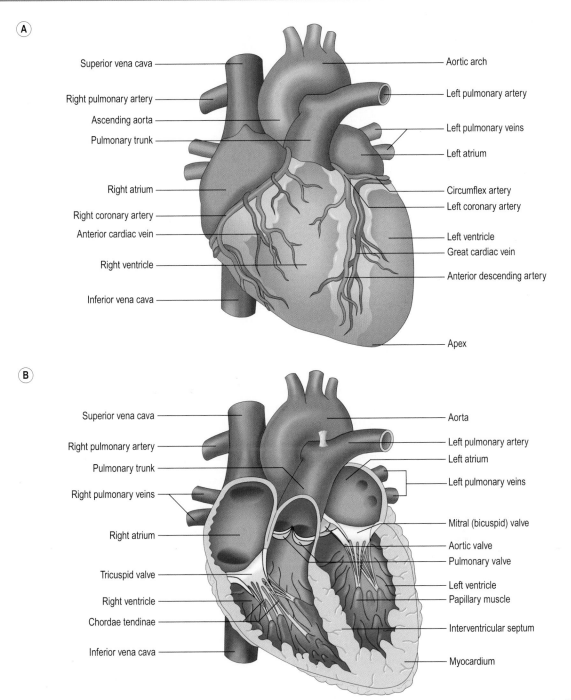

(A)

Superior vena cava

Right pulmonary artery

Ascending aorta

Pulmonary trunk

Right atrium

Right coronary artery

Anterior cardiac vein

Right ventricle

Inferior vena cava

Aortic arch

Left pulmonary artery

Left pulmonary veins

Left atrium

Circumflex artery

Left coronary artery

Left ventricle

Great cardiac vein

Anterior descending artery

Apex

(B)

Superior vena cava

Right pulmonary artery

Pulmonary trunk

Right pulmonary veins

Right atrium

Tricuspid valve

Right ventricle

Chordae tendinae

Inferior vena cava

Aorta

Left pulmonary artery

Left atrium

Left pulmonary veins

Mitral (bicuspid) valve

Aortic valve

Pulmonary valve

Left ventricle

Papillary muscle

Interventricular septum

Myocardium

Fig. 11.1 **The heart.** (A) Surface view showing major blood vessels leading into the heart and the coronary vessels. (B) Frontal section showing the heart chambers and valves.

Information box 11.1   **Character of the apex beat**

Historically, the character of the apex beat was attributed considerable diagnostic importance:

- A 'tapping' apex beat implies mitral stenosis, the tapping representing a palpable first heart sound
- A dynamic (or 'thrusting') apex beat is consistent with a volume loaded left ventricle due to severe aortic or mitral regurgitation
- A 'heaving' apex beat implies left ventricular hypertrophy due, for instance, to hypertension or aortic stenosis.

The ready availability of echocardiography, which provides accurate diagnostic information regarding valve disease and ventricular size and function, means that differentiating between these apex beat characters is now of limited clinical relevance.

Various pathologies can affect one or more of the heart valves resulting in restricted opening ('**stenosis**') or leakage of blood backwards ('**regurgitation**') through the valve. Valvular disease reduces the efficiency of the heart. The main causes and clinical consequences are described in Clinical box 11.2.

Heart sounds and murmurs

Auscultation of the heart through a stethoscope applied to the chest wall reveals distinct sounds that are related to specific events during the cardiac cycle. The dominant sounds in healthy adults are the **first and second heart sounds** which are produced by the closing of the AV and semilunar valves,

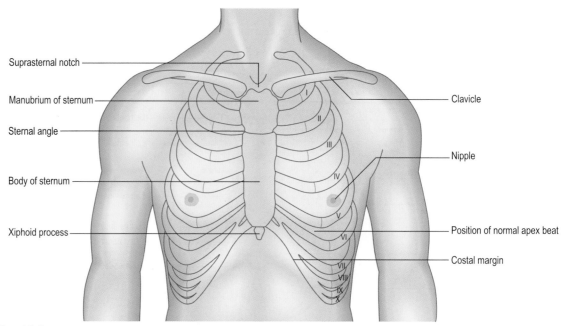

Fig. 11.2 **Surface anatomy of the chest (male).**

Clinical box 11.2   **Causes and clinical consequences of valvular heart disease**

Either a single valve or multiple valves may be affected in valvular heart disease. The most common congenital valve defect is a bicuspid aortic valve. This predisposes to aortic stenosis, which may present in childhood but more frequently presents in middle age. The abnormal flow patterns through the valve promote premature calcification, thickening and fusion of the valve cusps. Congenital valve abnormalities are often associated with other congenital defects. There is an increased incidence of bicuspid aortic valve in patients with coarctation, for example, and in tetralogy of Fallot, pulmonary stenosis (which may be at the infundibular level) occurs together with a ventricular septal defect and overriding of the aorta.

Degenerative valve disease, such as 'senile' calcific aortic stenosis, has overtaken rheumatic fever as the most common cause of valvular heart disease. Other infective causes of valve disease include endocarditis, HIV, and (rarely these days) syphilitic aortic valve disease. Systemic diseases, such as connective tissue disorders (e.g. systemic lupus erythematosus), the HLA-B27 spondarthopathies (e.g. ankylosing spondylitis), carcinoid syndrome, hypertension and aortic dissection can also cause valve defects.

Left-sided (i.e. mitral and aortic) valve disease is more common than right-sided (tricuspid and pulmonary) valve defects. Valvular stenosis or regurgitation results in turbulent blood flow which causes noises called murmurs which can be heard using a stethoscope (see Fig. 11.4).

The clinical consequences of valvular heart disease depend upon which valve is affected and upon the severity of the valve lesion. Stenosed valves cause a pressure load on the proximal chamber, which responds by hypertrophying, whereas regurgitant valves result in a volume load on the affected ventricle, which responds by dilating. If the valve lesion is severe enough, the end result of either pathophysiology is failure of the affected ventricle:

- **Aortic stenosis** causes a pressure load on the left ventricle while **aortic regurgitation** and **mitral regurgitation** cause a volume load on the left ventricle. They cause symptoms of left heart failure such as dyspnoea, orthopnoea and paroxysmal nocturnal dyspnoea. Pleural effusion may also develop.
- **Mitral stenosis** results in an elevated left atrial pressure which is the main cause of breathlessness. Chronic elevation of the left atrial pressure can cause pulmonary hypertension and right ventricular failure.
- Severe right-sided valve lesions cause right heart failure either through right ventricular volume overload (**pulmonary regurgitation**, **tricuspid regurgitation**), right ventricular pressure overload (**pulmonary stenosis**) or raised systemic venous pressure (**tricuspid stenosis**). Right heart failure is characterised by ankle swelling, fatigue and breathlessness with signs of raised jugular venous pressure, peripheral oedema, hepatomegaly and ascites.

---

respectively (Fig. 11.4A). These '**lubb**' and '**dub**' sounds mark the beginning and end of systole. The flow of blood through the heart and the opening of normal heart valves are usually silent. Added sounds occur due to the opening of abnormal valves. Turbulent blood flow produces sounds called **murmurs**. Murmurs may be physiological or 'innocent', or pathological. Innocent murmurs are usually ejection murmurs due to turbulent blood flow across normal semilunar valves; they are more common in the young, during pregnancy or fever, and in anaemic patients. Pathological murmurs are caused by valve disease (Fig. 11.4) or congenital heart defects (see Embryology, below). Sounds related to particular valves are heard best at different sites on the chest wall which are given the names of the relevant valve (Fig. 11.5). These locations

do not correspond to the positions of the valves but rather to where the sounds are transmitted most distinctly. Because of the way that the pulmonary artery and aorta wrap around each other as they leave the heart the aortic area is found not on the left, but over the right 2nd intercostal space with the pulmonary area over the left 2nd intercostal space. The tricuspid area is located over the 4th intercostal space at the left sternal border and the mitral area is at the apex of the heart.

The type and location of murmurs and the presence of added sounds provides information about the underlying pathology. Clinical box 11.3 describes the heart sounds and the most common added sounds while Clinical box 11.4 describes the most common murmurs.

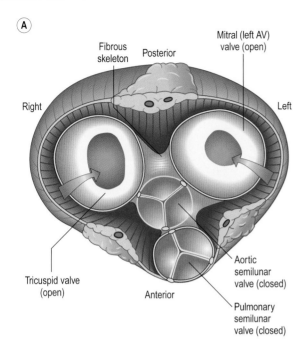

(A)

Mitral (left AV) valve (open)

Fibrous skeleton

Posterior

Right

Left

Tricuspid valve (open)

Anterior

Aortic semilunar valve (closed)

Pulmonary semilunar valve (closed)

(B)

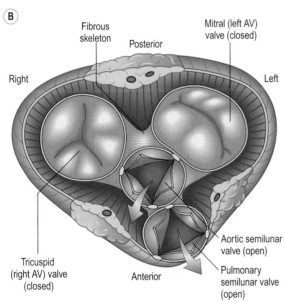

Fibrous skeleton

Posterior

Mitral (left AV) valve (closed)

Right

Left

Tricuspid (right AV) valve (closed)

Anterior

Aortic semilunar valve (open)

Pulmonary semilunar valve (open)

Fig. 11.3 **Transverse section of the heart showing the atrioventricular (AV) (mitral and tricuspid) and semilunar (aortic and pulmonary) valves.** Superior view with the atria and vessels removed. *Arrows* indicate direction of blood flow. (A) When the heart is filling with blood the AV valves are open and the semilunar valves are closed. (B) When blood is leaving the heart the semilunar valves are open and the AV valves are closed.

THE HUMAN CIRCULATION

The adult circulation comprises two vascular networks, a **pulmonary circulation**, which carries deoxygenated blood to the lungs to be oxygenated, and a **systemic circulation**, which delivers oxygenated blood to the tissues and organs (Fig. 11.6). The heart is the pump that drives the blood through the two circulations.

(A) Heart sounds

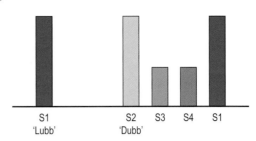

S1 'Lubb'   S2 'Dubb'   S3   S4   S1

(B) Aortic or pulmonary stenosis

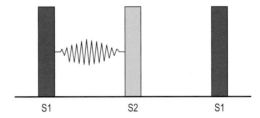

S1   S2   S1

(C) Aortic or pulmonary regurgitation

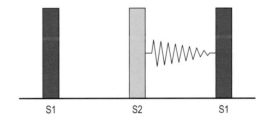

S1   S2   S1

(D) Mitral or tricuspid stenosis

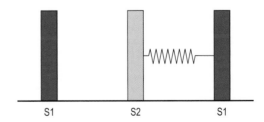

S1   S2   S1

(E) Mitral or tricuspid regurgitation or ventricular septal defect

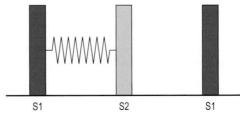

S1   S2   S1

Fig. 11.4 **Heart sounds and murmurs.** (A) The heart sounds. (B) Ejection systolic murmur. (C) Early diastolic murmur. (D) Mid-diastolic murmur. (E) Pan-systolic murmur.

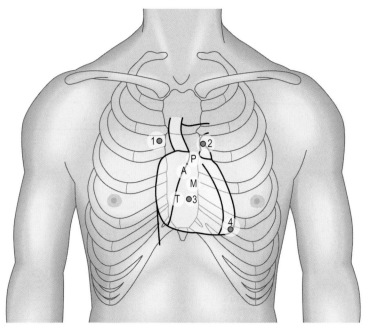

Fig. 11.5 **Surface positions and auscultatory areas for the four heart valves.** The letters A (aortic), P (pulmonary), T (tricuspid) and M (mitral) indicate the surface positions of the heart valves. Sounds arising from the four heart valves are usually heard best at the areas marked 1 (aortic), 2 (pulmonary), 3 (tricuspid) and 4 (mitral).

Clinical box 11.3 | **Heart sounds and added sounds**
(Fig. 11.4A)

- **The first heart sound (S1)** is generated by the closure of the AV valves. The sound is best heard near the apex of the heart.
- **The second heart sound (S2)** is produced by the closure of the semilunar valves. It is best heard towards the base of the heart. Because right ventricular ejection takes longer than left ventricular ejection, closure of the pulmonary valve usually occurs fractionally later than closure of the aortic valve. During inspiration, when increased venous return further prolongs right ventricular ejection, the aortic (A2) and pulmonary (P2) components of the second heart sound may be audible as two separate sounds. This is called **physiological splitting** of the second heart sound. Aortic stenosis, which delays emptying of the left ventricle and can produce a single component S2 or reversed splitting of S2. **Fixed splitting** of S2 is characteristic of an atrial septal defect.
- A **third heart sound (S3)** occurs in early diastole at the end of rapid ventricular filling, soon after the opening of the AV valves. It is best heard at the apex of the heart. It is a normal finding in children and young adults but it can indicate heart failure in older subjects.
- A **fourth heart sound (S4)** occurs in late diastole and is due to the rapid ventricular filling caused by atrial systole. It is sometimes found in healthy elderly subjects, but in younger people it usually indicates the presence of a non-compliant ventricle due to hypertensive heart disease, aortic stenosis, or hypertrophic cardiomyopathy.
- An **opening snap** occurs in early diastole in patients with mitral stenosis. It is a high pitched sound heard at the cardiac apex which reflects forced opening of the thickened mitral valve leaflets due to raised left atrial pressure.
- An **ejection click** occurs with valve opening in early systole in patients with a stenotic but pliable aortic valve.
- A **systolic click** occurs in mid systole in some patients with mitral valve prolapse. It is thought to be due to the abrupt halting of the prolapsing leaflet.

Clinical box 11.4 | **Murmurs in valvular heart disease**
(Fig. 11.4B–E)

There are two main types of valvular heart disease:
- **Stenosis**, in which the valve opening is restricted, producing an obstruction to blood flow
- **Incompetence or regurgitation**, in which the valve does not close properly and blood leaks backwards through the valve.
  The resulting murmur depends upon the timing within the cardiac cycle of forward flow through the stenotic valve or backward flow through the regurgitant valve:
- **Aortic stenosis**: turbulent blood flow occurs during the ventricular ejection (systolic) phase as blood passes through the restricted valve. The murmur is therefore called an **ejection systolic murmur**, which occurs between S1 and S2. Maximal flow, and therefore the peak intensity of the murmur, occurs in mid systole (Fig. 11.4B). It is best heard in the aortic area or at the left sternal edge and it radiates to the carotid arteries.
- **Aortic regurgitation**: blood flows backwards through the aortic valve immediately after its closure. The murmur is therefore an **early diastolic murmur**. It is a high pitched noise which is heard best at the left sternal border during held expiration.
- **Mitral stenosis**: produces **a mid-diastolic murmur**, the turbulent flow arising as blood flows forward through the restricted mitral valve. In sinus rhythm, pre-systolic accentuation of the murmur may be noticed during atrial systole. The murmur is low pitched and heard best at the apex with the patient leaning on their left side.
- **Mitral regurgitation**: the back flow of blood into the left atrium during ventricular systole produces a long murmur that lasts throughout systole, called a **pan-systolic murmur** (Fig. 11.4C). It is loudest at the apex and radiates to the axilla.
  Right-sided valve pathology produces the same type of murmur as the equivalent left-sided lesion but the location of the murmur is different. Pulmonary stenosis produces an ejection systolic murmur and pulmonary regurgitation produces an early diastolic murmur, both heard best in the pulmonary area. Tricuspid stenosis causes a mid-diastolic murmur and tricuspid regurgitation causes a pan-systolic murmur at the left sternal edge.

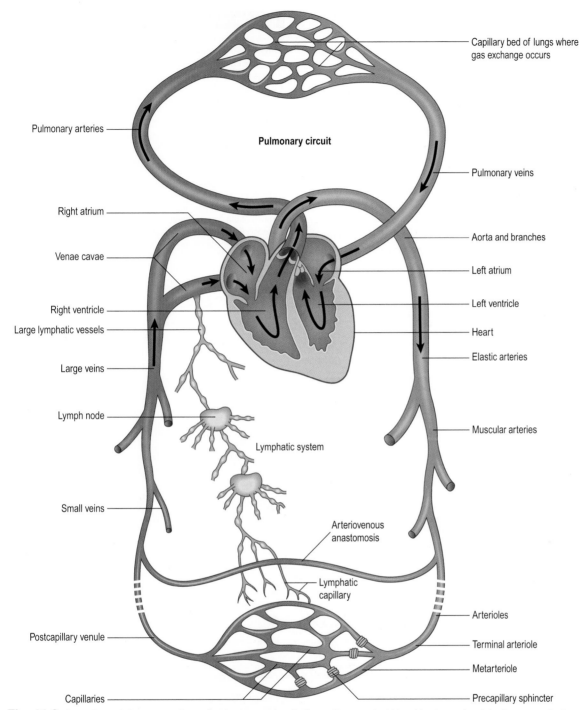

Fig. 11.6 **Overview of the systemic and pulmonary circulations.** Oxygenated blood is shown in *pink*, deoxygenated blood in *blue*, and the lymphatic system is *green*.

The pulmonary circulation

Oxygen-depleted blood is transported from the tissues to the right atrium via the superior and inferior venae cavae, before flowing through the tricuspid valve into the right ventricle. The right ventricle then pumps the blood via the pulmonary trunk into the right and left pulmonary arteries, which divide into the pulmonary lobar arteries to supply the lungs. A network of pulmonary capillaries facilitates the diffusion of oxygen from the alveoli into the blood and of carbon dioxide from the blood into the alveoli. Chapter 13 (The respiratory system) describes the process of gaseous exchange in detail. Oxygenated blood is drained by pulmonary capillaries into four pulmonary veins that transport blood to the left atrium.

Reduced tissue oxygen concentration (hypoxia) generally leads to vasodilatation in response to tissue need for O_2, a form of **metabolic hyperaemia** (action or functional hyperaemia). Pulmonary arterioles, however, constrict in response to hypoxia, reducing blood flow to poorly ventilated lung tissue. Well ventilated alveoli are perfused better, which facilitates O_2 uptake into the blood (see Ch. 13). The regulation of blood flow in capillary beds is discussed in detail later. The pulmonary capillary bed has a lower resistance to blood flow than systemic capillary beds, so it functions at lower pressures (about 10 mmHg). The vasoconstrictor response in the lungs to chronic hypoxia can cause pulmonary hypertension and right heart failure (Information box 11.2).

The systemic circulation

The systemic circulation is more complex than the pulmonary circulation, supplying different parts of the body in a number of regional circuits (Fig. 11.7). It carries oxygenated blood away from the heart in the arterial system, and returns de-oxygenated blood to the heart via the venous system.

The arterial system

The **ascending aorta** carries oxygenated blood away from the left ventricle, and almost immediately gives rise to the left and right **coronary arteries** (see Regional circulations, below). The ascending aorta then curves upwards and back-wards as the **arch of the aorta** or **aortic arch** (Fig. 11.8A),

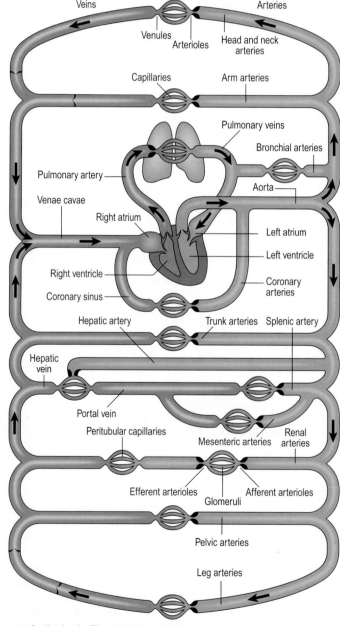

Fig. 11.7 **Circulatory routes in the body.** The diameter of the arterioles at the beginning of the capillary bed controls blood flow through the capillaries, and hence regulates blood flow. Vessels carrying oxygenated blood *pink*, vessels carrying deoxygenated blood *blue*.

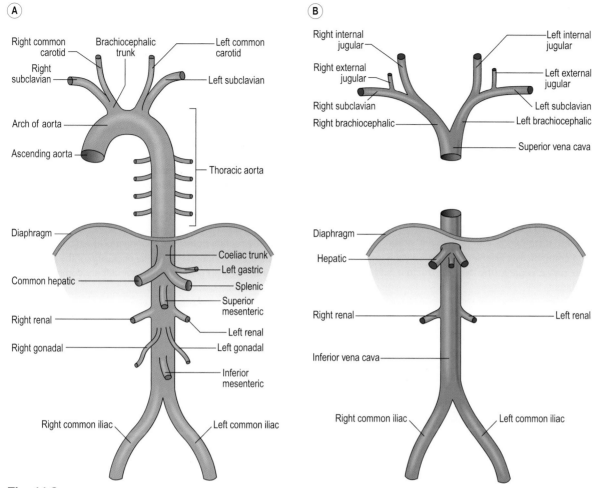

Fig. 11.8 (A) Major branches of the aorta. (B) Major tributaries of the superior and inferior venae cavae.

before turning downwards as the **thoracic** (or **descending**) **aorta** from the level of T4. Below the diaphragm (at T12), the thoracic aorta becomes the **abdominal aorta,** which bifurcates at about the level of L4 into the left and right **common iliac arteries**.

Aortic arch

Three main branches from the aortic arch supply blood to the head and neck, including the brain, upper limbs and part of the thoracic wall. The brachiocephalic artery divides into the right subclavian artery and the right common carotid artery, which supply the right arm and the right side of the head and neck, respectively. The left common carotid artery supplies the left side of the head and neck, and the left subclavian artery supplies the left arm. Each subclavian artery gives rise to an internal mammary artery which runs downwards behind the ribs and supplies blood to the anterior thoracic wall. Information box 11.3 describes a useful clinical application for these arteries.

Thoracic aorta

The thoracic aorta occupies the posterior mediastinum, beginning to the left of the vertebral column, but becoming more central as it descends, until it is just in front of the thoracic vertebrae as it passes through the diaphragm to become the abdominal aorta. Small, paired arterial branches supply the bronchi, pericardium, mediastinum, oesophagus, and upper surface of the diaphragm. Pairs of intercostal arteries branch out from the posterior aspect of the thoracic aorta to supply the intercostal muscles.

Information box 11.3	Use of internal mammary artery for coronary artery bypass graft surgery

The internal mammary arteries provide excellent natural conduits for the cardiac surgeon to use during coronary artery bypass graft surgery. One or both arteries are mobilised, their side branches are tied off to ensure maximal blood flow down the main artery to the heart, before the lower end is anastomosed to one of the native coronary arteries beyond its diseased segment. Most commonly, the left internal mammary artery is used as a graft to the left anterior descending artery. Internal mammary artery grafts have been shown to have much higher patency rates than venous bypass grafts at 5 and 10 years post-surgery, presumably because they are naturally better equipped than veins to deal with the much higher pressures in the arterial system compared with the venous system.

Abdominal aorta

The abdominal aorta carries oxygenated blood to the abdominal organs (Fig. 11.8A). The paired phrenic arteries supply the inferior surface of the diaphragm. The coeliac artery then emerges and divides into:

- The common hepatic artery, which supplies part of the liver and gives rise to the right gastric artery (gastro-epiploic artery) near the pylorus, supplying the pyloric part of the stomach and gives off branches to the lower oesophagus and duodenum
- The splenic artery which supplies the spleen

■ The left gastric artery which supplies the superior part of the lesser curvature of the stomach, with branches to the lower oesophagus. Branches anastomose with the right gastric artery.

The superior mesenteric artery emerges from the anterior surface of the abdominal aorta to supply the lower part of the duodenum, the small intestine, the large bowel to the splenic flexure and the pancreas. The next branches are the paired renal arteries that supply the kidneys, and the gonadal arteries. The inferior mesenteric artery arises from the anterior surface of the abdominal aorta to supply the large bowel from the splenic flexure to the upper part of the rectum.

Common iliac arteries

At its distal end, the abdominal aorta bifurcates into the common iliac arteries which supply the lower limbs and the pelvic organs: the bladder, rectum and reproductive organs.

Peripheral arterial pulses

When blood is ejected from the left ventricle it produces pulsations in the arterial circulation that can be palpated at various points on the body surface (Fig. 11.9). Examination of these pulses can provide information about the heart rhythm and stroke volume. In patients with aortic valve disease, the pulse character can indicate the severity of the valve lesion. Reduced or absent arterial pulses usually indicates atherosclerotic arterial disease proximal to the assessed pulse. The most commonly examined arterial pulses are:

■ The **radial pulse**: its ready accessibility in the wrist means that it is the pulse which is used routinely to assess the heart rate and rhythm. A 'collapsing' or 'water hammer' radial pulse indicates a wide pulse pressure which often accompanies severe aortic regurgitation.

■ The **brachial pulse**: the sounds produced by turbulent blood flow induced by partial occlusion of the brachial artery by a sphygmomanometer cuff are commonly used to measure blood pressure.

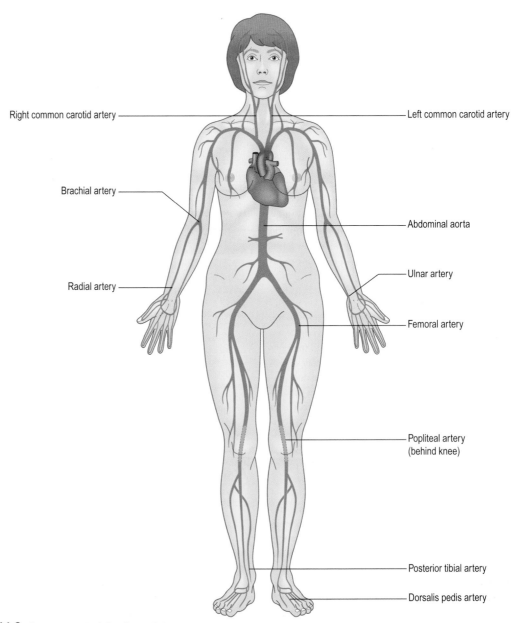

Right common carotid artery

Brachial artery

Radial artery

Left common carotid artery

Abdominal aorta

Ulnar artery

Femoral artery

Popliteal artery (behind knee)

Posterior tibial artery

Dorsalis pedis artery

Fig. 11.9 **Common arterial pulse points.**

- The **carotid pulse**: the 'slow rising' pulse of severe aortic stenosis is assessed by palpating the carotid artery.
- The **femoral, popliteal, posterior tibial and dorsalis pedis pulses**: these pulses are palpated in order to assess blood flow to the lower limbs, which may be impaired due to atherosclerosis and/or thrombosis.

The venous system

Most veins carry deoxygenated blood away from tissues and organs towards the heart. The exceptions are the pulmonary veins (which carry oxygenated blood from the lungs to the left atrium), the umbilical vein (which carries oxygenated blood in the umbilical cord from mother to foetus; see Embryology, below), and the hepatic portal vein (see Regional circulations, below).

The main vein draining blood from an organ often runs alongside the main artery that supplies oxygenated blood to the organ, and shares the name. The main veins in the body are illustrated in Figure 11.8B. Venous return to the heart is mainly through the superior vena cava, the inferior vena cava and the coronary sinus, all of which drain into the right atrium:

- **Superior vena cava**: this drains deoxygenated blood from the upper body. The subclavian arteries drain the upper limbs. The external jugular veins drain the scalp and the deep parts of the face, and drain into the subclavian veins. The internal jugular veins drain the brain, superficial part of the face and the neck. The subclavian veins and the internal jugular veins merge to form the brachiocephalic veins. The two brachiocephalic veins then join to form the superior vena cava. The ayzgos vein collects deoxygenated blood from much of thorax via the intercostal veins and it also empties into the superior vena cava.
- **Inferior vena cava**: this drains deoxygenated blood from parts of the body supplied by the abdominal aorta. It is formed at its inferior end by the confluence of the common iliac veins, which drain the lower limbs and pelvic organs. The inferior vena cava receives the renal veins and the hepatic veins before emptying into the right atrium.
- **Coronary sinus**: this drains deoxygenated blood from the heart. The major veins of the heart coalesce to form the coronary sinus on the posterior aspect of the heart. It drains directly into the right atrium close to the tricuspid valve annulus.

Jugular venous pulse

The internal jugular veins drain into the right atrium via the brachiocephalic veins and the superior vena cava (see Fig. 11.8B). These veins are free of valves so venous pulsations produced by changes in right atrial pressure during the cardiac cycle are transmitted unimpeded to the internal jugular veins. This **jugular venous pulse** is assessed with the patient reclining at 45°. The height of the venous pressure wave in the internal jugular veins measured in centimetres vertically from the sternal angle is the **jugular venous pressure** (JVP). The JVP is used clinically to assess right atrial pressure. The JVP is normally < 4 cm above the sternal angle. If the JVP is low due, for example, to dehydration or acute haemorrhage, the jugular venous pulse can be seen only if the person is at a lower reclining angle. Conversely, if the pressure in the right atrium is very high due, for example, to heart failure, visualisation of the top of the waveform may require the patient to be sitting upright.

Table 11.2	Blood flow (mL/min) to different organs at rest and during exercise		
	At rest	Strenuous exercise	Change
Brain	750	750	None
Heart	250	750	3-fold increase
Muscle	1250	12 500	10-fold increase
Skin	500	2000	4-fold increase
Kidney	1100	550	Halved
Abdominal organs	1400	700	Halved
Other	600	400	Reduced by one-third
Total	5850	17 650	3-fold increase

Regional circulations

There is considerable variation in the blood flow to different organs and tissues depending on their physiological function and metabolic requirements (Table 11.2). The presence of separate regional circuits allows independent regulation of blood flow to these organs and tissues, with the brain and heart taking priority over other organs. Some specialised systemic circulations are described here.

The coronary circulation

The coronary circulation consists of three main arteries which supply the heart muscle with oxygenated blood and a network of veins which run adjacent to the main arteries and drain deoxygenated blood to the right atrium via the coronary sinus (see Fig. 11.1A). The **right coronary artery** arises in the right aortic sinus before coursing down the right atrioventricular groove. It provides the main arterial supply to the right ventricle, and also supplies blood to part of the interventricular septum, and to both atria. The **left coronary artery** arises in the left aortic sinus as the **left main stem** before it divides into two branches, the **circumflex artery**, which passes down the back of the heart in the left atrioventricular groove, and the **anterior descending** (or **anterior interventricular**) **artery**, which runs down the anterior interventricular groove. They supply both atria, the rest of the interventricular septum and most of the left ventricle, the circumflex artery supplying the posterior and posterolateral aspects of the left ventricle and the anterior descending artery supplying the anterior wall, anterolateral wall and apex. The left and right coronary arteries and their main branches are referred to as epicardial arteries because they lie on the outer (epicardial) surface of the heart.

Coronary artery anatomy varies between individuals. The **dominant coronary artery** is the one which gives rise to the **posterior descending branch**, which supplies blood to the inferior wall of the left ventricle – in about 90% of individuals the right coronary artery is dominant and in about 10% of people the circumflex artery is the dominant vessel. There are extensive anastomoses between the left and right coronary arterial circulations which, in the healthy state, are functionally closed. However, should one of the major arteries become blocked, these anastomoses may open to become functionally useful **collaterals** which allow blood to flow from the open artery to the blocked one. The maintenance of blood flow through collaterals may limit the size of myocardial infarction or, in some cases, prevent infarction altogether.

Coronary blood flow

The oxygen requirement of the heart (and therefore its blood flow) varies according to the rate and force of cardiomyocyte contraction (see Cellular structure and function of the heart), which in turn responds to the metabolic requirements of the body. The important features of coronary blood flow include:

- Its coupling to the heart's demand for oxygen. In the normal heart, coronary blood flow increases with increased myocardial activity and O_2 consumption through metabolic (active or functional) hyperaemia. Adenosine, a product of ATP metabolism, is thought to be the main metabolic vasodilator.
- Its regulation through adrenoceptor-mediated vasoconstriction and vasodilatation. Basal tone in the arterioles is maintained by sympathetic vasoconstrictor nerves, which release norepinephrine (noradrenaline) onto α-adrenoceptors. During exercise, however, circulating levels of epinephrine (adrenaline) increase, which acts preferentially on $β_2$-adrenoceptors to produce vasodilation that reinforces the metabolic vasodilatation.
- Its pulsatile pattern, with the majority of flow occurring during diastole (Fig. 11.10). This relates to the compression of the small branches of the coronary arteries by ventricular contraction and the release of this compression during diastole.
- Its susceptibility to disruption through the development of coronary artery atherosclerosis (see Ischaemic heart disease, below).

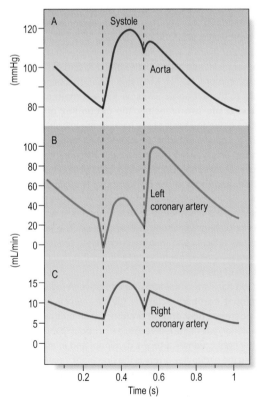

Fig. 11.10 **Blood flow in the coronary arteries during the cardiac cycle.** (A) Pressure in the aorta; (B,C) flow in the coronary arteries.

The cerebral circulation

The brain is an organ with a high metabolic rate as it is active all the time, even during sleep. Despite accounting for only 2% of total body weight, the brain receives about 15% of resting cardiac output, and accounts for 20% of total oxygen consumption (considerably more than the heart). The grey matter is very sensitive to hypoxia and, at normal body temperatures, damage can occur within 5 minutes of an interruption to its oxygen supply. The cerebral circulation is discussed in detail in Chapter 8. The special features of the cerebral circulation include:

- A remarkably constant cerebral blood flow over a wide range of mean arterial pressures (60–160 mmHg). This is achieved through the brain's capacity to regulate its own blood supply through **autoregulation** with very little control by extrinsic nervous input. Several theories have been proposed to explain the autoregulation of cerebral blood flow:
  - Humeral theory: the waste products of metabolism regulate cerebral blood flow. Increased pCO_2 (hypercapnia) causes cerebral vasodilation, and hypocapnia leads to vasoconstriction. The effect of increased pCO_2 decreases with age. The effect of O_2 is less marked, low pO_2 producing modest vasodilatation.
  - Myogenic theory: cerebral blood flow is regulated by the degree of stretch in the walls of the cerebral arteries (see below).
  - Neurogenic theory: cerebral arterioles respond to perivascular nerve stimulation; this effect is thought to be small.
  - Increased regional cerebral blood flow in relation to increased metabolic activity. For example, blood flow to motor and sensory regions of the brain increases with exercise.
  - Its reliance on end arteries (an end artery provides the sole blood supply to a segment of tissue) to provide the arterial supply to the brain. While the surface pial arteries form a collateral network (see Ch. 8) so that occlusion of one vessel does not necessarily interrupt blood flow, the deep penetrating and parenchymal arterioles are end arteries so that the occlusion of one arteriole leads to interruption of blood flow to the segment of brain that it supplies, causing infarction of the supplied tissue.
  - Intracranial blood vessels lined by endothelium which has tight intracellular junctions that join the inner vascular surface into a membranous sheet to form the **blood–brain barrier**. This barrier has a protective function, tightly regulating the exchange of nutrients, lipid soluble small molecules and water, while preventing the transport of toxins, drugs and large molecules. The blood–brain barrier may be breached in patients with inflammatory processes, infection, cerebral neoplasms and cerebral infarction (see Ch. 8).

The hepatic circulation

The liver receives arterial blood from the hepatic artery but the greater proportion (approximately 70%) of its blood supply comes through the **hepatic portal system**. This system comprises the veins which drain blood from the small bowel, from where nutrients (and toxins) are absorbed, before being transported to the liver in the hepatic portal vein. This supply to the liver is therefore in series (rather than in parallel) with the supply to the digestive tract, defining it as a 'portal system'. The nutrients absorbed from the gut are metabolised in the liver before being transported to the heart via the hepatic veins and inferior cava, and then on to the rest of the body. The liver also plays an important role in the removal of toxins which are absorbed from the gastrointestinal tract. The portal system ensures that venous blood from the gastrointestinal tract is delivered directly to the liver, where toxins are metabolised without prior circulation to the rest of the body, so protecting against their entry into the systemic circulation (see also Ch.15).

The skeletal muscle circulation

The metabolic requirements of skeletal muscle vary enormously, increasing dramatically during exercise, and blood flow increases in order to meet these demands (Table 11.2). The functional characteristics of skeletal muscle are discussed in Chapter 9. The main features of skeletal muscle blood flow are summarised below:

- At rest, not all skeletal muscle capillaries are perfused, but when oxygen requirements increase, the number of perfused capillaries increases. This is known as **capillary** or **vascular recruitment**.
- Skeletal muscle blood flow can be increased 20–50 fold (from 1–4 mL/min/100 g to 50–100 mL/min/100 g) during exercise compared with rest.
- Perfusion varies between different muscle types; muscles that perform rhythmic, coordinated contraction, containing predominantly phasic, white, fast twitch muscle fibres increase their flow rates during exercise to a much larger extent than the muscle groups which maintain posture and comprise mostly tonic, red muscle fibres.
- Skeletal muscle blood flow is regulated by local tissue and endothelial factors, and by sympathetic innervation (see Ch. 4, The autonomic nervous system). Local factors which are produced as a consequence of tissue hypoxia, including K^+, CO_2, H^+ (from lactic acid) and adenosine, increase blood flow through metabolic hyperaemia. Sympathetic stimulation produces vasoconstriction. The local factors override sympathetic effects during exercise.

The cutaneous circulation

The skin is the largest organ in the body, accounting for about 16% of total body weight. It forms a protective outer covering for the body which is responsible for sensory input and vitamin D synthesis. It also performs a key role in **thermoregulation** (see Ch. 1, Homeostasis). The cutaneous circulation comprises two important vascular structures (Fig. 11.11):

- **Capillary loops**, which extend into the dermal papillae. The tone in their supplying arterioles is responsible for autoregulation and reactive hyperaemia.
- An extensive **venous plexus** comprising wide vessels which run beneath the dermal papillae. The venous plexus receives blood through direct vascular communications with the arterial circulation called **arteriovenous anastomoses** (**AVAs**). The tone in the AVAs is under the control of the sympathetic nervous system with little influence from local metabolic factors. These vessels are responsible for thermoregulation and are most prevalent in the skin of the hands, feet and face.

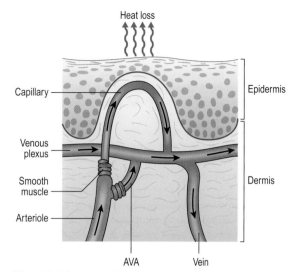

Fig. 11.11   The cutaneous circulation. Blood can flow either through the capillary loops or via the arteriovenous anastomoses (AVAs) into the venous plexus. The diameter of the AVAs is controlled by sympathetic vasomotor discharge.

Heat loss through the skin is by radiation, convection, conduction and evaporation. Effective thermoregulation by the skin is dependent upon its ability to achieve large variations in rates of blood flow, the greater the flow, the greater the potential for heat loss, and vice versa. Features of the cutaneous circulation which facilitate thermoregulation include:

- A dual control system for the rate of cutaneous blood flow which is responsive to metabolic activity and ambient temperature.
- Blood flow at neutral temperatures (10–12 mL/min per 100 g tissue) which exceeds the low metabolic requirements of the skin by 10 to 20 times. This means that blood flow can be reduced without compromising organ function.
- The ability to achieve large increases in flow rates (up to 200 mL/min per 100 g tissue) through the venous plexi when the AVAs are open.

Core temperature is monitored by receptors in the hypothalamus. At normal body temperatures, sympathetic activity keeps the AVAs closed. In response to high ambient temperatures, sympathetic discharge is reduced which relaxes the vascular smooth muscle in the AVAs. This increases blood flow in the venous plexi and promotes heat loss through the skin. In the cold, sympathetic discharge is increased which constricts the AVAs and reduces cutaneous blood flow and heat loss through the skin.

EMBRYOLOGY

The human heart begins as a tube developed from embryonic mesenchymal germ cells that differentiate into:

- Mesothelium, which forms the outer covering of the heart, the pericardium
- Endothelium, which becomes the inner lining of the heart, the endocardium, the blood vessels and lymphatics
- Myocardium, which forms the heart muscle.

At about 17 days after fertilisation, mesenchymal angiogenic cell clusters form on either side of the embryo. These cell clusters join up to form endothelial tubes. The tubes start to fold, and begin to fuse, completing the fusion by about 22 days after fertilisation. The inner layer of the fused tube develops into the endocardium and the outer layer into the myocardium. The embryonic heart starts beating at about 23 days post conception.

Development of the blood vessels and blood, **angiogenesis**, begins at about 3 weeks' gestation. Haemangioblasts differentiate from the embryonic and extra-embryonic mesoderm to form clusters, or **blood islands**. The blood islands extend and fuse, forming two populations of cells, the **angioblasts** which grow into networks of vascular tubes (blood vessels) and **haemopoietic stem cells** which migrate to the haemopoietic tissues, predominantly the bone marrow, liver and spleen. Blood develops within the blood vessels from about 5 weeks. The vascular tubes also grow towards the heart, completing the foetal vascular system.

DEVELOPMENT OF THE HEART

The embryonic heart tube enlarges, continues to fold, and develops bulges which become the future heart chambers (Fig. 11.12A). As the tube folds, it adopts an S-shape, bringing the atria above the ventricles (Fig. 11.12B):

- **Sinus venosus**: precedes the primitive atrium and is present only in the human embryonic heart. Part of it forms the coronary sinus, the vein that collects deoxygenated blood from the myocardium before draining into the right atrium, and part of it becomes incorporated into the adult right atrial wall. The sinus venosus also forms the sinoatrial node.

- **Primitive atrium**: develops into the adult atria.
- **Primitive ventricle**: separated from the primitive atrium by the atrioventricular canal; gives rise to part of the left ventricle.
- **Bulbus cordis** and **truncus arteriosus**: as the heart tube folds into its S-shape (Fig. 11.12B), the bulbus cordis migrates to lie in front (ventral) of the primitive ventricle with which it fuses to form the future ventricles. The truncus arteriosus forms the ascending aorta and the pulmonary trunk.

Clinical box 11.5 describes some of the abnormalities that arise through defective cardiac development. Information box 11.4 summarises some of the complications that may occur as a result of congenital heart defects. Despite these potential complications, recent years have seen a considerable improvement in the prognosis of patients with congenital heart disease. This has been realised by more accurate diagnosis, facilitated by better echocardiographic resolution, which can now often be made in utero. New diagnostic techniques such as magnetic resonance imaging (MRI) have proved helpful in complex cases. Early definitive surgical repair has become the treatment of choice for many defects and surgical techniques continue to evolve.

The chambers of the heart

The chambers are formed during the fourth and fifth weeks after conception. Their formation is determined by the direction of blood flow once the embryonic heart starts beating. The **endocardial cushions** (also known as the **atrioventricular cushions**) are a subset of cells that develop in the **atrioventricular canal**, separating the atria from the ventricles (see Fig. 11.12A). The cushions initially function as a sort of

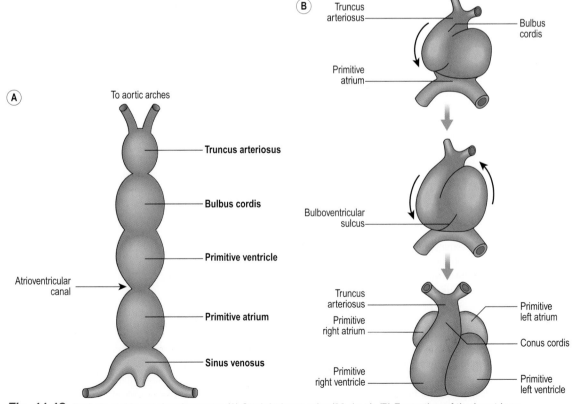

Fig. 11.12 **Early foetal heart development.** (A) Straight heart tube (22 days). (B) Formation of the heart loop.

Congenital heart abnormalities occur in about 6–8/1000 live births. Developmental defects may occur during:

- Fusion of the septum primum and septum secundum: atrial septal defects
- Development of the interventricular septum: ventricular septal defects
- Fusion and remodelling of the endocardial cushions: tricuspid and mitral valve defects, persistent atrio-ventricular canal, tricuspid atresia
- Partitioning of the bulbus cordis and truncus arteriosus: transposition of the great arteries, aortic or pulmonary valve defects, Fallot's tetralogy.

  Causes of congenital heart defects may be genetic or environmental:

- Genetic mutations or deletions leading to congenital heart defects may arise de novo or be inherited. Genetic disorders of connective tissue, such as Marfan syndrome, are associated with mitral and aortic valve abnormalities. Large chromosome abnormalities, the commonest being trisomy 21 (Down syndrome) are associated with congenital heart defects, but smaller chromosomal abnormalities may also lead to heart defects.
- Environmental causes of congenital heart disease include maternal infections, such as rubella and toxoplasmosis, drug and alcohol misuse, and maternal systemic illness such as diabetes mellitus and systemic lupus erythematosus.

Congenital heart defects can cause:

- **Obstruction to flow** (e.g. coarctation, right ventricular outflow tract obstruction – pulmonary valvular stenosis, infundibular, pulmonary arterial, left ventricular outflow tract obstruction – valvular, subvalvular, supravalvular)
- **Flow or 'shunts' through abnormal connections or 'holes'** (e.g. ventricular septal defect, atrial septal defect, patent ductus arteriosus). The pressure in the systemic circulation or 'left' side of the heart is higher than in the pulmonary circulation or 'right' side of the heart, so blood flow through holes is usually from left to right. The size of the shunt is determined by the relative resistance to flow in the two circulations. Large shunts result in volume overload on the ventricle receiving the additional blood flow, which causes ventricular dilatation and cardiac failure. Large shunts through the pulmonary circulation result in pulmonary hypertension and changes in the pulmonary vessel wall structure characterised by muscular hypertrophy and reduced luminal area, which exacerbates the pulmonary hypertension. Ultimately, large shunts may result in a pulmonary artery pressure which exceeds the systemic pressure, shunt reversal and **cyanosis** – this is called '**Eisenmenger syndrome**'.
- **Paradoxical emboli**, which are related to the right to left shunting of blood through defects. Thrombotic material in the venous circulation may be transported into the arterial circulation, bypassing the usual 'filter' provided by the lungs. The most common site for embolism is the brain. Polycythaemia in cyanotic patients predisposes to the initial formation of venous thrombus.
- **Brain abscesses**, which are also related to right to left shunting of blood. If the blood contains bacteria, then it can travel to the brain without the usual filtering of material in the lungs.
- **Endocarditis**, which is related to the turbulent blood flow which occurs in most patients with congenital heart disease.
- **Arrhythmia**, both supraventricular and ventricular, which are due to chamber dilatation and scarring. These are common even after surgical repair and are often poorly tolerated because of the limited haemodynamic reserve.

valve and later form the tricuspid and mitral valves. They also fuse and remodel to divide the primitive atrial and ventricular canals into left and right.

The atria

Division of the primitive atrium into left- and right-sided chambers is a process that continues until birth (Fig. 11.12B).

- Within the atrial canal, the **septum primum** grows from the roof of the primitive atrium towards the endocardial cushions, but leaving a temporary gap at its inferior margin called the **foramen primum**. A new opening, the **foramen secundum**, forms in the middle of the septum primum as it merges with the endocardial cushions to close the foramen primum.
- A semilunar shaped septum to the right of the septum primum, the **septum secundum**, also descends from the roof of the primitive atrium; the free edges form the **foramen ovale**. These foramina allow blood to flow from the right to the left atria, bypassing the high pressure foetal pulmonary circulation.
- The two septae fuse in their overlapping portions but leave an unfused flap of tissue of the septum primum over the foramen ovale which allows blood to flow across the septum.
- At birth, the foramen ovale closes to complete the formation of the interatrial septum.

  Atrial septal defects (ASDs) arise from abnormal developmental of the interatrial septum. Secundum ASDs are the most common variety and are caused by failure of the foramen secundum to close. Primum ASDs arise due to failure of the foramen primum to close. Failure of the foramen ovale to close is described in Clinical box 11.6.

The ventricles

The heart tube continues to fold and the bulge designated for the primitive ventricle develops into the future ventricles (Fig. 11.12B). Tissue grows upwards from the midline of the floor to form the **interventricular septum**, which separates the primitive ventricle into two chambers. The interventricular septum fuses with the endocardial cushion at about 7 weeks' gestation, which completes the formation of the basic structure of the heart as a four chambered organ. The interventricular foramen appears in the septum, allowing blood to flow

Failure of the flap of tissue which arises from the septum primum and which covers the foramen ovale to fuse with the septum secundum after birth results in a **patent foramen ovale (PFO)**. This is a common finding, occurring in about 20% of the general population. Blood does not normally flow from the left atrium to the right atrium because the higher left-sided pressure pushes the tissue flap against the septum. However, increases in right atrial pressure, such as on release of the Valsalva manoeuvre, can result in transient opening of the flap and right to left flow across the septum. This creates the potential for paradoxical embolism which has stimulated considerable debate over whether or not PFOs play a role in the aetiology of otherwise unexplained cerebral infarction or migraine. Randomised controlled trials in patients with prior stroke or transient ischaemic attack, and in patients with migraine, however, failed to demonstrate a reduction in the recurrence rate of stroke or improvement in migraine symptoms, respectively, in patients who were randomised to PFO device closure.

from right to left, bypassing the pulmonary circulation. This is later closed by non-muscular tissue to form the membranous part of the interventricular septum. Congenital ventricular septal defect is discussed in Clinical box 11.7.

The great arteries

Cells from the truncus arteriosus and the bulbar cordis develop into the truncal and bulbar ridges, respectively (Fig. 11.12B). These ridges grow inwards and spiral around each other before they fuse to form the aorto-pulmonary septum which separates the heart tube into the aorta and pulmonary trunk. The future semilunar aortic and pulmonary valves develop from endocardial cushions in the truncus arteriosus. Transposition of the great arteries occurs when the developing aortic and pulmonary arteries do not spiral correctly (Clinical box 11.8). Tetralogy of Fallot is an important and complex developmental defect of the heart which is due to anterior and cephalad deviation of the outlet septum (Clinical box 11.9).

Clinical box 11.7   **Congenital ventricular septal defect**

Failure of normal development of the interventricular septum results in a **ventricular septal defect (VSD)**. VSD is the most common congenital heart defect and it most frequently affects the membranous septum. The VSD results in a left-to-right and causes a systolic thrill and a pan-systolic murmur at the left sternal edge. Small defects have little physiological effect and may close spontaneously in childhood due to overgrowth of ventricular muscle. Large shunts place a volume load on the left ventricle and increase the pressure in the pulmonary arteries with subsequent thickening of the walls of the pulmonary arterioles and a progressive increase in the pulmonary vascular resistance. Eventually, the development of severe pulmonary hypertension results in reversal of the shunt with the development of cyanosis due to deoxygenated blood entering the systemic circulation – **Eisenmenger syndrome**. VSDs, like other communications between the systemic and pulmonary circulations, are at risk of **endocarditis** and **paradoxical embolism**. Surgical closure prior to the development of pulmonary hypertension is the treatment of choice for large defects.

Clinical box 11.8   **Transposition of the great arteries**

In this developmental abnormality of the great arteries, the outflow of the left ventricle is into the pulmonary artery and the outflow of the right ventricle is into the aorta. Patients with this condition can only survive if there is a shunt, either an atrial or ventricular septal defect, or a patent ductus arteriosus, otherwise the deoxygenated blood entering the right ventricle would be ejected into the aorta with no route to the lungs. The shunt allows blood entering the right ventricle from the periphery to pass through the shunt into the left ventricle, from where it is ejected into the pulmonary circulation. Similarly, blood draining from the pulmonary veins can pass through the shunt and enter the aorta.

Transposition is usually diagnosed in the first week of life due to cyanosis and failure to thrive. The right ventricle is incapable of maintaining the high pressures of the systemic circulation and inevitably fails. The administration of PGE_1 to maintain the patency of the ductus arteriosus or a percutaneous atrial septostomy to increase an atrial shunt may help to maintain the circulation pending corrective surgery in the first month of life. Arterial switch surgery is now performed in which the great arteries are transposed back to their correct ventricles and the coronary arteries are reattached to the aorta.

Clinical box 11.9   **Tetralogy of Fallot**

Fallot's tetralogy is the commonest cyanotic congenital heart defect with an incidence of about 1:3600 live births. It is associated with chromosomal deletion abnormalities. It has four main features:
- Right ventricular outflow tract obstruction
- A ventricular septal defect
- An overriding aorta: misalignment of the aorta, which straddles the VSD and receives blood from both ventricles
- Right ventricular hypertrophy.

The right ventricular outflow tract obstruction encourages shunting of blood through the VSD to the left ventricle, bypassing the lungs. This leads to hypoxaemia with failure to thrive, fatigue, breathlessness, dizziness and progressive cyanosis. Patients might instinctively squat during transient exacerbation of symptoms, which increases systemic vascular resistance and increases blood flow through the lungs.

Unoperated, patients die before the age of 40. Palliative procedures connect a systemic artery to one of the pulmonary arteries in order to increase blood flow to the lungs. The Blalock–Taussig shunt, for example, connects the left subclavian artery to the pulmonary artery. Surgical repair between the age of 6 and 18 months is now the treatment of choice and dramatically improves the prognosis.

DEVELOPMENT OF THE VASCULATURE

The foetal arterial system develops from about 4 weeks of gestation from the aortic arch. The venous system develops from about 4 to 8 weeks of gestation and empties into the sinus venosus (Fig. 11.12A).

The foetal circulation

The foetus relies on the **fetoplacental circulation** for nutrients and oxygen (Fig. 11.13A). The fetoplacental circulation includes the placenta, the blood vessels in the placenta, which carry blood to and from the foetus, and the umbilical cord, which consists of the two umbilical arteries and one umbilical vein. The foetal circulation is different from the circulation after birth because the lungs are collapsed and non-functioning. Blood bypasses the high pressure pulmonary circulation and nutrients and oxygen are supplied to the foetus by the mother via the placenta. Foetal haemoglobin has a higher affinity for oxygen than adult haemoglobin so that oxygen in the maternal circulation can diffuse to the foetus (see Ch. 12). Oxygenated blood is carried by the uterine arteries to the placenta, from where nutrients and oxygen diffuse to the chorionic villi before entering the umbilical vein (see Ch. 10). The umbilical vein therefore carries oxygenated blood from the placenta to the foetus, about half of which enters the liver and the other half passes through the **ductus venosus**, which allows it to join the inferior vena cava without being deoxygenated by the liver. The inferior vena cava also receives deoxygenated blood from the lower part of the foetus before joining the right atrium. Deoxygenated blood from the cerebral, coronary and pulmonary circulations and the limbs drains into the right atrium via the superior vena cava

In the foetal heart, most of the blood passes from the right to the left atrium through the foramen ovale, then into the left ventricle, bypassing the pulmonary circulation. From the left ventricle, blood is pumped via the aorta to the brain, heart and upper limbs. Some of the blood from the superior vena cava passes to the right ventricle and into the pulmonary artery. There is, however, a connection between

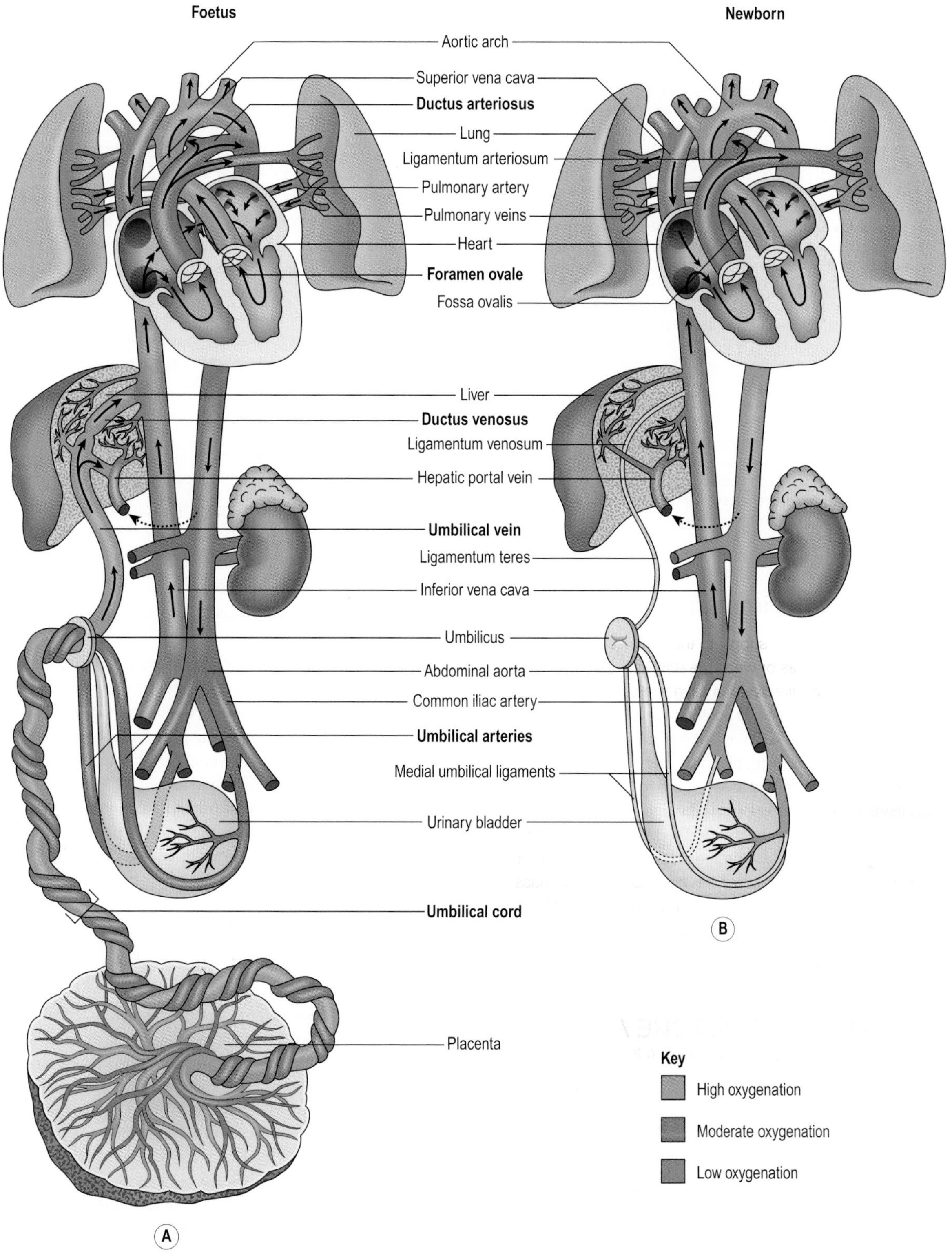

Fig. 11.13 Comparison of the foetal and newborn circulation. (A) Foetal circulation before birth. The ductus venosus allows blood to bypass the liver. The ductus arteriosus and foramen ovale allow blood to bypass the lungs. (B) After birth these close allowing the normal adult circulation to develop.

the pulmonary artery and the aorta, the **ductus arteriosus**, which channels most of this blood away from the pulmonary artery (the lungs are non-functioning) to the aorta, to supply the lower limbs and viscera. The descending aorta therefore carries deoxygenated blood; the reverse of the adult

circulation (see later). From the aorta, blood passes through the internal iliac arteries to the umbilical arteries to rejoin the placenta, where CO_2 and other waste products of metabolism are removed from the foetus and enter the maternal circulation.

The neonatal circulation

At birth, maternal blood supply to the neonate is cut off when the placenta separates or when the umbilical cord is clamped. The neonatal lungs take over the oxygenation of blood, and the foetal circulation assumes its adult pattern (Fig. 11.13B). At the baby's first breath, the lungs are inflated and pulmonary vascular resistance falls, allowing blood to flow freely into the lungs. The left atrial pressure increases relative to the right atrial pressure, leading to the closure of the foramen ovale. At the same time, the rise in oxygen tension in the blood leads to a fall in prostaglandins (PGE$_1$) causing the closure of the ductus arteriosus. These closures prevent the circulation from bypassing the lungs. Clinical box 11.10 describes the defect when the ductus arteriosus fails to close properly.

CELLULAR STRUCTURE AND FUNCTION OF THE HEART

The heart is a hollow, muscular organ whose function is to pump blood and the nutrients it carries around the body. The heart must generate a force sufficient to overcome the resistance to flow presented by the circulation. The heart is designed to function efficiently through the regular and coordinated contraction of its chambers. Two types of cells are needed for this: cardiomyocytes, which make up the atria and ventricles, and pacemaker cells, which regulate the rate and rhythmic beating of the heart.

STRUCTURE OF HEART MUSCLE

The myocardium is involuntary striated muscle. Individual cardiomyocytes are joined together by special adherent discs, the intercalated discs, to facilitate contraction. The sarcoplasmic reticulum is specially adapted with T-tubules for the storage and release of calcium, which is needed for cardiac muscle contraction.

Cardiomyocytes

Electrical signals pass readily between cardiomyocytes through gap junctions so that the heart contracts as a coordinated unit, a functional syncytium. Cardiac muscle contraction (unlike skeletal muscle contraction) is involuntary. The contractile proteins of cardiomyocytes and other muscle types are discussed in Chapter 9. Like skeletal muscle, cardiac muscle is striated by alternating thin actin filaments and thicker myosin filaments (Fig. 11.14). The actin filaments form I bands that appear lighter and the myosin filaments are labelled A bands which are darker on electron microscopy. The H band, or zone, contains only myosin filaments. Z and M lines are insertions of the actin and myosin filaments, respectively. In contrast to skeletal muscle filaments which are straight and long, cardiomyocytes may be branched, and are smaller.

Intercalated discs

Intercalated discs are adhering structures that stick individual cardiomyocytes together to form the functional syncytium that contracts regularly and rhythmically. They occur at the Z line and support synchronised cardiac muscle contraction. Three types of adhering junctions are described:

- Anchor sites for actin, known as **fascia adherens**. They transmit contractile forces.
- **Desmosomes**, also known as **macula adherens**, which are localised cell to cell adhesions (cytoplasmic bridges) randomly arranged on the lateral sides of the sarcolemma. They provide structural support and bind cardiomyocytes together to stop separation during contraction, and resist shearing force.
- *Gap junctions*, formed from transmembrane proteins known as connexins, which allow action potentials to pass between cardiomyocytes to enable coordinated contraction.

T-tubules and sarcoplasmic reticulum

Transverse or T-tubules are deep invaginations of the sarcolemma which allow depolarisation of the membrane to penetrate the muscle fibre. Compared with skeletal muscle (see Ch. 9), T-tubules in cardiomyocytes are less prevalent, larger and wider. They run along the Z disc where they form diads with the terminal cisternae of sarcoplasmic reticulum (SR) (Fig. 11.14).

    T-tubules are important for the excitation and contraction of cardiac muscle. They contain **L-type calcium channels** that are activated in response to electrical stimuli, allowing calcium, which is needed for muscle contraction, to enter the cardiomyocytes. Activation of the L-type calcium channels also opens the calcium-release channels on the SR, causing the release of its calcium stores; this process is called calcium-induced calcium release (CICR).

THE CONTRACTILE PROCESS

Cardiac muscle contraction

The contraction of cardiomyocytes is caused by the binding between actin and myosin filaments within the cell. The

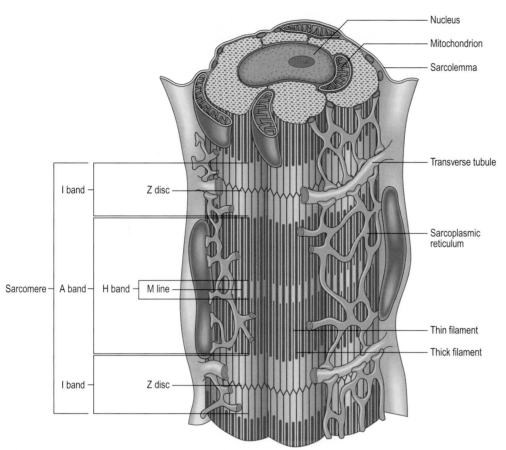

Fig. 11.14 **Cardiac muscle showing arrangement of transverse tubules, sarcoplasmic reticulum and the divisions of the sarcomeres.**

contractile process is dependent upon a rise in the intracellular concentration of calcium, which causes an interaction between calcium and troponin C. This leads to the formation of cross-links between the heads of the myosin filaments and the actin filaments. The cross-links act as the 'oar' and the myosin heads as the 'blade', as the myosin 'rows' over the actin filaments resulting in shortening of the muscle cell.

As for skeletal muscle, the strength of myocardial contraction, myocardial contractility, depends on the degree of stretch in the muscle fibres prior to contraction (see Ch. 9). The degree of binding also depends on the cytosolic (intracellular) calcium ion concentration, which increases in response to sympathetic nervous system stimulation.

As with the excitation–contraction coupling process in skeletal muscle, cardiac muscle contraction depends on a depolarisation/repolarisation cycle in the sarcolemma. Action potentials are propagated across the sarcolemma and deep into T-tubules by the activation of voltage dependent sodium channels allowing a rapid influx of Na^+ (Fig. 11.15) when the membrane is said to be **depolarised**. At the resting action potential, a small amount of K^+ leaks inward across the cell membrane (known as the inward rectifying current). The fast, Na^+ influx causes the sharp spike (A) in the action potential (electrical stimulus), which triggers the influx of extracellular calcium (C) into the myocyte via T-tubules. This in turn stimulates the mechanisms for calcium-induced calcium release from the sarcoplasmic reticulum. The rise in cytosolic calcium ion (Ca^{2+}) concentration causes the heart muscle to contract when the Ca^{2+} binds to the muscle protein troponin. Drugs which block the effect

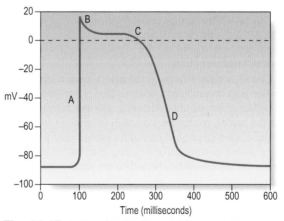

Fig. 11.15 **Action potential in cardiac ventricular myocytes.** A, Na^+ influx (fast inward); B, K^+ efflux (transient); C, Ca^{2+} influx (slow inward); D, K^+ efflux (delayed rectifier).

of calcium channels in the myocardium reduce the force of myocardial contraction (see Clinical box 11.11). This effect is called a negative inotropic effect.

Cardiac muscle relaxation

Following the wave of depolarisation through the heart muscle, potassium ions leave the cell, the action potential falls and the cell membrane returns to its resting state, known as **repolarisation**, and the heart muscle relaxes. The Na^+ channels are closed during this phase (Fig.11.15D, K^+ efflux, also known as the delayed K^+ rectifying current). Cardiac

---

Clinical box 11.11 **Therapeutic use of calcium channel blockers**

Calcium channel blockers can be used to reduce the entry of calcium into myocytes. Most of these drugs preferentially block L-type, voltage-gated calcium channels, targeting excitation–contraction coupling by blocking L-type calcium channel mediated MLCK (myosin light-chain kinase) activation. L-type calcium channels are not all the same, with different isoforms being present in vascular smooth muscle and the heart. Calcium channel blockers have different affinities for the different isoforms and therefore produce different pharmacological effects.

Classes of calcium channel blockers include:

- **Dihydropyridine derivatives**, e.g. **nifedipine**, **amlodipine** (vascular selective): these drugs cause relaxation of vascular smooth muscle cells resulting in peripheral vasodilatation. They reduce the work of the heart and blood pressure so can be used to treat angina and hypertension. The vasodilatory effects, however, may also produce side effects including hypotension, headache and peripheral oedema.
- **Non-dihydropyridine derivatives**:
  1. **Phenylalkylamines, e.g. verapamil** (cardioselective): acts mainly in the heart where it slows electrical conduction, lowering heart rate, and reduces myocardial contractility (a negative inotrope). These actions lower myocardial oxygen consumption which is useful in the treatment of angina. Verapamil's potent blockade of the AV node makes it valuable in the termination of nodal tachycardias and for the ventricular rate control of atrial arrhythmia.
  2. **Benzothiazepines, e.g. diltiazem** (intermediate selectivity between dihydropyridines and phenylalkylamines): some vasodilator effect and some effect on AV node.

---

muscle **relaxation** occurs with the removal of cytosolic Ca^{2+} by the calcium transporters, the Ca-ATPase pumps and the Na^+/Ca^{2+} co-transporter on the sarcolemma, into the extracellular fluid. Intracellular Ca^{2+} ions are also returned to the SR by Ca-ATPase pumps on the SR membrane for storage in the SR. Disturbances of plasma levels of calcium and potassium can lead to abnormalities in cardiac excitation (Clinical boxes 11.12 and 11.13).

As in skeletal muscle, a **refractory period** occurs between depolarisation and repolarisation of the sarcolemma. The Na^+ channels are inactivated until the full restoration of the resting membrane potential. In contrast to skeletal muscle, cardiomyocytes cannot be excited until the refractory period is completed, ensuring that the chambers of the heart are completely refilled before another contraction occurs.

Cardiac muscle metabolism

The constant work of the heart demands a high rate of oxygen consumption, which is 20 times greater than skeletal muscle, when at rest. A dense capillary network and large numbers of mitochondria facilitate continuous aerobic respiration. Under normal physiological conditions, energy substrates are derived from free fatty acids and triglycerides, glucose and a small amount of amino acids and ketone bodies. During ischaemia or starvation, lactate from anaerobic respiration may be used (see Ch. 3).

ELECTRICAL ACTIVATION OF THE HEART

Contraction of the heart is dependent upon depolarisation of the cardiomyocytes. Normal cardiac activation spreads from the atria to the ventricles and involves specialised cells with

---

Clinical box 11.12 **Effects of abnormal plasma potassium levels on cardiac excitation**

Most (95%) of the body's potassium (K^+) is in the intracellular space. The normal plasma (extracellular) concentration of K^+ is 3.5–5.0 mmol/L. Abnormalities in plasma K^+ concentration alter the resting membrane potential of cardiac myocytes which changes their excitability and the heart's susceptibility to arrhythmia.

Hyperkalaemia (elevated plasma K^+ level) lowers the K^+ gradient across the cardiomyocyte cell membrane. The resting membrane potential (which is negative) diminishes (becomes less negative) when the plasma K^+ concentration rises above 6.0 mmol/L, increasing cardiac excitation and the risk of serious cardiac arrhythmias, e.g. ventricular tachycardia. With further increases in K^+ concentration (>7 mmol/L), bradyarrhythmia and heart block may occur as voltage-dependent sodium channels become inactivated, reducing myocardial excitability. ECG changes seen in hyperkalaemia include peaked T-waves, reduced P-wave amplitude and prolongation of the QRS complex.

The commonest causes of hyperkalaemia are chronic kidney disease and drugs (e.g. ACE inhibitors, angiotensin receptor blockers and potassium sparing diuretics). It can also occur in Addison disease (hypoaldosteronism).

Hypokalaemia (low plasma K^+ level) increases the K^+ gradient across the cardiomyocyte cell membrane, causing hyperpolarisation (a more negative resting cell membrane), increasing the duration of the action potential and the refractory period and reducing cardiac excitability. Arrhythmias such as atrial fibrillation or flutter, ventricular ectopics, ventricular tachycardia and ventricular fibrillation may result. ECG changes in hypokalaemia include prominent U-waves, reduced T-wave amplitude, ST depression and prolongation of the PR interval.

Causes of hypokalaemia include excessive K^+ loss due to diarrhoea and vomiting (e.g. cholera, bulimia), diuretics and endocrine conditions such as Cushing syndrome and primary hyperaldosteronism. Treatment is by K^+ replacement and managing the cause.

Clinical box 11.13 **Effects of abnormal plasma calcium levels on cardiac excitation**

Calcium (Ca^{2+}) is the most abundant mineral in the body. The normal range for plasma Ca^{2+} concentration is 2.20–2.65 mmol/L. Calcium is a critical requirement for cardiac muscle contraction.

Hypocalcaemia is associated with prolongation of the QT interval and an increased risk of arrhythmia. A severe reduction in plasma Ca^{2+} concentration predisposes to heart failure. Causes of hypocalcaemia include hypoparathyroidism, vitamin D deficiency, malabsorbtion (e.g. in pancreatic disease, Ca^{2+} chelating drugs such as tetracyclines), renal disease and hyperventilation.

Hypercalcaemia is associated with a short QT interval. Extreme hypercalcaemia can cause cardiac arrest in systole. Causes include hyperparathyroidism, malignancies, sarcoid, vitamin D metabolism disorders (e.g. hypervitaminosis D), high bone turnover conditions and some endocrine neoplasias.

Hypocalcaemia is treated by calcium replacement. Hypercalcaemia is treated by hydration with intravenous saline, furosemide and, if necessary, bisphosphonates.

---

pacemaker activity and a specialised electrical conducting system. Heart rate and force of contraction is influenced by the autonomic nervous system.

Pacemaker cells

Contraction of cardiac muscle cells is triggered by depolarisation of their cell membranes. Cardiomyocytes, unlike skeletal muscle cells, are able to fire action potentials without nervous stimulation, a property known as **auto-rhythmicity**.

In patients with a normal heart rhythm (**sinus rhythm**), ventricular contraction is the end result of a spreading wave of depolarisation which is initiated by an action potential arising from pacemaker cells in a small area of tissue located in the posterior wall of the right atrium called the sinoatrial (SA) node. Cells in the SA node are less polarised than other myocytes, which makes them electrically unstable, the resting membrane potential being close to the threshold for triggering an action potential. Furthermore, between the end of one action potential and the beginning of the next, slow inward sodium and calcium currents and reducing outward potassium currents result in a gradual depolarisation of the cells in the SA node. This increased membrane potential is known as the **pacemaker potential** (or pacemaker current) (Fig. 11.16) that causes the cell membrane to reach threshold potential and fire off the next action potential.

The pacemaker potential provides cardiomyocytes with their property of auto-rhythmicity. The action potential firing rate determines the heart rate and this is determined by the slope of the pacemaker potential – the steeper the pacemaker potential, the more rapidly the threshold for an action potential is reached, and the higher the heart rate. Conversely, the flatter the pacemaker potential, the more time it takes for the next action potential to be triggered, and the slower the heart rate. While nervous stimulation of the heart is not necessary to trigger action potentials, the heart rate is modulated by the autonomic nervous system (see Nerve supply to the heart) and by some drugs. Effects on heart rate are known as **chronotropic** effects. Examples of drugs which have chronotropic effects and their clinical uses are discussed in Clinical box 11.14.

The cardiac conduction system

The main components of the cardiac conduction system, which initiates and propogates the spreading wave of depolarisation through the heart, are the **sinoatrial (SA) node**, the **atrioventricular (AV) node**, the **bundle of His**, the **bundle branches** and the **Purkinje fibres**. In sinus rhythm, action potentials generated by the SA node propagate through the atria, via gap junctions in the intercalated discs, along the three **internodal tracts**, to the AV node (Fig. 11.17). There is a delay of about 0.1 seconds at the AV node, which conducts slowly (Table 11.3), before the stimulus reaches the bundle of His. Depolarisation is then propagated to the ventricular myocardium through the bundle of His, the left and right

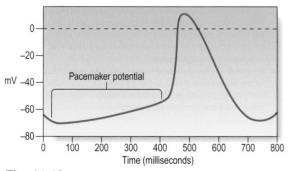

Fig. 11.16 **Pacemaker potential in the SA node.** Sinoatrial nodal cells show an unstable resting membrane potential due to a combination of slow inward sodium and calcium currents.

| Clinical box 11.14 | **Drugs whose actions are mediated through chronotropic effects** |

Drugs with chronotropic effects change heart rate either by their effect on the sinoatrial node or by affecting the nervous input to the heart. Positive chronotropes increase heart rate and negative chronotropes reduce heart rate (see also Ch. 4).

Drugs with negative chronotropic effects:
- Beta-blockers (e.g. atenolol, bisoprolol): block the effects of the sympathetic nervous system on the sinoatrial (SA) node and atrioventricular (AV) node. These actions are utilised for the treatment of angina and tachyarrhythmia, respectively.
- Digoxin: acts indirectly on the parasympathetic nervous system (vagus nerve) to slow conduction through the AV node. Used for rate control of atrial fibrillation.
- Some calcium channel blockers (e.g. diltazem, verapamil): reduce calcium influx, slowing conduction in the AV node. Used for the treatment of angina and tachyarrhythmias.
- Ivabradine, an SA node inhibitor: selectively blocks I_f channels in the SA node, reducing the slope of the pacemaker potential and thereby slowing the rate of sinus node discharge. Used to treat angina.

Drugs with positive chronotropic effects:
- Adrenergic agonists, e.g dobutamine, isoprenaline: stimulate β_1-receptors in the heart to increase heart rate and force of cardiac contraction. Used to treat heart failure, cardiogenic shock and bradyarrhythmia.
- Atropine: blocks parasympathetic stimulation (vagus nerve) and increases heart rate. Used to treat bradycardia.

---

bundle branches and the Purkinje fibres. This sequence of depolarisation facilitates efficient functioning of the heart (see Information box 11.5).

Cells in the heart other than the SA node have the capacity to initiate cardiac contraction though their spontaneous depolarisation. In normal circumstances, the SA node determines the heart rate because its inherent rate of discharge of 60–100/min is higher than the discharge rate of the other cardiomyocytes, which are therefore suppressed. However, if the SA node fails, or if there is blockade to electrical conduction before depolarisation reaches the AV node, the AV node initiates depolarisation at a rate of about 50 beats per minute (bpm). If the AV node also fails, then the Purkinje fibres take over the pacemaker function of the heart, stimulating ventricular depolarisation at a rate of about 30 bpm.

Nerve supply to the heart

The actions of the heart are modulated by the **autonomic nervous system** (see Ch. 4), with inputs from both the sympathetic and parasympathetic nervous systems. The autonomic nervous system influences heart rate and force of myocardial contraction. Figure 11.18 shows the autonomic effects on the pacemaker potential.

Parasympathetic supply

The heart receives parasympathetic input to the SA node via the right vagus nerve, and to the AV node via the left vagus nerve. Parasympathetic activity has a negative chronotropic effect, reducing the intrinsic myogenic heart rate from about 100 bpm to a resting rate of about 70 bpm. There is no parasympathetic input to the ventricles so the force of cardiomyocyte contraction is unaffected by parasympathetic activity.

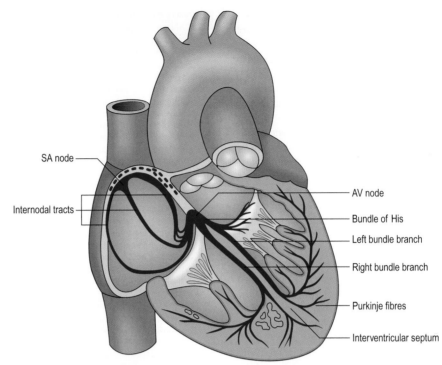

Fig. 11.17 **Conduction pathways of the heart.** Normally, excitation spreads from the sinoatrial (SA) node via internodal pathways to the atrioventricular (AV) node, from where it travels down the interventricular septum and across both ventricles.

Table 11.3	Conduction pathways in the heart	
Pathway	Duration (s)	Conduction velocity (m/s)
Sinoatrial node to atrioventricular node	0.04	1
Atrioventricular node to bundle of His	0.11	0.05
Bundle of His to Purkinje fibres	0.01	4
Purkinje fibres to ventricular myocytes	0.05	0.7

Vagal stimulation of the SA node decreases the pacemaker cell firing rate, whilst stimulation of the AV node slows conduction. This effect is mediated through the release of **acetylcholine** which causes a decrease in the intracellular second messenger **cyclic adenosine monophosphate** (cAMP). This reduces the activation of outward positive ion channels, which, in turn decreases the rate of depolarisation of the pacemaker potential. The initial resting membrane potential is also lowered moving it away from the threshold potential (Fig. 11.18C).

Sympathetic supply

The sympathetic nerve supply to the heart is via **cardiac nerves** which originate in spinal cord segments T1-T5 and which terminate on β_1-adrenoceptors in the plasma membranes of cardiomyocytes and on the cells of the SA and AV nodes. Sympathetic stimulation increases both the force of cardiac contraction and the heart rate. These effects arise through the release of **norepinephrine** from the sympathetic nerve terminals which leads to an increase in intracellular cAMP. Cardiomyocyte depolarisation is accelerated to reach the firing threshold faster (Fig.11.18B). The action potential

Information box 11.5	Efficient functioning of the heart through coordinated depolarisation of the atria and ventricles

Efficient functioning of the heart requires:
- **Time for the ventricles to fill to ensure an adequate stroke volume**: this is aided by slow conduction through the atrioventricular node which delays the transmission of the depolarisation wave from the atria to the bundle of His, prolonging diastole and time for ventricular filling.
- **Coordinated contraction of the atria before the ventricles**: in sinus rhythm, atrial contraction at the end of diastole augments ventricular filling, prior to ventricular contraction. Atrial contraction coordinated with ventricular contraction in this way is called atrioventricular concordance. The correct timing of atrial contraction before ventricular contraction is dependent upon conduction through the AV node. If conduction through the AV node fails (producing second or third degree heart block), AV concordance is lost and the atria and ventricles contract independently of each other. AV concordance is also lost in atrial arrhythmia such as atrial fibrillation when there is no coordinated atrial depolarization or contraction.
- **Contraction of the ventricles from their apex to base**: this is necessary for the efficient ejection of blood from the ventricles into the great arteries and is achieved through the sequential spread of the depolarisation wave through the Purkinje network. The action potentials are sustained to prevent relaxation until the whole myocardium has depolarised and contracted.
- **A period of muscle relaxation in order to allow filling of the chambers**: this is achieved through temporary inactivation of voltage dependent sodium channels which renders the cardiomyocytes refractory.

is shortened, and conduction through the AV node quickens to produce the positive chronotropic effects. The positive inotropic effects are the result of increased calcium concentrations in the cardiomyocytes due to increased calcium influx. In addition, the relaxation period is shortened due to the

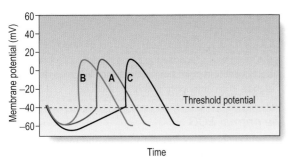

Fig. 11.18 **Autonomic effects on the heart.** (A) Control; (B) sympathetic stimulation; (C) parasympathetic stimulation.

β-Adrenoceptor antagonists, or '**β-blockers**', are an important group of drugs which are used to treat a number of cardiovascular conditions including angina, hypertension and heart failure. Their therapeutic actions are through blockade of the β_1-adrenoceptors in the heart which causes a reduction in heart rate and myocardial contractility. This reduces myocardial oxygen requirements, which is especially useful in the treatment of angina.

Some (non-selective) β-blockers also act as β_2-adrenoceptors producing unwanted side effects. Blockade of β_2-adrenoceptors in the lungs and peripheral arteries, for example, can cause bronchospasm and claudication, respectively. β-Blockers which preferentially block β_1-adrenoceptors, such as atenolol and metoprolol, cause fewer side effects.

more rapid uptake of intracellular Ca^{2+} into the SR for storage (see above).

β-Blockers inhibit the action of the sympathetic nervous system on the heart which is useful in the treatment of a number of clinical conditions (Information box 11.6, see Clinical box 11.14).

Adrenal medulla

The actions of the heart are also modulated by catecholamines released from the adrenal medulla. Sympathetic activation causes the secretion of epinephrine and, to a lesser extent, norepinephrine into the bloodstream. Their systemic effects are complex, and include increased blood flow to skeletal muscle, increased glycogen breakdown and glucose availability in skeletal muscle, and bronchodilatation. The main effects on the heart are produced through the stimulation of β_1-adrenoceptors which results in increased heart rate and myocardial contractility.

Electrocardiography

Electrocardiography involves the recording of the electrical activity of the heart from the body surface. The heart rate and rhythm can be determined, and information can be inferred about the size and position of the heart chambers, the thickness of the myocardium, the integrity of the conduction system, and the effects of drugs on the heart. It is particularly valuable in diagnosing the heart rhythm in patients with palpitation or syncope, and in diagnosing acute myocardial infarction or ischaemia in patients who have chest pain.

The ECG

The **electrocardiogram** (**ECG**) records the amplitude and direction of the wave of depolarisation as it spreads through the heart in relation to recording electrodes attached to both arms and legs, while another six electrodes, called the **chest or precordial leads**, are placed at specific positions on the chest (Table 11.4 and Fig. 11.19). The potential difference

Table 11.4	Placement of the ECG chest leads
Chest lead	**Position**
V_1	Fourth intercostal space, just right of the sternum
V_2	Fourth intercostal space, just left of the sternum
V_3	In between V_2 and V_4
V_4	Fifth intercostal space, mid-clavicular line
V_5	Anterior axillary line, level with V_4
V_6	Mid-axillary line, level with V_4 and V_5

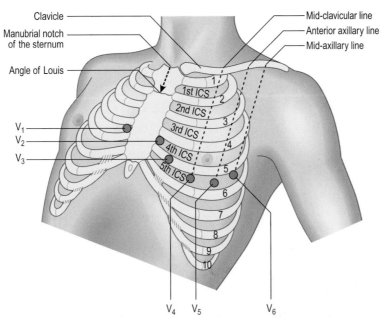

Fig. 11.19 **Positions of ECG chest leads.** ICS, intercostal space; ribs numbered 1–10.

Table 11.5	The 12-lead ECG	
Lead	**Positive electrode**	**Negative or reference electrode**
Bipolar leads		
I	Left arm	Right arm
II	Left leg	Right arm
III	Left leg	Left arm
Augmented unipolar leads		
aVR	Right arm	Zero (left arm + left leg)
aVL	Left arm	Zero (right arm + left leg)
aVF	Left leg	Zero (left arm + right arm)
Unipolar leads		
V_1–V_6	See Fig. 11.19	Zero (all three limb leads)

between electrodes is measured. Signals of 1 mV or more can be reliably detected by this method.

The ECG used routinely in clinical practice interrogates the heart from 12 different directions to produce the 12-lead ECG (Table 11.5 and Fig. 11.20). Two types of leads are used, bipolar and unipolar:

- Leads I, II and III are the standard bipolar limb leads that record the potential difference between two limb leads. Lead II, for example, records the difference between the left leg (+) and the right arm (−).
- The augmented unipolar limb leads, aVL, aVR and aVF, use the same electrodes as leads I, II and III, but record with respect to zero rather than to another limb.
- Leads V_1–V_6 are the precordial (or chest) leads, are unipolar, and record with reference to zero, estimated from connecting together the three limb leads.

The way in which the different leads 'look' at the heart can be illustrated by **Einthoven's triangle** (Fig. 11.20). This shows the positions of the three standard limb leads with the heart at its centre. The limb leads interrogate the heart in the vertical (coronal) plane whereas the chest leads interrogate the heart in the transverse plane.

- Leads I–III look at the electrical activity of the heart parallel to each side of the triangle.

- Leads aVR, aVL and aVF look at the heart from the points of the triangle.
- Leads V_1–V_6 look at the heart from six positions around the chest wall. Because the zero reference point is equivalent to a point behind the heart, this records signals in an anterior to posterior direction.

The normal ECG

Depolarisation activity moving towards the recording electrode produces an ECG signal with a positive deflection. Conversely, repolarisation moving towards the electrode produces a negative deflection (Table 11.6). The electrical activity of the heart shown by the ECG is related to the different phases of contraction and relaxation of the heart muscle. The different deflections from the baseline, described here for lead II, are labelled as follows (Fig. 11.21):

- The **P wave** is produced by depolarisation of the atria. It is a positive deflection as the wave of depolarisation moves towards the positive electrode.
- The **QRS complex** represents depolarisation of the ventricles. This is a complex signal which comprises:
  - Q: depolarisation of the interventricular septum from left to right
  - R: depolarisation of the main mass of the ventricles
  - S: depolarisation of the area of the heart near the base.

The voltages are large in comparison with the other ECG deflections because of the large muscle mass and the rapidity of depolarisation. The QRS complex therefore hides the electrical activity produced by atrial repolarisation, which occurs simultaneously.

Table 11.6	Determinants of ECG deflections	
Type of signal	**Direction of movement**	**Deflection of ECG**
Depolarisation	Towards electrode	Positive
Repolarisation	Towards electrode	Negative
Depolarisation	Away from electrode	Negative
Repolarisation	Away from electrode	Positive

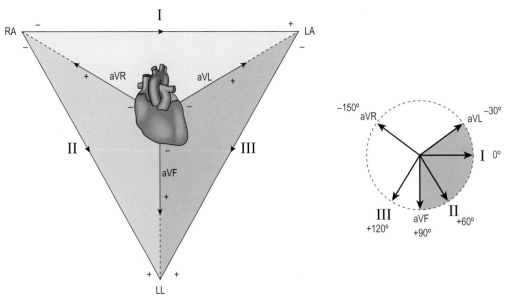

Fig. 11.20 Einthoven's triangle. Recordings from the different limb leads interrogate the heart from six different directions in the coronal plane. LA, left arm; RA, right arm; LL, left leg. The normal electrical axis of the heart is between −30° and +90°.

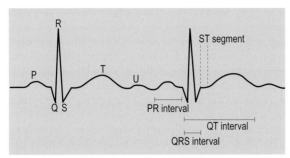

Fig. 11.21 Normal ECG tracing (lead II) in sinus rhythm.

- The **T wave** represents ventricular repolarisation. This is a positive wave because, although it is produced by repolarisation, it is moving away from lead II as the ventricles repolarise from the apex towards the base (Table 11.6). Although the muscle mass is large, its repolarisation is relatively slow which accounts for the lower amplitude and longer duration of the T wave compared with the QRS complex.
- The **U wave** is a deflection of low amplitude which is sometimes visible after the T wave. It is of uncertain origin but may be due to repolarisation of the Purkinje fibres. Prominent U waves are associated with hypokalaemia.

On the normal ECG, the **ST segment** is **isoelectric**, i.e. it has a zero potential. ST segment elevation is characteristic of an acute coronary artery occlusion (ST elevation myocardial infarction) though it may also be caused by pericarditis, a left ventricular aneurysm, or be a normal variant. ST depression is the hallmark of myocardial ischaemia but can be caused by ventricular hypertrophy or digoxin.

The **PR interval** corresponds to the time taken for excitation to spread across the atria, through the AV node and down the bundle of His. The spread of excitation from the atria to the ventricles is slowed by the AV node (Table 11.7), allowing the atria to complete their contraction before ventricular depolarisation occurs (Information box 11.5). If there is damage to this conduction pathway then the PR interval is prolonged and, in extreme cases, the transmission may be blocked entirely producing heart block (see Conduction disorders, below).

The electrical axis of the heart

The mean direction of the ventricular depolarisation wave is called the **electrical axis** of the heart. The true electrical

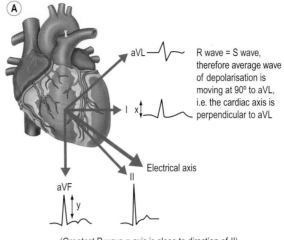

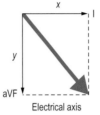

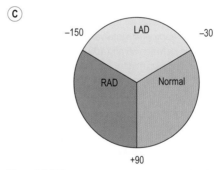

Fig. 11.22 Calculating the electrical axis of the heart.
(A) Calculation of the electrical axis by inspection; (B) x and y represent the heights of the QRS complex in leads I and aVF, respectively; (C) normal axis; LAD, left axis deviation; RAD, right axis deviation.

axis of the heart is a three dimensional vector. Inspection of the six ECG limb leads allows calculation of the electrical axis of the heart in the two dimensions of the coronal plane (Fig. 11.22). The axis lies at 90° to the isoelectric lead, the lead which has roughly equal QRS deflections above and below the isoelectric line, giving a net deflection of zero. The electrical axis can be estimated most accurately by plotting the height of the QRS complex (with respect to the isoelectric ST interval) from leads I and aVF on a diagram that represents the directions of the two leads and calculating the resultant vector (Fig. 11.22B). A normal axis is usually close to lead II although it may be anywhere between −30° and +90° (see Fig. 11.20 and Clinical box 11.15). The axis provides information about the conducting system of the heart and about the size and position of the contracting heart muscle.

Table 11.7	Timing of the normal ECG	
	Duration (s)	**Corresponds to**
P wave	0.11	Atrial depolarisation
PR interval	0.12–0.20	Atrial depolarisation, atrioventricular conduction, spread through bundle of His, bundle branches to Purkinje fibres
QRS interval	0.06–0.10	Ventricular depolarisation
QT interval	Varies with heart rate (see note below)	Ventricular depolarisation and repolarisation

Note: the QT interval is usually expressed as QTc which equals QT divided by the square root of the RR interval ($QTc = QT/\sqrt{RR}$). However, as a rough guide the normal QT interval should be less than half the RR interval.

The normal electrical axis of the heart is between −30° and +90°. The electrical axis of the heart may alter during breathing and it tends to be more vertical in tall thin subjects. An abnormal axis ('axis deviation') can be caused by abnormalities in the structure of the heart or by conduction disorders:

- **Left axis deviation** is when the electrical axis of the heart is between −30° and −150°. Causes include:
  - Left anterior fascicular block (also called left anterior hemiblock) where conduction is defective in the anterior fascicle of the left bundle
  - Q-wave inferior myocardial infarct
  - Primum atrial septal defect.
  Isolated left ventricular hypertrophy or left bundle branch block does not usually cause left axis deviation.
- **Right axis deviation** occurs when the electrical axis of the heart is between +90° and 180°. Causes include:
  - Right ventricular hypertrophy
  - Pulmonary embolism
  - Secundum atrial septal defect
  - Dextrocardia
  - Q-wave lateral myocardial infarction, which can lead to loss of left ventricular tissue
  - Left posterior fascicular block (also called left posterior hemiblock) where conduction is defective in the posterior half of the left bundle.
  Isolated right bundle branch block does not cause right axis deviation.

Cardiac arrhythmias

A detailed understanding of the shape, size and timing of the ECG components is crucial to the correct diagnosis of heart rhythms. In **sinus rhythm**, each atrial depolarisation is conducted normally to the ventricles so the ECG shows that every P wave is followed at an appropriate interval by a QRS complex. The normal heart rate is between 60 and 100 bpm (Fig. 11.23A). Heart rhythms other than sinus rhythm are called **arrhythmias**.

Sinus rhythm at a rate of more than 100 bpm is called **sinus tachycardia** (Fig. 11.23B), and at a rate of less than 60 bpm it is called **sinus bradycardia**. Sinus tachycardia is a normal physiological response to exercise, anxiety and pain, and it can be a sign of infection, shock or acute respiratory failure. Sinus bradycardia is physiological during sleep and in trained athletes but it can also be caused by sino-atrial node disease, drugs (ivabradine, β-blockers, calcium blockers and digoxin), hypothyroidism and hypothermia. If the rate of sino-atrial node discharge falls below about 40–50 bpm, the AV node takes over the pacemaker function within the heart to generate a **nodal bradycardia** (Fig. 11.23C). These bradycardias are frequently asymptomatic but profound bradycardias can cause dizziness or syncope when they require a pacemaker if there is no reversible cause.

Sinus arrhythmia is present when there is a noticeable increase in the sinus rate during inspiration and a decrease during expiration. These changes in heart rate are particularly noticeable in children and young adults and are due to phasic changes in the nervous input to the SA node from the vagus nerve.

A different variation in heart rhythm is produced by the occurrence of **ectopic beats** or extrasystoles. These are caused by the aberrant firing of a group of cells before the SA node's next scheduled discharge. So long as the aberrant discharge is conducted to the ventricles, it will cause a premature ventricular contraction which will be seen on the ECG as an early QRS complex. When the SA node does subsequently fire, the myocytes are in the refractory phase so they do not depolarise. There is therefore a compensatory pause before the SA node

is ready to depolarise again and trigger the next ventricular contraction. This next beat may be felt by the patient as a big beat or thump because the ventricular filling time is prolonged and the stroke volume is increased. Ectopic beats may arise from the atria or from the ventricles. Ventricular ectopic beats produce an abnormally wide QRS complex because ventricular depolarisation does not occur through the Purkinje fibres and is therefore slow. Atrial ectopic beats are conducted to the ventricles through the normal pathways so the QRS complex is normal. Ectopic beats are common and usually benign, particularly in the presence of a structurally normal heart.

Most sustained cardiac arrhythmias are **re-entrant tachycardias**. These occur when recurring circles of depolarisation result in repeated re-excitation of myocytes the moment they emerge from the refractory period, a phenomenon known as **re-entry**. These re-entry circuits can arise in the atria or in the AV node resulting in supraventricular tachycardias or in the ventricles causing ventricular tacharrhythmia. Supraventricular arrhythmias are not normally life threatening. They usually present with palpitation, but they can provoke shortness of breath or chest pain, particularly in patients who have concomitant coronary artery disease, ventricular disease or valve disease. By contrast, ventricular tachyarrhythmias are life-threatening emergencies which require careful assessment and expert management in order to reduce the risk of arrhythmic death.

Atrial fibrillation (**AF**) is the most common sustained cardiac arrhythmia. Its prevalence increases with age, affecting approximately 0.5%, 5% and 10% of subjects aged <50, 70 and 80 years, respectively. It occurs when multiple small re-entry circuits travel around the atria producing fibrillatory waves at a rate of 300–600/min. These waves are disorganised and fail to trigger atrial depolarisation and functional atrial contraction. The slow conduction of the AV node protects against extremely rapid ventricular rates. Furthermore, only a minority of wavelets are of sufficient amplitude to be conducted through the AV node. The chaotic pattern of the wavelets means that those large enough to be conducted to the ventricles arise at irregular intervals. These phenomena account for the characteristic ECG features of AF – an isoelectric line distorted by fibrillatory waves but no regular P wave activity, and irregularly spaced QRS complexes (Fig. 11.23F). The most important clinical impact of AF relates to its causative role in thromboembolic stroke. Most patients who have AF should receive anticoagulant therapy, which has been shown to reduce the risk of stroke in this group by about two thirds.

Atrial flutter has a number of features in common with atrial fibrillation – it is more common in older patients, it is associated with an increased risk of thromboembolic stroke which indicates the need for anticoagulation in most patients, and while the flutter waves are larger and more organised than the fibrillatory waves of AF, they remain insufficient to stimulate effective atrial contraction. The flutter waves circulate around the atria at a rate of approximately 300/min. In most patients, AV node refractoriness prevents one to one conduction of flutter waves to the ventricles which protects against very rapid ventricular rates. However, the AV node can usually conduct every second flutter wave so the ventricular rate is frequently about 150 bpm in untreated patients.

In **atrioventricular nodal re-entrant tachycardia** (**AVNRT**), the re-entry circuit is between the atrium and the AV node. Conduction proceeds normally through the bundle of His producing a narrow complex tachycardia with a ventricular rate of about 180–220 bpm. This arrhythmia typically occurs in young adults.

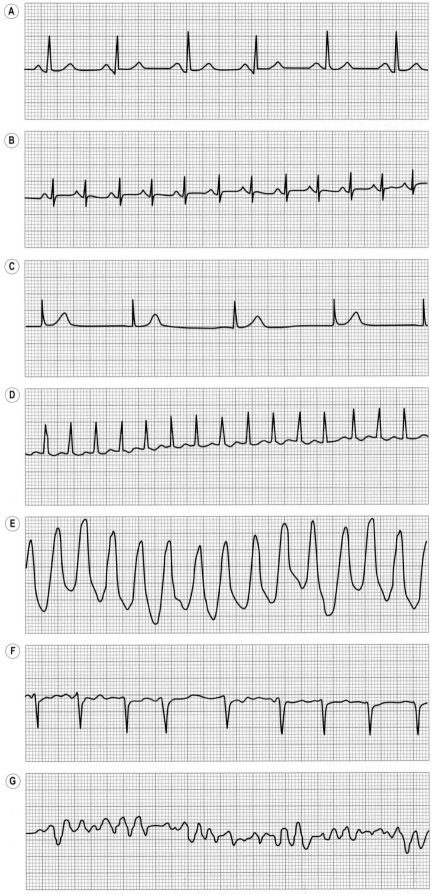

Fig. 11.23 **ECG examples of heart rhythm.** (A) Normal sinus rhythm; (B) sinus tachycardia; (C) nodal bradycardia; (D) supraventricular tachycardia; (E) ventricular tachycardia; (F) atrial fibrillation; (G) ventricular fibrillation.

Atrioventricular re-entrant tachycardia (AVRT) is a supraventricular tachycardia which can be difficult to distinguish from AVNRT on the ECG. It occurs in patients who have an abnormal, rapidly conducting electrical connection between the atria and ventricles called an **accessory pathway**. During the tachycardia, the re-entry circuit comprises antegrade (forward) conduction through the AV node and retrograde (backward) conduction through the accessory pathway. In sinus rhythm, ventricular depolarisation begins early via the accessory pathway (**pre-excitation**), but progression of the depolarisation wave through the ventricles is slow because it is not spread through the Purkinje system. This gives rise to a short PR interval and a slurred upstroke to the QRS complex which is called a **delta wave**. Conduction which occurred more slowly through the AV node now 'catches up' as it accelerates through the normal conducting system and rapidly completes depolarisation of the ventricles. The remainder of the QRS complex is therefore normal. Subjects who have evidence of pre-excitation on the ECG have **Wolff–Parkinson–White syndrome (WPW)**. The absence of pre-excitation on the ECG does not exclude the presence of an accessory pathway – antegrade conduction through the accessory pathway may be intermittent or absent in which case the accessory pathway is 'concealed', but the potential for arrhythmia remains. The development of atrial fibrillation is a particular concern in patients who have an accessory pathway, its short refractory period facilitating the conduction of atrial depolarisation waves to the ventricles. The patients are therefore vulnerable to very rapid ventricular rates which can degenerate into ventricular fibrillation. Pre-excited AF gives rise to an irregular tachycardia with broad QRS complexes due to the presence of delta waves.

Ventricular tachycardia (VT) is a life-threatening arrhythmia which causes a broad complex tachycardia of about 180–230 bpm (Fig. 11.23E). It is usually associated with left ventricular disease caused by ischaemic heart disease, dilated cardiomyopathy, or hypertrophic cardiomyopathy, but it can occur in structurally normal hearts when it more often arises from the right ventricular outflow tract. VT causes a reduction in cardiac output which may manifest as dizziness or syncope, angina, breathlessness, or cardiac arrest. Sustained VT causing haemodynamic compromise should be treated by direct current cardioversion.

The most dangerous arrhythmia is **ventricular fibrillation (VF)**. The fibrillating ventricles achieve no useful cardiac output and immediate cardiac arrest occurs, which is fatal unless electrical defibrillation is performed. The high voltage which passes through the heart has the effect of putting all the myocytes into the refractory period simultaneously. In many cases, the first cells to fire will be the pacemaker cells, which can then re-establish an organised heart rhythm. VF usually occurs in the context of severe myocardial ischaemia or myocardial infarction (MI) so patients with suspected MI require continuous ECG monitoring. The ECG shows a totally disorganised rhythm without recognisable QRS complexes (Fig. 11.23G). Patients who are at high risk of VT or VF remote from acute MI should receive an implantable cardioverter defibrillator.

Anti-arrhythmic drugs

The drugs used to treat cardiac arrhythmias, anti-arrhythmic drugs, affect heart rate and rhythm either by blocking ion channels that open during the action potential or by blocking the receptors that control heart rate. Clinical box 11.14 describes some of the drugs that affect heart rate. The **Vaughan–Williams classification** (Table 11.8) describes the effect of anti-arrhythmic drugs on the cardiac action potential. Anti-arrhythmic drugs, particularly class I and III agents, should be used with caution because their influence on the cardiac action potential paradoxically makes them pro-arrhythmic, patients with left ventricular disease being at highest risk.

Drugs which slow conduction in the AV node such as beta-adrenoreceptor antagonists (β-blockers), calcium blockers and digoxin are used to control rapid ventricular rates in patients with atrial fibrillation and atrial flutter. Class IA or IC anti-arrhythmic agents such as flecainide can be used to terminate acute AF and to maintain sinus rhythm in patients with paroxysmal AF. AVNRT or AVRT is usually terminated by intravenous adenosine or by intravenous verapamil. The management of ventricular arrhythmia is a complex area; sustained VT causing haemodynamic compromise requires urgent electrical cardioversion. Intravenous amiodarone or β-blockers can be used in patients with VT who are not haemodynamically compromised.

Therapeutic ablation is an option for tachyarrhythmias which are not adequately controlled by medical therapy. In this procedure, the arrhythmia is first mapped by an electrophysiological study. Then the arrhythmia substrate, for example an accessory pathway in AVRT, is destroyed by the application of heat energy (radiofrequency ablation) or cold energy (cryo ablation) to the endocardium.

Conduction disorders

Heart block (sometimes referred to as atrioventricular block) occurs when conduction through the AV node, the bundle of His, or the bundle branches is slow or completely interrupted (Fig. 11.24). This can be caused by fibrosis of the conduction

Table 11.8	Vaughan–Williams classification of anti-arrhythmic drugs		
Class	**Type of drug**	**Action**	**Examples**
Ia	Na$^+$ (open) channel blocker	Lengthens action potential	Quinidine, disopyramide
Ib	Na$^+$ (inactivated) channel blocker	Shortens action potential	Lidocaine, mexiletine
Ic	Na$^+$ (open) channel blocker	Slows upstroke and conduction speed	Flecainide
II	β-Adrenoceptor antagonist	Acts on sinoatrial node to block increases in the slope of the pacemaker potential and at the AV node to slow conduction	Propranolol, atenolol
III	K$^+$ channel blocker	Prolongs the action potential by slowing repolarisation	Amiodarone, sotalol
IV	Ca^{2+} channel blocker	Reduces conduction predominantly at the atrioventricular node	Verapamil, diltiazem

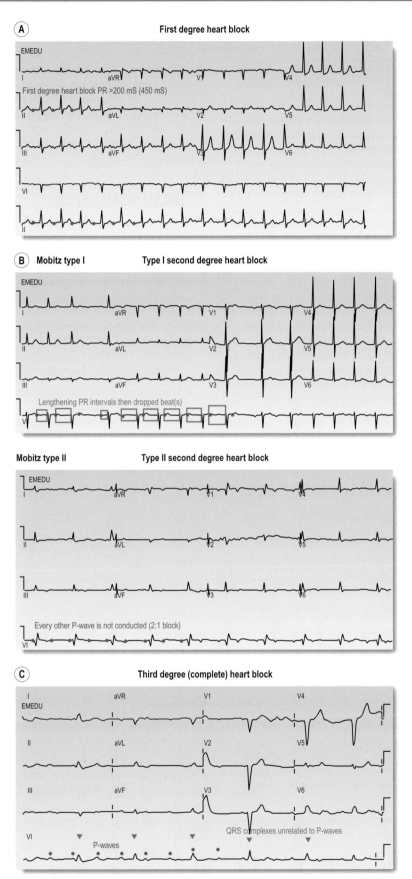

Fig. 11.24 **Heart block.** (A) First degree heart block; PR interval >200 ms. (B) Second degree heart block. Mobitz type I second degree heart block (Wenckebach): P wave conduction is intermittent; PR interval increases until a QRS complex is dropped. Mobitz type II second degree heart block: PR interval is constant, but not all P waves conduct to the ventricles. (C) Third degree (complete) heart block. There is complete failure of conduction of atrial depolarisation to the ventricles. Atrial and ventricular contraction are independent of each other. Here, the atrial rate is 86 bpm and the ventricular rate is 37 bpm.

system, drugs such as β-blockers, calcium blockers and digoxin, and acute myocardial infarction:

- **First-degree heart block** is defined by a PR interval longer than 200 mS. It is due to slowed conduction through the AV node.
- **Second-degree heart block** occurs when not every atrial depolarisation is transmitted to the ventricles. The ECG shows that some P waves are not followed by a corresponding QRS complex. There are two types of second-degree AV block; in Mobitz type I (also called the Wenckebach phenomenon), the PR interval becomes progressively longer until a P wave is not followed by a QRS complex. The PR interval then resets to normal and the cycle repeats itself. In Mobitz type II, the conducted beats have a constant PR interval. It is common for there to be a regular pattern of non-conducted P waves, for example every second P wave failing to trigger a QRS complex.
- **Third-degree (complete) heart block** occurs when there is total interruption of the transmission of electrical activity from the atria to the ventricles. The SA node continues to discharge P waves at a rate of 60–100 bpm. However, this has no impact on the ventricles, which contract at their own inherent rate of 30–40 bpm. The ECG shows no relationship between the P waves and QRS complexes.

Ventricular escape rhythms are unreliable, putting the patient at risk of ventricular standstill. Patients who have high grade (Mobitz type II or third degree) heart block should therefore be treated with a permanent pacemaker.

Failure of conduction in one of the bundle branches causes bundle branch block (Fig. 11.25). The QRS complexes are broad, reflecting slowed depolarisation in the affected ventricle. **Right bundle branch block** is present as a normal finding in about 5% of the population but it may also be caused by atrial septal defects, pulmonary embolism or coronary artery disease. **Left bundle branch block** is usually pathological and is caused by hypertension, aortic stenosis, hypertrophic or dilated cardiomyopthy, and coronary artery disease.

THE CARDIAC CYCLE

The coordinated sequence of events within the heart which culminates in the ejection of blood from the ventricles is known as the **cardiac cycle**. Each cycle comprises periods of cardiac chamber contraction, during which blood is expelled from a chamber – **systole** – and periods of myocardial relaxation, during which a chamber refills with blood – **diastole**. When unqualified, these terms refer to ventricular activity. The timing of ventricular systole and diastole can be determined from the ECG (Fig. 11.26A) and from the heart sounds (Fig. 11.26B and Clinical box 11.3).

The forward flow of blood through the heart requires:

- A pressure gradient from proximal to distal, which propels blood forwards
- An open inlet valve and a closed outlet valve during chamber filling
- A closed inlet valve and an open outlet valve during chamber contraction.

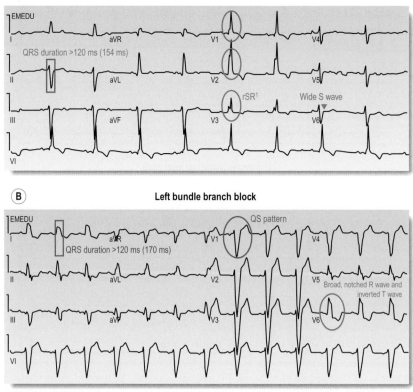

Fig. 11.25 **Bundle branch block.** (B) Left bundle branch block: wide QRS complexes (>120 ms), negative "QS" waves in leads V_1-V_3, notched or slurred R waves and T wave inversion in leads I, aVL, & V_5-V_6. (A) Right bundle branch block: wide QRS complexes (>120 ms), rSR¹ pattern in lead V_1, prominent S wave in lead V_6.

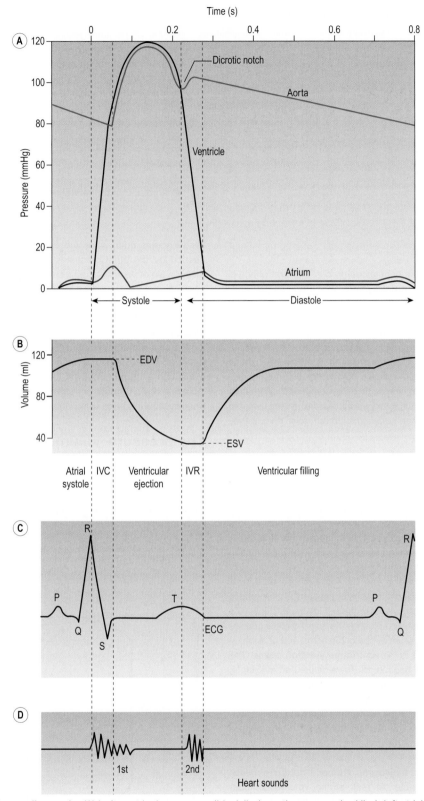

Fig. 11.26 The cardiac cycle. (A) Left ventricular pressure (*black line*), aortic pressure (*red line*), left atrial pressure (*blue line*); (B) left ventricular volume; (C) electrocardiogram (ECG); and (D) heart sounds. IVC, isovolumetric contraction; IVR, isovolumetric relaxation.

The opening and closing of the valves is determined by pressure changes in the heart related to chamber blood volume and myocardial contraction and relaxation. Valves open when the pressure in the proximal chamber exceeds the pressure in the distal chamber or vessel and they close when the pressure in the distal chamber or vessel falls below the pressure in the proximal chamber. There are five phases in each cardiac cycle (Fig. 11.26 and Table 11.9).

Table 11.9   Phases of the cardiac cycle

Phase of the cardiac cycle	Mitral and tricuspid valve position	Aortic and pulmonary valve position	Cardiac chamber physiology
Atrial systole	Open	Closed	Atria contract, blood is pumped into the ventricles
Isovolumetric ventricular contraction	Closed	Closed	Ventricular volumes unchanged, but ventricles begin to contract resulting in rapid rise in ventricular pressures
Ventricular systole (ejection)	Closed	Open	Ventricles contract fully and eject blood into the aorta and pulmonary artery
Isovolumetric ventricular relaxation	Closed	Closed	Ventricular volumes unchanged, ventricles relax. Rapid decrease in ventricular pressures. The atria are filling (atrial diastole)
Ventricular diastole (ventricular filling)	Open	Closed	Ventricles relaxed and passively fill with blood from the atria. Atrial contraction signals return to phase 1 of the cycle

Atrial systole

The cardiac cycle is a continuous process. Its first phase is arbitrarily defined by **atrial systole**, which occurs just after the P wave on the ECG (Fig. 11.26A). In sinus rhythm, atrial contraction occurs towards the end of ventricular diastole to augment ventricular filling (see Fig. 11.26D). In patients with AF, in whom atrial systole is absent, cardiac output can be reduced by 15–30%. Patients with 'stiff' ventricles (e.g. those with hypertensive heart disease, hypertrophic cardiomyopathy or aortic stenosis) are particularly dependent upon atrial augmentation for satisfactory ventricular filling and they are especially at risk of haemodynamic compromise should they develop AF.

Ventricular systole

Following atrial systole, the ventricles depolarise to initiate ventricular systole. This can be timed by the R wave of the QRS complex (Fig. 11.26A). As the ventricles contract, the intraventricular pressures rise rapidly above the atrial pressures, closing the mitral and tricuspid valves and preventing backflow of blood into the atria. The aortic and pulmonary valves are also closed during the initial phase of systole so the intraventricular volumes are constant – this phase is called **isovolumetric contraction** (Fig. 11.26C, D). The semilunar valves open and blood flows into the great arteries when ventricular pressure exceeds the aortic and pulmonary artery pressures; this is the **ventricular ejection phase**. The atria are relaxed and begin to fill. Towards the end of systole, the ventricular blood volumes are reduced, ventricular pressures fall until they are lower than the aortic and pulmonary artery pressures, when the semilunar valves close and ventricular systole ends. The **dicrotic notch** is the dip followed by a small rise in the aortic pressure trace that coincides with aortic valve closure.

Stroke volume is the volume of blood ejected from each ventricle during systole. At rest, stroke volume is about 70 mL. The ventricles do not empty completely; instead they contain about 50 mL blood at the end of systole, an amount known as the **end-systolic volume** (ESV).

Ventricular diastole

The ventricles are relaxed during diastole. Initially the AV valves and the semilunar valves are closed and ventricular volumes are constant – this phase is called **isovolumetric relaxation** (Fig. 11.26C, D). Ventricular pressures fall rapidly,

the AV valves open when the ventricular pressures are exceeded by the atrial pressures, and ventricular filling, the main phase of ventricular diastole, begins. This can be timed by the end of the T wave on the ECG. The flow of blood from atria to ventricles is predominantly a passive process and the majority of ventricular filling has occurred before the onset of atrial systole.

The **end-diastolic volume** (EDV) is the volume of blood in the ventricles at the end of ventricular filling. In normal hearts, this is about 120 mL, but both the EDV and the ESV may be influenced by a number of factors including myocardial contractility, afterload and valvular regurgitation (see below).

The pressure–volume loop

The changes in left ventricular (LV) pressure and volume which occur during the cardiac cycle are illustrated by the **pressure–volume loop** in Figure 11.27. The right ventricle will show a similar plot at lower pressures.

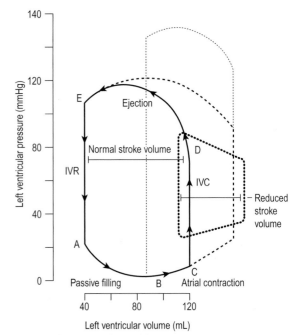

Fig. 11.27 Pressure–volume loop of the left ventricle. IVC, isovolumetric contraction; IVR, isovolumetric relaxation. For description of A–E, see text. *Solid line*, normal function; *dashed line*, increased end-diastolic volume (EDV); *dotted line*, increased EDV and increased arterial pressure.

During LV diastole:

- The ventricle fills passively when the mitral valve opens (A)
- The ventricle relaxes and distends so that its volume increases but pressure falls (A to B)
- A small rise in both LV pressure and volume occurs at the end of diastole when the atrium contracts (B to C).

During LV systole:

- Pressure increases at the start of systole due to isovolumetric contraction when the aortic valve is still closed (C to D)
- Opening of the aortic valve (D) and ventricular ejection leads to a decrease in ventricular volume
- Ventricular pressure falls abruptly with the closure of the aortic valve (E) due to isovolumetric relaxation and the loop returns to its original position (E to A)
- The distance between AE and CD represents the stroke volume.

The efficiency of the ventricle can be assessed from its pressure–volume loop. Increased venous return (e.g. during pregnancy, exercise, inspiration) or aortic or mitral regurgitation increases EDV but, so long as myocardial contractility is normal, stroke volume is increased (Fig. 11.27, *dashed line*) by the effects of 'pre-stretch' (see Starling's law, below). If, however, myocardial contractility is reduced due to dilated cardiomyopathy or prior myocardial infarction, for example, stroke volume is reduced and EDV and ventricular end-diastolic pressure are increased (Fig. 11.27, *dots*). If the afterload (the force against which the ventricle must contract) is increased by raised arterial pressure or raised systemic vascular resistance then the whole curve is shifted to the right (Fig. 11.27, *dotted line*). The ESV is raised and there is an increase in EDV but the stroke volume is reduced.

CARDIAC OUTPUT AND HEART FAILURE

Cardiac output (CO) is the volume of blood ejected by the heart in 1 minute. The heart must generate a cardiac output sufficient to meet the metabolic demands of the body. If it cannot achieve this without elevated filling pressures, or if cardiac output is low at normal filling pressures, then **heart failure** is present.

At rest, CO is approximately 5 L/min. However, CO varies widely between individuals, depending on body size and cardiac function, and within individuals, according to their metabolic requirements. CO can be corrected for body surface area when it is called the cardiac index. The cardiac index for an average-sized man at rest is about $2.8–3 \, \text{L/min/m}^2$. CO is dependent upon stroke volume (SV) and heart rate (HR) with the following relationship:

Cardiac output = stroke volume × heart rate

In sinus rhythm, heart rate is determined by the rate of discharge of the SA node. This is regulated by the autonomic nervous system with inputs from both sympathetic and parasympathetic fibres. At rest, acetylcholine released by parasympathetic fibres slows the pacemaker potential of the SA node, reducing heart rate. During physical activity or emotional stress, sympathetic fibres release norepinephrine, speeding up the pacemaker potential and increasing heart rate. Epinephrine and norepinephrine released from the adrenal medulla under sympathetic stimulation also increase the heart rate. An increase in heart rate results in a propor-

tional increase in cardiac output, if the stroke volume remains unchanged.

Stroke volume is dependent upon three main factors: preload, myocardial contractility and afterload. Preload is the degree to which myocardial muscle fibres are stretched prior to contraction. Myocardial contractility is the strength of contraction of the myocardium for a given preload. Afterload is the resistance which must be overcome for the ventricles to eject blood.

Preload

Preload can be thought of as the pressure which primes the ventricle in readiness for contraction. It is directly related to venous return and central venous pressure, and it is commonly referred to as the 'filling pressure'. In the absence of disease of the AV valves, venous pressure is equivalent to ventricular end-diastolic pressure. The amount of stretch in myocardial muscle fibres prior to contraction increases as venous pressure and ventricular end-diastolic pressure increases. The relation between stroke volume and preload is described by **Starling's law** (Fig. 11.28). An increase in preload stretches the cardiomyocytes prior to contraction, which results in greater force of contraction and an increase in stroke volume. However, there is a point at which a further rise in preload results in no further increase in stroke volume, and in fact stroke volume decreases if the muscle is overstretched. Cardiac output is directly related to stroke volume so, if heart rate is unchanged, an increase in preload increases cardiac output, within the limits described above.

Myocardial contractility

The stroke volume at a given preload, and the increase in stroke volume achieved for a given increase in preload, is dependent upon myocardial contractility. More contractile hearts achieve a larger stroke volume at any given preload and they have a steeper Starling's curve (see Fig. 11.28), achieving a greater increase in stroke volume for a given increase in preload. Conversely, hearts with lower contractility have a flatter Starling's curve. Myocardial contractility is increased by sympathetic activation and positive inotropic drugs (*blue line*) and reduced by acidosis, myocardial ischaemia and negative inotropes such as β-blockers and

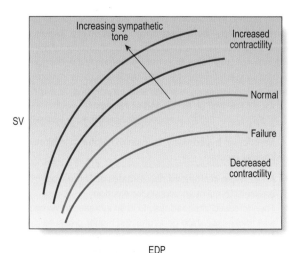

Fig. 11.28 Starling's curves. SV, stroke volume; EDP, end-diastolic pressure.

calcium channel blockers (*red line*). The failing heart also has a shallow Starling's curve – in the early stages of heart failure, an increase in preload produces a small increase in stroke volume, but as myocardial contractility decreases, further increases in end-diastolic pressure cannot be managed by the failing ventricle. This results in raised pulmonary and systemic venous pressures which promotes pulmonary oedema and peripheral oedema, respectively, due to increased net filtration of plasma in the capillaries.

Afterload

In order to eject blood, the heart must overcome the resistance to flow, or afterload, in the cardiovascular system. For the left ventricle, the afterload comprises the systemic vascular resistance (SVR), which is dependent upon the vascular tone in the systemic arterial circulation and the systemic arterial blood pressure. For the right ventricle, the afterload is the pulmonary vascular resistance, which is determined by vasoconstrictor tone in the pulmonary circulation and by the pulmonary artery pressure. If the pressure in the aorta is increased, left ventricular stroke volume is reduced and ESV is increased (Fig. 11.27). This is because the rate of cardiac myocyte contraction reduces as afterload increases but the ejection time is unchanged. If the ESV is increased, the blood remaining in the heart increases the EDV of the next beat and Starling's Law means that the stroke volume of the following beat will be increased. This is sufficient to maintain cardiac output but a high afterload increases the work of the heart and if the cardiomyocytes become overstretched due to a chronically raised afterload, heart failure occurs.

The effectiveness of ventricular ejection is also affected by wall tension and heart size. The relationship between the pressure (*P*) inside a sphere, wall tension (*T*) and the radius (*r*) is described by **Laplace's law:**

$$P = 2T / r$$

Although not spherical, a similar relationship exists in the ventricles. As ventricular volume (*r*) increases, the efficiency of ventricular ejection decreases because a greater tension is needed in the ventricular wall to maintain the pressure for ejecting blood.

Ventricular hypertrophy

The heart muscle responds to a chronic increase in afterload like any other muscle which repeatedly contracts against an increased load – by **hypertrophy** or becoming thicker. The hypertrophy is due to an increase in the thickness of the individual myocytes rather than through hyperplasia, an increase in the number of myocytes. Wall thickness (*h*) is inversely related to wall stress (δ), the wall tension per muscle width), so Laplace's law can be expressed as follows:

$$\delta = P \times r / 2h$$

Ventricular hypertrophy is initially helpful in maintaining ventricular ejection;

- An increase in afterload necessitates an increased pressure to maintain ventricular ejection
- The increased afterload results in an increase in ventricular wall thickness, which generates the higher pressure
- The inverse relation between wall thickness and wall stress means that the ventricular hypertrophy maintains a normal wall stress despite the increased ventricular pressure.

Ventricular hypertrophy has two important negative consequences. Firstly, myocardial oxygen requirements are increased and, secondly, compliance, or the ability of the heart muscle to stretch, is reduced. Reduced compliance impairs ventricular filling and increases ventricular end-diastolic pressure for a given end-diastolic volume. Increased left ventricular end-diastolic pressure is transmitted to the left atrium and pulmonary veins. This predisposes to pulmonary oedema even in the presence of maintained left ventricular contractility. Systemic arterial hypertension and aortic stenosis are the most common causes of an increase in afterload on the left ventricle. If right ventricular end-diastolic pressure is increased, this causes an increase in right atrial and central venous pressure, which promotes the development of systemic oedema. The most common cause of increased right ventricular afterload is pulmonary arterial hypertension.

In the long term, the hypertrophied ventricle may not be able to compensate for an increased afterload and heart failure occurs. The increased ventricular end-diastolic volume causes an increase in end-diastolic pressure beyond the 'tipping point' of the Starling curve, reducing ventricular contractility. The increased end-diastolic volume ultimately results in ventricular dilatation and, according to Laplace's law, wall stress also increases in relation to the dilated ventricle (as a consequence of the increased *r*).

Causes of heart failure

In the large majority of cases, heart failure occurs due to a reduced cardiac output. In **systolic heart failure**, this is due to reduced contractile function of the ventricle. By contrast, in **diastolic heart failure** (also called heart failure with preserved systolic function), systolic ventricular function is normal or near normal but the ventricle is non-compliant and 'stiff', which results in reduced left ventricular filling. Rarely, heart failure is due to the inability of the heart to maintain a high cardiac output demanded by increased metabolic requirements (e.g. in severe anaemia or thyrotoxicoisis) or by a large arteriovenous shunt. This is termed high output heart failure.

The causes of heart failure can be grouped according to the underlying mechanism for heart failure (Table 11.10). The most common causes of heart failure are ischaemic heart disease, hypertension, cardiomyopathies and valve disease. In ischaemic heart disease and dilated cardiomyopathy, the primary mechanism is reduced left ventricular contractility, Starling's curve is shifted downwards (Fig. 11.28, *red line*) and there is a lower stroke volume for any EDV. In hypertension and aortic stenosis, the main problem is an increased afterload on the left ventricle (see above), but the consequent development of left ventricular hypertrophy also causes reduced compliance and left ventricular filling. Aortic and mitral regurgitation place an additional volume load on the left ventricle, which ultimately causes it to fail.

Pathophysiological mechanisms activated by heart failure

The body continuously monitors parameters which are vital to its normal functioning, such as blood pressure and renal blood flow. Several cardiovascular reflexes and neurohormonal pathways are activated by heart failure in an attempt to restore the body's functions to normal (Information box 11.7). These homeostatic mechanisms are the same as those activated by hypovolaemic shock (see below). In hypovolaemic

Table 11.10	Causes of heart failure
Mechanism	**Condition**
Reduced myocardial contractility	Ischaemic heart disease
	Dilated cardiomyopathy
	Myocarditis
Increased afterload (pressure overload)	Hypertension
	Aortic stenosis
	Mitral stenosis
	Pulmonary hypertension
Increased preload (volume overload)	Aortic regurgitation
	Mitral regurgitation
	Left to right shunts
Restricted filling	Hypertrophic cardiomyopathy
	Restrictive cardiomyopathy
	Constrictive pericarditis
Arrhythmia	Severe tachycardias
	Severe bradycardias
High output states	Severe chronic anaemia
	Thyrotoxicosis
	Systemic arteriovenous fistula

Information box 11.7 **Pathophysiological mechanisms activated in heart failure**

- **Activation of the sympathetic nervous system**. Reduced blood pressure results in increased sympathetic outflow from the brainstem. This stimulates cardiac β-adrenoreceptors which helps to restore cardiac output through an increase in heart rate and myocardial contractility. Blood pressure is maintained through α-adrenoceptor-mediated vasoconstriction.
- **Stimulation of the renin–angiotensin–aldosterone system**. Reduced renal perfusion results in increased secretion of renin which promotes the synthesis of angiotensin II and aldosterone. Angiotensin II causes vasoconstriction and aldosterone increases salt and water retention.
- **Increased venous return** through venoconstriction and sodium and water retention increases venous pressure and thereby cardiac output according to Starling's law.

shock, maintenance of blood pressure and blood volume is central to homeostasis and this is achieved through vasoconstriction, tachycardia and salt and water retention. In acute heart failure, these mechanisms may help to maintain cardiac output and blood pressure, but their chronic activation is responsible for many of the symptoms and signs of heart failure. In the long-term, vasoconstriction increases afterload and myocardial work and increased circulating levels of catecholamines may have a direct toxic effect on the myocardium.

Activation of the renin–angiotensin–aldosterone system causes salt and water retention through the action of aldosterone on the distal convoluted tubule in the kidneys. The low cardiac output of the failing heart is unable to cope with the increased blood volume without an increase in venous pressures. High venous pressures translate into an increased hydrostatic pressure, which tends to force water out of the capillaries. In the lungs, this results initially in interstitial oedema and, at higher pulmonary venous pressures, in alveolar oedema and pleural effusions. Pulmonary venous pressure is increased further by lying down which accounts for the classical heart failure symptoms of orthopnoea and paroxysmal

nocturnal dyspnoea. High systemic venous pressure promotes the formation of peripheral oedema, liver congestion, and ascites. The increased pressure in the right atrium supports a taller column of blood than normal, which extends from the right atrium up into the internal jugular veins. This is visible clinically as an elevated jugular venous pressure (JVP).

Treatment of heart failure

The cause for heart failure should be identified and treated. For example, patients who have ischaemic heart disease should receive secondary prevention therapy including antiplatelet therapy and a statin. Left ventricular function may be improved in selected patients with viable myocardium by myocardial revascularisation. Hypertensive patients should have their blood pressure controlled. Corrective valve surgery is indicated for patients whose heart failure is caused by a primary valve lesion.

The main symptomatic treatment for heart failure is with loop diuretics such as furosemide. These promote salt and water loss and aim to restore a normal circulating volume and venous pressure. Angiotensin converting enzyme (ACE) inhibitors, angiotensin II receptor blockers, β-blockers and aldosterone antagonists has been shown to improve prognosis in patients with systolic heart failure. They all target some aspect of the maladaptive physiological mechanisms which are activated by heart failure (Information box 11.8).

Information box 11.8 **Mechanism of action for drugs used to treat heart failure**

- **Inhibition of sympathetic activation:** β-adrenoreceptor antagonists (β-blockers), e.g. bisoprolol, metoprolol slow release and carvedilol, improve survival in patients with systolic heart failure. They reduce heart rate, prolong diastole and thereby increase ventricular filling. Ivabradine is a newer drug which slows the heart by directly inhibiting the sinoatrial node and this has also been shown to improve prognosis.
- **Inhibition of the renin–angiotensin–aldosterone system:** angiotensin converting enzyme (ACE) inhibitors, e.g. ramipril, and angiotensin II receptor blockers (ARBs), e.g. candesartan, reduce afterload through the inhibition of the production and action, respectively, of angiotensin II, a potent vasoconstrictor. ACE inhibitors reduce the conversion of angiotensin I to angiotensin II while ARBs inhibit the effect of angiotensin II at receptor level. Aldosterone antagonists, e.g. spironolactone, bind to the aldosterone-dependent Na^+/K^+ exchange pump in the distal convoluted renal tubule. This promotes sodium and water excretion. These three classes of drug have been shown to improve survival rates in systolic heart failure.
- **Reduction in preload:** loop diuretics, e.g. furosemide, inhibit sodium and water reabsorption in the distal limb of the loop of Henle, reducing blood volume, venous return and preload. The reduction in hydrostatic pressure in the capillaries encourages reabsorption of fluid from the extracellular space, reducing pulmonary and peripheral oedema. Diuretics are the mainstay of treatment for symptoms of 'volume overload' but they have not been shown to influence prognosis in heart failure
- **Increased myocardial contractility**: digoxin, which is extracted from the foxglove (*Digitalis* sp.), inhibits the Na^+/K^+-ATPase of the plasma membrane. The increase in intracellular sodium concentration changes the activity of the Na^+/Ca^{2+} exchange pump so that the intracellular calcium concentration rises. This promotes the release of calcium from the sarcoplasmic reticulum during excitation-contraction coupling, thus increasing muscle contractility.

Clinical box 11.16	Cardiac resynchronisation therapy for heart failure

Cardiac resynchronisation therapy, or CRT, is a treatment which is indicated in patients who have symptomatic (New York Heart Association class II–IV) heart failure, a left ventricular ejection fraction <35%, and a broad QRS complex on their ECG. The treatment is based on the theory that patients in this group not only have impaired systolic function, but the bundle branch block also indicates dyssynchronous ventricular contraction which can be resynchronised by implantation of a biventricular pacemaker. This procedure involves the transvenous placement of a pacing lead in the right ventricle (as for a standard pacemaker), but a second 'ventricular' pacing lead is also placed in a branch of the coronary sinus which runs on the posterior aspect of the heart and which can therefore be used to pace the left ventricle. The ventricle which demonstrates delayed depolarisation is paced and pacemaker programming can be optimised by studying the effects of different atrioventricular and interventricular delays on echocardiographic parameters of cardiac haemodynamics. Randomised controlled trials of CRT and medical therapy compared with medical therapy alone have shown symptomatic and prognostic benefits from CRT in severe left ventricular dysfunction but only some patients respond to the treatment. The challenge remains to identify the patients who are most likely to benefit from CRT.

Not only do these drugs reduce mortality rates, they also reduce symptoms and hospital admissions. Some patients who have severely impaired systolic left ventricular function (left ventricular ejection fraction <35%) also benefit from a pacemaker-based therapy called cardiac resynchronisation therapy (or CRT; see Clinical box 11.16).

No treatment has yet been shown to improve the prognosis in patients who have heart failure with preserved systolic function. Treatment of these patients is directed towards symptom relief with diuretics. AF is common in these patients, who should be anticoagulated to reduce their risk of thromboembolic stroke.

BLOOD VESSELS

The circulatory system transports nutrients and metabolites to and from the tissues and organs through a network of blood vessels (Fig. 11.29A) that comprises:

- Arteries, which carry blood away from the heart
- Capillaries, which enable the exchange of nutrients and metabolites between blood and tissues
- Veins, which carry blood from the tissues and organs back to the heart.

THE VESSEL WALL

Arteries and veins have a similar basic structure which comprises a vessel wall made up of three layers, the tunica intima, tunica media and tunica adventitia, around a central lumen (Fig. 11.29B). The main difference between the two types of vessel is that the tunica media is considerably thicker in arteries than in veins.

- **Tunica intima:** the innermost and thinnest layer that lines the lumen. It is composed of a single layer of endothelium which is in contact with the blood and a thin layer of subendothelial connective tissue. This is surrounded by the **internal elastic lamina**, a layer of circularly arranged elastic fibres. Movement of blood cells and large molecules out of the circulation is prevented by **tight junctions** between the endothelial cells. Endothelial cells secrete many substances which affect vasoconstrictor tone and vascular permeability. They also play an important role in blood clotting (see Ch. 12) and in the growth of new blood vessels.
- **Tunica media:** this middle layer is the muscular component of the vessel wall, and the thickest layer in arteries. Smooth muscle cells are arranged in circular and spiral layers which are supported by elastic fibres

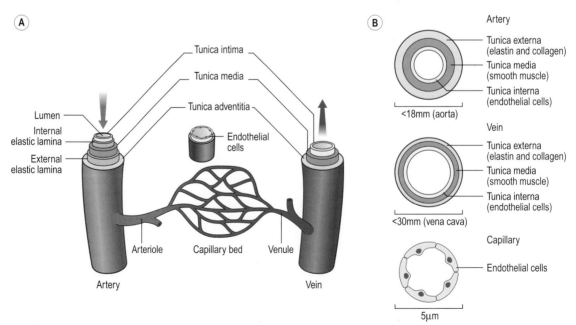

Fig. 11.29 **(A) The overall network of blood vessels. (B) Structure of arteries, veins and capillaries.** The tunica media is thicker in arteries than in veins. Capillary walls consist of a thin layer of endothelium and lack smooth muscle.

and collagen. Vascular smooth muscle is supplied by sympathetic nerve fibres which regulate the caliber of the vessel. Sympathetic vasoconstrictor tone is a key determinant of arterial blood pressure and capacitance of the systemic veins. The tunica media is separated from the outer layer by a thick layer of elastic tissue called the **external elastic lamina**.

- **Tunica adventitia:** also known as the **tunica externa**, this outermost layer is comprised entirely by connective tissues. It is the thickest of the three layers in veins. In larger blood vessels, the tunica adventitia contains small blood vessels known as **vasa vasorum** which supply the vessel wall with oxygen and nutrients.

Capillaries have a much thinner wall which is made up of a thin layer of endothelium, some connective tissue and a basement membrane (see below). They lack smooth muscle.

Arteries

Arteries receive blood at high pressure from the heart and distribute it around the body in a network comprised by three types of vessel:

- Elastic or conducting arteries
- Muscular or distributing arteries
- Arterioles.

The different functions of these vessels are reflected by the composition of their arterial wall (Fig. 11.30).

Elastic arteries are the large (1–2 cm diameter) vessels that leave the heart. The aorta and pulmonary arteries and their major branches expand when blood is ejected during ventricular systole and recoil when the pressure falls during diastole. This transforms the intermittent cardiac ejection into a smooth arterial blood flow to the periphery, maintaining diastolic pressure at about 80 mmHg. The tunica media contains a large number of elastic fibres which enables the expansion while the tunica adventitia is mainly collagen which prevents overstretching. These arteries are known as conducting arteries because their large lumen provides low-resistance pathways which conduct blood from the heart to medium-sized arteries.

Muscular arteries are small to medium (1 mm – 1 cm diameter) vessels whose main role is the distribution of blood to target organs. They have a thicker tunica media which

contains a higher proportion of smooth muscle than elastic arteries. This enables tight regulation of blood flow through rapid changes in vessel calibre in response to metabolic demands for energy.

Small arteries and arterioles are the terminal branches of the arterial system. They control local blood to the tissues and provide the **peripheral resistance** in the circulation. The larger (100–500 μm diameter) arterioles contain all three layers in their walls, but the smaller (20–30 μm diameter) ones that lead to capillary beds contain only smooth muscle around the endothelial lining. The contractile tone in this muscle is regulated by metabolites, hormones and the sympathetic nervous system (see below). End products of metabolism, e.g. nitric oxide (NO), cause relaxation of vascular smooth muscle, leading to local vasodilatation and increased blood flow to match energy requirements.

Veins

Microscopic venules drain blood from capillary beds and merge with progressively larger veins before entering the heart as the vena cavae. The walls of veins contain less muscle than arteries because they do not have to withstand the much higher pressures of the arterial system. The tunica adventitia, however, is thick which provides veins with a large degree of stretch. This enables them to act as blood reservoirs, the volume of which can be altered to regulate the effective circulating volume. The venous system contains about 70% of blood volume so constriction of these capacitance vessels can produce a large increase in venous return and cardiac output.

Upon standing, gravity creates a tendency for blood to pool in the veins of the legs. The veins of the legs contain semi-lunar valves which are formed from the tunica intima. They allow the forward flow of blood towards the heart, but prevent the back flow of blood due to gravity. Defects in these valves and/or increased pressure in the veins can lead to overstretching of the vessel walls, resulting in incompetence of the valves. Backflow of blood causes distended veins known as varicosities or varicose veins. Venous return from the legs is aided by the rhythmical muscular activity which occurs during walking, when the squeezing of the veins due to muscle shortening forces blood towards the heart (Fig. 11.31).

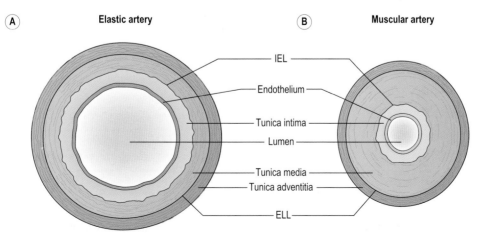

Fig. 11.30 **Structure of (A) elastic and (B) muscular arteries.** EEL, external elastic lamina; IEL, internal elastic lamina.

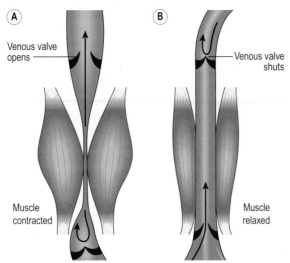

Fig. 11.31 **Skeletal muscle pump**. When the muscle contracts, blood is pushed towards the heart (A); when the muscle relaxes the vein refills from below (B). Competent valves ensure unidirectional blood flow.

ATHEROSCLEROSIS

The most common pathology to affect the arteries is **atherosclerosis**. This is a disease of large- and medium-sized arteries which involves the accumulation of lipid-rich material in the tunica intima. The fundamental pathological finding is the **atherosclerotic** or **atheromatous plaque**. This consists of a cholesterol core covered by a fibrous cap on its luminal side (Fig. 11.32). It is asymptomatic in its early stages of development. Clinical manifestations occur when arterial blood flow is reduced by stenotic plaques or by episodes of plaque rupture (see below). Atherosclerosis is the pathology that underlies coronary heart disease (CHD), carotid artery disease and peripheral arterial disease. Atherosclerotic conditions are therefore a common cause of death and morbidity.

Evolution of the atherosclerotic plaque

The first visible stage in the formation of atheromatous plaques is the development of **fatty streaks,** areas of yellow discolouration on the luminal aspect of the aorta and other large arteries. Fatty streaks are present in most individuals at 1 year of age, and cover about 10% of the aorta by 10 years. In some individuals, these streaks show no further development, whereas in others they develop into plaques by about 30 years of age. Genetic and environmental factors are important in determining which individuals develop atherosclerosis. Some degree of atherosclerosis is an almost universal occurrence in people from Western societies. Exposure to Western diets and a higher prevalence of smoking has resulted in increasing rates of atherosclerotic conditions in developing countries.

Three main stages are involved in the development of atherosclerotic plaques:

1. Endothelial damage
2. Uptake of modified **low-density lipoprotein (LDL)** particles, adhesion and infiltration of macrophages
3. Smooth muscle proliferation and formation of the fibrous cap.

Endothelial damage

Damage to the luminal endothelium is thought to be a key early event in plaque formation. Several factors have been implicated in this process:

- Shear stress – plaques do not occur uniformly throughout the arterial system; they are more common at points where arteries branch, where blood flow is turbulent and levels of shear stress on the endothelium are high (Fig. 11.33). Shear stress is also increased by hypertension, one of the main risk factors for the development of atherosclerosis.
- Toxic damage - e.g. by the chemicals in cigarette smoke.
- Exposure to high concentrations of LDL-cholesterol – such as in familial and other forms of hypercholesterolaemia.
- Glycosylation of proteins – in diabetes mellitus.

Uptake of modified LDL particles, adhesion and infiltration of macrophages

Damaged endothelium loses its ability to restrict the movement of circulating lipoproteins from the blood into the subendothelial layers of the artery wall. Lipoproteins carry lipid and other products around the body. They are categorised into five major classes depending on their

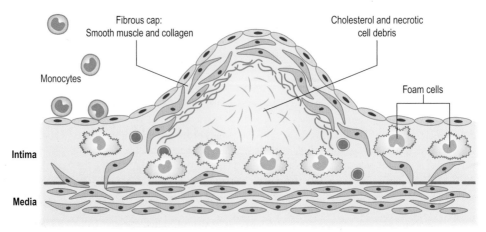

Fig. 11.32 **An atheromatous plaque.** The fibrous cap overlies the cholesterol-rich core. Rupture of the cap exposes collagen and stimulates thrombus formation.

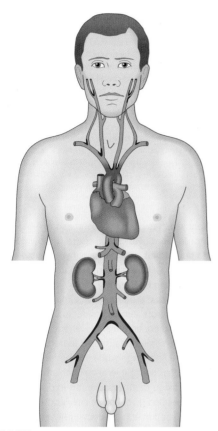

Fig. 11.33 **Common sites of atheroma formation,** shown in *blue*.

Table 11.11	Different types of lipoprotein	
Lipoprotein	**Main constituents**	**Notes**
Chylomicrons	Triacylglycerols (90%)	Carry dietary lipids from the intestine to the peripheral tissues from where their remnants go to the liver
VLDL (very-low-density lipoprotein)	Triacylglycerols (50%)	Produced in the liver from endogenous lipids which are carried to peripheral tissues
IDL (intermediate-density lipoprotein)	Cholesterol (30%)	Produced from VLDL remnants, these are then converted to LDL
LDL (low-density lipoprotein)	Cholesterol (50%)	Produced from IDL, carries cholesterol from the liver to peripheral tissues
HDL (high-density lipoprotein)	Phospholipid (30%), cholesterol (30%)	Transport cholesterol from peripheral tissues to the liver

source, size, lipid constituents and associated apoproteins (Table 11.11) (see also Ch. 3). They are modified through the action of lipoprotein lipases, which remove fatty acids, reduce the size of the lipoproteins, and increase the proportion of cholesterol, phospholipid and protein. Low-density lipoproteins have a high concentration of cholesterol, which they transport from the liver to the tissues, while high-density lipoproteins (HDL) transport cholesterol from the tissues to the liver.

LDL enters the artery wall through damaged endothelium. LDL is prone to **oxidation** by reactive oxygen species such as those produced by smoking, and **glycation** by the high glucose levels which occur in diabetes mellitus. The presence of modified LDL in the artery wall stimulates the overlying endothelial cells to express inflammatory mediators which attract inflammatory cells. Adhesion molecules bind monocytes which then cross the endothelium where they are transformed into macrophages.

Under normal conditions, macrophages ingest LDL using LDL-receptor-mediated endocytosis. The LDL receptor on the cell surface recognises apolipoprotein B-100, which is present in lipoproteins VLDL, IDL and LDL. The levels of LDL are controlled by a negative feedback mechanism, by which internal accumulation of LDL downregulates the LDL receptor numbers, reducing LDL uptake. By contrast, modified LDL is taken into phagocytic macrophages via a scavenger receptor which is not subject to downregulation of its surface numbers. High concentrations of modified LDL therefore result in its unrestricted uptake by the subendothelial macrophages, where it accumulates in large droplets known as **foam cells**. Lipids are released from foam cells when they die and accumulate in the subendothelial space.

Smooth muscle proliferation and formation of fibrous cap

The development of a mature plaque is caused by growth factors released by the damaged endothelial cells and macrophages. These growth factors cause the proliferation of smooth muscle cells which cover the plaque on its luminal aspect, and the deposition of collagen in the intima. The internal elastic lamina is broken down and pressure on the media causes muscle atrophy and an increase in collagen. Some smooth muscle cells become foam cells by the uptake of modified LDL.

In the early stages of plaque development, the arterial wall expands outwards to accommodate the accumulated lipid without encroaching into the vessel lumen – this is called positive remodelling. As the volume of plaque increases, however, it bulges inwards, reducing the luminal area (Fig. 11.32). The point of narrowing of the vessel lumen is called a stenosis. If the stenosis is severe enough to obstruct blood flow, then it may cause **ischaemia** – episodes during which the delivery of oxygen to a tissue is insufficient to meet its metabolic demands. Ischaemia of the myocardium caused by atherosclerotic narrowings of the coronary arteries causes chest pain called **angina** while stenoses in the arteries supplying the lower limbs causes ischaemic leg cramps provoked by walking called **claudication**.

Plaque rupture

The fibrous cap separates the plaque's lipid core from the bloodstream. The cap is prone to fissuring, erosion, or rupture, which exposes the lipid core to the blood. This triggers platelet activation and aggregation, and thrombus formation (see Ch. 12). If the thrombus causes complete occlusion of the affected artery, the usual result is infarction (cell death) of the supplied tissue or organ. Sub-occlusive thrombus may cause acute ischaemia or, if parts of the thrombus break off (**embolise**) to block smaller, distal arterial branches, small areas of infarction may arise. Through these mechanisms, episodes of plaque rupture are responsible for acute cardiovascular events; plaque rupture events in the coronary arteries are responsible for unstable angina and myocardial infarction while strokes and transient ischaemic attacks are caused by plaque events in the carotid arteries. Only a minority of plaque ruptures are manifest clinically and healed plaque ruptures are responsible for episodes of acute progression of atherosclerotic stenoses. Plaques which have a thin fibrous cap, a large lipid pool and a large inflammatory cell infiltrate are at greatest risk of rupture.

Risk factors for atherosclerosis

A number of factors have been identified which increase the risk of developing atherosclerotic conditions such as coronary heart disease. These can be divided into non-modifiable factors and factors that can be altered or even eliminated through drug treatment or lifestyle changes.

Non-modifiable risk factors

Risk factors for atherosclerosis that cannot be modified by drug treatment or changes in lifestyle are:

- **Age**: advancing age is the single most important risk factor for the development of atherosclerotic conditions. However, it is clear that many factors modulate the effect of age – young subjects in their 30s can develop myocardial infarction, while vascular disease is not an inevitable occurrence in the elderly.
- **Gender**: men are at higher risk than women of the same age. The risk in women increases after the menopause and the coexistence of diabetes removes much of the premenopausal protection. It is presumed that there is a hormonal basis for the different risks in men and women but the exact reasons are not known. Randomised trials of hormone (oestrogen) replacement therapy have not shown a reduced risk of cardiovascular events in postmenopausal women.
- **Family history**: a history of CHD in first degree relatives increases the risk of CHD by about 60%. It is thought that many different genes contribute to the increased susceptibility.
- **Racial origin**: individuals from South Asian countries (Bangladesh, India, Pakistan and Sri Lanka) have an increased risk of atherosclerotic diseases which is not accounted for by their higher rates of diabetes mellitus.

Modifiable risk factors

The following risk factors for atherosclerosis can be modified favourably by lifestyle changes and/or drugs with the expectation of reducing cardiovascular risk:

- **Lipids**: cardiovascular risk is directly related to levels of serum LDL cholesterol and inversely related to levels of serum HDL cholesterol. Western diets, diabetes mellitus and genetically inherited lipid disorders such as **familial hypercholesterolaemia** (Clinical box 11.17) are important influences on lipid concentrations. Lipid profiles can be improved through dietary modification but it was not until the advent of statin drug therapy that large reductions in LDL cholesterol could be achieved on a consistent basis.
- **Smoking**: one of the main risk factors for premature CHD, smoking increases reactive oxygen species which damage the endothelium. Nicotine is also toxic to endothelium. Smoking increases LDL, reduces HDL and increases the thrombogenicity of blood. Smoking cessation is one of the most effective measures for reducing risk in individuals and at a population level.

| **Clinical box 11.17** | **Familial hypercholesterolaemia** |

Disorders of lipid metabolism can lead to premature coronary heart disease (see Ch. 3, Clinical box 3.19). The most common lipid disorder is **familial hypercholesterolaemia**, which is an inherited autosomal dominant condition. Mutations of the gene for the LDL receptor, located on chromosome 19, cause a reduction in the number of LDL receptors. LDL cholesterol uptake in the liver is reduced and circulating levels of LDL (and intermediate density lipoprotein – IDL) are elevated. Heterozygotes for the mutation have a prevalence of about 1 in 500, they typically have a plasma cholesterol concentration >7.5 mmol/L and develop CHD aged <55. Homozygotes occur with a frequency of one per million population, they have a cholesterol >10 mmol/L and develop vascular disease as children or young adults.

- **Hypertension**: has been proposed as the most important risk factor for cardiovascular disease worldwide. Closely linked to cerebrovascular disease, hypertension is also a risk factor for CHD. Risk is reduced by effective blood pressure lowering treatment.
- **Diabetes mellitus**: the protective effect against atherosclerosis from female gender is lost in diabetes. In both sexes, diabetic patients without prior myocardial infarction have similar death rates to non-diabetic patients of the same age who have had a prior myocardial infarction. Several mechanisms underlie the predisposition to atherosclerosis in diabetic patients: increased glycation of cellular proteins (advanced glycation end products), a typical pattern of dyslipidaemia (raised LDL cholesterol, low HDL cholesterol, raised triglycerides), endothelial dysfunction and increased thrombogenicity all contribute. **Insulin resistance** without diabetes also increases risk. Good blood glucose control reduces the microvascular complications of diabetes but the evidence for a reduction in CHD events is disappointing.
- **Obesity**: the individual contribution of obesity to the risk of atherosclerotic conditions is confounded by its association with other key risk factors such as insulin resistance, diabetes and hyperlipidaema. Central obesity, in particular, where large amounts of fat are stored around the abdominal organs, however, appears to be a risk factor for atherosclerosis independent of raised blood glucose and lipid concentrations.
- **Lack of exercise**: the same confounding issues exist for a sedentary lifestyle. However, exercise favourably alters the LDL:HDL balance, lowers blood pressure, reduces insulin resistance and improves general cardiac function.

Markers of risk

Several other factors are associated with the occurrence of atherosclerotic events independent of the conventional risk factors described above. However, a causative role in the pathogenesis of atherosclerosis has not been established. They are currently best considered to be markers of risk:

- **Increased plasma C-reactive protein**: inflammation is considered to play an important role in the aetiology of atherosclerosis. Inflammatory cells are present in atherosclerotic plaques and pathological examination of ruptured plaques shows an intense inflammatory infiltrate. CRP concentration is associated with the occurrence of CHD, ischaemic stroke and cardiovascular death. In one trial, a reduction in the rate of cardiovascular events was achieved in patients with an elevated high sensitivity CRP but no established atherosclerotic disease by potent statin therapy.

- **Increased plasma homocysteine**: observational studies showed an association between high levels of plasma homocysteine and premature CHD. Randomised trials, however, have not demonstrated any protective effect from reducing plasma homocysteine concentration through the administration of B vitamins or folate.
- **Increased plasma fibrinogen**: similarly, increased plasma levels of fibrinogen have been associated with the occurrence of atherosclerotic cardiovascular events but interventions to lower fibrinogen have not been shown to affect prognosis.

Prevention and treatment of atherosclerosis

As many of the risk factors for atherosclerosis are modifiable by changes in lifestyle and/or drug therapies, this disease process is ideally suited to preventive strategies. Measures aimed at the prevention of a disease or its clinical manifestations are called **primary prevention** whereas the prevention of disease progression or recurrent clinical events in patients who already have the disease is called **secondary prevention**.

Increasing efforts are being made to prevent the development of atherosclerosis and subsequent heart disease at a population level. Government initiatives include increased taxation and public information campaigns aimed at reducing smoking, increasing exercise and healthy eating (five portions of fruit or vegetables per day, as well as reducing dietary fat and sugar intake). The substantial decrease in cardiovascular mortality rates in Western Europe over the last 30 years has probably been largely due to reduced rates of smoking. The increasing prevalence of obesity and diabetes, particularly in younger age groups, however, is a threat to the improved health of Western populations.

These same lifestyle measures should be employed in individual subjects in order to prevent the development of atherosclerotic vascular disease. In individuals who are at high risk for the development of vascular disease in whom lifestyle measures prove insufficient, drug therapy can be used for primary prevention. Individual risk factors have their own thresholds above which treatment is indicated. For example, a persistently raised blood pressure >160/90 mmHg requires anti-hypertensive therapy, and a total cholesterol:HDL ratio >6 requires lipid lowering therapy to reduce cardiovascular risk. Below these treatment thresholds, the decision regarding whether or not to advise primary prevention therapy is determined by the patient's overall cardiovascular risk, which can be estimated using charts which incorporate age, sex, smoking status, cholesterol:HDL ratio and blood pressure. More sophisticated, web-based cardiovascular risk calculators such as QRISK-2 are now available which include important additional risk factors like premature CHD in a first degree relative, racial origin and postcode as a marker of social deprivation. The current UK guidelines recommend drug therapy for primary prevention for individuals whose 10-year risk of an adverse cardiovascular event (stroke, heart attack, or death) exceeds 20%. Diabetic patients should be treated with primary preventive drug therapy irrespective of their estimated risk because they are known to be at high risk of adverse cardiovascular events. Whether or not primary preventive drug therapy should be given more widely, e.g. to all subjects over a certain age, is not clear (see Information box 11.9).

Information box 11.9 | **Universal primary prevention using a 'polypill'**

Many patients do not know they have atherosclerosis until they have a heart attack or stroke. In a significant proportion of patients, the first presentation of CHD is a fatal myocardial infarction. It has therefore been suggested that large numbers of people without obvious heart disease should take a statin to reduce their risk of developing atherosclerosis. A further development on this idea is the 'polypill', which contains a statin and three anti-hypertensive drugs in low dose with or without aspirin. One such combination pill reduced LDL cholesterol by 39% and blood pressure by 12%. The investigators hypothesised that the administration of this polypill to everyone aged over 50 in the UK would save thousands of lives and prevent many more non-fatal heart attacks and strokes.

The mainstay of primary and secondary preventive drug therapy is **statin cholesterol lowering therapy**. Statins comprise a group of drugs, such as simvastatin and atorvastatin, which lower LDL cholesterol by 30–50% through the inhibition of 3-hydroxy-3-methylglutaryl-coenzyme A (HMG-CoA) reductase in the cholesterol synthetic pathway. This leads to a reduction in cholesterol in the hepatocytes, which triggers an increase in the numbers of LDL receptors on their cell surfaces, increasing LDL uptake in the liver. Numerous large scale primary and secondary prevention clinical trials have shown that statins decrease the risk of myocardial infarction, stroke, or cardiovascular death by about 25% though the absolute risk reduction is greatest in patients who are being treated for secondary prevention. The reduction in risk is proportional to the decrease in LDL cholesterol achieved. The mechanism of risk reduction from statins is thought to be through plaque stabilisation; statin-treated patients have plaques which have thicker fibrous caps, a lower proportion of cholesterol in the core and fewer inflammatory cells, all morphological features which are associated with a reduced likelihood of plaque rupture.

Anti-platelet therapy such as aspirin is effective secondary preventive therapy and is recommended for all patients who have evidence of atherosclerosis and no contraindications to its use. The role of anti-platelet therapy in primary prevention continues to be debated. Other therapeutic and preventive measures should be used to optimise blood pressure (see above) and to treat diabetes.

Non-atherosclerotic arteriosclerosis

Arteries can be affected by two non-atherosclerotic conditions. In arteriolosclerosis, the walls of small arteries and arterioles are affected by the accumulation of plasma proteins and lipids. In contrast to atherosclerosis, the intima, media and basement membrane are involved in the pathological process. The thickening has a glassy appearance and is also called hyaline arteriosclerosis. This type of arterial disease is a prominent feature of systemic hypertension. The inability of the vessels to dilate and the reduction in lumen size cause distal ischaemia. The proximal increase in pressure exacerbates the hypertension and increases the risk of developing atherosclerosis.

Mönckeberg's sclerosis or **medial calcific sclerosis** is an idiopathic condition of the elderly. Large and medium-sized arteries develop areas of calcification in the vessel wall. The rigidity of the vessel is increased but this is of limited consequence as there is no narrowing of the lumen. The calcified arteries may be noted as an incidental finding on X-ray.

ISCHAEMIC HEART DISEASE

Ischaemic heart disease (IHD) can be defined as any manifestation of atherosclerotic narrowing of the coronary arteries (**coronary artery disease**, CAD). Atherosclerosis of the coronary arteries is frequently asymptomatic, particularly in its early stages. However, as the disease progresses to cause severe coronary artery luminal narrowing, the myocardium is at risk of **ischaemia** – episodes of insufficient oxygen delivery to meet its metabolic demands. At rest, myocardial blood flow is usually sufficient unless the artery diameter is reduced by more than 80% (Fig. 11.34, line 'a'). However, less severe coronary artery stenoses may be sufficient to cause myocardial ischaemia as myocardial oxygen requirements increase, typically during exercise (Fig. 11.34, line 'b').

Ischaemic heart disease may be manifest clinically as **angina**, **acute coronary syndromes**, heart failure, arrhythmia, or sudden death (see later for heart failure and arrhythmias). IHD is a major cause of death in the Western world. Over two-thirds of deaths from IHD occur outside hospital, often with few or no prior symptoms.

Angina

The hallmark of symptomatic myocardial ischaemia is **angina** (or **angina pectoris**). This is typically experienced as a pain or discomfort in the central chest which may radiate to the arm(s), neck, jaw, or teeth. Angina is usually described as 'crushing', 'tight' or 'heavy' but it may cause breathlessness or an ill-defined sensation which the patient finds difficult to describe.

Stable angina

Stable angina is provoked by exertion ('exertional angina') or emotion, and is exacerbated by the cold (due to peripheral vasoconstriction which increases afterload) or exercising after a meal ('post-prandial angina', in which blood is diverted from the heart to the gut). Symptoms are relieved by rest and sublingual nitrate within a few minutes. They are predictable and *stable*, with no recent deterioration.

Stable angina is usually related to one or more severe coronary artery stenosis which does not impair blood flow at rest, but which prevents the normal increase in coronary blood flow, which is necessary to meet the increased metabolic demands of the myocardium during exercise. The diagnosis of stable angina due to CAD is discussed in Clinical box 11.18. Much less commonly, angina is caused by conditions other than CAD, such as hypertensive heart disease, aortic stenosis, or hypertrophic cardiomyopathy. In these conditions, the mismatch between oxygen demand and delivery arises due to the increased oxygen requirements of the hypertrophied left ventricle.

Variant angina

Variant angina, also known as **Prinzmetal's angina**, is a rare condition in which vasospasm of the coronary arteries occurs at rest, often in the early hours of the morning. It is thought to be caused by an exaggerated response to vasoconstrictors such as epinephrine and 5-hydroxytryptamine. The classical presentation is with typical anginal pain associated with, often profound, ST elevation which resolves spontaneously or in response to the administration of nitrates. Coronary angiography reveals no severe stenosis to account for the ischaemia. The treatment is with vasodilators such as calcium-channel blockers and nitrates. The use of cocaine can cause a similar presentation or full blown myocardial infarction due to coronary vasoconstriction.

Treatment of angina

The aims of treatment in angina are to prevent myocardial infarction and death, and to reduce or abolish symptoms. The key aspects of management are risk factor modification, evidence-based medical therapy (see Information box 11.10) and, in some cases, myocardial revascularisation (see Information box 11.11). Patients who smoke must stop and the treatment of hypertension, diabetes and hyperlipidaema should be optimised, where relevant.

Acute coronary syndromes

The acute coronary syndromes (ACS) comprise unstable angina, non-ST elevation myocardial infarction (non-STEMI), and ST elevation myocardial infarction (STEMI). They share a common pathophysiology which involves coronary atheromatous plaque erosion or rupture, platelet activation, coronary thrombus formation and distal embolisation of platelet-rich material. The ensuing myocardial ischaemia is manifest clinically as 'unstable' chest pain, usually occurring at rest.

Unstable angina

Unstable angina is defined by new onset angina at a low workload or at rest, or by deterioration in pre-existing angina so that it occurs at a lower level of exertion and/or at rest. The ECG may be normal or show ST segment depression, and blood tests for cardiac biomarkers such as troponin T or I are normal, excluding myocardial infarction. Patients are managed along similar lines to those with non-STEMI (see below).

Myocardial infarction

Myocardial infarction occurs when heart muscle necrosis arises due to myocardial ischaemia. The diagnostic criteria for myocardial infarction have changed in recent years due to the availability of new cardiac biomarkers, called **troponins**, which have higher sensitivity and specificity for the detection of cardiac muscle damage than the traditional enzyme markers of **creatine kinase**, **aspartate transaminase** and **lactate**

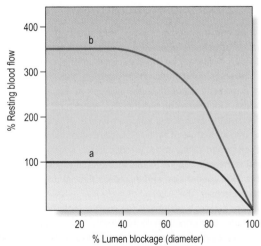

Fig. 11.34 **Blood flow is reduced by decreasing lumen diameter:** a, resting blood flow; b, maximal blood flow.

Clinical box 11.18   Diagnosis of stable angina

Patients who describe symptoms typical of angina and who have a high likelihood of underlying coronary artery disease (CAD) can be diagnosed based on the history alone. Where there is diagnostic uncertainty, investigations are performed to determine whether or not the patient has underlying CAD to support a diagnosis of angina. The most readily available test for CAD is the **exercise ECG**, during which the patient walks on a treadmill or cycles on an exercise bike in order to stimulate increased myocardial oxygen requirements. The development of ST segment depression during exercise is taken as a marker of myocardial ischaemia consistent with underlying CAD. It is now recognised, however, that the diagnostic accuracy of the exercise ECG is limited so it has been superseded by investigative modalities which diagnose CAD more accurately.

These can be divided into tests which image the coronary arteries directly ('anatomical' tests) and those which look for the presence of myocardial ischaemia ('functional' tests) (Table 11.12). The appropriate application of these tests depends upon the probability of underlying CAD, which can be determined from the patient's age, gender, risk factors and symptoms (Fig. 11.35). Patients at high risk of CAD (older patients, with risk factors and/or typical symptoms) should proceed directly to **invasive coronary angiography**, while patients at low or intermediate risk of CAD (younger patients, particularly females, few or no risk factors, non-typical symptoms) should undergo either **CT imaging**, **nuclear myocardial stress perfusion imaging**, **cardiac magnetic resonance stress perfusion imaging** or **stress echocardiography**.

Table 11.12   Diagnostic tests for coronary artery disease

Test	Advantages	Disadvantages
Exercise ECG	Widely available Cheap	Limited sensitivity and specificity Significant proportion of patients cannot complete test
CT calcium scoring	Non-invasive Safe in renal failure	Can 'miss' significant non-calcified disease No assessment of severity of stenoses
CT coronary angiography	High accuracy for identifying unobstructed coronary arteries Can identify non-obstructive coronary atheroma which is not apparent on invasive angiography or perfusion imaging Assessment of ventricular function	Involves radiation exposure (though this is greatly reduced by modern scanners) Heavy coronary calcification obscures stenoses Limited ability to differentiate between moderate and severe stenoses Risk of contrast nephropathy
Nuclear stress myocardial perfusion imaging	Most evidence linking results to prognosis Safe in renal failure Assessment of ventricular function and viability	Radiation exposure Extracardiac activity and artefact can compromise interpretation
Magnetic resonance stress myocardial perfusion imaging	Assessment of anatomy, valves, ventricular function and viability No radiation exposure	5–10% failure rate due to claustrophobia Contraindicated in patients with older pacemakers/ICDs Limited availability Expensive hardware
Stress echocardiography	Assessment of valves, ventricular function, viability No radiation exposure Safe in renal failure	Interobserver variability in image acquisition and interpretation Less sensitive for detection of mild/single vessel disease
Conventional angiography	Gold standard for stenosis severity Prelude to revascularisation	Invasive Radiation exposure Risk of contrast nephropathy

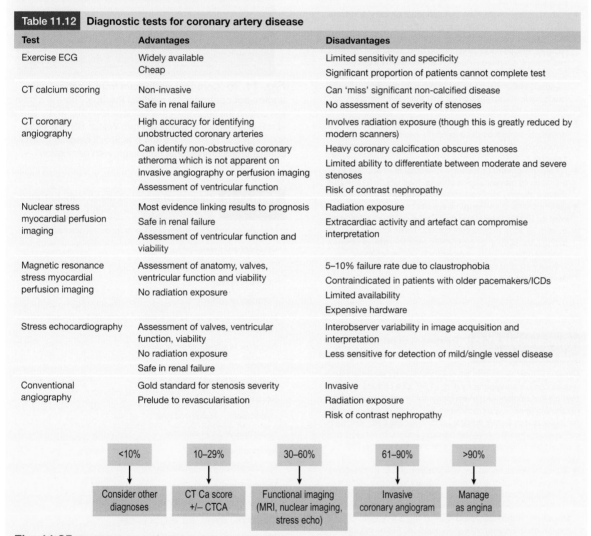

Fig. 11.35   Diagnostic testing for angina based on the pre-test probability of coronary artery disease. Recommendations of the National Institute for Clinical Excellence, UK, 2010. Ca, calcium; CTCA, CT coronary angiogram; MRI, stress perfusion MRI.

dehydrogenase. **Troponin T** and **troponin I** form part of the contractile apparatus within myocytes and they can be detected in the blood following very small amounts of myocardial injury. They do not indicate the mechanism of injury so, in order to differentiate myocardial infarction from the other causes of myocyte injury (Table 11.13), the diagnosis of myocardial infarction requires evidence of new myocardial cell death together with a clinical scenario in keeping with acute myocardial ischaemia; most commonly this is manifest by prolonged anginal chest pain unresponsive to sublingual nitrate.

Non-ST elevation myocardial infarction

In **non-STEMI**, the ECG is normal or shows ST depression or T-wave inversion, but no ST segment elevation, distinguishing it from STEMI. The blood troponin T or I concentration is elevated, differentiating it from unstable angina. The absence of ST elevation indicates a low probability of acute total occlusion of an important coronary artery. Patients do not therefore need to undergo immediate coronary angiography unless they have evidence of ongoing myocardial ischaemia. Unstable angina and non-STEMI are collectively known as

Information box 11.10 — Treatment of angina – medical therapy

Patients with angina should be treated with the following medical therapy:

- Low dose (75 mg) **aspirin** – reduces the acute event rate through the inhibition of platelet thrombi forming on atherosclerotic plaques. **Clopidogrel** is an alternative anti-platelet agent which can be used in patients who are intolerant to aspirin.
- **Statin therapy** – indicated in all patients with IHD irrespective of their blood cholesterol concentration. Reduces the risk of stroke, heart attack and death by about 25%.
- An **angiotensin converting enzyme (ACE) inhibitor**, if left ventricular systolic function is impaired, for long-term prognostic benefit.
- A short acting nitrate such as **sublingual glyceryl trinitrate (GTN)** – effective at relieving angina attacks. Acts by releasing NO, which causes vasodilation of both arteries and veins. This reduces venous return and preload, and peripheral resistance and thereby afterload. The main action of GTN therefore is to reduce myocardial oxygen demand. Blood flow through stenosed vessels is not affected because the obstruction is fixed, but it will increase blood flow through other arteries, which may increase collateral flow.
- A **β-blocker** – the first line anti-anginal agent – prevents ischaemic attacks by decreasing the heart rate and myocardial contractility, thus reducing myocardial oxygen demand.
- A **calcium-channel blocker** – instead of or in addition to a β-blocker to prevent angina attacks. Mechanism of action is through slowing the heart and vasodilatation.
- Other classes of **anti-anginal agents** can be used in patients who fail to tolerate first line drugs or who require additional therapy to achieve symptom control. These include long acting nitrates such as **isosorbide mononitrate**, potassium channel openers such as **nicorandil**, sodium channel blockers such as **ranolazine**, and sinus node inhibitors such as **ivabradine**.

Information box 11.11 — Treatment of angina – myocardial revascularisation

Patients whose symptoms are not controlled by medical therapy require coronary angiography (Fig. 11.36) as a prelude to **myocardial revascularisation** for symptom relief. Myocardial revascularisation is also recommended on prognostic grounds for patients with severe coronary artery disease (left main stem disease, proximal three-vessel disease, and multi-vessel disease involving the proximal left anterior descending artery). The procedures used are:

- **Percutaneous coronary intervention (PCI)**: this involves the dilatation of one or more coronary stenoses using a balloon catheter passed to the heart through the radial or femoral artery. In >90% cases a stent, a wire mesh structure, is then deployed against the artery wall, which minimises the risk of re-stenosis. Following stent deployment, patients require treatment with dual anti-platelet therapy, usually aspirin and clopidogrel, to prevent stent thrombosis.
- **Coronary artery bypass graft surgery (CABG)**: in this operation bypass grafts are anastomosed onto the diseased coronary arteries distal to the segment of narrowing. The graft may comprise a piece of long saphenous vein harvested from the leg, in which case the proximal end is anastomosed to the aorta. Alternatively, one or both of the internal mammary arteries may be used, in which case the proximal end of the graft remains part of the native arterial circulation arising from the subclavian artery. Internal mammary artery grafts have superior long-term patency rates compared with vein grafts.

In general, CABG is favoured in patients with widespread, diffuse coronary disease while PCI is ideal to treat focal segments of severe coronary narrowing.

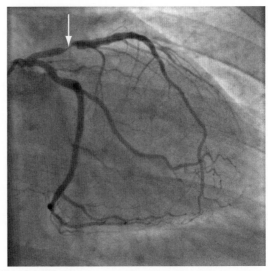

Fig. 11.36 **Coronary angiogram from a patient with angina not controlled by medical therapy.** There is a severe stenosis in the proximal left anterior descending artery (*arrow*) which is amenable to stenting. From Walker BR et al (eds) 2014 Davidson's principles and practice of medicine, 22nd edn. Churchill Livingstone, Edinburgh, with permission.

Table 11.13 — Causes of elevated blood concentrations of troponin T or troponin I

Myocardial ischaemic necrosis due to 'primary' coronary event

Coronary plaque rupture

Coronary stent thrombosis

Coronary spasm

Coronary embolism

Myocardial injury due to 'secondary' ischaemia unrelated to acute coronary event

Tachy- or brady-arrhythmia

Shock

Respiratory failure

Severe anaemia

Hypertrophic cardiomyopathy

Hypertensive heart disease

Aortic stenosis

Myocardial injury unrelated to ischaemia

Myocarditis

Cardiac contusion, ablation, or defibrillator shocks

Cardiotoxic agents, e.g. anthracyclines

Myocardial injury of multifactorial or indeterminate aetiology

Heart failure

Stress (Takotsubo) cardiomyopathy

Cardiac infiltration, e.g. amyloidosis, sarcoidosis

Cardiac surgery

Percutaneous coronary intervention

Pulmonary embolism

Renal failure

Strenuous exercise

Acute neurological conditions, e.g. cerebral infarction or haemorrhage

(Modified from ESC/ACCF/AHA/WHF Expert Consensus Document on the Universal Definition of Myocardial Infarction, 2012)

Treatment of non-ST elevation acute coronary syndromes

The risk of recurrent adverse cardiac events following NSTEACS varies widely between patients. It can be stratified by readily available clinical variables such as ECG findings and cardiac biomarker release, risk being increased in patients with ST segment depression and/or troponin elevation. Formal risk scores such as 'GRACE' are increasingly used to help guide clinical decision making (see Clinical box 11.20). Randomised controlled trials have shown that rates of death, recurrent myocardial infarction and rehospitalisation are reduced in intermediate or high risk patients by 'invasive management' comprising coronary angiography and myocardial revascularisation, where appropriate, compared with medical therapy alone.

Clinical guidelines recommend that myocardial revascularisation is undertaken within 72 hours of hospital admission. Patients with a GRACE score >140 should be treated within 24 hours and patients in the very highest risk group (those with refractory ischaemia, severe heart failure, ventricular arrhythmia, or haemodynamic instability) should be taken to the catheter laboratory as soon as possible (<2 hours). Conversely, there is no evidence for the routine invasive management of low risk patients, who may therefore be managed medically in the first instance, with refinement of their risk stratification by stress myocardial perfusion imaging.

Irrespective of their predicted clinical risk category, patients with NSTEACS should receive the following medical therapy to reduce their risk of death and recurrent non-fatal ischaemic events:

- **Aspirin** 300 mg loading dose followed by 75 mg maintenance therapy
- A second anti-platelet agent, which could be **clopidogrel, ticagrelor, or prasugrel**, taken for at least 1 year
- An antithrombin, either **fondaparinux**, a **factor Xa inhibitor** or, where not available, a **low molecular weight heparin such as enoxaparin**, administered for 2–5 days
- A **β-blocker**, which is the first line anti-ischaemic agent and lowers event rates after myocardial infarction
- Patients with recurrent ischaemia or visible thrombus at coronary angiography should receive a **glycoprotein IIb/IIIa receptor antagonist** (a potent anti-platelet agent) for up to 48 hours
- **Statin therapy** is indicated indefinitely
- An **ACE inhibitor** is indicated in patients with left ventricular dysfunction.

Risk stratification of patients with non-ST elevation acute coronary syndromes – the GRACE score

The Global Registry of Acute Coronary Events (GRACE) Investigators assessed the clinical factors which were associated with an adverse prognosis in a registry of 27 406 patients with non-ST elevation acute coronary syndromes. They identified eight variables which predicted in-hospital death and death at 6 months, which they incorporated into a formal risk calculator, the GRACE score:

- Age
- Killip class (a heart failure score, I–IV)
- Heart rate
- Systolic blood pressure
- Serum creatinine concentration
- ST segment deviation (Y/N)
- Cardiac arrest on admission (Y/N)
- Elevated serum cardiac biomarkers (Y/N).

The continuous variables are split into six or seven subdivisions, each of which is awarded a point allocation commensurate with the level of risk associated with those clinical characteristics. The influence of the individual variables was different on the risk of in-hospital death and death at 6 months so the scores are different for each model. Calculation of the total score allows patients to be stratified into tertiles of risk (low, intermediate and high), which aids clinical decision making:

Predicted mortality following non-ST elevation ACS in relation to GRACE risk score

Risk category (tertile)
GRACE risk score
In-hospital death rate

Low
  ≤108
  <1%
Intermediate
  109–140
  1–3%
High
  >140
  >3%

Risk category (tertile)
GRACE risk score
6-month death rate

Low
  ≤88
  <3%
Intermediate
  89–118
  3–8%
High
  >118
  >8%

(Data from European Society of Cardiology guidelines for the management of acute coronary syndromes in patients presenting without persistent ST-segment elevation, 2011.)

the non-ST elevation acute coronary syndromes (NSTEACS), the management of which is described in Clinical box 11.19.

ST elevation myocardial infarction

The diagnostic **ST segment elevation** in **STEMI** indicates acute occlusion of one of the three main epicardial coronary arteries or its major side branch. In the absence of effective treatment, the ECG infarct pattern evolves through a series of changes over the next few days (Fig. 11.37). Tissue death occurs within 15–30 minutes of vessel occlusion and, if the artery remains blocked, the entire region of heart muscle supplied by the artery dies. Patients with large infarcts have an adverse prognosis. The treatment of STEMI is described in Clinical box 11.21.

Complications of myocardial infarction

In the year after an ACS, the death rate is about 10% and the rate of death, recurrent MI or re-admission to hospital is approximately 30%. The death rate is highest within the first 10 days of STEMI and lowest in patients with unstable angina. For patients who survive beyond 30 days, the mortality rate is slightly higher following non-STEMI compared with STEMI so that by one year the survival rates are similar between these two groups.

The most common life-threatening complication of MI is **ventricular fibrillation** (VF) (Table 11.14). The risk of VF is greatest within the first few hours of acute coronary occlusion and VF is responsible for most of the deaths that

occur before patients reach hospital. VF can usually be restored easily to sinus rhythm by electrical defibrillation so it is vitally important that people who develop sustained chest pain contact the emergency medical services quickly and that they are placed on continuous ECG monitoring once the ambulance crew arrives. The greatest opportunity to save lives in the acute management of MI is in patients with chest pain calling for help earlier.

Mortality rates for patients who survive to reach hospital have halved in recent years and now stand at about 5%. However, patients who suffer major damage to their left ventricular muscle have an adverse prognosis, patients who present in **cardiogenic shock** faring worst of all with an in-hospital mortality rate of 35–50%. Left ventricular damage predisposes to **heart failure**, and patients with severe left ventricular systolic

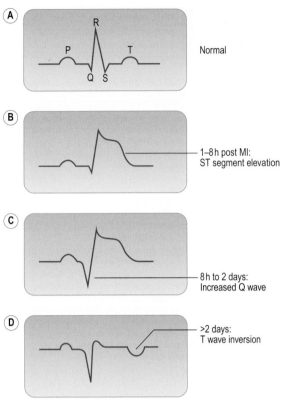

Fig. 11.37 Evolution of typical changes in the ECG following ST elevation myocardial infarction. Classically, there is ST elevation post MI with a series of changes over the next few days.

Clinical box 11.21 **Treatment of ST elevation myocardial infarction**

The main aim of treatment in STEMI is to restore blood flow to the ischaemic myocardium as rapidly as possible in order to limit the size of the infarct, so improving long term prognosis. Treatment which aims to restore blood flow in the infarct-related artery is called **reperfusion therapy**.

The first available reperfusion therapy involved the administration of a drug which promotes clot lysis through the activation of plasminogen to plasmin. This is called **thrombolytic therapy** and it reduces the mortality rate after STEMI by about 25%. Reperfusion therapy can also be achieved mechanically by emergency or '**primary' percutaneous coronary intervention** (**PCI**). Randomised controlled trials have shown that primary PCI is superior to thrombolytic therapy, treatment with PCI reducing rates of death, stroke and recurrent myocardial infarction by a further 25%. Prognosis is directly related to time from symptom onset to reperfusion therapy so it is important that clinical pathways deliver patients with STEMI rapidly to the PCI centre. Treatment guidelines recommend that patients who present within 12 hours of STEMI are managed with PCI so long as this can be delivered by an expert team within 120 minutes of first medical contact. Patients who present later than 12 hours and who have ongoing chest pain and persisting ST elevation may also benefit from PCI. Thrombolytic therapy is reserved for situations in which primary PCI cannot be delivered in a timely fashion.

The medical therapy which should be administered to improve prognosis is similar to patients for non-STEMI (see Clinical box 11.9) except that anti-thrombins such as fondaparinux are not needed and there is evidence (from the thrombolytic era) that the early administration of ACE inhibitors is beneficial.

Table 11.14	Complications of acute myocardial infarction
Infarct-related	
Ventricular arrhythmia	Early (within 12 hours): unrelated to infarct size; good prognosis if successfully treated
	Late (after 12 hours): more common in large infarcts, more likely to recur. Manage with β-blocker and ICD
Bradyarrhythmia	Sinus bradycardia, nodal rhythm, and heart block all common after inferior infarction; usually self-limiting. Advanced conduction disorders after anterior infarction reflect infarct size; more likely to be permanent and to require a pacemaker
Heart failure	Usually due to severe left ventricular systolic dysfunction due to large infarct. Prognosis improved by β-blockers, ACE inhibitors, aldosterone antagonists and ICD
Pericarditis	Early (first few days): related to inflamed pericardium adjacent to infarct. Causes pleuritic chest pain and pyrexia. Treat with NSAIDs
	Late (2–12 weeks): an autoimmune response to the infarct called Dressler syndrome. Treat with NSAIDs, and steroids if persistent
Ventricular rupture	Post-infarct VSD usually causes a low output state. Some patients can be supported through the acute episode to undergo surgical repair
	Rupture of a papillary muscle causes pulmonary oedema and cardiogenic shock due to acute severe mitral regurgitation – often rapidly fatal
	Ventricular free wall rupture invariably causes sudden death. Very occasionally the rupture is subclinical, contained by thrombus and soft tissue (a pseudoaneurysm), and is only recognised on echocardiography during routine follow-up or when the patient represents with heart failure or ventricular arrhythmia
Left ventricular aneurysm	Due to replacement of the myocardium by scar tissue. The muscle is non-viable and the LV wall is thin. Most commonly affects the left ventricular apex. Suspect in patients with persisting ST elevation. Either asymptomatic, or presents with left ventricular failure, ventricular arrhythmia, or thromboembolic episodes
Stroke	Due to thromboembolism arising from left ventricular thrombus or atrial fibrillation. Cerebral infarction after myocardial infarction should prompt echocardiography to search for LV thrombus. Anticoagulation is indicated
Venous thromboembolism	The post infarct period carries an increased risk of DVT and PE due to reduced mobility and a temporary increase in blood coagulability. Patients whose mobilisation is delayed should receive prophylactic low molecular weight heparin
Treatment-related	
Bleeding	Related to anti-platelet agents or thrombolytic therapy – gastrointestinal, intracranial
	Related to primary PCI – arterial access site haematoma, retroperitoneal haematoma
Other complications of PCI	Stroke, renal failure due to contrast nephropathy, contrast allergy

dysfunction (left ventricular ejection fraction <35%) at least 4 weeks after their infarct are at increased risk of sudden arrhythmic death and benefit prognostically from the implantation of an **implantable cardioverter defibrillator (ICD)**.

Much lesser degrees of heart muscle damage can cause cardiogenic shock if the dead muscle ruptures, causing either a **ventricular septal defect** (when the intraventricular septum is affected) or severe **mitral regurgitation** (when rupture of one of the papillary muscles causes a flail mitral leaflet). Rupture of the ventricular free wall invariably causes sudden death due to cardiac tamponade. These complications tend to occur within the first 10 days of infarction when the dead tissue is invaded by neutrophils, and there is breakdown of the old tissue and its replacement with scar tissue. During this process the tissue becomes very soft and prone to rupture. The inflamed tissue can cause **pericarditis** in the hours and days after myocardial infarction or develop several weeks later as an autoimmune phenomenon (**Dressler syndrome**). The inflamed luminal ventricular wall in combination with relative stasis of blood in the region of the infarct predisposes **to left ventricular thrombus** formation, which can embolise to the brain to cause cerebral infarction. Replacement of muscle by non-contractile scar can result in **aneurysm** formation, where the scarred tissue balloons outwards during systole. Early treatment with ACE inhibitors and β-blockers reduces the risk of problems related to the adverse consequences of left ventricular remodelling.

THROMBOEMBOLISM

The most serious condition to affect the venous system is **venous thromboembolism**. In this condition, a thrombus forms in the venous system before dislodging or **embolising** from the vessel wall and travelling through the circulation to lodge in one or more branches of the pulmonary artery (see below). Thromboembolism also occurs in the arterial circulation, with different causes and clinical consequences to venous thromboembolism (Information box 11.12).

Thrombus formation

A **thrombus** is a solid mass formed in the circulation from the constituents of blood. There are two main types, **white thrombus** and **red thrombus**, though these represent two ends of a spectrum, and many thrombi contain mixed elements.

- In the arterial circulation, thrombus most commonly forms in association with atherosclerotic plaques when the overlying endothelium is damaged due to plaque rupture, fissuring or erosion. They contain large quantities of platelets, which gives them a whitish colour, and they are therefore referred to as white thrombi.
- Red thrombus is composed mostly of fibrin and trapped red cells. This is the type of thrombus which occurs in static or slowly moving blood so it occurs in the venous system and in the left atrium in patients with atrial fibrillation.

More than 150 years ago, Virchow proposed three factors which predispose to venous thrombosis (**Virchow's triad**). It was subsequently recognised that these factors also confer an increased risk of thrombus formation in arteries:

- Abnormal blood flow
- Abnormal blood constituents
- Abnormal vessel wall.

Information box 11.12 **Arterial thromboembolism**

Arterial thromboembolism occurs when a piece of thrombus travels from its site of formation to a more distal part of the arterial circulation. The most common sites of thrombus formation within the arterial system are:
- The left atrium – in patients with atrial fibrillation, mitral stenosis, or a mitral valve prosthesis
- The left ventricle – in patients with dilated cardiomyopathy, left ventricular aneurysm, or following acute myocardial infarction
- The carotid arteries – at the site of carotid artery stenosis
- The abdominal aorta – within an abdominal aortic aneurysm
- The lower limb vasculature – within iliac, femoral, or popliteal artery aneurysms.

Occlusion of the arterial system by the embolus cuts off the oxygen supply to the subtended tissue resulting in ischaemia and, if this is prolonged, tissue infarction. Emboli from the heart may travel to any part of the arterial circulation while thrombus arising in an artery can embolise to an arterial branch distal to its site of origin. The most commonly affected organs or tissues are the brain, an upper or lower limb, and the intestine. The respective clinical consequences are:
- Stroke or transient ischaemic attack
- Acute ischaemia of a limb or digit
- Intestinal infarction.

Paradoxical embolism occurs when a thrombus which originated in the venous system passes into the arterial system through a connection, such as an atrial septal defect. Rather than cause a pulmonary embolus as for most emboli arising in the venous system, this causes arterial occlusion. Paradoxical embolism should be suspected when an arterial thrombotic event occurs in patients known to have congenital heart disease or when it occurs soon after a DVT.

At least one of these factors can be identified as the underlying pathophysiological mechanism in most of the patient groups who are at increased risk of venous thrombosis (Table 11.15). Immobility and heart failure predispose to thrombosis in the deep veins of the leg through stagnation of blood in these vessels. About 20% of cases of venous thrombosis are the result of inherited abnormalities of clotting factors, such as factor V Leiden. This is an autosomal dominant condition which renders clotting factor V insensitive to breakdown by activated protein C. Abnormal cellular composition of the blood such as polycythaemia (too many red cells) or thrombocytosis (too many platelets) also renders

---

Table 11.15 **Risk factors for venous thrombosis**

Reduced mobility
Trauma, fractures, or surgery
Active cancer
Age over 60
Critical care admission
Dehydration
Known prothrombotic disorder
Obesity
Medical comorbidities – heart disease, respiratory disease, metabolic disease, acute infection, inflammatory disease
Personal history or first degree relative with a history of DVT or PE
Use of hormone replacement therapy
Use of oestrogen containing contraceptive pill
Pregnancy
Varicose veins with phlebitis

it hypercoagulable. Vessel wall injury due to trauma or inflammation attracts platelets and inflammatory cells, which initiate clotting pathways. The increased risk from pregnancy is multifactorial – venous obstruction, reduced mobility and increased circulating levels of oestrogen all contributing.

Deep vein thrombosis

The most common site for venous thrombosis is within the deep veins of the legs. Thrombi tend to form in the calf vein sinuses behind the flaps of venous valves where the initial event is platelet adhesion (Fig. 11.38A). Activated platelets attract other platelets and release pro-coagulant factors which initiate the clotting cascade. Fibrin and red cells are

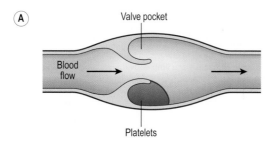

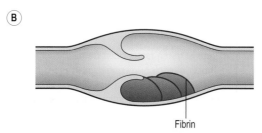

Fig. 11.38 **Evolution of venous thrombosis.** (A) Platelets aggregate behind the valve pocket. (B) Fibrin and red blood cells stabilise the clot. Subsequent layers of platelets form a distinctive coral-like structure.

incorporated into the thrombus in layers which alternate with platelets. In cross-section, these layers are visible as **lines of Zahn** (Fig. 11.39). If a vein becomes completely occluded with thrombus, then blood flow proximal to the point of occlusion becomes static, which predisposes to further thrombus formation. The thrombus can propagate along the vessel to form long lengths of clot.

The leg affected by deep vein thrombosis (DVT) is congested with venous blood which makes it painful, swollen and warm. DVT often occurs after periods of immobility or acute illness (Table 11.15 and Information box 11.13). The main complication of DVT, pulmonary embolism, is one of the most common causes of potentially avoidable death in patients admitted to hospital. All patients who are admitted to hospital should therefore have their risk of venous thrombosis assessed and preventive measures instituted. It is common practice to provide patients with compression stockings to reduce venous pooling in the legs and to mobilise patients as soon as possible following surgery. Patients who are at moderate or high risk of DVT should be treated with daily injections of low molecular weight heparin to reduce the coagulability of the blood and the risk of DVT.

Information box 11.13 | **DVT and long-haul air travel**

DVT can be caused by the long periods of immobility that occur during long-haul air travel. Airlines are being asked to provide more leg room and passengers are encouraged to exercise their calf and foot muscles and to take occasional walks along the aisle of the aircraft to reduce venous pooling in the leg veins. Dehydration may play a role in the increased risk, so drinking plenty of water or soft drinks is advisable. Alcohol intake should be limited as it can lead to dehydration. In patients who are at high risk of DVT, the use of compression stockings, low-dose aspirin or low molecular weight heparin can be considered to reduce the risk.

Pulmonary embolism

When a portion of thrombus breaks off from within the deep veins of the legs and travels through the great veins and the right side of the heart to lodge in the pulmonary circulation,

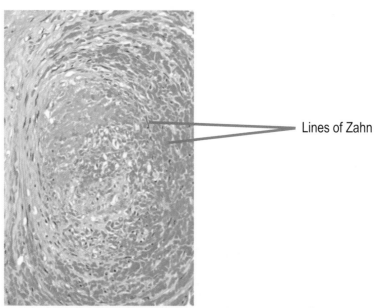

Lines of Zahn

Fig. 11.39 **Micrograph of a thrombus.** The lines of Zahn are the alternating lighter bands of fibrin platelets and darker bands red blood cells. From User: Nephron @ Wikimedia Commons.

this causes a **pulmonary embolus**. The embolus blocks the blood flow in the pulmonary vessel. This can have a number of consequences which depend upon the size of the pulmonary vessel that is blocked and on the cardiorespiratory reserve of the patient. A large pulmonary embolus which occludes the main pulmonary artery or one of its major branches typically causes the sudden onset of:

- Chest pain
- Breathlessness and hypoxia
- Syncope
- Haemodynamic collapse due to acute right heart failure.

Occlusion of a smaller, more peripheral pulmonary artery usually presents with:

- Pleuritic chest pain
- Haemoptysis due to alveolar haemorrhage.

Pulmonary embolism causes hypoxia by a ventilation–perfusion mismatch which arises from reduced or absent flow in the occluded artery. The diagnosis is confirmed by CT pulmonary angiography. Management is aimed at the prevention of further embolic episodes. In the acute phase, this is achieved with low molecular weight heparin, followed by oral anticoagulation for 3–12 months. Patients with large pulmonary emboli causing hypotension or right heart strain on echocardiography should be treated with thrombolytic therapy to rapidly dissolve the clot.

Non-thrombotic emboli

Not all emboli are caused by thrombus. The term embolus applies to any substance that travels in the blood resulting in occlusion of a vein or artery. Emboli can be produced by:

- **Air**: introduced during insertion of vascular devices, infusions of fluid, surgery, or dialysis.

- **Nitrogen**: the 'bends' results from the formation of nitrogen bubbles in the bloodstream and tissues following a period at high atmospheric pressure without sufficient time for decompression. It predominantly affects divers.
- **Fat**: following trauma, usually involving fractures.
- **Cholesterol**: from atheromatous plaques, often precipitated by arterial instrumentation such as during angiography.
- **Cells**: from metastasising tumours, atrial myxoma, or vegetations in endocarditis.
- **Amniotic fluid**: during labour.
- **Medical devices**: during percutaneous insertion of devices into the circulation, such as transcatheter aortic valve prosthesis, atrial septal defect closure device, or left atrial appendage occluder device.

THE MICROCIRCULATION

The **microcirculation** is the place where substances are exchanged between the tissues and the blood. Oxygen and nutrients are released from blood to the tissues and carbon dioxide and other waste products of metabolism diffuse from tissues into the blood. The microcirculation consists of the very smallest blood vessels in the body (Fig. 11.40):

- Pre-capillary arterioles
- Capillaries
- Post-capillary venules
- Lymphatic capillaries and collecting ducts.

Capillary structure

Capillaries are the main place of substance exchange. They are the smallest blood vessels, measuring 5–10 μm in diameter and 0.3–1 mm in length. Capillaries are thin walled,

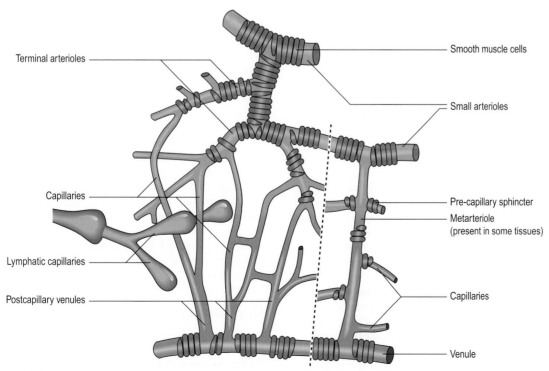

Fig. 11.40 **Anatomy of the microcirculation.**

Terminal arterioles

Capillaries

Lymphatic capillaries

Postcapillary venules

Smooth muscle cells

Small arterioles

Pre-capillary sphincter

Metarteriole (present in some tissues)

Capillaries

Venule

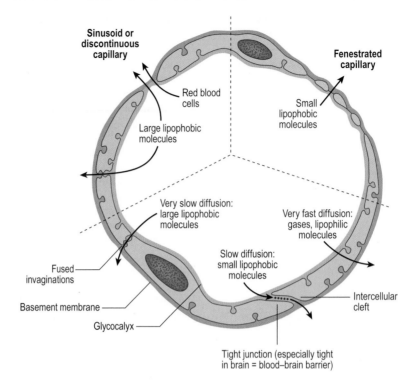

Fig. 11.41 **Different types of capillary.**

consisting of a single layer of endothelial cells and a basement membrane. Microscopic spaces between the cells facilitate the passage of substances across the capillary membrane. There are three types of capillary, each with different structures, which determine the substances which diffuse across them, and their rate of diffusion (Fig. 11.41):

- **Continuous capillaries** are lined by a continuous layer of endothelial cells which are joined by **tight junctions**. A basement membrane surrounds the whole capillary. Small molecules are able to diffuse across the basement membrane through the tight junctions. Continuous capillaries are the commonest capillaries found in skin, skeletal muscle and fat. They are important in maintaining the integrity of the blood–brain barrier, which protects the brain from toxic molecules.
- **Fenestrated capillaries** contain pores or fenestrations in their endothelial cells measuring 20–100 nm in diameter. The fenestrations are spanned by a diaphragm which allows the diffusion of small molecules (ions, water) and limited amounts of protein. Fenestrated capillaries are prevalent in tissues where substantial filtration or absorption takes place. They are primarily located in the renal glomeruli, endocrine glands, intestinal mucosa and pancreas. The fenestrations in the capillaries on the renal tubules lack a covering membrane, which allows large volumes of solute to be exchanged between blood and urine (see Ch. 14).
- **Sinusoidal or discontinuous capillaries** are a specialised form of 'leaky' fenestrated capillary. They contain large fenestrations in the endothelial cells measuring 30–40 μm in diameter, and pores in the basal lamina which allow the passage of red and white blood cells and proteins. They are found in parts of the body which manufacture or process blood cells

such as the liver, spleen and bone marrow. Their large, irregularly shaped lumen promotes slow blood flow which facilitates the movement of blood cells between blood and tissue. The release of blood from the surface of the liver and spleen is prevented by a peritoneal lining while bone marrow is encapsulated in compact bone.

The capillary bed

The capillary bed is formed by a complex network of branching capillaries which arise from **pre-capillary (terminal) arterioles**. At their distal end, the capillaries converge to form **post-capillary venules** (Fig. 11.40). Blood flow into the capillary bed is controlled by the tone in the vascular smooth muscle in the pre-capillary arterioles. In some tissues, capillaries arise as branches from small arterioles called **metarterioles** which provide a direct channel between arterioles and venules at the opposite ends of the capillary bed. Blood flow into the capillaries is then controlled by **pre-capillary sphincters** (rings of smooth muscle) at the inlet to the capillaries). Relaxation of the pre-capillary sphincters allows blood to flow into the capillaries. By contrast, when the pre-capillary sphincters are closed, blood flows directly from the pre-capillary arteriole to the post-capillary venule through the metarteriole, bypassing the capillary bed.

Capillary exchange

Capillary exchange involves the transport of micronutrients and waste products of metabolism blood and interstitial fluid. With the exception of plasma proteins, which are large in size, most substances and small molecules in plasma are able to cross capillary walls. There are two main mechanisms for the transport of substances across the capillary endothelium:

- Diffusion
- Active membrane transport.

Diffusion

Diffusion, or passive movement down a concentration gradient, is the main mechanism by which water and dissolved substances, or **solutes**, move across the capillary membrane. The rate of diffusion of solutes across the capillary membrane is described by Fick's law, and is directly related to:

- the permeability of the capillary membrane
- the surface area available for diffusion
- the size of the concentration gradient.

The permeability of the capillary membrane varies according to the type of capillary and the physical properties of the substance (see below). Permeability is high in the kidney due to the preponderance of fenestrated capillaries which allow solutes to pass readily from the blood into the urine for excretion. Capillary permeability in the brain is low due to the properties of continuous capillaries so that the neurons are protected from fluctuations in blood chemistry (the 'blood–brain barrier').

The concentration gradient is defined by the concentration of solute on either side of the membrane and the distance over which the solute must diffuse. Diffusion is increased by a large difference in concentrations on either side of the membrane and by a small diffusion distance.

Free diffusion

Lipid soluble compounds such as oxygen, carbon dioxide, cholesterol and other non-protein bound lipids diffuse freely across the capillary endothelium (see also Ch. 3). They do not require pores to cross the membrane so the surface area available to them for diffusion is high.

Channel-based diffusion

Small lipid-insoluble molecules, such as water, ions, glucose, some amino acids and urea, require specialised channels in order to diffuse across the capillary membrane. Water passes through specific channels in the membrane called **aquaporins**, while gaps between cells called **small pores** allow the passage of water, glucose, urea and amino acids (see also Ch. 14).

Except under disease conditions where capillary membrane permeability is increased, large, lipid insoluble molecules, such as albumin, remain in plasma and do not cross the capillary membrane.

Active membrane transport

In addition to diffusion, lipid insoluble molecules may also move across the capillary membrane by active membrane transport systems. **Transcytosis** (or **pinocytosis**) involves the invagination of one side of the capillary membrane to form a vesicle containing water and solutes (Clinical box 11.22). The vesicle is moved across the capillary membrane and the substances are released on the opposite side in a process which consumes energy. Specific substances can be taken up through **receptor-mediated endocytosis**. Examples include the absorption of insulin in the gut, the transport of immunoglobulins and the transport of iron by transferrin. It is an important mechanism for the transport of macromolecules

---

Clinical box 11.22 Clinical importance of transcytosis

Transcytosis may play a part in pathogenesis, where bacteria may exploit this mechanism for transporting macromolecules across cells. It has been demonstrated that some bacteria invade the human body by transcytosis across the intestinal epithelium and the blood–brain barrier. The toxin secreted by *E. coli* 0157, the entero-haemorrhagic strain of *Escherichia coli*, has been shown to transcytose into the intestinal mucosa.

Transcytosis may have a role in therapeutics. Owing to the impermeable nature of the blood–brain barrier, administered therapeutic agents cannot cross the barrier to reach their targets. Except in disease, when the blood–brain barrier is disrupted, antibiotics such as penicillin are ineffective (see Ch. 4). It may be possible to exploit transcytosis as a transport mechanism for moving drugs across the blood–brain barrier.

---

across the blood–brain barrier (see Ch. 8). The transport of large lipid-insoluble molecules involves membrane transport, discussed in detail in Chapter 2.

Influence of blood flow on capillary exchange

The rate of blood flow in the capillary has an important influence on the capacity for capillary exchange, its effect varying according to the permeability of the solute. The equilibration of concentrations across the capillary membrane for substances with a high permeability occurs quickly so that exchange finishes before the blood has reached the end of the capillary. This is called **flow-limited diffusion** because there is 'spare capacity' for diffusion, which can be accessed by increasing the flow rate. Increased flow delivers more solute per unit time, and equilibration occurs more distally in the capillary compared with lower flow rates. Flow-limited diffusion occurs in the lung, where O_2 and CO_2 are exchanged very rapidly between blood and alveoli, meaning that exchange can be increased by increasing pulmonary blood flow. By contrast, for solutes with a low permeability, equilibration of their concentrations on either side of the endothelium does not occur by the time blood reaches the end of the capillary. In these circumstances, capillary exchange is maximal at low rates of blood flow, allowing the solute more contact time with the capillary membrane. This is called **diffusion-limited diffusion**.

Water exchange

Water diffuses freely across the capillary membrane. Its movement is determined by the balance between hydrostatic and oncotic pressures in the intravascular and extravascular spaces (see also Ch. 1, Water and electrolytes: homeostatic control of body fluids):

- **Hydrostatic pressure**: water moves down pressure gradients from areas of high pressure to areas of low pressure
- **Oncotic pressure**: water moves by osmosis from areas of low solute concentration to areas of high solute concentration.

Starling forces

The blood and the extracellular fluid each generate a hydrostatic pressure and an oncotic pressure which act along the length of the capillary (Fig. 11.42A). These forces are known

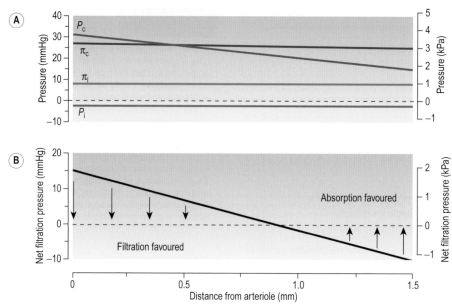

Fig. 11.42 **Starling forces and filtration pressure.** (A) Starling forces along a capillary; (B) net filtration pressure along a capillary. For explanation of abbreviations see text.

as Starling forces. They each have an effect on the tendency for water to move into or out of the capillary:

1. **Hydrostatic pressure of blood**: this equates to the blood pressure within the circulation. At capillary level, this is dependent upon the tone in the pre-capillary arteriole. At the proximal end of the capillary, the hydrostatic pressure (P_c) is about 32 mmHg, falling to about 17 mmHg at its distal end. **The hydrostatic pressure of blood forces water out of the capillary**.
2. **Hydrostatic pressure of interstitial fluid**: this is a small negative pressure of about −3 mmHg. The negative pressure is thought to be related to lymphatic drainage of extracellular fluid. **The hydrostatic pressure of interstitial fluid (P_i) tends to draw water out of the capillary**.
3. **Oncotic pressure of plasma**: the electrolytes and other small molecules in plasma account for most of its osmotic pressure. However, their concentrations in plasma and extracellular fluid are equal so they do not influence the capillary exchange of water. It is the large proteins in plasma called **colloids** (60–80 g/L), e.g. albumin, which are not usually found in the extracellular fluid, that account for the difference in osmotic pressure between the blood and the extracellular space. This pressure, known as the **colloid osmotic pressure** or **oncotic pressure** (π_c) is normally about 27 mmHg. **Plasma oncotic pressure draws fluid into the capillaries**.
4. **Oncotic pressure of interstitial fluid**: produced by the proteins in the interstitial fluid (20–30 g/L); this is usually about 8 mmHg. **The oncotic pressure of interstitial fluid (π_i) tends to draw water out of capillaries**.

Filtration and resorption

The movement of water into or out of the capillary is determined by the net effect of these four forces. The largest pressures and therefore those with the most influence on the movement of water are the capillary hydrostatic pressure

and the plasma oncotic pressure. The plasma oncotic and interstitial pressures remain virtually constant throughout the length of the capillary whereas the capillary hydrostatic pressure is highest at its arteriolar end before falling progressively due to the vascular resistance of the capillary.

At the arteriolar end of the capillary, the plasma oncotic pressure tends to draw water out of the capillary but its effect is opposed and exceeded by the greater effect of the capillary hydrostatic pressure. The net result is movement of water out of the capillary or **filtration** (Fig. 11.42B). Towards the venous end of the capillary, the decrease in hydrostatic pressure results in a reduction in the net filtration pressure, which favours movement of water into the capillaries (**reabsorption** or **resorption**).

Capillary blood flow determines the capillary hydrostatic pressure and it is therefore a major determinant of whether or not there is net filtration or net resorption, and its amount. In a well perfused capillary, the net filtration pressure is high throughout the capillary and there is net filtration (Fig. 11.43A). When vasoconstriction occurs, hydrostatic pressure falls at both ends of the capillary. If the fall is large enough, resorption occurs at the venous end of the capillary and, if this exceeds filtration in the arteriolar end of the capillary, net resorption results (Fig. 11.43B). In the chronically vasoconstricted state, a new steady state is established which favours net filtration at lower capillary filtration pressures (Fig 11.43C).

Under normal conditions, there is a very small excess of filtration over resorption in the capillaries. Despite only about 0.2–0.3% of plasma being filtered in most capillary beds, the large volume of plasma that passes through them leads to a filtrate of about 12 L per day. Most of this is resorbed and the remainder of the filtered fluid is removed from the interstitial space by the lymphatics. Filtration is much higher in the capillaries of the kidney where about 20% of the plasma is filtered (see Ch.14). This produces a daily filtrate volume of approximately 800 L, more than 99% of which is reabsorbed from the tubules.

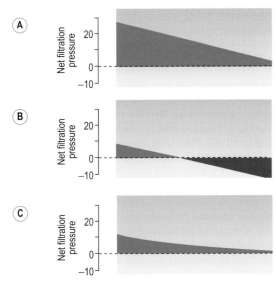

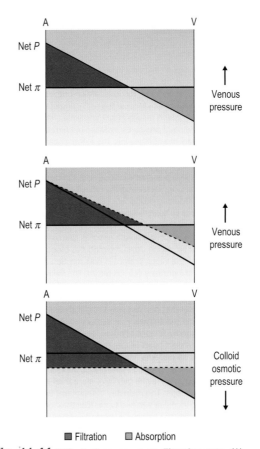

Fig. 11.43 Changes in pressure across the capillary.
(A) Well-perfused capillary; (B) vasoconstriction – early transient; (C) vasoconstriction – later steady-state. *Blue* shows net filtration and *red* net absorption.

Fig. 11.44 Effect of pressure on filtration rate. (A) Normal pressure. (B) Increased net filtration due to raised venous pressure (*dotted line*). (C) Reduced osmotic pressure (*dotted line*). Normal pressures are shown by the *black lines.* Net filtration is filtration (*red area*) minus absorption (*green area*).

Oedema

When the equilibrium between Starling forces is disturbed so that net capillary filtration exceeds the capacity for lymphatic drainage, water accumulates in the interstitial space. This produces swelling of the tissues called **oedema**. This can occur in many different conditions, and cause localised oedema or more generalised swelling, but the underlying mechanism is always one of the following:

- Increased capillary hydrostatic pressure
- Decreased plasma oncotic pressure
- Increased capillary permeability
- Reduced lymphatic drainage.

Increased capillary hydrostatic pressure

An increase in venous pressure increases the hydrostatic pressure at the venous end of the capillary. The hydrostatic pressure gradient favours filtration (*red area*) rather than absorption (*green area*) over a longer length of capillary and net filtration is increased (Fig. 11.44A, B). This mechanism is responsible for water diffusing into the tissues of the lungs (increased pulmonary venous pressure) to cause cardiogenic pulmonary oedema and in the legs (increased systemic venous pressure) in right heart failure (see Information box 11.14).

Decreased plasma oncotic pressure

A low plasma protein concentration due to hypoalbuminaemia reduces the plasma oncotic pressure, the main factor which tends to draw water into the capillary. Reabsorption is therefore reduced and net filtration is increased (Fig. 11.44C). Hypoalbuminaemia can be caused by protein-energy malnutrition (Ch.16), malabsorption, reduced production of albumin in chronic liver disease (Ch. 15), or by albumin loss through the kidneys in nephrotic syndrome (Ch. 14). The low plasma oncotic pressure applies to the whole circulation so excess water filtration occurs in many tissues and is manifest clinically as peripheral oedema, pleural effusions, pulmonary oedema, ascites, and pericardial effusion.

Increased capillary permeability

Increased capillary permeability results in the loss of protein from the plasma into the interstitial space. This increases the oncotic pressure of the interstitial fluid which promotes net filtration. Capillary leak is one of the manifestations of severe life-threatening infections and inflammatory conditions (Ch. 6) and of burns.

Reduced lymphatic drainage

Obstruction to the lymphatic drainage causes the accumulation of fluid and protein in the interstitial space. This results in non-pitting oedema (lymphoedema) in the area drained by the affected lymphatics, most commonly the upper or lower limb. Lymphatic obstruction is caused by:

- Infiltration by tumour cells, such as breast cancer
- Destruction by cancer treatments – either radiotherapy or surgical excision
- Destruction of lymphatic channels following deep vein thrombosis.
- Parasitic infiltration by nematodes leading to elephantiasis (see also Ch. 6).

Heart failure leads to elevated pressures in the venous circulation. Several mechanisms contribute to this. The reduced stroke volume causes an increase in end diastolic volume and pressure which is transmitted backwards to the atria and their feeding veins. In addition, the low cardiac output reduces renal perfusion causing activation of the renin–angiotensin—aldosterone system which results in salt and water retention.

The elevated venous pressures increase net filtration of fluid through the capillary membranes into the extracellular space and are the main cause of oedema in heart failure. In (untreated) left heart failure, the pulmonary venous pressure is raised. When the pulmonary venous pressure exceeds about 20 mmHg, fluid accumulates in the lung, increasing the diffusion distance for blood gases and reducing pulmonary compliance. One of the common symptoms of heart failure is breathlessness (**dyspnoea**) which is made worse by lying down (**orthopnoea**). Patients may also be woken by severe breathlessness (**paroxysmal nocturnal dyspnoea**). Lying down redistributes blood from the leg veins to the central veins, promotes reabsorption of fluid from the extremities and increases venous return. The failing heart cannot cope with the increase in preload, and the pulmonary venous pressure rises. Many patients with this condition have to sleep with the upper part of their body upright so that more fluid remains in the lower extremities. Pulmonary oedema can be seen on X-rays as a butterfly-shaped shadow (see Ch. 13, Fig. 13.8).

In patients with right heart failure, the systemic venous pressure is raised, so oedema occurs in the periphery. This is most obviously seen as swelling in the ankles and feet. Patients with severe chronic heart failure can have more than 10 L of excess fluid in their legs. The mainstay of treatment for oedema is diuretics, which increase salt and water loss through the kidneys. This reduces the blood volume and systemic venous pressure which shifts the balance of filtration at the capillary level in favour of reabsorption. The diuretic therapy maintains an increased urine output which ensures that the reabsorbed fluid is excreted from the body.

MECHANICS OF BLOOD FLOW

The heart pumps blood continuously around the cardiovascular system. The mechanics of blood flow describe the pressure changes in the blood vessels that carry blood around the body, and the forces that influence the circulation of blood.

Pressure and vascular resistance

Blood flows through a system from high pressure to low pressure. The rate of blood flow is directly related to the **pressure difference** and is inversely related to the **resistance** in the system. In the systemic circulation, the mean pressure falls from approximately 90–100 mmHg in the aorta to about 25 mmHg in the capillaries, to almost zero in the venae cavae (Fig. 11.45). The driving pressure for flow through the systemic circulation is therefore very close to the aortic pressure, or mean arterial blood pressure.

The resistance in the systemic circulation is the resistance from all of the blood vessels in the systemic vasculature, the **systemic vascular resistance** or SVR. The greatest resistance is presented by the small arteries and arterioles, which are therefore known as the resistance vessels of the circulation. The resistance of a vessel is inversely related to the radius. A small change in radius therefore produces a large change in resistance to flow.

In the absence of abnormal connections between the systemic and pulmonary circulations, blood flow through the two circuits must be equal. The pressure gradient in the pulmonary circulation is much lower than in the systemic circulation (mean pulmonary artery pressure about 20 mmHg, 10 mmHg in the pulmonary capillaries, and 0–5 mmHg in the pulmonary veins) but the pulmonary vascular resistance is much lower so the flow rate is the same.

Velocity of blood flow

The cardiovascular system is a closed system so the blood flow must equal the cardiac output, which is about 5 L/min at rest. As the flow divides between arterial branches, blood velocity changes. The velocity (v) of blood flow in different vessels is related to cardiac output (CO) and to the total cross-sectional area of the vessels (A) as follows:

$$v = CO / A$$

For a given flow through a single tube, if the tube becomes narrower the velocity increases. However, if the total

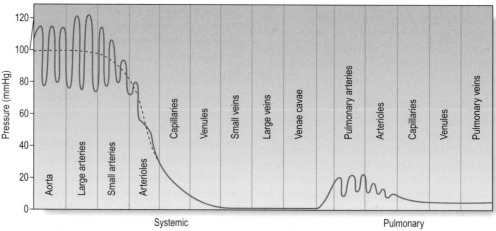

Fig. 11.45 **Pressure changes in the systemic and pulmonary circulations.** Most of the resistance to flow in the systemic system occurs at the arterioles. Pressures in the pulmonary system are much lower.

Table 11.16	Velocity of blood flow and cross-sectional area in the vasculature (approximate values for a resting human with a cardiac output of 5 L/min)		
Type of vessel	Total cross-sectional area (cm^2)	Velocity of blood flow (cm/s)	Relative velocity
Aorta	5	17	1
Large arteries	9	9.3	0.6
Small arteries	40	2.1	0.13
Capillaries	3000	0.03	0.002
Small veins	100	0.8	0.050
Large veins	30	2.8	0.17
Vena cava	7	12	0.7

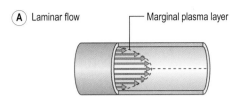

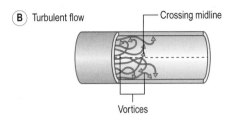

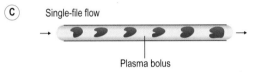

Fig. 11.46 Types of blood flow. (A) Profile of laminar flow with marginal plasma layer. (B) Turbulent flow showing eddies. (C) Bolus flow in capillaries.

flow divides to pass through a number of tubes then the velocity depends on the sum of their cross-sectional areas. If the total area is increased then the velocity decreases and vice versa. The total cross-sectional area of the arterial tree increases as the aorta branches progressively to finally deliver blood to the capillaries. This produces an inversely proportional reduction in the velocity of blood, which reaches its lowest in the capillaries (Table 11.16). As blood travels back towards the heart the total cross-sectional area of the converging veins decreases and velocity increases. The low velocity in the capillaries increases contact time of blood with the capillary membrane and facilitates the exchange of substances between blood and tissues.

Types of blood flow

Two main types of flow occur in tube-like structures such as blood vessels, **laminar flow** and **turbulent flow**. **Bolus flow** occurs in capillaries (Fig. 11.46).

Laminar blood flow

Laminar flow is characterised by concentric layers (or laminae) of blood which move smoothly down the length of a blood vessel. Blood flows fastest at the centre of the vessel (Fig. 11.46A), where there is least resistance. Through most of the circulation, laminar flow is the norm.

Turbulent blood flow

Turbulent flow occurs when flow is disrupted (Fig. 11.46B) to produce eddies and whirls rather than flow which is parallel to the walls of the blood vessel. This typically occurs at arterial branch points or through narrowed vascular segments. Turbulent flow in arteries may be audible on auscultation as a **bruit**, and in the heart as a **murmur** (see below, Heart sounds and murmurs). Common sites for bruits are over the carotid arteries, femoral arteries and renal arteries in patients with atherosclerotic disease.

Bolus flow

In most capillaries, red cells travel singly with a small amount (bolus) of plasma separating the cells – this is known as **bolus flow** (Fig. 11.46C). This is because the red cells

(erythrocytes) are slightly larger than the capillary diameter and have to squeeze through the capillaries in single file. In conditions where the erythrocyte membrane is defective and the cell is distorted, as in sickle cell disease (see Ch. 12, Haematology), the red cells can be trapped in the capillaries leading to occlusion and distal ischaemia.

Control of blood flow

Blood flow to different organs or tissues is regulated by the resistance in the small arteries and arterioles that supply the relevant vascular bed (SVR). Changes in the luminal area of these vessels by contraction or relaxation of the vascular smooth muscle in their walls is the main way in which blood flow is regulated. Resistance to flow is increased by vasoconstriction and decreased by vasodilatation.

Structure of vascular smooth muscle

Vascular smooth muscle cells, or **vascular myocytes**, are concentrated in the tunica media of the vessel wall (see above). They are spindle shaped, non-striated, involuntary muscle cells joined by gap junctions (Fig. 11.47). Vascular myocytes contain a single nucleus. Like cardiomyocytes and skeletal muscle, they contain the contractile proteins actin and myosin, but the sarcoplasmic reticulum is less extensive and, in contrast to cardiomyocytes, they do not contain troponin. **Caveolae** are invaginations of the cell membrane which increase the cell surface area in order to facilitate the movement of calcium from the extracellular fluid for contraction. The ends of the actin filaments are connected to the inner surface of the cell membrane by **dense bodies**. Intermediate filaments provide further integrity to the cell structure by cross linking dense bodies and through separate connections to the cell wall.

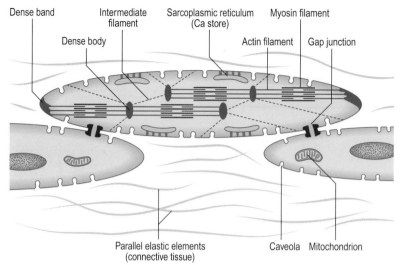

Dense band   Intermediate filament   Sarcoplasmic reticulum (Ca store)   Myosin filament

Dense body   Actin filament   Gap junction

Parallel elastic elements (connective tissue)   Caveola   Mitochondrion

Fig. 11.47 Structure of a vascular myocyte showing dense bodies and intermediate filaments.

Vascular smooth muscle contraction

As with other types of muscle, vascular smooth muscle contraction occurs due to the shortening of actin and myosin bundles (see Ch. 9 for details of actin and myosin) through increased overlap of their filaments. The dense bodies are pulled together so that the whole myocyte shortens. This is an involuntary process which consumes ATP. The contractile process in vascular smooth muscle is dependent upon a rise in the intracellular concentration of calcium but, unlike in cardiac muscle, this is caused by the **phosphorylation of myosin** rather than in an interaction between calcium and troponin C. The phosphorylation of myosin occurs by a cascade of calcium-dependent interactions:

1. Calcium diffuses into the cell from the interstitial fluid through calcium channels (see Chs 2 and 4) or is released from internal cellular stores in the sarcoplasmic reticulum
2. Calcium binds to four sites on **calmodulin**, a calcium-binding protein (see Ch. 9)
3. The enzyme **myosin light-chain kinase** (**MLCK**) is activated by calcium-bound calmodulin
4. MLCK phosphorylates the light chains of the myosin heads
5. Phosphorylated myosin heads form cross-bridges with the actin filaments
6. The rowing action of the myosin cross-bridges acts through the myosin heads to pull the actin filaments alongside the myosin chain, shortening the actin–myosin complex and therefore the vascular myocyte.

Unlike skeletal muscle, vascular smooth muscle is not capable of rapid contraction. However, its function in providing **vascular tone**, a basal state of low level contraction, is supported by two important properties. Firstly, vascular smooth muscle can maintain contraction for long periods and secondly, this can be achieved without consuming large amounts of ATP. This is partly because the cross-bridges between actin and myosin row much more slowly over each other during active contraction than in skeletal muscle and partly because a state of tension which fixes the cross-bridges in position can be achieved which does not consume energy. This basal vascular tone allows either vasoconstriction or vasodilatation through muscle contraction and relaxation, respectively, depending upon the requirements of the supplied tissues.

Excitation-contraction coupling of smooth muscle

The activation of MLCK links the rise in intracellular calcium ion concentration to vascular smooth muscle contraction. MLCK can be activated by an increase in intracellular calcium ion concentration which is produced by two different mechanisms called electromechanical coupling and pharmacomechanical coupling (Fig. 11.48).

Electromechanical coupling is responsible for the initial contraction of vascular smooth muscle (Fig. 11.48A). It is partly related to the opening of **voltage-sensitive calcium channels** (**VSCCs**), mainly L-type calcium channels, by action potentials causing depolarisation of the cell membrane. Spread of the depolarisation from cell to cell is aided by gap junctions between cells.

- The activation of **MLCK** and phosphorylation of myosin leads to the initial contraction of vascular myocytes
- Inhibition of **myosin light chain phosphatase** (**MLCP**). This enzyme breaks down MLCK and causes relaxation. The sustained high levels of intracellular calcium ions, however, activate rhoA kinase, which inhibits its action and maintains muscular contraction.

Pharmacomechanical coupling (Fig. 11.48B) involves the continuous entry of calcium into the myocyte through voltage-independent channels, called **receptor-operated non-selective cation channels** (**ROCs**). This diffusion of calcium is related to the much higher concentration of calcium outside the cell than in the cell and results in the activation of MLCK and smooth muscle contraction. The mechanism occurs particularly in large arteries which do not fire action potentials. Intracellular calcium is then removed by one of the following mechanisms:

- Pumped into the interstitium by Ca^{2+}-ATPase present on plasma membrane.

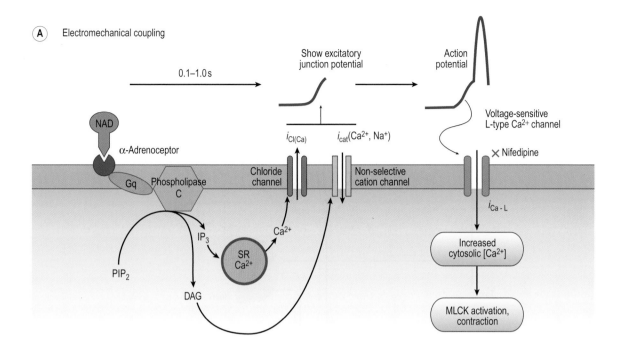

A Electromechanical coupling

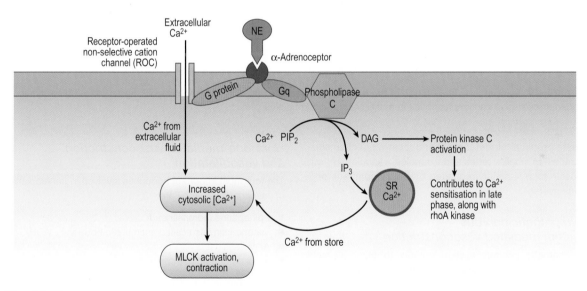

B Pharmacomechanical coupling

Fig. 11.48 **The pathways involved in the two phases of contraction in smooth muscle cells.** NE, norepinephrine (noradrenaline); IP$_3$, inositol trisphosphate; DAG, diacylglycerol; MLCK, myosin light chain kinase; MLCP, myosin light chain phosphatase; MLC, myosin light chains; PIP$_2$, phosphatidylinositol 4,5-bisphosphate; SR, sarcoplasmic reticulum. Not all the intermediate steps are shown. From Levick JR 2003 An introduction to cardiovascular physiology, 4th edn. Arnold, London, with permission.

- Returned to calcium stores by Ca^{2+}-ATPase present on the sarcoplasmic reticulum.
- Driven by the large sodium gradient across the cell membrane, intracellular calcium is exchanged for extracellular calcium by sodium/calcium co-transport. The excess intracellular sodium is removed by Na^+/K^+-ATPase.

The therapeutic use of drugs which disrupt the entry of calcium into myocytes through the blockade of calcium channels (calcium channel blockers) to inhibit vascular smooth muscle contraction is described in Clinical box 11.11.

Regulation of flow in small arteries and arterioles

The degree of contraction in vascular smooth muscle cells can be influenced by many different factors, including sympathetic nervous system output, hormones,

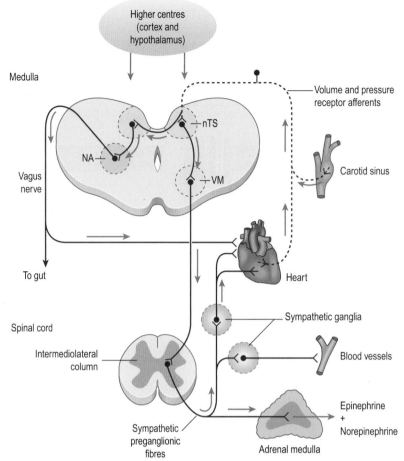

Fig. 11.49 **Sympathetic innervation of the heart, blood vessels and adrenal medulla.** nTS, nucleus tractus solitarius. *Dotted arrows* show sensory feedback from the heart and carotid sinus.

waste products of metabolism and local vasoactive substances. In small arteries and arterioles, vascular smooth muscle tone is mainly regulated by the sympathetic nervous system.

Sympathetic nervous system mediated vasoconstriction

Sympathetic nervous system outflow to blood vessels is controlled by the **nucleus tractus solitarius (nTS)** in the medulla (Fig. 11.49, see also Ch. 8). Afferent sensory inputs from the heart and carotid sinus provide information about blood volume and blood pressure, respectively, which together with higher cortical influences, determines sympathetic outflow. Efferent fibres originating in the nTS synapse in the **rostral ventrolateral medulla** (located near the midline of the medulla), which sends excitatory and inhibitory fibres to pre-ganglionic neurons of sympathetic ganglia in the dorsal horn of the spinal cord. Preganglionic fibres innervate the adrenal medulla and postganglionic neurons innervate the heart and blood vessels. Sympathetic nerve fibres terminate in the adventitia and the outer tunica media of the artery wall. These fibres contain multiple (up to 1000) varicosities (vesicles) which contain neurotransmitters that are released close to the surface of the myocytes. The principle sympathetic neurotransmitter is norepinephrine (with co-release of ATP and neuropeptide Y) which acts on **α-adrenoceptors** to cause **vasoconstriction**.

Hormone-mediated vasoconstriction and vasodilatation

The four most important hormones involved in the regulation of vasoconstrictor tone are:

- Epinephrine (adrenaline)
- Vasopressin (also called antidiuretic hormone – ADH)
- Angiotensin II
- Atrial natriuretic peptide (ANP).

Epinephrine is released from the adrenal medulla in response to sympathetic nervous system activation. It acts on both α- and β-adrenoceptors, but it is more active on β-adrenoceptors. β-Adrenoceptors predominate on vascular smooth muscle in skeletal muscle, the liver and cardiac muscle, where epinephrine causes **vasodilatation** (Fig. 11.50). Amongst its many other effects throughout the body, epinephrine also acts on β-adrenoceptors in the heart to increase heart rate and contractility, and thereby cardiac output. In tissues where α-adrenoceptors predominate on vascular smooth muscle, epinephrine causes vasoconstriction.

The actions of vasopressin, angiotensin II and ANP are discussed in detail in Chapter 14 (The renal system). Their main role is in the control of blood volume but they also affect vascular tone. The effects of **vasopressin** on blood flow are seen if blood volume becomes very low when it acts on V_1 receptors to cause **vasoconstriction** in all tissues, except the coronary and cerebral vessels. In the latter tissues, vasopressin stimulates the release of NO, resulting in vasodilatation to

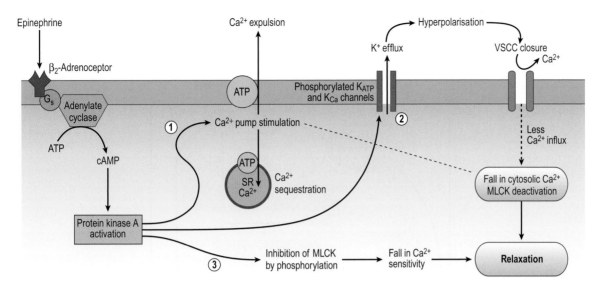

Fig. 11.50 **Vasodilation of smooth muscle by epinephrine (adrenaline).** G_s, G protein type s; cAMP, cyclic adenosine monophosphate; VSCC, voltage-sensitive calcium channel; MLCK, myosin light chain kinase; MLC, myosin light chains. From Levick JR 2003 An introduction to cardiovascular physiology, 4th edn. Arnold, London, with permission.

maintain perfusion to the heart and the brain. **Angiotensin II** is a potent **vasoconstrictor**, which acts through several mechanisms:

- Direct action on vascular myocytes to stimulate contraction
- Central action increasing sympathetic vasoconstriction
- Presynaptic action to increase norepinephrine release.

ANP is a **vasodilator**, acting by increasing cGMP levels in smooth muscle in a similar manner to NO.

Non-adrenergic autonomic nervous system mediated vasodilatation

In some tissues, such as male external genitalia, vagina and ovaries, vasodilator postganglionic parasympathetic fibres release acetylcholine and non-adrenergic, non-cholinergic (NANC) transmitters, including NO, neuropeptide P and vasoactive intestinal peptide (VIP). The blood vessels of sweat glands are innervated by sympathetic fibres that release acetylcholine causing vasodilatation and an increase in the production of sweat (see Ch. 4).

Receptor-mediated differential effects of catecholamines

The contrasting effects of norepinephrine and epinephrine in different vascular beds are entirely dependent on the receptor population of the particular smooth muscle (Table 11.17). While epinephrine and norepinephrine act on both α- and β-adrenoceptors, norepinephrine, released from sympathetic nerves, has a higher specificity for α-adrenoceptors, while epinephrine, the main catecholamine released from the adrenal medulla, is more active on β-adrenoceptors. It is the specific type of receptor that is activated, rather than the substance which activates it, that is critical in determining the response:

Vasoconstriction by catecholamines

Through electromechanical and pharmacomechanical coupling, the catecholamines norepinephrine and epinephrine cause vasoconstriction by binding to α-adrenoceptors, a type of G-protein-coupled receptor (see Ch. 4) (Fig. 11.51 and see Fig. 11.48B).

Table 11.17	Important endogenous vasoconstrictors and vasodilators
	Receptors activated*
Vasoconstrictors	
Norepinephrine epinephrine	α-Adrenergic
Endothelin	ET_a
Angiotensin II	AT1
Vasopressin	V_1
Thromboxane A_2	TP
Vasodilators	
Epinephrine norepinephrine	$β_2$-Adrenergic
Adenosine	A_2
Bradykinin	Bradykinin₁ and bradykinin₂
Prostacyclin	IP
Nitric oxide	Guanylate cyclase

* All the receptors shown here are types of G-protein-coupled receptors (GPLR) except for guanylate cyclase, which is an intracellular enzyme.

- The enzyme phospholipase C, linked to α-adrenergic receptors via the G protein, G_q, generates the second messengers **inositol trisphosphate (IP₃)** and **diacylglycerol (DAG)** from the membrane lipid PIP₂ (phosphatidylinositol 4,5-bisphosphate) (see Ch. 4)
- Calcium from intracellular sarcoplasmic reticulum is released by IP₃ to increase intracellular calcium, and also opens **calcium-activated chloride channels** in the plasma membrane
- Depolarisation occurs as the result of the efflux of chloride from the cell through the channels
- Voltage-sensitive calcium channels (VSCCs) open in response to depolarisation. Positive feedback in cells with large numbers of VSCCs leads to more VSCCs opening and a steep rise in intracellular calcium
- The influx of calcium activates MLCK, leading to contraction.

DAG generated with IP₃ activates **protein kinase C**, which is also calcium-dependent, can inhibit MLCP, thus increasing the sensitivity to calcium.

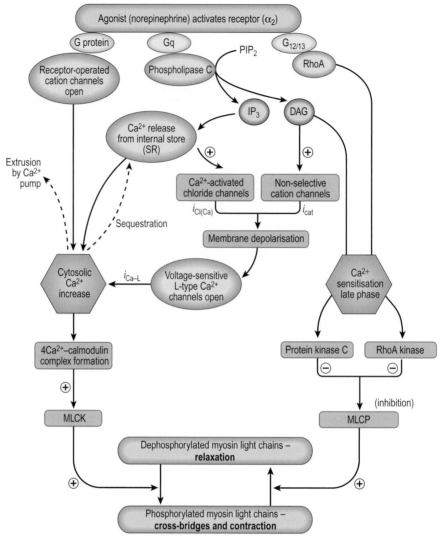

Fig. 11.51 **Vasoconstriction of smooth muscle by catecholamines.** G_q, G protein type q; PIP_2, phosphatidylinositol bisphosphate; IP_3, inositol trisphosphate; DAG, diacylglycerol; MLCK, myosin light chain kinase; MLCP, myosin light chain phosphatase. From Levick JR 2003 An introduction to cardiovascular physiology, 4th edn. Arnold, London, with permission.

Vasodilatation by catecholamines

Epinephrine causes vasodilation in some tissues, e.g. skeletal and cardiac muscle, liver (Fig. 11.50). Acting through G-protein linked β_2-adrenergic receptors, activation of the G protein G_s increases intracellular second messenger cAMP that activates protein kinase A (PKA) leading to the relaxation of vascular myocytes and vasodilatation (see also Ch. 3):

- PKA stimulates Ca^{2+}-ATPase which pumps calcium into the sarcoplasmic reticulum and out into the interstitium, lowering intracellular calcium concentration.
- Membrane K^+ channels open through phosphorylation by PKA, leading to hyperpolarisation, preventing the opening of VSCCs.
- MLCK is inactivated through phosphorylation by PKA, decreasing calcium sensitivity.

The fall in cytosolic Ca^{2+} leads to MLCK deactivation, and muscle relaxation.

Regulation of flow in the microcirculation

One of the key functions of the microcirculation is the delivery of oxygen and other nutrients to the tissues and the removal of CO_2 and other waste products of metabolism from them. Blood flow to the microcirculation changes in response to the metabolic needs of the tissues through vasoconstriction or vasodilatation. In contrast to the main resistance vessels of the circulation which are under the control of the sympathetic nervous system, the tone of the pre-capillary arterioles is determined predominantly by local factors which reflect local tissue blood flow requirements. In some circumstances, such as during exercise or shock, local tissue requirements may be temporarily over-ridden by the more urgent requirements of specific vascular beds, such as skeletal muscle (exercise), or for generalised vasoconstriction (to maintain arterial blood pressure in shock). The local factors which control blood flow at the capillary level are:

- Autoregulation
- Metabolic byproduct vasodilators
- Local vasoactive hormones.

Autoregulation of blood flow

Over a wide range, changes in arterial blood pressure do not affect the blood flow through most vascular beds (except in the pulmonary circulation) (Fig. 11.52). In response to

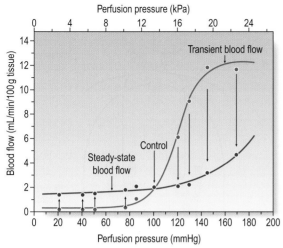

Fig. 11.52 **Autoregulation of blood flow.** When the perfusion pressure is changed there is a transient change in flow but this rapidly reverts to the steady-state.

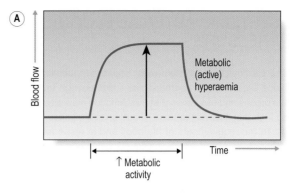

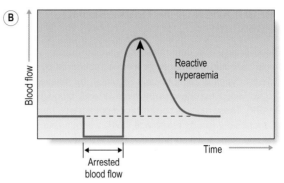

Fig. 11.53 **(A)** Metabolic and **(B)** reactive hyperaemia.

increased perfusion pressure, the flow initially increases but falls back towards baseline. This autoregulation of blood flow is believed to be mediated through mechano-sensitive ion channels in the myocyte plasma membrane which are activated by stretch in the artery wall. These cause the myocytes to depolarise, increasing the influx of calcium through voltage-sensitive calcium channels, which increases contraction and reduces flow.

Metabolic byproduct vasodilatation

A number of byproducts and other consequences of metabolism cause local vasodilatation. The main **metabolic vasodilators** are:

- Elevated CO_2
- Low O_2
- Acidosis
- Increased phosphate ions and adenosine (from the breakdown of ATP)
- Increased osmolality
- Increased K^+ (as a result of increased action potential frequency in nerves and muscles).

These factors cause vascular smooth muscle relaxation and increased blood flow by a variety of mechanisms including receptor activation, hyperpolarisation and stimulation of ion transport. This is known as **active hyperaemia** (**metabolic hyperaemia**, or **functional hyperaemia**) (Fig. 11.53A). Active hyperaemia may be a response to tissue hypoxia, generating vasodilator metabolites such as K^+, NO, CO_2 and adenosine. This is visible when hyperaemia occurs in the skin, giving the clinical appearance of **erythema** (redness).

It is important to note that pulmonary arterioles constrict in response to hypoxia rather than vasodilate. This diverts blood away from poorly ventilated lung (see Ch. 13) so that more blood is available to perfuse the ventilated areas of lung.

Reactive hyperaemia occurs following temporary interruption of tissue blood flow. The interruption of blood flow deprives the tissues of O_2 and nutrients, a phenomenon known as tissue **ischaemia**, which, if prolonged, can lead to permanent tissue damage or death (necrosis). Ischaemia could be transient, lasting a few seconds, or prolonged up to several hours. During this time, metabolic vasodilators

accumulate in the tissues, which increases blood flow above normal when it is restored (Fig. 11.53B).

Local vasoactive hormones

The vascular endothelium produces a number of hormones which have local effects on vasoconstrictor tone:

- Nitric oxide (NO) is a vasodilator which is synthesised in endothelial cells by the enzyme **nitric oxide synthase** (**NOS**) from the amino acid L-arginine, stimulated by increased calcium in the endothelial cell. This can be caused by a number of factors including shear stress on the endothelium. NO diffuses across the plasma membrane into the tunica media, where it diffuses into the smooth muscle cells, activating the cytoplasmic enzyme guanylate cyclase. Guanylate cyclase produces the second messenger cyclic guanosine monophosphate (cGMP). cGMP activates protein kinase G (PKG). It is thought that PKG causes relaxation in similar ways to protein kinase A (see above).
- The amino acid peptide **endothelin** (ET-1) is a vasoconstrictor formed and released in response to angiotensin II, ADH, cytokines and shearing forces on the vascular endothelium. It has a prolonged vasoconstrictor action that may have a role in maintaining capillary basal tone. Release is inhibited by NO, ANP and eicosanoids.
- Prostaglandins (prostanoids and eicosanoids), e.g. prostacyclin (PGI_2), thromboxanes and leukotrienes, are vasodilators with local effects (paracrine hormones). Their primary functions are related to inflammation and haemostasis (see Ch. 6).
- Other local vasodilator hormones include histamine, bradykinin, serotonin (5-HT) and platelet activating factor.

SYSTEMIC ARTERIAL BLOOD PRESSURE

The cardiovascular system must maintain systemic arterial blood pressure within certain limits – high enough to perfuse the organs and tissues so that they function normally, but not so high that it damages them. Blood pressure varies according to the requirements of the body and in response to different physical and psychological stimuli; it increases during exercise, anxiety and stress and decreases during rest and sleep. Blood pressure tends to rise with age as the elasticity of the arteries decreases.

REGULATION OF ARTERIAL BLOOD PRESSURE

Blood pressure is determined by cardiac output and systemic vascular resistance. Its level is monitored by various different types of receptor and regulated by reflexes which are activated by changes in mean arterial blood pressure (MABP). These reflexes control blood pressure by modulation of systemic vascular resistance (SVR), venous return, heart rate and myocardial contractility. They are the:

- Baroreceptor reflex
- Chemoreceptor reflexes
- Cardiopulmonary reflexes.

Baroreceptor reflex

The **baroreceptor reflex** arc sends information about the pressure in the aorta and carotid arteries to the brainstem, which modulates output of the sympathetic and parasympathetic nervous systems to the heart and blood vessels in order to maintain the blood pressure within the normal range. The degree of stretch in the aortic arch and carotid sinuses is monitored by sensory nerve endings called **baroreceptors** (Fig. 11.54). They respond to stretching of the arteries by firing action potentials which are transmitted along afferent fibres in the vagus and glossopharyngeal nerves to cell bodies in the petrous and nodose ganglia before their axons terminate in the nucleus tractus solitarius.

Baroreceptors have static and dynamic responses (Fig. 11.55). At normal blood pressure, they fire action potentials at a constant, moderate rate (S1). When blood pressure increases, their discharge rate increases (D1) proportional to the rate of increase in the blood pressure (**dynamic response**). This burst of firing is transient, but if the higher level of blood pressure is sustained, the baroreceptor discharge rate (S2) is maintained at a level higher than the initial base rate (**static response**). By contrast, when blood pressure falls, baroreceptor activity ceases (D2), before resuming at a rate slower than baseline activity (S1).

There are two types of baroreceptors in the aortic arch and carotid sinus:

- **A fibres** are active at mean arterial blood pressures above about 50 mmHg. The firing rate of these large, myelinated fibres increases rapidly in response to increases in MABP until their saturation point is reached at about 150 mmHg (Fig. 11.56, *red line*). They are responsible for refining blood pressure control at levels within and close to the normal range.

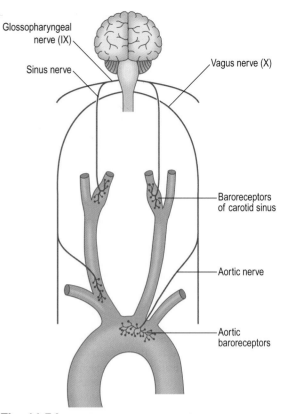

Fig. 11.54 **Arterial baroreceptors.** Afferent sensory fibres from the aortic and carotid baroreceptors have their cell bodies in the petrous and nodose ganglia and synapse in the nucleus tractus solitarius.

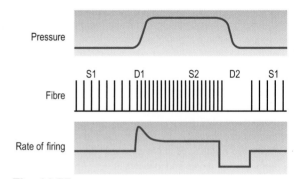

Fig. 11.55 Dynamic (D) and static (S) responses of baroreceptors.

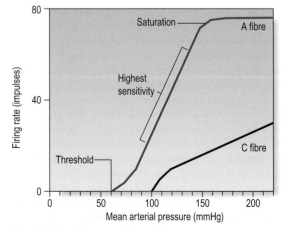

Fig. 11.56 Different types of baroreceptor signal different ranges of blood pressure.

- **C fibres** are activated at MABPs above about 100 mmHg. They have a lower firing rate than A fibres and are less sensitive to changes in pressure but their firing rate continues to increase in relation to rising blood pressure without an upper saturation level. (Fig. 11.56, *black line*). C fibres are small and unmyelinated, they are the more numerous type of baroreceptor, and they are principally involved in the regulation of high blood pressures.

Baroreceptor activity stimulates parasympathetic output from the nucleus tractus solitarius to the heart via the vagus nerve and reduces sympathetic output to the heart and vasculature. This leads to a reduction in MABP through:

- A decrease in heart rate and myocardial contractility, which reduces cardiac output
- A decrease in vasoconstrictor tone, which reduces SVR.

By contrast, reduced baroreceptor activity (in response to a fall in blood pressure) produces the opposite effects, resulting in reduced parasympathetic output and increased sympathetic output. Heart rate, myocardial contractility and vasoconstrictor tone are all increased. Venoconstriction in the gastrointestinal tract and liver increases the central venous blood volume, which increases venous return to the heart and thereby stroke volume (Starling's law). The baroreceptor reflex responds rapidly to changes in blood pressure and is particularly important in maintaining blood pressure in acute hypotension. Other reflexes and hormonal responses involved in the regulation of blood pressure effect changes which take longer to modulate blood pressure.

Chemoreceptor reflexes

In normal conditions, the chemoreceptor reflexes are primarily involved in the control of breathing (see Ch. 13). Groups of sensory cells (**chemoreceptors**) adjacent to the aorta and carotid sinuses called the **aortic and carotid bodies**, respectively, send impulses to the brainstem in response to changes in the blood concentration of oxygen, carbon dioxide and hydrogen ions, which modulates function of the respiratory centre. However, the concentration of these chemicals is not only dependent upon respiratory function; during severe hypotension, poor perfusion of the lungs and the body tissues results in low blood levels of oxygen (hypoxaemia) and high levels of carbon dioxide (hypercapnia) and hydrogen ions (acidosis). This is a potent stimulus to the chemoreceptors, which send impulses to the brainstem resulting in an increase in sympathetic nervous system output. In turn this results in systemic vasoconstriction which helps to maintain central blood pressure. The chemoreceptors also stimulate the respiratory centre to increase the respiratory rate in an attempt to improve oxygenation and to blow off carbon dioxide to compensate for the metabolic acidosis.

Cardiopulmonary reflexes

Cardiopulmonary receptors are a diverse group of receptors which are located in the heart, the great veins and pulmonary arteries, and in the lungs. They have vagal afferent fibres and contribute to the reflex control of central sympathetic outflow mediated by changes in thoracic blood volume and pressure.

Increases in central venous volume and pressure activate **mechanoreceptors** in the atria and vena cava in response to wall stretch. Increased afferent signalling results in sympathetic stimulation of the SA node and a reflex tachycardia. This is called the **Bainbridge reflex**, the purpose of which may be to move blood rapidly from the venous circulation into the systemic arterial circulation during exercise. This reflex also decreases renal sympathetic activity, which reduces renin secretion and thereby increases urine output, a mechanism which acts more slowly than adjustment of heart rate to regulate central blood volume and blood pressure. Other mechanoreceptors supplied by small non-myelinated afferents are stimulated by increased atrial and ventricular volumes and pressures to produce bradycardia and vasodilation.

Chemoreceptors in the walls of the heart which have unmyelinated vagal and sympathetic fibres are stimulated by bradykinin and prostaglandins, released by ischaemic heart muscle, to produce bradycardia and vasodilatation. The sympathetic fibres are responsible for signaling the pain associated with myocardial infarction and angina.

Juxtapulmonary (J) receptors in the lungs are activated by lung expansion resulting in an increase in heart rate and vasodilatation.

Central regulation of cardiovascular reflexes

The afferent nerve fibres from the baroreceptors and other cardiovascular receptors which mediate the cardiovascular reflexes terminate in the nucleus tractus solitarius (nTS) in the medulla. Neurons in the nTS send outputs to:

- Other areas of the **medulla,** which control autonomic output
- The **hypothalamus,** which receives inputs from the cerebral cortex
- The **cerebellum,** which coordinates muscular activity.

The **nucleus ambiguous** and the **dorsal motor nucleus** in the medulla contain the cell bodies of the parasympathetic vagal preganglionic neurons which, when activated, slow the heart. Inputs to the ventrolateral medulla control efferent neurons which mediate sympathetic output. These connections allow the cardiovascular reflexes to be modulated centrally in response to stimuli such as pain, temperature and alerting stimuli, such as sudden noises. The hypothalamus is responsible for the 'fight or flight' response. This response to danger causes an increase in heart rate, blood pressure and blood flow to skeletal muscle, preparing the body for action.

Regulation of the baroreceptor reflex

The level of blood pressure which is considered to be 'normal' and which results in a balanced output in parasympathetic and sympathetic nervous system activity is not fixed. During exercise, for example, the blood pressure around which the baroreceptor reflex operates at a neutral level is raised centrally to allow cardiac output to increase to meet the increased demands of the body. A sustained increase in pressure can also cause the baroreceptors to re-set to a higher pressure. This is thought to be an important mechanism in hypertension, where the slightly higher blood pressure becomes accepted as the level for neutral baroreceptor activity. If this happens repetitively, blood pressure lowering mechanisms are not activated until higher and higher blood pressures are reached.

Long-term control of blood pressure

The baroreceptor reflex and other cardiovascular reflexes respond rapidly to acute changes in blood pressure to effect short-term control measures, predominantly through alterations in heart rate and vasoconstrictor tone. Different mechanisms which act through hormonal pathways to modulate blood volume and blood vessel tone are important in the long-term regulation of blood pressure (see also Ch. 14). The most important hormones involved in the control of blood volume are:

- Vasopressin
- Angiotensin II
- Aldosterone
- Atrial natriuretic peptide (ANP).

Vasopressin

The main role of **vasopressin**, also known as **antidiuretic hormone (ADH)**, is to maintain normal blood osmolality, which it achieves through regulation of body water content. Vasopressin is produced by the **supraoptic** and **paraventricular** nuclei of the hypothalamus, prior to its storage in the posterior pituitary gland. The hypothalamus contains **osmoreceptors** which sense changes in blood osmolality and regulate the release of vasopressin from the posterior pituitary; an increase in blood osmolality stimulates vasopressin release while a decrease in blood osmolality inhibits vasopressin release. Vasopressin acts on the kidney to promote water retention, the increased blood volume acting to dilute solute concentration and restore normal osmolality. This is effected through the binding of vasopressin to V_2 receptors in the cells of the collecting duct. This increases the concentration of intracellular cAMP which, in turn, stimulates a conformational change in the luminal membrane which increases the water permeability of the collecting duct. Water reabsorption is increased and the urine is concentrated.

Vasopressin release is also stimulated by a low blood volume through the cardiopulmonary reflexes. If blood volume is dangerously low, restoration of blood volume is prioritised over regulation of osmolality and vasopressin is released irrespective of the blood osmolality.

Angiotensin II

Angiotensin II is a key component of the **renin–angiotensin–aldosterone system**, a hormone pathway which is central to the regulation of blood pressure and blood volume. The pathway is activated by three different stimuli:

- A fall in the perfusion pressure to the kidney (due to hypotension or renal artery stenosis)
- Stimulation of β_1-adrenoceptors on juxtaglomerular cells by circulating epinephrine or sympathetic nerve stimulation
- A reduction in sodium concentration in the distal tubule.

Any of these stimulate the release of **renin** from the **juxtaglomerular cells** in the kidney glomerulus. Renin is a proteolytic enzyme that activates **angiotensinogen** to produce **angiotensin I**. Angiotensin I is cleaved by **angiotensin converting enzyme (ACE)** in the lungs to produce its active form, **angiotensin II**. Acting on AT1 receptors, angiotensin II causes systemic vasoconstriction and an increase in blood pressure, and constriction of the efferent renal arterioles to maintain glomerular filtration rate. It also stimulates the release of aldosterone promoting the retention of salt and water in the kidneys, it has a direct effect on the proximal tubules to increase sodium reabsorption, it stimulates the release of vasopressin, and it stimulates the thirst centre, actions which all tend to increase blood volume.

Aldosterone

Aldosterone is a steroid hormone that is released from the adrenal cortex in response to stimulation by angiotensin II. Its release is therefore promoted by any of the causes of activation of the renin–angiotensin–aldosterone system. Aldosterone promotes Na^+ reabsorption and K^+ secretion in the distal tubules of the kidneys. It acts on nuclear receptors to increase the synthesis of Na^+/K^+-ATPases on the abluminal side of the distal tubular cells. These cells enable the transport of more sodium into the renal medulla at the expense of potassium. As well as being stimulated by angiotensin II, aldosterone release is also stimulated by reduced blood volume, reduced plasma sodium, trauma and stress.

Atrial natriuretic peptide

Atrial natriuretic peptide (ANP) and the closely related **brain natriuretic peptide (BNP)** are released by atrial myocytes in response to atrial stretch. This is an indication of elevated atrial pressure and blood volume. ANP produces effects opposite to vasopressin, angiotensin II and aldosterone, *increasing* salt and water excretion by the kidney in order to lower blood volume. ANP causes:

- An increase in glomerular filtration rate by relaxing the afferent glomerular arterioles while constricting the efferent arterioles, thus increasing the hydrostatic pressure in the capsule
- Reduced sodium and water reabsorption in the tubules
- Inhibited release of vasoconstrictors including angiotensin II, aldosterone and endothelin.

Circulating levels of ANP, and especially BNP, are raised in patients with heart failure reflecting activation of this system as a homeostatic mechanism to correct the increased blood volume. Measuring the blood concentration of BNP is a useful test to help diagnose heart failure in difficult cases.

Orthostasis

Orthostasis means the maintenance of standing upright. On moving from supine to vertical about 500 mL of blood moves from the central veins into the veins in the legs as a result of gravity. The increased blood volume in the legs during orthostasis increases pressures below the heart and decreases pressures above the heart. The fall in blood pressure in the upper part of the body immediately activates the baroreceptor reflex causing an increase in heart rate and vasoconstriction which compensates for the reduction in venous return, and in stroke volume and cardiac output which would otherwise occur. SVR increases and MABP rises by about 10 mmHg. When these normal physiological responses fail, blood pressure falls rather than rises on standing, which is called **orthostatic (or postural) hypotension**. The mechanisms involved in fainting are similar to those which cause orthostatic hypotension (Information box 11.15).

SHOCK

Adequate perfusion is essential in order to maintain oxygen delivery to the tissues. Under-perfused cells become **hypoxic** (starved of oxygen) and, if this under-perfusion persists, they

---

Information box 11.15 | **Mechanisms involved in fainting**

Fainting is caused by failure of the physiological mechanisms which maintain arterial blood pressure, and therefore cerebral perfusion, in the upright position. It usually occurs in subjects who have been standing for a prolonged period. The sympathetic tone which causes venoconstriction suddenly falls, blood pools in the veins in the legs reducing venous return to the heart, and cardiac output and arterial blood pressure fall. The reduction in sympathetic output means that the parasympathetic nervous system is dominant. The vagal effect on the heart prevents the corrective tachycardia which usually occurs in response to hypotension as part of the baroreceptor reflex and the heart rate is often abnormally slow. Reduced cerebral perfusion causes lightheadedness and, if the fall in blood pressure is large enough, syncope results. Consciousness following a faint is typically regained within seconds as the recumbent position aids venous return to the heart, restoring cardiac output and cerebral perfusion, and the failure in sympathetic tone is usually short lived. Fainting is sometimes referred to as **vasovagal syncope** because of the role of the parasympathetic nervous system in its aetiology.

---

eventually die. Tissue perfusion may be inadequate due to a local reduction in blood flow as, for example, when acute occlusion of a coronary artery results in infarction of the myocardium. However, when there is a widespread failure of perfusion to meet the metabolic demands of the body, this condition is called **shock**. The clinical syndrome of shock is characterised by hypotension and failure of the key body organs. There are five different types of shock:

- Hypovolaemic
- Cardiogenic
- Vasodilatory
- Anaphylactic
- Neurogenic.

Hypovolaemic shock

A reduction in blood volume leads to hypovolaemic shock. This can be caused either by blood loss (haemorrhage) or by a reduced plasma volume. **Haemorrhage** may be 'external', when the blood loss is visible from open wounds such as lacerations or amputations, or 'internal', when the bleeding is contained within the body. Causes of internal bleeding include pelvic fractures, ruptured abdominal aortic aneurysm, or traumatic liver or splenic injury. Large volumes of blood may be lost internally before the diagnosis is made so a high index of suspicion is required in patients who are at risk of internal bleeding such as patients who have suffered major trauma. The volume and rate of blood loss and the haemodynamic reserve determine the clinical consequences of haemorrhage. The more rapid the blood loss and the lower the haemodynamic reserve, the greater the likelihood of shock. Arterial bleeding is usually more serious than venous bleeding, the higher pressure in the arterial system compared with the venous system resulting in a higher rate of blood loss. Nevertheless, venous haemorrhage can still be fatal.

Most healthy subjects can tolerate the loss of 10% (500 mL) blood volume without developing symptoms or signs of shock, the body's homeostatic mechanisms compensating effectively for the reduced intravascular volume. The loss of 20–30% of blood volume over a short period of time, however, produces **shock**. The reduced blood volume is partially compensated for by increased activation of

homeostatic mechanisms, but the patient will have signs of shock such as tachycardia and cool peripheries (see below and Fig. 11.57). The loss of 30–40% (up to 2 L) of blood volume causes decompensated shock. The patient is hypotensive and tachycardic with signs of organ failure. This is fatal unless treated urgently and aggressively.

Hypovolaemia due to **reduced plasma volume** can be caused by dehydration due to inadequate oral intake of fluid or by increased extracellular fluid losses from the gastrointestinal tract or kidneys, or by loss of plasma.

- Dehydration due to **inadequate oral intake** is most common in children and the elderly, groups who may be dependent upon others to provide them with fluid. Fever and hot weather increase insensible extracellular fluid loses through sweat and predispose to dehydration. Elderly subjects who cannot get up following a fall or who become confused for any reason are at particular risk of dehydration due to inadequate oral intake of fluid.
- **Gastrointestinal losses of extracellular fluid** occur through persistent vomiting, diarrhoea, or gastrointestinal obstruction. Infective causes of diarrhoea such as **cholera** can result in massive losses of water and electrolytes and are an important cause of hypovolaemic shock in the developing world. Oral rehydration therapy (see Ch. 2, Clinical box 2.11), which consists of water, sodium chloride, potassium, citrate and glucose, has been shown to be effective in maintaining plasma volume and reducing mortality in patients with diarrhoea.
- Increased **renal losses of extracellular fluid** occur in hyperglycaemic states (diabetes mellitus), adrenocortical failure, diabetes insipidus and in over-diuresis.
  - In **hyperosmolar hyperglycaemic state** (previously called hyperosmolar non-ketotic coma), the high tubular glucose concentration exceeds the reabsorptive capacity of the kidneys resulting in an osmotic diuresis and dehydration. The plasma sodium concentration and plasma osmolality are high. Plasma viscosity is increased predisposing to venous thromboembolism.
  - In **adrenocortical failure**, there is reduced synthesis of adrenocortical hormones including aldosterone. This results in reduced sodium and water reabsorption from the distal tubule of the kidney and therefore increased sodium and water loss (see Ch. 10). Primary autoimmune adrenocortical failure is called **Addison disease**.
  - **Diabetes insipidus** occurs when vasopressin (ADH) release from the posterior pituitary gland is abnormally low (cranial diabetes insipidus) or its action on the kidney is reduced (nephrogenic diabetes insipidus). Both result in failure of water reabsorption in the kidney, and predispose to dehydration and hypernatraemia.
- **Plasma loss** can result from **burns** due to increased capillary permeability – the greater the body surface area affected, the greater the potential for blood volume loss. **Gastrointestinal obstruction** involves several mechanisms for hypovolaemia with large volumes of extracellular fluid secreted into the bowel lumen and plasma loss arising from increased capillary filtration **into the abdomin**al cavity from the swollen bowel wall.

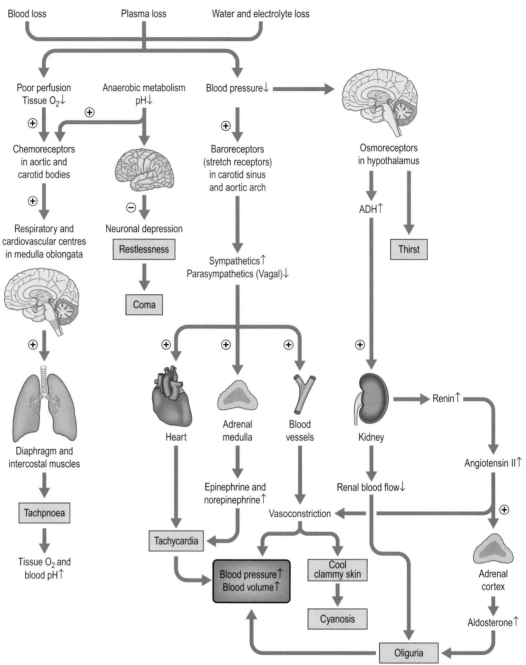

***Fig. 11.57* Shock: homeostatic mechanisms, signs and symptoms.** Homeostatic mechanisms are activated by shock to restore blood volume and tissue perfusion. The heart responds by an increase in rate (tachycardia) and stroke volume. Respiration increases both in rate (tachypnoea) and depth in response to the fall in pH (acidosis). Reduced glomerular perfusion due to falling blood volume and blood pressure triggers the release of renin from the juxtaglomerular apparatus, activating the renin-angiotensin-aldosterone system (see Ch. 14). The direct action of falling pH on the cerebral cortex leads to restlessness and coma. ADH, antidiuretic hormone (vasopressin).

Cardiogenic shock

Cardiogenic shock is present when there is failure of adequate perfusion of the tissues and organs due to a primary failure of cardiac function. It can be caused by any of the causes of heart failure (Table 11.10). In Western societies, the most common cause is acute myocardial infarction, when occlusion of one of the major epicardial coronary arteries results in such a large amount of myocardial damage that the heart cannot maintain a sufficient cardiac output to adequately perfuse the body's major organs. The patient has low blood pressure and pre-renal failure. Occlusion of the left anterior descending artery causes left ventricular failure and pulmonary oedema. If the occluded vessel is a dominant right coronary artery or dominant circumflex artery, there may be damage to the right ventricle, which becomes a non-contractile conduit resulting in a low output state without pulmonary oedema. Other causes of cardiogenic shock include pump failure due to myocarditis or dilated cardiomyopathy, acute valvular regurgitation due to endocarditis or aortic dissection, and cardiac tamponade (see Clinical box 11.1).

Vasodilatory (septic) shock

Vasodilatory shock is characterised by a vasodilated state and leaky capillaries, which manifest clinically as hypotension and oedema. Leakage of fluid into the lungs predisposes to adult respiratory distress syndrome (ARDS, see below and Ch. 13). Vasodilatory shock is usually caused by a severe systemic bacterial infection when it is commonly referred to as **septic shock**. It can also be caused by poisoning by carbon monoxide or nitrogen and a number of other chemicals such as cyanide the oral anti-diabetic drug metformin, or follow long-lasting shock of any cause.

In vasodilatory shock, the sympathetic nervous system and the renin–angiotensin system are activated but the vascular smooth muscle fails to contract. Systemic vascular resistance and blood pressure consequently fall. The release of endotoxins and the actions of cytokines are two key factors involved in the aetiology of vasodilatory shock. They cause the opening of ATP-sensitive potassium channels and potassium leaves the cell. The cell membrane becomes hyperpolarised which prevents the opening of voltage-dependent calcium channels and reduces the amount of calcium that is available for vascular smooth muscle contraction. In addition, nitric oxide levels are increased through the cytokine-induced activation of nitric oxide synthase. Nitric oxide increases intracellular cGMP and opens calcium-dependent potassium channels in the cell membrane which hyperpolarises the cell and prevents vascular smooth muscle contraction. After a prolonged period of shock, vasopressin levels fall due to depletion of pituitary gland stores. As well as promoting water retention, vasopressin has a vasoconstrictor effect so its reduced levels contribute to the vasodilated state.

Anaphylactic shock

Anaphylaxis is a serious allergic reaction which occurs minutes to hours after exposure to the causative allergen (see also Ch. 6). The clinical syndrome of anaphylaxis frequently includes shock, when it is termed **anaphylactic shock**. Anaphylaxis is caused by a **type I hypersensitivity reaction**, in which previous exposure to the allergen stimulates the formation of specific IgE antibodies. These antibodies bind to F_c receptors on mast cells and, when cross-linked by later repeat exposure to the allergen, they cause mast cells to degranulate. The clinical manifestations of anaphylaxis are related to the consequent release of inflammatory mediators from mast cells including histamine, leukotrienes, prostaglandins and platelet activating factor. These affect multiple body systems but some of the most common clinical features are itching and hives, hypotension due to profound vasodilatation, breathlessness due to bronchoconstriction and laryngeal oedema, which can threaten patency of the upper airway.

Anaphylactic shock can be caused by a wide range of allergens including nuts, bee stings, or drugs, particularly antibiotics. Several fatal cases of anaphylaxis to penicillin occur each year in the UK, often when the drug is administered in error to a patient who is known to be allergic to the drug. These deaths are avoidable and patients should always be asked whether or not they are allergic to penicillin before it is administered.

Rapid treatment of anaphylactic shock is necessary to prevent death. Intramuscular epinephrine should be administered to reverse the vasodilatation and bronchoconstriction and intravenous fluid is given to fill the expanded intravascular space. Airway management may be required in some cases. An antihistamine and hydrocortisone are also administered, but act more slowly to block the ongoing inflammatory response.

Anaphylactoid reactions are clinically indistinguishable from anaphylaxis. However, they are idiosyncratic reactions to a substance rather than a type I hypersensitivity reaction. They do not require prior exposure to the antigen. The treatment is the same as for anaphylaxis.

Neurogenic shock

Neurogenic shock occurs when there is a failure of sympathetic outflow due to spinal cord injury or damage to the brainstem. Unopposed vagal tone results in vasodilatation. Blood pools in the venous system, which reduces venous return and cardiac output.

Sympathetic outflow from the cord occurs between levels T1 and L2. Neurogenic shock does not usually occur with cord injuries below T6. High injuries produce bradycardia due to loss of sympathetic supply to the heart. Neurogenic shock can be simulated by general anaesthesia which depresses the vasoconstrictor activity of the brainstem while spinal anaesthesia also tends to cause hypotension through inhibition of the autonomic sympathetic outflow below the level of block.

Homeostatic mechanisms activated by shock

The body is equipped with several homeostatic mechanisms which are activated by shock in order to restore blood volume and tissue perfusion. These mechanisms are predominantly the cardiovascular reflexes and hormone systems which regulate blood pressure. The compensatory mechanisms activated by hypovolaemic shock are summarised in Figure 11.57. Most are common to all types of shock and these mechanisms are partly responsible for the clinical features of shock.

The decreased stretch in the aorta and carotid sinuses caused by low blood volume and blood pressure reduces the afferent input from the **baroreceptors** to the brainstem which results in decreased vagal output and increased sympathetic output. The heart rate is increased which helps to maintain cardiac output and the veins are constricted which helps to maintain venous return, Peripheral arterial vasoconstriction supports the blood pressure and helps to preserve blood flow to the heart and brain at the expense of other organs. In the early stages of shock, these compensatory responses may be sufficient to maintain arterial blood pressure within the normal range. Furthermore, hypertensive patients may experience a significant drop in blood pressure before it falls below normal. For these reasons, blood pressure by itself is a poor indicator of the reduction in blood volume and an elevated heart rate is a more sensitive sign of hypovolaemia.

The **renin–angiotensin–aldosterone system** is activated in shock by reduced renal perfusion and by increased renal sympathetic stimulation. This promotes vasoconstriction through the generation of angiotensin II, and helps to maintain blood volume through the action of aldosterone on the distal tubule to increase sodium and fluid reabsorption.

Reduced blood volume activates the **cardiopulmonary reflexes**. Stimulation of the mechanoreceptors in the great vessels is reduced which causes the release of vasopressin from the pituitary gland. This promotes water retention and thirst.

Reduced tissue perfusion increases anaerobic metabolism which results in the production of lactic acid. The low blood pH activates the **chemoreceptor reflexes**, with increased signalling to the respiratory centre in the brainstem and an increase in the respiratory rate. Carbon dioxide is blown off to achieve respiratory compensation for the metabolic acidosis. Central sympathetic output is also increased by this reflex.

Clinical signs of shock

In hypovolaemic shock, **hypotension** arises as the direct consequence of a reduced blood volume. The other clinical signs of hypovolaemic shock, however, are the effect of the compensatory mechanisms described above. Sympathetic stimulation causes **tachycardia** and vasoconstriction gives rise to **cool peripheries**. The sympathetic activation also causes an increase in sweating but the poorly perfused skin is cool so the sweat does not evaporate, resulting in the patient feeling **clammy**. The metabolic acidosis stimulates the respiratory centre causing **tachypnoea.** A low urine output (**oliguria**) is the result of aldosterone and vasopressin release.

In vasodilatory shock, anaphylactic shock and neurogenic shock, the primary abnormality is profound vasodilatation. It is not compensated for by peripheral vasoconstriction so the skin is typically warm. Bradycardia may occur in neurogenic shock due to unopposed vagal stimulation of the heart.

Decompensated shock and multi-organ failure

In decompensated shock, the body's compensatory mechanisms are insufficient to prevent a progressive deterioration in blood pressure and tissue perfusion. This results in a vicious circle of body system failures. At a MABP between 50 and 70 mmHg, the perfusion of the **heart** is significantly reduced. This, together with a myocardial depressant factor released from the pancreas during severe shock, impairs myocardial contractility and reduces cardiac output. Reduced tissue perfusion increases anaerobic metabolism and acid production. However, the ability of the kidneys to excrete hydrogen ions is reduced by inadequate renal perfusion so acid accumulates in the blood. **Acidosis** further reduces myocardial contractility which, in turn, lowers cardiac output and blood pressure, and myocardial and tissue perfusion.

At this stage of shock, the severe reduction in peripheral perfusion results in **vascular stasis**. Local vasodilators are released which increase endothelial permeability and fluid and proteins move into the interstitial space reducing blood volume and causing generalised oedema. Blood agglutinates in the capillaries which become blocked. This compounds the already reduced perfusion to the tissues and organs, the tissues subtended by the blocked capillaries become critically ischaemic and small areas of infarction result. This ischaemic injury further reduces function of the body's organs and contributes to the multi-organ failure that occurs in life-threatening cases of shock. Furthermore, widespread intravascular coagulation results in consumption of clotting factors and platelets giving rise to a bleeding disorder called **disseminated intravascular coagulation (DIC)**.

In the **brain**, neuronal function is depressed and the patient is confused or obtunded. Reduced functioning of the vasomotor centre in the medulla reduces sympathetic output and the compensatory vasoconstrictor and heart rate response to shock fails. At MABP less than about 50 mmHg, the ischaemic brainstem neurons make a final attempt to increase arterial blood pressure by an intense sympathetic discharge called the **central nervous system ischaemic response**.

All of the body's organs are at risk of ischaemic injury during shock. The liver and the kidney tubules, however, are particularly prone to ischaemic injury because they receive their blood supply via portal systems, in which the blood pressure and oxygen saturations are already reduced compared with other organs. Damage tends to be less at the arteriolar end of the capillary bed. In the liver, the centres of the liver lobules are the last to receive blood and suffer the most damage. **Ischaemic hepatocellular damage** causes the release of the liver enzymes alanine aminotransferase (ALT) and aspartate aminotransferase (AST) into the circulation so their concentrations in the blood are markedly elevated. Severe liver dysfunction is manifest by a bleeding diathesis related to the reduced production of coagulation factors, which can be detected by a prolonged prothrombin time. **Renal failure** is caused by **acute tubular necrosis (ATN)** which results in oliguria or anuria, rising blood concentrations of potassium and creatinine, and metabolic acidosis.

In the **lungs**, leakage of fluid and inflammatory cells from the capillaries into the interstitial and alveolar spaces causes **adult respiratory distress syndrome (ARDS)**. The affected areas of the lungs are not ventilated and oxygenation of the blood is reduced resulting in respiratory failure (see Ch. 13). Patients are severely hypoxic and chest X-rays show lung infiltrates. Also called **non-cardiogenic pulmonary oedema**, ARDS is differentiated from cardiogenic pulmonary oedema by the presence of a normal or low pulmonary capillary wedge pressure. ARDS is associated with a high mortality rate.

Cellular damage in shock

Some tissues are more sensitive than others to the effects of hypoxia. For example, skin can be deprived of blood flow for many hours before it is damaged whereas the brain is damaged after only a few minutes because of its high metabolic rate. In shock, tissue hypoperfusion is multifactorial, but whatever the cause, cellular damage is ultimately related to an inadequate supply of ATP, which arises because of reduced aerobic metabolism and a consequent reduction in ATPase activity. The Na^+/K^+-ATPase in the cell membrane is a large consumer of ATP so it is particularly sensitive to its reduced supply. Reduced functioning of the Na^+/K^+-ATPase results in an increase in the intracellular concentration of Na^+. Decreased Na^+/Ca^{2+} exchange and Ca^{2+}-ATPase activity leads to an increase in intracellular Ca^{2+} concentration, which saturates the regulatory proteins and causes mitochondrial dysfunction. Proteases released into the cytoplasm by lysosomes destroy intracellular proteins. The increase in intracellular cations leads to an influx of Cl^- and, by osmosis, an increase in cell water. The structural and functional integrity of the cell is compromised before swelling of the cell results in cell death by lysis.

Treatment of shock

Shock is a clinical syndrome rather than a diagnosis. It always has an underlying cause which needs to be identified and treated. For example, hypovolaemic shock due to a bleeding duodenal ulcer requires the administration of an intravenous proton pump inhibitor and upper gastrointestinal endoscopic treatment, whereas vasodilatory shock due to pneumonia requires intravenous antibiotic therapy.

Supportive therapy

Irrespective of the cause of shock, its initial management is the same as for any critically ill patient. The need for continuous monitoring of haemodynamic and other parameters requires management in a high dependency or intensive care unit. The aims of treatment are to ensure patency of the airway, satisfactory oxygenation, and the restoration of blood pressure and cardiac output. Patients who are unable to protect their airway require intubation. Patients who remain hypoxic despite high flow mask oxygen therapy, due to ARDS for example, require intubation and ventilation. Although the major problem in shock is tissue hypoxia, oxygen therapy may not have a significant effect in increasing oxygen levels in the tissues; in many cases the oxygenation of blood in the lungs is normal or near normal and it is the delivery of oxygen to the tissues that is reduced. Furthermore, the acidic environment in the tissues promotes the release of oxygen from haemoglobin due to the rightward shift in the oxygen-dissociation curve. Patients who develop severe renal failure require renal replacement therapy by haemofiltration. This is effective at removing excess fluid and correcting acidosis.

Fluid replacement

In most cases of shock, a vital element of treatment is the restoration of a low circulating blood volume to normal through the administration of intravenous fluid. The fluid chosen depends partly on the cause of shock; where possible, the replacement fluid should be of similar composition to the fluid lost. For example, in haemorrhagic shock, the best treatment is usually the transfusion of cross-matched red cells. However, cross-matched red cells are rarely available immediately so the initial rapid correction of circulating blood volume is achieved by the administration of an electrolyte solution (crystalloid) or a plasma substitute (colloid) (Information box 11.16). In an emergency, uncross-matched, group O Rhesus negative blood can be transfused pending the availability of cross-matched blood (see Ch. 12). In hypovolaemic shock due to plasma loss (e.g. in burns), colloid is the most appropriate replacement fluid. In shock caused by extracellular fluid loss (e.g. due to diarrhoea), the restoration of circulating volume should be achieved using crystalloid.

In most cases of cardiogenic shock, such as following massive anterior myocardial infarction, the filling pressures are high rather than low and inotropic and/or mechanical support plus diuretic therapy are required rather than fluid replacement. Hypotension following an inferior or inferoposterior myocardial infarct, however, is typical of infarction involving the right ventricle, when increasing the filling pressure of the right heart through fluid administration improves cardiac output. In some cases, the volume status of the patient is uncertain despite careful clinical assessment. In this group of patients, invasive measurement of the pulmonary capillary wedge pressure by means of a Swan–Ganz pulmonary artery catheter might be useful. The finding of a low pulmonary capillary wedge pressure indicates hypovolaemia and the requirement for fluid replacement.

Information box 11.16	Replacement fluids

Replacement of the fluids lost in pathological processes is an essential part of resuscitation. The choice of fluids for replacement should be based on the cause of fluid loss.

Crystalloid solutions

- Electrolyte solutions contain water and salts (e.g NaCl) in concentrations that are iso-osmolar with blood. These may also contain sugars such as dextrose and glucose, and lactate. They are called crystalloid because they are true solutions and pass freely across semi-permeable barriers, e.g. capillary endothelium. Normal saline solution contains 0.9% sodium chloride, which provides 154 mmol/L of both sodium and chloride ions, giving a total of about 300 mOsmol.
- A disadvantage of saline solutions is that they move freely from the vasculature into the interstitial fluid: so to increase blood volume by 1 L, 3 L of saline must be transfused. Care must be taken not to administer too much fluid because overload can lead to pulmonary oedema and heart failure. However, dextrose solutions also increase intracellular volume as dextrose is taken into cells and water follows osmotically.

Colloid solutions

- These are not true solutions; they are suspensions of particles. They include blood and plasma and a variety of synthetic preparations. Synthetic colloids are suspensions of high molecular-weight compounds, e.g. dextrans (40–70 kDa), derivatives of gelatine (30–35 kDa) and albumin.
- Because the particles are too large to pass through the capillary endothelial layer, the colloid osmotic pressure increases and fluid remains within the vasculature, which increases circulating volume rapidly.
- In **vasodilatory shock** or in **advanced shock,** endothelial permeability is increased. Thus the colloids can leak out of the vasculature, increasing the interstitial fluid volume and interstitial oncotic pressure. This leads to **oedema**, which is particularly dangerous if it occurs in the lungs because it reduces gas exchange.

Sympathomimetic drug treatment

If restoration of the circulating volume fails to correct the low blood pressure, shock can be treated using drugs which increase **cardiac contractility** and/or change **systemic vascular resistance**. Most of the drugs used in the treatment of shock act on adrenoceptors to increase the action of the sympathetic nervous system, and are therefore sometimes called **sympathomimetic agents**.

- **Epinephrine (adrenaline)** acts predominantly on β-receptors at low doses, which increases the force and rate of cardiac contraction (via β_1-receptors) and decreases peripheral vascular resistance (via β_2-receptors on skeletal and heart muscle vasculature). At higher doses, it acts on α-receptors to produce vasoconstriction.
- **Norepinephrine (noradrenaline)** acts mainly on α-receptors causing vasoconstriction, so it is particularly useful in vasodilatory shock.
- **Dopamine** acts on α- and β-receptors as well as at dopaminergic D_1 and D_2 receptors. D_1 receptors are postsynaptic and produce vasodilation. D_2 receptors are presynaptic and inhibit norepinephrine release. At low doses, dopamine produces vasodilation, particularly in the renal, coronary and cerebral circulations. Low dose dopamine is often used to augment renal blood flow but a protective effect on renal function has not been demonstrated. Some patients benefit from vasodilation because of the reduction in afterload, which is particularly important in patients with heart failure. At intermediate doses, dopamine binds to β_1-adrenoceptors which increases cardiac contractility. At high doses,

α-adrenoceptor-mediated vasoconstriction predominates as dopamine is converted to epinephrine.

- **Dobutamine** is an analogue of dopamine whose greatest affinity is for β_1-receptors. It is therefore useful to increase myocardial contractility in cardiogenic shock. It is frequently used in combination with the vasoconstrictor properties of norepinephrine in vasodilatory shock.

The appropriate use of sympathomimetic agents requires considerable clinical experience. In critically ill patients, the choice of drug and its dose adjustment is aided by invasive or non-invasive measurements of cardiac output, systemic vascular resistance, and pulmonary capillary wedge pressure.

Potential adverse consequences of these drugs include:

- Sinus tachycardia and risk of arrhythmia.
- Increased myocardial oxygen requirements due to the increased force and rate of cardiac contraction. This is a particular consideration in patients with ischaemic heart disease in whom myocardial ischaemia may be exacerbated.
- Digital ischaemia due to severe peripheral vasoconstriction.
- Hypotension, if the predominant effect is vasodilation.

Prognosis in shock

The prognosis in shock is dependent upon the patient's age and baseline function of their key organs; pre-existing impairment in the function of the heart, brain, kidneys, liver, or lungs predisposes to an adverse outcome. The cause of shock and whether or not it can be corrected, for example, stemming haemorrhage or treating infection, together with the point at which treatment is initiated are also important. Once multiorgan failure has developed, the prognosis is poor.

HYPERTENSION

Hypertension is defined by the presence of persistently elevated blood pressure. It is a common disorder that leads to morphological and functional changes in the heart and systemic arterioles. The increased afterload on the heart results in left ventricular hypertrophy and the increased pressure in the arterioles results in thickening of their walls and a reduced lumen. These changes increase the risk of stroke, heart failure, renal failure and retinopathy, with a direct relation between the risk and the level of blood pressure. Hypertension is also a risk factor for coronary artery disease, peripheral vascular disease, aortic aneurysm and aortic dissection. On its own, hypertension is symptomless which means that it frequently goes undetected until complications arise. Crucially, the lowering of raised blood pressure is effective at preventing complications which makes it important to screen subjects periodically for high blood pressure and to treat it effectively when it is diagnosed.

Diagnosis of hypertension

The level of blood pressure above which hypertension should be diagnosed remains the subject of considerable debate. Blood pressure is a continuous variable which is normally distributed across a wide range of values. The relation between blood pressure and cardiovascular complications persists down to blood pressures of 115/75 mmHg or lower, levels which would be considered 'normal'. Furthermore, blood pressure varies with age, systolic values in particular tending

Table 11.18	Classification of blood pressure			
Stage	**Blood pressure (mmHg)**			
	Systolic		**Diastolic**	**Ambulatory daytime average**
Stage 1 hypertension	140–159	± or	90–99	≥135/85
Stage 2 hypertension	160–179	± or	100–109	≥150/95
Severe hypertension	≥180	± or	≥110	

(National Institute for Health and Clinical Excellence; Clinical guideline 127; Hypertension. The clinical management of primary hypertension in adults; 2011.)

to increase as individuals get older as a consequence of reduced compliance in the large arteries. The selection of a single value to define hypertension is therefore problematic and somewhat arbitrary. However, a blood pressure persistently ≥140/90 mmHg is generally considered to be abnormal (Table 11.18).

Hypertension should not be diagnosed on the basis of a single elevated blood pressure measurement, which could be raised due to the patient's anxiety about being at the doctor's surgery or in the outpatient clinic (**white coat hypertension**). Several blood pressure readings should be taken on separate occasions and some clinical practice guidelines now recommend that, where feasible, ambulatory (24 hour) blood pressure monitoring should be performed to confirm the diagnosis.

Aetiology of hypertension

Hypertension can be divided into two types. By far the most common type is **primary** or **essential hypertension** in which there is no apparent underlying cause. In about 5% of cases, a specific cause can be found for hypertension, when it is known as **secondary hypertension**.

The aetiology of essential hypertension is incompletely understood. Genetic factors are thought to be important in determining who develops hypertension because of its greater prevalence in Afro-Caribbean subjects and in those with a family history of the condition. Other factors which are associated with the development of essential hypertension include:

- Advancing age
- Low birth weight
- Low socio-economic status
- High salt diet
- Obesity
- Sedentary lifestyle
- Excessive alcohol intake
- Stress and anxiety.

In common with many conditions, essential hypertension is probably triggered by one or more environmental factor in a genetically susceptible individual.

Pathophysiology of hypertension

Several mechanisms have been proposed, but no single mechanism has been found, to explain all cases of essential hypertension. It seems clear that different mechanisms operate in different individuals. The most credible pathophysiological mechanisms are:

- **Increased sympathetic drive:** the level of sympathetic nervous system output from the medulla is one of the key determinants of vasomotor tone and blood pressure. A primary increase in sympathetic output, causing increased vasomotor tone, has been postulated as one of the underlying mechanisms for essential hypertension. Chronically high levels of stress may contribute to increased sympathetic drive in some patients. Another possible explanation for a chronically high sympathetic drive is an abnormality in the setting of the baroreceptor reflex in which lower than expected baroreceptor activity for a given level of blood pressure indicates to the brain that the blood pressure is too low, resulting in increased sympathetic nervous system output to 'correct' the blood pressure.
- **Activation of the renin–angiotensin–aldosterone system:** this hormonal system is another of the key regulators of blood pressure. Its activation promotes vasoconstriction through angiotensin II and sodium and water retention through aldosterone. Blood renin concentrations tend to be elevated in hypertensive patients who are white and aged less than 55 years. This mechanism may be less important in older patients and in Afro-Caribbean patients in whom blood renin concentrations tend to be normal or low.
- **Increased blood volume:** the observation that a high salt intake increases blood pressure and a low salt intake lowers blood pressure implicates increased blood volume as a causative mechanism in some cases of hypertension. Furthermore, diuretics are effective blood pressure lowering medications, though it is not clear that their antihypertensive effect is related to blood volume reduction.

Secondary hypertension

The most common cause of secondary hypertension is chronic kidney disease. Renovascular disease, a variety of endocrine disorders, drugs and coarctation of the aorta account for most of the remaining cases (Table 11.19). An identifiable cause for hypertension is more likely in patients who are younger than 40 years of age, and in those with resistant or malignant hypertension. Selective testing for secondary causes of hypertension should be considered in these groups and in those patients who have symptoms or signs suggestive of an underlying cause. When a cause for hypertension is identified, its treatment frequently does not render the blood pressure normal, particularly when the hypertension is longstanding. This may be because the cardiovascular reflexes and hormonal systems which regulate blood pressure have recalibrated to accept as normal a higher level of blood pressure.

Hypertension due to chronic kidney disease

Chronic kidney disease (CKD) accounts for 2–4% of cases of hypertension. The majority of patients with CKD stage ≥III (estimated glomerular filtration rate <60 mL/min) have hypertension. Cardiovascular death rates are high in patients with CKD. Effective blood pressure lowering reduces both the rate of kidney disease progression and the rate of cardiovascular complications in this high risk group.

The main mechanism of hypertension in CKD is impaired sodium excretion, which increases blood volume and cardiac output. However, vasoconstriction has also been implicated in the aetiology of CKD-related hypertension. This is due to several factors including increased renin secretion, sympathetic activation, increased endothelin production and reduced nitric oxide release. CKD is not only the most common cause of secondary hypertension, it is also one of the most frequent complications of hypertension. All patients with hypertension should therefore have blood taken to measure their creatinine concentration and glomerular filtration rate, and their urine analysed for protein and blood.

Renovascular hypertension

Renovascular hypertension is caused by renal artery stenosis. Reduced renal perfusion stimulates the release of renin with consequent activation of the renin–angiotensin–aldosterone system. Angiotensin II causes vasoconstriction and aldosterone promotes salt and water retention.

Renal artery stenosis is usually caused by atherosclerosis. It occurs most commonly in middle-aged or elderly patients with peripheral vascular disease and/or diabetes. Less frequently it is due to fibromuscular dysplasia, an abnormality of the connective tissues of the artery wall, which typically presents in females under the age of 30. Renal artery stenosis is under-diagnosed. It should be suspected in young patients without a family history of hypertension (fibromuscular dysplasia), in resistant hypertension, in patients with abdominal bruits, in patients with unexplained episodes of sudden ('flash') pulmonary oedema, and in patients with deteriorating renal function after ACE inhibitor or angiotensin II receptor blocker (ARB) treatment.

In renal artery stenosis, maintenance of glomerular filtration becomes dependent on angiotensin II-induced constriction of the efferent glomerular arterioles so ACE inhibitors and ARBs should be used with caution. Angioplasty has proven disappointing as a treatment for hypertension in atherosclerotic renal artery stenosis in contrast to fibromuscular dysplasia where it is often curative.

Endocrine causes of hypertension

Endocrine hypertension is due to the excessive release of hormones which influence the regulation of salt and water balance, blood volume and blood pressure (see Ch. 10).

- A **phaeochromocytoma** is a catecholamine-producing tumour that secretes epinephrine and norepinephrine. The majority arise in the adrenal medulla but about 10% have an extramedullary location. The elevated blood pressure is related to stimulation of cardiac β_1-adrenoceptors by epinephrine which causes an increase in heart rate and cardiac contractility and of α-adrenoceptors in the systemic vessels

Table 11.19	Main causes of hypertension	
Type	**Proportion of hypertensive patients**
Essential hypertension	95%
Secondary hypertension	
Renal parenchymal	2–4%
Renovascular	1%
Phaeochromocytoma	0.2%
Coarctation of the aorta	0.1%
Primary hyperaldosteronism	0.1%
Cushing syndrome	0.1%

by norepinephrine causing vasoconstriction. Phaeochromocytomas are uncommon, accounting for <0.1% cases hypertension, but they should be suspected in hypertensive patients who complain of palpitation, headache, anxiety and sweating. Tachycardia and impaired glucose tolerance are common features. The diagnosis is made by the finding of elevated levels of metepinephrine and normetepinephrine on 24 hour urine collection and by tumour imaging.

- **Primary hyperaldosteronism** is caused either by bilateral adrenal hyperplasia or by an aldosterone-secreting adenoma of the adrenal gland (**Conn syndrome**). Aldosterone promotes sodium and water retention at the expense of potassium loss so hypokalaemia is usually present. Blood testing shows an inappropriately high concentration of aldosterone and suppressed renin and imaging identifies the adrenal hyperplasia or tumour.

- **Cushing syndrome** is due to an excess of adrenocortical hormones such as cortisol. Most patients with Cushing syndrome have hypertension, which arises due to the intrinsic mineralocorticoid activity of cortisol, activation of the renin–angiotensin–aldosterone system and increased vasoconstriction. In Cushing disease, increased adrenal production of cortisol is stimulated by an excess of adrenocorticotropic hormone (ACTH) release from a pituitary tumour. Other causes of Cushing syndrome are the long-term use of exogenous corticosteroids for medical purposes such as rheumatoid arthritis or asthma, ectopic ACTH secretion from a lung carcinoma, and cortisol release from an adrenal tumour. Early morning blood cortisol levels are high and are not suppressed by the administration of dexamethasone (the dexamethasone suppression test).

- **Acromegaly** is due to the over-production of growth hormone by a pituitary tumour. Growth hormone has anti-natriuretic actions which contribute to the high prevalence of hypertension in acromegaly. The diagnosis is suspected from the typical enlarged facial features and is confirmed by elevated blood concentrations of growth hormone and by imaging of the pituitary gland.

Drug-induced hypertension

In clinical practice, the most widely prescribed drugs which elevate blood pressure are oestrogen-containing oral contraceptive agents, non-steroidal anti-inflammatory drugs (NSAIDs) and selective cyclo-oxygenase (COX)-2 inhibitors. Oestrogens increase the synthesis of angiotensinogen, the precursor to angiotensin II, causing vasoconstriction. NSAIDs inhibit COX-1- and COX-2-mediated prostaglandin synthesis. COX-1 generated prostaglandins increase renal perfusion through vasodilatation while COX-2 generated prostaglandins have natriuretic effects. NSAIDs and selective COX-2 inhibitors, therefore, promote salt and water retention, while NSAIDs also tend to be vasoconstricting. Not only can these drugs cause or exacerbate hypertension, they also blunt the effect of anti-hypertensive therapy, particularly diuretics and those agents which act on the renin–angiotensin–aldosterone system.

Monoamine oxidase (MAO) inhibitors are drugs which increase the availability of neurotransmitters for release from sympathetic nerve terminals and can be used to treat depression and parkinsonism. Their clinical use is in decline, however, because of an interaction with tyramine, which can cause episodes of acute hypertension. Tyramine is a naturally occurring monoamine found in some foodstuffs (some cheeses, yeast products and red wine) which promotes the release of norepinephrine, dopamine and serotonin. In normal circumstances, these neurotransmitters are broken down by MAO after they have been reabsorbed into proximal nerve terminals, and ingested monoamines, including tryamine, are broken down by MAO in the gut. In patients who are taking MAO inhibitors, however, tyramine breakdown in the gut is inhibited allowing it to be absorbed and this may result in the release of sympathetic neurotransmitters and a surge in sympathetic activity.

Coarctation of the aorta

Coarctation of the aorta is a congenital narrowing of the aorta, usually just distal to the origin of the left subclavian artery. It is frequently associated with a bicuspid aortic valve. Hypertension is related to reduced renal blood flow and activation of the renin–angiotensin–aldosterone system. The cardinal clinical sign of weak and delayed femoral pulses (radio-femoral delay) should be looked for in all young patients with hypertension. Collaterals may be palpable through the chest wall and chest X-ray may show rib notching. The diagnosis is confirmed by CT or MRI. Contemporary treatment is by endovascular stenting but this does not always result in normalisation of the blood pressure.

Pregnancy-induced hypertension

Pre-existing hypertension is usually detected during the first half of pregnancy. **Gestational hypertension** is new hypertension presenting after 20 weeks. **Pre-eclampsia** is present when patients with gestational hypertension develop proteinuria. It affects approximately 5% pregnancies. The aetiology of pre-eclampsia is uncertain, but it is thought to be caused by the release of placental factors into the maternal circulation in response to defective placental implantation. The risk of pre-eclampsia is increased in expectant women who have a history of pre-eclampsia in a previous pregnancy, CKD, autoimmune disease, diabetes mellitus, or chronic hypertension, and in women aged >40 years, in first pregnancies and in obese women. Pre-eclampsia may cause symptoms of headache, visual disturbance, chest pain, vomiting and swelling of the face, feet and hands. It is associated with increased rates of intra-uterine growth retardation, prematurity and foetal death. A blood pressure >160/110 mmHg or pre-eclampsia associated with a blood pressure >150/100 mmHg requires hospital admission for blood pressure control and to prevent the development of **eclampsia**, a syndrome of severe hypertension, fits and haematological and biochemical abnormalities. Eclampsia is one of the most frequent causes of maternal death in the developed world.

Malignant hypertension

The adverse effects of hypertension on the arterioles and the organs they supply are usually slowly progressive over many years. However, in rare cases the blood pressure rises rapidly and damages the walls of the arterioles (causing fibrinoid necrosis) and target organs within weeks or even days. This is known as **malignant hypertension**. The blood pressure is usually >220/120 mmHg and the clinical syndrome can also include headache, confusion, chest pain, pulmonary oedema, renal failure, visual loss, haemolytic anaemia, thrombotic episodes and disseminated intravascular coagulation. Loss of autoregulation of cerebral perfusion at these high levels of blood pressure is responsible for many of the cerebral manifestations while blockage of small arterioles by the deposition of fibrin is responsible for the thrombotic episodes. It requires immediate treatment to prevent irreversible blindness, renal damage and cerebral injury.

Treatment of hypertension

All patients with hypertension should receive advice about lifestyle measures to lower their blood pressure and to reduce their overall cardiovascular risk. Where relevant, these measures might include:

- Weight loss
- Reduced salt intake
- Reduced alcohol consumption
- Increased aerobic exercise
- Smoking cessation.

Anti-hypertensive drug therapy produces the greatest risk reductions in patients who have the highest levels of blood pressure, and in patients who have lower levels of blood pressure but who have a high overall cardiovascular risk. Patients in whom anti-hypertensive therapy is recommended can be divided into three groups:

- BP >160/100 mmHg (or ambulatory day time average BP >150/95 mmHg)
- BP >140/90 mmHg (or ambulatory day time average BP >135/85 mmHg) plus established cardiovascular disease, target organ damage, diabetes mellitus, or CKD
- BP >140/90 mmHg (or ambulatory day time average BP >135/85 mmHg) plus a 10-year estimated risk of adverse cardiovascular events ≥20%.

Target organ damage comprises left ventricular hypertrophy, hypertensive retinopathy, or hypertensive nephropathy. Established cardiovascular disease refers to cerebrovascular disease, ischaemic heart disease, heart failure, or peripheral vascular disease.

Ten-year cardiovascular risk assessment may underestimate the lifetime risk of cardiovascular events in patients less than 40 years of age. Young patients with BP 140–159/90–99 mmHg may therefore warrant anti-hypertensive therapy in the absence of target organ damage or other cardiovascular risk factors.

The classes of drugs used most commonly to treat hypertension are listed in Table 11.20. The drug of choice depends upon the patient's age, race and co-existing conditions.

Patients with left ventricular dysfunction and/or ischaemic heart disease should be treated with an ACE inhibitor and a β-blocker. In the absence of any pre-existing conditions, the first line anti-hypertensive agents are ACE inhibitors or angiotensin II receptor blockers and calcium-channel blockers. There are theoretical reasons for particular drug choices in different groups of patients. White patients who are aged less than 55 years of age are most likely to have 'high renin' hypertension so blockade of the renin–angiotensin–aldosterone system through an ACE inhibitor or an angiotensin II receptor blocker is the first choice for these patients. In contrast, older patients or Afro-Caribbean patients tend to have 'low renin' hypertension and respond better to a calcium-channel blocker such as amlodipine, which works through vasodilation. If blood pressure is not controlled on one anti-hypertensive agent then further agents are added in stepwise fashion until an acceptable level of blood pressure control is achieved.

The optimal or 'target' blood pressure for patients with hypertension has not yet been established. It is known that the rate of cardiovascular events in population cohorts is directly related to blood pressure above levels of about 115/75 mmHg. However, there appears to be a J-shaped relationship with higher event rates at blood pressures below about 100/60 mmHg. Furthermore, it has not been established that lowering blood pressure aggressively in individual patients improves outcomes compared with a more conservative treatment target. Current guidelines recommend a target of <140/90 mmHg for most patients and <140/85 mmHg in diabetic patients. Many patients require at least two anti-hypertensive agents to achieve these targets. In pregnant women, blood pressure should be kept below 150/100 mmHg. Angiotensin converting enzyme inhibitors and angiotensin II receptor blockers should be avoided during pregnancy because they are associated with an increased risk of congenital abnormalities.

Resistant hypertension

Resistant hypertension is defined as hypertension which is uncontrolled despite at least three anti-hypertensive agents at maximal tolerated dose. Ambulatory blood pressure monitoring is extremely helpful in clarifying the response to treatment and in diagnosing white coat hypertension. The principal causes of resistant hypertension are:

- Incorrect measurement of blood pressure (using too small a cuff, for example)

Table 11.20 Drugs used to treat hypertension

Class of drug	Example	Mode of action
ACE inhibitors	Ramipril Perindopril	Block production of angiotensin II leading to reduced vasoconstriction
Angiotensin II receptor blockers	Losartan Irbesartan	Block angiotensin II receptors reducing vasoconstriction. Often used in patients who cannot tolerate ACE inhibitors
Calcium-channel blockers	Amlodipine Nifedipine	Block entry of calcium into vascular smooth muscle, resulting in vasodilatation. May also affect entry of calcium into cardiac myocytes
Thiazide & thiazide-like diuretics	Bendrofluazide Indapamide	Initial reduction in blood volume by increasing sodium (and water) excretion. Later fall in TPR by unknown mechanism/s
α-Blockers	Doxazosin	Inhibition of α-adrenoceptors on vascular smooth muscle to produce vasodilatation
β-Blockers	Bisoprolol Atenolol	Initial reduction in heart rate and contractility, and inhibition of renin release. Sustained reduction in blood pressure by unknown mechanism/s
Aldosterone antagonists	Spironolactone	Promotes sodium loss in the distal renal tubule

ACE, angiotensin-converting enzyme; TPR, total peripheral resistance.

- White coat hypertension
- Non-compliance with treatment
- Concomitant drug use (e.g. NSAIDs, sympathomimetics, oral contraceptives, over-the-counter drugs and herbal supplements)
- Excess sodium intake
- Excess alcohol intake
- Obesity
- Chronic kidney disease (CKD)
- Secondary hypertension.

Treatment options in resistant hypertension include aldosterone antagonists such as spironolactone and α-adrenoceptor antagonists such as doxazosin. Loop diuretics may be more efficacious than thiazide diuretics, particularly in patients with renal failure. An innovative therapy which has recently been shown to be effective in the treatment of patients with resistant hypertension is renal sympathetic denervation. This treatment reduces the sympathetic nervous activity to and from the

---

Information box 11.17   **Renal sympathetic denervation**

This is a new treatment for resistant hypertension in which a flexible radiofrequency ablation catheter is introduced into the arterial system via the femoral artery. The catheter is then passed into each renal artery in turn and bursts of radiofrequency energy are delivered to the luminal walls of the renal arteries at points 5 mm apart to disrupt the nerves. In the Symplicity HTN-2 trial, renal sympathetic denervation lowered average blood pressure by 33/11 mmHg at 6 months compared with controls in patients whose average starting blood pressure was 178/97 mmHg despite five anti-hypertensive agents. The longevity of these impressive early results is uncertain and renal denervation therapy is currently reserved for patients who have very high blood pressure (e.g. clinic values >160/110 mmHg) confirmed by ambulatory monitoring despite multiple agents.

---

kidneys, so reducing activation of the renin–angiotensin–aldosterone system and direct sympathetic actions on the heart and blood vessels, respectively (Information box 11.17).

12

Haematology

Drew Provan, Adrian C. Newland and Denise Syndercombe Court

The haemopoietic system	**567**
Blood and its constituents	567
Stem cells and their role in haemopoiesis	570
Blood cell production and the bone marrow microenvironment	570
Red cells	**571**
Transcription factors in erythropoiesis	571
Growth factors in erythropoiesis	571
Stromal molecules in erythropoiesis	572
Transport of oxygen by haemoglobin	573
Transport of carbon dioxide	574
The red cell membrane	575
Haemoglobin	575
Red cell enzymes are required to maintain red cell components	576
Maintenance and recycling of red cells	576
Anaemias	576
Oncogenesis and disorders of blood cell production	**589**
Normal blood production relies on coordinated gene expression	590
Oncogenesis	590
The lymphoid system	590
Myeloproliferative diseases	591
Myelodysplastic syndromes	592
Leukaemias	592
Lymphomas	595
Plasma cell disorders	596
Haemostasis and thrombosis	**596**
Normal haemostatic mechanisms	596
Coagulation factor disorders	601
The thrombocytopenias	602
The thrombophilias	603
Blood groups and transfusion medicine	**604**
Definition of a blood group	604
Blood group antigens	604
Antibody production	604
Blood group systems in transfusion medicine	604
Blood transfusion	608
Non-red-cell transfusion	610

THE HAEMOPOIETIC SYSTEM

BLOOD AND ITS CONSTITUENTS

Blood is one of the body's largest tissues, comprising a mixture of cells within a fluid (plasma). Blood permeates all organs and tissues, distributing essential organic and inorganic substances. It maintains homeostasis and body temperature, carries oxygen, acts as a buffering system and has many other functions. Definitions and explanations of many of the terms that are used throughout the chapter are given in Table 12.1.

Blood plasma

Plasma makes up about 60% of our blood volume and is a complex mixture of water (90%) absorbed from the gut, proteins (8%), molecules such as glucose, and a variety of other dissolved or bound chemicals.

Blood cells

The average adult has around 24×10^{12} red cells (making up a third of the total number of cells in the body), which live for around 120 days with a daily death rate of 2×10^{11} cells. This equates to the breakdown of 400×10^{12} haemoglobin molecules *per second* (Information box 12.1).

The ratio of the volume of red cells to total volume of blood is the **packed cell volume** (**PCV**) or **haematocrit**,

---

Information box 12.1   **Key features of blood**

A 70 kg man will have approximately:
- 5 L of blood:
  - 60% as plasma
  - 40% as cells – referred to as the packed cell volume (PCV).
  The main blood cell types and their quantities are:
- Red blood cells: 4.5–6.5×10^{12}/L (3.9–5.8×10^{12}/L females)
- White blood cells: 4–11×10^9/L
- Platelets: 150–400×10^9/L.

---

which is usually between 0.36 and 0.52 (men 0.42–0.53; women 0.36–0.45). Disturbances of normal PCV or haematocrit occur in a variety of situations (see Clinical box 12.1).

Red cells (erythrocytes)

Red cells are biconcave disc-shaped cells that lack a nucleus, since this is extruded while the cell is maturing in the bone marrow (Fig. 12.1). The reason why red cells have no nucleus is not known. Perhaps the cells are consequently more pliable and can travel through small blood vessels more easily. This cannot be the complete answer, however, since birds have red cells that contain nuclei. The diameter of a red cell is around 6.7–7.7 μm. The principal function of red cells is to carry oxygen and carbon dioxide round the body. The biconcave shape provides an increased surface area compared with a sphere, making gas exchange faster, and is maintained by a complex cytoskeletal system.

Table 12.1	Terms used in haematology
Term	**Explanation**
-aemia	Of the blood
Anisocytosis	Red cells of different sizes
APTT	Activated partial thromboplastin time
Bite cell	Irregular red cells with indentations that look like bites
Blast	Primitive blood cell
-cyte	Cell
ESR	Erythrocyte sedimentation rate
Haemoglobinuria	Red urine due to presence of haemoglobin from lysed red cells
Hyperplasia	Abnormal cellular increase
Hypochromic	Red cells with reduced haemoglobin
Leucopenia	Reduced white cell numbers
Macrocytic	Red cells that are larger than normal
MCH	Mean (red) cell haemoglobin in picograms (pg)
MCHC	Mean cell haemoglobin concentration in %
MCV	Mean cell volume in femtolitres (fL)
Megaloblast	Red cell precursor (blast) in bone marrow that is abnormally large (megalo)
Microcytic	Red cells that are smaller than normal
Normocytic	Red cells of a normal size
-osis	Too much
Pencil cells	Elongated red cells
-penia	Not enough
-philia	Affinity for
Poikilocytes	Red cells with abnormal shape
Polychromasia	Red cells showing a bluish tinge because they contain little haemoglobin
PT	Prothrombin time
Reticulocytes	Young red cells containing ribosomal remnants that can only be seen with reticulum stains – an increase in reticulocytes in blood is an indicator of increased red cell production
Spherocytes	Small red cells with no central pallor
Target cells	Red cells which appear pale but have a central dark area making them look like targets due to an increased surface membrane to volume ratio
Thrombocytopenia	Reduced platelet numbers
TT	Thrombin time

White blood cells (leucocytes)

There are several types of white blood cell (Fig. 12.1), but those most numerous in peripheral blood are neutrophils and lymphocytes. Other cell types found in blood, but in smaller numbers, are eosinophils, monocytes and basophils. Some cells engulf foreign particles – they are phagocytic, e.g. neutrophils, eosinophils and monocytes/macrophages – while others are non-phagocytic, such as lymphocytes. White cells that have granules visible in their cytoplasm (neutrophils, eosinophils and basophils) are often referred to as granulocytes. White cells are an important part of the immune system, whose role is to protect the body from invading pathogens.

Clinical box 12.1	Variations in packed cell volume

Packed cell volume (PCV), or haematocrit, may be raised or lowered owing to a number of mechanisms related to red cell production (erythropoeisis) and size, discussed later in the chapter, and a variation in plasma volume (see also Fig. 12.23). The main factors that give rise to significant changes in haemocrit are:

Raised PCV:
- Increased red cell production (erythropoiesis): as in polycythaemia (see later), chronic obstructive pulmonary disease (COPD) (see Ch. 13); increased circulating erythropoietin in hypoxia (see Chs 13 and 14), including use of erythropoietin (EPO) or anabolic, androgenic steroids by professional athletes.
- Increased red cell size (macrocytosis): when haemoglobin transports carbon dioxide (see Ch. 13), the formation of bicarbonate in plasma causes water to be taken up by red cells, so that cells increase in size. This is most likely to occur when there is CO_2 retention, as in COPD. Macrocytosis can also occur in hypothyroid disease and various forms of macrocytic anaemia (see later).
- Reduced plasma volume, as in dehydration (see below), and loss of plasma from the circulation for whatever reason, such as in severe burn injuries.

Lowered PCV:
- Reduced red cell production: as in iron deficiency (see later) or in chronic renal disease (Ch. 14). It also occurs when there is an increased demand for iron, as in pregnancy, which affects erythropoiesis.
- Reduced red cell volume: mainly seen where there is significant blood loss, which may be acute or chronic.
- Increased plasma volume: fluid overload, as a risk in parenteral feeding (Ch. 16).

Neutrophils

Neutrophils are the commonest white cell found in peripheral blood (50–70% total white cells) with a lifespan of around 8–10 hours. Their appearance in the peripheral blood is extremely dynamic. Characteristically, the nucleus has two to five lobes. The cytoplasm has granules that contain proteolytic enzymes used to break down ingested material, such as pathogenic bacteria. The function of neutrophils is primary defence against bacteria and fungi. This defence is non-specific as neutrophils do not recognise specific antigens in the same way as other cells of the immune system, such as lymphocytes.

Neutrophils are attracted to sites of infection by chemo-attractant chemicals to which they are very sensitive. Chemoattractant molecules include bacterial cell wall proteins and endothelial cell molecules, such as leukotrienes. The cells have receptors for a variety of adhesion molecules, such as fibronectin and complement, and migrate towards the site of infection.

Killing of ingested bacteria within neutrophils involves a variety of mechanisms including oxygen-dependent pathways. The various neutrophil granules contain several different proteins that fulfil the different functions of adhesion and bacterial killing; their release (neutrophil degranulation) is stimulated by leukotrienes and chemoattractants. The azurophilic granules contain enzymes that kill bacteria, such as lysozyme and myeloperoxidase, and others that facilitate the process, such as by increasing membrane permeability. The killing mechanism involves superoxide O_2^-, hydrogen peroxide (H_2O_2) and other oxygen species, generated from O_2 and NADPH:

$$2O_2 + NADPH \rightarrow 2O_2^- + NADP^+ + H^+$$

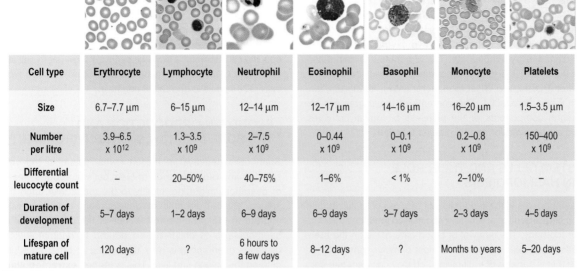

Cell type	Erythrocyte	Lymphocyte	Neutrophil	Eosinophil	Basophil	Monocyte	Platelets
Size	6.7–7.7 μm	6–15 μm	12–14 μm	12–17 μm	14–16 μm	16–20 μm	1.5–3.5 μm
Number per litre	3.9–6.5 x 10^{12}	1.3–3.5 x 10^{9}	2–7.5 x 10^{9}	0–0.44 x 10^{9}	0–0.1 x 10^{9}	0.2–0.8 x 10^{9}	150–400 x 10^{9}
Differential leucocyte count	–	20–50%	40–75%	1–6%	< 1%	2–10%	–
Duration of development	5–7 days	1–2 days	6–9 days	6–9 days	3–7 days	2–3 days	4–5 days
Lifespan of mature cell	120 days	?	6 hours to a few days	8–12 days	?	Months to years	5–20 days

Fig. 12.1 **Blood cells.** Redrawn from Young B, Woodford P, O'Dowd G, et al 2013 Wheater's functional histology: a text and colour atlas, 6th edn. Churchill Livingstone, Philadelphia, with permission.

Most of the O_2^- is converted into H_2O_2, which reacts with myeloperoxidase and halides in the neutrophils producing a series of toxic chemicals that are thought to kill the ingested microorganisms. A recent study in mice has suggested that the proteins cathepsin G and elastase are more important in this respect. Further, lactoferrin within the neutrophils binds iron, essential for bacterial growth, which therefore has a bacteriostatic effect.

Monocytes and macrophages

Monocytes are larger than neutrophils and make up around 5% of our circulating white cells. The nucleus is characteristically kidney shaped (indented) and there are usually vacuoles within the cytoplasm. Monocytes contain granules that store acid hydrolases and myeloperoxidase. Monocytes and macrophages can ingest pathogenic material, degrade it and present peptides or peptide fragments to T lymphocytes. Because of this function, monocytes and macrophages are called **antigen-presenting cells**, since they present antigen to these T cells. Monocytes circulate for about 10 hours in the blood before they mature into tissue macrophages. Their main role is to kill intracellular microorganisms, such as *Listeria*, mycobacteria and some fungi.

Eosinophils

Eosinophils make up 1–6% of the total white cells in a healthy individual and have a striking orange appearance due to the cytoplasm that takes up eosin dye when blood films are stained. Eosinophils circulate in the peripheral blood for 4–5 hours and then make their way to the tissues, where their main function is to provide defence against helminth (worm) parasitic infestations. Certain cytokines stimulate the increased production of these cells (**eosinophilia**).

Basophils

These dark-staining cells are present in peripheral blood in very small numbers (up 0.2% of total white cell count).

Basophils possess granules that contain a variety of mediators of inflammation including histamine, leukotrienes and proteases. **Mast cells**, found in the tissues, are very similar to **basophils**, but it is thought that they are not so closely related and they express different receptors. Both basophils and mast cells possess receptors for the Fc portion of IgE, and after activation by IgE the cells degranulate, spilling their granule contents into the peripheral blood.

Lymphocytes

Most lymphocytes are small cells, roughly the same size as a red cell, with a round nucleus and very little cytoplasm. Lymphocytes make up 20–40% of all white blood cells. Their lifespan is much longer than the other white cells. Some may live for many years and act as 'memory' cells. There are two main types of lymphocyte, indistinguishable microscopically, called **B and T lymphocytes**. Functionally these have very different roles. Other types of lymphocyte, including **natural killer (NK) cells** have also been identified and these take part in antibody-dependent cellular cytotoxicity reactions.

Platelets

These small cells (Fig. 12.1) are actually fragments of **megakaryocytes** that bud off in the bone marrow before entering the peripheral blood, and are non-nucleated. Megakaryocyte nuclei are large polyploid structures with chromosome contents between diploid (2N) to 64N, where N is a single set of chromosomes. Such polyploid status is achieved through a process termed nuclear endoduplication, where there is successive doubling of the chromosome content in the absence of cell division. A single megakaryocyte can generate around 3000 platelets, of which 20–30% are pooled in the spleen. In health, the peripheral blood platelet count is 150–400 × 10^9/L but this fluctuates, for example following heavy exercise, 'stress' and throughout the menstrual cycle.

The main role of platelets is to plug a small hole in the blood vessel wall (primary haemostasis): when blood vessels are damaged the platelets form a primary plug, which stops or slows down bleeding, while the clotting cascade generates fibrin to seal off the damaged area. In health, platelets live for 10–12 days. Platelets have no nucleus but contain two types of granule: **dense bodies** and α **granules**. Dense bodies contain adenosine diphosphate (ADP), adenosine triphosphate (ATP), 5-hydroxytryptamine (5-HT), calcium and pyrophosphate. The α granules contain platelet factor (PF) 4, β-thrombospondin, platelet-derived growth factor (PDGF), von Willebrand factor (vWF), fibrinogen, factor V and fibronectin. The contents of these granules are integral components of the platelet's biological activities, and are required for normal platelet function.

STEM CELLS AND THEIR ROLE IN HAEMOPOIESIS

Haemopoiesis is the production of new red cells, white cells and platelets, all of which have specialised functions throughout the body. The renewal of blood cells relies on the **stem cells**. Stem cells represent the most primitive form of blood cell that is capable of multiplying and they can generate cells of any lineage, e.g. red cell, granulocyte, lymphocyte and other cell types. Once a stem cell has begun to differentiate as it matures, it will no longer be able to produce new stem cells. There is a delicate balance in the bone marrow between stem cell multiplication (i.e. renewal) and differentiation. This is necessary because if there are insufficient numbers of stem cells, the number of mature cells falls. The mechanisms controlling stem cell renewal and differentiation are poorly understood but probably involve the **bone marrow stroma** and cytokines or other hormones interacting with stem cells. The stroma is the supporting network or matrix and is capable of passing signals to stem cells, as well as controlling various replicative pathways and differentiation events.

Stem cells are multipotent

There appear to be several types of stem cell, some more primitive (multipotent, or pluripotent) than others. A multipotent cell can differentiate into any cell type since the cell has not become committed to any specific lineage (Fig. 12.2).

There is a major difficulty in agreeing what constitutes a stem cell when looking at bone marrow in a stained preparation, since these are indistinct cells and look rather unremarkable, resembling small lymphocytes. Stem cells can, however, be detected using monoclonal antibodies against specific cell membrane proteins such as CD34 (stem cell antigen) and CD38 (an activation marker). Stem cells are typically CD34 positive and CD38 negative.

BLOOD CELL PRODUCTION AND THE BONE MARROW MICROENVIRONMENT

Stem cells derive from mesenchymal tissue in the yolk sac, forming **blood islands** of stem cells at about 6 weeks of gestation, migrating initially to the foetal liver, then the spleen. By 6–7 months of development the stem cells migrate to the bone marrow, which is the principal site of haemopoiesis in children and adults. In haematological diseases haemopoiesis may take place at other sites, including the spleen and liver. This is termed **extramedullary haemopoiesis**.

Regulation of haemopoiesis

The bone marrow stroma

The marrow stroma provides the ideal environment for growth and development of stem cells. The stroma comprises blood vessels and specific supporting cell types including fat cells, fibroblasts, endothelial cells, macrophages and sinusoids. The stromal cells maintain the delicate cellular balance of the bone marrow by secreting a variety of hormones and other molecules such as collagen, fibronectin, thrombospondin and glycosaminoglycans, in addition to growth factors, or **cytokines**.

Growth factors

Coordination of the various growth factors is controlled by hormone production and their interaction with specific receptors on the developing cells (Table 12.2). Hormones or growth factors that play a major role in the growth and

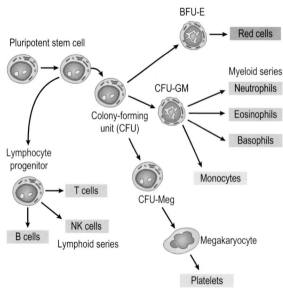

Fig. 12.2 Growth factors act on stem cells and early progenitor cells to stimulate haemopoiesis. BFU-E, erythroid burst-forming unit; CFU, colony-forming unit; GM, granulocyte macrophage; Meg, megakaryocyte; NK, natural killer.

Table 12.2	Growth factors and their function
Growth factor	**Function**
Stem cell factor (SCF)	In the foetus: helps haemopoietic cells move from the yolk sac to liver and then bone marrow
	After birth: needed at all stages for normal blood cell production
Interleukin 3 (IL-3)	With other growth factors acts on early progenitors to produce mature red cells, granulocytes, monocytes and platelets
Granulocyte-macrophage colony-stimulating factor (GM-CSF)	Like IL-3 but acts to produce neutrophils, eosinophils and monocytes
Granulocyte colony-stimulating factor (G-CSF)	Similar to GM-CSF but directed mainly at producing neutrophils
Monocyte colony-stimulating factor (M-CSF)	Targeted at monocyte growth and development
Erythropoietin (Epo)	Responsible for erythroid cell development
Thrombopoietin (Tpo)	Responsible for megakaryocytic development

differentiation of myeloid and erythroid cells are called **colony-stimulating factors** (**CSFs**), and those that are responsible for lymphocyte development are **lymphokines**. They are all glycoproteins.

Some growth factors act on more than one lineage; others act only on a single pathway, or at a particular state of haemopoiesis, stimulated by the acquisition of specific receptors on the cell surface. Usually more than one growth factor is involved in each stage of maturation (Fig. 12.3).

Haemopoietic receptors

The various growth factor receptors are distinct from other types of cell surface receptors, but, individually, are similar in structure and span the plasma membrane. Once receptors are bound by a growth factor they are activated, forming a dimeric complex with another receptor unit. These complexes can activate tyrosine kinase, which signals the start of cell division.

Chromosome 5 carries many of the receptor genes in a small area on the long arm and deletions in this region are associated with the development of acute leukaemia.

Growth factors are also synthesised for therapeutic use (Clinical box 12.2).

RED CELLS

The main function of red cells is delivery of oxygen from the lungs to the tissues. The bone marrow produces approximately 10^{10} cells per hour in order to maintain a steady state, but must be able to adapt rapidly to maintain oxygen delivery in situations where blood is lost.

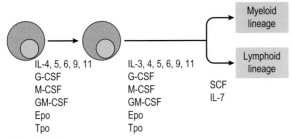

Fig. 12.3 Many growth factors are required in concert to drive differentiation of stem cells. IL, interleukin; G-CSF, granulocyte colony-stimulating factor; M-CSF, monocyte colony-stimulating factor; GM-CSF, granulocyte-macrophage colony-stimulating factor; Epo, erythropoietin; Tpo, thrombopoietin; SCF, stem cell factor.

Clinical box 12.2   Therapeutic use of growth factors

Advances in molecular biology have meant that many growth factor genes have been cloned and sequenced, enabling the synthetic production of these molecules for therapeutic use. Because of the concern of inducing leukaemia if growth factors that act early in haemopoiesis are given, there is more emphasis on the clinical use of growth factors that act late and are lineage specific. Important clinical growth factors in use are:

- G-CSF – for treatment of patients with neutropenia.
- Epo – used especially to treat anaemia associated with renal disease. rEpo is manufactured by inserting the relevant DNA sequence into a host cell, such as a bacterium, leading to a 'recombinant' rDNA that codes for the protein.

The production of red cells from stem cells is driven by various transcription factors that further influence the expression of growth factors and adhesion molecules necessary for cell differentiation.

TRANSCRIPTION FACTORS IN ERYTHROPOIESIS

Tal-1/SCL

This factor is thought to be important at very early stages of erythropoiesis, at the multipotent or myeloid-erythroid stem cell level. Studies in mice have shown that disrupting the gene for this factor results in uterine death with no blood production, whereas an overexpression leads to increased erythroid differentiation.

Rbtn2/LMO2

This protein, rhombotin 2, seems to form a complex with Tal-1/SCL and is of similar importance, as mice lacking the gene also cannot produce blood and die in utero.

GATA-2

Laboratory animals, such as zebra fish, provide the opportunity for much molecular research. GATA-2 expression in this animal is associated with areas of haemopoiesis. Also found on multipotent stem cells, increased expression of GATA-2 leads to proliferation of these cells, and a reduction results in a loss of haemopoiesis.

GATA-1

While GATA-1 is found in association with multipotent progenitors and several blood cell lineages, its absence leads to a failure of erythroid cell production with cells not developing beyond the primitive proerythroblast. The interaction between GATA proteins and another transcription factor, **PU.1**, appears to influence whether uncommitted stem cells commit to either the erythroid or myeloid lineages; overexpression of PU.1 leads to cells developing down the myeloid lineage.

GROWTH FACTORS IN ERYTHROPOIESIS

Committed erythroid cell production begins with the primitive **erythroid burst-forming unit** (**BFU-E**). With a combination of growth factors the erythroid progenitors divide to form **erythroid colony-forming units** (**CFU-E**) that subsequently develop sequentially into **proerythroblasts** (the earliest recognisable erythroid cell), **erythroblasts**, **normoblasts** and **reticulocytes**, where the nucleus is then extruded to form the mature red cell over about 5 days. Erythropoiesis may speed up in certain clinical conditions (Information box 12.2).

The most important of the growth factors is **erythropoietin** or **Epo**, which appears to be essential for the differentiation of the CFU-E progenitors. Other growth factors involved in erythropoiesis include SF (Steel factor) – 'Steel mutant' mice are very anaemic – interleukin (IL)-3, GM-CSF, insulin and activin.

Erythropoietin controls the red cell mass

The rate of production of red cells is governed by erythropoietin, a glycosylated protein of 165 amino acids produced by the kidney (90%), and to a lesser extent by the

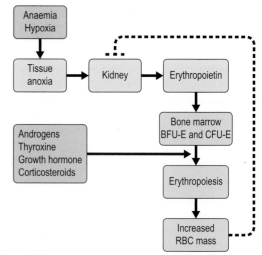

Fig. 12.5 **Oxygen levels are sensed by the kidney, which then modulates Epo production in combination with other hormones.** BFU-E, erythroid burst-forming unit; CFU-E, erythroid colony-forming unit; RBC, red blood cell.

liver. Glycosylation is a **post-translational modification** and adds sugar molecules to the protein, which helps prolong its half-life.

The body has no stores of erythropoietin and its regulation is at the gene transcription (i.e. mRNA) level. This means that when Epo is needed the DNA must be transcribed into mRNA, which is then translated into protein. The **hypoxia-inducible factor-1** (**HIF-1**) has two subunits, α and β. The α form interacts with oxygen sensors to activate Epo transcription. It is seen only in hypoxic (low oxygen) situations; when oxygen levels reach a high level a molecule hydroxylates HIF-1α, which then binds to **von Hippel–Lindau** (**VHL**) **protein**, activating a ligase complex that destroys HIF-1α so that Epo transcription is rapidly stopped.

The kidney responds to reduced oxygen tension with production of erythropoietin by the interstitial peritubular cells, resulting in a higher rate of red cell production by stimulating proliferation of BFU-E and CFU-E. As the number of red cells increases, so does the oxygen delivery to the tissues and erythropoietin production falls (Fig. 12.4). It is believed that erythropoiesis is controlled by the kidneys because the kidney represents the only organ in which oxygen consumption parallels blood flow.

Epo production involves a negative feedback loop

As the number of red cells increases, and the red cell mass rises, oxygen is delivered more easily to tissues. The kidney senses this increase in oxygen delivery and erythropoietin levels drop. Where oxygen levels are low (**hypoxia**), erythropoietin levels rise, leading to increased red cell production until oxygenation levels return to normal. In effect, this is a simple feedback loop (Fig. 12.5). An abnormal increased

production of erythropoietin leads to the clinical condition of polycythaemia (Information box 12.3).

STROMAL MOLECULES IN ERYTHROPOIESIS

In addition to haemopoietic cells the bone marrow stroma contains endothelial cells, fibroblasts, macrophages and associated stromal proteins. The stroma appears to have several functions that are essential for cell differentiation and facilitating release of cells from the marrow.

■ Adhesion proteins, such as **fibronectin**, bind to the **very late antigen** (**VLA**) on erythroid cells; as the cell differentiates into a reticulocyte the adhesion is lost. Interaction between VLA on erythroid cells and the **vascular adhesion molecule** (**VAM-1**) is also thought to be important.
■ **Macrophage deoxyribonuclease II** may be instrumental in the ability for red cells to lose their nuclei.
■ Cells must pass through small endothelial pores in order to enter the blood and need to be flexible. Only mature cells have that flexibility.

Other hormones that influence haemoglobin production

Although erythropoietin is the main hormone controlling red cell production, other hormones such as corticosteroids, androgens, growth hormone and thyroxine also play a role.

Red cell production during life

■ Babies are born with very high red cell counts and high haemoglobin levels, since foetal haemoglobin binds oxygen very tightly, shifting the **oxygen dissociation curve** to the left. This is a normal physiological adaptation.
■ Soon after birth the haemoglobin and red cell count drop and children have an overall lower red cell count and haemoglobin level than adults.

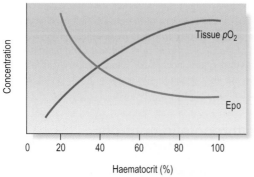

Fig. 12.4 **Erythropoietin (Epo) levels are driven by tissue oxygenation, in an inverse relationship.**

Secondary polycythaemia results from an increased production of erythropoietin, leading to increased red cell production. It can be due to a number of causes:

Cause	Reasons	Explanation
Decreased oxygen concentration	High altitude	Low ambient oxygen concentration
	Sleep apnoea (stopping breathing while asleep)	Hypoventilation of the lung alveoli
	High levels of carboxyhaemoglobin from carbon monoxide exposure	Exposure to smoking or exhaust fumes
Impaired blood perfusion of the kidneys	Blocked or thickened renal arteries	
	Renal failure	
	Renal transplantation	
Increased stimulation of Epo	Tumours secreting Epo	
	Chuvash polycythaemia	Mutation in VHL gene, preventing Epo production from being switched off
	Blood doping	Self-administration of rEpo by athletes resulting in an increase in red cells, and thus the oxygen carrying capacity

- After puberty, under the hormonal control of the androgen testosterone, males have higher haemoglobin levels than females.
- Finally, elderly people have lower haemoglobin levels than their younger counterparts, but males retain a higher level in comparison with elderly females.

TRANSPORT OF OXYGEN BY HAEMOGLOBIN

At rest an adult uses around 0.25 L of oxygen per minute. Oxygen consumption and carbon dioxide production increase dramatically with exercise. In general, oxygen is not particularly soluble in water and requires a carrier molecule to transport it from the lungs to the tissues. Respiratory pigments serve this purpose, and in humans take the form of **haemoglobin** and **myoglobin**. In both of these molecules oxygen molecules are bound to Fe^{2+} within the haem moiety.

- **Myoglobin** is found predominantly in muscle and is made up of a single globin protein chain with an associated haem group, which has an iron core (Fe^{2+}). Oxygen binds to myoglobin and easily saturates the molecule, resulting in a hyperbolic curve (Fig. 12.6).
- **Haemoglobin**, by comparison, is a tetramer (two α-like and two β-like globins) each subunit of which has an associated haem group (Fig. 12.7).

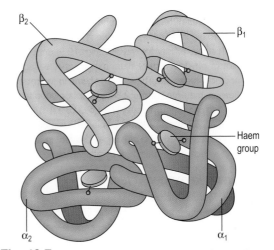

Fig. 12.7 **A haemoglobin molecule is made up of two α and two β globin chains and four haem groups.**

The oxygen dissociation curve

Binding of oxygen to the first haem is quite difficult, but as each haem takes up an oxygen molecule, the binding of subsequent oxygen molecules becomes easier, resulting in a sigmoid-shaped curve, which flattens out when haemoglobin becomes saturated with oxygen (Fig. 12.8). At the steepest part of the curve a small change in oxygen tension (pO_2 concentration) results in rapid release or uptake of oxygen (reflected in the large change in haemoglobin oxygen saturation). This ensures rapid delivery to the tissues where oxygen tensions are lower.

When blood returns to the lungs, carbon dioxide will diffuse out into the alveoli to be breathed out. Blood pCO_2 will be reduced, and pH will increase (becoming more alkali) – due to a decrease in blood carbonic acid. The curve will shift to the left and, at any given alveolar pO_2, the amount of oxygen that binds to haemoglobin will increase.

At the capillaries, carbon dioxide diffuses in from the tissues – the curve shifts to the right as the blood becomes more acidic and oxygen will be displaced from haemoglobin, delivering oxygen to the tissues.

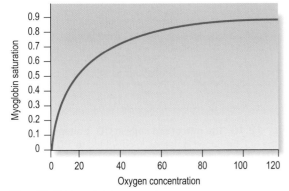

Fig. 12.6 **Myoglobin saturation curve.**

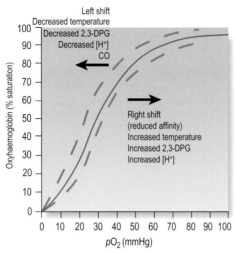

Fig. 12.8 The oxygen dissociation curve.

In order to function as an oxygen carrier, haemoglobin needs a high affinity for oxygen in the lungs and a low affinity for oxygen in the tissues. Haemoglobin exists in two principal tertiary forms, dependent on local environmental factors: **relaxed** (R), with high oxygen affinity, and **tense** (T) in the absence of oxygen, with a low affinity for oxygen (Fig. 12.9). Induced by lower levels of oxygen in the tissue, oxygen is released from the haemoglobin molecule. The α and β chains in the molecule rotate, allowing the entry of the 2,3-diphosphoglycerate (also known as 2,3-biphosphoglycerate) (2,3-DPG or 2,3-BPG) molecule. This then produces a lower affinity of haemoglobin for oxygen and increases the rate of oxygen delivery in active tissues. This is reflected in Figure 12.8 by a 'shift to the right'.

Role of acid in oxygen release

Under acidic conditions the equilibrium between deoxyhaemoglobin and oxyhaemoglobin shifts in favour of deoxyhaemoglobin. This is termed the **Bohr effect** and is very useful in physiological terms, since oxygen will dissociate from haemoglobin when muscle tissue is acidic. The acidity occurs during exercise when carbohydrates are metabolised to lactic acid in an anaerobic reaction. This is shown by the oxygen dissociation curve shifting to the right under the influence of H⁺ ions.

At any pO_2 level the oxygen saturation of blood is much lower in a right shifted curve, reflecting the move of oxygen into the tissues. Typically the partial pressure of oxygen in body cells is about 40 mmHg, when the haemoglobin saturation will be around 70%. At this same partial pressure, when the curve is shifted to the right, the haemoglobin saturation reduces to around 60% as oxygen is released.

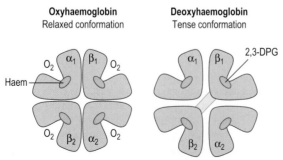

Oxyhaemoglobin
Relaxed conformation

Deoxyhaemoglobin
Tense conformation

Fig. 12.9 **Oxygenated and deoxygenated haemoglobin molecules.** 2,3-DPG, 2,3-diphosphoglycerate.

Role of 2,3-DPG in oxygen release from haemoglobin

2,3-DPG is a byproduct of glycolysis and present in red cells at the same concentration as haemoglobin. The binding of more 2,3-DPG to haemoglobin promotes the release of oxygen to the tissues.

Levels of 2,3-DPG rise during exercise, altitude and anaemia, shifting the oxygen dissociation curve to the right, ensuring that oxygen is off-loaded more easily.

TRANSPORT OF CARBON DIOXIDE

Carbon dioxide is taken from the tissues where it is produced, and eventually ends up in the lungs where it is breathed out. CO_2 carriage is more complex than oxygen transport. Figure 12.10 illustrates this.

- In the tissues, CO_2 is produced from catabolic reactions and enters the red cell where the enzyme carbonic anhydrase converts it to **carbonic acid** (H_2CO_3). The release of oxygen from oxyhaemoglobin buffers the acidic carbonic acid by taking up H⁺ ions and releasing bicarbonate, HCO_3^-, which diffuses back into the plasma and is carried in the venous circulation back

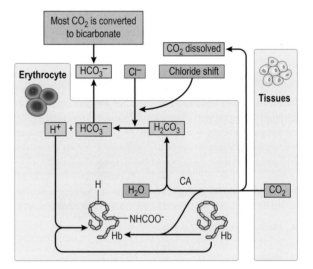

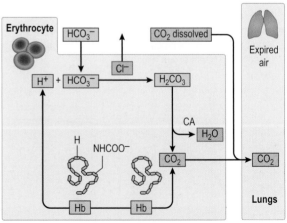

Fig. 12.10 **The role of red cells in CO_2 transport.** Most of the CO_2 produced in tissues is converted to HCO_3^- for transport to the lungs: approximately 20% of the total amount is transported bound to haemoglobin as carbamino groups, and small amounts are transported as dissolved gas in plasma. CA, carbonic anhydrase.

to the lungs. The movement of HCO_3^- into the plasma is counterbalanced by the movement of chloride ions (Cl^-) into the red cell (**chloride shift**). This exchange maintains electro-neutrality.

- About 10% of CO_2 is transported as **carbamino haemoglobin**, where it is covalently linked to the N-terminal valine residues of the haemoglobin subunits:

$$CO_2 + HbN \rightarrow HbNH\,COO^- + H^+$$

Thus further H^+ ions are available, in addition to those released from carbonic acid. Not all are taken up by haemoglobin and thus venous blood plasma is more acidic (reflected by the higher pCO_2 and lower pO_2) than arterial blood.

On arrival at the lungs, the reduced haemoglobin is oxygenated and this results in release of H^+ ions. For HCO_3^- to move back into the red cell, the negatively charged chloride ion must take its place, and the H^+ ions react with HCO_3^- to produce H_2CO_3 again. Here the carbonic anhydrase catalyses the reverse reaction, releasing H_2O and CO_2 gas, which then diffuses out of the capillaries to be expired through the lungs.

THE RED CELL MEMBRANE

Like most cell membranes of higher organisms, the red cell membrane is a lipid bilayer made up of phospholipids, cholesterol and glycolipids. The protein compartment contains about 10–15 major proteins and many minor proteins, including band 3 protein (anion exchange channel) and glycophorins.

The cell membrane and cytoskeleton are responsible for maintaining the disc shape of the red blood cell, but at the same time must allow great flexibility in order to allow the red cells to travel through blood vessels that are much narrower than the red cell diameter.

Spectrin

This is the major structural protein. It is 100 nm long, is highly pliable, and comprises two subunits, α and β. Each subunit is made up of tandem repeats (106 amino acid repeats). The subunits are aligned side by side and form heterodimers, cross-linked at their tail ends by **actin** filaments. The membrane cytoskeleton is linked to integral proteins in the lipid bilayer by **ankyrin** and **protein 4.1**. Ankyrin binds to β spectrin near a self-association site and links it to the cytoplasmic portion of band 3. This meshwork of proteins, which underlies the plasma membrane, restricts the lateral mobility of the integral proteins.

We know that these are important molecules since mice lacking spectrin or ankyrin have gross haemolysis (increased red cell breakdown). In humans, diseases such as **hereditary spherocytosis** and **hereditary elliptocytosis** are caused by defects in the red cell membrane (see Inherited anaemias, below).

HAEMOGLOBIN

Haemoglobin molecules each comprise four polypeptides, two α-like and two β-like globin molecules, in addition to a haem group, which is synthesised in the mitochondria.

The main adult haemoglobin is **HbA**, which comprises two α globin and two β globin polypeptide chains ($\alpha_2\beta_2$). Other important haemoglobins found in adults are **HbA$_2$** ($\alpha_2\delta_2$) and **HbF** ($\alpha_2\gamma_2$).

Coordinating haemoglobin production throughout life

Different types of globin molecule are produced at varying stages of human development. After conception the human embryo produces three types of early Hb called haemoglobins **Gower 1**, **Gower 2** and **Portland** (Table 12.3). The structure of these molecules follows the same rules as all Hb molecules, namely two α-like globin molecules linked to two β-like globin molecules to produce the familiar tetrameric structure.

The genes for all globins related to α globin are found on chromosome 16, the β-like globins are found on chromosome 11, and the order of the different genes on each of the chromosomes reflects the order in which different haemoglobin molecules are produced during embryonic development.

Figure 12.11 illustrates the arrangement of α-like globin genes on chromosome 16 and the β-like globin genes on chromosome 11. Three pseudogenes ψ (psi) are also present on chromosome 16 and one pseudogene on chromosome 11.

- From left to right, ζ (zeta) is the first α-like globin to be produced in the embryo by the ζ gene. After ζ expression stops, α is switched on (so-called ζ–α switch), resulting in the production of α globin chains.
- On chromosome 11 the arrangement of β-like globins follows the order (from left to right) ε (epsilon) $\rightarrow$ γ (gamma) $\rightarrow$ δ (delta) $\rightarrow$ β, which mirrors the β-like globin chains produced during development. There are two γ genes, Gγ and Aγ, differing only by one amino acid, guanine and alanine, respectively, at position 136.

As the embryo develops into a foetus, production of ζ stops and α is produced instead. α-Globin combines with γ chains and produces $\alpha_2\gamma_2$, which is also called **foetal haemoglobin**

Table 12.3	Embryonic haemoglobin	
Haemoglobin Gower 1 $\zeta_2\varepsilon_2$	**Haemoglobin Gower 2** $\alpha_2\varepsilon_2$	**Haemoglobin Portland** $\zeta_2\gamma_2$
Two ζ (zeta) chains	Two α chains	Two ζ (zeta) chains
linked to	linked to	linked to
Two ε (epsilon) chains	Two ε (epsilon) chains	Two γ (gamma) chains

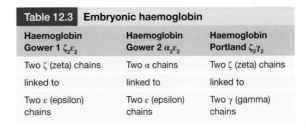

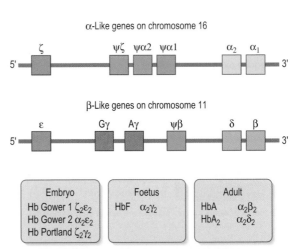

Fig. 12.11 Arrangement of globin-producing genes on chromosomes and haemoglobins formed during human development.

or **HbF**. Both G and A forms are produced. HbF is the main haemoglobin type in the foetus leading up to birth.

After birth, γ chain production drops and both δ and β chains are produced. The main adult Hb is **HbA** ($\alpha_2\beta_2$) although small amounts of **HbA$_2$** ($\alpha_2\delta_2$) and **HbF** ($\alpha_2\gamma_2$) are produced.

The mechanisms underlying the switch are, at least in part, physiological. We know that HbF ($\alpha_2\gamma_2$) binds oxygen much more tightly than adult Hb (oxygen dissociation curve shifts to the left). This ensures adequate oxygen delivery to the developing foetus, which has to extract its oxygen from the mother's circulation. After birth the lungs expand, the oxygen is derived from the air the baby breathes and β chains are produced instead of γ, leading to an increase in adult Hb ($\alpha_2\beta_2$).

RED CELL ENZYMES ARE REQUIRED TO MAINTAIN RED CELL COMPONENTS

The red cell contains a number of enzymes whose role is to provide energy for metabolic reactions. In addition, the red cell must maintain haemoglobin and red cell membrane integrity. Oxygen transport does not require energy but, in order to survive for around 120 days, the red cell membrane requires regular maintenance and this relies on energy. The following maintenance processes require energy:

- Red cell membrane integrity
- Red cell enzymes and haemoglobin sulphydryl groups must be maintained in reduced form
- Red cell shape (biconcave disc)
- Haem iron must be kept in reduced (Fe^{2+}) form
- K$^+$ and Ca^{2+} gradients.

If there is insufficient energy the red cell cannot maintain these functions, ionic gradients fail and the red cell adopts a spherical shape (**spherocyte**). These abnormal cells are quickly removed by the spleen and by other reticuloendothelial (phagocytic) cells. In addition, during a normal day, about 2% of the total body haemoglobin becomes oxidised to form **methaemoglobin**. The latter cannot combine with oxygen and is functionally useless, requiring energy to re-reduce it to its functional form. Abnormally increased methaemoglobin compromises tissue oxygenation (Information box 12.4).

Glucose is the main source of red cell energy

Glucose is metabolised mainly via the glycolytic pathway (see Ch. 3), which uses glucose in a series of steps that do not require oxygen (**anaerobic**).

One mole of glucose generates 2 moles of ATP, with lactate and pyruvate as the end-products of the pathway. NADH, required to maintain Hb in the reduced ferrous form, is produced in the glycolytic pathway. About 10% of the glucose is metabolised in the **pentose phosphate pathway**

(also called the **hexose monophosphate shunt**) and results in the generation of NADPH, a cofactor required to maintain glutathione on the red cell membrane in its reduced form.

Since red cells lack a nucleus there is no capacity for further gene transcription. Instead the red cell must maintain its cell membrane and haemoglobin molecules using only the mRNA and enzymes it already contains. The red cell probably has enough mRNA to manufacture enzymes for a few days after losing its nucleus and leaving the bone marrow, but for most of its life it will rely on the preformed red cell enzymes for all these housekeeping functions.

MAINTENANCE AND RECYCLING OF RED CELLS

Fate of old red cells

Normal red cells live for around 120 days, showing signs of age towards the end of this time:

- Become more rigid
- Glycolysis slows down
- ATP levels fall
- Membrane lipid levels reduce
- Cell gradually desiccates
- Haemoglobin cross-links to spectrin
- Antibodies are produced against neoantigens (new antigens) that have been revealed by ageing.

The markers of senescence are poorly understood but it is likely that increasing red cell rigidity, caused by a reduction in normal red cell enzyme function, and immune reactions, mark red cells for destruction by the reticuloendothelial system. Old red cells are phagocytosed and digested by macrophages found throughout the reticuloendothelial system, and particularly within the spleen.

Recycling of red cell components

At the end of their life, red cells are broken down (around 1% each day) and most constituents are used in the production of new red cells (Fig. 12.12).

- Free haemoglobin is released into plasma and binds avidly to **haptoglobin (Hp)**, an 85 kDa α2 glycoprotein present in plasma. The HpHb complex is rapidly cleared by the liver. Excess haemoglobin can result in its excretion in the urine (Information box 12.5).
- Iron from the haem group is released and recycled via plasma **transferrin**, which passes the recycled iron to developing red cells in the marrow (these cells expressing transferrin receptors).
- The haem porphyrin ring is broken down and generates unconjugated **bilirubin**, which is transported bound to albumin. After processing by liver hepatocytes, bilirubin becomes conjugated and excreted as **urobilinogen** in urine and through the gut.

ANAEMIAS

General features of anaemia

The term **anaemia** implies a reduction in red cell haemoglobin concentration, in comparison with that found in a population of similar age and sex (Table 12.4). Anaemia is not a diagnosis in itself as there is always an underlying cause.

Information box 12.4	Toxic chemicals and methaemoglobin

Exogenous chemicals can increase the rate of auto-oxidation to methaemoglobin. Gold and aluminium metal workers have been shown to have an increased proportion of their haemoglobin present in this inactive form. Tissue oxygenation will be compromised with increasing amounts of methaemoglobin being present in red cells.

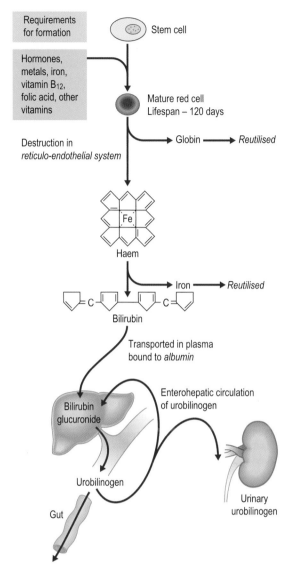

Requirements for formation

Hormones, metals, iron, vitamin B$_{12}$, folic acid, other vitamins

Stem cell

Mature red cell
Lifespan – 120 days

Destruction in *reticulo-endothelial system*

Globin → *Reutilised*

Fe

Haem

Iron → *Reutilised*

Bilirubin

Transported in plasma bound to *albumin*

Bilirubin glucuronide

Enterohepatic circulation of urobilinogen

Urobilinogen

Gut

Urinary urobilinogen

Fig. 12.12 Steps in the production and breakdown of red blood cells.

Information box 12.5   Haemoglobinuria

When haemoglobin concentrations in plasma rise, for example in haemolytic anaemia where large numbers of red cells are ruptured, the haptoglobin level in plasma drops as they mop up the excess free haemoglobin.

The haptoglobin–haemoglobin (HpHb) complex is too large to be filtered through the kidney glomeruli, but once the haptoglobin levels drop, as the protein is used up, free haemoglobin in plasma can be filtered easily, resulting in haemoglobinuria, where the urine becomes red in appearance.

Table 12.4   Clinical indications of anaemia

Signs more likely	Signs less likely
Severe anaemia	Mild anaemia
Elderly	Younger patients
Sudden drop in haemoglobin concentration	Gradual drop in haemoglobin
Other pathologies, e.g. cardiorespiratory disease	Absence of other diseases

---

Mostly the signs and symptoms of anaemia simply reflect a reduction in haemoglobin concentration, and hence delivery of O$_2$ to the tissues. These may be minimal or even absent, especially if the anaemia is mild and the individual is physically fit.

Anaemia in an adult male is defined as having a haemoglobin level of less than 13.5 g/dL and in a female of less than 11.5 g/dL. Anaemia is the commonest blood disorder worldwide, affecting some 30% of the world population.

Signs and symptoms may be general, and found in all types of anaemia, or specific and limited to specific causes of anaemia. The signs and symptoms of anaemia may reflect the fact that less oxygen is being delivered to tissues, or may be the result of the compensatory mechanisms that try to restore oxygen delivery towards normal (Table 12.5).

Physiological adaptations to anaemia

The body is equipped with a variety of mechanisms that are able to offset the effects of a reduced haemoglobin level and these explain, in part, why individuals with reduced haemoglobin may have very few symptoms. As discussed earlier, 2,3-DPG binding to β globin shifts the oxygen dissociation curve to the right, making haemoglobin offload oxygen to tissues more easily. With increased 2,3-DPG, oxygen delivery may increase by 40%.

Tissues and perfusion

The total blood volume in anaemia is generally much the same as normal, but blood may be diverted from less vital tissues, such as the skin and kidney, to more vital organs such as the heart, brain and muscle in an attempt to increase the flow of oxygen to sites which need it for energy production.

Cardiovascular system

As the haemoglobin drops to below 7–8 g/dL, the output of blood from the heart is increased, with an increase in heart rate and stroke volume. This is usually well tolerated, unless the individual has coexisting cardiovascular disease, such as coronary heart disease, in which case **angina** (heart pain) may develop or worsen.

Table 12.5   Symptoms and signs of anaemia

Symptoms of anaemia	Signs
Tiredness	Pallor, e.g. seen by looking at palmar creases, nail bed, conjunctivae (all generally unreliable in the assessment of anaemia)
Fainting	Rapid heartbeat (**tachycardia**)
Shortness of breath	Bounding pulse
Worsening of heart-related pain (**angina**) or pain in limbs (**claudication**)	Systolic flow murmur
Rapid heartbeat (**palpitations**)	Cardiac failure
	Retinal haemorrhages

Classification of anaemia

(1) Using the mean cell volume (MCV)

As with most diseases, anaemias may be:

- **Acute** (sudden) or **chronic** (of long standing)
- Inherited or acquired
- Primary or secondary.

Classification of anaemias on the basis of the red cell size is also useful and helps the clinician to select investigations that are likely to determine the underlying cause (Table 12.6).

The MCV in anaemia may be **normocytic**, **microcytic** or **macrocytic** and will be associated with differing conditions. For example:

- Normocytic anaemia is associated with **renal failure**
- Microcytic anaemia is associated with **iron deficiency**
- Macrocytic anaemia is associated with **vitamin B$_{12}$ deficiency**.

Table 12.6	Causes of different forms of anaemia according to red cell volume	
Small red cells		
MCV <76 fL		
Microcytic	Iron deficiency	
	Thalassaemia	
Normal sized red cells		
MCV normal		
Normocytic	Acute blood loss	
	Anaemia of chronic disease, e.g. infections, malignancy, connective tissue diseases	
	Renal failure	
	Hypothyroidism	
	Bone marrow infiltration with leukaemia, or other cancers	
Large red cells		
MCV >96 fL		
Macrocytic	Megaloblastic marrow	Vitamin B$_{12}$ or folate deficiency
	Normoblastic marrow	Alcohol
		Myelodysplasia

(2) Acquired or inherited

There are many reasons for developing anaemia. These can be due to acquired or inherited conditions. While some are discussed in some detail (shown in bold in Table 12.7), the reader is advised to consult a specialist haematological text for more information about other causes.

Acquired anaemias due to deficiencies

Iron deficiency

Iron is one of the commonest elements on the earth but, despite this, iron deficiency is the commonest cause of anaemia worldwide. Iron is a key component of haemoglobin and without iron there is a defective synthesis of haemoglobin, resulting in red cells that are both microcytic and **hypochromic**.

Iron metabolism

Iron plays a major role in many metabolic processes, but carriage of oxygen by haemoglobin, where it is the core component, is the most important.

The average adult contains 3–5 g of iron, of which two-thirds is in the oxygen-carrying molecule haemoglobin. A normal Western diet provides about 15 mg of iron daily, of which only 5–10% is absorbed (~1 mg), principally in the proximal end of the small intestine where the acidic conditions help its absorption in the ferrous form. The body can increase its iron absorption if there is increased demand, e.g. in pregnancy, lactation, growth spurts and iron deficiency. Table 12.8 lists the average daily iron requirements.

Iron is absorbed by enterocytes in the duodenum. Iron must be in the ferrous (Fe^{2+}) form. Ferric (Fe^{3+}) iron is converted to Fe^{2+} by the ferric reductase enzyme Dctyb (duodenal cytochrome b) on the enterocytes' brush border. Divalent metal transporter 1 (DMT1) transports iron across the enterocyte's cell membrane and into the cell.

The protein ferroportin is responsible for regulation of iron in the circulation. This protein has been shown to be responsible for the anaemia of chronic disease.

Once absorbed from the bowel, iron is transported across the mucosal cell to the blood, where it is carried by the protein **transferrin** to developing red cells in the bone marrow.

Table 12.7	Causes of acquired and inherited forms of anaemia			
Acquired anaemia			**Inherited anaemia**	
Deficiencies	**Iron** **Vitamin B$_{12}$** **Folate**		**Red cell membrane defects**	e.g. Hereditary spherocytosis
Blood loss	**Acute or chronic**		**Red cell enzyme defects**	e.g. Glucose-6-phosphate dehydrogenase deficiency
Anaemia of chronic disease	**Chronic infections, chronic inflammatory diseases, renal failure and malignancies**		**Globin abnormalities**	e.g. Sickle cell anaemia Thalassaemia
Haemolysis	**Immune: auto-immune, e.g. autoimmune haemolytic anaemia (AIHA); allo-immune, e.g. haemolytic disease of the newborn (HDN)** Non-immune: red cell fragmentation syndromes		Other rare inherited disorders	e.g. Fanconi anaemia
Marrow infiltration	E.g. leukaemia, lymphoma, cancers radiation, fibrosis		Other disorders (inherited or acquired)	e.g. Sideroblastic anaemia
Aplastic anaemia	E.g. red cell aplasia, cytotoxic therapy			

Table 12.8	Average daily iron requirement
Daily dietary iron requirements	mg/24 hours
Male	1
Adolescence	2–3
Female (menstruating)	2–3
Pregnancy	3–4
Infancy	1

Our bodies have two main types of iron store:

- **Ferritin**, a readily accessible source of iron (protective since free iron is toxic), and
- **Haemosiderin**, an insoluble form of storage iron found mainly in macrophages.

Iron loss

Only around 1 mg of iron a day is lost from the body in urine, faeces, sweat and cells shed from the skin and gastrointestinal tract. Menstrual losses of an additional 20 mg a month and the increased requirements of pregnancy (500–1000 mg) contribute to the higher incidence of iron deficiency in women of reproductive age. Humans have no specific mechanism for eliminating iron from the body other than the passive mechanisms listed above. In the adult male, 90% of cycling iron is that released from old recycled red blood cells.

Iron is transported by **transferrin** to developing red blood cells where it is reused. Some 20 mg iron is recycled daily for erythropoiesis, and several milligrams are required to replenish the haem and non-haem iron of cycling tissue cells. Figure 12.13 illustrates the uptake of iron by the cells. The transferrin receptor (TfR) expressed on the cell surface binds transferrin (Tf) when bound to two iron atoms. The Tf-TfR complex is internalised, iron dissociates, moves into cytosol, and Tf-TfR recycles to plasma and dissociates. Unbound transferrin, measured as the **total iron binding capacity (TIBC)**, in plasma will be increased when iron levels are low.

Iron homeostasis: regulation of ferritin and transferrin receptor levels

Iron balance relies on two proteins that readily take up iron:

- **Transferrin**, responsible for iron transport and the recycling of iron. The amount of iron delivered to a red cell precursor also depends on the balance of monoferric and diferric transferrin forms. Normally the affinity of TfR for diferric forms is greater than for monoferric forms, which begins to wane when the supply of iron diminishes.
- **Ferritin**, a protein that safeguards iron entry into the body, and maintains surplus iron in a safe and readily accessible form. Ferritin is one of the substances that can be measured in order to make a diagnosis of iron deficiency anaemia (Clinical box 12.3).

When iron is in short supply transferrin receptor levels are upregulated, encouraging more iron to be taken up by the cells and incorporated into haemoglobin molecules, and ferritin levels fall. Conversely, when iron is abundant, ferritin levels rise with a concomitant fall in transferrin receptor concentration. Thus there appears to be close coordination of expression of the genes encoding ferritin, transferrin receptor and the haem biosynthetic enzymes.

Studies of the iron regulatory proteins, **IRP**, have provided an insight into the mechanisms of this coordinated response.

- Ferritin messenger RNA (mRNA) has a 5′ untranslated region (5′UTR) which contains a stem-loop structure, termed the **iron responsive element (IRE)**. The IRE is recognised by **IRP-1**, a soluble polypeptide which has a similar amino acid sequence to the TCA (or citric acid) cycle enzyme aconitase. In the absence of iron, IRP-1 represses ferritin mRNA translation and blocks the attachment of initiation factors for translation.
  - The active site of IRP-1 is a [4Fe–4S] cluster; when cytoplasmic iron levels are high the cluster is complete. In this form IRP-1 cannot bind to mRNA, and thus the ferritin message is translated and more ferritin produced.
  - However, if cytoplasmic iron levels are low, IRP-1 will bind mRNA, resulting in prevention of translation of the ferritin message. Ferritin is therefore reduced.
- IRP-1 also controls the expression of the **transferrin receptor (TfR)** gene, located on chromosome 3 close to the gene encoding transferrin. The 3′UTR region of the TfR gene contains five potential stem-loop structures that are very similar to the ferritin IRE. These conserved regions of the TfR mRNA bind the same protein as the IRE of ferritin, with resulting stabilisation of the message and increased levels of TfR in iron deficient states.

Clinical box 12.3   Diagnosis of iron deficiency anaemia

The concentration of ferritin in plasma is a good indicator of iron stores, and low levels are only seen in deficiency. Normally the levels are about 40–200 ng/mL and virtually everyone with levels below 15 ng/mL is iron deficient although deficiency might be suspected at any level below normal. This test shows high sensitivity, but specificity is not so good if a 15 ng/mL level is used as a cut-off point.

Measurement of soluble transferrin receptor concentration has both high sensitivity and specificity for identifying iron deficiency.

Diagnostic test sensitivity and specificity

A test that has high sensitivity (is very good at detecting a disease that is present) and high specificity (is very good at detecting when a disease is not present) will have few false positives or false negatives, and so a negative result (soluble transferrin receptor concentration normal) is a very good pointer to the disease (iron deficiency) not being the cause of the anaemia.

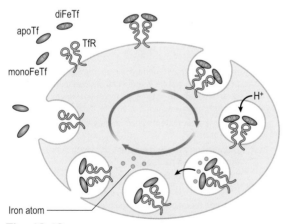

Fig. 12.13 Schematic representation of cellular iron uptake. Tf, transferrin; TfR, transferrin receptor; monoFeTf, transferrin bound to 1 iron atom; diFeTf, transferrin bound to 2 iron atoms; apoTf, transferrin lacking bound iron.

Causes of iron deficiency

Diet alone is seldom the sole cause for iron deficiency anaemia in developed countries except when it prevents an adequate response to a physiological challenge, e.g. pregnancy. Table 12.9 lists various causes.

Laboratory findings in iron deficiency

A full blood count and blood film is used to investigate the anaemia, but abnormalities typical of iron deficiency can also be seen in other disorders, such as the globin chain disorder, thalassaemia. Measurements of iron binding proteins can help confirm the diagnosis: Table 12.10 lists typical features and Figure 12.14 shows a blood film from a patient with iron deficiency.

As the iron supply reduces there is greater preference for monoferric transferrin, allowing a greater number of erythroid precursors to continue to receive iron, albeit in lower amounts, in an attempt to compensate for the developing anaemia and consistent with the fact that the MCV reduces before the haemoglobin decreases.

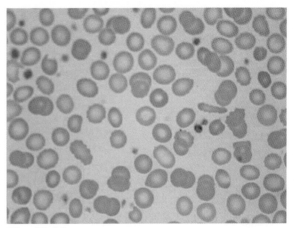

Fig. 12.14 **Typical blood film in chronic iron deficiency anaemia.** Note the pale red cells with pencil (elongated) cells seen in this patient.

Megaloblastic anaemia

In **megaloblastic anaemia** there is an impairment of DNA synthesis, but not RNA synthesis, and the **megaloblastic** cells are characteristically large because they are unable to divide by mitosis. The nucleus also has an immature appearance.

Although we are primarily concerned in this chapter with blood cells, megaloblastic changes will affect *all* actively dividing cells, including those of the gut lining. Megaloblastic red cells in the bone marrow will give rise to **macrocytic** red cells in the peripheral blood.

The terms 'megaloblastic' and 'macrocytic' are often used as though they mean the same thing; however, 'macrocytic' simply implies that the red cells are larger than normal (the MCV is >96 fL). There are other instances where the red cells are macrocytic, while the marrow cells are completely normal: for example, chronic alcohol ingestion may give rise to a raised MCV through a toxic effect, but in these cases the cells in the marrow are normal.

Why are vitamins B$_{12}$ and folate important?

All actively dividing cells require DNA synthesis in order to undergo mitosis. The metabolic pathways involved in replication

Table 12.9	Causes of iron deficiency
Causes of iron deficiency	
Blood loss	Heavy periods are the most likely cause in young females
Gastrointestinal	Bleeding peptic ulcer
	Inflammatory bowel disease
	Carcinoma of stomach, colon or rectum
	Abnormal blood vessels in gut (angiodysplasia)
	Malabsorption, e.g. coeliac disease
Dietary	Vegans
	Elderly
Infection	Hookworm infestation is commonest worldwide cause
Normal	Physiological demands, e.g. growth spurts in children
	Pregnancy

Table 12.10	Laboratory findings in iron deficiency	
Source	**Finding**	**Explanation**
Blood count	Low Hb concentration	Insufficient precursor iron
	Low red cell indices, MCV and MCH	
Blood film	Microcytic hypochromic red cells	A reduced rate of haemoglobin synthesis due to lack of precursors results in more cell division time as red cells develop until they reach the critical haemoglobin concentration – resulting in smaller cells
		Lower levels of haemoglobin in the cells make them appear pale
	Pencil cells	Unbalanced surface membrane to cytoplasmic volume due to reduced haemoglobin
	Target cells	Decreased cytoplasmic volume due to reduced haemoglobin
Biochemical	Low serum ferritin. Normal levels do not exclude iron deficiency as ferritin is an acute phase protein that may be raised for other reasons	Low iron represses ferritin production
	Low serum iron	Reduced iron availability
	Increased serum total iron-binding capacity (TIBC)	More free transferrin available to bind to iron

of DNA are complex, and involve both **vitamin B$_{12}$** and **folate** within the same pathway; hence a deficiency of these substances results in the same clinical picture.

Vitamin B$_{12}$ (cobalamin, Cbl)

The **cobalamins** are compounds that have three main components:

- A corrin nucleus (a porphyrin-like structure around a cobalt atom)
- A nucleotide
- A β group linked to cobalt. The β group may be cyanide (in cyanocobalamin), hydroxyl (hydroxocobalamin), methyl (methylcobalamin) or ado (adenosylcobalamin).

Vitamin B$_{12}$ is only manufactured by microorganisms and is ingested through eating meat and dairy products from animals contaminated with these bacteria. Vegans therefore need to take supplements to avoid a deficiency in this vitamin. The average Western diet provides about 5 µg per day and the total liver store is about 2–5 mg, which is sufficient for about 3–4 years in the absence of vitamin B$_{12}$.

1. In the *stomach*, **Cbl** is released from non-specific binding proteins due to the acid environment.
2. Cbl then binds to pepsin-resistant **R protein**.
3. In the *duodenum*, trypsin digests the R protein and vitamin B$_{12}$ is then bound to **intrinsic factor** (**IF**), which is produced by gastric parietal cells.
4. Once it reaches the terminal *ileum*, the **cobalamin-IF** complex binds to a receptor, named **'cubulin'** after the **CUB domains** that make up most of the protein. A CUB domain is a highly conserved sequence consisting of 110 amino acid residues and found in many regulatory proteins, but in a particularly high concentration in this protein.
5. Cbl dissociates from IF and the Cbl is transported by **transcobalamin II** (**TC II**), which carries the B$_{12}$ into the *portal circulation.*
6. TC II binds to specific receptors on the cell surface and is internalised. Then Cbl is released and the transport protein is degraded by cellular enzymes. Within the liver cell, Cbl acts as a coenzyme in the complex pathway leading to DNA synthesis.

Tetrahydrofolate (THF) is the biologically active form of folate. Its role is to acquire and donate carbon atoms to biosynthetic pathways that make thymidine nucleotides and methionine, an essential amino acid.

- Folate, in the form of **5-methyl-tetrahydrofolate** (**5-methyl-THF**) transfers a carbon atom through action of the **methyl-transferase** enzyme to Cbl, and then on to **homocysteine** to form the amino acid, **methionine** and then **S-adenosyl methionine**.
- **S-Adenosyl-methionine** is needed to donate a methyl group to maintain the protein **myelin**.
- Free THF is then used to transfer a single carbon atom through a series of folate coenzymes to **deoxyuridine monophosphate** (**dUMP**), thus producing **thymidylate** (**TMP**), required for nucleotide synthesis.
- TMP formation also involves the transfer of two hydrogen ions, producing **dihydrofolate** (**DHF**) which must be reduced to THF by **dihydrofolate reductase** (**DHFR**). THF can then enter the metabolic cycle again.

There are two main consequences of a **B$_{12}$ deficiency**:

1. A lack of *S*-adenosyl-methionine methylation is associated with demyelination of nerves and peripheral neuropathy.
2. A block in the production of THF means that 5-methyl-THF accumulates, and folate coenzymes needed for nucleotide biosynthesis are limited (the **methyl trap hypothesis**). This produces a pseudofolate deficiency, with an anaemia that resembles that seen in true folate deficiency. In B$_{12}$ deficiency, treatment with folate will, therefore, correct the anaemia, but not the neuropathy.

Figure 12.15 shows a simplified DNA synthesis pathway, illustrating the role of vitamin B$_{12}$ and folate in this process.

Causes of vitamin B$_{12}$ deficiency

Reduced absorption, rather than dietary deficiency, is the commonest cause of vitamin B$_{12}$ deficiency in the UK. The most severe cases, resulting in a condition known as **pernicious anaemia**, are due to an autoimmune condition in which the lining of the gut atrophies. This results in a loss of the intrinsic factor production, required for absorption of B$_{12}$ (see Ch. 16).

Vitamin B$_{12}$ deficiency also can occur after total or partial gastrectomy, and may also be seen in association with other bowel diseases or dietary deficiency.

Folate

The other key player in DNA synthesis is **folate**, derived from folic acid. Folate comprises three components:

- Pteridine component
- Para-aminobenzoic acid component
- An L-glutamine residue.

Folates are found in green vegetables, and are easily destroyed by cooking (see Ch. 16). The average requirement in adults is 100 µg per day (diet provides about 250 µg daily) and the liver can store 8–20 mg. Compared to Cbl, the body stores of folate are therefore quite small, and will only last about 4 months if supply stops.

Folate is absorbed in the upper small intestine, and the dietary form is predominantly polyglutamates. The polyglutamic form has a side chain of multiple glutamic acids joined in peptide linkages and this side chain must be cleaved before absorption can occur. The monoglutamate form is therefore most easily absorbed and can enter cells either by diffusion or by being taken up by specific folate-binding proteins. This form is employed therapeutically.

Causes of folate deficiency

The most common cause of folate deficiency is nutritional, due to poor diet and/or alcoholism. Table 12.11 lists these and other causes.

Laboratory findings in B$_{12}$ and folate deficiency

Clinically B$_{12}$ and folate deficiencies present with a macrocytic, megaloblastic anaemia, which may be mild or severe (Hb < 6.0 g/dL) but only B$_{12}$ deficiency produces neurological changes. Table 12.12 lists typical features of these diseases.

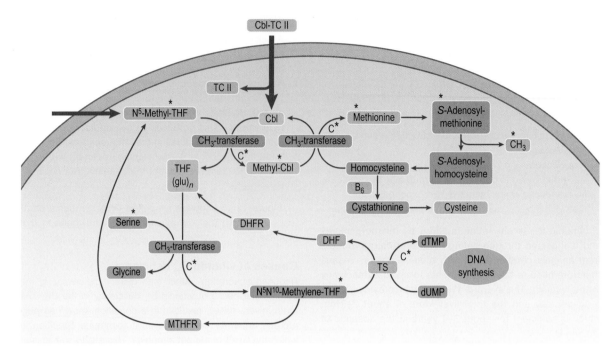

Fig. 12.15 **Cobalamin-folate metabolism.** *Indicates the carbon atoms that are transported through a series of biochemical reactions. TC II, transcobalamin II; Cbl, cobalamin; THF, tetrahydrofolate; DHF, dihydrofolate; DHFR, dihydrofolate reductase; MTHFR, methylene tetrahydrofolate reductase; TS, thymidylate synthase; dUMP, deoxyuridine monophosphate; dTMP, deoxythymidine monophosphate. Redrawn with permission from Israel LG, Israel ED 2002 Mechanisms in hematology, 3rd edn. Core Health Sciences, Canada.

Table 12.11	Causes of folate deficiency
Poor nutrition	Seen in poverty, old age, alcoholics
Increased requirements for folate, or excessive loss	Pregnancy (rapid growth of foetus), malignancy (increased cell turnover), chronic red cell haemolysis (increased red cell production)
Malabsorption	Coeliac disease, Crohn disease and other malabsorptive states
Drugs	Phenytoin, barbiturates, valproate (anti-epileptics), oral contraceptives
Antifolate drugs	Methotrexate (cytotoxic drug), trimethoprim (antibiotic), pentamidine (anti-protozoal drug)

Acquired anaemias due to blood loss

Acute blood loss

When large volumes of blood are lost from the body in a short space of time there are general features of volume depletion:

- Increased heart beats (**tachycardia**)
- Low blood pressure.

The haemoglobin concentration will be normal for several hours following the bleed; in fact a full blood count taken immediately after the bleed will be normal because red cells and plasma are lost together. Anaemia only develops once the blood volume has been restored through the movement of fluid from the extravascular to the intravascular space. The MCV remains normal and so this anaemia may be described as **normocytic**.

Chronic blood loss

In the developed world this is the most common cause of iron deficiency anaemia. Examples might be unrecognised loss from a bleeding gastric ulcer, or heavy menstruation.

Acquired anaemias due to chronic disease

Anaemia of chronic disease (ACD)

This is very common in medical practice and generally reflects the presence of other underlying disease, such as chronic infection (e.g. tuberculosis, osteomyelitis), chronic inflammation (e.g. rheumatoid arthritis, systemic lupus erythematosus (SLE)) or malignancy. By definition the anaemia is normocytic.

Mechanism of ACD

Why should the presence of a chronic disorder induce anaemia? Previously called **reticuloendothelial block**, since there is abundant iron in the bone marrow macrophages, the iron is not, however, passed to developing red cells.

The molecular and cellular mechanisms are still poorly understood, but appear to be multifactorial.

- In chronic renal failure the erythropoietic drive does not seem to be able to release iron from the reticuloendothelial system at the expected rate, which could be due to a depressed response to erythropoietin.
- In other cases the problem may be due to disruption of iron metabolism in the developing red cells.
- Key molecules involved in iron uptake are the transferrin receptor, ferritin and the red cell enzyme, 5-aminolaevulinic acid synthase. These are controlled, post transcription, by iron regulatory proteins that bind to mRNA when intracellular iron is low and it is possible

Table 12.12	Laboratory findings in B_{12} and folate deficiency		
Source	B_{12} deficiency	Folate deficiency	Explanation
Blood count	Reduced haemoglobin, often severe		Ineffective erythropoiesis
	Raised MCV (often severe)		Due to cells being unable to divide efficiently
	Leucopenia and thrombocytopenia		Due to reduced DNA synthesis
Blood film	Oval macrocytes		DNA synthesis is impaired, but not RNA synthesis and so there is a build-up of cytoplasmic components in a slowly dividing cell
	'Tear drop' poikilocytes		Often seen when there is an abnormal proliferation of cells within the bone marrow
	Basophilic stippling and Howell–Jolly bodies		Nuclear activity remnants (see Table 12.14)
	Hypersegmented neutrophils		Disordered nuclear maturation
Bone marrow	Erythroid hyperplasia and giant neutrophil precursors		Poor conversion of deoxyuridate to thymidylate, which leads to slowing of DNA synthesis and delayed nuclear maturation
	Atypical nuclear chromatin		Due to disordered nuclear maturation
Biochemical	Reduced serum B_{12}	Reduced serum folate	Folate cannot be used for nucleotide synthesis
	Increased serum folate	Reduced red cell folate	
	Increased serum iron		Increased iron turnover in response to megaloblastosis
	Increased iron stores		Iron from effete cells cannot be used because of block in DNA synthesis
	Increased lactate dehydrogenase (LDH)		Increased cell death
Immunological	Gastric parietal cell antibodies		Autoimmune condition leading to reduced intrinsic factor production
	Intrinsic factor antibodies		Autoimmune condition blocking Cbl attachment to intrinsic factor, or the attachment of the complex to receptors in the ileum

that cytokines (inflammatory mediators), such as tumour necrosis factor (TNF)-α, could interfere with this process.

- Inflammatory cytokines also upregulate ferritin synthesis, diverting iron into storage, rather than release.

Diagnosis of ACD

Diagnosis may be difficult because of the varying causes but generally there is a mild normocytic anaemia often associated with increases in acute phase proteins, such as ferritin and **C-reactive protein (CRP)** and an increased **erythrocyte sedimentation rate (ESR)**, due to inflammatory changes in plasma proteins.

If the process is longstanding, the picture may resemble iron deficiency, but the patient will *not* respond to iron therapy.

Anaemias due to haemolysis

Haemolytic anaemias are disorders in which the red cells are destroyed faster than normal; i.e. they have a reduced lifespan. Anaemia occurs because the bone marrow cannot produce sufficient new red cells to keep pace with the rate of destruction. Instead of 120 days, red cells may live for as little as 20 days. Consequently, in haemolytic anaemias, red cell breakdown will be increased and red cell production will be increased as a response to the anaemia. If the bone marrow can increase erythropoiesis sufficiently the patient may not even be anaemic.

Haemolytic anaemias may be acquired (and due to immune or non-immune processes) or inherited. Whatever the cause of the red cell breakdown there are metabolic consequences that are reflected in the clinical and laboratory picture. Figure 12.16 illustrates these.

Acquired autoimmune haemolytic anaemia (AIHA)

These anaemias are characterised by:

- Autoantibodies (i.e. antibodies directed against the individual's own antigens)

  or

- Complement, which attaches to red cells and either causes destruction via macrophages in the reticuloendothelial system within the spleen (mainly IgG coated red cells), or the liver (mainly complement coated red cells), resulting in an extravascular breakdown of red cells.

Red cells become coated with antibody, most often IgG. These antibodies react with Fc receptors on the macrophages leading to phagocytosis of the red cells. If the phagocytosis is incomplete the remaining portion of the red cell continues to circulate as a spherocyte (note that phagocytosis is usually complete if complement is involved) (Fig. 12.17).

The autoantibodies are of various types: 'warm', in which haemolysis occurs at normal body temperature; 'cold', in which haemolysis occurs at low temperatures, and the condition may be idiopathic (of unknown cause) or associated with other diseases. Some anaemias appear to be drug induced, leading to complement-induced haemolysis.

Most of the red cell breakdown takes place in the spleen causing it to enlargen from the debris (**splenomegaly**). Removal of the spleen (**splenectomy**) can resolve the anaemia.

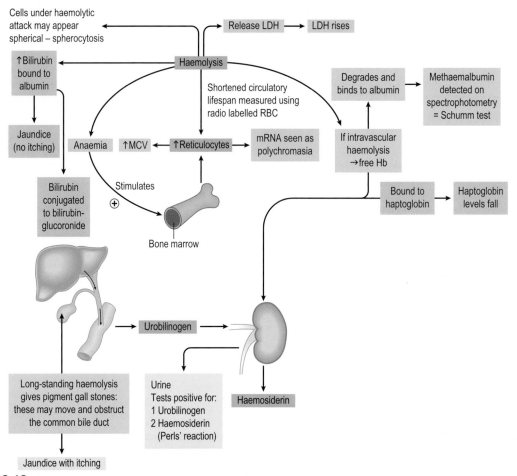

Fig. 12.16 **Metabolic effects of increased red cell breakdown.** LDH, lactate dehydrogenase; MCV, mean cell volume; RBC, red blood cell.

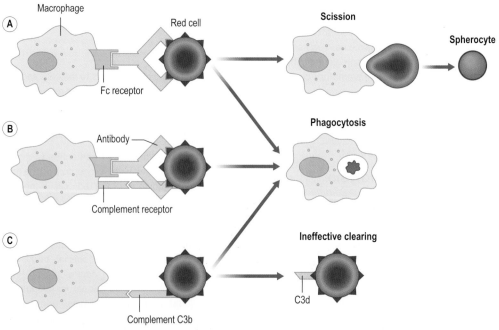

Fig. 12.17 **Extravascular haemolysis is due to interaction of antibody-coated cells with cells in the reticuloendothelial system, predominantly in the spleen.** (A) Spherocytes result from partial phagocytosis. (B) Complete phagocytosis may occur and this is enhanced if there is complement as well as antibody on the cell surface. (C) Cells coated with complement only are ineffectively removed and circulate with C3d or C3b on their surface.

Laboratory findings in AIHA

Examination of a blood film shows features typical of haemolytic anaemia: spherocytes and polychromatic red cells (Fig. 12.18). Table 12.13 details other features associated with AIHA.

Other acquired anaemias

Anaemia can also be caused by a variety of other mechanisms that interfere with either red cell production or the normal lifespan of the red cell.

Non-immune haemolytic anaemias

Paroxysmal nocturnal haemoglobinuria (PNH) is a rare defect of red cells that makes cells vulnerable to destruction by **activated complement**. The breakdown of red cells reveals itself in dark-coloured urine (**haemoglobinuria**), particularly evident in the morning when urine is more concentrated, although it was originally thought to be due to red cell breakdown at night due to increased acidosis – hence nocturnal and paroxysmal (intermittent). PNH is caused by a mutation in the **pig-A** (phosphatidyl inositol glycan complementation group A) gene, which makes a protein that anchors complement-protective proteins to the red cell surface.

Mechanical red cell fragmentation

This can occur in several conditions:

- Artificial heart valves – damaged valves can shear the red cells

- **Microangiopathic haemolytic anaemia (MAHA)** – in some conditions the microenvironment that the red cells encounter may produce fragmentation
- **March haemoglobinuria** – caused by traumatic exercise (such as prolonged marching in a military exercise)
- Heat – burns where red cells are exposed to heat over 47°C will result in the cells being fragmented
- **Malaria** – parasite-infected red cells are fragmented.

Marrow infiltration

When the marrow is taken over by clonal expansion of a particular cell, such as can occur in leukaemia, normal red cell precursors are squeezed out.

Marrow failure

Aplastic anaemia – is caused by a failure of the *pluripotent stem cells*. This failure can affect all blood cell precursors, or just one line, as in **red cell aplasia**. It can be caused by a variety of drugs, but is often the intentional consequence of the therapeutic use of certain cytotoxic drugs.

Rare inherited anaemias

Fanconi's anaemia is an autosomal recessive disease that results in skeletal, skin and organ abnormalities, as well as an aplastic anaemia. Several genes on different chromosomes are involved in making a complex essential for DNA repair.

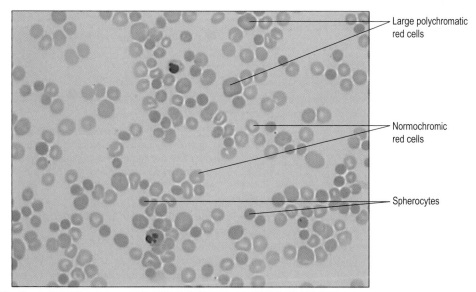

Large polychromatic red cells

Normochromic red cells

Spherocytes

Fig. 12.18 Blood film from patient with autoimmune haemolytic anaemia. Note the presence of spherocytes and polychromatic cells.

Table 12.13	Laboratory findings in AIHA	
Source	**Finding**	**Explanation**
Blood count	Reduced haemoglobin	Destruction of red cells
	Increased reticulocytes	Response of bone marrow to haemolysis
Blood film	Spherocytes	Due to a partial loss of the red cell membrane, possibly during partial phagocytosis stimulated by antibodies on the cell surface
	Polychromatic cells	Young red cells or reticulocytes produced in response to the haemolysis
Biochemical	Increased lactate dehydrogenase (LDH)	Released from red cells as a result of the haemolysis
	Decreased haptoglobin (Hp)	Haptoglobin binds free haemoglobin and the HpHb complex is removed by the reticuloendothelial system
Other	Positive direct antiglobulin test (DAT)	Detection of red cells coated with antibody or complement

Individuals with this condition have cells that are hypersensitive to genotoxic agents, such as mitomycin. Cells are seen to have increased chromosome breaks.

Inherited anaemias

Hereditary anaemias are virtually all haemolytic in nature and may be classified by the pathological process causing decreased red cell lifespan. These can be separated into three major groups of disorders affecting:

- Red cell membrane
- Red cell enzymes
- Haemoglobin molecule.

Clinical and laboratory findings reflect those seen in the acquired haemolytic disorders but may be more severe and can be associated with some specific findings.

Red cell membrane disorders

The red cell membrane is a typical lipid bilayer containing integral membrane proteins. These externally carried glycoproteins are responsible for the various blood group systems. Internally these integral proteins are bound to a protein cytoskeleton, which is responsible for the maintenance of the shape and flexibility of the red cell.

The principal cytoskeletal proteins identified are **spectrin**, **ankyrin**, **actin** and **protein 4.1**, of which spectrin is by far the most abundant. **Hereditary spherocytosis** and **hereditary elliptocytosis** represent a group of disorders in which there are deficiencies or dysfunction of these skeletal proteins.

Hereditary spherocytosis

Spectrin deficiency is the most common cause of hereditary spherocytosis and leads to instability in the red cell cytoskeleton, producing spherocytes. Different point mutations result in different forms of the disease:

- Mutations of **α spectrin** result in a recessive condition.
- Mutations of **β spectrin** are seen in families that show an autosomal dominant inheritance.

The reason for the difference in inheritance manifestation is because α spectrin synthesis normally occurs in excess, unlike β spectrin synthesis, with unwanted chains being degraded. Individuals who are heterozygotes will therefore normally produce enough α spectrin to balance the normal β spectrin production.

The laboratory findings are similar to other haemolytic anaemias with many of the red cells showing the characteristic spherical or elliptical shape. Often the MCV will be increased, because of the high prevalence of larger reticulocytes. The MCHC may also be increased because spherical cells can hold more haemoglobin than disc-shaped normal red cells. The increased haemoglobin breakdown will result in increased serum bilirubin in plasma, urobilinogen in urine and stercobilinogen in faeces. Special tests help to confirm the diagnosis (Clinical box 12.4).

Red cell enzyme disorders

Although haemolytic anaemia can be the result of defects in any of the red cell enzymes, only three disorders are common: **glucose-6-phosphate dehydrogenase (G6PD) deficiency**, **pyruvate kinase (PK) deficiency** and **pyrimidine 5′ nucleotidase deficiency**.

Clinical box 12.4	Diagnosis of hereditary spherocytosis

Osmotic fragility is the test used to detect spherocytosis. The degree of red cell lysis (rupture) caused by incubating red cells in sodium chloride solutions of various strengths is measured. Curves are drawn for normal and test samples and the mean corpuscular fragility (MCF) is calculated (Fig. 12.19). This is the saline concentration at which 50% lysis occurs. Normal red cells remain intact until the saline concentration reaches 50% and lysis increases as the solution becomes more hypotonic. Spherocytes, with their lower surface area to volume ratio, lyse more readily.

In normal subjects the curve is steep and symmetrical, whereas in spherocytic anaemias the span and shape of the curve is altered and, characteristically, in hereditary spherocytosis, a long tail of highly fragile cells will be seen.

Radioactive studies may also be helpful:

- Red cell lifespan – this can be determined by labelling the patient's red cells with radioactive chromium and measuring loss of radioactivity over time
- Red cell destruction sites – this will often be combined with the former, the body being scanned for hot spots of radioactivity where cells are being destroyed.

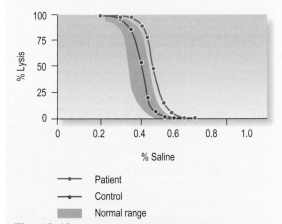

— Patient
— Control
— Normal range

Fig. 12.19 Osmotic fragility test. The patient's red cells are more prone to rupture (lysis) than the control red cells at the same saline concentration because the patient's red cells are spherical rather than disc-shaped.

Glucose-6-phosphate dehydrogenase deficiency

G6PD deficiency is the commonest red cell enzyme defect leading to haemolytic anaemia. The enzyme plays an important role as part of the pentose phosphate pathway (hexose monophosphate shunt) reducing NADP to NADPH (see also Ch. 3).

NADPH maintains glutathione in its reduced form, protecting the red cell from oxidative damage by detoxifying hydrogen peroxide produced by bacteria and certain drugs. G6PD is the only source of NADPH in red cells and a fully functioning biochemical pathway is needed to keep the red cell intact.

Oxidative damage leading to a haemolytic crisis may be caused by various factors:

- Drugs such as analgesics, antimalarials (primaquine) and antibiotics
- Ingestion of fava beans
- Sepsis.

G6PD deficiency is inherited in an X-linked recessive manner, so males are affected more frequently than females, although females who are heterozygous may still show features of the disorder. The condition is commonest in the tropics, ancestrally because of mutations that offer protection against *P. falciparum* malarial infections, but has become increasingly common in northern Europe, the UK, and North and South America.

The disease is extremely variable in terms of both its phenotype and genotype, with several hundred variants already described. Many of the mutations are point mutations in the 18 kilobase structural gene for G6PD found at Xq28. Three major forms of G6PD deficiency exist:

- G6PD A
- G6PD A−
- G6PD Mediterranean.

The last variant is the most severe form and associated with acute haemolytic crises. Patients may have a mild anaemia or are asymptomatic until they experience an oxidative 'stress' that results in an acute attack.

In addition to the typical findings associated with haemolytic anaemia the red cells often show particular characteristics:

- **Heinz bodies** are seen with particular stains where haemoglobin has been rendered unstable due to oxidant damage
- **Bite cells** are thought to result from the processing of cells through the spleen and removal of Heinz bodies.

Haemoglobin disorders

These may be due to structural abnormalities of the haemoglobin molecule, e.g. **sickle haemoglobin**, or due to defective and imbalanced globin chain production, e.g. **thalassaemia**.

Sickle cell disease

Sickle cell disease results from a single base change in the β globin gene, resulting in a change of amino acid number 6 glu→val due to the point mutation GAG→GTG. The resultant haemoglobin produced by the β^S gene is referred to as **HbS**.

Red blood cells containing the sickle haemoglobin elongate under conditions of reduced oxygenation, and form characteristic sickle shaped cells. These do not flow well through small vessels, and are more adherent than normal RBCs to vascular endothelium, leading to vascular occlusion and **sickle cell crises**. Sickling is initially reversible but red cells become progressively more rigid due to membrane defects. Sickled red cells have reduced lifespan and result in chronic haemolysis.

The sickle gene is widespread throughout Africa, the Middle East, parts of India and the Mediterranean. In the Afro-Caribbean population of the UK, the gene is found in 10% of individuals. Screening programmes offer early diagnosis of this and other inherited disorders of haemoglobin (Clinical box 12.5). Despite the deleterious nature of the sickle gene it

has remained at high frequency because heterozygous carriers have increased resistance to malaria.

Sickle cell disease is generally due to homozygous HbSS ($\alpha_2\beta^S_2$), but may also be due to interactions with other abnormal haemoglobins, such as:

- **HbC** (resulting in HbSC, $\alpha_2\beta^S\beta^C$)
- **β thalassaemia** (resulting in HbSβ⁺ thalassaemia, $\alpha_2\beta^S\beta^+$thal or β° thal)
- **HbD** (resulting in HbSD, $\alpha_2\beta^S\beta^D$).

All of these produce significant symptoms but SS and Sβ° are the most severe. The parents of individuals with HbSS sickle cell disease are both carriers of the β^S gene, i.e. they usually both have **sickle cell trait**.

Elevated foetal haemoglobin levels are beneficial

Adult Hb comprises **HbA** ($\alpha_2\beta_2$), which makes up the majority of Hb, along with **HbA₂** ($\alpha_2\delta_2$). Sickle cell disease is not detected at the time of birth since the main haemoglobin in early life is **HbF** ($\alpha_2\gamma_2$), which does not contain the β chain. When γ chain production diminishes and β globin production increases, sickle cell disease becomes apparent and is normally diagnosed before the age of 2 years.

Precipitants of sickle cell disease

Sickle cell disease is highly variable. Many patients have few symptoms, since HbS has reduced O_2 affinity and oxygen is given up more easily, although they are often severely anaemic. The anaemia is chronic, however, and patients are generally well adapted until an episode of decompensation occurs, resulting in a sickle cell crisis and an accompanying severe haemolytic anaemia (Fig. 12.20).

Precipitants include:

- Infection – leading to acidosis
- Dehydration – such as a result of exertion or hot weather, or secondary to a viral illness or excessive vomiting, leading to plasma hypertonicity and acidosis in its extreme
- Cold – leading to vasospasm and local tissue hypoxia.

Laboratory findings in sickle cell disease

Table 12.14 summarises the laboratory findings associated with sickle cell disease.

Specialist tests are also available to confirm the presence of haemoglobin S:

- Sickle test screen – the presence of HbS produces a turbid appearance when blood is left in a dilute solution of potassium dihydrophosphate. This test will not discriminate between sickle cell trait and homozygous disease and will not detect other abnormal haemoglobins.
- Haemoglobin electrophoresis (Information box 12.6) – confirmation of a homozygous state requires haemoglobin electrophoresis, which will show 80–95% sickle Hb ($\alpha_2\beta^S_2$) with no normal HbA ($\alpha_2\beta_2$). Foetal haemoglobin ($\alpha_2\gamma_2$) may be elevated to about 15% (range 5–15%). The parents will have features of sickle cell trait.

The thalassaemias

This group of disorders arises as a result of diminished or absent production of one or more globin chains. The net result is unbalanced globin chain production. Globin chains

---

Clinical box 12.5   Screening for the sickle gene

The identification of individuals who carry the sickle gene, and other inherited abnormal haemoglobins, is important in order to reduce morbidity and mortality. Screening tests are undertaken on adults at risk who may experience problems under anaesthesia, and for genetic counselling.

Infants with sickle cell disease are normally healthy at birth because of the high levels of foetal haemoglobin. The early recognition of affected infants is important in order to make plans for their care. Use of prophylactic penicillin and comprehensive care has reduced the mortality among children with sickle cell disease in their first 5 years from approximately 25% to less than 3%.

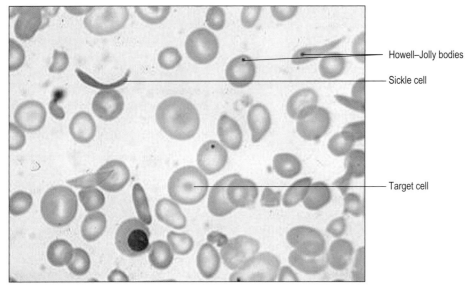

Howell–Jolly bodies

Sickle cell

Target cell

Fig. 12.20 **Blood film of sickle cell crisis.** The blood film shows several sickle cells as well as a nucleated red cell, target cells and cells with inclusion bodies (Howell–Jolly body).

Table 12.14	Laboratory findings in sickle cell disease	
Source	**Finding**	**Explanation**
Blood count	Low haemoglobin (6–9 g/dL)	Destruction of sickled red cells
	High reticulocytes (20–39%)	Increased bone marrow production of red cells
Blood film	Sickle cells	Haemoglobin S aggregates and distorts cell shape
	Target cells	Decreased cytoplasmic volume due to reduced haemoglobin
	Basophilic stippling and Howell–Jolly bodies	Evidence of nuclear remnant from cells undergoing rapid erythropoiesis
	Polychromatic cells and nucleated red cells	Immature red cells released from the bone marrow to compensate for the acute anaemia

in excess precipitate within red cells, leading to chronic haemolysis.

Thalassaemias occur at high frequency in parts of Africa, the Mediterranean, Middle East, India and Asia, and are found mostly in areas where malaria is endemic. Like the sickle gene, inheritance of thalassaemia probably offers some protection against malaria.

Thalassaemia is further classified after the gene affected, e.g. in α thalassaemia, the α globin gene is altered in such a way that either α globin synthesis is reduced (α^+) or abolished (α°) from red blood cells. The severity varies and depends on the type of mutation or deletion of the α globin or β globin gene. The consequence of impaired production of globin chains leads to red cells being microcytic and hypochromatic.

α Thalassaemia

α Thalassaemia is generally caused by large deletions within the α globin complex (compared with β thalassaemia, which is usually due to point mutations). There are two α globin genes on each chromosome 16, making a total of four α globin genes per cell (the normal person is designated $\alpha\alpha/\alpha\alpha$). Like sickle cell anaemia, patients can have:

■ Mild α thalassaemia where one ($\alpha-/\alpha\alpha$ **silent α thalassaemia**) or two ($\alpha-/\alpha-\alpha$ **thalassaemia trait**) α globin genes are affected; severe α thalassaemia if three ($\alpha-/-$ **Haemoglobin H disease**) or four ($-/-$ **Haemoglobin Barts hydrops foetalis**) of the genes are affected.

■ In its mild form those with α thalassaemia have no symptoms and no treatment is required.

■ Patients with HbH disease may have some features of red cell haemolysis, but treatment is not normally required. Up to 40% of the haemoglobin is HbH (β_4) and the remainder HbA, HbA$_2$ and HbF.

■ When all four α globin genes are affected no functioning α globin genes remain. The γ chains form tetramers (γ_4) which bind oxygen very tightly, resulting in poor tissue oxygenation – the oxygen dissociation curve is shifted to the left. Most of the haemoglobin is Hb Barts (γ_4) with small amounts of HbH (β_4). Inheritance of this severe condition usually results in a stillbirth at 34–40 weeks, gestation, or the baby dies soon after birth. Haemoglobin Barts hydrops foetalis is a common cause of stillbirth in South East Asia.

β Thalassaemia

Most **β thalassaemias** are due to single point mutations in the β globin gene and are not as deleterious as α thalassaemia (Clinical box 12.6).

■ Normally there are two copies of the β globin gene per cell, one inherited from each parent. An abnormality in one β globin gene results in the asymptomatic **β thalassaemia trait** – the patient has increased HbA$_2$ ($\alpha_2\delta_2$).

■ If both β globin genes are affected the patient has **β thalassaemia major** and most of the haemoglobin will be HbF ($\alpha_2\gamma_2$).

Information box 12.6   Haemoglobin electrophoresis

Haemoglobin electrophoresis is an electrical method for separating molecules on the basis of overall electrical charge. Electrophoresis allows the separation of different haemoglobins providing they have differing charges (if different types of Hb have the same charge these will move together on the gel and cannot be distinguished). Electrophoretic methods in current use are:

- Cellulose acetate (at pH 8.6)
- Citrate agar (at pH 6.0)
- Isoelectric focusing (IEF)
- High-performance liquid chromatography (HPLC).
    Some haemoglobin variants travel together through one type of gel and must be separated using another type of electrophoresis. There is no single electrophoretic method that allows each different type of haemoglobin molecule to be identified – usually two techniques are required to be absolutely certain that the haemoglobins have been fully separated.

Cellulose acetate electrophoresis
This is a common test which, although fairly old, is still used (Fig. 12.21). Different haemoglobins that have the same net charge will run together on the gel, e.g. HbS will run in the same band as HbD (hence cannot be distinguished using this method). Similarly HbG and HbC will run with HbE. In order to separate these bands the electrophoresis needs to be repeated using an acid pH (citrate agar).

Citrate agar
This is very similar to cellulose acetate but uses a pH gradient to separate different haemoglobins. HbD and HbG cannot be distinguished from HbA with this method but HbS will be distinguished from HbD.

Isoelectric focusing (IEF)
IEF is a high resolution method for separating different Hb molecules and the basic principle of the test relies on the fact that all proteins and amino acids have a pH at which their net charge is zero (**isoelectric point**). At this pH there is no net movement in the presence of an externally applied electric field. The Hb

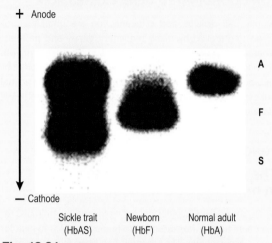

Fig. 12.21 Cellulose acetate haemoglobin electrophoresis of blood from a patient with sickle cell trait (HbAS), a newborn baby (HbF) and a normal adult (HbA).

molecules are subjected to a pH gradient. This method has the advantage of high resolution but is more expensive than standard electrophoresis.

High-performance liquid chromatography (HPLC)
HPLC is used for analysis of haemoglobin molecules. Haemoglobins are passed through a matrix column and eluted from the column at varying times, and their absorbance measured. Detection of standard haemoglobin variants is simple and the technique has the added advantage that novel haemoglobin variants can be detected. HPLC can separate proteins that cannot be resolved using other techniques.

Clinical box 12.6   Thalassaemia

Infants with this disease fail to thrive once HbF has declined and suffer severe anaemia needing lifelong blood transfusion (every 4–6 weeks) to suppress ineffective erythropoiesis and stimulate normal growth and development in childhood. They will suffer from an enlarged liver and spleen (due to production and destruction of red cells by these organs) and iron overload (leading to heart failure, endocrine dysfunction and chronic hepatitis) and are likely to need injections of desferrioxamine to chelate the excess iron.

- To date more than 150 mutations have been identified. These may result in reduced β globin synthesis (β^+) or absent β globin production (β°).

Laboratory findings in the thalassaemias
The findings depend on the severity of the disease.

- α Thalassaemia shows limited changes in red cell indices. In contrast, individuals with β thalassaemia have a significantly reduced MCV and increased red cell count.
- In the more severe disease (HbH disease, or β thalassaemia major) anaemia can be severe (Hb 3–9 g/dL) and the blood film shows changes that reflect this:
    - Microcytic hypochromic cells (because of the severe imbalance of globin chain synthesis)
    - Increased reticulocytes, polychromasia and nucleated red cells (due to the bone marrow response to the severe anaemia)
    - Poikilocytosis, especially in β thalassaemia, seen because the excess α chains precipitate, distorting the cells and damaging the cell membrane, leading to intravascular haemolysis.

ONCOGENESIS AND DISORDERS OF BLOOD CELL PRODUCTION

In health, the bone marrow regulates the number of cells in the peripheral blood to match requirements. Our bodies make sufficient red cells to transport oxygen to our tissues. White cell numbers are maintained to provide defence against infection and platelet numbers are adequate for normal primary haemostasis. However, the bone marrow may malfunction and produce excess numbers of cells (**myeloproliferative diseases**), or the bone marrow may produce cells that are functionally defective, a large proportion of which are destroyed within the marrow, leading to low numbers in the circulation (**myelodysplastic syndromes**). Finally, in extreme cases the marrow may produce excess numbers of malignant cells that spill out into the peripheral blood whilst within the marrow they suppress the production of normal cells (**leukaemias**).

NORMAL BLOOD PRODUCTION RELIES ON COORDINATED GENE EXPRESSION

Normal cell division and differentiation are complex processes, controlled by many regulatory genes and proteins. When these processes go wrong we see disordered growth of bone marrow cells. Why these events occur is poorly understood but we have learned a great deal by studying animal leukaemia models, in addition to examining haematological malignancies in humans.

ONCOGENESIS

The search for oncogenes in human blood disease

When **oncogenes** (cancer genes) were found in animals, researchers turned their attention to human cancers to look for similar associations. The research has been fairly rewarding in the case of solid tumours (lung, breast, colon and others) but undoubtedly the most significant advances have been made in blood disorders. Some leukaemias, such as **chronic myeloid leukaemia** (**CML**), have been intensively studied and CML is arguably the paradigm of human haemopoietic malignancy. Through the efforts of many clinicians and scientists we know much about this disease at the molecular level. This molecular knowledge has been used to full advantage, and we now have treatment aimed at specifically deactivating molecular targets implicated in the disease.

Oncogenes and tumour suppressor genes

Neoplasia is a process whereby uncontrolled growth occurs, and results from a loss of the normal process governing coordinated cellular growth. Two major classes of gene have been implicated, namely **oncogenes** and **tumour suppressor genes**.

Oncogenes

Oncogenes appear to cause malignancy through their direct effects. This group of genes includes growth factors, growth factor receptors and DNA binding proteins. Such genes are part of our normal genetic makeup and serve useful purposes, although, as **proto-oncogenes**, by definition they have the potential to become oncogenes. Once altered, through mutation or other processes, such as chromosomal translocation or viral activation, they become oncogenes, which have detrimental effects on cell growth and differentiation. Human cancers often involve the activation of one or more oncogene along with a loss of tumour suppressor gene(s).

Mutations

Point mutations induced by mutagens, such as UV light and ionising radiation, can lead to the production of oncogenes from their normal counterparts.

Chromosome translocations

Translocation of DNA from one chromosome to another, or within the same chromosome, can result in novel fusion genes. The best studied example is the **Philadelphia chromosome** (Fig. 12.22) (t(9;22)) in which **ABL** from chromosome 9 becomes fused to **BCR** on chromosome 22. The resulting *BCR-ABL* fusion gene, through its gene product

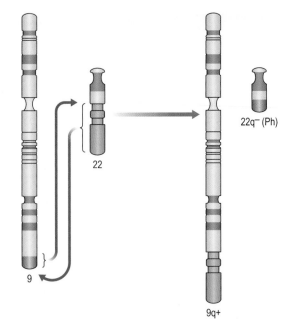

Fig. 12.22 The Philadelphia chromosome (Ph). The long arm (q) of chromosome 22 has been shortened by the reciprocal translocation with chromosome 9.

(BCR-ABL protein), gives rise directly to the typical phenotype seen in chronic myeloid leukaemia (CML). This disease occurs because *BCR-ABL* is a tyrosine kinase and its action results in uncontrolled growth of haemopoietic cells.

Viral activation

Viral genes may become incorporated into the host chromosomes, directly stimulating adjacent genes. In addition, viruses may pick up pieces of host DNA and transduce these into the next host, inducing cancer by this mechanism. Animal experiments have shown that the **Rous sarcoma virus** (**RSV**) in chickens may pick up the **ras oncogene** from one host and transmit it into another host, inducing **sarcoma** (a cancer of the mesoderm – bone, cartilage, muscle) in the new host.

Tumour suppressor genes

Tumour suppressor genes are implicated in a variety of malignant disorders, including myelodysplasia (MDS), leukaemia and lymphomas (Information box 12.7).

Tumour suppressor genes are able to result in malignancy through *loss or inactivation* (compare this with oncogenes, which induce malignancy through their activity). It seems that, under normal circumstances, tumour suppressor genes suppress uncontrolled cell growth, or at least they are key players in the regulation of cell growth. Uncontrolled cell growth will result if the suppressive effect is lost. Many tumour suppressor genes have now been identified that are associated with diseases such as **familial retinoblastoma** (cancer of the eye in children), **Wilm's tumour** (a kidney cancer in children) and **familial adenomatous polyposis** (leading to colon cancer).

THE LYMPHOID SYSTEM

The lymphoid system is found throughout the body (Clinical box 12.7) and acts to protect the body from foreign antigens. Specialised tissues have different functions and neoplastic transformations within the tissues lead to a variety of associated diseases.

| Information box 12.7 | Retinoblastoma gene – a tumour suppressor gene |

The retinoblastoma (RB) gene, found on chromosome 13, was the first gene to be studied in detail. Retinoblastoma is a childhood cancer occurring in 1 in 20 000 children. Two forms are found, namely sporadic and familial. From family studies it appeared that 'two hits' were required to develop the malignant disorder. Inactivation of one RB gene was not sufficient to trigger the disease since the other RB gene was still functioning. If, however, the second RB gene was also inactivated then disease occurred.

| Clinical box 12.7 | Lymphoid tissues in the body |

- The **tonsils** are lymphoid tissues found at the back of the throat.
- The **thymus** gland is prominent in children and lies in front of the trachea, from the level of the cricoid cartilage (at the level of the top of the oesophagus and C6 – the sixth cervical vertebra), running down behind the sternum.
- The **mediastinum** is the area between the two pleural cavities, which hold the lungs. The thymus is found in this area, along with the oesophagus, the trachea, the pericardial cavity, holding the heart, and the great arteries and veins of the heart.
- **Lymph nodes** are areas where lymphatic vessels join at various parts of the body. The lymphatic vessels carry tissue fluid around the body and generally lie alongside arteries. As arteries pulsate, fluid is moved in one direction, the reverse being prevented by the presence of valves. The lymphatics are important because it is through this fluid that malignant cells can spread and involve other organs.

Primary lymphoid tissues

In the bone marrow, primitive cells (**stem cells**) are stimulated by **cytokines** to mature into blood cells that enter the peripheral circulation. Lymphocytes are programmed in primary lymphoid tissue:

- **Pre-B lymphocytes** mature to form **B cells** in the bone marrow, which then circulate within the secondary lymphoid tissues.
- **T lymphocytes** are attracted to the **thymus** gland by chemotactic factors. Self-antigens enter through the capsule that surrounds the gland and come into contact with lymphocytes, where thymus epithelial cells promote the different steps of T cell differentiation and maturation. This is done through direct contact, allowing presentation of antigens (presentation of the **major histocompatibility complex**) enabling the recognition of 'self', and through hormonal influence, producing **helper T cells** and **cytotoxic T cells** (see also Ch. 6).

Secondary lymphoid tissues

Lymph nodes are collections of cells, surrounded by a capsule, that are placed in areas of the body through which body fluid drains. Macrophages that line the sinuses beneath the capsule collect antigens present within fluid. Within the nodes lie the cortex, composed of follicles, and in the centre is the medulla. Different areas of the nodes have different functions:

- **B cells** proliferate in the follicles in response to antigen sensitisation.

- **T cells** differentiate and proliferate in the inter-follicular region, also in response to antigens.
- **Plasma cells** are present in the medulla and positioned close to the sinuses to facilitate delivery of immunoglobulins to react with foreign antigens.
- **Mucosa-associated lymphoid tissue** (**MALT**) is found along mucosal surfaces to protect antigen entry through this route. **Tonsils** are an example of MALT tissue. They are similar to lymph nodes but are filled mainly with B cells. Their position in the nasopharynx means they are suited to detect antigens within breathed-in air.

MYELOPROLIFERATIVE DISEASES

This is a diverse group of conditions with one feature in common: they are all **clonal** proliferations that may eventually (after several years) transform into acute leukaemia. The clinical and laboratory features reflect the predominant cell type in each.

The myeloproliferative diseases

- **Polycythaemia rubra vera** – proliferation of red cells
- **Essential thrombocythaemia** – proliferation of platelets
- **Myelofibrosis** – proliferation of myeloid cells
- **Chronic myeloid leukaemia** – proliferation of leukaemic myeloid cells.

Polycythaemia

Polycythaemia is an increase in haemoglobin concentration, packed cell volume (PCV) and red cell count. Depending on whether there is a real increase in the red cell mass (RCM) or a reduction in plasma volume, polycythaemias fall into two major groups:

- Absolute erythrocytosis (true increase in red cell mass)
- Relative erythrocytosis (RCM normal but plasma volume reduced).

The three main groups (Fig. 12.23) are:

- **Primary proliferative polycythaemia** (PPP; also called polycythaemia rubra vera, PRV)

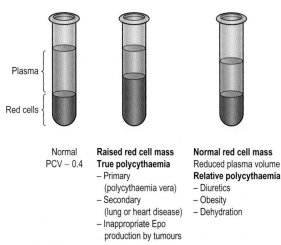

Normal
PCV ~ 0.4

Raised red cell mass
True polycythaemia
– Primary
  (polycythaemia vera)
– Secondary
  (lung or heart disease)
– Inappropriate Epo
  production by tumours

Normal red cell mass
Reduced plasma volume
Relative polycythaemia
– Diuretics
– Obesity
– Dehydration

Fig. 12.23 **Different types of polycythaemia.** PCV, packed cell volume.

- **Secondary polycythaemia** – due to an increase in erythropoietin which may be physiological and appropriate, or produced inappropriately by a variety of tumours
- **Relative polycythaemia**, which is also called **apparent polycythaemia** – due to a reduced plasma volume making the red cell count relatively higher than normal.

Polycythaemia rubra vera

In **PRV** there is an absolute erythrocytosis (a true elevation of the red cell mass) often accompanied by an increase in granulocytes and platelets. The underlying cause is unknown but is likely to be due to acquired genetic changes in the stem cell leading to disturbance of the normal cellular growth pattern.

Cell culture studies have shown that the red cell precursors are more sensitive than normal to a variety of growth factors, including **Epo** and **thrombopoietin** (**Tpo**). Precursor red cells are usually critically dependent on Epo. Cellular proliferation is believed to be driven through protein phosphorylation, and the tumour suppressor gene, SHP-1, appears to be a suitable candidate influencing this process; SHP-1 interacts with a variety of growth factor receptors including that of Epo.

The disease is generally found in older people with non-specific and variable symptoms, often resulting in PRV being unrecognised. Once diagnosed it is often treated by:

- Venesection – removal of a unit of blood at regular intervals to relieve symptoms
- Chemotherapy (hydroxyurea) – to control thrombocytosis and risk of vascular complications
- Allopurinol – to block uric acid production.

Essential thrombocythaemia

Essential thrombocythaemia is a malignant clonal disorder affecting the bone marrow megakaryocytes. These increase in number and produce excess platelets. As with PRV, this disorder is commoner from middle age onwards. Thrombosis and haemorrhage may occur; the former occurs because there are excess platelets, and haemorrhage may result from interference in platelet function.

Myelofibrosis

Myelofibrosis is an uncommon myeloproliferative disease in which there is megakaryocyte hyperplasia in the bone marrow, with intense bone marrow fibrosis. Extramedullary haemopoiesis (production of blood at unusual sites) in the spleen, liver and at other sites is common.

MYELODYSPLASTIC SYNDROMES

The **myelodysplastic syndromes** (**MDS**) comprise clonal stem cell disorders characterised by abnormal blood cell development. There is a highly proliferative bone marrow but with peripheral blood cytopenia. This is caused by the cells within the bone marrow being destroyed before being released into the circulation. Although the bone marrow is trying to produce adequate numbers of cells, these are largely defective. This leads to anaemia, with reduced white cell and platelet counts.

Some forms of MDS have a tendency to transform into acute leukaemia, and MDS was previously termed **pre-leukaemia**. However, many patients never develop leukaemia so this term has been abandoned. MDS is probably the commonest haematological neoplasm, with an incidence of about 1:10 000, and is primarily a disease of the elderly.

Overall, 5q– (a deletion in the long arm of chromosome 5) is the commonest cytogenetic finding in MDS and constitutes a separate clinical syndrome, usually affecting elderly females, and carries a good prognosis. Mutations of p53 have also been found and are associated with a poor prognosis and increased tendency to progress to acute leukaemia.

LEUKAEMIAS

Leukaemia literally means 'white blood', so-called because of the enormous numbers of white cells in the peripheral blood in patients with leukaemia at diagnosis. Classically, the leukaemias are divided into **acute** and **chronic** forms:

- **Acute leukaemia** tends to present more dramatically, and must be treated early or death will occur within a short period of time
- In general, **chronic leukaemia** is more indolent (slow growing) and in some cases may not require therapy for years.

In both acute and chronic leukaemias there is progressive accumulation of abnormal white blood cells in the bone marrow or other organs, which spill out into the peripheral blood. There is progressive bone marrow failure with a reduction in the other normal cell types. Patients therefore tend to also have a reduced number of red cells (producing anaemia) and megakaryocytes (leading to low platelets and bleeding).

Acute leukaemia is uncommon and may occur at any age. There is a peak in early childhood and a progressive increase with age. The overall incidence is 4/100 000 per year. Leukaemias are categorised into either **childhood** (<15 years) or **adult** disease.

The acute leukaemias

Childhood and adult acute leukaemias differ in their frequencies, with **acute myeloid leukaemia** (**AML**) primarily a disease of adults and **acute lymphoblastic leukaemia** (**ALL**) affecting mainly children. Their response to treatment is also quite different; for example, children with ALL would be expected to be cured if treated, whilst adults with ALL do badly. The reasons for these age-related differences are complex and not fully understood. The acute nature of the disease is experienced through:

- Tiredness, shortness of breath and anaemia – due to reduced red cells
- Increased susceptibility to infection – due to reduced white cells
- Bruising or bleeding – due to reduction in platelets
- Bone pain in children – accumulation of leukaemic cells in long bones
- Respiratory and neurological symptoms – due to large numbers of white cells in the peripheral blood causing hyperviscosity and sludging of the blood.

Table 12.15   Causes of acute leukaemia

Implicated agent	Mechanism	Examples
Ionising radiation	Induces genetic damage to haemopoietic progenitor cells. The peak incidence is 7–8 years after exposure	X-ray workers Post-atomic bomb survivors Irradiation used as part of therapy for Hodgkin disease, non-Hodgkin lymphoma, and other cancers
Chemical agents	DNA damage	Benzene and its derivatives Alkylating agents (anti-cancer drugs)
Genetic factors	Unstable chromosomes	Down syndrome (trisomy 21) Fanconi's anaemia
Viruses	Some may integrate their DNA into the host and influence (e.g. upregulate) regulatory genes	Evidence exists for the role of viruses in causing leukaemia in animals but less so for humans. One human disease for which a virus has been shown to be causative is acute T cell leukaemia/lymphoma (ATLL), which is induced by the virus HTLV-1

Incidence and causes

As with many malignancies the underlying causes are not fully elucidated. However, there are environmental and genetic factors that predispose to the development of acute leukaemia; these are shown in the Table 12.15.

Laboratory findings

While it may be clear from the blood film that the patient has an acute leukaemia, differentiation between the myeloid and lymphoid forms are likely to need specialist tests.

Examination of the bone marrow will usually show an increased cellularity with most of the cells being abnormal blast cells. The blood film reflects the contents of the marrow with reduced numbers of normal red cells, white cells and platelets (because there is limited room in the marrow for the normal lineages), and immature white cells (leukaemic blast cells). Specialist tests are used to provide a formal diagnosis (Clinical box 12.8).

Chronic leukaemias

Chronic myeloid leukaemia (**CML**) and **chronic lymphocytic leukaemia** (**CLL**) have very little in common, apart from the fact that they are chronic in nature. Both may be discovered by chance.

Chronic myeloid leukaemia

CML is an uncommon clonal stem cell disorder making up 15% of all leukaemias. Presentation is more common in adults between the ages of 40 and 60 years. CML is characterised by a high white cell count, of granulocytic lineage, and the presence of the **Philadelphia chromosome** (**Ph**). There are two different forms of the resulting **BCR-ABL** mutation, depending on where the join to the 3′ end of BCR is placed. One type, seen in about 30% of patients, is associated with a more rapid progression of disease. The mutation leads to transcription of proteins with high **tyrosine kinase** activity. Tyrosine kinases are important in cell growth and differentiation. CML was the first human malignancy shown to be associated with a specific chromosome translocation.

CML has three main phases: **chronic phase**, which lasts about 5 years before progressing to an **accelerated phase**, with increased numbers of blast cells, and finally **blast crisis**.

Table 12.16   Clinical features of chronic leukaemia

Chronic myeloid leukaemia	Chronic lymphocytic leukaemia
Non-specific – tiredness, fatigue and weight loss	
Abdominal discomfort – due to enlarged spleen and/or liver	
Progressive anaemia – due to marrow infiltration	
Gout – due to increased cell turnover producing high levels of uric acid	
Mild fever, night sweats – due to hypermetabolism	Enlarged lymph nodes – due to clonal B cell production
	Petechiae – pin point blood spots in the skin – due to reduced platelets
	Increased infection rate – due to reduced immunoglobulin

The crisis resembles an acute leukaemia; there may be features of acute myeloid leukaemia in 80% of cases and lymphoid in 20%. Frequently there is evidence of other cytogenic abnormalities, such as another Ph-positive clone, trisomy 8, 9, 19 or 21, loss of one chromosome 17, or deletion of the Y chromosome.

Chronic lymphocytic leukaemia (CLL)

CLL is the commonest adult leukaemia in Western societies with a peak incidence in patients aged between 60 and 80 years of age, and a male to female ratio of 2:1. CLL is a slow-growing disorder characterised by progressive accumulation of neoplastic cells in the bone marrow, spleen, liver and lymph nodes. In some cases there is bone marrow failure with marked reduction in the normal cell lines. Both disease and treatment complications are causes of death. Table 12.16 summarises the clinical features of CLL (and CML).

The cause is largely unknown and most cases of CLL are of B cell lineage, their maturation arrested. Although the cells look like mature lymphocytes, examination of cell surface antigens reveal some differences and the cells have very low levels of surface immunoglobulin. Cytogenic abnormalities are also common: about 50% have a deletion of 13q, and other deletions or trisomy may be seen.

An overexpression of **BCL2** is seen in the disease. This proto-oncogene is a suppressor of **apoptosis** (programmed cell death) and thus the affected cells have a longer lifespan.

Research has shown that somatic mutation of the variable regions of the immunoglobulin heavy chain genes (IgH V region genes) predicts a favourable outcome, whereas

Clinical box 12.8 Diagnosis of acute leukaemia

Cytochemistry

Blood films are stained with different stains to detect specific proteins, carbohydrates and lipids that are characteristic of certain cell lineages (Fig. 12.24).

Immunophenotyping using flow cytometry

This technique has improved the diagnosis of leukaemia and other haematological disorders. It uses a panel of powerful monoclonal antibodies (MAbs) to determine the presence or absence of specific antigens on the surface (or inside) leukaemic cells. The MAbs are very sensitive and specific and will only bind to one target antigen. We now know the pattern of expression of antigens on the cells of most leukaemias, making it relatively easy to determine whether blast cells are lymphoid or myeloid.

Leukaemic cells are incubated with a variety of MAbs after which they are passed through a fluorescence activated cell sorter (FACS) machine. The FACS plots forward and side scatter and provides a guide to positivity or negativity for the antigens tested (Fig. 12.25).

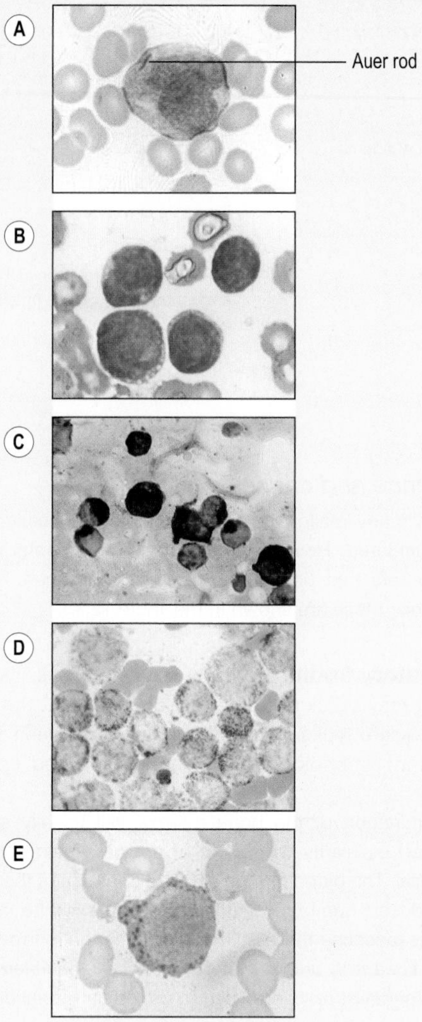

Fig. 12.24 **Cytochemical staining for acute leukaemia helps to distinguish between different forms of leukaemia.** (A) AML blast with Auer rod (top left) (May–Grunwald–Giemsa stain). (B) ALL blasts (May–Grunwald–Giemsa stain). (C) AML blasts: Sudan black stains lipids black. Lipids are rarely seen in lymphocytes. (D) ALL blasts: acid phosphatase positive staining in T cell subsets in ALL. (E) ALL blasts: Periodic acid–Schiff (PAS) stains glycogen red in ALL blasts. Glycogen is not present in normal lymphocytes.

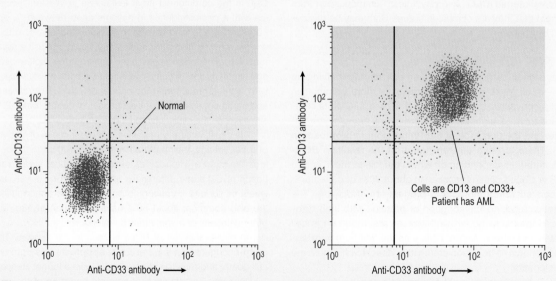

Fig. 12.25 **Flow cytometry using different monoclonal antibodies to cell surface molecules can distinguish between normal (*left*) and acute myeloid leukaemia (AML) (*right*).**

Normal

Cells are CD13 and CD33+
Patient has AML

Table 12.17	Laboratory findings in chronic leukaemia
Chronic myeloid leukaemia	Chronic lymphocytic leukaemia
White count very high, up to >100 × 10⁹/L, reduced haemoglobin	
Mainly granulocytic with full range of precursors (Fig. 12.26A)	Mainly mature looking lymphocytes with 'smear' cells. These are produced when the blood film is made (Fig. 12.26C)
Bone marrow hypercellular – mostly granulocytes (Fig. 12.26B)	Bone marrow has increased number of small lymphocytes

patients in whom the IgH V genes are not mutated fare less well. The reason for the influence of IgH V gene mutational status on survival is that B CLL lymphocytes, in which the IgH V genes are mutated, have passed through the lymph node germinal centres and are by definition more competent. By contrast, those with unmutated IgH V genes are pre-germinal.

Laboratory findings

In chronic leukaemia the white cell count is very high, typically greater than 100 × 10⁹/L, and the types reflect the disease (Table 12.17). In myeloid leukaemia the full range of precursors are seen in the blood, and the bone marrow is hypercellular (Fig. 12.26A, B), whereas in lymphoid leukaemia the cells appear mature but are often accompanied by 'smear' cells, produced when the blood film is made (Fig. 12.26C).

LYMPHOMAS

Lymphomas are malignancies affecting lymphoid tissue, i.e. lymphocytes, and comprise the **non-Hodgkin lymphomas (NHLs)** and **Hodgkin disease**.

Non-Hodgkin lymphoma (NHL)

In **NHL** there is a clonal expansion of lymphoid cells, mostly of B cell origin. Several different mechanisms are thought to be involved.

Chromosome translocations

Different chromosomal translocations and molecular rearrangements influence the pathology and disease prognosis.

- t(14;18) involves an apoptotic inhibitor oncogene, *bcl-2*, leading to its overexpression, and is particularly associated with **follicular lymphoma**
- t(11;14) leads to overexpression of the cell cycle regulator, *bcl-1*, associated with **mantle cell lymphoma**
- t(8;14) leads to movement of the *c-myc* proto-oncogene and results in its deregulation, leading to cell proliferation, associated with **Burkitt** and **human immunodeficiency virus (HIV)-infection associated lymphomas**
- t(2;5) links two genes (*NPM*) and (*ALK1*) and produces a new protein which is found in associated **anaplastic large cell lymphomas**

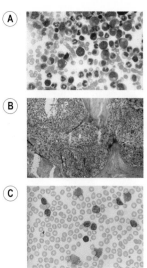

Fig. 12.26 Chronic leukaemia. (A) CML blood film: note the large numbers of granulocytic cells, in particular neutrophils, at all stages of development. (B) CML bone marrow trephine biopsy showing a packed marrow with granulocytic cells similar to those are found in the peripheral blood. (C) CLL blood film showing numerous mature-looking lymphocytes, with 'smear' cells.

- t(11;18) links an apoptosis inhibitor gene with the *MALTI* gene and produces a protein that is associated with **MALT lymphomas**.

Viral infection

Viral infection can lead to chronic antigenic stimulation and dysregulation of cytokines, resulting in B or T cell proliferation. Several viruses are implicated and their geographical locations may influence the prevalence of different disease expression:

- Epstein–Barr virus (EBV)
- Human T cell leukaemia virus type 1 (HTLV-1)
- Hepatitis C virus (HCV)
- Kaposi's sarcoma-associated herpes virus (KSHV).

Other implicated factors

- Environmental: chemicals (organic solvents, pesticides, hair dye, etc.) or radiation exposure
- Immunodeficiencies: congenital (severe combined immunodeficiency disease); acquired (acquired immune deficiency syndrome (AIDS)); induced (immunosuppressive therapy)
- Chronic inflammation of MALT tissues
- *Helicobacter pylori* infection.

Hodgkin disease

Hodgkin disease is less common and potentially curable. There are two incidence peaks: one in young adults, and the second in older individuals. The cause is unknown but **EBV infection** may have a role. The annual incidence is 2–3 per 100 000. **Reed–Sternberg cells** (Fig. 12.27) are characteristically seen when lymph nodes are biopsied. These cells are B lymphocytes that originate in the lymph node germinal centre but have lost the ability to produce antibodies.

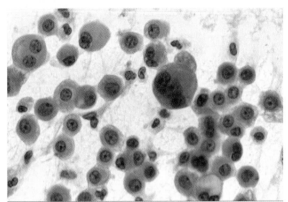

Fig. 12.27 **Reed–Sternberg cells in Hodgkin disease.** These cells appear as abnormal giant and often multinucleated cells.

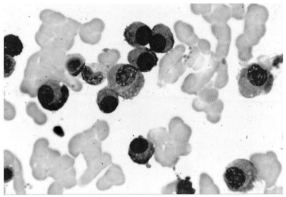

Fig. 12.28 **Plasma cells showing characteristic features:** an eccentric nucleus; very dark blue cytoplasm; a paler region close to the nucleus (perinuclear halo).

PLASMA CELL DISORDERS

Plasma cells are terminally differentiated B cells (cannot divide any further) whose main role is the production of antibody. Plasma cell diseases include:

- Monoclonal gammopathy of undetermined significance
- Multiple myeloma
- Plasmacytoma
- Plasma cell leukaemia.

Multiple myeloma

Myeloma has an incidence of 4 per 100 000 individuals, with 2500 new cases in the UK each year. The incidence increases with age and most patients are over 60 years of age; the disease is rare in individuals under the age of 40 years. For reasons not understood, myeloma is commoner in black Americans, although a role for susceptibility genes is suspected. Genetic associations and environmental chemical exposure have both been linked to development of the disease.

The malignant **plasma cells** accumulate in the bone marrow and suppress normal cell production. Most myelomas produce large quantities of **monoclonal immunoglobulin** (i.e. antibody molecules that are identical, as opposed to the normal polyclonal pattern seen in health).

Clinical feature of multiple myeloma

About 60% of patients have bone disease and bone pain is a common presenting factor. Bones are destroyed due to activation of osteoclasts by cytokines such as TNF-α and IL-1α, produced by the neoplastic cells. The osteoclasts also make and secrete IL-6, which is a growth factor for plasma cells.

Almost 30% of patients experience renal failure. Damage to the kidneys may be by direct injury to the tubules by proteins, amyloidosis (deposition of insoluble protein in the tissues) or plasmacytoma interference (soft tissue mass of plasma cells).

In addition, the patients also experience anaemia (multifactorial), infection (due to defective humoral and cellular immunity) and neurological problems (from hyperviscosity, producing headaches and hazy vision, or from spinal cord compression).

Table 12.18	Laboratory features of multiple myeloma	
Source	**Finding**	**Explanation**
Blood count	Reduced haemoglobin	Plasma cell proliferation interferes with normal cell production
Blood film	Plasma cells	Overproduction of malignant cells
Other	Very high erythrocyte sedimentation rate (ESR)	See Information box 12.8
Biochemistry	Abnormal urea and electrolytes	If renal impairment or renal failure is present
	Raised serum calcium	Excess calcium from bone destruction
	Monoclonal globulin in electrophoresis	Malignant plasma cells produce a single gamma globulin
	Bence Jones protein in urine	Free light chains from the excess abnormal globulin

Laboratory features of multiple myeloma

While patients might have experienced symptoms of anaemia and bone pain these may be have been dismissed as something common in the older patient, which is the key target group for this disease, and diagnosis could be delayed. A blood film may well, however, reveal the presence of characteristic plasma cells (Fig. 12.28). Table 12.18 lists other typical findings.

HAEMOSTASIS AND THROMBOSIS

NORMAL HAEMOSTATIC MECHANISMS

The haemostatic system is designed to ensure that there is no major leakage of blood following injury and consists of a complex system of proteins and enzymes. In health, any local bleeding is arrested by an interaction between platelets and blood vessel endothelial cells, followed by a cascade of coagulation factors. Any defect in these may result in bleeding or thrombosis.

This is a laboratory test undertaken by placing anticoagulated blood in a narrow vertical tube. Red cells fall through the plasma under gravity, dropping only a few millimetres in an hour under normal conditions (Fig. 12.29).

A non-specific test with high rates (high ESR) being associated with acute and chronic inflammation (including infections and cancer), autoimmune diseases and multiple myeloma (due to the changes in plasma proteins), anaemia (due to the reduction in red cell content), sickle cell disease (due to the shape of the red cells). It is particularly useful in the diagnosis of **temporal arteritis** (chronic inflammation of the large arteries of the head) and **polymyalgia rheumatica** (shoulder and pelvic joint stiffness).

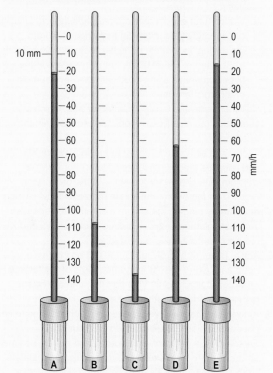

Fig. 12.29 Erythrocyte sedimentation rate (ESR): the rate at which red cells precipitate (in a Westergren tube) in mm/h. The rate increases in inflammatory diseases. Blood samples A and E show normal ESR, B, C and D show greatly increased ESR; each division is 10 mm.

The role of the endothelium and platelets in the maintenance of haemostasis

Endothelial cells line all blood vessels and these play a central role in preventing unwanted thrombosis. The endothelium provides an effective barrier between the thrombogenic subendothelial cells and the blood coagulation factors. Agents produced by endothelium include:

- **Thrombomodulin** – protein involved in thrombin control
- **Heparan sulphate** – a naturally occurring heparin that leads to inhibition of thrombin
- Enzymes that degrade platelet-derived molecules, such as ADP, the latter encouraging platelets to aggregate
- **Prostacyclin** and **nitric oxide (NO)**, which are potent inhibitors of platelet aggregation, discouraging platelets from sticking to the vessel wall.

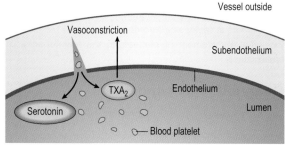

Fig. 12.30 Early involvement of platelets and blood vessel subendothelium. Platelets are attracted to subendothelial material when the endothelial layer is breached, plugging the gap and stimulated to release substances that enhance vasoconstriction in order to further reduce blood loss from the vessel. TXA$_2$, thromboxane A$_2$.

When tissue damage occurs, the subendothelium is exposed to blood cells, including platelets. Figure 12.30 illustrates the components involved.

1. Prostacyclin concentration is lower in the subendothelium than in the endothelium.
2. Lower levels of prostacyclin, along with collagen and other subendothelial molecules, attract platelets causing them to stick, producing a platelet plug.
3. **Thromboxane A$_2$** and **serotonin** are released from the activated platelets. These are vasoconstrictors, serving to reduce the vessel lumen and thus also blood flow and loss.

For minor breaches in vessel integrity these events may be sufficient for repair, but in severe breaches, or high flow, more is needed.

Platelets do not have a nucleus and so have limited ability to provide energy for their necessary functions. Glycogen stores and mitochondria within platelets provide energy through **microtubules** to change their shape, facilitating aggregation, and allowing release of substances from **dense** and **α granules** present within the platelet cytoplasm.

1. Platelets adhere to the connective tissue through a glycoprotein receptor (**GpIb-Ix**) in combination with von Willebrand factor (**vWF**), located in association with type VI collagen microfibils in the subendothelium
2. More platelets adhere to the site, binding to each other through the **GPIIa-IIIb** platelet receptor in combination with the plasma protein **fibrinogen**
3. Platelets are discouraged from extending along the vessel wall by the high concentration of **prostacyclin** in the intact endothelium
4. At this point, although platelets have changed shape and aggregated together, this action is reversible and platelets can return to normal and be released back into the circulation
5. Once granule release takes place the aggregation becomes irreversible.

Amongst other substances, **ADP**, **thrombin** and **thromboxane A$_2$** are released. These serve to recruit even more platelets to the site and thrombin acts to change fibrinogen into fibrin, thereby helping to stabilise the platelet plug. **Platelet factor 4** and the structurally related **β-thromboglobulin** promote clotting by neutralising heparin and heparin-like substances.

Platelet factors are also an integral part of the coagulation cascade that is subsequently stimulated by the release of tissue factor and thrombin. Figure 12.31 illustrates the initial involvement of platelets in the maintenance of haemostasis.

Coagulation cascade

This comprises two main components:

- **Coagulation** – production of the blood clot, in order to arrest bleeding
- **Fibrinolysis** – to dissolve the clot once it has served its purpose.

Most of the clotting factors are present in the circulation as inactive proteins called zymogens, probably a safety feature to prevent unwanted blood clotting. These inactive proteins require activation, usually by other clotting factors, to an active form in order to take part in a coagulation reaction.

Figure 12.32 shows the entire coagulation cascade, which comprises intrinsic and extrinsic pathways. Both of these terms are somewhat dated, and we no longer view the cascade in this manner. Nonetheless, it does help explain some of the tests used to detect coagulation cascade abnormalities.

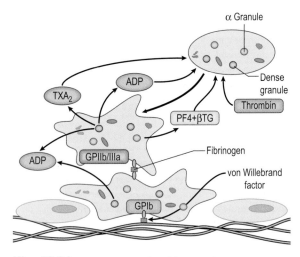

Fig. 12.31 **Platelet–vessel wall interactions.**

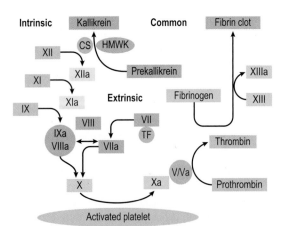

Fig. 12.32 **The coagulation cascade.** Clotting factors are indicated with roman numerals and their active forms by the 'a'. For example, VIII is inactive factor VIII, and VIIIa is the active form. TF, tissue factor; CS, contact surface; HMWK, high-molecular-weight kininogen.

The cascade is normally triggered by local damage, which brings coagulation factors into contact with negatively charged phospholipid surfaces and non-endothelial surfaces.

The intrinsic pathway

Prekallikrein, high-molecular-weight kininogen (HMWK), calcium ions, phospholipids from platelets and clotting factors XII, XI, IX, VIII and X are required for this pathway, which is initiated on exposure to a negatively charged non-endothelial surface, such as collagen, finally resulting in the production of factor Xa.

1. Contact phase components convert prekallikrein to kallikrein.
   a. The contact exposure is often a phospholipid (usually phosphatidylethanolamine) that originates from circulating lipoprotein particles such as chylomicrons, VLSLs and oxidised LDLs, found in excess in the hyperlipidaemia associated with the development of atherosclerosis.
2. Kallikrein activates factor XII to factor XIIa, which also stimulates more kallikrein production to maintain the cascade.
3. Factor XIIa activates factor XI to produce factor XIa and releases bradykinin (a vasodilator) from HMWK.
4. Calcium ions and factor XIa activate the proenzyme factor IX to factor IXa, the serine protease activity being released by binding of calcium to vitamin K-dependent γ-carboxyglutamate (gla) residues (factors II, VII and X are also gla-containing proenzymes).
5. Active factor IX hydrolyses factor X at an internal arg-ile bond and, along with other components of the **tenase complex** (calcium ions, VIIIa and IXa, and activated platelets) produces activated Xa.
6. Activated platelets have exposed phosphatidylserine and phosphatidylinositol residues on their surface.
7. Factor VIII is a cofactor, and is activated to VIIIa by small amounts of thrombin, released from activated platelets, although the high levels of thrombin produced in the clotting cascade cleave VIIIa, limiting the extent of the coagulation cascade.

The extrinsic pathway

The cascade is initiated by tissue factor (TF), also known as factor III, and also involves the serine protease factor VII present in plasma. TF is a protein present on subendothelial cells, such as smooth muscle cells.

1. Factor VII is activated by thrombin to factor VIIa, and also further activated by factor Xa from the intrinsic pathway
2. Factor VIIa and its cofactor, TF, is involved in the activation of factor X to Xa, in the same way as factor IXa.

The common pathway

The two pathways converge with the production of factor Xa. Production of a clot further involves factors II, I and XIII.

1. Factor Xa cleaves prothrombin (factor II) at two sites to form a two-chain active thrombin molecule (factor IIa), each chain being held by a single disulphide bond on the surface of activated platelets within a prothrombinase complex.
2. The prothrombinase complex is similar to the tenase complex and involves the phospholipids on activated platelets, calcium, prothrombin, factor Xa and factor Va as a cofactor.

3. Factor V is activated to factor Va by small amounts of thrombin, like factor VIII.

4. Thrombin reinforces the clotting cascade by further activating factor XI, VIII and V and also converts fibrinogen (factor I) to form the fibrin clot.

5. Fibrinogen is composed of three pairs of polypeptides, linked with disulphide bonds. The polypeptides have residues that have a high negative charge, making fibrinogen soluble in plasma. Activation with thrombin releases the polypeptides for monomers that spontaneously aggregate to form a weak fibrin mesh.

6. Thrombin also activates factor XIII to form factor XIIIa (transglutaminase) which cross-links the fibrin with covalent bonds between glutamine and lysine residues to consolidate the clot.

Natural anticoagulants are required to maintain the balance

In addition to the possession of a highly effective coagulation mechanism there needs to be an anticoagulant system in place to maintain the homeostatic balance. The body has several molecules that serve this purpose:

- **Thrombomodulin**, a glycoprotein present on endothelial cells that combines with thrombin
  - The thrombomodulin-thrombin compound activates **protein C** to protein Ca
  - Protein Ca and its cofactor, **protein S**, degrade factors Va and VIIIa
- **Antithrombin** combines with its substrates, which include factor Xa and thrombin, to limit action of the coagulation pathways
- **Heparin cofactor II** inhibits thrombin.

Both antithrombin and heparin cofactor II are stimulated by **heparin**, which is used clinically as an anticoagulant.

The fibrinolytic system

After a blood clot has served its purpose it requires breaking down in order to restore normal flow in the blood vessel. The fibrinolytic system is responsible for this activity and, much the same as the coagulation cascade, consists of a series of coordinated enzyme reactions.

The key player in the whole process is **plasmin**. The zymogen (inactive proenzyme) **plasminogen** must first be converted, through activators, to plasmin, whose main role is to break down fibrin molecules, in addition to coagulation factors V and VII. This leads to the release of **fibrin degradation products (FDPs)**.

The largest fragment produced by fibrin degradation is **fragment X**, generated by plasmin cleavage of the terminal α and β chains of the fibrin molecule. Fragment X is then cleaved by plasmin to form two fragments Y and DXD. Finally, through further enzyme cleavage, **D-dimers** are produced (D-D). D-dimers represent in vivo lysis of fibrin rather than fibrinogen. This is important clinically since laboratories used to measure FDPs for the diagnosis of disorders such as **disseminated intravascular coagulation (DIC)**, but FDPs cannot distinguish between fibrin and fibrinogen degradation. The newer D-dimer assay is now used as a measure of in vivo fibrinolysis since D-dimers represent only fibrin degradation.

Clinical consequences of fibrin degradation products

Apart from FDPs being used as indicators of continuing thrombosis/haemostasis, they have major functional consequences for haemostasis itself, contributing to the ongoing intravascular coagulation that is seen in **disseminated intravascular coagulation (DIC)**.

Fibrin breakdown products possess antithrombin activity, and they interfere with normal polymerisation of fibrin monomers. The larger of the fragments, X and Y, are the most inhibitory. These fragments also coat platelets and interfere with normal platelet function, thereby worsening the haemorrhagic tendency.

Plasminogen activators: tissue and urinary plasminogen activator

Tissue plasminogen activator (tPA) is a glycoprotein produced by endothelial cells. tPA is found in blood and most body fluids. The binding of tPA to fibrin leads to cleavage of plasminogen, producing plasmin. Excess tPA in the blood is rapidly cleared by the liver. Synthetic tPA is used therapeutically to treat patients who may be experiencing a heart attack (Clinical box 12.9).

Urinary plasminogen activator (uPA) is made by the renal tubules and collecting ducts. The molecule has many similarities to tPA but its primary role is not clear; it appears to be involved in cell signalling but may also be involved in the breakdown of fibrin clots deposited in the excretory ducts.

Clinical box 12.9   **Clot-busting drugs**

The understanding of the physiology of clot breakdown has led to the development of drugs serving the same purpose. These are useful where thrombosis has occurred within a vessel, causing life-threatening consequences. One example of this is in **myocardial infarction**. In this situation a thrombus occludes one or more of the coronary arteries, compromising blood flow to the heart muscle.

Streptokinase is an example of an agent that can be administered in the acute situation in order to break down the clot and restore blood flow.

- Streptokinase is isolated from β-haemolytic streptococci, and is a polypeptide that binds to plasminogen, which then undergoes a change in conformation.
- The active site of plasminogen is exposed and the molecule then resembles plasmin (although it is not plasmin, since no cleavage of plasminogen has occurred; however, functionally it acts as though it *is* plasmin).

Streptokinase is used therapeutically, but has several disadvantages:

- Its half-life is very short.
- The streptokinase-plasminogen complexes degrade fibrin *and* fibrinogen, which is undesirable (increases bleeding).
- Streptokinase is very antigenic and can cause severe allergic reactions. This occurs because streptokinase is derived from bacteria to which most individuals have been exposed.

Human tissue plasminogen activator (tPA) was shown to have advantages over streptokinase:

- Not antigenic
- 1% lower mortality at 12 months
- *But* – more patients were likely to have an early stroke after treatment with tPA, compared with streptokinase.

Fibrinolysis inhibitors

- Fibrinolysis inhibitors are required in vivo to prevent prolonged or unwanted degradation of fibrinogen. Several natural inhibitors have now been described, including **plasminogen activator inhibitor** 1 and 2 (PAI-1, PAI-2), α_2-antiplasmin, adhesion molecules and thrombin-activated fibrinolysis inhibitor.
- Free tPA and uPA are rapidly inhibited by PAI of which PAI-1 is the most important. PAI-1 is made by endothelial cells of blood vessels and is also found in platelet α granules. Increased levels of PAI-1 predispose individuals to thrombosis and are one cause of thrombophilia.
- Free circulating plasmin is inhibited by α_2-antiplasmin.
- Thrombin binds to and releases G protein protease activated receptors (PARs) that signal release of interleukins (IL-1 and IL-6) to increase the secretion of intercellular adhesion molecule-1 (ICAM-1) and vascular cell adhesion molecule-1 (VCAM-1) – increasing platelet activation and leucocyte adhesion.
- Thrombin activates **thrombin-activated fibrinolysis inhibitor** (**TAFI**), which impairs plasminogen activation, and therefore also fibrinolysis.

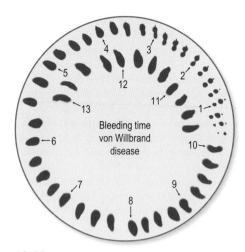

Fig. 12.33 **Bleeding time record in a patient with von Willebrand disease.** It took more than 13 minutes for this patient to stop bleeding.

Assessment of the coagulation system

Over the years a number of tests have been developed that help to determine which component of the haemostatic mechanism is functioning incorrectly.

Full blood count and film

A full blood count will detect any abnormalities in platelet number. A high platelet count will not necessarily mean that there is no danger from bleeding. A blood film is useful to confirm the automated platelet count and also allows the morphology of the platelets to be assessed – some inherited platelet disorders are associated with large platelets.

The bleeding time

This crude test is useful for assessing the in vivo function of the platelets, since platelets are responsible for providing the first line of defence in bleeding. By inflicting controlled depth incisions into the skin using a template bleeding time device, bleeding is induced (Fig. 12.33). Platelets plug up the defect in the blood vessels and the bleeding will stop, usually within 9 minutes. If platelet function is defective, or if the platelet number is low, bleeding will occur for much longer. Platelet function may also be abnormal due to inherited disorders or drug ingestion (e.g. aspirin). The bleeding time is prolonged in von Willebrand disease, not because the platelets are abnormal, rather their adhesion through an abnormal or absent vWF receptors is inhibited.

Coagulation tests

These are used to determine the function of the intrinsic and extrinsic components of the coagulation system. Blood is taken from the patient and placed into tubes containing sodium citrate. The normal functioning of the coagulation cascade requires calcium. Citrate binds calcium, and blood taken into citrate is therefore anticoagulated and will not form a clot until further calcium is added (Fig. 12.34).

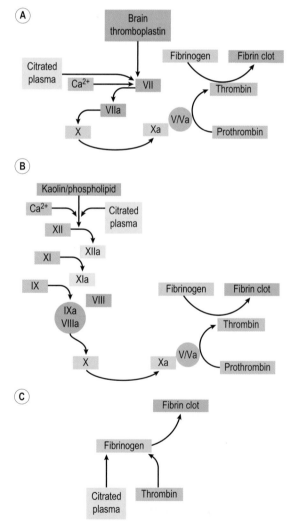

Fig. 12.34 **(A) Principle of the prothrombin time. (B) Principle of the activated partial thromboplastin time (APTT). (C) Principle of the thrombin time.**

The principal tests in current use are:

- **Prothrombin time (PT)** – used to assess the extrinsic pathway (Fig. 12.34A). Calcium is added to plasma to replace that removed by citrate anticoagulant and brain thromboplastin is added to substitute for tissue factor. Clotting normally takes 12–15 seconds and the test time is compared with a standard normal control in a ratio – the **international normalised ratio (INR)**. The test is used to assess liver function and monitor **warfarin** therapy.
- Factors II (prothrombin), VII, IX and X are all produced in the liver and so will be reduced in liver disease. Factor VII (in the extrinsic pathway) has the shortest half-life and the decrease more readily detected in the PT test.
- Warfarin as an anticoagulant:
  - Prothrombin and factors VII, IX and X are produced in the liver and require vitamin K for their production.
  - Warfarin competes with sites that bind vitamin K and thus interferes with the production of these clotting factors.
- **Activated partial thromboplastin time (APTT)** – used to assess the intrinsic pathway (Fig. 12.34B). Calcium is added to plasma to replace that removed by citrate anticoagulant, then kaolin and phospholipids are added to substitute for contact factor. Clotting normally takes 25–36 seconds. The test is used to check for most factor deficiencies and monitor **heparin** therapy.
- **Heparin as an anticoagulant**:
  - Heparin binds to, and activates, anti-thrombin III in plasma which inhibits the production of factor Xa and thrombin in the common pathway, reducing the ability to clot.
  - Heparin is not absorbed through the gut and so cannot be given parenterally.
  - Heparin has a short half-life (1 hour) and so must be given continuously or regularly.
- **Thrombin clotting time (TCT)** – used to assess the common pathway (Fig. 12.34C). Calcium is added to plasma to replace that removed by citrate anticoagulant, then thrombin is added to substitute for the products of the intrinsic and extrinsic pathways and to assess the conversion of fibrinogen to fibrin. The test is used to check for **disseminated intravascular coagulation (DIC)** but will also be prolonged in the presence of **heparin**.
- **Correction tests** – if the clotting time is prolonged. The patient's plasma is mixed 50:50 with normal plasma containing all clotting factors. If *correction* occurs, this implies that the patient's sample has a **factor deficiency**. If addition of normal plasma *fails to correct* the prolongation, this would tend to indicate that a **clotting factor inhibitor** is present. The inhibitor interferes with the normal clotting pathway.
- **Coagulation factor assays** to determine the actual deficiency.

COAGULATION FACTOR DISORDERS

Coagulation factor disorders may be inherited or acquired.

Inherited disorders

Inherited disorders include:

- Haemophilia A (factor VIII deficiency)
- Haemophilia B (factor IX deficiency)
- von Willebrand disease (vWD)
- Inherited platelet disorders.

Haemophilia A

Haemophilia A is an inherited X-linked disorder where mutations within the factor VIII gene lead to defective function of the factor VIII-C molecule in the coagulation cascade, although about a third of diagnoses are new mutations. A large number of different genetic mutations have been described in this gene which has 26 exons and 25 introns at 28q on the X chromosome, leading to different manifestations of what is, nevertheless, a significant bleeding diathesis. About 40% of diagnoses are due to a major inversion of part of the tip of the long arm of the X chromosome, one break point of which is situated within intron 22 of the gene.

As a key protein in the intrinsic pathway, deficiency of factor VIII leads to prolongation of the APTT coagulation screening test, whereas the PT test is normal. Haemophilia A affects 1 in 5000 males and the disease is classified according to the factor VIII level.

Males, who only have one X chromosome, are the main sufferers of this condition, with females generally only having one of their X chromosomes affected. Such females are referred to as **carriers**, and their male children will have a 50% chance of having haemophilia. Female children of the union of a male haemophiliac with a female carrier will also have a 50% chance of having haemophilia.

Haemophilia B (Christmas disease)

Haemophilia B is an inherited X-linked disorder, where mutations within the factor IX gene leads to defective function of the factor IX molecule in the coagulation cascade. Like haemophilia A, about a third are new mutations. While most mutations are point mutations, at various sites, a variety of other mutations have been described. The original factor IX deficient subject, Mr Christmas, was a severely deficient patient whose mutation was cys-206-ser.

Like haemophilia A, a deficiency in factor IX leads to an abnormal APTT with a normal PT. Haemophilia B, however, is not as common, affecting about 1 in 30 000 males. The pattern of disease in males, with female carriers, is identical to that in patients with haemophilia A. In 2009 this was discovered to be the cause of the blood disorder that affected many of the royal families in Europe.

Clinical and diagnostic features of haemophilia

Patients with very low factor levels, who experience repeated and painful bleeds into their joints and muscles, are given factor replacement. Originally the factors were produced from plasma pooled from a large number of individuals. This led to a large number of haemophiliac patients also being infected with HIV in the 1970s and 1980s. Since 1998, children have only received recombinant factors. Porcine factor replacement is also used.

Typically, in severe disease, factor levels are less than 1% of normal levels. The APTT screening test is prolonged, but the bleeding time is normal (because primary platelet plug formation is not affected).

Von Willebrand disease

Von Willebrand disease (vWD) is an autosomal dominant inherited disorder associated (although some forms are recessive) with a deficiency in circulating vWF. The *vWF* gene is found on chromosome 12 and a variety of quantitative and qualitative defects have been described that result in reduced expression of vWF. vWF is a large glycoprotein, released, in response to stimuli, from platelet storage granules and endothelial cells. vWF has two major roles:

- Mediating platelet adhesion to sites of vascular injury (see Fig. 12.31)
- Binding and stabilising factor VIII.

vWD is the most common inherited bleeding disorder. Clinically it affects about 125 per million people and leads to a mild bleeding disorder affecting males and females equally. Bleeding is typically seen in mucocutaneous tissues (skin and mucous membranes) because of the high capillary density; these tissues particularly depend on the efficient formation of platelet plug to stop bleeding.

Because of its links to factor VIII, low levels of vWF, like haemophilia A, also result in a prolonged APTT test and reduced factor VIII clotting activity. Unlike haemophilia A, patients have a prolonged bleeding time because of a failure in platelet–vessel wall interaction.

Inherited platelet disorders

The best known of these are:

- Glanzmann's thrombasthenia
  - Autosomal recessive inheritance
  - Abnormality in platelet GpIIb–IIIa interaction (see Fig. 12.31) preventing platelet aggregation.
- Bernard Soulier syndrome
  - Autosomal recessive inheritance
  - Reduced complex of GpIb, factor IX and factor V, which serves as a receptor for vWF, leading to lack of platelet plug formation (see Fig. 12.31).

Acquired disorders

A range of acquired platelet and clotting factor disorders have been described that are often associated with other diseases. For example, **acquired haemophilia** is the result of stimulation and production of an autoantibody that reduces factor VIII levels (factor VIII inhibitor).

THE THROMBOCYTOPENIAS

Thrombocytopenia, a reduction in platelet count, may be caused by:

- Impaired production
- Increased destruction
- Altered distribution.

Patients with thrombocytopenia are likely to have the following clinical features:

- Pin-point skin haemorrhagic spots (**petechiae**) that result from capillary bleeds (Fig. 12.35). These red spots do not 'blanch' when pressed.
- Bruising and mucous membrane bleeding resulting in **epistaxis** (blood from nose), **melaena** (blood in faeces) and **menorrhagia** (heavy periods).

Thrombocytopenia caused by impaired platelet production

This can be drug induced, or the result of a bone marrow failure. For example, cytotoxic drugs that are myelosuppressive

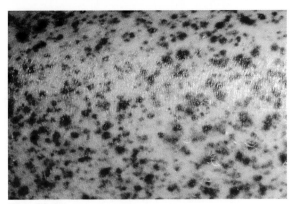

Fig. 12.35 Skin with petechial haemorrhages.

will inhibit megakaryocyte stem cells, and hence may cause thrombocytopenia.

Aplastic anaemia is an uncommon disorder with an incidence of 2–5 per million population per year. When the bone marrow is examined there are hardly any cells present and this is reflected in a lack of all the mature cells in the blood. The cells, when seen, appear morphologically normal. The lack of platelets in this condition results in problems with primary haemostasis.

Thrombocytopenia caused by increased platelet destruction

These may be immunological or non-immunological in origin.

Non-immune causes of thrombocytopenia
Disseminated intravascular coagulation
Disseminated intravascular coagulation (**DIC**) is characterised by excessive activation of the coagulation cascade and may be triggered by the release of tissue thromboplastins that contain a high concentration of phospholipids following trauma, surgery, mismatched blood transfusion and a variety of other triggers, such as premature separation of the placenta (**abruptio placenta**). Unrecognised and untreated DIC can lead to uncontrolled bleeding as all the clotting factors are used up, and may result in death.

Thrombocytopenia due to an altered distribution, or dilution
In health, the **spleen** may pool up to one-third of the total platelet mass, but in disease states this may rise to 90%. If the spleen is removed there is a large rise in the platelet count. Platelets can pool in the spleen in conditions such as liver cirrhosis and this leads to a relative thrombocytopenia.

Massive transfusion, when a patient's total blood volume is replaced over a short time period, may lead to thrombocytopenia. The degree is largely related to the amount of blood transfused, but the mechanism is *not* purely dilutional since there appears to be an element of platelet consumption as well.

Immune causes of thrombocytopenia
The more important immune-mediated causes of thrombocytopenia are:

- Neonatal alloimmune thrombocytopenia (NAIT)
- Post-transfusion purpura (PTP)
- Immune thrombocytopenic purpura (ITP)
- Drug-induced thrombocytopenia
- Heparin-induced thrombocytopenia (HIT).

Platelet antigens can be platelet specific, or shared with other cells. Important shared antigens include human leucocyte antigen (HLA) class I and ABH (blood group A and B) antigens. Platelet-specific antigens fall into five well-defined human platelet antigen (HPA) groups: HPA-1, HPA-2, HPA-3, HPA-4 and HPA-5, each of which has an 'a' and a 'b' allele. Because some platelet glycoproteins carry antigenic sites that play a major role in platelet function, platelet alloantibodies may not only cause thrombocytopenia but also affect primary haemostasis.

Immune thrombocytopenic purpura

In **immune thrombocytopenic purpura** (**ITP**), platelets are coated with anti-platelet autoantibodies and removed prematurely by the reticuloendothelial system, leading to a reduced peripheral blood platelet count. In some cases, self-reactive T cells may causes lysis of megakaryocytes with the bone marrow. It is thought to be due to an inappropriate response to an environmental trigger, such as infection or vaccination. The cause, however, is unknown and the clinical course is variable and unpredictable. ITP has an incidence of around 60 new cases per million population per year.

- Childhood ITP generally leads to an illness that is seasonal, typically follows a trivial viral infection or vaccination, and in most cases is transient, requiring no treatment. There is spontaneous recovery in 80% of cases.
- In most cases of adult ITP the platelet glycoprotein (Gp) antigen targets are GpIIb/IIIa and GpIb/IX.

Heparin-induced thrombocytopenia

Thrombocytopenia in patients treated with heparin is fairly common, but in most cases has no serious consequences. Heparin-induced thrombocytopenia (HIT) is caused by the production of antibodies against heparin–PF4 complexes. In some patients an immune response is induced, leading to platelet activation and thrombin generation, and rarely can result in large thromboses or massive bleeding due to the consumption of platelets and clotting factors.

THE THROMBOPHILIAS

Thrombophilias are conditions associated with excessive clotting. The coagulation system is a delicately balanced series of coagulation and fibrinolytic events and a defect or deficiency in one of the natural anticoagulants (e.g. **protein C or S**) will swing the balance towards thrombosis. There are two principal types of hypercoagulable state:

- Inherited – where the patient has a specific defect in one of the natural anticoagulant mechanisms
- Acquired thrombophilia – which represents a heterogeneous group of disorders associated with an increased risk of thromboembolism.

Thromboembolism is responsible for nearly 50% of all adult deaths in the UK and thrombophilia plays an important role. Inherited thrombophilias should be considered in all patients under 40–50 years of age who experience a venous thrombosis.

The inherited thrombophilias

Table 12.19 summarises the prevalence and incidence of thrombotic events among individuals with an inherited thrombophilia.

Table 12.19 Inherited thrombophilias

Inherited disorders	% in population	% with thrombosis
APCR: factor V Leiden mutation	3–8 of Caucasians	20–25
Prothrombin G20210A	2–3 of Caucasians	4–8
Antithrombin deficiency	1 in 2000–5000	1–1.8
Protein C deficiency	1 in 300	2.5–5.0
Protein S deficiency	Unknown	2.8–5.0
Hyperhomocysteinaemia	11	13.1–26.7

Protein C deficiency

Protein C is a vitamin K-dependent glycoprotein that acts as one of the major regulatory inhibitory proteins of the coagulation system. Protein C is activated to form activated protein C on endothelial surfaces by the **thrombin thrombomodulin complex**. Protein C acts as an anticoagulant by degrading activated factors V (Va) and VIII (VIIIa).

Protein C deficiency is inherited as an autosomal dominant disorder. Affected heterozygotes have protein C levels of around 50%. Some 75% of affected individuals have venous thromboembolism in young adulthood.

Protein S deficiency

Protein S was isolated and characterised in Seattle (hence protein S). It is a non-enzymatic cofactor of activated protein C. Like protein C, protein S is a vitamin K-dependent protein and is synthesised by the liver endothelial cells and it is also found in α granules of platelets. Inherited protein S deficiency is autosomal dominant.

Activated protein C resistance

Dahlback and others described APCR in 1993 as a mechanism for recurrent thrombosis. They described patients whose plasma exhibited a poor response to activated protein C in an APTT assay. A mutation in the factor V gene (**factor V Leiden**) was identified as the major cause. Factor V Leiden is a point mutation at the site at which activated protein C cleaves factor Va; this mutation makes the Va molecule biochemically resistant to inactivation by activated protein C.

Factor V Leiden deficiency has been demonstrated in more than 20% of thrombotic patients and has a prevalence of around 5% in the general population. APCR therefore may represent the commonest cause of inherited thrombophilia. Patients who co-inherit protein C deficiency are at an even greater risk of thrombosis.

The acquired thrombophilias

A large number of conditions are associated with thrombotic events, but the most important are shown in the following list, in order of the risk involved:

- Femoral and tibial fractures
- Hip, knee, gynaecological or prostate surgery
- Adenocarcinoma
- Chronically elevated factor VIII
- Oral contraceptives
- Pregnancy
- Hormone replacement
- Homocysteinaemia due to vitamin deficiency
- Anti-phospholipid syndrome.

Anti-phospholipid syndrome

Anti-phospholipid syndrome (**APS**) is the most common acquired thrombotic disease and is associated with antibodies in the form of **lupus anticoagulant** or **anti-cardiolipin antibody**. These antibodies are not thought to be directed at the phospholipids, but to proteins bound to the phospholipids, such as β_2-glycoprotein I.

The mechanisms producing the thrombotic events are not clear but bound β_2-glycoprotein I normally inhibits some activated clotting factors, inhibits activation of protein C and decreases serotonin release from platelets, decreasing platelet activation. Auto-antibodies directed against this protein may, therefore, induce a procoagulant effect.

Lupus anticoagulant

This is due to an antiphospholipid antibody (IgG or IgM or both) but is often recognised because it prolongs the phospholipid-dependent APTT clotting assay. Although seen in about 25% of patients with **SLE**, a generalised autoimmune condition, the term is a misnomer since it occurs frequently in patients with no evidence of SLE and is seen in association with other autoimmune disease, drugs, infections, malignancy and in many otherwise normal individuals.

Anti-cardiolipin antibody

Discovered in the 1980s, these antibodies to combinations of phospholipids and serum proteins, such as β_2-glycoprotein I or prothrombin, have been associated with thrombotic events of the APS.

BLOOD GROUPS AND TRANSFUSION MEDICINE

DEFINITION OF A BLOOD GROUP

In its widest sense this can just mean an observation of characteristics in blood that differ between individuals. When we refer to a **blood group**, it is usually used in a much more restricted sense.

Three characteristics define a blood group: a variation (or **polymorphism**) detected in the blood; the variation is seen in a protein, glycoprotein or glycolipid on a blood cell surface membrane (usually a red cell); the protein, glycoprotein or glycolipid are also antigens (can produce antibodies that bind to the antigen).

BLOOD GROUP ANTIGENS

Blood group antigens are generally found only on the red cell, but some are also found throughout the body. The antigens are usually made by the red cells but some are adsorbed on to the red cell from plasma.

Antigens are generally:

- Proteins, produced by blood group genes.
- Carbohydrates on glycoproteins or glycolipids. The blood group genes produce glycosyltransferase enzymes that produce the different antigenic variants.

It is not known why there are different blood groups, but those that have reached a significant frequency in the population have probably provided individuals with a selective advantage. Some blood groups are associated with resistance to parasitic infections (Duffy blood group). It has been suggested that the exploitation by microorganisms allowing them

to invade red cells occurs through receptors on glycoproteins and glycolipids. Polymorphisms may simply be chance mutations that have had a selective advantage because the parasite cannot interact with the altered receptor. The selective factors may no longer exist but the polymorphisms will remain until other selective factors interact with them.

ANTIBODY PRODUCTION

Antibodies are produced by B lymphocytes when an antigenic structure is recognised as foreign (i.e. non-self) by the immune system – for example by transfusion of blood cells with different red cell antigens on their surface. Usually macrophages, dendritic cells or other antigen-presenting cells 'process' the antigen, which generally involves digesting it into smaller subunits and presenting it to a T cell. The T cells, in turn, instruct the B cells to make antibodies against the antigenic substance.

BLOOD GROUP SYSTEMS IN TRANSFUSION MEDICINE

Knowledge of blood groups is of key importance in providing safe blood and blood products for transfusion, as well as minimising the risk of diseases such as haemolytic disease of the newborn. It is the interaction between an antigen and its antibody, and the effect of that interaction on the red cells that defines whether a blood group system is seen as being clinically important.

There are 30 different blood group systems, controlled by single, or related clusters of genes, and over 600 blood group antigens have been defined. The most important blood group systems in transfusion medicine are **ABO** and **Rhesus**, although others may also produce clinically important antibodies.

The ABO system

The genes for ABO are inherited in a Mendelian manner, giving rise to a variety of different types (**phenotypes**). Blood group 'O' is so called because it lacks both A and B (more like 'zero').

ABO antigens

The ABO system is sugar, rather than protein, based. **H substance** is the precursor of the A and B antigens and whether a person produces A or B antigens is dependent on which enzyme he or she inherits.

The *FUT 1* (*H/h*) and *FUT 2* (*Se/se*) genes on chromosome 19 give rise to the enzyme **H-fucosyltransferase** which leads to the production of the H antigen. Most people have the H antigen on their red cells.

People without H are rare and this is the result of various genetic changes in the FUT 1 gene. The earliest description was of a group of people without H from India – they were said to have the **'Bombay' type**. Other genetic changes that result in no H antigen (h) have been described since.

The FUT genes act in different tissues:

- FUT 1 is active in tissues of endodermal and mesodermal origin
- FUT 2 is active in tissues of ectodermal origin and produces the soluble H antigen found in secretions, such as urine and saliva, of those 80% of people who have inherited the Se form of the gene – referred to as being 'secretors'.

A and B genes are found on chromosome 9 and code for two different **glucosyltransferases**. The action of the enzymes produced by A and B genes on the H antigen (**H substance**) dictates which blood groups are produced:

■ If there is *no* active enzyme, the H antigen is modified and is described as the O allele (**blood group O**).
■ Action of **α1,3-*N*-acetyl-D-galactosaminyltransferase** on the H antigen modifies it to the A antigen, producing the A allele (**blood group A**).
■ Action of (**α1,3-*N*-D-galactosyltransferase** on the H antigen modifies it to the B antigen, producing the B allele (**blood group B**).
■ Inheritance of both enzymes from their parents will result in red cells that express both antigens (**blood group AB**).

ABO blood groups can be determined by mixing the red cells with serum containing antibodies to A and B. For example, anti-A antibody will agglutinate A cells, but not B cells or O cells. Figure 12.36 illustrates this.

The antigens we *detect* on the red cells determine the **phenotype** of the individual. Antigens A and B are each recognised by agglutination with the respective antibody, but the O antigen is defined by a lack of agglutination with anti-A and anti-B, and so is not detected in the presence of cells carrying the A or B antigens.

■ An individual who is blood group O must have inherited the 'O' allele from both parents, and will have an OO **genotype**.
■ An individual who is blood group A must have blood that agglutinates with anti-A, and therefore must have inherited the 'A' allele from one parent, but we are unable to tell from the agglutination test whether he will also have inherited an 'A' allele (genotype AA) or an 'O' allele (genotype AO) from the other parent. Table 12.20 illustrates the possible genotypes of people with each blood group.
■ As we inherit half our genes from one parent, and half from the other, sometimes our red cells have a different phenotype from our parents. For example, a father with genotype AO (phenotype A) and a mother with genotype BO (phenotype B) can produce children who are phenotype A (genotype AO), phenotype B (genotype BO), phenotype AB (genotype AB) or phenotype O (genotype OO).
■ Sometimes the genotypes that a person must have can be inferred from knowledge of the blood groups of their true parents. For example, a mother and father who are both blood group O (phenotype O, genotype OO) can only produce children with a phenotype O (genotype OO).
■ The frequency of different blood groups differs between populations.

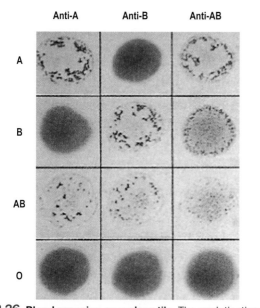
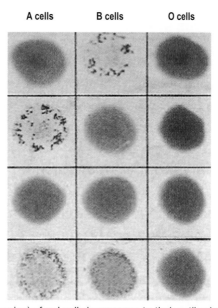

Fig. 12.36 **Blood grouping on a glass tile.** The agglutination (clumping) of red cells in response to their antibody is clearly shown on the tile and illustrates the potential seriousness of this reaction occurring within a person. In the left half is shown the interaction between red cells from a person of blood group A, B, AB and O (shown down the left side of the tile) and serum containing the anti-A, anti-B and anti-AB antibodies. In the right half is shown the interaction between serum or plasma from a person of the various blood groups, with group A, group B and group O red cells. (The terms 'serum' and 'plasma' are sometimes used interchangeably, but strictly 'serum' is used when blood is placed in a glass tube without anticoagulants and clots, the clotting factors within the plasma having been used up.)

Table 12.20	ABO blood group phenotypes, antigens, defining antibodies and blood group genotypes			
ABO blood group (phenotype)	Frequency in UK Caucasians (%)	Antigens on red cells	Agglutinated by	Genotypes
O	44	O	None	OO
A	45	A	Anti-A	AO or AA
B	8	B	Anti-B	BO or BB
AB	3	AB	Anti-A and anti-B	AB

- In comparison with the UK, blood group O is more common in America (particularly south and central), and in some parts of Africa.
- Blood group A is quite prevalent in Europe, particularly Scandinavia.
- Higher levels of blood group B are found in central Asia, and across Europe the frequency declines from east to west.
- Knowledge of these different distributions has implications for planning of blood stocks for transfusion in a multiracial community.

Changes in blood groups

Many rare variants of ABO groups have been described but do not change within an individual.

- Loss of A activity – apparent changes in ABO blood group are sometimes observed in patients with leukaemia, with patients who are group A losing ability to agglutinate with anti-A. Lower expression of the antigen is usually associated with a reduction in A- or B-glucosyltransferase.
- **Acquired B** – a weak B antigen develops on group A cells and is associated with digestive tract disease. The phenomenon is likely to be due to a bacterial deacetylation of *N*-acetylgalactosamine

The Rhesus system

The **Rhesus (Rh) blood group** system is more complex than ABO and is the second most important blood group system in terms of blood transfusion practice because of its high **immunogenicity** (the ability of an antigen to elicit an immune response). In all there are around 50 Rh antigens but only five are common, namely D, C, c, E and e. We use the term **Rh positive** for individuals who are Rhesus (D) positive, which is the case in 83% of Caucasians and higher for Africans and Asians, and **Rh negative** for those individuals who do not have the D antigen.

The Rh antigens function as transmembrane proteins with an apparent ion exchange function and they possibly also act as CO_2 transporters.

Inheritance of the Rh genes puzzled scientists for many years and it was originally proposed (the **Fisher–Race theory**) that there were possibly either three closely linked genes (C, D and E) or multiple alleles of a single gene (**Wiener's Rh-Hr theory**). In 1986 Tippett proposed a new model, and subsequent molecular analysis in the 1990s has shown this to be more accurate. There appear to be at least two Rh genes, **RHD** expressing D, and **RHCE** expressing C or c, and E or e, both found close to each other on chromosome 1.

Some eight different **haplotypes** have been defined consisting of a 'C or c', 'D or no-D' and 'E or e' components. (A haplotype is the configuration of the genes on one chromosome.) Note that the d antigen has not been found; we now know that 'd' represents deletion (not mutation) of D. Anti-d therefore cannot exist. Haplotypes are shown in the Table 12.21 in Fisher–Race and Wiener nomenclature, with their relative population frequencies. In the Fisher–Race system **D** is used for Rh positive and **d** for **no-D**, or Rh negative. In the Weiner system the presence of D is indicated by **R**, and no-D by **r**.

Examination of Rh-family genes has helped in the understanding of human evolution. Like humans, chimpanzees and gorillas have the two Rh genes, RHD and RHCE, whereas

Table 12.21	Rh haplotypes and relative population frequencies			
CDE (Fisher-Race)	**Rh-Hr (Wiener)**	**UK Caucasian**	**Black African**	**South-East Asian**
CDe	R¹	0.42	0.06	0.73
cDE	R²	0.14	0.12	0.19
CDE	Rᶻ	<0.01	<0.01	<0.01
cDe	R⁰	0.03	0.59	0.03
Cde	r'	0.01	0.03	0.02
cdE	r"	0.01	<0.01	<0.01
cde	R	0.39	0.20	0.02
CdE	rʸ	<0.01	<0.01	<0.01

other primates have only one, suggesting that the gene duplication happened in the common ancestor some 8–11 million years ago.

The human ancestral Rh haplotype is thought to be **cDe**, the other haplotypes developing from a point mutation, gene conversion or deletion, each followed by rarer recombination events, reflecting the rarer haplotypes. Note that this particular haplotype is very common in black African communities (about 60%) compared with less than about 3% in non-African populations – supporting the 'Out of Africa' origin of modern human populations.

The presence or absence of the D antigen, D+ or D–, is what is normally referred to as Rhesus positive or (Rh+) or Rhesus negative (Rh–). The frequency of D+ is close to 100% in the Far East, with about 95% of black Africans also being D+. The frequency is lowest among Europeans and in white North Americans is at a minimum of 82%. Recent research suggests that the D deletion in Rh– homozygotic or heterozygotic individuals offered a balanced selective advantage with improved neuropsychometric reaction times across much of Europe, whereas the presence of the D antigen is more protective in populations with latent toxoplasmosis. This parasitic cat infection, transmitted to humans through consumption of undercooked meat, was prevalent across Africa and Asia, but rare in Europe in prehistory, because of its low cat population, maintaining the advantage of D+ in the former continental masses.

Production of antibodies to blood group antigens

Antibodies can be 'natural', not needing exposure to non-self blood group molecules through transfusion or pregnancy, or 'immune' where such exposure is required. Both types of antibody are encountered in transfusion medicine.

ABO blood group system antibodies

Anti-A and anti-B antibodies are almost always present in the serum of people lacking these antigens, other than newborn infants. We know from animal work that bacterial proteins resembling A and B molecules present in food result in the production of anti-A and anti-B. Chickens, which normally develop anti-B within a few months after hatching, fail to produce anti-B if kept in a sterile environment. Because these antibodies arise naturally they are called 'naturally occurring' antibodies. The antibody molecules are IgM in contrast with 'immune' antibodies, which are usually IgG. IgM antibodies are large and cannot cross into the foetal circulation.

These ABO antibodies are generally detected from around 3 months of age and appear to be the result of immunisation by epitopes (antigen components) of bacterial, viral or plant origin, which are similar to A and B glycoprotein antigens present in the environment. People of blood group O don't actually have *both* antibodies: it is thought likely that people of blood group O develop an antibody (anti-A, B) that recognises a structure common to both A and B antigens. Table 12.22 lists these naturally occurring antibodies.

Rh blood group antibodies

In contrast with the ABO blood group system, immune reactions, produced as a result of exposure to a foreign antigen through blood transfusion or pregnancy, may lead to the production of **immune IgG antibodies**. Antibodies produced against Rh system antigens are an important example of IgG antibody development. IgG antibodies react best in the warm.

Rh(D) is the most important of the Rh antigens since it is extremely immunogenic, probably because it is more different in its amino acid makeup in comparison. This means that very few Rh(D) positive cells are required to induce anti-D formation if given to an Rh(D) negative individual. Development of antibodies can result in serious reactions to blood transfusion and anti-D is the principal cause of **haemolytic disease of the newborn (HDN)** (Clinical box 12.10).

Other blood group systems

There are too many to discuss in detail but a few will be mentioned that are particularly important in transfusion and neonatal medicine:

- Kell
- Duffy
- I/i
- HPA (a non-red cell system).

Kell

Like Rhesus, **Kell** is highly immunogenic. **Anti-K** is generally caused through blood transfusion and may also arise in pregnancy. Anti-K is common because the K gene is only present in about 9% of Caucasians, and is even rarer in the black and East Asian populations. Its production may result in subsequent transfusion reactions.

A woman who is herself Kell negative, carrying a foetus which is Kell positive, may develop IgG anti-K antibodies. IgG is the only immunoglobulin that can cross the placenta and anti-K may lead to haemolytic disease of the newborn, much as in Rh incompatibility. All women of child-bearing age are now given Kell negative blood in order to reduce the incidence of Kell associated HDN.

Table 12.22	Antibodies found in people of different ABO blood groups	
ABO group		**Antibodies in serum**
O		Anti-A, B
A		Anti-B
B		Anti-A
AB		None

Clinical box 12.10   **Haemolytic disease of the newborn**

HDN describes a situation in which there is incompatibility between the mother and the foetus, and leads to a destruction of the newborn infant's red cells. Several blood group antigens are implicated in severe HDN: in North America and Europe the disease is most commonly due to Rh(D), but in South America, Africa and Asia, ABO incompatibility is an important cause.

Any person who is Rh(D) negative and exposed to Rh(D) positive red cells, for example, will most likely make anti-D. Such exposure may occur through:

- Transfusion
- Pregnancy (by leakage from the foetal circulation)
- During birth delivery
- Amniocentesis and other obstetric investigations
- Termination of pregnancy.

In HDN, the exposed mother's immune system will generate IgG antibodies against the D antigen that they do not possess. Since IgG can cross the placenta, the mother's IgG anti-D will attack foetal Rh(D) positive red cells, causing haemolysis within the foetus.

With severe haemolysis there can be:

- Significant anaemia
- Significant rise in foetal bilirubin levels – the baby appears jaundiced
- Irreversible brain damage (**kernicterus**) due to unconjugated bilirubin being deposited in the basal ganglia
- Massive oedema (**hydrops foetalis**) due to abnormal transport of water
- Perinatal death.

Of women who develop this antibody, about 20% lose their infants in their first affected pregnancy and this rate increases further in subsequent pregnancies. For this reason, exposure to Rh(D) positive blood through blood transfusion in women who may become pregnant is avoided wherever possible.

Rhesus HDN is not common today, however, due to the introduction in 1967 of **anti-D prophylaxis** programmes (Fig. 12.37):

- Pregnant women are checked during pregnancy for the presence of anti-D (and other antibodies) and, if detected, are measured serially in order to check whether the antibody levels are rising.
- To prevent Rhesus HDN, pregnant women who are Rh(D) negative are now given anti-D injections during pregnancy at 28 and 34 weeks, to mop up any foetal cells that might enter the circulation. This prevents the immune system from forming antibodies and thus protects the foetus.
- Rh(D) negative women who subsequently deliver a Rh(D) positive child are given a further injection within 72 hours of the birth.

This programme has been very successful: before its introduction there were around 1.6 perinatal deaths per 1000 births; this had dropped to around 1 death per 10 000 births by 1986.

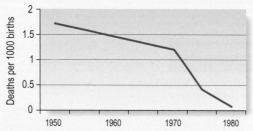

***Fig. 12.37* Fall in perinatal death rate following introduction of anti-D prophylaxis.** Perinatal death rates fell between 1950 and 1970 because of better medical care, but the introduction of the policy for anti-D immunoglobulin prophylaxis (100 μg) within 72 hours of birth led to a dramatic fall in the death rate.

Duffy

There are two main antigens in the **Duffy (Fy)** system, namely **Fya** and **Fyb**.

Individuals may have either Fy(a+b−) or Fy(a−b+), or both, Fy(a+b+). A GATA-1 transcription factor binding site upstream of the Duffy gene has produced a mutation that prevents expression of the Duffy glycoprotein on red cells. This mutation, **Fy(a−b−)**, is extremely common in the black population due to natural selection because of **malaria** exposure. Individuals with this phenotype are refractory to the malarial parasite *Plasmodium falciparum*, and resistant to *Plasmodium vivax* infection, which requires an interaction between the parasite and the Duffy glycoprotein to invade red cells.

Antibodies to the Fy antigens may arise through transfusion or pregnancy. They can lead to:

- Delayed transfusion reactions, i.e. haemolysis occurring several days after an incompatible red cell transfusion
- HDN.

I/i

These are interesting since different antigens are present at different stages of development.

- **i** is found on cord blood (taken from the placental cord at birth) or the red cells of neonates (I is absent)
- Adult red cells have mainly **I** with little i.

Antibodies against I are naturally occurring IgM antibodies that react best in the cold. IgM anti-I may be found in diseases such as **cold haemagglutinin disease** characterised by cold-induced haemolysis. Pneumonia caused by *Mycoplasma pneumoniae* may give rise to antibodies with anti-I specificity.

Platelet antigens

Blood cells such as platelets and neutrophils have antigens specific for these cell types. Platelet antigens include **human platelet antigen** (HPA)-1, HPA-2, HPA-3, HPA-4 and HPA-5; in addition, each can have an a or b allele. These are relevant to disorders such as **neonatal alloimmune thrombocytopenic purpura** (**NAITP**; see Clinical box 12.11).

BLOOD TRANSFUSION

Whereas blood transfusion is normally considered to be a transfusion of red cells, and originally that meant whole anticoagulated blood, today donated blood is processed to produce the separate different components that might be required for medical or surgical purposes, e.g. red cells, white cells, platelets, fresh frozen plasma, heat-treated plasma, and other more specialised fractionations of whole blood.

Blood has never been an unlimited resource and blood transfusion can no longer be considered as a safe process. The aims of good transfusion medicine should always be to limit unnecessary exposure to blood products and there is good evidence to show that much of the blood transfusion that has been considered normal in the past – for example to raise the haemoglobin to normal in a patient who is anaemic after a surgical operation, in order to increase the oxygen carrying capacity of the blood – is ineffective in the latter terms and therefore unnecessary and risky to the patient. Recommended transfusion triggers are haemoglobin levels less than 7 g/dL and never greater than 9 g/dL in critically ill patients. Blood transfusion is not an appropriate treatment for iron deficiency anaemia.

Guidelines for safe transfusion

Sometimes blood transfusion is indicated, and great care must be employed to reduce the associated risk, not only in *what* is transfused, but *how* the process of blood provision is managed in order to ensure that the blood is of the highest quality (Clinical box 12.12).

Management of the blood transfusion process

A survey of UK blood transfusion in 1993 identified an incidence of blood being transfused to the wrong patient for 1 in 30 000 units of blood. Over 18 months there were 111 incidences of **incompatible transfusion** and 12 of these patients died as a result. The deaths were as a result of errors in:

- Collection or labelling of the sample for blood grouping
- Laboratory error
- Failure of final pre-transfusion checks.

In the UK these incidences are monitored by the Serious Hazards of Transfusion (SHOT) initiative. Between 1996 and 2011 almost 10 000 transfusion related events have been recorded, with more than 50% of these being preventable and relate mainly to wrong patient identification, although there is a key role in education, competency and knowledge and clinical/laboratory handover. Although the risk of death

---

Clinical box 12.11 | **Neonatal alloimmune thrombocytopenic purpura**

In **NAITP**, the mother and foetus are incompatible in terms of their platelet antigens.

- The mother lacks the platelet antigen present in the foetus and makes an IgG antibody against it
- The IgG crosses the placenta and destroys the foetal platelets causing marked thrombocytopenias
- The foetus may bleed in utero (e.g. intracerebral), but more commonly the disorder is diagnosed after birth
- The antigen most commonly implicated is **HPA-1a**
- NAITP affects 1 in 2000 live births and makes up 20% of neonatal thrombocytopenias.

Clinical box 12.12 | **Avoiding transmission of variant Creutzfeldt–Jakob disease (vCJD) through blood transfusion**

In the UK, the blood transfusion service has introduced a number of measures in order to protect individuals from possible transmission of vCJD. These include:

- Withdrawal and recall of any blood components, plasma derivatives or tissues obtained from any individual who later develops vCJD (December 1997)
- Import of plasma from the US for fractionation to manufacture plasma derivatives (October 1999)
- Leucodepletion (removal of white cells) of all blood components (Autumn 1999)
- Importation of clinical fresh frozen plasma from the US for patients born on or after 1 January 1996 (introduced in Spring 2004)
- Deferral of donors who have received a blood transfusion in the UK since 1980 (announced March 2004, implemented April 2004).

and major morbidity from transfusion is very low in the UK in 2012, the majority remain and should be preventable.

Transfusion reactions

Transfusion reactions may be:

- **Haemolytic** – due to an antigen–antibody reaction as a result of an incompatible transfusion, resulting in severe or fatal intravascular haemolysis.
- **Non-haemolytic** – due to damaged blood products that release high levels of cytokines, leading to fever and rigor. Usually benign.
- **Allergic** reactions (IgE mediated) – leading to rashes and itching. Benign.
- **Anaphylactic** reactions (IgA mediated) in certain patients. Potentially, but rarely, fatal.
- Transfusion of antileucocyte antibodies – leading to **transfusion-related acute lung injury (TRALI)**. Can be fatal.
- Due to **volume overload** – leading to acute pulmonary oedema. Outcome depends on the other conditions.
- Transfer of **bacteria** – leading to endotoxaemia (as a result of free bacterial toxins) and septicaemia. Potentially fatal.

Although acute transfusion reactions relating to anaphylaxis, bacterial infections and pulmonary complications are currently the most common cause of transfusion-related morbidity, **haemolytic transfusion reactions** are the most preventable. The transfusion of an antigen into someone who does not possess that antigen results in the recognition of that antigen, either by production of an antibody against it, or by reaction between an already pre-existing antibody (ABO antibodies, or immune antibodies stimulated as part of a previous antigen exposure). The consequences of the antigen–antibody reaction will depend on the particular immunogenic response, but some responses are extreme and will be determined as the result of an **incompatible transfusion**. These incompatibilities can result in shock, kidney failure and death.

The most severe reactions are caused by IgM antibodies, such as seen in **ABO incompatibility**, particularly when group A or group AB blood cell antigens are transfused into group O recipients. For example:

- If blood of group A is transfused to a group O person then the anti-A in the group O plasma will react with the transfused A cells – an antigen–antibody reaction.
- The antigen–antibody reaction also activates **complement**, which rapidly ruptures the incompatible cells (**haemolysis**), resulting in haemoglobin being released into the plasma (**haemoglobinaemia**).
- Ruptured cell membrane debris activates the coagulation pathway within blood vessels (**disseminated intravascular coagulation – DIC**).
- DIC can lead to **renal failure** and **death**.

Group O blood, if transfused into a group A, B or AB patient, does not normally produce a reaction because the blood is transfused as red cells, without the plasma that would normally contain the anti-A and anti-B found in group O plasma, and the recipient antibodies do not react against the O antigen. Hence group O blood has been referred to as being **universal donor** blood. In contrast, plasma from a group O individual, for example given as a fresh frozen plasma (FFP) preparation to provide clotting factors, *will* contain the anti-A and anti-B antibodies, and should not be given

to a group A or B individual. Use of the 'universal donor' term (and **universal recipient** for someone of blood group AB, who can theoretically receive red cells from any ABO group donor) is discouraged as this only really applies to red cells and hence transfusion practice now recommends the use of ABO identical components.

IgG antibody–antigen reactions that might be seen in incompatible blood group Rh, Kell, Duffy, Kidd and Ss (MNSs blood group) transfusions, in particular, where the relevant antibody has previously been stimulated, produce a milder, but still clinically significant reaction.

Misinterpretation of the cause of anti-D antibodies found in pregnant women and subsequent inappropriate surveillance is a further significant cause of transfusion related mortality and morbidity.

Tests used in transfusion medicine

Blood grouping

For transfusion purposes we are normally only concerned with:

- **ABO blood group** – because of the danger of incompatibility to the patient
- **Rh(D) blood group** – particularly in women because of the danger of subsequent HDN.

Other blood groups may become important to consider if a person develops an antibody to a particular antigen, since it is then important not to expose someone to that antigen again to avoid transfusion reactions.

Before automation, blood grouping was carried out using glass tiles and polyclonal antisera derived from human blood (see Fig. 12.36). A whole panel of antisera was required, each one recognising different blood group antigens. This type of grouping technique was carried out by placing drops of red cells of unknown group (e.g. the patient) onto the tile, after which one drop of antiserum was added. The red cells and antiserum were mixed on the tile and agglutination (clumping of red cells) noted. Agglutination occurs when there is a positive reaction.

Nowadays automated blood grouping machines are available that can perform blood group typing on large numbers of samples efficiently and safely. The results are read by computer (Fig. 12.38) and stored within blood group databases. Accuracy is provided through rigorous operating procedures and use of bar codes for computerised verification. Transfusion of group-compatible blood should never proceed until the ABO group has been confirmed.

The antibody screen

Antibody screening exposes the patient's plasma to pools of red cells which contain *all* the common blood group antigens in all the important blood group systems. Use of cells from blood group O ensures that the naturally occurring ABO antibodies are not picked up. Thus agglutination will indicate the *presence of an immune antibody*. Once the particular antibody has been defined using a series of different antigen pools, compatible blood, without the antigen, can be provided. If the patient is pregnant, or has had a transfusion within the previous 3 months, plasma for screening must be taken within 3 days of the intended transfusion event, in order to detect recent antibody production.

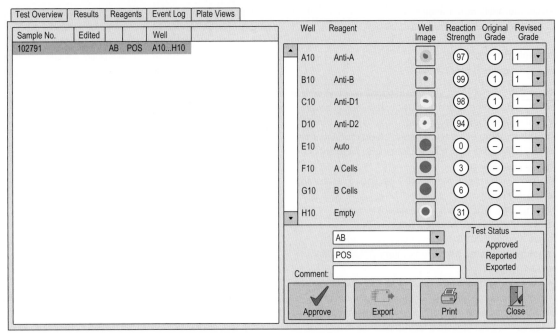

Fig. 12.38 Automated blood group typing. A computer generated output from an automated blood grouping instrument of a patient who is blood group AB Rh(D) positive, showing images of the reaction and the automated interpretation of the results.

While antibodies, such as those IgM antibodies found in the ABO blood group system can easily be detected by simple mixing of serum and red cells at room temperature, another strategy has been developed to detect the smaller IgG antibodies, such as those seen after immunisation in the Rhesus system. This is known as the **antiglobulin test**.

The antiglobulin test

This test was devised by Coombs in 1945 and until recently was known as the **Coombs test** but has now been renamed the **antiglobulin test** (Fig. 12.39). Coombs recognised that red cells can be coated with antibody but fail to show agglutination in the test tube (in vitro). The reason for this is because the antibody molecules are too small to link the red cells and cause agglutination. This occurs mainly with IgG molecules.

Coombs' strategy was to generate another antibody (an anti-IgG antibody) that would bind to any human antibody already present on the red cells, bound to its respective antigen, and agglutinate these. This test is called the **direct antiglobulin test** (**DAT**) since it detects antibody *bound* to the surface of the red cells. The **indirect antiglobulin test** (**IAT**) detects the presence of antibody in the patient's serum (i.e. free unbound antibody) in a two-stage test. In other words it detects immune antibodies in the patient that have been stimulated by exposure to a foreign antigen. This is the basis of the **antibody screen**.

The cross-match (compatibility test)

The **cross-match** is designed to ensure that any blood transfused into a recipient is compatible with the recipient and will not cause a transfusion reaction. Transfusion reactions occur when there is a blood group antibody in the recipient's serum which reacts with the transfused red cells. In order to detect this, red cells from the donated blood (intended for transfusion) are mixed with some of the recipient's serum.

- Agglutination indicates a positive reaction
- No agglutination indicates a negative reaction.

Only when there is a negative reaction between the two can the blood be issued and transfused into the recipient. Because ABO antibodies are potentially always present it is usually *only ABO compatibility* that is being tested. Only where the antibody screen indicates that immune antibodies are present do we need to cross-match donor cells with recipient plasma for other blood group antigens. Antibodies that will usually result in clinically important transfusion reactions include those from the Rh, Kell, Duffy, Kidd and Ss (MNSs) blood groups.

While cross-matching implies the physical mixing of the patient's serum and the red cells to be transfused, in the UK an 'electronic' cross-match is often performed. Provided the antibody screen is negative at the time then the patient can simply be transfused with ABO compatible red cells – and generally, for the good reasons referred to above, Rh(D) compatible cells as well. Electronic cross-matching can only be used where the systems of information technology and labelling are safe and robust.

NON-RED-CELL TRANSFUSION

A variety of other components of blood are used for administration to patients in certain circumstances.

Platelet transfusion

Platelet transfusion is indicated to prevent or treat haemorrhage that may be the result of thrombocytopenia or platelet function defects. Platelets are expected to be at a very low level ($<10 \times 10^9$/L) before platelet transfusion is needed. Prophylactic transfusion may also be recommended at such low levels in conjunction with bone marrow failure, to provide surgical cover, or to treat medical emergencies, such as DIC or immune thrombocytopenias.

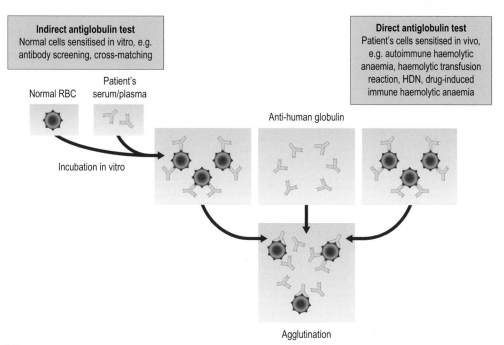

Fig. 12.39 **Principles of the antiglobulin test.** HDN, haemolytic disease of the newborn.

White cell transfusion

Transfusion of white cells in the form of **bone marrow** or **stem cells** is undertaken for bone marrow transplant to treat conditions such as leukaemia. White cell engraftment occurs after bone marrow ablation, where a patient's marrow is destroyed (along with its cancer cells) and replaced with that from a compatible donor.

Frozen plasma and plasma concentrate transfusion

Fresh frozen plasma (**FFP**) and concentrates such as **cryoprecipitate** may be transfused. Indications for **FFP** administration include **DIC**, if there is active bleeding. It is never indicated to reverse **warfarin anticoagulant therapy**, unless bleeding is very severe. A **pathogen-reduced plasma** (**PRP**), sourced from counties with a low incidence of bovine spongiform encephalopathy (BSE), is recommended for all children born after 1995. **Octoplas** is a new therapeutic preparation of FFP, processed to inactivate any viruses that might be present and is given to reduce the incidence of TRALI.

Cryoprecipitate is the cryoglobulin fraction of fresh frozen plasma and is particularly rich in FVIII, vWF, FX111, fibronectin and fibrinogen. It is usually used in conditions where fibrinogen levels are low (**hypofibrinogenaemia**).

13

The respiratory system

Gavin Donaldson

Introduction	613
Epidemiology of respiratory disease and its social impact	614
Smoke and respiratory disease	614
Classification of common respiratory diseases	614
Obstructive pulmonary disease	615
Restrictive pulmonary disease	615
Anatomy of the respiratory system	615
Anatomy of the upper airways	616
Gross anatomy of the lungs	617
Anatomy of the pulmonary circulation	623
Surface anatomy of the respiratory system	626
Mechanics of breathing	627
The diaphragm and other muscles used in breathing	627
Pulmonary pressure changes during ventilation	628
Pulmonary ventilation	629
Work of breathing	631
Principles of gas exchange	636
Diffusion	636
Partial pressures of gases in air	637
Partial pressures of gases in alveoli and blood	637
Carriage of oxygen by the blood	637
Respiratory pigments	638
Carriage of carbon dioxide by the blood	639
Carbon dioxide dissociation curve	639
Disturbances of acid–base balance	639
Matching lung ventilation to lung perfusion	640
Ventilation–perfusion ratio	641
Control of breathing	642
The respiratory centre	642
Respiratory receptors	642
Higher centre control of breathing	645
Energy production and oxygen consumption	645
Respiratory quotient as an indication of metabolic fuel	645
Methods for estimating energy consumption	645
Challenges to normal respiration	646
Exercise	646
Altitude	646
Breath-holding	647
Diving	647
Diver's reflex	648
Drowning	648
High oxygen levels	648
Carbon monoxide poisoning	648
Respiratory failure	648
Causes of respiratory failure	648
Lung defences against infection	650
The upper airways	650
Conducting airways	650
Innate immunity	650
Inflammatory responses	651
Development of the lungs and changes in the newborn	651
Early lung development	651
Stages in lung maturation	651
Respiratory system changes at normal delivery	653
Respiratory distress syndrome of the newborn	653

INTRODUCTION

The primary function of the respiratory system is to move air into the lungs to supply oxygen for the metabolic processes of the body whilst removing sufficient carbon dioxide to maintain the acid–base balance of the blood. Breathing involves actively drawing air in (inspiration) through the nose, mouth and trachea into the lungs, and expulsion of air (expiration). In the lungs, oxygen and carbon dioxide move across the barrier between air and blood, made up of lung tissue (alveolar wall) and capillaries, by simple diffusion. The rate of diffusion depends on the lung surface area, wall thicknesses and partial pressure difference (i.e. concentration gradient of oxygen and carbon dioxide). This process is called gaseous exchange. In general, respiratory diseases interfere with the efficient operation of this process.

The lungs also carry out other functions apart from gaseous exchange:

- Expulsion of air from the lungs to produce sound and speech (phonation)
- Conversion of angiotensin I to angiotensin II in the regulation of blood pressure and volume
- Local production of surfactant (a phospholipid) to lower surface tension in the alveolar cells
- Act as a reservoir of blood
- Filtration of small blood clots from the blood to prevent them entering the systemic circulation
- Synthesis of arachidonic acid metabolites, the eicosanoids that play an important part in the body's defence mechanisms in inflammation and homeostasis
- Inactivation of norepinephrine (noradrenaline), bradykinin, 5-hydroxytryptamine (5-HT) to prevent constriction of the airways
- Secretion of immunoglobulin (mainly IgA) into bronchial mucus in response to allergic challenges

- Maintenance of acid–base balance – by excretion of carbon dioxide
- Phagocytosis of unwanted viruses and bacteria.

EPIDEMIOLOGY OF RESPIRATORY DISEASE AND ITS SOCIAL IMPACT

Respiratory disease is an important cause of mortality and morbidity at all ages. In 1999, chronic obstructive pulmonary disease (COPD) was the fifth leading cause of death globally (4.8% of total deaths), and acute lower respiratory infections were the second most common cause of death in Africa (10.3% of total). Worldwide, the prevalence of chronic obstructive lung diseases is projected to be the fourth leading cause of death by 2030. Tuberculosis is also increasing in incidence and prevalence, particularly related to the compromised immune systems in individuals with human immunodeficiency virus/acquired immune deficiency syndrome.

In the UK, asthma is a common chronic disease in children, but mortality from asthma is confined to the elderly with only a small proportion occurring in children (3 per million aged 0–14 years and 158 per million in those aged 75+). In adults, chronic obstructive lung diseases are important causes of sickness absence from work, reduced quality of life, disability and hospital admissions (Table 13.1).

Acute upper respiratory tract infections (common colds) occur frequently, with two to four episodes per year in adults and six to eight episodes per year in children. These infections result in absenteeism from school and work, and are costly in terms of the purchase of 'over-the-counter drugs'. The inflammatory processes and symptomatic deterioration triggered by upper respiratory tract infections account for a substantial number of hospital admissions and mortality at all ages.

SMOKE AND RESPIRATORY DISEASE

Much of adult respiratory disease is tobacco related (Fig. 13.1) in the developed world. Cigarette consumption became well established during the First World War, but did not become popular among women until the Second World War. The Tobacco Advisory Council in the UK estimated that, in 1948, 65% of men and 41% of women smoked manufactured cigarettes, and that, by 1996, these figures had fallen

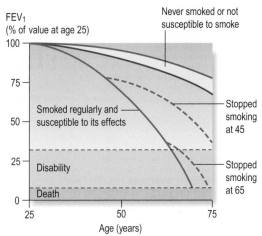

Fig. 13.1 Influence of smoking on airflow limitation. FEV_1, the forced expiratory volume in 1 second, is a sensitive indicator of lung function and reductions in FEV_1 can indicate respiratory disease.

Clinical box 13.1	Chronic obstructive pulmonary disease

COPD is a chronic respiratory disease which has the symptoms of:
- Productive cough
- Wheeze
- Shortness of breath, especially on exertion.

The airways become obstructed with forced expiratory volume in 1 second (FEV_1) <70% of predicted and FEV_1/forced vital capacity (FVC) ratio <0.7. This obstruction is not relieved by bronchodilators.

COPD gets progressively worse and usually occurs in smokers, although a few cases (5%) occur in non-smokers. While most patients with COPD are smokers and severity is related to the number of cigarettes smoked, the susceptibility of individual smokers varies widely. About 50% of smokers do not develop any significant deficit and only 15% will get clinically significant COPD.

---

to 29% and 28%, respectively. This decrease has been in all age groups except those aged 20–24, where there has been a steady increase since 1988. However, as a consequence of people smoking in the 1940 and 1950s, deaths attributed to COPD, which is overwhelmingly caused by smoking, are currently rising to such an extent that this disease has recently risen to being the fourth leading cause of mortality worldwide.

In the developing world, smoke from biomass fuels used in cooking has been associated with the development of COPD. In a rural districts of China with 88% of households using biomass fuel compared to 1% in an urban district, the prevalence of COPD was 12% compared to 7% in the whole population, and 7% compared to 3% in non-smoking women respectively (Clinical box 13.1).

CLASSIFICATION OF COMMON RESPIRATORY DISEASES

The classification of respiratory diseases is difficult as patients may have one or a combination of diseases or conditions. A useful way of thinking about respiratory diseases is to consider them to be of two main types: obstructive and

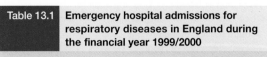

Table 13.1	Emergency hospital admissions for respiratory diseases in England during the financial year 1999/2000
	No. of admissions
Chronic obstructive pulmonary disease, excluding asthma, in patients aged 65 years and over	75 600
Asthma in children	28 500
Lower respiratory infections, pneumonia and acute bronchitis	97 000
Pneumonia in patients aged 65 years and over	47 200
Acute bronchitis in children	21 800
Total	182 800

Chronic lung diseases
- **COPD**: a chronic, slowly progressive disease characterised by a fixed airflow obstruction that cannot be reversed by bronchodilator therapy. Commonly associated with smoking.
- **Asthma**: a pulmonary disease characterised by reversible airway obstruction, airway inflammation, and bronchospasm to a variety of stimuli.
- **Emphysema**: destruction of the alveolar walls leading to enlarged air spaces.
- **Atelectasis**: collapsed areas of lung with reduced or no gas exchange.
- **Bronchiectasis**: irreversible dilation of the bronchial walls caused by destruction of the muscle and elastic tissue. The bronchi are dilated, inflamed and easily collapsed resulting in airflow obstruction
- **Pulmonary fibrosis**: development of excess fibrous connective tissue (fibrosis) in the lungs (idiopathic, occupational, etc.).

Acute lung diseases
- **Acute bronchitis**: acute inflammation of the trachea and bronchi. Characterised by sputum (phlegm) production.
- **Pleurisy**: inflammation of the pleura.
- **Pneumonia**: acute inflammation of lung substance, usually bacterial.
- **Pneumothorax**: free air between the visceral and parietal pleurae.
- **Pulmonary embolism**: obstruction of blood flow in a section of the lung which prevents perfusion and gas exchange.
- **Adult respiratory distress syndrome** (**ARDS**): an inflammatory response which causes non-cardiogenic pulmonary oedema leading to hypoxaemia and respiratory failure.

restrictive. Also both types can be chronic or acute in onset (Information box 13.1).

- **Obstructive pulmonary disease**, where the overall volume of the lungs available for gas exchange is unchanged, but there is *obstruction* to the flow of gases along the airways.
- **Restrictive pulmonary disease** is less common than obstructive disease. The available lung volume for gaseous exchange is reduced, or *restricted*, but there is no obstruction to airflow.

OBSTRUCTIVE PULMONARY DISEASE

Obstructive pulmonary disease is due to narrowing of the airways that conduct air into and out of the lungs. This may be caused by:

- Inflammation of the lining of the airways, particularly of the smaller airways, when the lining swells and causes blockage
- Mucus plugs obstructing the lumen of the airways, which occurs in acute or chronic infections when there is excessive mucus secretion
- Constriction of the smooth muscles in the walls of the airways, causing airway narrowing. The commonest example is asthma
- Loss of tissue surrounding the airways that provides a supporting structure to keep the airways open. The loss of tissue allows the airway to collapse (particularly on expiration).

Common examples of obstructive pulmonary disease are asthma, COPD, chronic bronchitis and emphysema (Clinical box 13.2).

- **Emphysema**: is due to the breakdown of the alveolar membranes giving rise to large spaces called emphysematous bullae, common in chronic obstructive pulmonary disease (COPD).
- **Bronchiectasis**: results from inflammatory destruction of bronchi leading to irreversible bronchial dilation. Clinically characterised by a chronic cough with production of large amounts of purulent sputum. Common in COPD and emphysema.
- **Occupational lung diseases**: may develop as the result of prolonged exposure to dust particles and fumes at work. Coal miners' pneumoconiosis, asbestosis and silicosis are probably the best known.

RESTRICTIVE PULMONARY DISEASE

Restrictive pulmonary diseases are due to reduced total lung capacity (TLC), but airflow and airway resistance are normal. Restriction may be caused by:

- Intrinsic lung disease, when lung tissue (parenchyma) is destroyed, which reduces lung volume. Chronic inflammation with scarring and fibrosis (interstitial fibrosis) destroys air spaces, thereby reducing lung volume. In acute situations (infection or toxic inhalation), the air spaces become filled with inflammatory exudates and debris.
- Extrinsic disorders of the muscles of respiration, the chest walls, connective tissue, pleura or the nerve supply that impair movement during inspiration. The inability of the chest to expand for whatever reason mechanically restricts ventilation.

Examples of restrictive pulmonary disease are kyphoscoliosis (a spinal defect), pneumothorax (puncture and collapse of the lung), pulmonary embolism (blockage of the blood supply), adult respiratory distress syndrome (due to inhalation of fumes) and idiopathic pulmonary fibrosis (believed to be caused by endogenous or environmental stimulation of alveolar epithelial cells and aberrant epithelial cell repair and associated with various genetic factors, such as a mutant telomerase) (Clinical box 13.3).

Pulmonary fibrosis is characterised by the development of stiff lungs caused by the thickening of the alveolar walls with the proliferation of fibroblasts and the laying down of abnormal levels of collagen. Severe fibrosis could result in ipsilateral deviation of the trachea (and mediastinum).

It is caused by many different factors among which are dust and/or gas inhalation, infection, drug side effects and sarcoidosis. Two occupational causes are inhalation of coal dust or asbestos fibres.

ANATOMY OF THE RESPIRATORY SYSTEM

The respiratory system consists of the **upper respiratory tract** (Fig. 13.2), which is concerned mainly with **conduction** of gases from the atmosphere to and from the lungs, and the **lower respiratory tract**, which is partly

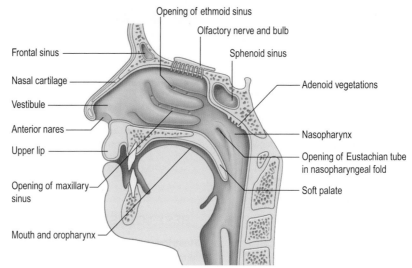

Opening of ethmoid sinus

Olfactory nerve and bulb

Sphenoid sinus

Frontal sinus

Nasal cartilage

Vestibule

Anterior nares

Upper lip

Opening of maxillary sinus

Mouth and oropharynx

Adenoid vegetations

Nasopharynx

Opening of Eustachian tube in nasopharyngeal fold

Soft palate

Fig. 13.2 **Upper respiratory tract.**

concerned with conduction and mainly with **gaseous exchange**. The upper airway or the upper respiratory tract is made up of the:

- Nasal cavity
- Pharynx
- Larynx.

The lower respiratory tract consists of:

- Conducting airways
- Respiratory airways.

The **conducting airways** are made up of the trachea, main bronchi and those bronchioles which make up branches 1–16 of the **tracheobronchial tree** (see below and Fig. 13.5). They are lined with specialised ciliated pseudostratified columnar (or columnar) epithelial cells, macrophages, goblet cells, Clara cells and glands, with cartilage and smooth muscle in the walls. This part of the respiratory tract is not concerned with gaseous exchange (non-respiratory). These air passages have the function of:

- Protecting the lower airways by removing dust particles, atmospheric pollutants and other debris from the airways
- Humidifying and warming inspired air.

The **respiratory airways**, where gaseous exchange takes place, consist of the smaller bronchioles which are branches 16–23 of the tracheobronchial tree and the alveoli.
The alveoli:

- Are where the alveolar walls form the thinnest possible barrier between the air and the blood
- Consist of type I (squamous epithelium) and type II (cuboidal) alveolar cells (also called pneumocytes)
- Contain macrophages, lymphocytes and granulocytes.

Gaseous exchange of oxygen and carbon dioxide takes place at the interface between the alveoli and the pulmonary circulation (see Fig. 13.7). This interface is known as the **alveolar–capillary barrier**. The **pulmonary circulation** and the **pulmonary lymphatics** provide the blood supply and fluid drainage of the lungs, respectively. The alveoli have a very extensive blood supply and extracellular fluid is drained from the alveoli by the lymphatics.

ANATOMY OF THE UPPER AIRWAYS
(Clinical box 13.4 **and** Information box 13.2**)**

Nasal cavity

Air is drawn into the lungs via the **nasal cavity** (Fig. 13.2) and passes highly vascular nasal mucous membranes, which, with the exception of the nasal entrance, are covered by ciliated columnar epithelium. These nasal membranes moisten the entering air, remove large particles of dust and can warm it sufficiently to raise the temperature of the inspired air from 6°C to 30°C. Inhaled air is then fully humidified and warmed to body temperature (37°C) as it travels through the trachea. Expired air is always below body temperature because it

---

Clinical box 13.4   **Relieving airway obstruction**

If a person chokes and an obstruction lodges in the trachea, the victim will become greatly distressed, be unable to speak and rapidly become cyanosed. Mouth-to-mouth resuscitation is of no use. An attempt should be made using the Heimlich manoeuvre to dislodge the object. Stand behind the victim, encircle the lower abdomen below the ribcage with your arms, and give a short forced squeeze forcing the diaphragm into the thorax. If you are on your own, with no time to get help, try slumping forward over the edge of a chair back so that the abdomen is forced upwards.

   Laryngotomy is a procedure performed when the airway is blocked above the vocal cords (foreign body, swelling or tumour). A stoma (orifice) is made in the midline, in the cricothyroid membrane below the thyroid prominence.

Information box 13.2   **Common respiratory reflexes**

- **Gasping**: application of cold water to the skin during a cold shower will cause gasping followed by hyperventilation.
- **Sneezing**: this is the sudden expiratory blast through the nose produced by irritation of the nasal mucosa and stimulation of the nasal branches of the maxillary nerve, which is the second division of the trigeminal nerve (cranial nerve V). Droplets may spread to 5 m, making this a significant mode of spread for many respiratory infections.
- **Hiccups**: this term refers to the repetitive spasmodic contraction of the diaphragm and external intercostal muscles during which the glottis closes suddenly and further entrance of air into the chest is prevented, thus producing the characteristic sound and sensation.

gives up heat when it leaves the nasal passages. This **counter-current exchange system** prevents excessive heat loss from the body core.

Pharynx

The **pharynx** is divided by the soft palate into an upper **naso-pharyngeal** and a lower **oropharyngeal** region. The area contains lymphoid structures such as the **adenoids** and **tonsils**. The airway can be opened during anaesthesia or emergency resuscitation by tilting the head backwards at the atlanto-occipital joint (between C1 and skull). The airway can also be opened by protruding the jaw to lift the tongue forward. A partial blockage of the airways by the tongue, uvula or soft palate during sleep leads to turbulence in airflow which is heard as snoring.

Larynx

The **larynx** (Fig. 13.3) consists of a number of articulated cartilages, vocal cords, muscles and ligaments, which keep the airway open during breathing and closed during swallowing. It can remain closed and withstand the highest pressures generated by the thorax (90 cmH$_2$O) prior to sudden release during **coughing**. It is innervated by the laryngeal nerve.

Trachea

The **trachea** begins at the lower border of the cricoid cartilage of the larynx, at the level of the sixth cervical vertebra. It has a mean diameter of 1.8 cm and a length of 11 cm. It is supported by C-shaped cartilaginous rings to prevent kinking during head and neck movement. It can, however, be compressed by moderate external pressure of between 50 cmH$_2$O and 70 cmH$_2$O or by internal pressure from a haematoma (blood collection) following surgery or accident.

GROSS ANATOMY OF THE LUNGS

The two lungs (Fig. 13.4) are divided into lobes:

- The **right lung** is divided into three lobes: upper, middle and lower
- The **left lung** has only two lobes: upper and lower.

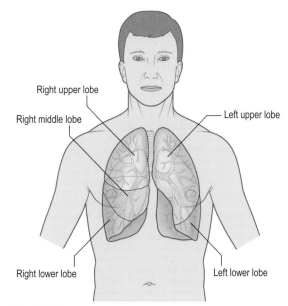

Right upper lobe
Right middle lobe
Left upper lobe
Right lower lobe
Left lower lobe

Fig. 13.4 **Gross structure of the lungs,** showing the lobes and fissures.

Invaginations of the **pleurae** (see below) separate the lobes of the lungs. The upper and lower lobes are separated by an **oblique fissure**, the right middle lobe being further demarcated by the **horizontal fissure**. Each lobe is further divided into **bronchopulmonary segments**, which in turn are divided into pyramidal lobules with their apices towards the **bronchiole** (see below) that supplies them. Divisions of the bronchioles eventually end in the blind, balloon-like **alveoli**. The bronchopulmonary segments are separated by fibrous septa, which are extensions of the pleura.

The tracheobronchial tree

The trachea divides into two bronchi. The right **bronchus** is wider than the left and makes a smaller angle with the trachea. The right bronchus is therefore more likely to receive

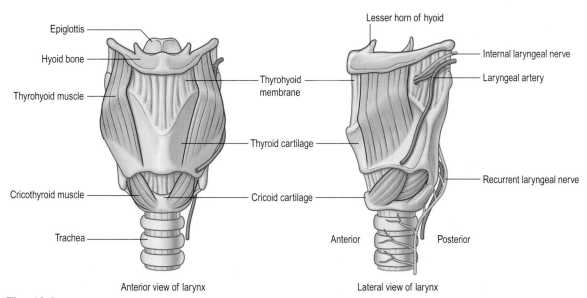

Epiglottis
Hyoid bone
Thyrohyoid muscle
Cricothyroid muscle
Trachea
Thyrohyoid membrane
Thyroid cartilage
Cricoid cartilage

Anterior view of larynx

Lesser horn of hyoid
Internal laryngeal nerve
Laryngeal artery
Recurrent laryngeal nerve
Anterior   Posterior

Lateral view of larynx

Fig. 13.3 **Views of the larynx.**

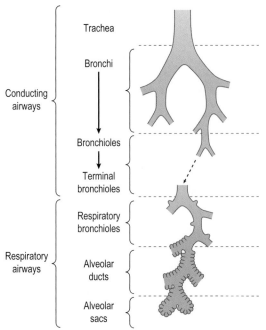

Fig. 13.5 **The tracheobronchial tree.** There are about 23 orders of branching from the trachea to the alveoli. Only the smallest respiratory bronchioles and the alveoli are involved in gas exchange.

inhaled foreign bodies. After the trachea has divided into two main bronchi, it continues to subdivide (Fig. 13.5) into four lobar bronchi, 16 segmental bronchi, and thereafter into small bronchi, **terminal bronchioles**, **respiratory bronchioles** and **alveolar ducts**. Eventually, 23 generations of division result in about 8 million **alveolar sacs**. These sacs form the last generation of blind air passages and, from each, about 17 **alveoli** arise. These alveoli account for about half of the 250–300 million alveoli, the others arising directly from the alveolar ducts. They have a total surface area of about 75 m² (adult male).

The trachea, bronchi and bronchioles are tubular structures that are designed for conducting air. Their walls consist of an outer fibrous layer with supporting pieces of **cartilage**, and **bronchial smooth muscle**. The bronchial smooth muscle is arranged in clockwise and anticlockwise helical bands and there is a matrix of elastic tissue supporting the muscles. The lumen of the airways decreases in size with progressive numbers of divisions in the tracheobronchial tree:

- As the airways get smaller, the supporting cartilage, which maintains the rigidity of the walls so that the larger airways remain patent during expiration, gradually disappears so that the proportion of muscle increases.
- The walls of the bronchioles consist of smooth muscle, collagen and reticular fibres for support. There is *no* cartilage in bronchiolar walls. Bronchial smooth muscle occupies as much as 20% of the walls of the smallest bronchioles.
- With further divisions, the bronchiolar muscle layer becomes progressively thinner.
- The airways are lined with **epithelium** containing ciliated and goblet cells (see below), with a **submucosa** containing mucus-secreting cells. These cells function to ensure that inhaled air is adequately humidified and irritants or foreign bodies are trapped in the mucus and then removed from the airways.

- The lining of the tracheobronchial tree also contain **endocrine cells** – the Kulchitzky or APUD (amine precursor uptake and decarboxylation) cells containing 5-HT. These cells are capable of secreting hormones that have an effect on smooth muscle.
- As the bronchioles become smaller, the epithelium becomes progressively thinner until it is only one cell thick, containing mostly ciliated cells, very few goblet cells and non-ciliated Clara cells (see below).

From the trachea, as far down as the smallest bronchioles, the functions of the air passages are solely conduction and humidification, but beyond this point there is a gradual transition to the function of gas exchange and so the covering of smooth muscle stops.

Breath sounds

Breath sounds are caused by movement of air through the trachea, bronchi and alveoli. They can be heard using the diaphragm of a stethoscope (use a bell in patients with lots of hair on their chest) and can be used to diagnose a number of respiratory conditions. Normal breath sounds are:

- Vesicular, i.e. inspiratory breath sounds are longer than expiratory sounds (which are very brief) with no distinct gap between the end of inspiration and the beginning of expiration
- Loudest over the upper lobes anteriorly.

Breath sounds may be loud in a thin healthy subject, or soft in patients with emphysema, or have a prolonged expiratory phase when the airways are narrowed, as in asthma. Pulmonary disease will often result in abnormal breath sounds (Information box 13.3).

Information box 13.3 **Abnormal breath sounds**

- **Bronchial breathing**: inspiration and expiration are of equal length, with a short gap in between. These sounds mimic the sound heard over the trachea or between the scapulae at the level of the fourth thoracic vertebra where the trachea bifurcates. Bronchial breathing is heard over areas of consolidation (pneumonia), collapse, bronchiectasis or fibrosis because of narrowing of the airways.
- **Reduced or absent breath sounds**: when there is severe narrowing of the airway (severe asthma), extensive lung damage (e.g. emphysema) over a pleural effusion, a pneumothorax or when there is no air going in to that part of the lung because of an obstruction such as a neoplasm.
- **Expiratory wheezes**: heard in airways obstruction, e.g. asthma and chronic bronchitis/chronic obstructive pulmonary disease (COPD). The wheezes may vary in tone and sound: high pitched when there is narrowing of numerous small airways, or harsh and monophonic in obstruction of a single large airway, e.g. bronchial cancer. Wheezes are not always heard in airways obstruction, e.g. in asthma when the airflow is very restricted.
- **Crackles**: brief crackling sounds, fine or coarse, which may be caused by the opening of previously closed airways. Early inspiratory crackles are heard when there is diffuse airflow limitation, as in COPD, and late inspiratory crackles occur in pulmonary oedema, fibrosis and bronchiectasis.
- **Pleural rub**: heard as a creaking or rubbing, and sometimes palpable, occurs with inflammation, often accompanied by pain.
- **Stridor** is an inspiratory wheeze which is audible without a stethoscope. It is louder over the larynx and indicates an upper airway obstruction. This may indicate a life-threatening condition, especially in children, where the epiglottis can compromise the airway.

Vocal resonance

The sound of spoken words (e.g. 99) is heard as an indistinct resonance. Intensity reflects the conductivity of the lung substance; for example, when there is consolidation of the lungs with pneumonia the sounds are heard much more clearly.

Specialised tracheobronchial cells

The tracheobronchial tree is lined by cells that have a protective function. Their defensive actions remove dust and other noxious particles, and destroy invading bacteria.

Cilia and macrophages

From the nose to the bronchioles, the respiratory tract is lined by ciliated columnar epithelium cells. Where these border the tract, they each have several hundred cilia 1–5 µm long and 0.3 µm wide. The cilia beat synchronously about 20 times per minute with a rapid forward movement followed by a slower return movement. They sweep particles and mucus towards the main bronchi and trachea, which are finally expelled from the airway by coughing.

The lower respiratory tract also contains macrophages. Smaller particles (<10 µm diameter) which may reach the alveoli are phagocytosed by macrophages and eventually eliminated via the trachea (by coughing) and the gastrointestinal tract (i.e. swallowed). Alveolar macrophages vary from 15 µm to 30 µm in diameter and there are an estimated 16 macrophages per alveolus in the human lungs. Macrophages also immobilise and destroy bacteria. In some disease (e.g. COPD) defects in phagocytosis may be associated with bacterial colonisation of the lungs.

Goblet cells and the mucociliary escalator

Goblet cells are found predominately in the epithelium from the nose to the bronchi. They are columnar, tapering towards the base. Their function is the secretion of mucus, a sticky, gelatinous substance composed of glycosylated proteins. Mucus is relatively impermeable to water, forming a layer, like a gelatinous 'blanket', around the cilia of the epithelial cells. Under normal circumstances, the tips of the cilia extend into the mucus layer. Movement of the cilia then sweeps the mucus upwards. This process is called the mucociliary 'escalator' (Fig. 13.6). Along with the cilia, mucus is part of airways defence. Inhaled particles, macrophages, cell debris and bacteria are trapped in the sticky mucus to be swept away on the **mucociliary escalator**. The mucociliary escalator can

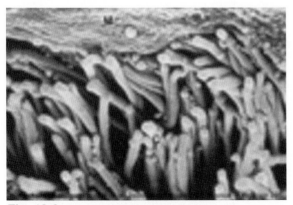

***Fig. 13.6* The mucociliary escalator.** Scanning electron micrograph of the respiratory epithelium showing large numbers of cilia overlaid by a mucus 'raft'.

be slowed by anaesthetics, airborne pollution, bacterial or viral infection or tobacco smoke.

Cilia may be slowed by genetic diseases that predispose to ciliary dyskinesia ('immotile cilia' syndrome due to a wide variety of autosomal recessive defects in the large number of cilia associated proteins); these diseases invariably result in chronic infections of the nose, sinuses and lower airways. Increase in mucus viscosity, for example by diseases such as cystic fibrosis, will also result in more frequent and often chronic infection of the airway (Clinical box 13.5).

Clara cells

Clara cells are found mainly in the distal conducting airways, the terminal bronchioles and alveolar ducts. They are nonciliated cells with a broad heterogeneity in their morphology. They have short microvilli, they possess large quantities of smooth endoplasmic reticulum and have a protruding apical cap that contains dense granules. These granules contain Clara cell secretory protein (CCSP) and a solution similar to lung surfactant. Their main functions are protective:

- Detoxification of inhaled noxious pollutants through secretion of cytochrome P450, for example (**xenobiotic metabolism**)
- Assist in the mucociliary clearance of environmental particles
- Control of inflammatory processes
- Provide a lung epithelial cell reparative reservoir through proliferation and differentiation to maintain the ciliated cell population.

There is evidence to suggest that the number of Clara cells are decreased after prolonged tobacco smoke inhalation. Clara cells are particularly vulnerable because of their high abundance in the air passages and through their xenobiotic function are particular susceptible to cytotoxic agents, such as naphthalene, which is a major component of tobacco smoke.

The alveoli

Alveoli are minute balloon-like structures at the end of the terminal bronchioles and alveolar ducts (Fig. 13.7A). Extremely thin layers of tissue, known as alveolar septa, form the walls between neighbouring alveoli. Each alveolus contains an

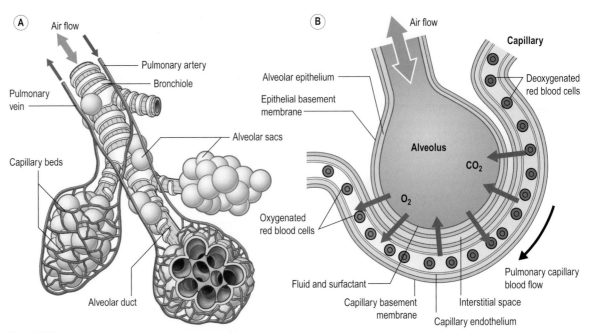

Fig. 13.7 **(A) Lung alveolar tissue and (B) its blood supply.**

alveolar space. Clusters of alveoli open into spaces, alveolar sacs, giving the appearance of tiny bunches of grapes. A few alveoli open directly into terminal bronchioles. The walls of some alveoli have holes, the pores of Kohn, which allow communication between adjoining alveoli or alveolar sacs.

The alveoli are the principle sites for **gaseous exchange**, where inspired gases enter the blood in the pulmonary circulation from the alveolar space and expired gases leave the pulmonary circulation to enter the alveolar space. The gap between the alveolar space and the pulmonary circulation, known as the **gas–blood barrier** (or the **alveolar–capillary barrier**), has to be extremely thin to allow rapid gaseous exchange.

The alveoli are regular polyhedrons between $70\,\mu m$ and $300\,\mu m$ in diameter. They are smaller in the more dependent

(lower) parts of the lungs than in the less dependent (upper) parts. At maximal inflation, as when taking the deepest possible breath in, these lower alveoli become larger so that the vertical gradient in size disappears.

Table 13.2 summarises the histological components of lung tissue.

The gas–blood barrier

The thinnest possible membrane between the alveolar spaces and pulmonary capillaries, the **gas–blood barrier**, facilitates rapid and efficient **gaseous exchange** (Fig. 13.7B). Gases such as oxygen have to diffuse across the gas–blood barrier to reach the blood. Carbon dioxide travels in the opposite direction.

Table 13.2	**Histological composition of respiratory tissue**							
Zone	Conducting 150 mL					Respiratory 2.0–3.0 litres (300 million alveoli)		
Generation	0–1	2–3	4–15		16	17–19	20–22	23
	Trachea and primary bronchi	Lobar and segmental bronchi	Small bronchi	Bronchioles	Terminal bronchioles	Respiratory bronchioles	Alveolar ducts	Alveolar sacs
Cartilage	Present	Present	Some present (patchy)	Absent	Absent	Absent	Absent	Absent
Smooth muscle	Present (bridging cartilage)	Present (helical plates aid active reduction of length and calibre)		Present (highest proportion relative to lumen diameter)		Present	Scattered delicate	
Goblet cells	Present (largest number at points of branching)		Scattered	Absent	Absent	Absent	Absent	Absent
Mucous and serous glands	Present	Abundant	Scattered	Few or absent	Absent	Absent	Absent	Absent
Ciliated cells	Present (fewer at points of branching)	Present	Present	Present → Few present (decreasing progressively)		Absent	Absent	Absent
Air flow	←←← Bulk flow →→------→-----→--→---→--→---→----→--------→					←←← Diffusion →------→------→------→		
Blood supply	Bronchial and pulmonary circulation					Pulmonary circulation (1000 capillaries per alveolus)		

The gas–blood barrier is only 0.5 μm wide, and consists of:

- Alveolar epithelium (type I and type II alveolar cells – see below)
- Fused membrane of the alveolar epithelial cells and capillary endothelium
- Vascular epithelium of the pulmonary capillaries (the capillary endothelial cells).

Once in the blood, gases still need to pass through the plasma, red blood cell wall and cytoplasm to reach the haemoglobin.

The total surface area of the gas–blood barrier is estimated to be 70–100 m² in the adult man. Gaseous exchange takes place by diffusion, when there is a gradient in pressures across the gas–blood barrier.

Cell types at the alveolar level

Gaseous exchange takes place at the alveoli, where oxygen is taken into the bloodstream, and carbon dioxide is off-loaded into the alveolar gases.

Capillary endothelial cells

Very thin-walled alveolar capillaries, lined with **capillary endothelial cells**, form a dense network in the alveolar walls. This gives a large surface area that facilitates rapid gaseous exchange between the pulmonary circulation and the alveoli. Each capillary endothelial cell has a thickness of only 0.1 μm except in its nuclear region, where it is wider to accommodate the nucleus. The cells abut loosely against each other and the junctions between cells are about 5 nm wide. These junctions permit the passage of large molecules, and macrophages can also pass easily through them. This is unlike the walls of most systemic capillaries, which do not allow migration of large molecules or cells.

Type I alveolar cells

The epithelial lining of alveoli consist mainly of **type I alveolar cells** (also known as **type I pneumocytes**). These are large, flat, squamous cells with few organelles and thin cytoplasm. They cover about 93% of alveolar surface area. Their primary purpose is air–blood gas exchange. The junctions between these cells are narrow (1 nm). This tightness is necessary for preventing the escape of fluid into the alveoli. Flooding the alveoli (alveolar oedema, see below) with fluid would prevent effective gaseous exchange by increasing the diffusion distance for gases.

Type II alveolar cells

Type II alveolar cells (**type II pneumocytes**) are domed cuboidal cells in the alveolar epithelium containing lamellar bodies that secrete **surfactant** (lipoproteins that act as 'wetting agents' as they have water-soluble and oil-soluble components, reducing tension at an interface of different composition). They cover only ~5% of the alveolar surface area. Pulmonary surfactant forms a thin film covering the whole alveolar surface. The film consists of:

- A basal layer mostly made up of protein
- A surface layer of a phospholipid, dipalmitoyl lecithin.

Surfactant is continuously synthesised and secreted by type II alveolar cells. It reduces alveolar surface tension throughout the lungs, in order to:

- Prevent the basically spherical alveoli from collapsing during expiration

- Decrease the effort needed to expand the alveoli at the next inspiration (increase **pulmonary compliance**).

Premature babies have a deficiency in surfactant production and hence have difficulties in expanding their lungs.

Macrophages

Alveoli also contain **macrophages**, which enter the alveolar lumen to phagocytose dust particles and bacteria. Macrophages are part of the pulmonary defence mechanism.

Collateral ventilation

As well as the main air pathways from the trachea through the bronchi and into the alveoli, other pathways link the different regions of the lungs and allow collateral ventilation. The pathways include the pores of Kohn and accessory bronchiolo-alveolar communications. These allow communication between adjacent alveoli, which equalises pressure and provides collateral ventilation. When small airways are blocked, these alternative pathways provide a means for maximising the use of all available alveoli.

The pleura

The outer surface of the lungs is covered by a membrane – the **visceral pleura**. This is separated by a thin fluid film from the **parietal pleura** which covers the thoracic walls and upper surface of the diaphragm. The pleural layers can only be separated by considerable force but can slide easily over each other (like two wet microscope slides). The space between the two layers is called the **pleural cavity** and contains a few millilitres of fluid that acts as a lubricant.

Pleurisy and other pleural conditions

Pleurisy is an inflammation of the pleura, which gives rise to sharp pain on inspiration. The inflammation and roughing of the pleura may be associated with a pleural rub (a creaking sound) at the lung bases, best heard posteriorly. The pain and rub disappear when the pleurae become separated by fluid.

Pleural effusion occurs when fluid fills the space between the visceral and parietal pleurae (Clinical box 13.6). It is more common at the lung bases, i.e. it is dependent on posture. The chest wall over the effusion is dull to percussion, sometimes 'stony dull'. Breath sounds at the site of effusion are reduced or absent and, if heard, are vesicular (lower pitch and quieter than bronchial breathing). **Empyema** is a collection of pus and occurs when a pleural effusion becomes infected.

A **pneumothorax** is the entrance of air into the pleural space which then prevents the lung from expanding. With a large pneumothorax, the trachea (and mediastinum) may be deviated contralaterally. The side of the chest containing the pneumothorax is resonant to percussion (see Clinical box 13.7). Breath sounds are reduced or absent.

Clinical box 13.6 **Chest drainage**

When structures within the chest are damaged, the pleural cavity may become filled with blood or air, compressing the lungs and heart. A polythene tube can be inserted between the ribs to drain the fluid or air. Chest drains are commonly inserted into the second intercostal space in the mid-clavicular line or the sixth intercostal space in the mid-axillary line.

Clinical box 13.7 | **Pneumothorax**

There are three types of pneumothorax:

- **Spontaneous**: this occurs without an obvious cause in a patient without an underlying respiratory disease. It typically occurs in tall thin young men and may be caused by the rupture of a localised defect. It often occurs without exertion but can be associated with the pressure changes due to diving or high-altitude flying.
- **Traumatic**: this occurs when air enters through a wound, usually a knife wound. It can also be caused by rib fractures.
- **Tension**: this occurs when air can enter the pleural space through a defect that acts like a one-way valve. Air moves into the space during inspiration but is trapped during expiration. The rise in pressure in the pleural space can displace the mediastinum affecting the central vessels and reducing cardiac performance. High pressures can result in cardiac tamponade – where the pumping of the heart is impaired.

Pulmonary lymphatics

The channels providing lymphatic drainage in the lungs lie in the interstitial spaces between the alveolar cells and the endothelial cells of the alveolar capillaries. These lymphatic channels drain into a network of lymph nodes that follow the tracheobronchial tree towards the hilum. In the normal, healthy state, pulmonary lymphatic drainage is highly efficient.

The alveolar surfaces are continually moistened by a net filtration of fluid. Any excess fluid is removed by the lymphatics. Under normal physiological conditions, these channels can hold up to 500 mL of fluid. Fluid will leak into the interstitial spaces giving rise to **pulmonary oedema** if excessive fluid filtration exceeds the capacity of the pulmonary lymphatic system. When pulmonary oedema is present, the pulmonary lymphatic channels become engorged, as do the hilar lymph glands. This will appear as a butterfly shadow on a chest radiograph (Fig. 13.8). As the left heart pressure increases (as in left heart failure), thickening of the interlobular

septa may be visible as horizontal linear shadows on a chest X-ray, known as Kerley B lines. These are more easily seen at the costophrenic angles (visualised junctions between the ribs and the diaphragm or pleura), but may disappear as the hydrostatic pressure increases further, leading to alveolar oedema.

Pulmonary oedema

The alveoli are the primary units for gaseous exchange in the lungs. They therefore have to be kept relatively 'dry' in order to facilitate rapid and efficient gaseous exchange. The normal balance between capillary hydrostatic pressure/interstitial hydrostatic pressure and capillary oncotic pressure/interstitial oncotic pressure has the overall effect of maintaining a net filtration of fluid to continually moisten the alveolar surface. Excessive accumulation of fluid in the pulmonary interstitial spaces (interstitial oedema) or alveoli (alveolar flooding) leads to pulmonary oedema. Pulmonary oedema may be produced by excess filtration from the pulmonary capillaries or normal filtration with impaired drainage of fluid:

- Increased capillary hydrostatic pressure
- Decreased oncotic pressure across the capillary membrane (rare)
- Increased capillary permeability (to both fluid and protein)
- Impaired lymphatic drainage.

In the blood surrounding the alveoli, the oncotic pressure (due to plasma proteins tending to pull water into the blood circulation) at about 25 mmHg normally exceeds the hydrostatic capillary blood pressure (10 mmHg) due to gravitation in the pulmonary circulation. However, there is a high protein concentration in the lungs, about 70% that of the plasma, which gives an oncotic pressure in the lungs of about 18 mmHg.

Thus, in conditions such as heart failure where there is even a small rise in left atrial pressures to 20 mmHg or above, there is an increase in pulmonary venous pressure, so net

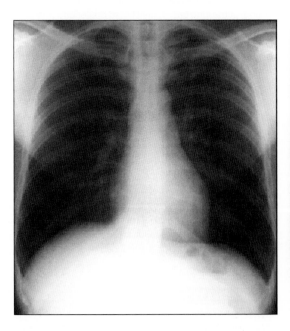

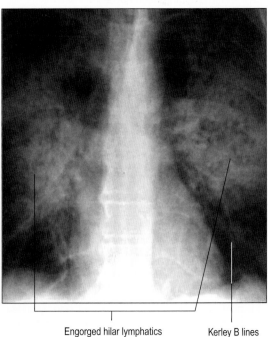

Engorged hilar lymphatics and glands   Kerley B lines

Fig. 13.8 **Appearance of the normal lung (left) and the lung in pulmonary oedema (right).** The shadowing in oedema typically has a 'butterfly' shape.

filtration exceeds the capabilities of the lymphatic drainage, and consequently pulmonary oedema occurs. Alveolar oedema occurs when the pulmonary venous pressure exceeds 30 mmHg.

ANATOMY OF THE PULMONARY CIRCULATION

The air pressure in the alveoli is close to atmospheric pressure; as the lungs expand the pressure becomes negative in relation to atmospheric pressure, drawing air in, reversing as the respiration muscles contract and the lung volume decreases, increasing the relative pressure difference and air leaves the lungs. To ensure maximum efficiency in oxygen transfer between alveoli and blood, the pulmonary circulation is at very low pressure in very thin-walled vessels facilitating transfer by simple diffusing down partial pressure gradients. The lungs have two sources of blood supply (Fig. 13.9) delivered by two separate sets of blood vessels:

- **Deoxygenated blood** from the systemic circulation is carried to the lungs by the pulmonary artery from the right ventricle. After successive divisions that follow the bronchi and bronchioles, the pulmonary artery ends as thin-walled pulmonary capillaries in the alveolar walls to form the alveolar–capillary complexes, where gaseous exchange takes place (see Fig. 13.7). Oxygenated blood is collected via the pulmonary venous circulation into the pulmonary veins, which empty into the left atrium for onward distribution.
- **Oxygenated blood** from the descending aorta supplies the bronchial circulation, carrying nutrients to the lungs via the bronchial arteries. Bronchial veins drain deoxygenated blood from the lung parenchyma, bronchial tree, pleura and nerves. Most of this blood is returned to the right side of the heart via the superior vena cava. Blood from the deeper lung parenchyma drains into the pulmonary vein, and is therefore returned to the left side of the heart, forming a right-left shunt.

Although the two sets of circulation through the lungs are considered to be separate, there are overlaps where there are communications between the pulmonary and bronchial vascular systems (right-to-left shunt, see below). In total, the pulmonary blood vessels contain about 24% of the body's total blood volume (about 1.2 L of a total blood volume of about 5 L). Their capacity is variable and decreases during expiration, thus affecting inflow into the left atrium and beat-to-beat output of the left ventricle.

Arteries

The main **pulmonary artery** divides into two arteries, one for each lung. Their resistance is about one-sixth of the resistance of systemic arteries that have the same blood flow. Structurally, the pulmonary artery is primarily elastic, with the muscular media layer of the arterial wall about half the thickness of equivalent systemic arteries. Maximum muscularity occurs in vessels about 200–100 μm diameter, but muscular tissue is lost as the vessels narrow from 100 μm to 30 μm diameter.

Pulmonary capillaries arise abruptly from the larger vessels (see Fig. 13.7B); each is about 8 μm in length and diameter. They form a dense network or sheet around the alveoli, with an estimated surface area of 30–50 m². A capillary is not confined to one alveolus but passes from one alveolus to another, and blood can traverse a number of alveolar septa before it reaches a venule.

The **bronchial arteries** enter each lung and their branches follow the larger bronchi and bronchioles. They supply arterial blood to bronchial smooth muscle as far as the respiratory bronchioles, the intrapulmonary nerves, nerve ganglia, pleura, interstitial lung substance, lymphoid tissue and vasa vasorum of the pulmonary artery. **Vasa vasorum** is the name for the blood vessels that supply the walls of large blood vessels such as the aorta.

Veins

Blood from the pulmonary capillaries drains into the pulmonary vein and thence into the left atrium. Blood from the bronchial arteries can either drain back to the heart via the true **bronchial veins** into the right atrium or via the **pulmonary vein** into the left atrium. Blood from the systemic circulation can therefore reach the pulmonary circulation by way of the bronchial vascular system. There are also connections (**anastomoses** or **shunts**) between these two circulatory systems at the capillary level. As the bronchial arteries are carrying oxygenated blood at systemic pressures and the drainage is via the low-pressure pulmonary venous system, the bronchial circulation becomes an arteriovenous shunt.

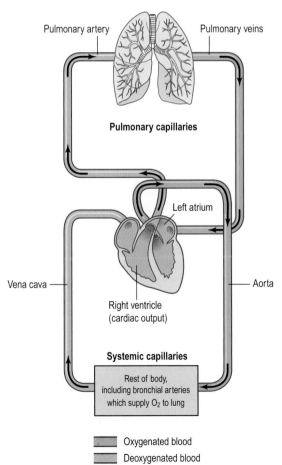

Pulmonary artery

Pulmonary veins

Pulmonary capillaries

Left atrium

Vena cava

Aorta

Right ventricle (cardiac output)

Systemic capillaries

Rest of body, including bronchial arteries which supply O₂ to lung

Oxygenated blood
Deoxygenated blood

Fig. 13.9 **Anatomy of the pulmonary circulation.** The alveoli have two supplies of blood, from the pulmonary artery and from the aorta.

Right-to-left (arteriovenous) shunts

Shunting of blood refers to the phenomenon whereby deoxygenated blood from the right side of the heart bypasses the ventilated areas of the lungs and enters the systemic circulation without effectively taking up oxygen and off-loading carbon dioxide. This lowers the partial pressure of oxygen in the arterial blood due to mixing of blood from various sources:

- Oxygen-depleted blood from the bronchial circulation entering the pulmonary vein and thus the left ventricle
- Congenital abnormalities of the heart where there is addition of deoxygenated blood from the right side directly to the left, e.g. **atrial septal defects (ASD)**; **Fallot's tetralogy (ventricular septal defect (VSD))**; failure to close the connection between the pulmonary artery and the descending aorta in the foetus, allowing the blood to bypass the non-functioning lungs, at birth, resulting in a **patent ductus arteriosus**
- Vascular anomalies such as pulmonary arteriovenous fistulas (direct connection between an artery and a vein)
- Coronary venous drainage directly into the left ventricle (Thebesian veins, or venae cordis minimae)
- Blood flow through diseased or damaged areas of the lungs that are poorly or not ventilated, where gaseous exchange is inefficient.

Pulmonary blood flow

Blood flow through the pulmonary artery is usually taken to be equal to cardiac output even though 1–2% of blood pumped out of the right ventricle bypasses the lungs via shunts. This relationship is the basis of direct (invasive) and numerous indirect (non-invasive) methods for estimating cardiac output using the **Fick equation** (see Clinical box 13.8). Table 13.3 lists the commonly used respiratory symbols.

The normal pulmonary blood flow or cardiac output in the average man at rest is 5 L/min or, when expressed as the cardiac index, 3.0 L/min/m^2 body surface area. Output from the right ventricle is not distributed equally to the two lungs: about 45% of deoxygenated blood passes through the left lung and 55% through the right. The time taken by blood to pass through the lungs from pulmonary artery to left atrium is about 5 seconds but the time blood spends in the alveolar–capillary complex during which gaseous exchange can take place is about 0.75 seconds. This may fall to 0.3 seconds during strenuous exercise, but the blood is still **fully saturated** in that time because **haemoglobin** has such a high affinity for oxygen.

Volume of blood in lungs

There is an estimated 100 mL of blood in the pulmonary capillaries. The pulmonary blood volume can vary under different conditions and therefore acts as a reservoir. This reservoir of blood is important in ensuring that the left side of the heart is filled during diastole. This ability of the lungs to store blood means that it can buffer minor irregularities in the output of the two ventricles.

Pulmonary arterial and venous pressure

Pulmonary arterial pressures are much lower than systemic arterial pressures, at about 25/8 mmHg (mean 11–15 mmHg) compared with 120/80 mmHg in the aorta. The pulmonary arterial walls are about half as thick as corresponding vessels

Clinical box 13.8   **Determining pulmonary blood flow or cardiac output (CO)**

- Blood is sampled from the aorta and pulmonary artery using catheters inserted into the heart.
- The concentration of oxygen (O_2) or carbon dioxide (CO_2) is measured in the respective arterial (a) and mixed venous (v) blood.

The **Fick principle** states that the rate at which oxygen is taken up from the atmosphere (O_2 consumption) is equal to the flow of blood passing through the lungs and the increase in oxygen concentration of blood passing through the lungs. Thus:

$$CO = \frac{O_2 \text{ consumption}}{a - v \; O_2 \text{ concentration difference}}$$

or

$$CO = \frac{O_2 \text{ production}}{v - a \; CO_2 \text{ concentration difference}}$$

- Normal O_2 consumption is 250 mL/min, the arterial O_2 concentration 190 mL/L blood and the venous O_2 concentration 140 mL/L blood
- Normal CO_2 production is 200 mL/min, the venous O_2 concentration 520 mL/L blood and the arterial O_2 concentration 480 mL/L blood

Using either O_2 consumption or CO_2 consumption should give the same answer.

$$CO = (250 \text{ mL / min}) / (190 - 140 \text{ mL / L blood})$$
$$= (250 \text{ mL / min}) / 50 \text{ mL / L}$$

or

$$CO = (200 \text{ mL / min}) / (520 - 480 \text{ mL / L blood})$$
$$= (200 \text{ mL / min}) / (40 \text{ mL / L})$$

Both of which give a pulmonary blood flow or cardiac output = 5 L/min.

in the systemic circulation. Pressures can be measured directly by inserting a catheter through a large leg vein via the left side of the heart, through the chambers into the pulmonary artery. Pressures inside the pulmonary artery are the same as in the right ventricle.

There are no valves between the left atrium and the pulmonary vein, so pressures in the left atrium are equivalent to those in the pulmonary vein and left atrial pressure may be taken as a measure of **pulmonary venous pressure**. Left atrial pressures are measured by inserting a catheter into the heart via an artery (normally the femoral artery). The mean left atrial pressure, equivalent to the pulmonary venous pressure, varies from 0 mmHg to 5 mmHg. This suggests that the pressure drop across the lungs is about 12 mmHg.

Pulmonary blood vessels

The pulmonary blood vessels are supplied by sympathetic vasoconstrictor fibres. Little is known about regulation of pulmonary vessel diameter, but there must be a certain level of resting tone since, during exercise, pulmonary resistances must decrease to accommodate a six-fold increase in pulmonary blood flow. Pulmonary blood vessels, unlike vessels in the systemic circulation, are constricted by hypoxia or acidosis. The response to hypoxia is non-linear and partly dependent on the carbon dioxide levels. Hypoxic vasoconstriction is very important as a means of diverting blood flow away from lung regions where the oxygen tension is low, to regions

Table 13.3 **Respiratory symbols**

Symbol	Definition	Example
p	Partial gas pressure	p_aCO_2, arterial CO_2 pressure
V	Gas volume	V_T, tidal volume
$\dot{V}$	Gas volume per unit time (flow)	$\dot{V}$ volume of expired air/min
F	Fractional gas concentration	FO_2, fractional concentration of O_2 in inspired gas
D	Diffusing capacity	DO_2, diffusing capacity of O_2 (e.g. 50 mL O_2/min/mmHg)
Q	Volume of blood	Q_c, volume of blood in pulmonary capillaries
$\dot{Q}$	Volume flow of blood per unit time	$\dot{Q}$ blood flow through pulmonary capillaries/min
C	Concentration of gas in blood	C_aO_2, mL O_2 in 100 mL arterial blood
S	% saturation of haemoglobin with O_2	S_vO_2, saturation of haemoglobin with O_2 in mixed venous blood
Gas symbols		
A	Alveolar gas	
B	Barometric	
D	Dead space gas	
E	Expired gas	
I	Inspired gas	
L	Lung	
T	Tidal gas	
Blood symbols		
a	Arterial blood	
v	Venous blood	
c	Capillary blood	

A bar (–) above any symbol indicates a mean value (P_cO_2, mixed venous pO_2). A dot (·) above any symbol indicates a time derivative.

where oxygen is available to be taken up by haemoglobin. Chronic hypoxia, as seen in COPD, will lead to pulmonary hypertension and the development of right heart failure (**cor pulmonale**) (Clinical box 13.9).

Clinical box 13.9 **Clinical conditions associated with defects in the pulmonary circulation**

Cor pulmonale is a condition in which there is right heart (ventricular) failure resulting from raised blood pressure in either the pulmonary arteries or the pulmonary veins – pulmonary hypertension. Right heart failure is caused by a primary disorder of the respiratory system, or it may be secondary to some other cardiopulmonary disease.

Chronic cor pulmonale is associated with right ventricular hypertrophy. Common causes include:
- Chronic obstructive pulmonary disease (COPD)
- Pulmonary fibrosis from whatever cause
- Cystic fibrosis
- Primary pulmonary hypertension
- Chronic thromboembolic pulmonary disease
- Obstructive sleep apnoea.

Right ventricular dilatation occurs in **acute cor pulmonale**. Acute cor pulmonale is reversible, and may occur with massive pulmonary embolism. Symptoms of cor pulmonale are mainly associated with right ventricular failure and the underlying lung disease. Physical signs are those of pulmonary hypertension and right ventricular failure, together with the underlying lung condition.

Pulmonary oedema occurs in left ventricular failure from whatever cause. Symptoms include:
- Shortness of breath (dyspnoea) on exertion
- Orthopnoea – dyspnoea when lying flat
- Paroxysmal nocturnal dyspnoea – acute shortness of breath while asleep, causing patient to wake from sleep.

The presence of bilateral fine, basal crackles on auscultation of the chest is the cardinal physical sign of pulmonary oedema.

Variations in pulmonary blood flow

Pulmonary blood flow varies during normal breathing. Intrathoracic pressure falls during inspiration, so that blood flows more readily through the veins. There is increased filling of the right ventricle and so increased right ventricular output. Pulmonary arterial pressure rises and pulmonary blood vessels engorge. However, pulmonary venous outflow falls, possibly because of the expansion in capillary volume, and there is a reduction in left ventricular filling and a slight fall in left systemic pressure.

During expiration the increased volume of blood in the lungs is expelled through the pulmonary veins with the result that the left ventricular output increases, causing a rise in systemic blood pressure. Simultaneously the higher intrathoracic pressure reduces the return of blood to the right ventricle and the mean pulmonary artery pressure falls.

Effect of gravity on pulmonary blood flow

Gravity has an effect on pulmonary blood flow. In the upright posture, the contents of the thorax are like a semi-liquid column. Due to gravity, the hydrostatic pressure in the lower part of the column is higher than in the upper part.

This higher blood pressure has the effect of increasing blood flow through the lower parts of the lungs by opening up the capillaries that are collapsed. As a result, the lower parts of the lungs are better perfused than the upper parts. These can be divided into three 'zones' (see section below, Uneven perfusion, and Fig. 13.24). At rest, and in the upright position, the upper zone capillary bed is closed, but it may open up during exercise due to increased oxygen demand, the mid-zone is open during pulmonary systole but closed during diastole, and in the lower zone the capillary bed is always open.

SURFACE ANATOMY OF THE RESPIRATORY SYSTEM

The surface anatomy of the respiratory system gives an indication of the underlying structures, and it is essential to know these surface markings when performing clinical examinations or procedures.

Larynx and trachea

The larynx is made up of the prominent **thyroid cartilage** (thyroid prominence: Adam's apple) and the **cricoid cartilage** just beneath it, and is palpable in the anterior part of the neck. Its complex structure reflects the variety of muscles attached to it. The vocal cords lie within the larynx behind the thyroid cartilage. The first of the cartilaginous rings of the trachea can be felt in the midline in the depths of the suprasternal notch. The trachea ends just right of the midline at the level of the sternal angle (see below).

Surface markings of the thorax

Anterior surface of the chest

The **clavicles** (collar bones) and the **sternum** (breastbone) form the single bony articulation (joint) between the upper limb and the thorax. The sternum is in two parts and can be felt throughout its entire length within the sternal furrow, situated between the **pectoralis major** muscles. The upper end of the body of the sternum is attached at a slight angle to the **manubrium**. The curved upper end of the manubrium and the medial ends of the clavicles form a recess called the **suprasternal notch**, where the cartilage of the trachea may be felt. The sternocleidomastoid muscles appear as oblique cords narrowing and deepening the notch. The **xyphoid process (xiphisternum)** is a tongue of cartilage at the lower end of the sternal body (Fig. 13.10).

The manubrium and body of the sternum are joined by the manubriosternal joint. The **sternal angle** (angle of Louis) is the angle made by this joint. The sternal angle can be seen

and felt and is used to mark the medial end of the costal (rib) cartilage of the second rib and further laterally the rib itself. All ribs may be counted from this point systematically down the chest wall from one rib to another, with the soft intercostal spaces between them. Ribs are numbered according to the vertebra to which they are attached posteriorly. **Intercostal spaces** are named after the rib above. The lower border of the pectoralis major at its attachment corresponds to the fifth rib. The vertical line that passes through the mid-point of the clavicle is the mid-clavicular line.

The costal margin is formed by the costal cartilages of the 7th to 10th ribs marking the lower border of the thorax. Posteriorly, the 11th and 12th ribs are usually separate from the costal margin. The 12th rib is small and is more difficult to feel because it is buried in bulky muscles.

Lateral surface of the chest

The anatomical term for the armpit is the axilla or axillary fossa. The upper part of the lateral chest wall lies in the space between the **axillary folds**, which come into prominence when the upper limb is raised above the head. The anterior fold is formed by the lower border of a large muscle, the pectoralis major. The posterior fold is formed by the tendon of the latissimus dorsi muscle as it passes round the lower border of the teres major muscle. The vertical line midway between the axillary folds is the mid-axillary line.

Posterior surface of the chest

The spinous processes of the 12 thoracic vertebrae are visible as plate-like knobs and can be felt, providing attachments for large muscles. The first palpable (and visible) spinous process is that of the seventh cervical vertebra (C7, vertebra prominens). The spinous processes of the first thoracic vertebrae are inferior (caudal) to the vertebra prominens. The spinous process of each thoracic vertebra lies immediately posterior to the body of the one below.

The scapula (Fig. 13.11) is a prominent landmark on the posterior wall of the chest, shaped to form a large surface for attachment of the powerful muscles that move the upper limb in relation to the thorax. It has a lower point (apex) and a spine that projects from its posterior surface.

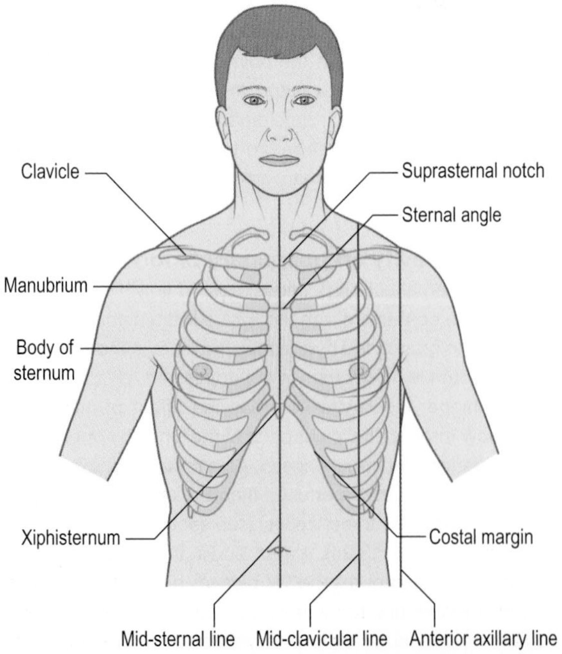

Clavicle — Suprasternal notch
— Sternal angle
Manubrium —
Body of sternum —
Xiphisternum — Costal margin
Mid-sternal line Mid-clavicular line Anterior axillary line

Fig. 13.10 Surface anatomy of the anterior chest (male).

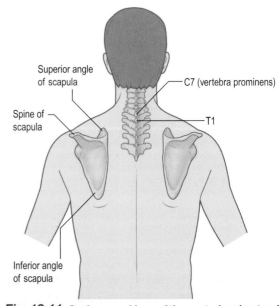

Superior angle of scapula
Spine of scapula
Inferior angle of scapula
C7 (vertebra prominens)
T1

Fig. 13.11 Surface markings of the posterior chest wall.

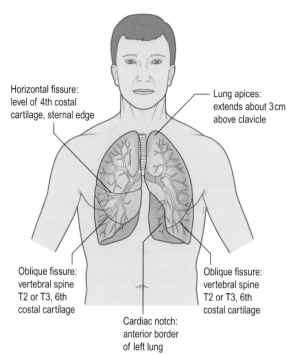

Horizontal fissure:
level of 4th costal
cartilage, sternal edge

Lung apices:
extends about 3 cm
above clavicle

Oblique fissure:
vertebral spine
T2 or T3, 6th
costal cartilage

Oblique fissure:
vertebral spine
T2 or T3, 6th
costal cartilage

Cardiac notch:
anterior border
of left lung

Fig. 13.12 **Surface markings of the lungs.**

The lungs and pleural cavity

The lungs lie inside the pleural cavity and almost entirely beneath the ribs. The apex of the lung and the pleural cavity which surrounds it extend slightly above the clavicles by about 3 cm. They then extend downwards to the diaphragm, and between the ribs and the diaphragm as the costodiaphragmatic recess. The surface markings for the lungs and pleura are similar except that the lungs do not extend below the vertebral level of T10 (Fig. 13.12).

MECHANICS OF BREATHING

Ventilation (movement of air into and out of the lungs) is produced by changes in the size of the thoracic cavity. When the cavity enlarges during inspiration, air flows into the lungs because at that instant the pressure in the atmosphere is greater than that in the lungs.

THE DIAPHRAGM AND OTHER MUSCLES USED IN BREATHING

The **diaphragm** is the main muscle of respiration. It is a dome-shaped sheet of skeletal muscle separating the thoracic and abdominal cavities and consisting of muscle fibres and a central tendinous portion. The fibres run upwards from their origin at the inner part of the thoracic cage and then arch towards the midline.

During normal, **quiet respiration**, the diaphragm contracts and moves downwards in inspiration and the parietal pleura attached to the diaphragm descends. This movement pulls down the visceral pleura so that the airways and alveoli expand and air is sucked into the lungs. The diaphragm

relaxes in expiration and the recoil of the elastic tissues in the lung expels air from the alveoli and airways. Movement of the **ribcage** also contributes to respiration by increasing the diameter of the chest, thereby increasing the thoracic volume and making the negative pressure in the lungs more 'negative', again causing air to be sucked in. The external intercostal muscles move the ribcage upwards and outwards to increase the lateral and anteroposterior diameter of the thorax. The joints between the posterior ends of the ribs and the transverse processes of the vertebrae enable the lower ribs to swivel upwards and outwards to increase the lateral diameter of the chest, while the anterior ends of the ribs move up and out to increase the anteroposterior diameter. The diaphragmatic movement contributes about 75% and movement of the ribcage contributes 25% to the increase in thoracic volume.

During **forced respiration**, when there is increased demand for oxygen, as in exercise or disease, **accessory muscles of respiration** come into play. These are muscles that are not primarily involved in respiration, but enlarge the ribcage in any way possible during inspiration to increase the amount of air, and therefore oxygen, breathed in (Fig. 13.13).

The neck muscles pull the ribcage upwards; the sternocleidomastoids will elevate the sternum while the scalenus major and minor muscles will elevate both the first two ribs and the sternum. The oblique, transversus and rectus abdominis muscles will pull the ribcage downwards. By fixing the shoulder girdle, the pectoralis major and latissimus dorsi muscles will pull the ribcage outwards.

These muscles can be seen hard at work in patients with respiratory distress (Clinical box 13.10) as in acute asthma or in athletes at the end of a hard race.

Inspiration

The diaphragm is the main muscle of **inspiration**. It has a motor nerve supply from cervical segments C3–C5 via the left and right phrenic nerves. The sensory supply is also through the phrenic nerve centrally and branches of the intercostal nerves peripherally. When stimulated, the diaphragm moves downwards, increasing the size of the thoracic cavity. This has the effect of making the negative intrapulmonary pressure more negative, and thus drawing air into the lungs. In **eupnoea** (normal breathing) the diaphragm may move by 1.5 cm, and in deep breathing it may show as much as a 7 cm excursion.

In spinal cord injuries, only breaks above C3–C4 will affect the phrenic nerve and result in apnoea (absence of breathing) and death. If the phrenic nerve is severed by accident but the spinal cord remains intact, ventilation can be adequately accomplished by contraction of the external intercostal muscles. The intercostal muscles are innervated by motor neurons from vertebrae T1–T12. The muscles move the chest wall upwards and outwards.

The position of the diaphragm varies with body posture. In an upright posture, the abdominal contents sink under gravity as does the diaphragm. The diaphragm also flattens out, increasing its cross-sectional area. Thus, in the upright posture, the diaphragmatic movement required to achieve expansion of the thoracic cavity is smaller than that required to achieve the same expansion in the supine posture, when the diaphragm is more dome-shaped. This partly explains

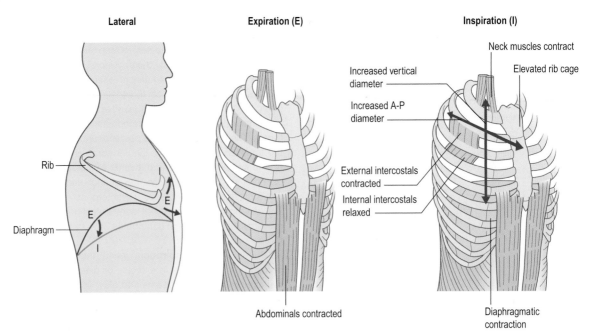

Lateral **Expiration (E)** **Inspiration (I)**

Neck muscles contract

Increased vertical diameter

Elevated rib cage

Increased A-P diameter

Rib

External intercostals contracted

Internal intercostals relaxed

Diaphragm

Abdominals contracted

Diaphragmatic contraction

Fig. 13.13 **Chest and rib movements contribute to chest expansion.** The accessory muscles assist in increasing chest capacity in forced respiration. A-P, anteroposterior.

Clinical box 13.10	Accessory muscles of respiration in respiratory distress

The use of accessory muscles of respiration is a sign of respiratory distress or failure. Breathing becomes laboured and the accessory muscles of respiration may be seen clearly in the neck and abdomen. Intercostal recession occurs because of the external intercostal muscles contracting to move the ribcage up and outwards. This is accompanied by tachypnoea and dyspnoea, and sometimes cyanosis is present.

why patients with respiratory diseases, particularly those diseases that involve respiratory muscle fatigue, prefer an upright posture.

Expiration

In quiet breathing, **expiration** is usually passive and results from the elastic recoil of the lungs and chest wall, and the inward pull of surface tension in the pleural space.

1. Muscles of the diaphragm and intercostals relax
2. Thoracic and intrapulmonary volumes decrease
3. Intrapulmonary pressures increase to about 1 mmHg above atmospheric pressure.

Forced expiration during maximal ventilation or against an obstruction is an active process: the abdominal muscles contract to increase intra-abdominal pressure. This movement forces the diaphragm upward and depresses the lower ribs, so decreasing the volume of the thoracic cavity and expelling air. Lung emptying can be enhanced by contraction of the internal intercostal muscles. This displaces the ribs down and back, which also decreases the volume of the thorax and expels air from the lungs.

The diaphragm, muscles of respiration and chest wall work together to expand the thorax and inflate the lungs during inspiration. These muscles reduce their effort, causing the thorax to contract, deflating the lungs during expiration.

PULMONARY PRESSURE CHANGES DURING VENTILATION

Intrapulmonary pressure

With expansion of the chest and the accompanying inflation of the lung, the pressure within the alveoli of the lungs, the **intrapulmonary pressure**, falls to about 3 mmHg below the atmospheric pressure. As the lungs fill, this gradient decreases, and by the end of inspiration the intrapulmonary pressure equals atmospheric pressure. During expiration, intrapulmonary pressures become positive relative to atmospheric (+3 mmHg) but return to atmospheric pressure once expiration is complete.

Intrapleural pressure

Intrapleural pressure refers to pressures within the pleural space, i.e. between the visceral and parietal pleural layers. These are normally sub-atmospheric (−4 mmHg) because of the elastic recoil of the lungs on one side, and desire of the ribs to move outwards on the other side, continually trying to separate the two layers. During normal breathing and movement of the diaphragm and ribcage, intrapleural pressures will fall or rise by about 5 mmHg relative to this sub-atmospheric pressure. A deep inspiration can drop the intrapleural pressures by as much as 30 mmHg below atmospheric. Intrapleural pressures can be measured by inserting the tip of a needle connected to a manometer into the pleural cavity. Less invasively, changes in intrapleural pressure can be measured by a balloon catheter in the oesophagus at the level of the mediastinum.

Maximal respiratory pressures

Maximal respiratory pressures are used to measure the strength of inspiratory and expiratory muscles. Muscle weakness will restrict maximal inspiration, whereas stiff lungs will stretch less for the same muscular effort. In disease conditions such as multiple sclerosis, poliomyelitis or spinal injuries, these pressures may be used to monitor the effectiveness of interventions to strengthen the respiratory muscles. The maximal expiratory pressures (PE_{max}) that can be developed are 150–200 cmH$_2$O at high lung volume, while maximal (negative) inspiratory pressure (PI_{max}) is 100 cmH$_2$O at low lung volumes.

PULMONARY VENTILATION

Pulmonary ventilation is the process for moving gases in and out of the lungs. In the healthy state, the amount of gas (or air) that can be accommodated will depend of the size of the lungs and thorax. Lung capacity is related to the age, sex, height and ethnicity of the individual. The amount of gas (or air) that can be moved with respiration is known as a lung volume, and will depend on inspiratory and expiratory effort and the lung capacity. Pulmonary disease will affect both lung capacity and volume. Pulmonary ventilation can also be referred to as the amount of gas moved in or out of the lungs per minute.

Lung volumes and capacities

The changes in the volume of the lungs during breathing can be measured with a spirometer. There are various types of spirometer: either mechanical, such as a rolling seal spirometer, or electronic, which integrate flow measured by a pneumotachygraph to calculate volume. Figure 13.14 shows the lung capacities and lung volumes recorded on a spirometer.

As a rule, lung capacities are made up from two or more 'volumes' (Fig. 13.15):

- **Total lung capacity** (TLC): the maximum amount of gas the lungs can accommodate. TLC is the sum of four 'volumes'.

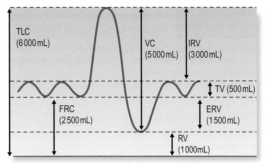

Fig. 13.15 **Lung volumes** can be considered as having various components. The figure shows lung volumes measured with a spirometer during quiet breathing with one maximum breath. Volumes shown are for an average-sized healthy young man. RV, residual volume; ERV, expiratory reserve volume; IRV, inspiratory reserve volume; TLC, total lung capacity; FRC, functional respiratory capacity; TV, tidal volume; VC, vital capacity.

- **Tidal volume** (TV): the amount of air inspired and expired at each breath at any level of activity. During normal, quiet breathing this is about 0.5 L, but TV can increase to 1 L or more during exercise and with training.
- **Expiratory reserve volume** (ERV): the amount of gas that could be expelled with maximum expiratory effort at the end of normal, quiet expiration – about 1.5 L.
- **Residual volume** (RV): the volume of air that still remains in the lungs – about 1.0 L.
- **Inspiratory reserve volume** (IRV): the amount of air that can be breathed in with a maximum inspiration from the end of a normal inspiration – about 3.0 L.
- **Forced vital capacity** (**FVC**) or **vital capacity** (**VC**) is the maximum possible breath that can be taken, typically 5 L. FVC (VC) is made up of three 'volumes':

$$FVC = TV + ERV + IRV$$

- **Functional residual capacity** (**FRC**): the volume of air left in the lungs at the end of normal quiet expiration when all respiratory muscles are relaxed. For a healthy, resting, recumbent young man (1.7 m^2 body surface) breathing at sea level, an average FRC would be 2.5 L.

$$FRC = RV + ERV$$

Total lung capacity (**TLC**) is equal to FVC plus RV, which is about 6 L:

$$TLC = FVC + RV$$

RV cannot be determined by the use of a simple spirometer, nor therefore can FRC because it is given as the sum of RV + ERV; other means have to be used (see Clinical box 13.11).

Dead space

Dead space is the volume of the respiratory tract not involved in gas exchange. The **anatomical dead space** lies between the mouth/nose entrance and the respiratory bronchioles where the tissue walls are too thick and blood vessels too few to allow diffusion of gases into the blood. Some air may also enter parts of the lungs where gaseous exchange is not fully efficient because these parts of the lungs are either relatively poorly perfused or relatively over-ventilated. The

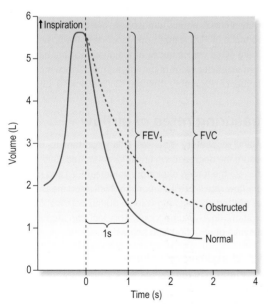

Fig. 13.14 **Lung volumes as measured using a spirometer.** Subjects breathe out as fast as possible from maximum inspiration. The volume expelled relates to lung capacity. The volume expelled in the first second (FEV$_1$) is used expressed as a percentage of the total forced expiratory capacity (FVC); in health this should be >80%.

This open-circuit method is based on the fact that air contains a fixed concentration (about 80%) of nitrogen (N_2) that is neither absorbed nor produced by the body. So, by washing all the N_2 out of the lungs and measuring its volume, the volume of air that was in the lungs can be estimated. That is:

Volume of gas in the lung (V)
× concentration of N_2 in the lung
= Volume of gas exhaled
× concentration of N_2 in gas exhaled

- To wash the N_2 from the lungs, the subject breathes O_2 (N_2-free) gas and breathes out through a turbine volume-flow meter for a few minutes. Normally 2 minutes are required in healthy adults but longer (7 minutes) may be necessary for people with asthma or emphysema.
- The expired gas is collected and its N_2 concentration measured and its volume determined.
  Example: If 40 L of expired gas was collected and it contained 5% nitrogen, then:

$$V \times 80/100 = 40 \times 5/100$$

$$V = 40 \times 0.05/0.80 = 2.5 L$$

If this test is begun precisely at the moment of complete and maximal expiration, then **RV** is measured, while if it is begun at the end of a normal expiration, **FRC** is measured.

- Ask a volunteer to breathe into a Douglas bag and measure the volume of air collected while counting the number of breathes exhaled into the bag. Calculate the tidal volume (TV).
- Measure the CO_2 concentration in the bag (F_ECO_2).
- Ask the volunteer to make a rapid and deep expiration into a Haldane tube (a tube about 1 m long and 2.5 cm diameter with a sample tap near the mouthpiece). Sample air with a syringe at the end of the expiration but before the volunteer removes their mouth, to prevent contamination by room air. Measure the CO_2 concentration of the sample gas (F_ACO_2).

$$DS = TV \times (F_ACO_2 - F_ECO_2)/(F_ACO_2) \text{ (Bohr equation)}$$

The underlying assumptions are that:
- The Haldane tube sample contains the last air to be expelled from the lungs and can be taken to be alveolar air
- Exhaled tidal volume is diluted by the air in the physiological dead space (DS), thus:

$$(TV - DS) \times \%CO_2 \text{ in alveolar air}$$
$$= TV \times \%CO_2 \text{ in expired air}$$

- Air in the dead space has 0% CO_2.

total volume of air not involved in oxygenation of blood is termed the **physiological dead space** and encompasses this and the anatomical dead space. In healthy people, the physiological dead space is identical to the anatomical dead space (Clinical box 13.12).

At rest, typically the respiratory rate (RR) is 12–15 breaths per minute and the tidal volume (TV) 500 mL (Clinical box 13.13). Therefore:

$$\text{Pulmonary ventilation} = RR \times TV$$
$$= 12 \times 500$$
$$= 6 L/min$$

- In emphysema, the loss of lung elastic recoil increases FRC so that the thorax is over-inflated. Expanding already over-expanded lungs also makes breathing in harder work.
- Conversely, a low FRC occurs in restrictive lung disorders. The increased lung stiffness in pulmonary oedema, interstitial fibrosis and other restrictive disorders decreases FRC.
- Space occupying intra-abdominal masses also reduce FRC, e.g. pregnancy, ascites and hepatosplenomegaly.
- Kyphoscoliosis, with deformity of the thoracic cage, leads to a decrease in lung volumes because a stiff, non-compliant chest wall restricts lung expansion.

Clinical signs of hyperinflation of the chest
The anteroposterior diameter of the thorax increases as the chest is continually over-inflated giving rise to the following characteristics:
- The 'barrel' shaped chest
- Relatively horizontal ribs
- Protruding abdomen
- Hyper-resonance on percussion.

However, not all of the breath can take part in gaseous exchange. About 150 mL of each breath fills the so-called anatomical dead space (DS). The volume of air that participates in gas exchange because it is in contact with perfused alveoli is termed the alveolar ventilation, and is less than pulmonary ventilation. Using the figures above:

$$\text{Alveolar ventilation} = RR \times (TV - DS)$$
$$= 12 \times (500 - 150)$$
$$= 4.2 L/min$$

In disease the physiological dead space will increase with pulmonary embolism or emphysema.

Functional residual capacity

Functional residual capacity (FRC) refers to the volume of air left in the lungs at the very end of normal expiration. At this stage, all the muscles of respiration are at rest, and the intrapulmonary pressure equals atmospheric pressure (see above). The importance of FRC is that it corresponds to the point where the outward elastic recoil forces of the chest wall are balanced by the inward elastic recoil of the lungs. This balance is changed in a number of respiratory diseases (Clinical box 13.13).

Measuring rates of airflow

In many respiratory diseases it is important to be able to measure the degree to which airflow is limited. Two measures of this are the forced expiratory volume (FEV_1) and peak expiratory flow rate (PEFR). A more sophisticated measure is flow rates plotted against lung volume during both inspiration and expiration: flow–volume loops. This test can identify the site of airways obstruction (see below).

Forced expiratory volume

A type of spirometer known as a vitalograph is commonly used to measure FEV_1, which is the amount of air that can be forcibly expelled from a maximal breath in 1 second. Vitalographs can also measure the FVC (Clinical box 13.14). Measurements of FEV_1 and FVC are related to expected values predicted from the height, age (see Clinical box 13.15), sex and ethnicity of the person (Fig. 13.16). The measured volumes will also depend on respiratory muscle strength;

- The patient should be upright (FEV_1 will be greater in the upright posture), a nose clip should be worn (but is not absolutely essential), a sterile mouthpiece should be used with the lips sealed firmly around it, and the patient verbally encouraged by the operator (because measurement is effort dependent) to fully empty their lungs.
- The patient is asked to make a maximal inspiration followed by a single, forced and long expiration.
- Patients with severe airflow limitation may have a prolonged forced expiratory time so any test should not be prematurely terminated. With a vitalograph-type spirometer the recording takes about 5 seconds in healthy people.

   Reductions in FEV_1 and forced vital capacity (FVC) can be used to distinguish between diseases (Fig. 13.17). Expression of FEV_1 as a percentage of the predicted FEV_1 is a good measure of airflow limitation and is used clinically in comparisons of disease severity between patients. In healthy people it is normally greater than 80%. The FEV_1/FVC ratio (or FEV_1 expressed as a percentage of FVC) is a useful measure of airway obstruction:

   - In patients with an obstructive lung disease (asthma, COPD, emphysema) the ratio is less than 0.7. Asthmatic patients with air trapping will have reduced FEV_1 and FVC, but FEV_1 as a percentage of FVC would also be reduced.
   - With a restrictive lung disease, i.e. interstitial lung disease, respiratory muscle weakness and thoracic cage deformities such as kyphoscoliosis (kyphosis: dorsal curvature; scoliosis: side-to-side curvature of the spine), both FEV_1 and FVC are reduced but the FEV_1/FVC ratio is normal (FEV_1 as a percentage of FVC is normal).

swimmers, divers and brass musical instrument players who exercise against a respiratory load typically have larger than expected FEV_1 and FVC. Differences between these two measurements also show variation in different lung diseases (Fig. 13.17). (See also Information box 13.4.)

Peak expiratory flow rate

Although not as good as spirometry for measuring airflow limitation, measuring **PEFR** with a peak flow meter is a convenient way by which patients can monitor their asthma or COPD at home (Clinical box 13.16). Wide diurnal variations occur in PEFR, with the highest readings in the evening and the lowest in the early hours of the morning. PEFR is less dependent on effort than the FEV_1 but only measures expiratory flow rate. The unit used is L/min or L/s.

Reversibility of airflow limitation

Measurements of FEV_1 and PEFR are made before and after inhalation of a bronchodilator (e.g. the β-adrenoceptor agonist salbutamol).

- In asthma, the airways constriction is reversible so that the FEV_1 and PEFR would be restored to normal after salbutamol.
- In COPD, typically the airways constriction is irreversible, or nearly irreversible. There would be <15%, or <200 mL/s, improvement in FEV_1 and PEFR after salbutamol.

WORK OF BREATHING

Breathing requires energy. About half of the work done during a respiratory cycle is dissipated during inspiration (as heat) to overcome resistance to airflow. The remaining energy is stored as potential energy in the elastic structures of the lungs and chest wall, and this stored energy is the driving force for normal expiration. The amount of work done is given by the area within the **flow–volume loop** that describes pressure and volume changes during inspiration and expiration (Fig. 13.18).

Flow–volume loops measure the velocity of air flowing through the airways in relation to the volume of air moved during inspiration or expiration. The measurements therefore reflect both the condition of the conducting airways and lung capacity. Analysis of flow–volume loops gives a better idea of where airflow limitation occurs in the lungs. Different pulmonary diseases give different flow–volume loops, so that an experienced chest physician is able to make a diagnosis from the shape of the loop.

In normal individuals, at rest, the work performed by the muscles of respiration is small at between 2% and 5% of the resting oxygen consumption, but with maximal hyperventilation, the work of breathing increases to about 30% of the resting oxygen consumption. The work of breathing increases disproportionately with increasing airflow because:

- As the speed of airflow increases, the air moves in whirls in the airway, rather than in parallel with the walls of the airway, creating 'turbulent flow' (see below)
- The resistance to airflow increases with turbulent flow, requiring the driving pressure for moving the air along to increase by the power of 2, thus increasing the work involved.

The work of breathing can also become much greater when the elastic property of the lung/chest wall, or airway resistance to airflow, increases. The elastic load will increase with lung 'stiffness', as in interstitial pulmonary fibrosis, while flow resistance will be increased with obstructive lung diseases. If the workload becomes too great, respiratory fatigue will develop. When respiratory fatigue develops, the muscles of respiration cannot ventilate the lungs sufficiently to satisfy oxygen requirements. Under these circumstances, patients often require mechanical ventilation unless pharmacological measures reduce their work of breathing.

Airway resistance

Airway resistance is the result of frictional forces opposing the flow of air. Under normal conditions, air flowing through the conducting airways is streamlined, known as **laminar flow**. There is very little resistance to laminar airflow; air at the centre of a tube moves faster than air near the walls of the tube. This is analogous to blood flow (see also Ch. 11).

Where the airways branch or become narrower, or when ventilation increases, the air flows in eddies and whirls rather

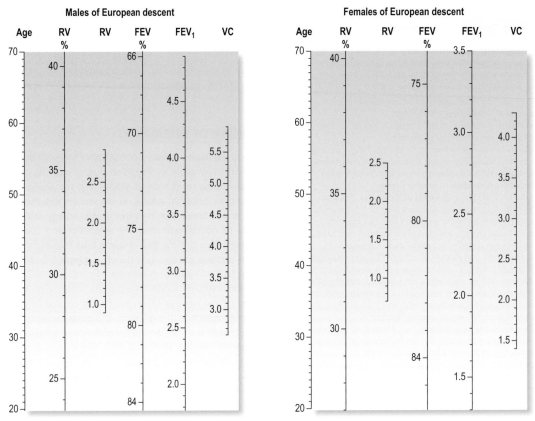

Fig. 13.16 Nomograms showing predicted airflow values for different ages. FEV, forced expiratory volume; RV, residual volume; VC, vital capacity. Percentages are related to the total forced expiratory volume (FEV); FEV$_1$, volume expelled in the first second.

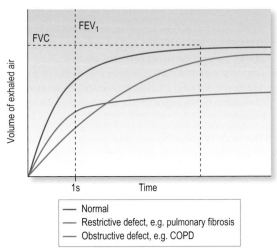

Fig. 13.17 Changes in the forced expiratory volume in 1 second (FEV$_1$) and the forced expiratory capacity (FVC) in obstructive and restrictive pulmonary disease. COPD, chronic obstructive pulmonary disease.

Information box 13.4 | **Measuring airflow limitation in chronic obstructive pulmonary disease**

Patients with COPD, as in asthma, experience periods of acute deterioration in symptoms and increased airway inflammation, with respiratory viruses being an important trigger. Exacerbations are an important cause of mortality, morbidity, excess winter hospital admissions and impairment of quality of life.

The best guide to the severity and progression of COPD is the change in forced expiratory volume (FEV$_1$) over time. FEV$_1$ normally declines after the age of 30, but this decline is accelerated in COPD.

- Stage I – mild: FEV$_1$/FVC < 0.7 and FEV$_1 \geq$ 80% predicted
- Stage II – moderate: FEV$_1$/FVC < 0.7 and 50% < FEV$_1$ < 80% predicted
- Stage III – severe: FEV$_1$/FVC < 0.7 and 30% < FEV$_1$ < 50% predicted
- Stage IV – very severe: FEV$_1$/FVC < 0.7 and FEV$_1$ < 30% predicted or FEV$_1$ < 50% predicted plus chronic respiratory failure.

There is evidence that acute exacerbations of COPD lead to an increased rate of FEV$_1$ decline. No drug treatment has yet been shown to affect the rate of FEV$_1$ decline.

---

than parallel to the walls of the tubes. The smooth laminar flow changes to **turbulent flow** and airway resistance is increased. Turbulent flow is also noisy, as demonstrated by an exhausted athlete at the end of a competition.

Airflow can be modelled in a way that is analogous to the flow of electricity, which can be described by Ohm's law where $R = V/I$ (V = voltage, I = current and R = resistance). In this model $R = P/F$ where resistance to flow (R) is equal to pressure (P) divided by flow (F) (Fig. 13.19).

Airway resistance must be overcome for air to flow. It is analogous to electrical resistance to the flow of electrical current. Greatest resistance is found close to the walls of the airways and least in the centre of the airways. The resistance for laminar airflow (without turbulence) is described by **Poiseuille's equation**:

$$\text{Resistance} = \frac{8 \times \text{length} \times \text{viscosity of gas}}{p \times (\text{radius})^4}$$

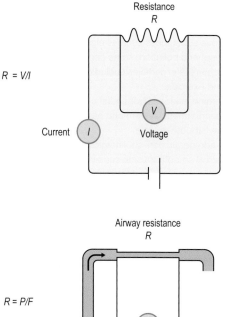

$R = V/I$

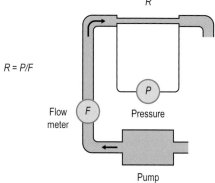

$R = P/F$

Fig. 13.19 **Analogy between electrical and airway resistance.**

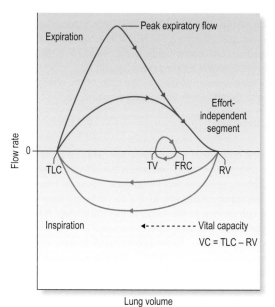

Fig. 13.18 **Normal flow-volume loop for increasing inspirations.** Both meet in a common effort-independent segment. A normal tidal volume (TV) breath is shown. TLC, total lung capacity; FRC, functional respiratory capacity; RV, residual volume.

This equation indicates that resistance to airflow increases dramatically as the airways narrow. In practice, most of the resistance to airflow in lungs is offered by the large airways, trachea and bronchi of more than 2 mm diameter (80–90%) rather than by the smaller airways. This is counter-intuitive because, usually, the narrower the tube the greater the resistance. However, resistance falls moving down the tracheobronchial tree because there are many smaller airways in parallel and thus the effective cross-sectional area is much larger at lower points in the tracheobronchial tree (see Fig. 13.5). In the trachea, which has a diameter of about 20 mm, the cross-sectional area is 3 cm². At generation 23 of the airways, at the level of the alveolar sac, the airways are only 0.4 mm in diameter, but the cross-sectional area is much greater at 4×10^5 cm² because there are so many of them (3×10^8). If this was not the case it would be virtually impossible to ventilate the alveoli.

Airway resistance can be increased by **bronchospasm** (constriction) in smaller, muscular airways, as in asthma, or by partial blockage of the airways with **increased mucus production**, as in chronic bronchitis. Airway resistance can also be increased by pressure due to:

- Structures outside the conducting airways, such as tumours, mediastinal masses or hilar lymph nodes

- Laryngeal spasm
- Blockage of the airways with gastric contents or blood
- Relaxation of the genioglossus muscle during anaesthesia causing the tongue to fall backwards
- Aspirated objects, such as peanuts and pretzels.

Asthma

In asthma the airways are obstructed, increasing resistance and reducing airflow. This obstruction has a number of causes including:

- Constriction of airway smooth muscle, in response to a wide range of stimuli which is usually reversible with bronchodilators.
- Inflammation of the bronchi producing oedema and plugging with mucus. Eosinophils and lymphocytes infiltrate the airways and the epithelium is damaged.

These factors cause pathophysiological changes that lead to airway obstruction and non-uniform ventilation. The triad of **bronchoconstriction**, **inflammation** and **secretion** is useful to bear in mind when considering the principles for appropriate treatment.

Bronchoconstriction

Typically, all asthma patients with active disease have hyper-responsive (hyper-reactive) airways. Bronchomotor tone is mainly under control of the parasympathetic system. The constriction is mediated by efferents from the vagus to ganglia in the walls of the small bronchi, from which short postganglionic fibres lead to nerve endings which release acetylcholine to act on muscarinic receptors in the bronchial smooth muscle, causing bronchoconstriction. Many different triggers can cause bronchospasm. Stimulants include:

- Noxious substances such as cigarette smoke, atmospheric pollution, some occupational sensitizers and chemicals, particles (including nebulised water), cold air and exercise
- Histamine, released from mast cells, which affects the parasympathetic system and has a direct action on airway smooth muscle
- Non-adrenergic non-cholinergic fibres that pass to bronchial smooth muscle can also cause constriction by releasing vasoactive intestinal polypeptide
- Some classes of drugs, such as non-steroidal anti-inflammatory drugs (notably aspirin) and β-adrenoceptor blocking drugs.

Inflammation and secretion

Many **inflammatory mediators** are found in the airway secretions of patients with asthma, causing mucus secretion, bronchoconstriction and gaps in the capillary endothelium. Leakage of protein into the interstitium leads to submucosal oedema, which narrows the lumen, increasing airway resistance, and contributes to bronchial hyper-responsiveness. Inflammatory mediators are released from mast cells, neutrophils and eosinophils.

Mast cells are activated by the attachment of the Fc portion of IgE and other complement fractions. This leads to a rise in intracellular calcium ions as calcium channels open, and the release of a range of mediators, primarily **histamine**, that are stored within granules inside the mast cells. Activation of mast cells will also lead to synthesis of arachidonic acid derivatives such as the leukotriene C4 that cause a slow but sustained contraction of bronchial smooth muscle (see Ch. 6).

Lung inflation and deflation

The force required for inflation and deflation of the lung depends on the stiffness of the lung and surface tension at the surface of the alveoli.

Pressure–volume relationship

During inflation and deflation the pressure around the lung changes with lung volume (Fig. 13.20). During inspiration, there is only a small volume change until a pressure of more than 5–6 mmHg is reached. Subsequent expansion is non-linear until complete expansion is reached at about 15 mmHg. During deflation, the curve is displaced to the left, so that the pressure at any volume is less on expiration than inspiration. This phenomenon, known as **hysteresis**, is attributed to the presence of surface tension at the interface of air and fluid lining the alveolar walls and the effect of surfactant.

Compliance

Compliance is a measure of how easily the lungs can be distended. The elastic properties of the lungs tend to pull them away from the thoracic walls, giving rise to a negative intrapleural pressure (Fig. 13.21). The strength of this elastic force is related to lung volume, so that more inflated lungs that are more stretched give rise to more negative intrapleural pressure. Lung **compliance** is the measure of the relationship between the inflating pressure and lung volume.

Compliance is defined as the ratio of the change in volume to the change in intrapleural pressure, i.e.:

$$\text{Compliance} = \frac{\Delta V}{\Delta P}$$

The changes in lung volume are measure by spirometry. The change in inflating pressure is the difference between atmospheric pressure and intrapleural pressure, measured by an oesophageal balloon, at the two different lung volumes. The compliance of the lungs is therefore lower if the lungs become stiff and less elastic, because ΔV is smaller, as in pulmonary fibrosis. In the healthy adult male it varies from $0.09\,\text{L/cmH}_2\text{O}$ to $0.26\,\text{L/cmH}_2\text{O}$. Compliance varies with lung volume, and can be estimated by determining the slope at any point of the pressure–volume curve in Figure 13.20 (see also Clinical box 13.17). Compliance in the newborn child is relatively low at only $0.005\,\text{L/cmH}_2\text{O}$ and the lungs are not easy to inflate. If there is not sufficient surfactant, as can be seen in premature babies, then inflation becomes even more difficult leading to respiratory distress (see below).

Compliance decreases with age. It is seriously reduced in emphysema, pulmonary fibrosis or pulmonary congestion as the elasticity of the lungs is lost. Lung elasticity can also be lost if the pleurae stiffen, for example with pleural plaques associated with asbestosis or with chest deformity (kyphoscoliosis) or if the skin tightens around the chest because of scars, e.g. from severe burns. A sustained external pressure is also sufficient to prevent expansion of the lungs, such as crushing in crowds or when buried under rubble or snow.

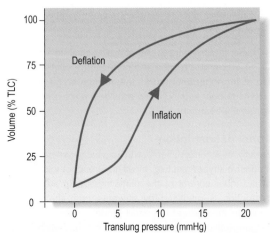

Fig. 13.20 **Pressure–volume relationship in the lung.**

Clinical box 13.17   **Conditions leading to problems in lung inflation**

Atelectasis is a failure of the lungs to expand. This is most commonly caused, whether acutely by foreign bodies or chronically by tumours, when complete obstruction of the airways prevents air inflating the alveoli. Air in this distal region is absorbed and the alveoli collapse. Secretions then accumulate and may become infected. If the lung remains collapsed, irreversible fibrosis occurs. Atelectasis may also be caused when compression, e.g. due to pleural effusion or pneumothorax, opposes inflation.

Bronchiectasis is the condition of permanently dilated bronchi with chronic infection. It is most commonly caused by severe respiratory infection (often in childhood) leading to permanently dilated bronchi, although it can also be caused by congenital abnormalities of the cilia which reduce the removal of mucus from the lungs.

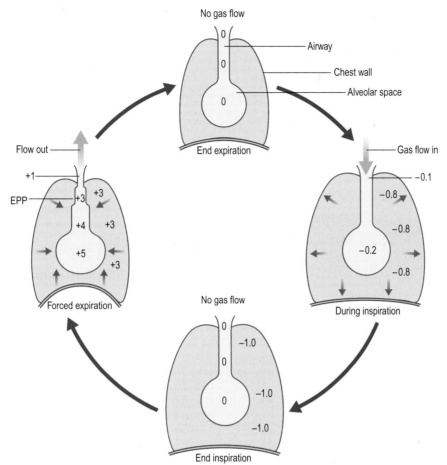

Fig. 13.21 **Pressure changes in the chest and lung in a supine individual during inspiration and forced expiration.** The pleural pressure around the airways is usually negative (less than atmospheric). During inspiration the chest wall expands and there is a greater negative pleural pressure, drawing air into the airways. At forced expiration, the pleural pressure may become positive, forcing air out. The equal pressure point (EPP) is where airway pressure equals pleural pressure.

Surface tension

Alveoli are nearly spherical structures, rather like tiny, interconnecting bubbles. The alveolar surfaces are covered with a thin film of fluid, and surface tension at the air–water interface produces forces that act to reduce the area of the interface. For example, in a soap bubble blown at the end of a tube, the surface contracts as much as it can, forming a sphere and thus minimising the surface area for a given volume. This surface tension generates a pressure inside the bubble that can be predicted using **Laplace's equation**:

$$P = 2 \times \text{surface tension} / \text{radius}$$

The surface tension in the alveolus is inversely proportional to its radius. At a constant surface tension, smaller alveoli would generate a greater pressure and might be expected to collapse into larger alveoli. Surfactant, however, differentially reduces surface tension more at lower volumes than at higher volumes, stabilising the alveoli and preventing collapse.

Experiments on foam generated from fluid extracted from alveoli show it to exert a very low surface tension. Surfactant reduces the surface tension of the thin liquid film covering the whole alveolar surface, where gaseous exchange takes place. This makes the lungs easier to inflate during inspiration, thus increasing compliance and reducing the effort needed for expansion.

Flow-related airway collapse

Air may be trapped behind a collapsed conducting airway during **expiration**. Airways beyond generation 11 in the tracheobronchial tree have no cartilage and hence no structural rigidity and rely on the elastic recoil of the surrounding tissue to prevent collapse.

When making a forced, rapid expiration, intrathoracic pressure must be raised well above atmospheric to generate the required flow rate. As air flows from the alveoli to the mouth, the pressure in the airway will drop due to airway resistance. Thus, at some point along the airway the forces maintaining airway patency match the intrathoracic pressure, and the pressure across the airway wall (the transmural pressure) is zero (Fig. 13.21). Further downstream, i.e. towards the mouth in expiration, the transmural pressure gradient is reversed and the airway collapses. This collapse is temporary, because the occlusion of the airway will increase the pressure behind it (i.e. upstream), raising the intra-airway pressure to open the airway again and restore airflow. This flow-related collapse during a forced expiration accounts for the brassy sound which is occasionally heard. A similar mechanism narrows large airways during coughing to increase the velocity and the scouring action caused by the rapidly moving exhaled air on the airway walls.

The 'collapse point' moves backwards (upstream), towards the smaller airways as the elastic recoil of the lungs is

- Carbon monoxide (CO) is commonly used to assess diffusing capacity. The patient breaths in a small amount of carbon monoxide (0.3% CO in air), holds breath for 10 seconds, and then exhales rapidly during which CO is measured.
- $D_LCO = VCO/(PACO - P_aCO)$
- $PaCO = 0$. There is no back-pressure because of the high affinity of haemoglobin for carbon monoxide

$$D_LCO = \frac{50 \text{ mL/min}}{2 \text{ mmHg}} = 25 \text{ mL/min/mmHg}$$

Normal range for oxygen at rest is 24–36 mL CO/min/mmHg
D_LCO:
- increases with exercise (recruitment and distension of pulmonary capillaries)
- lower in emphysema, interstitial lung disease (emphysema).

reduced with decreasing lung volume. Flow-related collapse in small air passages is common in certain diseases where there is loss of recoil pressure, particularly asthma and emphysema. Airway collapse over time can lead to hyperinflation of the chest because inhaled air is not as fully expired and is thus trapped within the lungs.

Closing capacity and posture

In the upright posture, the airways in the dependent, lowest, parts of the lungs are compressed and narrowed by the weight of the overlying tissues. In these regions, expiration will reduce the volume of air in an airway to a point where the airway closes. The lung volume at which this occurs is known as the **closing capacity**. In young adults, the closing capacity is less than FRC, but it becomes equal to FRC at an approximate age of 44 years in the supine posture and at 66 years in the upright posture. When the closing capacity exceeds the FRC, it begins to compromise gaseous exchange as airways collapse before the lungs are emptied.

PRINCIPLES OF GAS EXCHANGE

DIFFUSION

The movement of gases, principally oxygen and carbon dioxide, across the alveolar–capillary barrier takes place by simple diffusion. The rate of diffusion is related to the concentration gradient of the gases in solution on either side of the blood–gas membrane. The gases flow down a gradient, from a higher to a lower concentration. The fundamental law governing this situation is **Fick's equation**.

$$\text{Rate of diffusion } \frac{dn}{dt} = D \times A \times \frac{dc}{dx}$$

where dn/dt is the rate of linear diffusion (quantity n, time t), D is the diffusion coefficient (cm²/s), A is the surface area, dc is the difference in gas partial pressures and dx is the thickness.

The diffusion coefficient, or diffusion constant (D), is defined as the volume of gas (in mL) which diffuses through 1 cm²/min under a pressure of 1 mmHg. This is related to the size and shape of the gas molecules, so that D is proportional

to the gas solubility (S) but inversely proportional to the square root of the molecular weight of the gas (MW), i.e.

$$D(\propto)S/\sqrt{MW}$$

In the lungs, the efficiency of pulmonary diffusion will depend on the thickness of the alveolar–capillary membrane barrier (dx), which is only about 0.5 μm and may be as little as 0.2 μm in places. The alveolar–capillary barrier comprises the alveolar epithelium (~0.2 μm), a very thin tissue space with a common basement membrane and the capillary endothelium (~0.2 μm) (see Fig. 13.7B). Once across this barrier, oxygen needs to move through the plasma, enter the red blood cell and attach itself to the haemoglobin. The red blood cells are similar in size to pulmonary capillaries, and have to deform to squeeze through and are therefore in intimate contact with the capillary endothelium.

Pulmonary diffusion capacity

Pulmonary diffusion capacity is the ability of the lungs to transfer a gas, usually oxygen (O_2), or carbon dioxide (CO_2), across the alveolar–capillary membrane. The diffusing capacity for both oxygen (D_LO_2) and carbon dioxide (D_LCO_2) is difficult to measure, and therefore not often used clinically. The **single breath carbon monoxide (CO) diffusion test** is the more usual test of pulmonary diffusion capacity. Interpretation of D_LCO needs to be in the context of other clinical and physiological findings.

When it has been measured, oxygen diffusion capacity at rest varies between 15 mL/min/mmHg and 35 mL/min/mmHg. The average is about 20 mL/min/mmHg. The overall diffusion capacity of the lungs increases in exercise, to 65 mL/min/mmHg or more, due to dilatation of the capillaries and opening up of the closed capillary bed in the lung apex. In disease, diffusion capacity is reduced. Thickening of the alveolar–capillary interface can occur in scleroderma, asbestosis, pulmonary fibrosis, pulmonary oedema and sarcoidosis. Reduction of the area of the alveolar–capillary interface may occur through emphysema or surgery.

Measuring lung diffusion capacity – single breath CO testing (D_LCO)

Carbon monoxide (CO) is used in testing pulmonary diffusion capacity. It is a non-reactive gas which binds to haemoglobin with such a high affinity that virtually no CO will be released and diffuse back into the alveoli. In this test, a single breath from a volume of gas containing a known small quantity of carbon monoxide is inspired. The breath is held for 10 seconds, then rapidly and forcibly expired (as in measuring FVC). The expired gas is analysed to determine the amount of CO that was absorbed during the breath, from which the CO diffusing capacity (D_LCO) is calculated as:

$$V_{co}/(p_ACO - p_aCO)$$

but $p_aCO = 0$ because carbon monoxide is bound almost irreversibly to the haemoglobin.

The major types of lung disease causing decreased D_LCO include:

- Destruction of the lung parenchyma with a reduction in the surface area of the alveolar–capillary interface resulting in a reduction in gas transfer (particularly emphysema and possibly cystic fibrosis)

Table 13.4	Partial pressures of the various constituents of air under various conditions				
	Dry gas (%)	Partial pressure of dry gas, at sea level (mmHg)	Partial pressure of dry gas, at 4800 m (16 000 ft) (mmHg)	Partial pressure at sea level (mmHg), moist air at 37°C	Partial pressure of at 4800 m (16 000 ft) (mmHg) moist air at 37°C
Oxygen	21	160	84	150	74
Carbon dioxide	0	0	0	0	0
Nitrogen	79	600	316	563	279
Water vapour	0	0	0	47	47
Total	100	760	400	760	400

- Interstitial lung disease with thickening of the alveolar–capillary membrane causing a reduction in gas transfer, e.g. fibrosing alveolitis, asbestosis
- Pulmonary vascular disease particularly with vascular occlusion and a reduction in the pressure gradient across the alveolar–capillary interface, e.g. pulmonary embolism, pulmonary hypertension.

PARTIAL PRESSURES OF GASES IN AIR

Air is a mixture of oxygen (20.93%), carbon dioxide (0.03%), argon (0.93%), nitrogen (78.09%) and a number of other trace gases, but for all practical purposes, air can be thought to consist of 21% oxygen and 79% nitrogen (Table 13.4). If this mixture was enclosed in a sealed container, then it would exert a pressure as the molecules collide into the walls of the container. The total pressure exerted would be the sum of the separate pressures exerted by each of the gases. A **partial pressure** is therefore the pressure that one of these gases would exert if it occupied the same total volume alone. If the container was not pressurised, then the total pressure exerted by the gas mixture inside the container would equal the outside barometric pressure.

The concept of partial pressures also applies to liquids. Gas molecules will enter a liquid until the partial pressure in the liquid matches that in the surrounding air. The speed at which equilibrium is achieved depends on solubility and chemical binding. Gas volumes are typically stated to be dry or moist, and at:

- **STP**: standard temperature (20°C) and pressure (760 mmHg)
- **BTP**: body temperature, normally taken as 37°C, and atmospheric pressure
- **ATP**: atmospheric temperature and pressure.

The **partial pressure of a dry gas** can be calculated by multiplying its fractional concentration by the barometric pressure. Barometric pressure is the atmospheric pressure exerted by the weight of a column of air on the surface of a unit area at sea level, which is around 760 mmHg. For example, in air, oxygen has a concentration of 21% (a fractional concentration of 0.21). Its partial pressure at a barometric pressure of 760 mmHg is 0.21×760 or 160 mmHg. If the barometer pressure was to fall from 760 mmHg to 400 mmHg while ascending to an altitude of 4800 m (16 000 ft), the partial pressure of oxygen would fall proportionally to 84 mmHg.

When liquids vaporise they also contribute to the total pressure. **Water vapour** complicates the situation as its pressure is dependent on temperature. The partial pressure of gaseous components of humidified air must, therefore, be reduced so that their total will equal barometric pressure *less* water vapour pressure. For example, the vapour pressure of fully saturated air at 37°C is 47 mmHg. In moist air at normal body temperature, oxygen has a partial pressure of 0.21×(760 − 47) or about 150 mmHg.

Expired air is normally fully saturated with water at 37°C. Inspired air may not be fully saturated and the pressure it exerts will be less than at full saturation. The saturation of inhaled air depends on humidity, which is in turn dependent on climatic conditions.

PARTIAL PRESSURES OF GASES IN ALVEOLI AND BLOOD

In human respiration, the partial pressures of O_2 and CO_2 are of particular importance. Partial pressures in alveoli (p_A), sometimes known as **alveolar tension**, would obviously affect the efficiency of gaseous exchange by diffusion. There is a reciprocal relationship between $p_A O_2$ and $p_A CO_2$ so that CO_2 retention in the alveoli reduces $p_A O_2$ and less O_2 enters the blood. Arterial $p_a O_2$ is reduced, which in turn affects the oxygen-carrying capacity of the blood (see below). Normally, the alveolar–arterial oxygen difference ($p_{A-a} O_2$) is small, but increases with diseases that limit diffusion. Clinically, this can be influenced through increasing by a few percentages the concentration of inhaled O_2 or administering air under pressure (i.e. effectively increasing the barometric pressure).

CARRIAGE OF OXYGEN BY THE BLOOD

One of the functions of the circulation is to deliver O_2 to the tissues to sustain metabolism, and the demand for O_2 will vary according to consumption. For example, O_2 consumption will increase many times during exercise. The body has evolved an ingenious way for doing this efficiently, while minimising the effort needed by the heart. O_2 can be carried by blood in two ways:

- Dissolved in the plasma
- Combined with haemoglobin in the red blood cells.

The amount of O_2 dissolved in the plasma is quite small (0.3 mL per 100 mL of arterial blood and 0.13 mL per 100 mL of venous blood). So most oxygen is transported and stored by oxygenated **respiratory pigments**. Almost all of the O_2 is carried by **haemoglobin** in red blood cells, but some is combined with **myoglobin** in muscle. These two molecules each have different functions. Haemoglobin is the main transporter of oxygen to all tissues, whereas myoglobin carries the oxygen reserve for tissues that have variable demand for oxygen (see Ch. 11).

RESPIRATORY PIGMENTS

Haemoglobin and myoglobin both consist of protein chains, the **globin** portion, and a haem group which contains ferrous **iron**. The O_2 molecule combines with an iron molecule in the **haem** part of haemoglobin and myoglobin. Haemoglobin (Hb) and myoglobin (Mb) are structurally different, so that they can fulfil their different functions. Haemoglobin is made up of four subunits each containing one globin chain and one haem group; myoglobin consists of single globin and haem molecules. Haemoglobin therefore has the capacity to carry four molecules of O_2 whereas myoglobin can only carry one molecule of O_2. The presence of haemoglobin greatly increases the O_2-carrying capacity of the blood (see Ch. 12).

Oxygen dissociation curve

A distinction should be made between the O_2 content of the blood and O_2 saturation:

- O_2 **content** refers to the amount of O_2 carried by 1 L of blood
- O_2 **saturation** (S) is the percentage of O_2-carrying sites on the haemoglobin molecule occupied by O_2. Under normal physiological conditions, arterial O_2 saturation, S_aO_2, would be around 100%.

The saturation of haemoglobin depends on the partial pressure of oxygen, pO_2. This relationship is described by the O_2 dissociation curve, which has a sigmoidal or S shape (Fig. 13.22). This relationship ensures that blood is fully saturated with oxygen when it leaves the lungs, even with small reductions in atmospheric O_2, but can easily off-load it when it reaches tissues where the pO_2 is low.

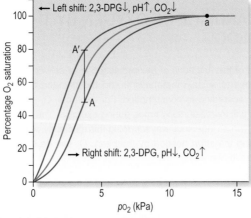

Fig. 13.22 **Oxygen saturation curve, with the Bohr effect and effect of 2,3-diphosphoglycerate (2,3-DPG).** In the tissues, where there is increased 2,3-DPG (a product of energy metabolism), CO_2 and [H^+] (i.e. pH is lower), the shift of the curve means that less O_2 can be carried by haemoglobin at the same pO_2 (A′ to A) and so O_2 is released to the tissues.

Haemoglobin

As discussed above, haemoglobin consists of four subunits of haem and globin. The alteration in the structure in one subunit and the breakage of salt bridges by binding with O_2 alters the structure of the other subunits, making it easier for more O_2 molecules to bind, until there are few haemoglobin molecules that are not fully saturated. Full saturation is not reached until the alveolar p_AO_2 exceeds 100 mmHg. This cooperative binding of O_2 greatly increases the efficiency of haemoglobin as the main O_2 transporter in the blood. O_2 uptake by haemoglobin is extremely rapid, and O_2 off-loading to tissues is even faster. A number of factors can favour unloading of O_2 when the surrounding tissues have a low pO_2, such as in exercising muscle. These include:

- Hydrogen ions
- Temperature
- 2,3-Diphosphoglycerate (2,3-biphosphoglycerate) (2,3-DPG/2,3-BPG).

Hydrogen ions (H^+) reduce haemoglobin affinity for O_2 by altering the haemoglobin structure so that it binds less easily with O_2. This is known as the **Bohr effect**. When tissue pH is reduced (i.e. a rise in H^+), as for example with the accumulation of lactic acid in exercising muscle, or the accumulation of CO_2 in solution from metabolic processes, O_2 dissociates more rapidly from haemoglobin so that the O_2 is unloaded to the tissues needing it (Fig. 13.22). Heat also reduces haemoglobin affinity for O_2. Working tissues generate heat so that more O_2 is given up to it at any pO_2. The haemoglobin affinity for O_2 is reduced by increasing the concentration of 2,3-DPG in the red cells, thus releasing O_2 more easily. 2,3-DPG is produced in response to hypoxia, as in anaemia and high altitude. 2,3-DPG is low in transfused blood and reduces the supply of oxygen to tissue (Information box 13.5).

Myoglobin

Myoglobin is found in muscles, particularly those involved in slow repetitive contractions, e.g. leg muscles or heart muscle of large mammals. Myoglobin has a single protein chain, contains one iron per molecule and its oxygen dissociation curve is a simple rectangular hyperbola. Myoglobin has a greater affinity for oxygen than haemoglobin, and can easily take up oxygen at the low oxygen pressures found in the body. It is 95% saturated at a pO_2 of 40 mmHg. It will rapidly release oxygen under hypoxic conditions. Myoglobin acts as an oxygen reserve when the oxygen demands of muscles are not met by the blood supply, such as when muscular contraction increases the muscles' cross-sectional area and compresses the local blood vessels.

CARRIAGE OF CARBON DIOXIDE BY THE BLOOD

CO_2 is the end-product of tissue metabolism, and has to be transported from the tissues to the lungs. CO_2 also has a role in the maintenance of normal acid–base balance, so that disturbance of CO_2 concentrations is the basis for respiratory acidosis or alkalosis (see below and Ch. 1). It diffuses across cell membranes more easily than O_2, and can be carried in the blood in three ways:

- In solution in plasma and the cytoplasm of red cells
- Combined with the protein subunits of haemoglobin and with other plasma proteins
- As bicarbonate in the plasma (Information box 13.6).

About 3 mL of CO_2 per 100 mL of blood is dissolved in the blood at a pCO_2 of 40 mmHg. A further 0.1–0.2 mL CO_2 per

100 mL blood will be in the form of carbonic acid, which is formed when CO_2 is dissolved in water:

$$CO_2 + H_2O \rightleftharpoons H_2CO_3$$

Carbon dioxide can also form neutral carbamino compounds with the amino acid subunits of haemoglobin and to a lesser extent with other plasma proteins. Carbon dioxide reacts with the amine (NH_2) groups of the protein. When deoxygenated, blood carries about 4 mL of CO_2 as carbamino per 100 mL of blood.

The remaining carbon dioxide (45 mL per 100 mL deoxygenated blood) is carried in the blood as hydrogen and bicarbonate ions (HCO_3^-). These are formed rapidly within the red blood cells by the enzyme **carbonic anhydrase** (CA), which catalyses the rapid formation of carbonic acid. Carbonic acid then dissociates into H^+ and HCO_3^-:

$$CO_2 + H_2O \rightleftharpoons H_2CO_3 \rightleftharpoons H^+ + HCO_3^-$$

Carbonic anhydrase is a zinc-containing enzyme that can be inhibited by cyanide and the enzyme acetazolamide. Much use has been made of acetazolamide in experimental investigations into the role of carbonic anhydrase in other organs – gastric mucosa, pancreas and renal tubular cells – but it also acts as a diuretic and is used in treatment of raised intraocular pressure (glaucoma) and altitude sickness.

CARBON DIOXIDE DISSOCIATION CURVE

At a given pCO_2, the degree of oxygen saturation will influence the CO_2-carrying capacity of the blood. In the lungs, as haemoglobin becomes fully saturated, CO_2 is displaced and therefore excreted, whereas in the tissues, the off-loading of O_2 from haemoglobin enables it to increase its affinity for CO_2 (Fig. 13.23).

Haemoglobin reacts more readily with CO_2 to form carbamino compounds as it off-loads O_2, increasing the CO_2-carrying capacity of blood. The opposite occurs as haemoglobin becomes oxygenated, with a decrease in CO_2-carrying capacity. This is known as **Haldane's effect**, and mirrors the Bohr effect for O_2. The overall relationship between carbon dioxide content and pCO_2 is curvilinear, but over the physiological range, i.e. between the extremes of arterial and venous blood (40 mmHg and 46 mmHg, respectively), it is essentially linear. The relationship is quite steep: approximately 0.7 mL CO_2 per 100 mL blood is unloaded for 1 mmHg drop in pCO_2. This ability to load or unload CO_2 with minimal change in pCO_2 helps to minimise the change in pH between arterial and venous blood.

DISTURBANCES OF ACID–BASE BALANCE

The physiology of renal and metabolic acid–base control is discussed elsewhere (Ch. 1) but it is intimately linked to respiratory acid–base control. Respiration is in part under regulation by the hydrogen ion concentration of the cerebral spinal fluid in the brain (see Control of breathing, below). This feedback system will cause hyperventilation to lower plasma pH or hypoventilation to increase plasma pH. Thus, in patients with metabolic disorders, ventilation can be used to quickly compensate for disturbances in acid–base balance. Conversely, chronic respiratory disease will lead to disturbance in the balance that can only be slowly compensated for by excretion or retention of hydrogen ions in the urine,

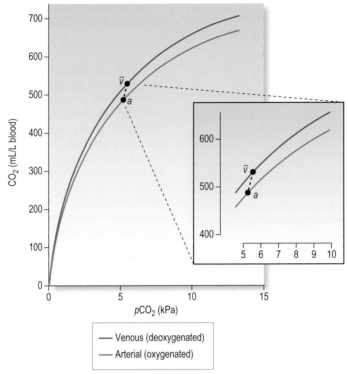

Fig. 13.23 The carbon dioxide dissociation curve. The ability of deoxygenated blood to carry more CO_2 than oxygenated blood is called the Haldane effect. The enlarged part of the curve shows how this effect 'steepens' the true physiological curve and enables deoxygenated blood in the tissues to pick up in excess of 50 mL more CO_2 per litre than it would if it remained oxygenated.

although most hydrogen ions are buffered in the urine by bicarbonate or phosphate, or converted to ammonia.

Hydrogen ion concentrations ($[H^+]$) in the blood are normally very low at about 40 nmol/L, i.e. 10^{-7} L, expressed by the term **pH**, which is the log 1/$[H^+]$. Water has a pH of 7 and is regarded as neutral. An increase in the hydrogen ion concentration in the blood, and thus lowering the pH to below 7, is described as **acidaemia** or **acidosis**, while a reduction (rise in pH) is described as **alkalaemia** or **alkalosis**. There are four classes of acid–base disorder depending on whether it causes acidaemia or alkalaemia, and whether the problem is caused by the respiratory system or a metabolic problem.

The four classes of acid–base disorder

Respiratory acidosis

- Is caused by retention of carbon dioxide: the blood p_aCO_2 rises and pH falls.
- Is associated with impaired efficiency of gaseous exchange. Common causes include type II respiratory failure in COPD and respiratory depression from drugs or paralysis of respiratory muscles (see below).

Respiratory alkalosis

- p_aCO_2 falls and pH rises.
- Causes are over-breathing (hyperventilation) which causes blood p_aCO_2 to fall as the fresh air drawn into the lungs favours the removal of CO_2 from the body. Hyperventilation can be due to hysteria, aspirin poisoning, cerebral diseases such as viral infection (encephalitis) or head injuries.

Metabolic acidosis

- Caused by excessive production of hydrogen ions, for example in diabetic ketosis or with increased lactic acid production following shock or in any situation where tissue perfusion is compromised.
- Can also occur with the loss of fluid rich in bicarbonate from the small intestines, e.g. because of diarrhoea or loss of intestinal contents through aspiration tubes or fistulae.
- Less common is loss of bicarbonate from the kidney due to a defect in its reabsorption.

There are characteristic breathing patterns in metabolic acidosis that develop as acidosis increases called **Kussmaul** respiration, consisting of very deep and gasping rapid but regular breathing.

Metabolic alkalosis

- Caused by excessive intake of bicarbonate in the treatment of peptic ulceration, or by loss of acidic fluids by vomiting gastric contents.
- Respiratory compensation is often slight, and it is rare to encounter a p_aCO_2 above 6.5 kPa (50 mmHg) even with severe alkalosis.

MATCHING LUNG VENTILATION TO LUNG PERFUSION

Ventilation is the movement of air in and out of the lungs. Specifically, alveolar ventilation refers to the movement of air in and out of the alveoli. The rate at which oxygen exchange can take place at the alveolus then depends on the blood flow through the alveolar tissues, called **perfusion**. The efficiency of gas exchange thus concerns both ventilation and perfusion.

VENTILATION–PERFUSION RATIO

In the healthy resting adult about 4 L of air ventilate the alveoli (V_A) and 5 L of blood pass through the lungs (Q) each minute. Hence, the mean ventilation–perfusion ratio (V_A/Q) is 4/5 or 0.8.

Uneven perfusion

In health, efficient exchange of gases between alveolar air and the blood would occur if alveolar ventilation matched the alveolar perfusion. However, blood flow through different parts of the lungs is uneven. In the upright position, blood flow is maximal at the lung bases, decreasing linearly to the apices. There is a 7–10-fold increase in perfusion at the bases relative to the apex of the lungs. This can be explained by the differences in hydrostatic pressure within the blood vessels in different parts, or zones, in the lungs (Fig. 13.24).

Zone 1 is at the top of the lungs where blood flow is poor, because the mean pulmonary artery pressure of 11–15 mmHg is barely sufficient to propel blood the 15 cm to the lung apices in an upright individual. Should pulmonary arterial pressure (p_a) fall below alveolar pressure (p_A), the capillaries would collapse and no blood flow would be possible. In this case, despite normal alveolar ventilation, there is no perfusion and gaseous exchange cannot take place. This

zone then becomes an alveolar dead space. This phenomenon occurs when pulmonary arterial pressure falls, e.g. due to blood loss. Perfusion is then dependent on the difference between p_a and p_A.

The effect of hydrostatic pressure increases pulmonary arterial pressure lower down in the upright lungs, in zone 2, where it exceeds alveolar pressure. Pulmonary venous pressure (p_v), however, is still below alveolar pressure. In this case, blood flow is determined by the pressure difference between the pulmonary artery and alveolus, with venous pressure being unimportant.

Here blood flow is determined by the arterial–venous pressure difference since both arterial and venous pressures are higher than alveolar pressure.

Pulmonary venous pressure only affects perfusion when it exceeds alveolar pressure, and this occurs in zone 3, the lung bases. Gravity, together with hydrostatic pressure, further raises arterial pressure, but venous pressure also rises due to gravity. Blood flow here is determined by the difference between arterial and venous pressure.

Uneven ventilation

The distribution of inspired air is also not uniform, with a 1.5–3-fold greater ventilation of the base in healthy individuals. This occurs because there are regional differences in **airway resistance** and **compliance** that influence the alveolar filling time in each region. The situation is further complicated by the time constants for alveolar filling being affected by the rate, duration and frequency of inspiration. Other factors affecting ventilation involve airway closure, the right bronchus being at less of an angle to the trachea than the left, and the conformation of the chest and diaphragm.

Ventilation–perfusion mismatch

Ideally, the amount of ventilation (V_A) to a given area of lung should be matched with the amount of blood perfusing (Q) that area for the efficient exchange of oxygen and carbon dioxide. The ventilation–perfusion ratio is commonly used to describe their mismatch. Because of the variations in perfusion and ventilation, the V_A/Q ratio varies from 3.3 at the apex of the lungs to 0.6 in the base. The effect of V_A/Q mismatch on gaseous exchange can be minimised. Localised hypoxia in under-ventilated areas of the lungs causes local vasoconstriction, so that blood is diverted to better ventilated areas. The importance of V_A/Q matching is illustrated by an often quoted example of one lung being ventilated but not perfused while the other is perfused but not ventilated. If this absurd situation arose suddenly, the individual would soon die from asphyxia. Clinical conditions leading to uneven ventilation include:

- Asthma
- COPD
- Emphysema
- Pneumothorax
- Pulmonary fibrosis.

Uneven blood flow may arise from:

- Anatomical shunts (right to left): blood flow through an area of lung with no ventilation due to airway obstruction or collapse
- Regional destruction of vascular beds by emphysema

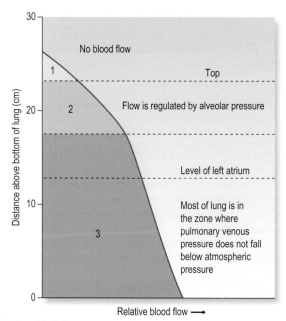

Fig. 13.24 Uneven distribution of blood flow in the lungs results in regional differences in gas exchange down the normal lung. Three zones can be identified. Zone 1 is where alveolar pressure exceeds capillary pressure and so no blood flow occurs. This will be very small and at the apices of the lung in normal healthy people. In zone 2, gas exchange will vary with the balance of alveolar pressure and capillary pressure. The latter increases in systole, forcing open more capillaries. In zone 3, the hydrostatic pressure in the column of blood above the heart is sufficient to keep the alveolar capillaries open throughout the respiratory cycle.

Clinical box 13.20   **Pulmonary embolism**

Pulmonary embolism is a condition in which blood clots migrate into the pulmonary arterial system, blocking the circulation and preventing deoxygenated blood from passing through the ventilated parts of the lungs. These areas of lung are ventilated, but not perfused, creating a **dead space** where gaseous exchange cannot take place. Many emboli originate from deep vein thrombi in the legs or pelvis and most of these lodge in the large or intermediate pulmonary arteries. Fat emboli can be released from fractured bones and usually end up in the smaller pulmonary vessels. Once lodged in the lung, the thrombi start to lyse but massive emboli can cause rapid death.

In order to prevent pulmonary emboli in patients undergoing surgery, deep vein thromboses are avoided by rapid mobilisation after the operation, the use of elastic pressure stockings to prevent vascular stasis and the prophylactic use of anticoagulants.

- Pulmonary embolism (see Clinical box 13.20) or tumour preventing blood flow to an area of the lung
- Increased pulmonary vascular resistance due to heart failure.

CONTROL OF BREATHING

The requirement for O_2 by the human body varies widely, being low during sleep and at rest, and rising during exercise. At the same time, CO_2 output also varies. Yet, despite these variations, the partial pressures of arterial O_2 and CO_2 are kept within narrow limits. The control of breathing for effective gas exchange in the lungs to maintain a normal p_aO_2 and p_aCO_2 is regulated by the nervous system.

Respiration is controlled by the nervous system, and like all neural systems the process has an afferent pathway, where receptors or sensors collect information to be relayed to:

- A central control in the brainstem
- An efferent, or effector pathway to the muscles of respiration.

The reflex control of breathing can, however, be overridden by higher, cortical centres when voluntary respiration becomes necessary (Fig. 13.25).

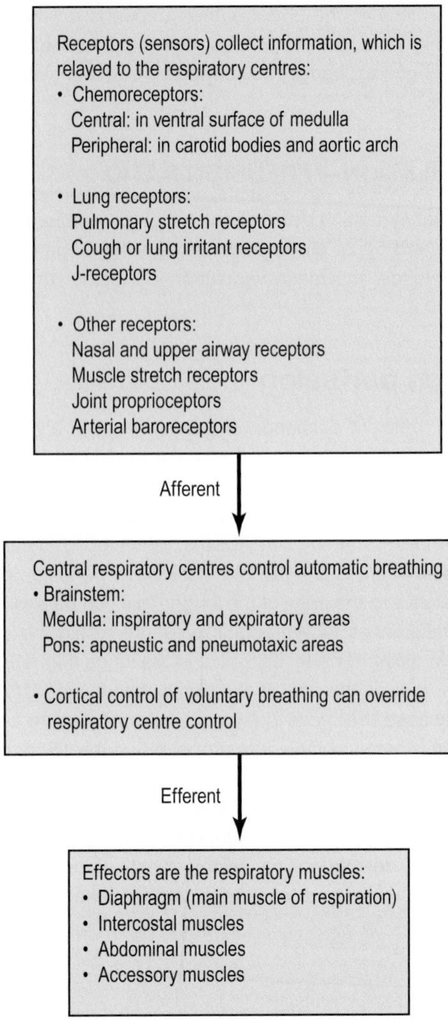

THE RESPIRATORY CENTRE

The **respiratory centre** is a collection of neurons situated in the **medulla** of the brainstem which control the **pattern of breathing**. This **primary centre** consists of a collection of separately arranged neurons that are capable of altering their firing threshold so that activity oscillates between them during inspiration and expiration. The neurons responsible for inspiration are in the dorsal medulla, and those for expiration are in the ventral medulla. The **primary centre** is under the influence of two centres in the pons:

- The **apneustic centre** (apneusis = prolonged inspiration or gasping inspiration) is located at the level of the area vestibularis in the lower pons. Impulses from the apneustic centre may stimulate the inspiration areas of the medulla.
- The **pneumotaxic centre** is located in the upper part of the pons. If the brain is transected just above this centre, inspiration and expiration take the same time, suggesting

Receptors (sensors) collect information, which is relayed to the respiratory centres:
- Chemoreceptors:
  Central: in ventral surface of medulla
  Peripheral: in carotid bodies and aortic arch

- Lung receptors:
  Pulmonary stretch receptors
  Cough or lung irritant receptors
  J-receptors

- Other receptors:
  Nasal and upper airway receptors
  Muscle stretch receptors
  Joint proprioceptors
  Arterial baroreceptors

Afferent

Central respiratory centres control automatic breathing
- Brainstem:
  Medulla: inspiratory and expiratory areas
  Pons: apneustic and pneumotaxic areas

- Cortical control of voluntary breathing can override respiratory centre control

Efferent

Effectors are the respiratory muscles:
- Diaphragm (main muscle of respiration)
- Intercostal muscles
- Abdominal muscles
- Accessory muscles

Fig. 13.25   **The component parts in the control of breathing.**

that the pneumotaxic centre inhibits inspiration. Cells in these centres in the pons therefore affect rhythm in the respiratory centre, but are not essential.

The drive for ventilation can be inhibited by depression of the respiratory neurons of the medulla by hypoxia, a wide variety of therapeutic drugs (opiates, barbiturates and anaesthetic agents) and inhibition of blood supply (by pressure, trauma, neoplasm or vascular catastrophe). Severe respiratory depression can lead to respiratory failure and eventually death. There is a wide range of different breathing patterns that are produced under different conditions (Information box 13.7).

RESPIRATORY RECEPTORS (Clinical box 13.21)

The neurons in the respiratory centre also respond to many afferent impulses arising from a wide variety of respiratory receptors. These receptors control ventilation by increasing or decreasing the volume of air breathed in or out, whereas the medullary centres control the patterns of respiration.

Respiratory chemoreceptors

There are two groups of chemoreceptors (Clinical box 13.22):

- Central chemoreceptors respond to changes in the pH of cerebrospinal fluid (CSF)

- Peripheral chemoreceptors respond to changes in the O_2 and CO_2 content in the blood.

Central chemoreceptors

The central chemoreceptors lie just below the anterolateral surfaces of the medulla, close to the origins of the glossopharyngeal (IX) and vagus nerves (X), but are anatomically separate from the medullary respiratory centre. They respond to changes in the pH of the surrounding CSF. A rising pH

(lowering the hydrogen ion (H^+) concentration) inhibits ventilation, whereas lowering the pH (rising H^+ concentration) stimulates it. The composition of the CSF is determined by blood flow and metabolic processes.

The **blood–brain barrier** separates the CSF from the blood. Hydrogen ions cannot pass through the blood–brain barrier, but CO_2 diffuses through it easily. CO_2 crossing the blood–brain barrier combines with water to form carbonic acid, which is then ionised to release H^+. CSF is relatively poorly buffered, so that CSF H^+ concentration is proportional to p_aCO_2.

Through this mechanism, a rise in p_aCO_2 (**hypercapnia**) would thus cause a rise in brain extracellular H^+ (fall in pH, acidosis), and increased ventilation. This central response to an increase in p_aCO_2 is relatively slow when compared to the response by peripheral chemoreceptors (see below). There is also considerable variation between people in the ventilatory response to CO_2. However, p_aCO_2 is the most important factor in the regulation of ventilation and 80% of the stimulus to ventilation originates in the medullary chemoreceptors.

Peripheral chemoreceptors

Peripheral chemoreceptors are located in:

- The carotid bodies, found above or near the bifurcation of the common carotid artery on either side of the neck
- The aortic bodies in the aortic arch.

The carotid and aortic bodies are surrounded by sinusoidal capillaries which allow the cells within them to be bathed directly by blood. Specialised cells called glomus cells (peripheral chemoreceptors similar in structure to neurons) in the small carotid bodies respond to hypoxia by releasing dopamine on to afferent nerves of the carotid sinus nerve which run to the glossopharyngeal nerve and thence to the medullary respiratory centres. Afferents from the aortic body run via the aortic nerve to the vagus.

The peripheral chemoreceptors respond rapidly, within 1–3 seconds, to falls in p_aO_2 (hypoxia) and pH, or rises in p_aCO_2 (hypercapnia), to increase ventilation. Experiments show that gas mixtures containing little O_2 will stimulate ventilation only if the nerves to these chemoreceptors are intact, suggesting that peripheral chemoreceptors respond to an O_2 deficit, whereas the central chemoreceptors do not.

The carotid bodies are extremely well perfused (2000 mL/min per 100 g tissue), although in absolute terms the blood flow through them is small (40 µL/min). Likewise, their O_2 consumption on a relative scale is high (9 mL/min per 100 g).

They undergo hypertrophy during chronic hypoxia such as in COPD or during acclimatisation to high altitude.

Lung receptors

Pulmonary stretch receptors

Pulmonary stretch receptors lie close to or in the smooth muscle of the bronchi and trachea. Whether they also exist in bronchiolar smooth muscle is less clear. The receptors are localised chiefly at the points of bronchial branching, where the smooth muscle is thickest. Drugs that increase bronchial tone increase stretch receptor discharge. Stretch receptors can also be found at the lower end of the trachea and the main bronchi.

The afferent fibres from pulmonary stretch receptors run in the vagus nerve in large myelinated fibres to send impulses to the respiratory centre. Inflating the lungs stimulates these receptors. Thus, during normal breathing, vagal impulse activity from stretch receptors increases with the onset of inspiration, dying down as expiration begins. Stimulation of the stretch receptors by maximally inflating the lungs in humans inhibits inspiration, thereby limiting tidal volume, and also slows respiratory rate. This so-called **Hering–Breuer lung inflation reflex** (first described in 1868) is important in situations in which an increased depth and rate of breathing is needed, such as during exercise, preventing over-inflation of the lungs. Although it is thought that this reflex is inactive in adult human beings until the tidal volume exceeds 1 L, the reflex produces an increase in respiratory frequency by shortening the time for inspiration. Thus the need to increase ventilation is satisfied. There is an added benefit in that the energy expenditure involved in breathing is minimised as deep breathing requires more energy than more frequent smaller volume breaths. There is evidence to suggest that this reflex is more important in infants.

Cough or lung-irritant receptors

Cough is a common symptom in a range of respiratory diseases and can be a useful diagnostic tool (Clinical box 13.23). It is a sudden explosive expiratory manoeuvre when an expiratory effort against a closed glottis is suddenly released. Coughing intends to clear material such as sputum from the airways. It also helps protect the lungs against aspiration. Coughing is caused by the stimulation of receptors by foreign bodies or sputum in the bronchi or trachea. Histological studies show that there are receptors throughout the airways from the trachea to the bronchioles which respond to foreign bodies and reflexively cause coughing.

Clinical box 13.23 **Different types of cough**

Different types of cough are characteristic of different conditions. Conditions such as pneumonia and chronic obstructive pulmonary disease (COPD) cause a productive cough. The cough may be intermittent or persistent, or may be worse in the morning or at night. Coughing can also be stimulated by non-respiratory causes such as gastro-oesophageal reflex or treatment with angiotensin-converting enzyme inhibitors. A productive cough (i.e. one with sputum) should not be suppressed as the mucus needs to be cleared. Mucolytics reduce the viscosity of the mucus, aiding clearance. Antitussives, such as codeine, suppress coughing by acting centrally. Expectorants are also intended to reduce the viscosity of the mucus and increase the fluid in the respiratory tract although their effectiveness is disputed.

Myelinated afferent fibres from the cough or lung-irritant receptors run in the vagus to the respiratory centre in the central nervous system. The receptors also respond to irritants, such as sulphur dioxide, but stimulation of these receptors in the intrapulmonary bronchi and the bronchioles does not cause coughing; hence these are named **lung-irritant receptors**. Stimulation of these receptors causes hyperpnoea (deep inhalation) and reflex bronchial or laryngeal constriction. The nose and upper airways contain receptors that respond to chemical and mechanical stimulation in a similar way to the lung-irritant receptors. Reflex responses include sneezing, coughing and bronchoconstriction. These reflexes need to be abolished with local anaesthetics when passing an endotracheal or nasogastric tube.

Haemoptysis

Haemoptysis occurs when there is bleeding from the airways. This can vary from streaks of blood in the sputum to massive bleeding. Bleeding usually arises from the bronchial circulation rather than the pulmonary circulation, unless trauma or erosion by a granulomatous or calcified lymph node or a tumour has damaged a major pulmonary vessel. Haemoptysis is a symptom described by patients, and needs to be distinguished from haematemesis (bringing up blood from the stomach). It is a serious symptom and must always be investigated.

J-receptors

The **J-receptors** (juxtacapillary receptors) lie in the alveolar walls, close to the capillaries. Impulses from these receptors travel along slowly conducting nerve fibres in the vagus nerve when the receptors are stimulated by the presence of interstitial fluid in the alveoli and by histamine and other inflammatory mediators. Their stimulation may be the cause of the dyspnoea and the rapid, shallow breathing in left ventricular failure and interstitial pulmonary disease.

Other receptors

There are other types of receptors located in parts of the body other than the respiratory system which can also respond to the need for more oxygen. Stimulation of these receptors leads to increased inspiration.

Muscle stretch receptors

Muscle stretch receptors are located in the **muscle spindles** of the diaphragm and the intercostal muscles. The intercostal muscles contain numerous muscle spindles whereas the diaphragm (the main respiratory muscle) is sparsely supplied. The spindles are richly innervated and lie in parallel with the muscle fibres. As the muscle is stretched so too are the spindles, leading to an increased rate of discharge of their action potential. The rate of increase is dependent on the rate of muscle movement; thus they can signal both instantaneous length and the velocity of stretch. These receptors reflexively control the strength of muscle contraction to increase the depth of breathing. They may give rise to dyspnoea when large breathing efforts are required, e.g. in airways obstruction or when breathing through a narrow tube.

Joint proprioceptors

The costovertebral joints contain mechanoreceptors that are sensitive to rib displacement. These **joint proprioceptors** are the thought to be the main site of impulses giving rise to the conscious sensation of lung distension since this sensation is still present when the vagus is severed and input from the pulmonary and intercostal stretch receptors is lost. These joint proprioceptors are involved in the sensation of dyspnoea arising from absence of chest movement during, e.g. breath-holding (see below). Impulses from the movement of the limbs may signal increased breathing during early stages of exercise.

Baroreceptors

A rise in blood pressure detected by the carotid or aortic sinus **baroreceptors** tends to depress respiration, causing hypoventilation or apnoea. The reverse occurs when blood pressure falls, leading to hyperventilation. The afferents run in the carotid sinus nerve or glossopharyngeal nerve.

HIGHER CENTRE CONTROL OF BREATHING

Breathing is voluntary to some extent, and, within limits, cortical activity can over-ride reflex control of ventilation. Voluntary hyperventilation (deep, rapid breathing) can blow off CO_2 to lower p_aCO_2, causing a rise in pH (alkalosis). The resultant alkalosis effectively leads to hypocalcaemia, which may cause tetany with muscle spasm in the hand and foot (carpopedal spasm). Hypoventilation or breath-holding is more difficult because the duration of breath-holding is restricted by either p_aCO_2 or p_aO_2 (see later). Breathing patterns can also be altered by emotions such as fear or anger.

ENERGY PRODUCTION AND OXYGEN CONSUMPTION

The primary function of respiration is to supply oxygen for the combustion of food stuffs and to remove carbon dioxide. This is described by the **respiratory quotient** (RQ), which is the ratio of the CO_2 production to the O_2 consumption (Information box 13.8). The RQ is affected by:

- Changes in acid–base balance from whatever cause
- Hyperventilation
- The type of food consumed (metabolic fuels).

Information box 13.8 | **Respiratory quotient changes with diet and ventilation**

- A person eating a mixed Western diet containing carbohydrates, fats and proteins will have an overall or average RQ of 0.85
- A highly physically active person on a predominately carbohydrate diet will have a higher RQ, closer to 1
- A diabetic patient will have a low RQ due to the increased utilisation of fats and decreased metabolism of carbohydrates.
  RQ can be affected by changes in pulmonary ventilation that are unrelated to food metabolism:
- Hyperventilation (voluntary hyperpnoea) will wash out excessive quantities of CO_2 from the body and RQ will rise above 1
- RQ will rise in acidosis and will fall in alkalosis from metabolic causes, because of the raised and lowered CO_2 excretion produced by respiratory compensation
- RQ will rise in severe exercise as lactic acid is produced and ventilation is overstimulated.

RESPIRATORY QUOTIENT AS AN INDICATION OF METABOLIC FUEL

If only carbohydrates are metabolised, e.g. glucose ($C_6H_{12}O_6$), the volume of CO_2 produced is equal to the volume of O_2 used, and the RQ is equal to 1.

$$C_6H_{12}O_6 + 6O_2 \rightleftharpoons 6CO_2 + 6H_2O$$

Thus

$$RQ = \frac{6CO_2}{6O_2} = 1$$

The metabolism of fatty acids alone gives an RQ of about 0.7. For example, stearic acid is converted in a two-stage process:

$$C_{17}H_{35}COOH + 8O_2 \rightleftharpoons 3C_6H_{12}O_6$$

$$C_6H_{12}O_6 + 6O_2 \rightleftharpoons 6CO_2 + 6H_2O$$

Overall, the reaction is

$$C_{17}H_{35}COOH + 26O_2 \rightleftharpoons 18CO_2 + 18H_2O$$

Thus

$$RQ = 18/26 \approx 0.7$$

The RQ for protein depends on the precise amino acid composition of the protein but RQ for the average protein is about 0.8. RQ can be used to calculate energy consumption in humans using indirect calorimetry (see below). This has clinical significance, as energy consumption increases or decreases in diseases such as hyperthyroidism or hypothyroidism.

METHODS FOR ESTIMATING ENERGY CONSUMPTION

Energy consumption in the healthy human varies according to their nutritional status and physical activity (see Ch. 16). This can be quantified as the **basal metabolic rate** (**BMR**) plus the additional energy needed in fuel metabolism and growth, to combat cold and for physical activity. It may be altered by disease processes, for example thyroid disease, when energy consumption could be increased or decreased by the effects of disordered hormone activity.

Basal metabolic rate

BMR refers to the minimum energy used by the body to maintain the essential activities of the brain, heart and lungs. BMR is commonly expressed as a fraction of the body's surface area. A person of average height 1.7 m and weight 70 kg has a surface area of 1.8 m^2. Before the discovery of immunoassays for thyroid hormones, BMR was the standard test for the diagnosis of hypo- and hyperthyroidism. There are two methods of measuring BMR:

- **Direct calorimetry** – which is based on the principle that energy expended by the body is eventually lost as heat
- **Indirect calorimetry** – which is based on the principle that energy consumption depends on oxygen consumption, which can be easily measured.

For a man the average BMR is about 46 W/m^2 and for women 42 W/m^2. The lower figure of women is probably due to their greater fat content and lower muscle mass. In newborn babies, for whom the surface area is not known, BMR is given by the oxygen consumption as 4.8 mL/min/kg. On the day after birth, it averages 6.6 mL/min/kg and then is about 7.0–7.2 mL/min/kg for the next 18 months. After that, BMR falls gradually with age.

CHALLENGES TO NORMAL RESPIRATION

EXERCISE

During exercise, both ventilation and oxygen consumption increase linearly with work load (Table 13.5). The severity of exercise is a subjective sensation which appears related more to the oxygen consumption than to the work done.

The mechanism by which ventilation during exercise is controlled is unclear. Arterial blood gases are substantially unchanged by exercise up to an O_2 consumption of 3 L/min at sea level, and so cannot easily explain the increased ventilation. This is not to say that chemoreceptors cannot feed into the respiratory control system, as administering pure O_2 during exercise will depress ventilation. Factors thought to play a role in regulating ventilation during exercise include:

- Feedback from joint proprioceptors
- The anticipation of exercise
- Increased venous return and cardiac output
- Rising core temperature
- Increased sensitivity of the peripheral chemoreceptors to oscillations in arterial pH and pCO_2.

In severe exercise, ventilation may be further increased by lactic acid from muscles lowering blood pH and the release of potassium ions from exercising muscles. This increased ventilation may actually lower p_aCO_2 as CO_2 is blown off. During heavy exercise, ventilation cannot supply sufficient O_2. The difference is made up by anaerobic metabolism, which produces lactic acid. The point when anaerobic metabolism starts is called the aerobic threshold. The threshold can be raised by physical training; available evidence suggests no difference in the benefit of continuous or intermittent training at the threshold.

The phenomenon of a **second wind** during exercise, which can be marked in untrained individuals, occurs when the initial dyspnoea and raised p_aCO_2 disappears. It coincides with increased body temperature and the onset of sweating.

Table 13.5	Oxygen consumption at different levels of activity
Exercise	**Oxygen consumption (mL/min)**
Rest	200
Brisk walking (5 km/h)	1000
Running (12 km/h)	3000
Severe exercise	4000
Elite rowers, for a brief period*	6600

*From Clark JM, et al. (1983) J Appl Physiol 55:440.

ALTITUDE

As a person ascends a mountain or in an aircraft, barometric pressure falls but the fractional concentration of oxygen and the saturated vapour pressure of the air remains constant (see Table 13.4). Thus, the inspired pO_2 falls according to:

$$\text{Inspired } pO_2 = 0.21 \times (\text{barometric pressure} - 47) \text{ mmHg}$$
$$= 74 \text{ mmHg}$$

Physiological responses to high altitude

Sudden exposure to high altitude, as in ascent in a hot air balloon or unpressurised aircraft, leads to acute, severe hypoxia and loss of consciousness. O_2 must therefore be provided in unpressurised aircraft for passengers above 3700 m (12 000 ft). Pilots are required to use oxygen above 3000 m to ensure safety.

During more gradual exposure to high altitude, as when climbing a mountain, the peripheral chemoreceptors are the first to respond to hypoxia, leading to hyperventilation. As CO_2 is washed out, p_aCO_2 is lowered, and consequently the pH of the blood and CSF rises (alkalosis). This hypocapnia places a brake on the ventilation response to the hypoxia, so that hyperventilation is less than would otherwise occur if p_aCO_2 remained normal.

In a few hours, active transport of bicarbonate out of the CSF brings the pH of CSF under control, but the kidneys take longer to excrete the bicarbonate and bring arterial pH under control. It should be remembered that haemoglobin without O_2 is also more alkaline and this adds to the alkalosis. Increased bicarbonate excretion leads to diuresis. Dehydration may occur. Water and electrolyte imbalance such as potassium deficiency and sodium retention could accompany mountain sickness (see below). In the longer term, hypoxia causes an increase in pulmonary vasoconstriction and may lead to pulmonary oedema. Hypocapnia, from hyperventilation, decreases cerebral blood flow giving rise to symptoms of cerebral dysfunction. Cerebral oedema may also occur, although the pathophysiology is not clear. Currently is it hypothesised that hypoxic stimulation of neurohumoral and haemodynamic receptors in the brain allow capillary leakage in the microvasculature, leading to development of oedema.

To compensate for the low alveolar pO_2, the body attempts to increase the blood O_2-carrying capacity by increasing red cell volume. Renal erythropoietin secretion increases so that haemoglobin concentrations rise from an average of 141 g/L to 196 g/L after 4 weeks (polycythaemia) (see also Ch. 12). Elite athletes may train at altitude to increase the oxygen-carrying capacity of their blood before returning to sea level to compete. At altitude, the accompanying increase in blood viscosity increases resistance to blood flow which may be offset by a general vasodilatation.

Acclimatisation to altitude

Over time, a series of integrated physiological adaptations takes place in people living at high altitudes to restore tissue oxygenation to normal levels: acclimatisation. This process includes:

- Hyperventilation
- Correction of persistent alkalosis

- Polycythaemia
- Increased cardiac output
- Increased tolerance for physical exercise.

Mountain sickness

The unacclimatised mountaineer becomes aware of breathlessness at about 2000 m (6600 ft) and may experience the symptoms of **mountain sickness** (headache, nausea, loss of appetite, difficulty in sleeping and performing exercise). At 5500 m, feelings of unreality, amnesia and dizziness become apparent. Disturbances to sleep arise from sleep apnoea, the commonest form of which is Cheyne–Stokes breathing, during which periodic apnoea occurs between periods of increasing tidal volume. Some people are more susceptible than others to the effects of high altitude, and symptoms vary among individuals. The clinical manifestations and severity of mountain sickness are therefore a spectrum of conditions.

BREATH-HOLDING

When a breath is held, p_aCO_2 and p_ACO_2 rise to a remarkably constant point termed the **breaking point**, when the respiratory chemoreceptors force the person to take a breath. Hyperventilation prior to breath-holding will reduce the p_aCO_2 though not increase p_aO_2 but will extend the breath-holding time, thus demonstrating the dominance of the CO_2 drive to ventilation. Mental determination can be another important factor in determining the breaking point, as can re-breathing into a bag, which overcomes the discomfort due to the absence of rhythmic chest movements.

Prolonging the held breath

The duration of apnoea in a breath-hold can be increased by **hyperventilation** which 'blows-off' CO_2 and lowers p_aCO_2. Thus there is a longer period before the p_aCO_2 rises sufficiently to trigger the central chemoreceptors, when the so-called CO_2 breaking point is reached and the person must take another breath. Hyperventilation prior to breath-hold diving carries the risk of fainting underwater since dangerous levels of hypoxia will be reached before the CO_2 drive forces breathing. There are unconfirmed reports of this occurring in synchronised swimmers so that emphasis is now placed on controlled breathing (optimal use of available breathing opportunities during prolonged aquatic exercise, which might mean breathing less often) rather than the more dangerous breath-holding. Any prolonged breath holding is dangerous, whether initiated by long distance or time underwater, or through cumulative oxygen deprivation associated with multiple short breath-holding sessions.

DIVING

The simplest method of diving is **breath-hold diving** (also known as 'free' diving), when the diver does not use any artificial aids to breathing and simply holds his or her breath. After breathing air, breath-holding times are normally limited to 60–75 seconds. Longer times can be achieved. It is unclear whether this is due to training or to an inherited ability.

Effects of pressure in free diving

The pressure exerted by water increases rapidly as greater depths are reached. During a breath-hold dive, lung volumes decrease as the external pressure rises according to Boyle's law. At a depth of 50 m a starting lung volume of 6.0 L would be reduced to 1.0 L. Lung volume should not be reduced below residual volume and collapse alveoli, so that further increases in water pressure during descent may lead to undesired effects. Conversely, lung volume will increase during ascent.

At a depth of only 1.6 m the increase in pressure will exceed 100 mmHg. At this point, the inspiratory muscles cannot overcome the external water pressure, so that, for some people, it becomes impossible to breathe in. This has important significance for diving while breathing air through a rigid hose, a snorkel. The length of the snorkel should therefore be limited for use near the surface (34 cm).

Effects of pressure during ascent from depth

At a depth equivalent to 2 atm the partial pressures of O_2 and CO_2 in the lungs will be doubled even though the percentage concentration remains unchanged. It is therefore possible that the tension of CO_2 in the lungs will be higher than that of the blood, which is incompressible. CO_2 will therefore pass in the reverse direction to normal. Oxygen will continue to enter the blood and maintain an adequate O_2 tension due to the affinity of haemoglobin for O_2 (the diver does not feel a lack of O_2). This constitutes a danger when returning to the surface, as on ascent the partial pressure of O_2 in the lungs may fall below that of the blood. Consequently, O_2 will leave the blood and pass into the lungs. This will lead to acute anoxia and may lead to unconsciousness. Another risk exists during escape from submarines. Air must be breathed out during ascent as the gases in the chest expand, otherwise lung rupture is almost certain.

Effects of pressure in deep diving

At greater depths using underwater breathing apparatus (aqua-lung or SCUBA) the air is supplied at the environmental pressure so that the normal pressure differential between the lungs and outside the chest wall is maintained. The risks of acute anoxia and lung rupture are, however, still present.

At very great depths, helium–oxygen mixtures are used (98% helium, 2% oxygen) but supplied at the environmental pressure. Only 1–2% O_2 is required because of the high partial pressures. Nitrogen is replaced by helium because of three properties of nitrogen:

- It is an anaesthetic and at 30 atm can cause full surgical anaesthesia
- It has increased solubility in tissues, which is a problem during decompression, when gas bubbles may be produced, variously known as the '**bends**' or 'chokes'
- Its density increases at pressure which hinders breathing.
- Nitrogen narcosis ('**narks**', raptures of the deep) may occur if breathing compressed air during deep diving (40 m), when loss of consciousness and drowning is preceded by euphoria.

Helium is not without problems. It increases voice pitch, making it squeaky, and so communication becomes difficult. Helium under pressure is a good conductor of heat and can cause hypothermia unless the diver's environment is heated. Slow decompression is also required to prevent the bends.

DIVER'S REFLEX

The diver's reflex is a response to hypoxia when oxygenated blood is directed to the brain. Observations in diving mammals, such as seals, show that during a dive, primary bradycardia (vagal in origin) and vasoconstriction directed to the skin, muscle, gastrointestinal tract and kidneys effectively 'shut down' the peripheral circulation, ensuring adequate O_2 to the heart, lungs and brain. However, ventilation drive is **suppressed**. This is contrary to the normal response to hypoxia, when hyperventilation occurs in response to the low p_aO_2 and raised p_aCO_2, with an associated secondary tachycardia. This reflex is triggered by submersion in cold water, and may in part explain survival in cases of near drowning in man (see below).

DROWNING

Most drowning victims eventually inhale water into the lungs, either before or after losing consciousness. In some cases, drowning will occur without inhalation when entry of cold water into the upper airways causes laryngeal spasm, closing the glottis, and producing apnoea, thus preventing the water from entering into the lungs. In fresh water, most of the water entering the lungs will move into the circulation causing haemodilution. Sea water is hypertonic with three times the osmolarity of blood and so will remain in the lungs and tend to draw fluid from the circulation to cause haemoconcentration. Both conditions lead to heart failure, which can complicate efforts to resuscitate victims of drowning. It is also usual for drowning people to swallow large quantities of water and then regurgitate or vomit, further complicating the drowning with acid aspiration.

There are remarkable accounts of survival of children for as long as 40 minutes in cold water. It is clear that reduction in cerebral metabolism by cooling is protective, but very rapid cooling (>1°C/min) would be required to lower metabolism before the anoxia caused brain cell death. Cooling by simple immersion would be too slow. Other factors which could better explain the survival of these children include reflex apnoea, reflex closure of the glottis or the diver's reflex.

HIGH OXYGEN LEVELS

The body most commonly has to deal with low oxygen levels. Prolonged exposure to high oxygen concentrations can cause disease because of oxygen toxicity. Exposure to oxygen at partial pressure in excess of 2 atm can occur during deep sea dives or during hyperbaric oxygen therapy.

Neurological oxygen toxicity

The central nervous system, especially the brain, responds adversely to too much O_2 and seizures are common. High levels of O_2 lead to the generation of damaging free radicals (see Chs 2 and 16).

Cellular oxygen toxicity

The use of inspired oxygen during mechanical ventilation is part of the routine care for treating critically ill or injured patients. However, there is some question as to the level of inspired oxygen that creates a toxic effect to the lungs and reduces their ability to produce surfactant.

Continuous exposure to high concentrations of oxygen can damage the lungs. This has to be taken seriously when giving continuous oxygen therapy: the lowest concentrations of oxygen for adequate arterial oxygenation should be used. Newborn babies can develop retrolental fibrosis leading to blindness if the incubator pO_2 is too high.

CARBON MONOXIDE POISONING

CO has a very high affinity for haemoglobin, about 250 times that of O_2. So it easily displaces O_2 to form HbCO and effectively reduces the amount of haemoglobin available for gas transport.

Low levels of HbCO (less than 2%) are normal, but smokers have 5–10% HbCO and significant amounts of HbCO are found in the blood of foetuses whose mothers smoke. Acute levels but below 20% are usually asymptomatic in individuals with no cardiorespiratory disease but levels above 60% may lead to coma. However, lower chronic exposure can lead to headaches and nausea and may lead to permanent neurological damage.

Treatment of CO poisoning is by 100% O_2 in order to displace the CO, although in some centres patients are treated with 100% O_2 in a high pressure chamber (hyperbaric oxygen) in order to displace the CO even faster.

RESPIRATORY FAILURE

Respiratory failure is when alveolar ventilation in not sufficient to maintain normal arterial blood gases. It is defined practically as:

- $p_aO_2 < 8\,kPa\ (60\,mmHg)$
  or
- $p_aCO_2 > 7\,kPa\ (55\,mmHg)$
  although the extreme limits of survival are:
- $p_aO_2 < 2.7\,kPa\ (20\,mmHg)$ and
- $p_aCO_2 > 11\,kPa\ (83\,mmHg)$.

CAUSES OF RESPIRATORY FAILURE

Respiratory failure occurs when either pulmonary gas exchange or the respiratory muscles fail, or both (see Clinical box 13.24). Disturbances in ventilation and perfusion in pulmonary disease lead to V_A/Q imbalance, so that the balance of p_aO_2 and p_aCO_2 becomes disrupted, with the ensuing disturbance in acid–base balance. There are two types of respiratory failure:

- **Type I** where p_aO_2 is low (**hypoxaemia**), and p_aCO_2 is normal or low
- **Type II** where p_aO_2 is low, and p_aCO_2 is high (**hypercapnia**).

Although type I and type II respiratory failure have distinct blood gas patterns, physiologically they represent a continuum. For example, mild to moderate right-to-left shunts could give rise to a type I respiratory failure where, although the p_aO_2 is low, the p_aCO_2 is maintained as normal or low through compensation by hyperventilation. However, as the lung disease progresses and larger areas of lung damage give rise to more severe right-to-left shunting, the central respiratory drive (hyperventilation) can no longer compensate for the rise in p_aCO_2 and hypercapnia ensues, giving rise to type II respiratory failure.

Type I respiratory failure

Type I respiratory failure occurs in **restrictive lung disease**, when there is a significant, and sometimes sudden, reduction in lung volume leading to acute hypoxaemia. This could be the result of right-to-left shunts, when unventilated parts of the lungs are perfused so that gaseous exchange does not take place effectively. Alternately, there is severe ventilation–perfusion (V_A/Q) mismatch. Clinical conditions leading to type I respiratory failure include those in which lung tissue is damaged or reduced, as in:

- Pneumonia
- Pulmonary oedema
- Adult respiratory distress syndrome (ARDS)
- Pneumothorax
- Fibrosing alveolitis (idiopathic pulmonary fibrosis) (normally chronic in form).

(See also Clinical box 13.17.)

Type II respiratory failure

Type II respiratory failure occurs mainly with **obstructive lung disease**. Arterial pO_2 is less than 8.0 kPa (60 mmHg) giving rise to hypoxia and arterial pCO_2 is greater than 7 kPa (55 mmHg) leading to hypercapnia while breathing air at sea level. Lung volumes can be unchanged, but airflow is reduced so that alveolar ventilation is reduced. The alveoli fail to adequately oxygenate the blood and excrete sufficient CO_2. The commonest cause is COPD. Other causes include asthma, chest wall deformity, respiratory muscle weakness and depression of the respiratory centre.

Asthma

There is currently no standardised definition of asthma. Its diagnosis is a clinical one but most diagnoses will include recurrent respiratory symptoms of wheezing, cough, difficulty in breathing and chest tightness. Descriptions include airway hyper-responsiveness (intermittent, reversible constriction of airways due to smooth muscle spasm) and mucosal inflammation. Excess mucus secretion leads to further narrowing of the airways, increasing airway resistance. Voluntary respiratory effort has to increase in order to expel air against increasing resistance and small airways collapse before tidal volume is expelled. This causes the FRC to increase, leaving over-expanded lungs (**hyperinflation**), which make inspiration more and more difficult.

These changes lead to varying degrees of airway obstruction and to ventilation that is uneven and patchy. Continued blood flow to some hypoventilated areas (right-to-left shunt) causes V_A/Q imbalance, resulting in **arterial hypoxaemia**. Early in an attack, a patient typically compensates by hyperventilating the unobstructed areas of the lung, resulting in a decrease in p_aCO_2 (type I respiratory failure). As the attack progresses, the capacity for hyperventilation is impaired by the increased FRC, more extensive airway narrowing and muscle fatigue. Hypoxaemia worsens, and p_aCO_2 begins to rise (hypercapnia), leading to respiratory acidosis. At this point, the patient is in type II respiratory failure.

COPD

The current GOLD (Global Initiative for Obstructive Lung Disease) guidelines describe COPD as a preventable and treatable disease, characterised by persistent airflow limitation that is usually progressive and associated with an enhanced chronic inflammatory response. The disease is a mixture of small airway disease (**obstructive bronchiolitis**) and parenchymal destruction (**emphysema**). The vast majority of cases are caused by cigarette smoking, severe atmospheric pollution and inhalation of smoke particles from burning biomass fuels. Other currently proposed risk factors include poor nutrition in utero and α_1-antitrypsin (AAT) deficiency (see below).

Small airways collapse easily due to destruction of pulmonary elastic tissue causing further obstruction. As with asthma, the FRC increases, giving rise to hyper-inflation of the chest. Furthermore, the effort required to ventilate the alveoli against increasing resistance gives rise to dyspnoea on exertion, where even speech becomes difficult in severe cases. As in asthma, airways obstruction causes inadequate ventilation. Destruction of alveolar walls leads to the formation of larger air sacs (emphysema, see below) that are inefficient for gaseous exchange. The varying combinations of airway disease and pulmonary emphysema lead to hypoxia of respiratory origin (hypoxic hypoxia) and hypercapnia, and thus chronic, type II respiratory failure of varying severity.

Emphysema

Emphysema is an enlargement of the alveolar sacs by the destruction of the alveolar walls. Large spaces called **bullae** form, which reduce the surface area for gas exchange. Bullae situated close to the visceral pleura can also rupture to cause a pneumothorax. The main cause of the enlargement is the destruction of elastin fibres in the lung tissue by the activity of the enzyme neutrophil elastase.

Emphysema occurs in about 20–30% of heavy smokers. A few patients with emphysema are deficient in AAT, which inhibits neutrophil elastase. Although it is not known why some smokers with normal levels of α_1-antitrypsin develop the disease and others do not, this is likely to be due to genetic differences in inflammatory and repair responses, or their modulation by other current or prior environmental insults. Cigarette smoke stimulates neutrophil influx with the release of excess elastases. Synergistic roles are suggested also for macrophage-derived matrix metalloproteinases (MMPs) and the resultant enzyme release overwhelms the protective antiproteases, exacerbated by associated free radicals from cigarette smoke that promote oxidative apoptosis.

There are different types of emphysema, according to the anatomical distribution of the damage:

- Centriacinar – begins in the bronchioles of the upper lungs and spreading peripherally. Associated with long generation smoking.
- Panacinar – predominant I in the lower lungs destroying alveolus. Associated with AAT deficiency (autosomal recessive)
- Paraseptal, or distal – involving all distal airway structures, ducts and sacs, localised around the lung septae or pleura. Associated with development of bullae but air flow is often otherwise preserved.

Clinical effects of respiratory failure

Hypoxia interferes with aerobic metabolism, so that cellular function is disrupted. Effects on the brain give rise to confusion and drowsiness, progressing to coma and death in severe cases. To compensate for the reduced p_aO_2, renal tubular cells increase erythropoietin production so that red blood cell numbers increase and the resultant polycythaemia increases the O_2-carrying capacity of the blood. Pulmonary vasoconstriction to divert blood from poorly ventilated parts of the lungs may lead to pulmonary hypertension and, eventually, cor pulmonale (see above).

Hypercapnia adds to the effects of hypoxia on the brain and also causes respiratory acidosis as the result of inadequate CO_2 excretion. In chronic respiratory failure (e.g. COPD), the respiratory centre becomes desensitised to hypocapnia, so that the central ventilatory drive from the elevated p_aCO_2 no longer operates. Renal retention of bicarbonate can, to some extent, compensate for the respiratory acidosis, but this takes time. The combination of hypoxia and acidosis could be fatal.

LUNG DEFENCES AGAINST INFECTION

Spread of germs by touching the nose and eyes with contaminated fingers and the inhalation of airborne microbes results in infections of the upper respiratory tract. This can progress to infection of the lower respiratory tract. Elaborate systems have evolved to defend the lungs but when activated these processes can also damage the lungs.

THE UPPER AIRWAYS

The nasopharyngeal airways trap particles >10 μm diameter and is relatively effective in filtering particles >5 μm diameter. The nasopharynx also absorbs soluble and reactive gases such as sulphur dioxide.

The nose and upper airways have two major defences against infection:

- The physical barrier of a continuously moving layer of mucus that lines the airway
- A local immune response involving phagocytic polymorphonuclear leucocytes and other leucocytes such as natural killer cells.

Respiratory infections are more common in winter, and airway cooling in winter may compromise both these

mechanisms of respiratory defence and predispose to respiratory infection by slowing the mucociliary escalator and the phagocytic activity of macrophages. Others factors may be of importance, such as staying indoors in cold weather as the greater proximity to other people makes more likely the spread of infections. Cross-infection explains the peak in general practitioner consultations and hospital admission of children with asthma, when they return to school after the summer vacation.

CONDUCTING AIRWAYS

Mucins and ciliary action

Particulates larger than 2 μm diameter become trapped in the viscous 5 μm thick mucus blanket that covers the airway epithelial cells. This mucus is formed from mucins, a group of glycosylated proteins. Mucins are synthesised by goblet cells in the surface epithelium and mucous cells in the submucosal layers. A sub-layer of water underlies the mucus layer and provides less resistance to the movement of cilia. The cilia are just long enough to catch the base of the viscous mucus layer and propel it forward (see Fig. 13.6). Each ciliated epithelial cell has about 200 cilia that beat at 12–14 strokes/s. Microbes can be cleared from the trachea within 30 min and from the distal airways with a half-time of hours. Cigarette smoking, bacterial or viral infection, anaesthetics and cold exposure can slow cilia or destroy airway epithelium, delaying clearance, and increase the likelihood of recurrent infection.

Other factors

The airways also secrete a number of factors that inhibit bacteria or limit the damage they cause. Lactoferrin is released by epithelial cells and by binding iron limits the growth of bacteria since a supply of iron is essential for the production of the bacteria's transport proteins. Lysozyme is secreted (10–20 mg/day) and catalyses the hydrolysis of bonds between bacterial cells walls.

INNATE IMMUNITY

With innate immunity, carbohydrates in the microbial cell wall identify the organism as harmful and it is destroyed by a system involving macrophages, natural killer cells, complement factors and defensins (see Ch. 6).

Destroying the invading organism

Pulmonary macrophages normally lie within the alveoli and airways and are derived mainly from monocytes that enter the lung from the circulation. There are four aspects to the microbicidal action of macrophages:

- Recognition
- Migration
- Ingestion and
- Secretion of mediators.

Macrophages recognise the microbe using surfaces receptors to specific carbohydrates, e.g. lipopolysaccharide (LPS), which is commonly found on Gram-negative bacteria, or mannose that is found in yeasts, mycobacteria and *Pneumocystis carinii*. Macrophages also have receptors for the third component of **complement**. Complement is present in bronchial fluid and when activated generates C3b, an opsonin that promotes receptor-mediated phagocytosis. The microbes are killed once recognised and engulfed, but killing is not fully activated until certain signals are received. These activation stimuli can be produced by the macrophages themselves, such as the release of interferon (IFN)-and IFN-β, induced by LPS, or the release of granulocyte-macrophage colony-stimulating factor or IFN-γ by natural killer cells.

Defensins

Oxidative and non-oxidative processes are used to kill the phagocytosed microbes, but macrophages are not as effective as monocytes or neutrophils, as they are deficient in myeloperoxidase (MPO), an essential part of the MPO–hydrogen peroxide–halide system. The non-oxidative mechanisms involve **defensins** that kill many Gram-positive organisms (*Staphylococcus aureus*) and Gram-negative species (*Escherichia coli*, *Klebsiella pneumoniae*) and fungi, and inactivate certain viruses.

Surfactant proteins

Also under the umbrella of innate immunity are type 2 alveolar cells that secrete **surfactant proteins** A and D which enhance the phagocytosis and agglutination of Gram-positive bacteria.

INFLAMMATORY RESPONSES

Macrophages are capable of dealing with low levels of bacterial infection and minimally virulent organisms. However, when the lungs are infected with numerous bacteria or virulent encapsulated organisms such as *Pseudomonas aeruginosa* or *Streptococcus pneumoniae*, the recruitment of polymorphonuclear neutrophils for containment and clearance is essential. Simply, the process is:

1. Bacteria or their products stimulate macrophage production of cytokines (tumour necrosis factor (TNF)-α, interleukin (IL)-1, IL-8, leukotriene B$_4$) or cause the production of complement activation products C5a and C3a. These molecules act as chemoattractants or stimulate production of further cytokine production by epithelial cells or fibroblasts.
2. The chemoattractants induce the migration of neutrophils from the capillaries into the alveolar space.
3. The neutrophils phagocytose the bacteria and kill them with a 'respiratory burst' of reactive oxygen metabolites such as hydrogen peroxide, hydroxyl radicals and singlet oxygen.
4. These reactive oxygen molecules are derived from the reduction of oxygen by an NADPH (nicotinamide adenosine dinucleotide phosphate (reduced form)) oxidase present in the phagocyte cytoplasm or from the synthesis of nitric oxide. Besides damaging the invading microbe, they are also toxic to the host cells.

Neutrophils also release the enzyme elastase, which produces a number of side effects: excessive mucus secretion, epithelial cell damage and a significant slowing of the beat frequency of the ciliated epithelium.

DEVELOPMENT OF THE LUNGS AND CHANGES IN THE NEWBORN

EARLY LUNG DEVELOPMENT

Embryonic phase

The earliest, embryonic, phase of lung development occurs at 4 weeks with the formation of the **lung bud** or **respiratory diverticulum**, an outgrowth on the ventral surface on the wall of the foregut just below the primordial pharynx (Fig. 13.26). This then divides into two buds which will eventually make up the two main bronchi. The right bud is slightly larger and is more vertically orientated, a relationship which persists in the adult. By the end of week 8 these main bronchial buds have further divided to produce the segmental bronchi, which will form the lobes, two on the left and three on the right. These buds continue to divide to form the bronchioles. By 24 weeks there are about 17 orders of branching, with the remaining seven orders developing after birth. The lung buds are closely associated with the visceral pleura that covers the lobes and each lung is covered with the parietal pleura, which encloses the pleural cavity.

STAGES IN LUNG MATURATION

Once the basic structure has been laid down the lung develops and matures in four phases which span a long period from 6 weeks post-conception to 8 years after birth. The four phases are:

- Pseudoglandular phase
- Canalicular phase
- Terminal saccular phase
- Alveolar phase.

Pseudoglandular phase (6–16 weeks in utero)

During the **pseudoglandular phase**, so called because the lung tissue resembles an exocrine gland, the lung consists of the terminal bronchi which are surrounded by connective tissue which contains capillaries. However, there are no respiratory bronchioles so there is no possibility of survival for foetuses born during this period. Towards the end of the pseudoglandular phase, the lumen of the bronchi starts to enlarge and the epithelia become thinner.

Canalicular phase (16–24 weeks in utero)

In the **canalicular phase**, the terminal bronchioles divided to form respiratory bronchioles which themselves divide to form alveolar ducts and the capillaries. At the end of the canalicular phase these can support some respiration, because the ends of some of these ducts have developed into **terminal saccules** (primordial alveoli with thin walls which are highly vascularised). However, foetuses born before 24 weeks may not survive due to the immaturity of other systems as well as poor respiratory function.

Saccular phase (24 weeks in utero to birth)

The **saccular period** is where the number of terminal saccules increases and the epithelium covering them thins to

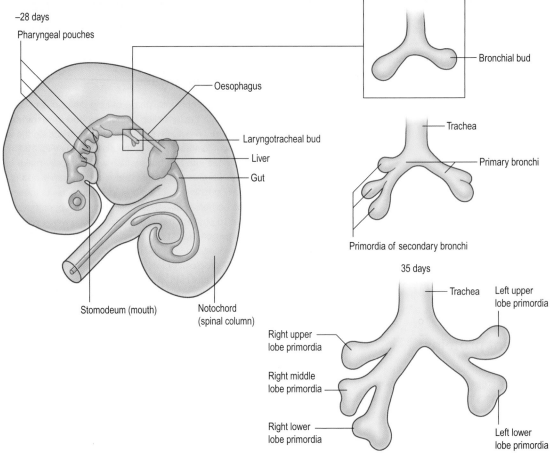

Fig. 13.26 **Early lung development.** The lung bud develops at 4 weeks as an outgrowth of the embryonic foregut (the laryngotracheal bud). The whole of the epithelium lining the entire respiratory tract is, therefore, derived from endoderm. This bud forms two subsections, with the smaller bud on the left initiating the asymmetry of the bronchi at this early stage. By 8 weeks the right and left segmental bronchi have formed and the pleura cover the lungs.

form the **blood–air barrier**. The epithelium differentiates into mainly type I alveolar cells (type I pneumocytes) although there are also type II alveolar cells (type II pneumocytes), which secrete surfactant. The capillary and lymphatic network develops around the terminal saccules, providing a short diffusion distance for dissolved gases.

The increases in surface area provided by the thinning of the epithelium and the increase in surfactant production, especially after week 30, mean that foetuses born in this period have much higher survival rates.

Alveolar phase (32 weeks–8 years)

The **alveolar phase** overlaps with the saccular phase as it depends on the definition of an alveolus. After 36 weeks the walls of the alveoli are so thin that the capillaries bulge into the alveoli. Most fully mature alveoli do not appear until after birth and form from the division of the terminal saccules which become the alveolar ducts. New alveoli arise by the formation of septa across the enlarging immature alveoli and the development of new capillaries. While there is a large increase in their number soon after birth, alveoli continue to be produced in large numbers for about 3 years and this process is complete by about 8 years of age.

Breathing movements with aspiration of amniotic fluid occur for several months before birth. These stimulate lung development and may help to condition the respiratory

muscles. Lung growth is also inhibited by lack of space and inadequate amniotic fluid (**oligohydramnios**).

Also see Information box 13.9 and Clinical box 13.25.

RESPIRATORY SYSTEM CHANGES AT NORMAL DELIVERY

At birth, passage through the pelvis expels much of the amniotic fluid contained within the lungs (although this does not occur with caesarean sections), the baby takes its first breath and the placental circulation ceases. Before the first breath, the alveoli are not inflated and their small size means that the surface tension is high, and pressures in the order of $30\,cmH_2O$ are needed to inflate an excised lung of a full-term baby. This presents little difficulty as the baby can develop pressures of $90\,cmH_2O$ during the first respiratory effort. Most babies take their first breath within 20 seconds of delivery. Rhythmic respiration of about 30 per minute (range 14–60) is reached within 90 seconds. Average tidal volume is $17\,mL$, with a crying vital capacity of 56–$110\,mL$. The stimulants to initiate respiration at birth are probably cooling of the skin and mechanical. The release of the compression caused by passage through the birth canal will also passively draw air into the lungs.

Inflation of the lungs and reduction of the hypoxic pulmonary vasoconstriction following the first breath causes a decrease in the resistance to pulmonary circulation. This coupled with the rise in the systemic circulation causes the right atrial pressure to fall below the left atrial pressure and results in closure of the foramen ovale, which is then followed by closure of the ductus arteriosus (see Ch. 11). The pulmonary capillaries and the relatively large lymphatic vessels in the foetal lung allow remaining fluid to be reabsorbed rapidly from the lungs. In stillborn infants this does not occur, so their lungs are filled with fluid, not air.

RESPIRATORY DISTRESS SYNDROME OF THE NEWBORN

Respiratory distress syndrome of the newborn (RDS) is usually caused by a deficiency in surfactant and often occurs in premature infants. The lungs contain a protein-rich fluid which has a glassy, membranous appearance. With low surfactant levels, lung compliance is decreased, and the work of inflating the stiff lungs is increased. In newborn infants, the ribs are more easily deformed (compliant) than the lungs, so breathing results in deep sternal retractions but poor air entry. Rapid, laboured, grunting respirations will usually develop immediately or within a few hours after delivery.

Surfactant production can be increased by the administration of corticosteroids, which stimulate lung development and surfactant production, although this is of little use in an emergency delivery. However, the administration of exogenous surfactant can also aid breathing and reduce the severity of RDS.

Newborn infants have a lower p_aO_2 than adults, 50–$70\,mmHg$ compared with $100\,mmHg$ in adults. At these levels the foetal haemoglobin is almost fully saturated due to the higher affinity for O_2 of foetal haemoglobin. While most cases of RDS in the neonate are due to prematurity there are rare cases because of other causes, including congenital absence of a component of surfactant.

14

The renal system

Girish Namagondlu and Alistair Chesser

Introduction   655
Functions of the kidney   655
Urine volume and composition   655
Balance of fluid intake and loss   656
Renal failure   656
Anatomy of the kidney   657
Gross structure   657
The nephron   659
Renal vasculature   659
Nerve supply to the renal tract   662
Development of the kidney   662
Permanent kidney   662
Renal function   663
Glomerular filtration and the production
of primary urine   664

Functions of the proximal convoluted tubule   665
Renal function tests   670
Renal control of fluid balance   674
Renal control of sodium balance   680
Diuretics   684
Renal control of acid–base balance   686
The urinary tract   690
Ureters   690
Gross structure of the bladder   691
Control of micturition   692
Renal diseases   692
General classification of renal disease   693
Onset of renal disease   693
Acute kidney injury   693
Chronic kidney disease   694
Renal replacement therapy   696

INTRODUCTION

The kidney is an essential organ for life and plays a central role in homeostasis. Homeostasis, originally defined by the great French physiologist Claude Bernard, refers to the stability and maintenance of the internal environment of the body – the so-called 'milieu intérieur' (see Ch. 1). Key renal functions may be deduced from what happens when the kidneys cease to function or fail.

FUNCTIONS OF THE KIDNEY

The functions of the kidneys may be summarised as:

- Homeostasis – consisting of filtration, when the blood is filtered to remove waste products of metabolism and toxic substances but retains essential nutrients, which is followed by reabsorption and secretion of water and essential electrolytes, to maintain acid–base balance, water (fluid) and electrolyte balance, and a normal blood pressure. Urine is produced in the process.
- Hormone secretion – independent of the endocrine system, the kidneys secrete erythropoietin to stimulate red cell production, renin as part of the blood pressure control mechanism, and the active form of vitamin D.

Therefore, the kidney:

- Controls the volume, osmolarity and acid–base balance of the plasma and extracellular fluid
- Controls the level of electrolytes in blood and extracellular fluid (ECF)
- Recovers all the small molecules filtered by the nephron, such as sugars and amino acids

- Excretes nitrogenous waste and 'fixed' acid from protein metabolism, mainly urea, uric acid and creatinine
- Excretes a variety of toxic metabolites and excess electrolytes and water
- Maintains red cell production by the secretion of the hormone erythropoietin
- Produces the active form of vitamin D and hence maintains calcium balance
- Controls blood pressure over the long term.

URINE VOLUME AND COMPOSITION

In a healthy person the kidneys form about 1.5–2 L of urine every 24 hours, which is equivalent to 1 mL/min entering the bladder. Urine composition differs from plasma:

- First, the levels of urinary nitrogenous waste products, mostly in the form of urea and ammonia, are much higher, whereas levels of protein, glucose and amino acids are all very much lower
- Second, although in any given 24 hours the total amount of any urinary constituent, such as salts (NaCl, KCl, $NaHCO_3$) and urea, are excreted at a fairly constant rate, the volume of water in which they are contained can vary widely, so that the amount of solute excreted is independent of the volume of urine.

Normally, urine is a slightly acidic, pale yellow fluid, with a pH of about 6. However, when large volumes of water are ingested, it can rapidly change to an almost colourless fluid, the excreted volume matching the intake and the osmolarity falling to a minimum of 50 mOsm. In contrast, if sweating is increased by hard exercise or if the water intake is restricted, the volume of urine will fall and a dark concentrated fluid is produced with an osmolarity which can rise to 1400 mOsm (Information box 14.1). Plasma has a constant osmolarity of approximately 285 mOsm.

Osmolarity measures the concentration of 'particles' that are capable of exerting osmotic pressure, so that the osmolarity of a solution reflects the number of 'particles' in a given volume of fluid that can exert an osmotic pressure across a membrane. The kidneys are vital in keeping the osmolarity of blood and the ECF constant. The kidneys are therefore a key element in the control of electrolytes and acid–base balance in the body. Sodium as NaCl and $NaHCO_3$ is conserved, whereas potassium is eliminated and 'fixed' acid is excreted in the form of ammonia and phosphate ions in the urine.

BALANCE OF FLUID INTAKE AND LOSS

In a healthy human being, the daily intake of water roughly equals loss in the steady state. The principal source of water is drinking water and other fluids and in food (oral), and most of the loss is in urine, via the kidneys. Some water is lost as 'insensible loss', via respiration, skin, sweating and faeces. Table 14.1 shows the approximate balance of the total intake and loss of water by the body over 24 hours and the electrolyte balance, and the factors that can disturb this balance.

RENAL FAILURE

In a person whose kidneys are beginning to fail, there is at first no detectable sign or symptom of damage, since human beings have a massive over-capacity in renal function. Few changes are seen until three-quarters of the normal renal function is lost (Clinical box 14.1). Symptoms appear late in renal failure and are usually:

- A result of waste product accumulation, mainly urea (uraemia), such as loss of appetite, lethargy, nausea, vomiting, weight loss, itching (uraemic frost), muscle cramps etc.
- The inability to excrete water (fluid overload) resulting in breathlessness, orthopnoea, oliguria, peripheral oedema.

An early feature of renal failure is a drop in the glomerular filtration rate (GFR) by all the nephrons (see later). There are several ways of measuring GFR. A commonly used method, which is easy and reasonably reliable, is estimating GFR by MDRD (modification of diet in renal disease) formula, which is based on age, sex, race, serum creatinine and popularly

Table 14.1 Water balance and factors which disturb the balance

Sources for the input of water	Litres	Sources of output	Litres
Water content in food	1.0	Urine osmotic load	0.7
Food metabolism	0.5	Urine from choice drinking	0.8
Drinking minimum	0.5	Lungs and airways	0.4
Drinking by choice	1.0	Skin insensible loss	1.0
		Faeces	0.1
Total	3.0	Total	3.0

Factors disturbing balance	Composition and route
Hyperventilation/fever	Loss of pure H_2O – diffusion through skin
Sweating	$H_2O + Na^+$, Cl^- – sweat glands and ducts
Air conditioning (dry air)	0.5–1 L per day pure H_2O – diffusion into lungs
Diarrhoea – cholera	20 L in 48 h Na^+, Cl^-, HCO_3^-, K^+ – small bowel/colon
Lactation – milk	Isotonic salts – milk secretion, breasts

known as eGFR (estimated glomerular filtration rate). In healthy individuals, the GFR is a very large volume of fluid – 125 mL/min in the young male (equivalent to 180 L per 24 h).

Blood urea and serum creatinine are commonly measured but are surrogate and late markers of renal failure (Figure 14.1). Levels only increase in the blood when 50% of the kidney function is lost. For a normal person on a mixed diet the level of plasma urea is about 5 mM and it does not begin to change until the GFR has fallen by about 75%. However, this response does depend on the diet – a high protein intake in a meat eater would cause the plasma urea to rise more rapidly in renal disease, whereas a vegetarian diet would delay this rise until an even greater loss of renal function had occurred. Often, prior to the rise in plasma urea, the blood pressure begins to increase to high levels at rest (hypertension) and this can be an early warning sign of renal problems (Clinical box 14.2).

Clinical box 14.1 Clinical consequences of renal failure

The consequences of renal failure are related to kidney functions other than fluid balance and excretion, which include:

- Hypertension – the kidneys secrete the enzyme renin in response to impaired renal perfusion. Renin activates angiotensin-converting enzyme (ACE) to convert angiotensin I to angiotensin II, which is a powerful systemic vasoconstrictor and stimulates aldosterone secretion to promote sodium and water retention (see below and Ch. 4). Chronic disruption of the renin–angiotensin–aldosterone system in renal failure leads to hypertension. Pharmacological treatment with ACE inhibitors is used in the management of hypertension (see below). Before the advent of effective hypotensive drugs, nephrectomy was performed to prevent renal hypertension.
- Cardiovascular disease – is the major cause of death in renal failure patients. Ischaemic heart disease is common and often a combination of arteriosclerosis and atherosclerosis. Incidence of cardiac arrhythmias and sudden cardiac death is increased in CKD.
- Anaemia – renal interstitial cells secrete erythropoietin, which stimulates red cell production (see Ch. 12). Destruction of renal tissue in CKD results in iron and erythropoietin deficiency.
- Vitamin D deficiency – the distal convoluted tubules secrete the enzyme 1α-hydroxylase. Naturally occurring vitamin D needs to

be hydroxylated to an active metabolite in the liver, then further converted by 1α-hydroxylase to produce the metabolically active 1,25-dihydroxychlolecalciferol (vitamin D_3). Chronic renal failure thus leads to disorders of bone (renal osteodystrophy), calcium metabolism and secondary hyperparathyroidism (see Chs 10 and 16).

- Hypoproteinaemia – the persistent and chronic urinary protein loss in chronic renal failure leads to hypoproteinaemia, which can lead to impaired protein binding with consequent adverse reactions from therapeutic agents (see Ch. 4), wasting and malnutrition (see Ch. 16).
- Other metabolic complications – e.g. defective excretion of urate leads to gout; defective insulin excretion may lead to hypoglycaemia in insulin-dependent diabetics.
- Other endocrine disorders – these may arise owing to defective protein binding of hormones consequent to hypoproteinaemia (e.g. thyroid hormone), or impairment of hormone action and excretion (e.g. hyperprolactinaemia leading to gynaecomastia in men, growth retardation secondary to complex defects of growth hormone secretion and action in uraemic children).
- Neurological complications – severe, persistent uraemia depresses cerebral function and may lead to convulsions (see also Ch. 3).

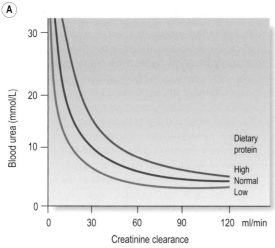
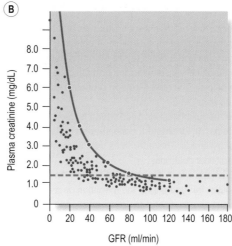

Fig. 14.1 (A) The relationship between blood urea concentration and creatinine clearance showing the effect of high, normal and low protein intakes. (B) Relationship between true glomerular filtration rate (GFR) (as measured by inulin clearance) and plasma creatinine concentration in 171 patients with glomerular disease. The *open circles* joined by the *solid red line* represent the relationship that would exist if creatinine were excreted solely by glomerular filtration; the *dashed line* represents the upper limit of 'normal' for plasma creatinine concentration of 1.4 mg/dL. In the patients (*dark dots*), variations in GFR between 129 and 60 mL/min were often associated with a plasma creatinine concentration that remained within the normal range due to increased creatinine excretion, which becomes saturated at a plasma concentration above 1.5–2 mg/dL; as a result, plasma creatinine concentration rises as expected with further reductions in GFR. Redrawn from Richards P, Truniger B 1983 Understanding water electrolytes and acid base balance. William Heinemann, London, with permission.

Clinical box 14.2 | **Renal failure**

Renal failure occurs when glomerular filtration is compromised from a variety of causes, but may also be the consequence of renal tubular function:

- Pre-renal – due to depressed renal vascular perfusion so that the hydrostatic filtration forces are reduced. Causes can be divided into:
  - True volume depletion, e.g. hypotension, dehydration, vomiting, diarrhoea, haemorrhage (gastrointestinal blood loss), shock
  - Decrease in 'effective' circulating blood volume, e.g. heart failure, liver failure, NSAIDs and ACE inhibitors.
- Renal – often called intrinsic renal disease and is due to disease of the nephron, the glomeruli and or microvasculature, or the tubules, e.g. microvascular disease as in diabetes mellitus (see Ch. 3), nephrotoxic drugs, acute tubular necrosis.
  - Renovascular
    - Macrovascular – renal artery stenosis, renal vein thrombosis
    - Microvascular – small vessel disease, e.g. diabetes mellitus, vasculitis.
  - Renal parenchymal
    - Glomerulonephritis – nephritic syndrome, rapidly progressive glomerulonephritis, nephrotic syndrome
    - Tubulointerstitial disease – ATN, tubulointerstitial nephritis.

- Post-renal – due to obstruction anywhere in the outflow system: the renal pyramid (calyces, pelvis), ureters, down to the bladder neck, or recurrent ascending infections (e.g. pyelonephritis). Renal failure may be acute or chronic:
- **Acute kidney injury** is the sudden deterioration of renal function, which is usually reversible over time. When severe, the consequent fluid and biochemical disturbances may be life-threatening and constitute a medical emergency. Management of acute renal failure is aimed to correct the fluid and biochemical imbalance during the time needed for renal function to recover. Dietary controls of electrolyte, nitrogen and water intake (see Ch. 16), pharmacological interventions (see Ch. 4) and dialysis to remove toxic products of metabolism and excess fluid may be necessary.
- **Chronic kidney disease** is a longstanding and progressive impairment of renal excretory function, which may be insidious in onset and should be diagnosed after at least 3 months of persistent renal failure. The biochemical abnormalities may be undetected for long periods. Causes of chronic renal failure may be congenital (see below) and include glomerular or vascular disease. Treatment is aimed at controlling the biochemical and fluid imbalances (including chronic dialysis), and at the cause, e.g. tight glycaemic control in diabetes mellitus, and to manage complications. Renal transplantation may ultimately be needed.

ANATOMY OF THE KIDNEY

GROSS STRUCTURE

The adult kidneys are two 'bean'-shaped structures weighing about 150 g each, lying on either side of the vertebral column (at about the level of T12–L3) in the midline, but outside the peritoneum in the abdominal cavity (retroperitoneal). The concave aspect of each kidney faces medially (towards the vertebral column). Each kidney normally measures 10–12 cm in length, 5–7 cm in width and 2–3 cm in thickness.

The kidneys are surrounded by three layers of tissue:

- Renal fascia (Gerota's fascia) – a thin, outer layer of fibrous connective tissue that surrounds each kidney (and the attached adrenal gland).
- Adipose capsule – a middle layer of fat tissue that cushions the kidneys.
- Renal capsule – an inner, thick, fibrous membrane. The thickness of the capsule is necessary to withstand the high tissue pressure of 10 mmHg generated within the tissue extracellular fluid by the filtration process.

The inside of kidney has three distinct regions:

1. Outer cortex borders the convex side and lies immediately under the capsule. It contains the renal corpuscles and tubules (apart from the 'hairpin' loop of Henle), blood vessels and the cortical collecting ducts (see below). The renal filtration processes take place in the cortex.
2. Inner medulla (see Fig. 14.2) which is deep to the cortex, contains 10–20 striated, cone shaped regions called renal pyramids. This alternates with an unstriated region called renal columns.
3. Renal sinus which lies adjacent to medulla and opens to the hilum (an opening in the medial aspect of the kidney) that allows passage of the renal artery and vein, nerve supply and ureters (Fig. 14.2).

Renal pyramids

In longitudinal section, the kidney is divided into a number of conical structures, the renal pyramids (see Fig. 14.2). The gross structure also reflects the highly organised microstructure with linear feature, the medullary rays, arranged into the inner and outer stripes. These are related to the capillary networks and to the straight tubular elements of the loop of Henle, the vasa recta and the collecting ducts (see below). The tip of each pyramid forms a papilla which is enclosed in a funnel-shaped extension of the renal pelvis, the calyx. It is these structures which collect the urine draining from the collecting ducts passing through renal papilla at the apex, into a minor calyx (usually 9–12) then into a major calyx (3–4) before passing through the renal pelvis into the ureters via the pelviureteric junction (PUJ). The walls of calyces, renal pelvis and ureters are

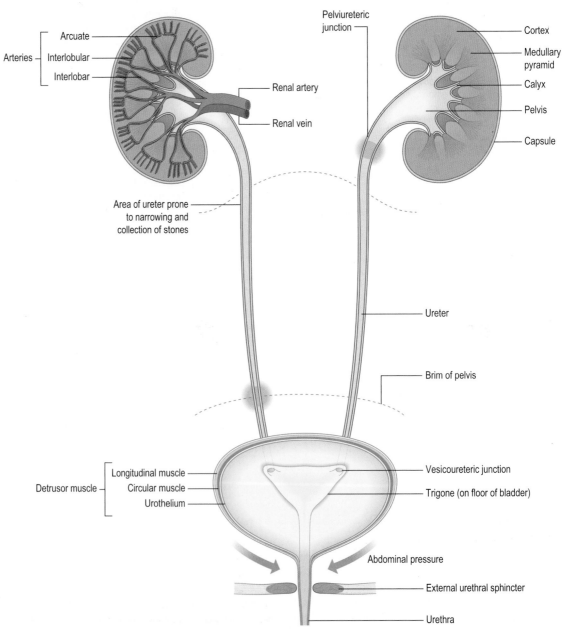

Fig. 14.2 **The major components of the urinary tract and bladder.** Note the pelviureteric junction, the brim of the pelvis and the vesicoureteric junction, which are sites where renal stones can lodge and impede urine flow, so causing back pressure and renal damage.

lined with smooth muscle, which produces peristaltic waves to carry urine down the ureter and into the bladder.

THE NEPHRON

The functional unit of the kidney is the nephron, of which there are some 1.5 million in each kidney. Each nephron consists of the renal corpuscle, where the primary urine is first formed, and the renal tubule, a highly coiled tube where the primary urine is modified. A simplified overall structure of the nephron is shown in Figure 14.3.

The renal corpuscle (renal glomerulus)

The renal corpuscle, the filter in the kidney sited in the cortex, consists of the glomerulus, which is a knot of capillaries attached to the mesangium, surrounded by the Bowman's capsule where fluid is forced out of the plasma into Bowman's space to form the glomerular filtrate. Bowman's capsule, also known as the glomerular capsule, elongates to become the renal tubule. Bowman's capsule has an inner layer formed by visceral epithelial cells (podocytes), which at the vascular pole is reflected to form the outer layer (parietal epithelial cells).

The renal tubule

The renal tubule is the reabsorptive part of the renal system. It is a highly convoluted structure, varying in size throughout its length, consisting of:

- Proximal convoluted tubule (PCT)
- Loop of Henle
- Distal convoluted tubule (DCT)
- Collecting ducts (CDs).

Although originating in the renal cortex, the renal tubule descends into the medulla as the hairpin loop of Henle (see below), which doubles back so that the distal convoluted tubule returns to the cortex ending next to the glomerulus of the same nephron.

Proximal convoluted tubule

The fluid formed by the glomerular capillaries flows from Bowman's space along the nephron into the highly coiled structure of the PCT. The PCT is grossly divided into pars convoluta (initial convoluted portion) and pars recta (straight portion) that descends into the medulla. The PCT is lined by cuboidal cells having fine densely packed microvilli (brush border) on the luminal side (urine side). Each cell is joined to the others around it, close to the luminal boundary, by an occluding band of tight junctions. The base of each cell (blood side) is inwardly convoluted in many folds which interdigitate with the cells around it. These structures enormously expand the surface of the cell for exchange processes. The cells are also densely filled with mitochondria, which are always present in cells that are metabolically active and use energy generated from glucose and oxygen.

Loop of Henle

After the PCT, the nephron then descends from the cortex towards the medulla via the hairpin loop of Henle. There are three types of loop:

- Loops from juxtaglomerular nephrons which are very long and extend all the way down to the renal pyramids (medulla).

- Loops from cortical nephrons which are short and only reach the cortex/medulla border. About 80% of nephrons have short loops.
- A few intermediate loops between the above types.

The functional reasons for the differences in the length of the loops are not fully understood but desert animals that produce a highly concentrated urine have the highest proportion of the long loops. The loop of Henle consists of several cell types; the bulk of this structure is the thin descending and thin ascending loops. The cells of this region are sparse in number, and are narrow with few infoldings on either face and few mitochondria. The loop of Henle is amazingly long, the length being about 1000 times the diameter, and if Figure 14.3 was drawn to scale, it would be as high as a 20-storey building! After the thin ascending loop, the next section undergoes a major change in structure becoming the thick ascending loop. The cells in this section are thick, complex and rich both in mitochondria and cellular inclusions which reflects their active transport functions.

Distal convoluted tubule

Fluid now leaves the loop of Henle and enters the DCT, which is in the renal cortex. Here, 10–15% of ions and fluid of the filtrate are recovered. Tubules from five to six nephrons then merge to form the larger collecting duct, which re-enters the renal medulla. Up to this point the fluid recovery is a fixed proportion of that which has been filtered, and is said to be constitutive.

Collecting ducts

The CDs are derived from a different embryological origin than the rest of the nephron, and are divided into a cortical section (CCD) and a medullary section (MCD). In these ducts the fluid recovery can be varied either to produce a dilute or a concentrated urine under the influence of the antidiuretic hormone (ADH), also called vasopressin (see below).

RENAL VASCULATURE

Each kidney is supplied by a large artery from the descending aorta and together they receive about 20% of the cardiac output (1.2 L/min). After circulating through the medulla and cortex, blood from renal capillaries is collected in renal venules and leaves the kidney via the renal vein to join the inferior vena cava. The kidneys also have a prominent lymphatic drainage.

The renal arteries enter the kidney on the medial surface of each kidney via the hilum, through which the renal artery enters and the veins and lymphatics exit; here also the renal nerves enter and leave the kidney.

Renal microvasculature

On entering the kidney, the renal artery divides to form interlobar vessels, which supply each pyramid. These then subdivide to form arcuate arteries and finally interlobular arteries supplying the grape-like glomerular capillaries (Fig. 14.4), where the renal filtrate is formed.

The arterial supply enters the start of the nephron at the blind-ended dilation, the Bowman's capsule, and divides into a knot of capillaries, the glomerulus. The glomerular capillaries are unusual in that they have an arteriole at the start of the capillary bed, the afferent arteriole, and a second arteriole, the efferent arteriole, at the end of the glomerulus, where the capillaries combine to emerge from Bowman's capsule.

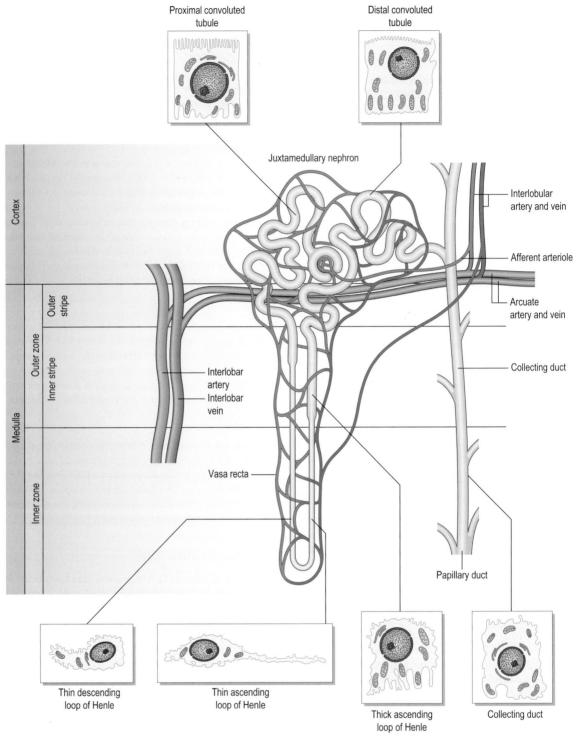

Proximal convoluted tubule

Distal convoluted tubule

Juxtamedullary nephron

Cortex

Outer stripe

Inner stripe

Outer zone

Medulla

Inner zone

Interlobular artery and vein

Afferent arteriole

Arcuate artery and vein

Interlobar artery

Interlobar vein

Collecting duct

Vasa recta

Papillary duct

Thin descending loop of Henle

Thin ascending loop of Henle

Thick ascending loop of Henle

Collecting duct

Fig. 14.3 **Structure of the nephron.** Primary urine formed within the glomerulus is modified during its passage along the kidney tubules before entering the collecting duct from where it goes to the bladder for excretion. The zones of the kidney are shown on the left hand side with the major blood vessels that supply the kidney. The nephron shown is the juxtaglomerular nephron, consisting of the proximal convoluted tubule (PCT), which dips deep into the medulla as the thin descending loop of Henle then bends acutely as the thin ascending loop of Henle and then becomes the thick ascending loop. The thick ascending loop of Henle emerges into the cortex to form the distal convoluted tubule (DCT). The DCTs merge to form the collecting duct which again descends into the medulla and forms the urine. The changing morphology of the tubule walls reflects the differences in permeability and function. The macula densa, a densely packed group of specialised cells lining the DCT, is at the top of the thick ascending loop of Henle, a key site for the control of sodium balance. Some nephrons only penetrate into the outer medulla, the cortical nephrons. It is thought the nephrons with the longest loops of Henle are responsible for forming the most concentrated urine.

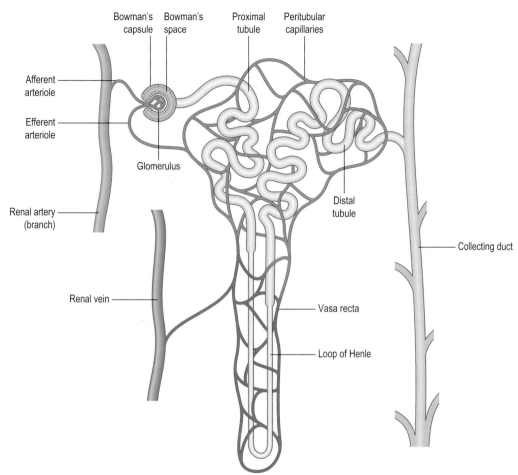

Fig. 14.4 **Renal vasculature.** The blood supply originates from the renal artery (*red*) and leaves via the renal vein (*blue*). Blood passes through two capillary beds, the glomerular capillaries followed by the vasa recta.

Peritubular capillaries

The glomerular capillaries reunite into an efferent arteriole which then divides again to form a second capillary bed becoming either the peritubular capillaries, which envelop both the proximal and distal convoluted tubules, or descend as looped capillaries into the medulla of the kidney as the vasa recta around the loop of Henle (see Fig. 14.4).

Blood flowing through the glomerular capillaries is under high pressure, whereas the tubular capillaries and vasa recta are under low pressure.

Glomerular filtration barrier

Filtration of the blood entering the glomerulus at the afferent arteriole relies on the permeability of the glomerular filtration barrier, which is formed inside out by (Fig. 14.5):

- Capillary endothelial cells with round to oval fenestrations (holes or pores) measuring 50–100 nm.
- Glomerular basement membrane (GBM) consisting of a fibrillar network of matrix proteins, rather like an irregular fishing net, but with holes of a fairly consistent size. Each of these 'holes' has negative charges on the surface of the matrix, so molecules with a similar charge would be repelled by these charges. In health, this prevents negatively charged molecules from being filtered out of the blood (see below). Matrix proteins consist of type IV collagen (α3, 4 and 5 chains), laminin, fibronectin, entactin,

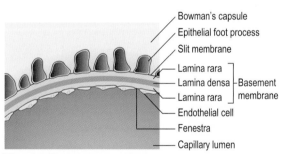

Fig. 14.5 **Glomerular capillary wall.** The structure of the glomerular capillary wall, which is the filtration pathway.

other negatively charged glycoproteins and sulphated glycosaminoglycans such as heparin sulphate.
- Podocytes have foot processes, which are finger-like projections of the capillary epithelium that interdigitate with each other, leaving between them filtration slits, that are bridged by an extracellular structure, the slit diaphragm. The foot processes enclose and strengthen the vessels, so enabling them to withstand the large filtration pressures which are needed to form the urinary filtrate.

Filtration through the glomerular capillary wall occurs along an extracellular pathway including the endothelial pores, the GBM, and the slit diaphragm. Thus formed filtrate enters Bowman's space and then pass through tubules. The main challenge for the glomerular capillaries is to combine selective leakiness with stability.

NERVE SUPPLY TO THE RENAL TRACT

The kidney is supplied via the renal plexus and the course is along the renal arteries to reach each kidney:

- Sympathetic nervous system triggers vasoconstriction in the kidney and reduces renal blood flow. This travels through T10–T11 levels of the spinal cord.
- Parasympathetic nerve supply is through the renal branches of the vagus nerve (cranial nerve X) and the function of this is not yet clear.

Nerve supply of the ureters is from the following sources:

- Renal plexus
- Aortic plexus
- Superior hypogastric plexus
- Inferior hypogastric plexus
- Testicular (or ovarian) plexus.

Nerve supply to the bladder is described in detail on pages 693–94. Nerve supply to the spinchters controlling urethral orifice is from pudendal nerve, pelvic splanchnic nerves and inferior hypogastric plexus.

DEVELOPMENT OF THE KIDNEY

In humans, the embryonic kidneys originate from the intermediate mesoderm (see Ch. 10). The reproductive organs and adrenal cortex also develop from the intermediate mesoderm. The tissues that are destined to become permanent kidneys are preceded by embryonic structures, most of which degenerate and atrophy before birth. Clinical box 14.3 describes some congenital abnormalities of the kidneys and urinary tract. There are three stages in the development of these embryonic structures:

- Pronephros
- Mesonephros
- Metanephros.

Clinical box 14.3	Congenital abnormalities of the kidneys and urinary tract

Congenital malformations of the kidneys and urinary tract (CAKUT) are relatively common. Many are asymptomatic and only detected during investigative (e.g. excretion urogram, ultrasound examination) or therapeutic procedures (e.g. laparotomy). Some conditions, however, lead to serious complications such as progressive renal failure, and require surgical interventions or even renal transplantation. The aetiology of the anomalies is generally unknown, but genetic mutation and chromosomal anomalies have been proposed. The congenital defects include:

- Defect in embryonic development owing to abnormal interaction between the ureteric bud and metanephric blastema, which may lead to **agenesis** (failure to develop), **hypo-** or **dysplasia** of the kidneys, **vesicoureteric reflux** (VUR) (see later, Clinical box 14.14) and congenital malformation of the ureters (ectopic or double ureters) among others.
- Hereditary autosomal dominant or autosomal recessive **polycystic kidney disease.**
- Embryological errors with one kidney failing to ascend (ectopic kidney) or the two kidneys fusing to form a **horseshoe kidney**, which is still functional and is only incidentally detected (Fig. 14.7E).

Pronephros

Cells that develop into the **pronephros** originate in the intermediate mesoderm. Structures known as the cervical nephrostomes, at the level of the fifth cervical to the third thoracic segments, grow as evaginations from the segments to fuse and extend in a caudal direction (downwards) to form a series of ducts, the **pronephric ducts** (or **nephric ducts**). Within the ducts, glomeruli develop. The pronephric ducts and glomeruli make up the pronephros. The Wolffian duct forms below the pronephric duct. The pronephros is not functional, and rapidly degenerates and disappears at an early stage.

Mesonephros

The **mesonephros** originates in the cell mass on the medial side of the Wolffian duct (from about the sixth thoracic to the third lumbar segment), developing into a series of tubules. One end of the tubules dilates and is invaginated by capillaries to form glomeruli. The mesonephros is functional until the fifth gestational week, but atrophies rapidly from the sixth week onwards.

Metanephros

The **metanephros** is destined to become the permanent kidney. It arises partly from the caudal end of the intermediate mesoderm and partly from the Wolffian duct. At about the fifth or sixth week of gestation, the Wolffian duct develops a diverticulum, the ureteric bud, which eventually becomes the renal pelvis and calyces (proximal and distal convoluted tubules, loop of Henle, collecting tubules), and the ureters. The ureteric bud invades the cell mass of the intermediate mesoderm, when cells from the mesoderm migrate over the ureteric bud and differentiate to eventually form the excretory part of the kidneys, the **nephrons** (the renal cortex, glomeruli). The metanephros migrates upwards to the lumbar region to take up the lumbar position of the adult kidney. The ureters elongate as the metanephros ascends.

PERMANENT KIDNEY

The ureteric buds bifurcate until the 32nd week producing 1–3 million collecting ducts (Fig. 14.6). At the tip of each is a metanephric tissue cap (metanephric blastema, containing cells capable of asexual division and differentiation, Fig. 14.6B) which forms the nephric vesicle (Fig. 14.6C). This eventually forms the Bowman's capsule and the rest of the nephron. As the vesicle elongates a capillary complex forms near one end and invaginates into the tubule to form the Bowman's capsule and glomerulus (Fig. 14.6D–F).

Between the sixth and ninth week the kidneys ascend to a lumbar site just between the adrenal glands (Fig. 14.7). By the 10th week the metanephros has evolved into the cortex and medulla, and each 'tree' of collecting ducts drains into a minor calyx and converges to form the renal papilla. Urine produced by the foetus is excreted into the amniotic fluid but kidney function is not necessary until after birth.

Congenital renal agenesis

Congenital renal agenesis leads to the absence of one (unilateral renal agenesis) or both (bilateral renal agenesis) kidneys at birth. Bilateral renal agenesis is rare, but incompatible with life. While in utero, the absence of foetal kidneys leads to a deficiency in amniotic fluid production (**oligohydramnios** or **anhydramnios).** Without amniotic fluid to cushion the foetus, the foetal facial and other features become 'squashed'. The combination of absent kidneys, oligohydramnios and

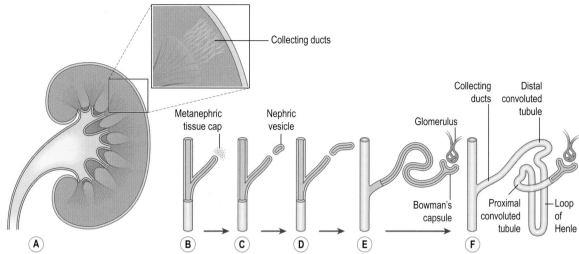

Fig. 14.6 Development of the renal collecting system and nephrons. (A) The ureteric buds continue to bifurcate until the 32nd week, producing 1–3 million collecting ducts (B–F). The tip of each collecting duct induces the development of a metanephric tissue cap, which differentiates into a renal vesicle. This vesicle ultimately forms a Bowman's capsule and the proximal and distal convoluted tubules and loop of Henle. Functional nephric units (of the type shown in (E)) first appear in distal regions of the metanephros at 10 weeks.

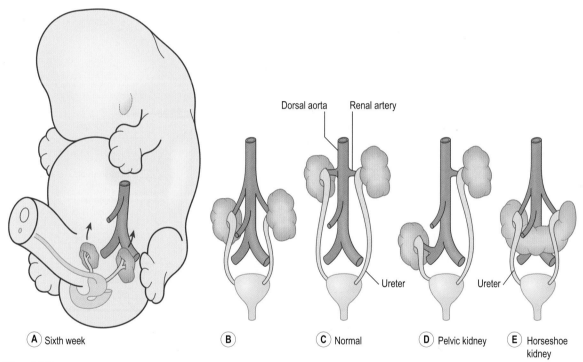

Fig. 14.7 Normal and abnormal ascent of the kidneys from the pelvis. (A–C) The metanephroi normally ascend from the sacral region of their definitive lumbar position between the sixth and ninth week. (D) Infrequently, a kidney may fail to ascend, resulting in a pelvic kidney. (E) If the inferior poles of the metanephroi make contact and fuse before ascent, the resulting horseshoe kidney catches under the inferior mesenteric artery.

characteristic features is sometimes referred to as **Potter syndrome** (also called **Potter's sequence, oligohydramnios sequence**). Unilateral renal agenesis is more common, but not life-threatening as long as the single kidney remains healthy.

Polycystic kidney disease

Polycystic kidney disease is characterised by multiple renal cysts (Clinical box 14.4). The autosomal dominant form of polycystic kidney disease (ADPKD) is a hereditary disorder presenting in adulthood, with associated other organ abnormalities

(e.g. liver cysts). Autosomal recessive polycystic kidney disease (ARPKD) is rare, thought to be due to gene mutation, and fatal in early childhood.

RENAL FUNCTION

In healthy individuals, the kidneys filter 180 L (125 mL/min) of fluid in 24 hours, excreting 1.5–2 L as urine (see above). They are also involved in the retention of essential nutrients

The pattern of inheritance for polycystic kidney disease is autosomal dominant (ADPKD), which means that each offspring has a 50% chance of inheriting the responsible mutation and, hence, the disease. ADPKD is a genetically heterogeneous condition that involves at least two genes. *PKD1* is located on 16p13.3 and accounts for most ADPKD cases (85%). *PKD2* is located on 4q21-q22 and accounts for 15% of ADPKD cases. ADPKD presents earlier in life. ADPKD1 is more severe than ADPKD2. The mean age of ESRD for patients with ADPKD1 and ADPKD2 is 53 years and 74 years, respectively.

Clinical features are usually loin pain, haematuria, urinary tract infections, renal stones, hypertension and progressive renal failure. Approximately 20–25% have polycystic liver, 10–15% have mitral valve prolapse and 5–50% have berry aneurysms. Differentiating features from other causes of multicystic disease is that ADPKD patients have bigger kidney size/volume and there is usually a strong family history.

Management involves analgesics, good control of BP, proteinuria and prompt treatment of UTIs.

- Filtration
- Reabsorption, which may be passive or selective
- Secretion.

Different parts of the nephron perform different functions. Figure 14.8 is a simplified diagrammatic representation of how the nephron functions.

GLOMERULAR FILTRATION AND THE PRODUCTION OF PRIMARY URINE

Urine is formed by the capillary hydrostatic pressure forcing the water and salts of plasma through the wall of the glomerular capillaries, most probably through the gaps between the endothelial cells and through the fenestrae (regions of thinning of the wall) in the capillary wall (Fig. 14.5). The fluid then passes between the epithelial podocytes, and between these structures lies the **basement membrane**. This is the filter bed of the kidney which holds back plasma proteins from passing into the nephron (see above).

From measurements of the permeability of molecules of different sizes, all molecules of less than 12 000 molecular weight are filtered into the nephron. This implies that all

such as protein and glucose; water, acid–base and electrolyte balance; and hormone secretion, as well as the excretion of waste products of metabolism. The complex processes concerned are:

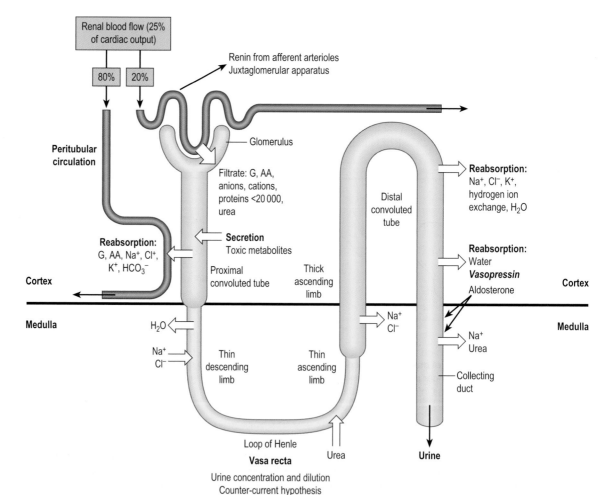

Fig. 14.8 Diagrammatic representation of major transport sites in the nephron. Apart from macromolecules, the glomerular filtrate contains glucose, amino acids, electrolytes such as Na^+, K^+, Cl^-, urea, bicarbonate and water. The PCT is the major site for reabsorption: 99% of the glucose is reabsorbed into the peritubular circulation, also essential nutrients and electrolytes. Bicarbonate reabsorption at the PCT affects renal acid–base homeostasis. Toxic metabolites, cations and anions are also secreted by the PCT. The loop of Henle is the major site for urine concentration according to the counter-current hypothesis. Further NaCl and water reabsorption takes place in the DCT and CT, controlled by vasopressin and aldosterone. PCT, proximal convoluted tubule; DCT, distal convoluted tubule; CT, collecting tubule; G, glucose; AA, amino acid; G, glucose; HCO_3^-, bicarbonate.

electrolytes, sugars, amino acids, vitamins, etc. pass easily into the Bowman's capsule and then must be recovered by the rest of the nephron, back into the plasma.

Pore size and macromolecules

If it is assumed that the 'holes' (pores) in the basement membrane are tiny cylinders in the wall of about 1.4 nm in diameter, as the size of the molecule approaches the diameter of the pore it will have less and less chance of being filtered. The size of a molecule is usually judged by its molecular weight (MW), but this can be misleading, since some molecules are spherical (globular) whereas others are long and thin. This latter group may get through into filtrate in small amounts by passing 'end on' through the pores, although from their molecular weight it could be assumed that they are far too large; this effect may explain why a small quantity of even the largest proteins do get filtered into the urine, although there may also be a small population of large pores.

However, the most critical factor that affects the filtration of a macromolecule is whether it has a surface charge. Haemoglobin (MW 67 000) escapes into the urine, whereas albumin (MW 62 000) although smaller is not filtered. This is related to the fact that although both molecules are globular proteins, albumin has a negative surface charge, so is held back by the repulsion of the charges on the fibrillar matrix of the basement membrane, whereas haemoglobin is not charged, so it can pass through relatively freely.

In disease states the surface charge on the fibrillar matrix can be disturbed and albumin now appears in the urine (albuminuria), which is a useful early warning sign of kidney injury.

Filtration forces

The hydrostatic pressure (HP) at the afferent arterioles as they enter the glomerulus is about 50 mmHg, which is about 15 mmHg higher than most other systemic capillaries. The capillary hydrostatic pressure only falls by 5 mmHg along the length of the glomerular capillary to 45 mmHg in the efferent arterioles. This large hydrostatic pressure and high permeability of the capillary walls causes a large fraction of fluid and small molecules to be filtered into the Bowman's capsule of the nephron. This 'outward' force is, however, balanced by the opposing pull of the plasma proteins which, being too large to pass through the wall, exert an osmotic force in the opposite direction to the hydrostatic pressure force. This is the colloid osmotic pressure (COP) or oncotic pressure of the plasma proteins and has a value of about 25 mmHg at the start of the glomerular capillaries. The COP gradually rises along the length of the capillary, as water and salts move out of the blood, so increasing the effective concentration of the plasma proteins. By about one-third along the length of the glomerular capillary, the COP has risen to about 35 mmHg.

In addition, the movement of fluid into the Bowman's capsule surrounding the capillaries causes a rise in hydrostatic pressure of about 10 mmHg in the tubular pressure within this space, since the exit into the rest of the nephron is narrow. These two pressures balance the hydrostatic pressure so only about 20% of the volume of the blood is filtered into the nephron, as shown in Figure 14.8. Note that in other systemic capillaries, the pressure in the extracellular fluid (ECF) is usually slightly negative (−0.5 mmHg).

The hydrostatic pressure of the blood draining from the glomerulus is 45 mmHg, as opposed to 12 mmHg in muscle capillaries. This high pressure is needed to drive the blood through the second capillary bed of the peritubular capillaries or through the vasa recta (see Fig. 14.4). The COP of the peritubular blood is also elevated to 30–35 mmHg, which also helps to draw fluid back into the peritubular capillaries.

Proteins

Proteins are mostly held back by the basement membrane. However, a small percentage is filtered and has to be recovered by the cells of the nephron as the filtrate passes down the renal tubule. This recovery is by the process of receptor-mediated endocytosis so the eventual loss of protein into the urine is small, usually about 50–80 mg per 24 hours.

FUNCTIONS OF THE PROXIMAL CONVOLUTED TUBULE

The first segment of the tubular portion of the nephron, the proximal convoluted tubule (PCT), has four main functions:

- It recovers some 70% of glomerular filtrate with respect to the filtered water and electrolytes
- It reabsorbs most of the filtered sugars, amino acids, nucleosides, other small non-electrolytes and low molecular weight proteins (e.g. retinol binding proteins, α and β microglobulins)
- It is the prime site for both the recovery of bicarbonate and the generation of new bicarbonate depending on the arterial pCO_2
- It secretes a number of organic acids and bases, as well as a wide variety of toxic and fat soluble molecules into the urine.

This latter function means that the level of these compounds is higher in the urine than in the blood capillaries (see below). Urinary organic acids and bases, toxic and fat soluble molecules can be in excess of endogenous molecules, from administered drugs or dietary sources. These functions involve a wide range of different types of transport and a large number of different carrier molecules (Fig. 14.9). Most of these processes require energy. The renal metabolic processes are aerobic, and consume large amounts of oxygen, almost equal to cardiac muscle.

Tight junctions

Each epithelial cell of the PCT is joined to those surrounding it by an occluding band of tight junctions close to the apical, or urine, side of the cells (rather like the plastic holding a 'six-pack' of soft drink cans); these junctions can vary in their 'tightness' or permeability. In the PCT they are 'moderately leaky', so although they slow the rate of passage of small molecules between cells, they do not permit steep gradients to be established between the lumen and the blood across the whole epithelium. Any concentration gradients established between the cells on the blood side of the PCT by the transport processes across the cell wall will osmotically draw fluid and some ions through these 'leaky' tight junctions. This process helps to recover water, salts and other small molecules back into the blood by a relatively low energy cost process. This recovery of water mainly aided by a member of cellular water channels called **aquaporins**. Aquaporin 1 (AQP-1) is localised in the apical and basolateral region of

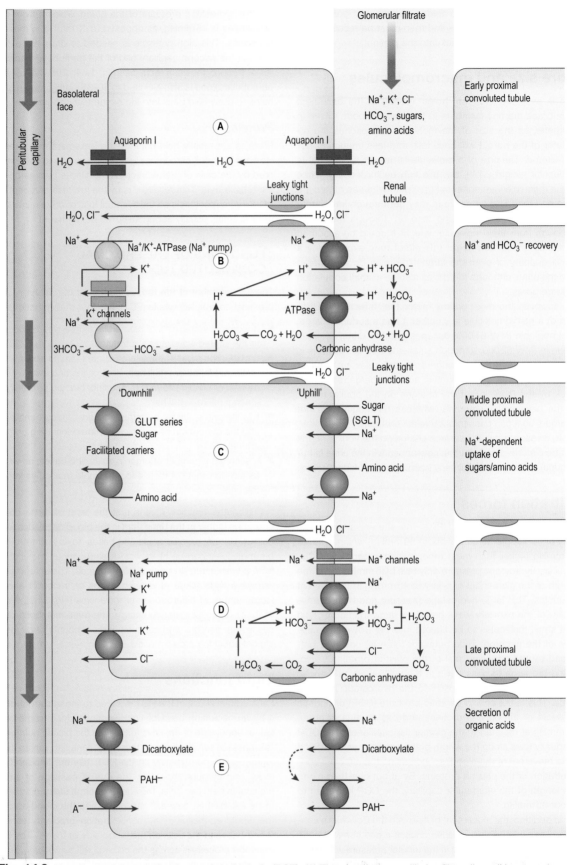

Fig. 14.9 **Functions of the proximal convoluted tubule (PCT).** (A) The glomerular capillaries filter all small ions, sugars and amino acids into the tubule at a rate related to their plasma concentrations and the GFR. (B) Filtered Na⁺ is recovered in exchange for H⁺ ions and by ATPase dependent H⁺ transport. (C) In the middle PCT sugars and amino acids are recovered by a Na⁺ dependent uptake into the cells of the PCT, then moved into the blood by facilitated downhill carriers such as the GLUT series. (D) In the late PCT Na⁺ is recovered by Na⁺ channels. (E) The transport pathway for organic anion secretion. See text for further details. GLUT, glucose transporter; SGLT, sodium coupled glucose transporter; PAH, para-aminohippuric acid.

the PCT epithelial cell membrane (Fig. 14.9A). AQP-1 is not regulated by vasopressin, whereas AQP-2 located in the apical plasma membrane and intracellular vesicles of collecting duct principal cells are regulated by vasopressin. The high permeability of the PCT enables a vast volume of fluid to be recovered at low energy cost. The PCT only uses about 5% of the total energy consumption of the kidney.

The sodium pump

The 'power house' which drives most of the processes in the kidney is the sodium pump (sodium–potassium pump, Na^+/K^+-ATPase pump), located in the basolateral membrane of the tubular epithelial cells. All cells in the body have the ability to pump sodium from inside the cell across the cell membrane into the ECF (see Ch. 1). The pump requires energy in the form of ATP, which is generated from oxygen and glucose. The pump must also have K^+ on the outside of the cell, and it usually pumps $3Na^+$ out of the cell for every $2K^+$ transferred in the opposite direction. Transport of sodium in PCT by this pump is an example of primary active transport (uphill against electrochemical gradient).

The walls of the epithelial cells of the PCT are polarised, which is to say they have functionally different properties on the luminal (urine) side compared with the blood side of the cell (Fig. 14.9B). The sodium pumps are only found on the blood side of the cell, as tight junctions between the epithelial cells maintain the differential distribution of membrane proteins between apical and basal membranes, and this difference enables the cells to transport ions and non-electrolytes from the urinary filtrate back into the blood.

A rise in intracellular Na^+ concentration increases sodium pump activity, to 'pump' Na^+ ions out of the cell into the ECF. The pumping of sodium out of the cell, and a gradient in the opposite direction for K^+, creates a potential energy gradient across the cell wall that can be used to recover many substances from the glomerular filtrate.

Carrier proteins

In the membranes of all epithelial cells are a number of carrier proteins which can move ions across the cell walls on either the lumen or the blood side of the cell. These carriers use the potential energy of the gradients of Na^+ or K^+ ions set up by the sodium pump to move ions either both in the same direction or one goes 'out' and the other comes 'in'. This arrangement maintains the balance of positive and negative charges across the cell wall, i.e.

- A +ve ion and −ve ion go out together (symport or co-transport) or
- A +ve ion goes 'out' in exchange for a +ve ion coming 'in' (antiport or counter-transport).

The arrangement of these carriers is also different on the two sides of the cell and often certain ions such as K^+ are recirculated, being carried into the cell by one carrier then passing back out again either via an ion selective channel or on another carrier. The overall effect of these carriers is to recover most of the filtered ions, as well as sugars and amino acids, from the tubular fluid back to the blood (Fig. 14.9B).

Ion channels

There are also membrane-spanning proteins which form ion channels that are selective for a specific ion which will move through a pathway formed by the transmembrane loops of protein. Ions move under the influence of the concentration gradient through these channels across the cell wall. Some ion channels can be in an 'open' state, which permits the ion to pass through, or a 'closed' state when the flow is impeded. These changes in opened or closed state, called 'gating', can be brought about by variation in the membrane potential or by ligands (chemical factors such as acetylcholine (ACh), cyclic nucleotides or G proteins) (see Ch. 4; Fig. 14.9B).

Recovery of bicarbonate by the PCT

Bicarbonate (HCO_3^-) is filtered at the same concentration as the blood, i.e. 24–26 mM, which represents some 4000 mM per 24 hours. The first segment of the PCT has cells which exchange Na^+ for H^+ ions using the Na^+ gradient to 'power' the process. This is an antiport process by which there is a balance in charge and is a major component in the recovery of filtered Na^+ (Fig. 14.9B). There is also an H^+-ATPase dependent process in this section which secretes the H^+ ions into the tubule but it is only a small part of the process and reduces the pH by the end of the PCT to 6.7.

The H^+ produced by these two processes reacts with the filtered HCO_3^- ions to form carbonic acid (H_2CO_3) which immediately dissociates non-enzymatically to form CO_2 and H_2O (see also Ch. 3). The CO_2, being lipid soluble, crosses the lumen side of the cell membrane where the enzyme **carbonic anhydrase** is present, both bound to the cell wall and in the cytoplasm. In the cell, carbonic anhydrase catalyses the formation of H_2CO_3 from CO_2 and H_2O, speeding up the reaction many-fold, so that H_2CO_3 rapidly forms inside the cell, which again dissociates to form H^+ ions and HCO_3^- ions (Fig. 14.9B).

$$CO_2 + H_2O \rightleftharpoons H_2CO_3 \rightleftharpoons H^+ + HCO_3^-$$

Most of the bicarbonate is thus reabsorbed, and the H^+ ions are excreted in the urine. This is an important process in the renal control of acid–base balance (see below and also Chs 1 and 3).

Some of the H^+ ions are fed into the Na^+/H^+ antiport process so help to recover Na^+ ions. The Na^+ and the HCO_3^- are extruded into the blood on the basolateral side of the cell by the Na^+/K^+-ATPase and by a $Na^+/3HCO_3^-$ carrier (see Fig. 14.9B). These processes recover the filtered HCO_3^- and about 30% of the filtered Na^+ water will osmotically accompany the process, so aiding the fluid and ionic balance. Inhibition of carbonic anhydrase activity thus promotes the excretion of Na^+ and water (see also Ch. 4). Acetozolamide is a carbonic anhydrase inhibitor.

Water

As ions are moved into the ECF on the blood side of the proximal tubular epithelium, both between cells via the 'leaky' tight junctions and into the basal infoldings, osmotic forces are generated which draw water through the cell and across the tight junctions (Fig. 14.9). The passage of water through the lipid bilayer of the cell membranes has been something of a puzzle. The PCT recovers some 67% of 180 L of the glomerular filtrate, which is about 120 L of fluid being recovered over 24 hours. Although the tight junctions between the cells can be classified as moderately 'leaky', the total surface area offered by this paracellular route between the cells would be inadequate to explain this vast movement of water. In addition, since water molecules are partly polar and have a negative charge it is difficult to envisage that this molecule could pass through a lipid bilayer.

Aquaporins

A chance finding from work on the protein content of the red cell membrane identified a special class of proteins – the aquaporins (AQPs). The AQPs are membrane-spanning proteins with the ability to form a specific channel for water through the cell membranes. About 10 classes of aquaporins have been identified, with AQP1 being most prevalent on both sides of the cells of the PCT, which explains the unexpected high water permeability of this tissue (Fig. 14.9). These molecules allow the osmotic gradient created by the movement of various electrolytes and non-electrolytes to exert a much greater force than could be predicted, and permit a relatively low expenditure of energy for the vast movement of fluid. The location of other AQPs, especially AQP2, which can be added to the luminal side of the collecting duct cells under the influence of antidiuretic hormone, will be discussed later.

Peritubular capillaries

The PCT and the DCT are enveloped in a dense capillary network, the peritubular capillaries (Fig. 14.4). The recovery of fluid into these capillaries is further aided by the raised COP of 30–35 mmHg of the blood draining from the glomerulus. This also draws water, salts and other molecules into the blood by the Starling mechanism so that by the time this blood passes into the veins it has a normal COP of 25 mmHg.

Sugars, amino acids and other small organic molecules

Sugars, amino acids and other small molecules are recovered from the glomerular filtrate by sodium-dependent carriers found on the luminal side of the PCT cell wall (Fig. 14.9C). Each of these carriers has a special site for the binding of Na^+ and a site for a specific molecular species. There are several carriers for sugars (Na^+-coupled glucose transporter (SGLT)), five for amino acids, others for ions and many nutrients, each of which are specific for their own molecule. Once both sites are occupied, the carrier undergoes transformation and the Na^+ and the other molecule on the carrier are now transferred into the cell. This process is termed co-transport and although it does not use energy directly, it does again use the steep gradient for sodium across the cell wall which has been generated by the Na^+ pump on the opposite side of the cell to 'power' the entry of the non-electrolyte 'up' their concentration gradient (Fig. 14.9C). This is secondary active transport (see also Chs 2 and 4).

The Na^+ dependent SGLT co-transport carriers will move their sugar molecules against a concentration gradient. In the first part of the PCT there are SGLT2 carriers, which have a low affinity for glucose, so they will work when there is a high sugar content in the lumen. In the later PCT segment, where the concentration of sugar is low, SGLT1 carriers, which have a high affinity for glucose, will move the sugar against a steep concentration gradient to recover molecules from the filtrate back into the blood.

Since these processes depend upon a finite number of carriers in the cell wall, a sudden large excess of a particular molecule present in the blood will increase the amount filtered

into the tubule and cause all the sites to become occupied. When this occurs the process is said to be saturated; the molecules are not fully recovered by the PCT, and will appear in the urine. This condition is seen in diabetes mellitus when glucose appears in the urine (glycosuria), leading to an osmotic diuresis (see also Ch. 3).

Facilitated carriers

Once inside the PCT cell wall, there are other carriers on the blood side for sugars and amino acids called facilitated carriers. This is a type of secondary active transport (see Chs 2 and 3). For sugars these are the GLUT series, with other series for amino acids, ions and other nutrients. These types of carrier move the non-electrolytes only down their concentration gradient into the ECF and then by diffusion into the blood. This type of carrier can also work in the opposite direction and carry sugars, amino acids and other molecules from the blood into the cell when the concentration gradient is reversed (Fig. 14.9C).

Sodium and chloride

The initial recovery of Na^+ is coupled to the Na^+/H^+ antiporter which in turn is dependent on HCO_3^- in the tubule to generate the H^+ ions. The first third of the PCT recovers most of the HCO_3^- ions, so that when its concentration in the tubular fluid falls, the recovery of Na^+ slows. However, to overcome this problem, the next section of the tubule has a Cl^-/HCO_3^- coupled exchange process, so here the HCO_3^- ions are returned to the tubular fluid to help recover Cl^- ions. Now the H^+/Na^+ antiport has more HCO_3^- to react with to help the recovery of more Na^+ ions as well as the Cl^- (Fig. 14.9D).

In this region there are also Na^+ channels which allow Na^+ to enter the cell and be recovered into the blood by the Na^+/K^+-ATPase. This would produce a large potential difference, but Cl^- ions pass through the leaky tight junctions into the intracellular spaces and balance the Na^+ ion charge. Water accompanies these processes so water and salt are recovered (Fig. 14.9).

Secretion of organic anions and cations

Renal tubules can secrete a wide variety of toxic metabolites, both ingested in the diet and produced as by-products of metabolism, including drugs. These are often organic lipid soluble anions and cations that can cross the cell membrane into the cell. These metabolites could accumulate in the cytoplasm, requiring a specific system of transport to eliminate the molecules from the circulation.

Organic anion transport

Organic anions are mostly weak aromatic and aliphatic organic acids with pKs generally of less than 7. The transporter systems to eliminate organic anions have a wide substrate specificity. At the pH of blood (7.4), these molecules are anions, whereas in the acid pH of the urine they become undissociated and lipid soluble. The renal tubules are able to secrete these compounds into the lumen so the urinary concentration of these molecules is higher than in the plasma. This is a basis for measuring renal plasma flow by the clearance method described below. Although this secretory mechanism is an advantage for the elimination of unwanted molecules, the broad specificity of the process means that many drug molecules will also be excreted. For example, this was a major problem with penicillin when the bulk of the administered dose was lost into the urine. Probenecid was found to competitively inhibit the secretion of penicillin, so that administration of probenecid together with penicillin maintained the plasma level of the antibiotic (see Ch. 4). Probenecid inhibits organic anion transporters

By the use of coloured organic acids the site of secretion was identified as the second S_2 segment of proximal tubules. The mechanism of PCT anion secretion is shown in Figure 14.9E and some examples of typical compounds are given in Table 14.2.

The SLC22A gene family codes for organic anion transporter (OAT) proteins. The OAT family plays the central role in renal organic anion transport. OAT1, OAT3, OAT4 and URAT1 are expressed in the proximal tubular cells of the kidneys. OAT1 and OAT3 mediate uptake of a wide range of relatively small and hydrophilic organic anions from plasma. URAT1 transports those organic anions from the cytoplasm of the proximal tubular cells into the lumen of the nephron. Other known substrates of OAT1 include para-aminohippurate (PAH), dicarboxylates, prostaglandins, cyclic nucleotides, urate, folate, diuretics, ACE inhibitors, antiviral agents, β-lactam antibiotics, antineoplastics, mycotoxins, sulfate conjugates, glucuronide conjugates, cystein conjugates, ochratoxin A, NSAIDs and uraemic toxins.

Para-aminohippuric acid

Hippurate is the prime organic anion secreted by the kidney and about 1 g per day is excreted in the urine. PAH is an amide derivative of the amino acid glycine and para-aminobenzoic acid. It is a model substrate for this process and on the basolateral side of the cell there is a two-stage process (Fig. 14.9E). The first step is the entry of dicarboxylates (α-ketoglutarate and glutarate) co-transported with sodium. The ubiquitous Na^+ pump maintains the low Na^+ in the cell, which enables this co-transport to proceed. Then the intracellular dicarboxylate exchanges with an organic anion, in this case PAH, which moves into the cell on the apical (luminal) side of the cell. The PAH is then exported into the lumen on the basolateral side in exchange for another anion such as chloride, urate or hydroxyl ions so the PCT can concentrate PAH to a much higher level than in plasma (200–300 times).

In plasma (pH 7.4), PAH with a pK of 3.8 is 99% ionised whereas in urine with a pH of 4.5, 83% is ionised. The non-ionised fraction can diffuse through the lipid cell membrane, so making the urine more acidic and increasing the secretion of PAH into the urine. This leads to a complete clearance of PAH on a single passage through the kidney.

In contrast, the excretion of some molecules such as probenecid, phenobarbital and salicylic acid can be increased by urinary alkalisation (see Ch. 4). This mechanism is a balance between the pK_a, the partition coefficient (K_p) and the pH, so that the excretion of some drugs such as barbital and urate are not increased by urinary alkalisation. PAH has been found to enhance the rate of excretion of water, Na^+, K^+ and HPO_2^- and this is seen in patients receiving massive doses of carbenicillin. This also occurs in starvation where there are increased organic acids derived from fat metabolism (see Ch. 3).

PAH is useful for the measurement of renal plasma flow (RPF) because it is secreted primarily by the renal tubules; only 20–30% is filtered by the glomerulus. PAH is completely filtered from plasma in the nephron and not reabsorbed by the tubules, in a manner identical to inulin. The clearance of PAH is reflective only of RPF to portions of the kidney that deal with urine formation, and thus underestimates actual RPF by about 10%.

PAH and drug dosage

When the glomerular filtration rate (GFR) falls to 10% or less of normal, hippurate accumulates in the blood and competes for the binding of several drugs such as salicylate, phenytoin, sulfonamides and furosemide. There will be an increased level of the unbound drug in the plasma with a greater therapeutic effect for a given dose. In contrast, when such patients are dialysed, the hippurate is removed so the protein binding now increases and the therapeutic effect of some drugs will be decreased and the dose must be adjusted to allow for this effect.

Efflux transporters and drugs

Efflux transporters are active transport systems that extrude drugs out of cells (see Ch. 4). They require energy to function. These efflux transporters have a broad range of specificity so can handle many molecules. The transport proteins can also be induced or upregulated, so account for the failure of some drugs to continue to act with repeated doses.

Table 14.2 Representative compounds secreted by the renal organic anion and cation transport systems

Anions		Cations	
Endogenous compounds	**Drugs**	**Endogenous compounds**	**Drugs**
Amino acids	Acetazolamide	Acetylcholine	Amiloride
Benzoate	Cephalothin	Epinephrine (adrenaline)	Amprolium
Bile salts	Chlorothiazide	Choline	Atropine
Cyclic AMP	Ethacrynic acid	Creatinine	Cimetidine
Long-chain fatty acids	Furosemide	Dopamine	Hexamethonium
Hippurate	Indometacin	Histamine	Mecamylamine
Hydroxybenzoates	Penicillin G	5-Hydroxytryptamine	Morphine
Hydroxyindoleacetic acid	Probenecid	Norepinephrine (noradrenaline)	Neostigmine
Oxalate	Saccharin	N-Methylnicotinamide	Paraquat
Prostaglandins	Salicylate	Serotonin	Quinine
Urate		Thiamine	Tetra-ethylammonium

This effect explains why some anti-cancer agents fail to work after the initial positive response, and may contribute to bacterial multidrug resistance.

Nephrotoxicity

Some drugs can damage the cells of the nephron as they accumulate within the cytoplasm and this nephrotoxicity is related to their uptake in the tubule cells by these processes and the lower ability of the cells to transport these drugs into the urine. Neonates are protected from this damage as their uptake transport system is poorly developed at this stage.

Organic cation transport

Many organic cations in the blood are excreted by the kidney where a series of organic cation transporters (OCT1–3) are expressed. These are electrogenic organic cation transporters with a broad specificity which suggests they are involved in the first step of secretion of the compounds, moving the molecules across the basolateral membrane. The exit across the brush border is accompanied by an organic cation/H^+ antiporter acting down the lumen/cell H^+ gradient established by Na^+/H^+ exchange. Table 14.2 gives some examples of these compounds (Clinical box 14.5). However, the detailed mechanism of their transport has not been well characterised and work is still in progress, although the structure of OAT and OCT has been identified.

RENAL FUNCTION TESTS

The symptoms of renal failure can masquerade under an amazing variety of clinical conditions, so it is essential to be able to screen patients using simple low-cost techniques before proceeding to more complex and expensive diagnostic tests.

Blood and urine tests

In routine blood tests a raised level of urea and creatinine are the first signs of possible renal problems, which can be confirmed by testing the urine, where increased levels of protein and tubular debris after centrifugation can often be found. Measurement of the urinary volume over 24 hours and the ability to form concentrated urine, when water intake is restricted, can also be used and will identify both problems within the kidney and of the water control mechanisms.

Relative density of urine
This can be measured by a number of methods.

Osmolality

Osmolality of urine depends on the number of particles present and be measured directly by the depression of freezing point with an osmometer. It is significantly increased in glycosuria but not influenced by temperature or protein.

Specific gravity

A more simple guide is to measure the specific gravity using a hydrometer, which compares the specific gravity of the test fluid with the specific gravity of pure water:

Specific gravity = density of test fluid/density of water

In pure water, the float will sink to a level of 1.000 on the hydrometer. With increasing density of the test solution, the scale on the hydrometer will float to a higher level which is related to the ionic content. Plasma has a specific gravity of 1.010 (285 mOsm). Urine can vary from a specific gravity of 1.035 (1400 mOsm), the most concentrated and dark, down to 1.005 (50 mOsm), the most dilute and pale. Note, however, since the density of fluids varies with temperature and hot fluids are less dense, it is essential to allow the urine to cool to the calibrated temperature of the hydrometer. In hot environments it is necessary to ensure that the hydrometer used is calibrated to the range of climatic temperature.

Although not frequently performed, measurement of the specific gravity of a urine specimen can give an indication of the efficiency of the renal control of fluid balance mechanisms (see below). If the specific gravity is >1.035, glycosuria should be considered and when it is >1.040 indicates the presence of extrinsic osmotic agents (e.g. contrast)

Refractometry

This is based on measurement of refractory index which depends on the size and weight of solutes and correlates well with osmolality.

Dry chemistry

Dry chemistry is incorporated into dipsticks and detects the presence of cations and protons by colour change.

Analysing urine

The history of urine analysis can be traced back to ancient Egypt where polyuria and haematuria were mentioned in medical papyri, and, by 400 BC, Hippocrates had observed the changes to the colour and odour of urine and its relation to disease. Healthy urine should be clear and a straw colour. Other colours can indicate the presence of drugs, blood haemoglobin or bilirubin. The odour of urine can reflect chemical conditions: a fruity odour or acetone in diabetes mellitus and a musty odour indicates hepatic disease, and ingestion of various dietary constituents such as garlic gives other odours. The various penicillins are excreted via the kidney and can impart a strong odour to the urine. By the end of the eighteenth century, the chemistry of urine analysis had progressed to various spot tests and then to test papers, which identify specific constituents present in the urine. Table 14.3 sets out the range of tests commonly in use, and their purpose.

Specialised spectrophotometers can be used to quantify the concentration of various constituents in urine.

Proteinuria

Physiologic proteinuria does not exceed 150 mg/24 hours for adults and 140 mg/m^2 in children. Urine dipstick is highly sensitive in detecting albumin (limit approx. 0.2 g/L). Dipstix allows rough quantification of urine from 0 to ++++. Urine dipstix does not identify globulin fraction of protein and can be negative in Bence Jones proteinuria (free immunoglobulin light chains in urine).

Clinical box 14.5 **Furosemide**

Furosemide is bound to plasma proteins and is not filtered so only passes into the tubule by these secretion processes. Indometacin, aspirin and probenecid compete with this step so reduce the diuretic action of this drug, although they do displace it from the protein binding which increases entry into the tubule by filtration (see Ch. 4).

Table 14.3   Urine tests and purpose

Range of tests	Uses
Specific gravity	To monitor drugs in athletes
pH 4.8–7.4	Acid–base disturbances
Leucocytes	Inflammatory disease of the kidney
Nitrite	Presence of bacteria
Protein (albumin)	Renal disease
Glucose	Diabetes mellitus renal threshold 8.3–10 mM
Ketones	Increased fat degradation, gastrointestinal infection in diabetes mellitus
Urobilinogen	Liver disease or increased haemolysis
Bilirubin	Liver damage, hepatitis, cirrhosis
Blood	Renal and post-renal bleeding

Clinical box 14.6   Interpretation of urine protein to urine creatinine ratio

Child under age 2 years
Normal ratio <0.5

Adults and children over age 2 years
Normal ratio <2 mg/mmol correlates with 0.2 g protein/day (i.e. 2 × 10 mg protein/day)
Nephrotic range >3.5 (correlates with 3.5 g protein/day)

Interpretation of urine albumin to creatinine ratio (ACR)
Microalbuminuria: ACR of 2.5–30 mg/mmol (men) and 3.5 to 30 mg/mmol (women)
Macroalbuminuria: ACR of >30 mg/mmol (this is approximately equivalent to PCR >50 mg/mmol, or a urinary protein excretion >0.5 g/24 h).

Protein quantification is expressed as g/L or g/24 h. 24 hour urine collections are time consuming and practically difficult, hence an alternative measure, the protein:creatinine ratio (PCR) on a random urine sample, has now been validated, widely accepted and used. First or early morning urine sample is more accurate (see Clinical box 14.6).

Proteinuria may be increased by a factor of 2–3 times by strenuous exercise or fever. Other causes of transient proteinuria include urinary tract infection, vaginal mucus, orthostatic proteinuria (occurs after patient has been upright for some time and is not found in early morning urine – this condition is uncommon in patients over 30 years old) and pregnancy. Causes of persistent proteinuria include:

- Primary renal disease – this may be glomerular (e.g. glomerulonephritis) or tubular
- Secondary renal disease – diabetes mellitus, hypertension, connective tissue diseases, vasculitis, amyloidosis, myeloma, congestive cardiac failure.

Renal handling of molecules

Simple estimates of renal function can be derived from changes in the way that the kidney handles molecules. The kidney can handle molecules in three ways:

- First, a molecule can be simply filtered and then passed unchanged into the urine (Fig. 14.10A).
- Second, it can be filtered then reabsorbed as it passes through the PCT, so the final concentration in the urine is less than in plasma (Fig. 14.10B).
- Finally, a molecule can be filtered and then more can be added to the urine by secretion in the PCT, making the concentration in urine higher than in plasma (Fig.14.10C).

These mechanisms can be studied by the use of a technique called clearance. Water being abstracted from the tubule will alter the concentration in the urine but its effect will depend on the transport of each molecule. Even molecules which are only filtered will be concentrated in the urine by this process.

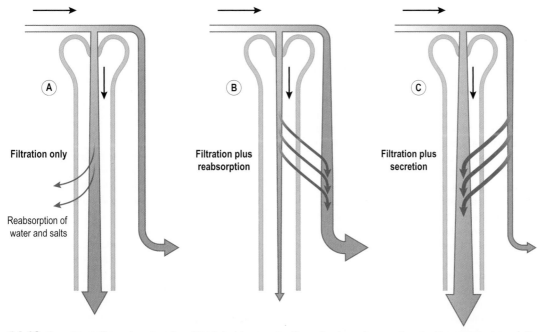

Fig. 14.10 Renal handling of molecules. (A) Molecules can be filtered only and not reabsorbed or secreted, but will still have an increased concentration in the urine due to the fact that fluid is recovered along the nephron. (B) Molecules that are filtered and reabsorbed will have a very low concentration in the urine. (C) Molecules that are filtered and secreted will have an elevated concentration in the urine and very low levels in the blood draining from the nephron.

Renal clearance

The clearance of a molecule is defined as 'volume of plasma cleared of that molecule per minute'. Since no molecule is fully cleared by the kidney, it is more a concept than a reality. It is a simple way of quantifying the handling by the nephron of various types of molecule. The most useful renal function which can be derived from a clearance measurement is the glomerular filtration rate (GFR).

If the renal excretion ($U_x \times V$), i.e. the concentration of a molecule in mM in the urine (U_x) multiplied by the volume of urine formed per minute (V), is measured and divided by the concentration of the molecule in plasma (P_x), we can gain some idea of how the nephron is handling the molecule. This is termed the clearance of a molecule.

The clearance of molecule x is expressed as:

$$C_x = (U_x \times V)/P_x$$

U_x = the concentration in the urine in mM
P_x = the concentration in plasma in mM
V = the volume of urine formed per min, i.e. mL/min.
The unit of clearance is mL/min.

Clearance of molecules that are only filtered

If a molecule is filtered and then passes unchanged into the urine, the clearance of such a molecule is an index of the effective glomerular filtration rate of all the nephrons, i.e. the glomerular filtration rate (GFR). The concentration of such a molecule will be raised in the urine, as it will remain trapped in the tubule after filtration, where some 99% of water and other constituents of the filtrate are mostly recovered as they pass along the tubule.

'Inulin' clearance as an index of GFR

In the past, 'inulin' (a plant starch) of molecular weight 5200, was used for testing renal clearance as a molecule that is filtered then passed unchanged into the urine. 'Inulin' is now no longer available and polyfructans are used instead. Inulin clearance, however, is still a benchmark against which all other methods are judged and the term 'inulin clearance', is still used. To perform a clearance test with 'inulin' (C_{in}), the bladder is first emptied and the 'inulin' injected intravenously as a bolus. Since this molecule is filtered, the level in the blood will rise to a peak value then fall with time, as shown in Figure 14.11A. The urine is collected for a set period and the concentration of 'inulin' in the urine and the volume formed in mL/min ($U_{in}V$) can be easily determined. The problem, however, remains to find a value of plasma which reflects the average concentration for the period (P_{in}). Various methods have been used to obtain a mean of this value of plasma concentration, including infusing a dilute 'inulin' solution to balance the renal loss as shown by the dotted line in Figure 14.11A, or calculating the area under the curve, but errors in this value have a large effect on the calculation of C_{in}.

Note that whatever level of 'inulin' appears in the blood the same level is filtered into the urine, so the relationship becomes a straight line with a slope of 45 degrees. Figure 14.11B shows that the clearance (C_{in}) of this molecule is independent of the blood level.

Values of 'inulin' clearance are in the range of 125 ± 30 mL/min for normal male subjects. This is the value taken as 'normal' GFR. Again, note that the range of C_{in} in normal subjects is quite large, i.e. ± 30 of the population mean value of 125 and depends on body size, age and sex. Females have a lower value than males with a mean of about 90 mL/min

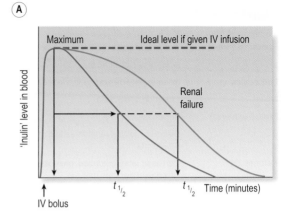

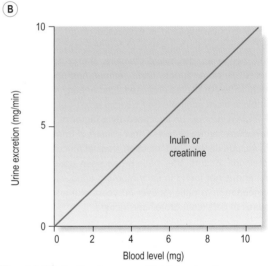

Fig. 14.11 Inulin clearance. (A) Molecules that are filtered only, such as 'inulin', can be re-used as an index of GFR. If 'inulin' is given as a bolus into the plasma the level rises rapidly to a maximum then 'falls' off with time as it is filtered. In renal failure the rate of 'fall' is much reduced and by measuring the time to reach a value that was half the maximum, an index of renal function can be derived from the fall off in plasma level. To get a true reading plasma level 'inulin' would have to be infused at a rate to match the filtered loss; since this is not known this is difficult to achieve. (B) Since the urine excretion matches the blood level, it indicates that this molecule is filtered only. IV, intravenous.

being taken as normal. Infants do not achieve adult GFR until they are about 4 years old and cannot fully concentrate their urine until the kidney has matured. With increasing age, renal function begins to decrease above the age of about 65–70.

Creatinine clearance

Creatinine is a breakdown product of muscle metabolism (creatine phosphate) and is usually produced at a constant rate by the body (depending on the muscle mass) so has a constant level in the blood. (Note: creatinine is a di-amino acid and must not be confused with creatine.) This molecule was thought to be a good marker for GFR since it is endogenous, i.e. occurs naturally in the circulation and the plasma concentration (P_{cr}) is relatively constant. Serum creatinine is affected by the level of GFR and by factors independent of GFR, including age, gender, race, body size, diet, certain drugs and laboratory analytical methods. This makes it a poor marker of true renal function.

Creatinine clearance, C_{cr}, gives values close to 'inulin', i.e. 125 mL/min, although there is a small component of secretion. However, the error caused by the raised value of urinary creatinine, U_{cr}, is balanced by a plasma chromogen which raises the value of P_{cr}, so the errors cancel.

Serum creatinine levels may vary from one laboratory to another, depending on the method used to measure. Usually for males (higher muscle mass) 60–80 µmol/L and is 40–60 µmol/L in females (lesser muscle mass). It is simple to measure and is elevated only in renal failure. Creatinine is mostly filtered but is secreted by proximal tubules as well.

Urea clearance

Urea is also a natural product, but it is reabsorbed and re-circulated in the kidney so gives values three-fifths of GFR; urea clearance, C_u, is about 80 mL/min. The ratio of C_{cr} to C_u can be used to reduce variation. C_u does, however, vary with water intake, so if the water intake is low even more is reabsorbed and the value of C_u falls.

Current methods for measuring renal clearance (half-life)

Figure 14.11A shows that the level of 'inulin' in plasma when injected as a bolus decreases with time as it is filtered through the kidney. If the kidney is damaged and GFR is depressed, the rate of 'inulin' filtration with time will be less, and the blood level will fall more slowly (*hatched line* Fig. 14.11A). This fact can then be used as an indication of renal function. An easily measured molecule, such as ^{51}Cr-EDTA (ethylene diamine tetra-acetic acid, molecular weight 300) is given as a bolus and then the blood level followed for a period of time by taking serial blood samples. EDTA is a molecule which strongly binds to chromium (Cr). ^{51}Cr is an isotope which emits gamma rays and is easy to count. Initially the counts in plasma samples will rapidly rise to a maximum then decrease over a period. The time can then be taken for the isotope level to fall to half of the maximum, which is the half-life ($t\frac{1}{2}$) for healthy subjects (Fig. 14.11A). With the progressive deterioration of renal function the $t\frac{1}{2}$ gradually increases, indicating loss of filtration capacity, and reflects the number of nephrons which are still functional. This method is quick and cheap and has largely replaced other clearance methods. It has limited clinical use apart from use in estimation of GFR in a potential kidney donor. It can be used in certain groups of renal failure patients with unreliable estimated GFR, e.g. amputees, extremes of body weight.

Clearance of molecules that are filtered and reabsorbed

Clearance of molecules that are filtered and reabsorbed is not used as a test, but gives an idea of one of the most important functions of the kidney (see Fig. 14.10A). Molecules such as glucose have a very low clearance (0.2 mL/min) since they are actively reabsorbed. The normal plasma level is 4–5 mM and only tiny amounts are found in the urine of normal subjects; however, as the blood level of glucose increases a point is reached – the renal threshold – when glucose appears in the urine at the same rate as 'inulin', etc. This is the result of the saturation of all the carrier sites; i.e. there is a limited number of sites for uptake and, if there is a large excess of glucose in the blood, they all become occupied and now the molecule passes through the PCT, as if it was only filtered. As can be

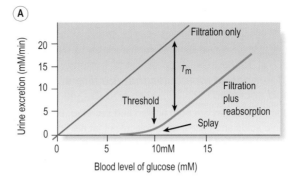

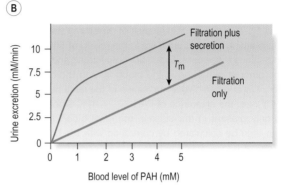

Fig. 14.12 **Clearance of molecules that are filtered and reabsorbed, such as glucose.** (A) Initially no glucose appears in the urine, as it is reabsorbed; however, once the plasma level exceeds the renal threshold glucose is filtered into the urine. This point is related to the availability of carriers to recover the filtered glucose, which eventually becomes saturated. Different nephrons vary in their saturation level so there is a splay in the threshold level. Once the threshold is exceeded, glucose is just filtered and the line is parallel to that of molecules which are only filtered. The displacement of this line gives an index of the tubular maximum, T_m, for the recovery of glucose. (B) For molecules which are filtered and secreted, the level in the urine is higher than in the plasma. This process will also saturate in most cases. Molecules such as para-amino hippuric acid (PAH) are virtually cleared from the plasma by these processes.

seen from Figure 14.12A, once the threshold is reached the behaviour of glucose parallels that of a molecule which is only filtered, such as creatinine.

The threshold is not a sharp point but has a 'splay' as different nephrons have a slightly different value for threshold. In the normal subject, the threshold is about 8–10 mM and so after a meal with a high sugar content, this value is exceeded for a short while, which explains why a small amount of glucose is found in the urine of normal people. The displacement of the glucose response, compared to that of a molecule that is only filtered, is expressed as the tubular maximum, T_m, and represents the total capacity of the kidney to reabsorb glucose. With diabetes mellitus, glucose in the urine is common due to the lack of insulin and high levels of glucose in the plasma, but as the disease progresses, microvascular complications lead to renal damage and a much elevated threshold for glucose. Now little glucose appears in urine, although the plasma levels may be 20 mM or greater (normal 4–5 mM). This is why urine testing for glucose in diabetes mellitus is now no longer used and has been replaced by measuring the glucose level in blood with various reagent strips which give an accurate colour change depending on the level of glucose in the blood. This colour is measured by various meters which now can respond in about 10 seconds or less.

Clearance of molecules that are filtered and secreted

Some molecules are both filtered and secreted, such as organic acids and bases, and molecules that are lipid soluble or are toxic and have been converted into glucuronides by the liver (see Ch. 4). With these compounds, more appears in the urine than in the blood as they are secreted into the tubule. As with sugars, this process saturates since there is a finite number of carriers. The process has both a threshold and T_m. The values for clearance of molecules such as PAH (para-amino hippuric acid) are in the region of 650–700 mL/min. Since these compounds are both filtered and secreted, the amount remaining in the blood leaving the nephron is very low and can give an indication of the renal plasma flow (RPF), i.e. the clearance of PAH, C_{PAH} = RPF. Since the PAH is only present in the plasma, the renal blood flow (RBF) can then be calculated by correction with the haematocrit (Hct), i.e.

$$RBF = C_{PAH} / 1 - Hct$$

Use of clearance methods to assess renal function

Renal blood flow (RBF) is about 1.2–1.4 L/min, i.e. one-fifth of cardiac output. Thus we can then, by relatively simple methods, obtain the effective GFR and RBF using clearance techniques. The ratio of GFR to RBF is called the filtration fraction (FF) and is about 0.10–0.15; i.e. 20% of the plasma passing through the kidney is filtered into the nephron.

$$FF = GFR/RBF = C_{in}/C_{PAH}$$

With the large number of patients with possible renal failure it is essential to take a detailed history and to be able to screen patients using blood tests and simple low cost techniques before proceeding to those which are more complicated and expensive.

Advanced clinical tests

If signs of renal failure are detected on simple testing, a variety of diagnostic tests can then be used to identify the site of the renal dysfunction, e.g. obstruction, by imaging, ultrasound, nuclear medical imaging, computed tomography scans or the gamma camera.

RENAL CONTROL OF FLUID BALANCE

The mechanisms which balance fluid intake with fluid loss are more precise than those for acid–base and electrolyte balance. The control of these processes resides in an osmoreceptive complex located in the hypothalamus (see Fig. 14.13A) and comprises the subfornical organ (SFO), the organum vasculosum of the lamina terminalis (OVLT) and the median pre-optic nucleus (MnPO), all of which input on to the magnocellular neurons of the supraoptic (SO) and paraventricular nuclei (PVN). The SO and PVN neurons can act both as osmoreceptors and also synthesise two peptide hormones – vasopressin and the reproductive hormone oxytocin.

Vasopressin

Vasopressin (or antidiuretic hormone, ADH) is a nonapeptide (nine amino acids) that has two cysteine residues in positions 1 and 6, linked by a disulphide bridge (see Fig. 14.13B). It has a short half-life of 15–20 minutes. Antidiuretic hormones evolved very early in evolution and are found in most animal species. In mammals, vasopressin is released from the posterior pituitary in response to a small rise in the osmotic pressure of the plasma usually caused by an increased rate of water loss. There is an inverse relationship between the plasma vasopressin level and the osmolarity of the urine (see Fig. 14.13C). Note, however, that although the volume and concentration of urine vary, the net loss of solute does not, and is maintained constant for a given period. There is thus a mechanism by which the water balance is separated from that of solute.

Water intake is regulated to maintain a physiological serum osmolality of 285 to 290 mOsm/kg. Normally, the level of vasopressin in the plasma is in the range 2–4 pg/mL and is rapidly increased as the plasma osmolarity changes. Osmotic threshold for vasopressin release is 280 to 290 mOsm/kg. Thirst plays an important role in water balance and only 2–3% change in plasma osmolarity can produce a strong desire to drink water. This precise matching of the plasma VP level to osmolarity is the central mechanism of water homeostasis (Fig. 14.14A,B). The normal response to a fall in water intake is a rise in plasma osmolarity, and within minutes an increase in the plasma vasopressin level.

Once vasopressin has been synthesised by neurons of the SO and PVN, it is then attached to the transport protein neurophysin as granules, which are then rapidly transported within 30 min to the posterior pituitary, down microtubules in the axons of the neurohypophyseal tract; here it is stored prior to release.

Bursts of action potentials in these axons of the neurohypophyseal tract, in response to a tiny rise in osmotic pressure, cause the release of vasopressin into the bloodstream. However, the slope of this response is steep, and in addition the gradient can be altered by the fluid volume of the extracellular fluid, which will increase or decrease the sensitivity of the response (see Fig. 14.13). Vasopressin can also be released in response to a fall in blood pressure, but the change in blood pressure must be of a much larger magnitude than that of osmolarity.

Vasopressin release

Release of ADH can be divided into:

- Inappropriate, when it is called syndrome of inappropriate ADH secretion (SIADH) and can only be diagnosed when renal, thyroid, adrenal, liver and cardiac function is normal. Causes are listed in Clinical box 14.7.
- Appropriate increase in vasopressin can be due to nephrotic syndrome, cardiac failure, cirrhosis, ascites, pregnancy, AV fistulae and hypovolaemia.

Vasopressin receptors

Figure 14.14C shows the cellular action of vasopressin. Vasopressin binds to three type of receptors (V1a, V1b and V2) with a variety of functions. V1a and V2 receptors are expressed peripherally and involved in the modulation of blood pressure and kidney function respectively, while the V1b and V1b receptors are expressed in the central nervous system.

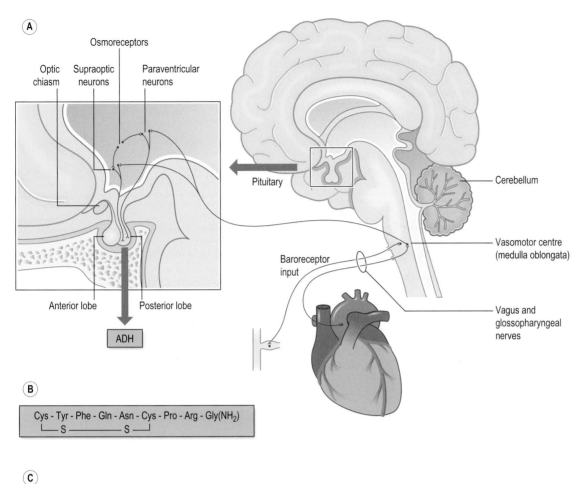

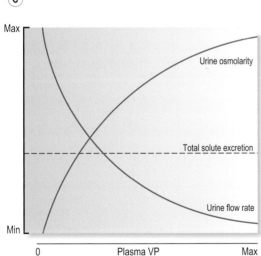

***Fig. 14.13* Vasopressin secretion.** (A) Anatomy of the hypothalamus and pituitary gland (mid-sagittal section) depicting the pathways of vasopressin (VP) secretion. Also shown are pathways involved in regulating VP secretion. Afferent fibres from the baroreceptors are carried in the vagus and glossopharyngeal nerves. The vasomotor centre includes the solitary tract nucleus. The closed box illustrates an expanded view of the hypothalamus and pituitary gland. (B) The amino acid sequence of vasopressin. (C) Relationship between plasma VP levels and urine osmolarity, urine flow rate and total solute excretion.

On reaching the kidney, vasopressin binds to specific V2 receptors located on the basolateral side of the principal cells of the cortical and medullary collecting ducts. V2 receptors are members of the G protein superfamily and, when stimulated by vasopressin, cause the activation of an intermediary G protein. This G protein activates a membrane-bound adenylate cyclase that catalyses the conversion of cytoplasmic ATP (adenosine triphosphate) to the second messenger cyclic AMP (cAMP) (see Ch. 4). The cAMP activates protein kinase A, which in turn phosphorylates myofilaments and myofibrils associated with vesicles in the cytoplasm close to the apical side of the tubular wall.

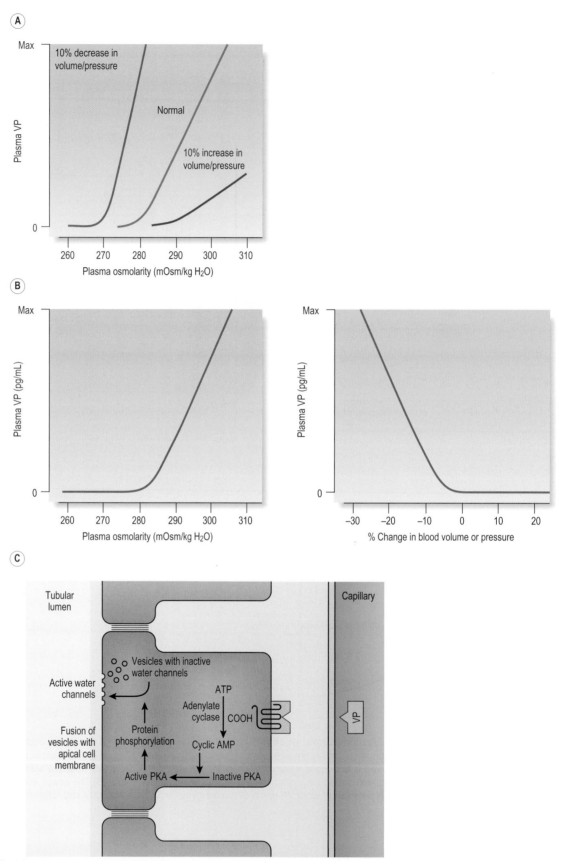

Fig. 14.14 **Action of vasopressin.** Interaction between osmotic and haemodynamic stimuli for vasopressin (VP) secretion. With decreased blood volume and pressure, the osmotic set point is shifted to lower plasma osmolarity values and the slope is increased. An increase in blood volume and pressure has the opposite effect. (A) Changes in VP secretion in response to plasma osmolarity variation. (B) Plasma VP levels in relation to plasma osmolarity to changes in blood volume or pressure. (C) Cellular action of VP.

Disease states related to renal fluid balance

Diabetes insipidus

Diabetes insipidus (DI), 'tasteless urine', is characterised by a high volume of dilute urine with haemoconcentration and polydipsia (excess drinking of water), caused by a lack of vasopressin, either from central hypothalamic damage (permanent DI) or from posterior pituitary damage (temporary DI). Temporary DI recovers because the neurons of the posterior pituitary regenerate. Causes include:

- Iatrogenic post-surgical or post-radiation (cranial)
- Trauma (i.e. head injury)
- Tumours
- Nephrogenic: V2 receptors on the collecting duct become unresponsive to vasopressin, which could be familial or idiopathic
- Psychological: 'hysterical water drinking'.

In normal subjects, water restriction is associated with an increase in the vasopressin level, and this will be paralleled by a rise in the urine osmolarity. DI caused by a hypothalamic lack of vasopressin will not show a rise in vasopressin with water restriction whereas renal insensitivity will show a rise in vasopressin but very little increase in the urine concentration. With the psychological syndrome there will be a normal rise of vasopressin and urine concentration.

Syndrome of inappropriate ADH secretion

The converse of DI is seen with excess vasopressin, known as the syndrome of inappropriate ADH secretion (SIADH), characterised by a low volume of concentrated urine and haemodilution. Causes include:

- Low fluid intake
- Ectopic oat cell carcinomas in the lung or pancreas that secrete vasopressin at an uncontrolled rate and are not responsive to the normal feedback inhibition with changes in osmolarity of the plasma
- Pulmonary lesions, e.g. tuberculosis, pneumonia
- Postoperative anuria.

Aquaretics (vasopressin receptor antagonists)

Tetracyclines

Demeclocycline, a tetracycline antibiotic, is sometimes used to block the action of vasopressin in the kidney in hyponatremia due to inappropriately high secretion of vasopressin (SIADH), when fluid restriction has failed.

Vaptans

A new class of medication, the 'vaptan' drugs, act by inhibiting the action of vasopressin on its receptors (V1A, V1B and V2). Vaptans have a role in treatment of euvolemic and hypervolemic hyponatremia. Examples of vaptans available for clinical use are conivaptan (unselective blocker of V1A and V2) and tolvaptan (selective V2 blockers).

When the intake of water is low or there is an increased loss of fluid, such as in hard exercise, the osmolarity of the extracellular fluid rises and the rate of urine production falls with a marked increase in urine concentration. In humans, this can rise to a plasma level of 1400 mOsm (normal plasma is about 285 mOsm). This ability to vary the urine osmolarity from as low as 50 mOsm to 1400 mOsm is independent of solute excretion, which must be kept constant to eliminate toxic metabolites. Vasopressin antagonists are used in the treatment of SIADH (see Clinical box 14.8).

Calculation of renal water excretion

The kidney can eliminate 'solute free' water to excrete excess water or can conserve water by concentrating the urine. This ability can be measured by using clearance techniques. The osmolar clearance (C_{osm}) is the volume of plasma cleared of solutes each minute or the volume required to excrete solutes at the concentration of solutes in plasma:

$$C_{osm} = (U_{osm}/P_{osm}) \times V$$

If the plasma osmolarity (P_{osm}) has the same value as urine osmolarity (U_{osm}), C_{osm} equals the urine flow (V) where V is the rate of urine production in mL/min. The free-water clearance (C_{H2O}) is the difference between the urine production rate and the osmolar clearance:

$$C_{H2O} = V - C_{osm}$$

A positive value indicates dilute (hypotonic) urine whereas a concentrated (hypertonic) urine gives a negative value.

In Table 14.4 it can be seen that the osmolar clearance stays constant although the urine osmolarity is varied. We can also calculate the amount of solute 'free' water excreted (C_{H2O}) or conserved by subtracting C_{osm} from the urine flow which is also shown in Table 14.4. This again emphasises the ability of the kidney to handle water and solute separately.

These vesicles contain water permeable channels made up of the pre-formed AQP2 protein. The vesicles have 'vesicle associated membrane proteins' (VAMP) on their surface which serve to 'dock' with specific sites on the apical membrane of these cells. The AQP2 proteins are then inserted into the membrane by exocytosis, which causes a rapid increase in the water permeability of the apical side of the cells.

On the basolateral side of the collecting duct cells, there are aquaporins 3 and 4 which maintain a high and continuous level of water permeability on this side of the cell. The insertion of AQP2 channels leads to a large increase in the trans-epithelial water flux within about 9 minutes, so that water is rapidly recovered from the tubule into the blood. The high colloid osmotic pressure of the blood in the peritubular blood vessels also aids the uptake of water in this direction. Once the osmotic pressure of the plasma returns to its normal value as water is reabsorbed, the level of vasopressin falls and the AQP2 channels are returned to the vesicles, and the water permeability of the apical wall rapidly falls within 30 minutes.

Table 14.4	**Free water clearance**		
Urine state	**Concentrated ($U_{osm} = 1200$)**	**Dilute ($U_{osm} = 150$)**	**Iso-osmotic ($U_{osm} = 300$)**
V (urine excreted)	0.5 mL/min	4 mL/min	2 mL/min
$C_{osm} = (U_{osm}/P_{osm}) \times V$	$(1200 \times 0.5)/300 = 2$ mL/min	$(50 \times 4)/300 = 2$ mL/min	$(300 \times 2)/300 = 2$ mL/min
C_{H2O}	$0.5 - 2 = -1.5$ mL/min	$4 - 2 = 2$ mL/min	$2 - 2 = 0$ mL/min
Result	Solute free water conserved	Solute free water lost	No loss of free water

Mechanism of urine concentration and dilution

The ability of the kidney to produce a dilute or concentrated urine resides in its unique morphological structure (counter-current mechanism).

Osmolarity gradient

There is a raised gradient of osmolarity from the cortex to the tip of the medulla, which has been demonstrated in animal experiments (Fig. 14.15). If the kidney is sliced horizontally down a renal pyramid, the osmolarity in the cortex is isotonic with the plasma, but as each slice is taken down the pyramid, the osmolarity increases, rising in desert rodents to some 5000 mOsm at the apex. How this is achieved is still a matter of some debate, but studies using isolated perfused segments of the loop of Henle have identified some clues to the processes.

The loops of Henle are very long structures which plunge into the medulla then return to the cortex and the DCT. Here the tubules from several loops then join together to form the large collecting ducts, which again descend to the medulla and then drain into the renal pelvis.

Vasa recta and counter-current hypothesis

Running in parallel to the tubules are the blood vessels of the kidney medulla known as **vasa recta** (Fig. 14.15). These structures gave rise to the counter-current hypothesis, derived from the chemical industry, which had to concentrate drugs such as penicillin which had been produced in large vats of dilute solution by bacterial fermentation. By having fluids with different solubility for the drug in one arm of a 'U' shaped tube, and using solvents which are immiscible flowing in the opposite direction, the drug is concentrated in one phase and can then be extracted.

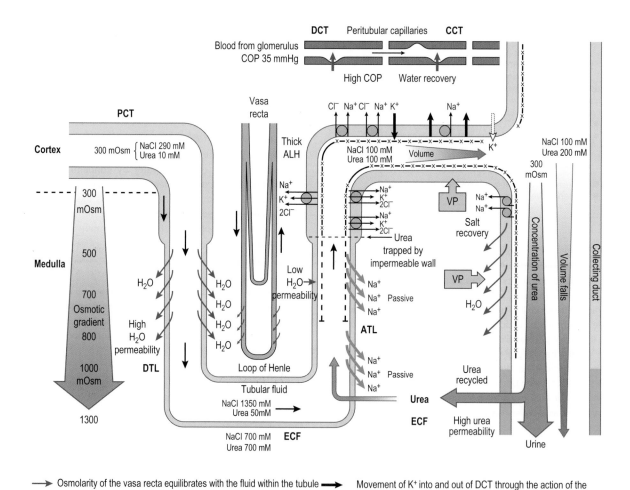

Fig. 14.15 Concentration of urine. On the left side is shown the osmotic gradient from the cortex to the medulla. Fluid passing down the water-permeable descending thin loop will lose fluid drawn out by the osmotic gradient and the tubular fluid becomes concentrated. After the turn in the loop of Henle the wall of the ascending thin loop has a low permeability to water and high salt and urea permeability. On reaching the thick ascending loop the powerful Na+/K+/2Cl− pump recovers ions so the fluid passing into the distal convoluted tubule (DCT) has a low ionic content. In the cortical collecting tube (CCT) water is recovered so the volume of fluid decreases further, but the concentration of urea increases as it is trapped in the tubule by the impermeable wall. As fluid descends the collecting duct, if vasopressin (VP) is present, water is withdrawn and a concentrated urine produced. In the last section of the collecting duct the wall becomes permeable to urea, which is recycled. PCT, proximal convoluted tubule; DTL, descending thin loop of Henle; ATL, ascending thin loop of Henle; ECF, extracellular fluid; ALH, ascending loop of Henle; COP, colloid osmotic pressure.

Transport properties of the loop of Henle

In the kidney, the counter-current mechanism is achieved by having tubules with fluid flowing in opposing directions but with different permeabilities of the tubular wall and different transport properties.

Water

The descending thin loops of Henle (DTL) have a high permeability to water (Fig. 14.16). This is reduced to a low value after the turn of the loop and the rest of the thin and thick ascending loops of Henle have a low permeability to water. This low permeability is also seen in the DCT. However, in the remainder of the tubule, in the cortical collecting duct (CCD) and the medullary collecting duct (MCD), there is a variable water permeability depending on the presence or absence of vasopressin; with vasopressin present, the permeability to water is high, and it is low when vasopressin is absent (indicated by the solid lines in Fig. 14.16).

The effect of fluid descending the DTLs is that water moves out into the interstitium and the remaining fluid in the

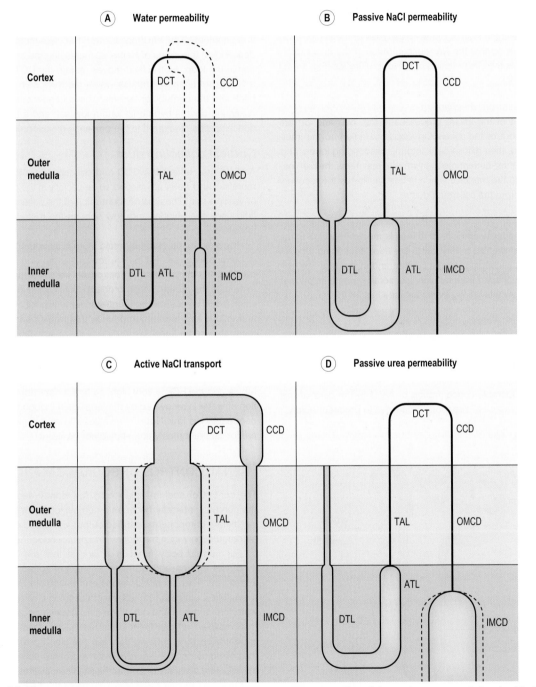

Fig. 14.16 Tubular permeability. Transport and passive permeability properties of the nephron segments involved in the dilution and concentration of urine. The width of the tubular segments is proportional to the magnitude of the parameter. The solid lines depict the situation in the absence of vasopressin. The dashed lines show the effect of vasopressin. DTL, descending thin loop; ATL, ascending thin loop; TAL, thick ascending loop; DCT, distal collecting tubule; CCD, cortical collecting duct; OMCD, outer medullary collecting duct; IMCD, inner medullary collecting duct. After Knepper MA, Rector FC 1991 Urinary concentration and dilution. In: Brenner BM, Rector FC (eds) The kidney. WB Saunders, Philadelphia, with permission.

tubules becomes concentrated (hypertonic) with a reduction in volume; this volume reduction is under the influence of the osmotic gradient shown in Figure 14.15. Note: the osmotic gradient is always present to some degree in both diuresis and antidiuresis.

Sodium and chloride
In Figure 14.17, it can be seen that the passive permeability to sodium also varies along the loop, being high in the outer medulla, but falling in the inner medulla, then rising to a high value in the thin ascending loop of Henle. For the rest of the loop, the passive permeability to Na$^+$ is low. In contrast, the active transport for Na$^+$ is greatly increased in the medullary thick ascending loop of Henle in response to the Na$^+$/K$^+$/2Cl$^-$ transporter so that the Na$^+$ concentration in the fluid rapidly falls; this is the site of action of the loop diuretics (Fig. 14.15) (see Ch. 4).

Counter-current mechanism
The result of the above processes is that Na$^+$ and Cl$^-$ are pumped out of the ascending loops of Henle into the interstitial fluid, then diffuse back into the descending loops. This is the counter-current mechanism that maintains the high osmolarity in the medulla, which in turn facilitates the recovery of water from the collecting ducts.

Urea
The permeability of the loop to urea is moderately high in the inner medulla, but is very low in the thick ascending loop, in the thin descending loops of Henle and in most of the collecting duct apart from the very last section where its permeability to urea is greatly increased (see Fig. 14.16).

Vasa recta
The vasa recta dips into the medulla and returns to the cortex. The osmolarity of blood in the vasa recta will equilibrate with the fluid within the tubule and supply the cells with oxygen and nutrients without destroying the osmotic gradient. There is a considerable concentration of AqP1 in the cells of this structure, which allows these processes to proceed rapidly.

Figure 14.15 shows that as fluid moves out of the descending thin loops of Henle into the interstitium, it is carried away by the vasa recta. Within the tubule, the fluid at the bottom of the loop has a high NaCl and urea concentration as water has moved out of the loop. In contrast, the extracellular fluid around the loop has a composition which is very different, with less NaCl and much more urea, than within the tubule. This difference is achieved by the differences in the wall permeability and the direction of the flow within the loop.

The diluting segment and the DCT
The thick ascending loop of Henle transport processes recover NaCl but leave behind urea; this is the so-called 'diluting segment'. The NaCl passes into the vasa recta and the descending thin loops of Henle, so increasing the concentration in the loop. As the fluid moves up into the DCT, there is a NaCl co-transport process which recovers salt and fluid back into the peritubular vessels. The fluid now entering the collecting duct is hypotonic with a low salt and a high urea concentration recovered in the presence of vasopressin.

Cortical collecting duct
As fluid now enters the CCD and descends into the MCD, more salt and water are recovered, especially in the presence of vasopressin. The urea concentration of the collecting duct fluid rises even higher and now acts as the main 'osmotic' molecule.

Towards the tip of the pyramid there is a sudden increase in permeability (see Fig 14.15) towards urea, and this high permeability allows urea to recirculate from the tubule and reinforces the concentration process. Note that in starvation, when blood urea is low, concentrated urine cannot be formed and fluid is lost, which compounds the problems for the already stressed subject.

If vasopressin is absent, the water permeability of the whole collecting duct is low so dilute urine is formed. However, in this state the gradient between the inside of the tubule and the ECF is very high, so that a considerable fraction of water is recovered by the loop, even though the water permeability is low. Note: The values shown in Figure 14.15 are for illustration only and should not be learnt.

RENAL CONTROL OF SODIUM BALANCE

The control of sodium balance by the kidney depends on the complex interplay between a number of factors, including dietary components, cardiac output and blood pressure, autoregulation within the kidney and neuroendocrine factors.

For normal body function it is vital that the osmolarity of the plasma and ECF are closely controlled to about 285 mOsm. This control depends on the sodium content of these fluids, which in turn will affect the volume of cells since water can move in and out of the cells depending on the osmotic gradient across the cell membrane. The plasma volume is controlled by a balance between the blood pressure and the colloid osmotic pressure of plasma proteins acting across the capillary walls according to the Starling equilibrium.

On a day-to-day basis, the volume of the ECF depends on sodium content, which is initially kept constant by the addition or excretion of water via the actions of vasopressin. Water can be rapidly lost or gained within 30 min by this mechanism if the osmolarity of plasma changes which, as we have seen, is independent of the control solute. Independent of this fluid homeostasis is the control of sodium balance

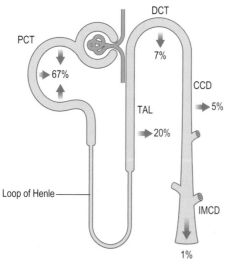

Fig. 14.17 Control of sodium balance. Segmental Na$^+$ reabsorption. The percentage of the filtered load of Na$^+$ reabsorbed by each nephron segment is indicated. PCT, proximal convoluted tubule; TAL, thick ascending limb; DCT, distal convoluted tubule; CDD, cortical collecting duct; IMCD, inner medullary collecting duct.

which is a much slower process, yet over a period of a few days maintains a balance between the sodium intake and sodium loss.

In a diet of natural foods, the content of sodium is relatively low and both humans and animals seek salt (NaCl), both for its value as an essential ion and to improve food flavour. Providing the diet contains 1–2 g of NaCl per day and exercise is moderate (sweat rate low), a human will stay in salt balance with this level of intake. With the added salt in modern processed foods, however, excess salt intake is now a major problem. When we are young, we can consume 100–200 g salt per day and simply excrete the excess salt which is termed **natriuresis** (Information box 14.2). As we age, the ability to excrete excess salt is lost and salt is retained.

Salt balance is mainly controlled via the kidney, but salt can be lost or retained by both the sweat glands and the colon. The hormone aldosterone, released from the adrenal cortex in response to a number of stimuli, can induce these tissues to conserve salt by the upregulation of channels and carriers.

Renal sodium handling

The kidney filters a huge amount of sodium into the renal tubules. Assuming that the GFR is about 180 L/day and the plasma Na^+ concentration is 145 mM, the renal filtration of Na^+ will be in the region of 26 000 mM of Na^+ per 24 hours. Of this vast amount, 99% must be reabsorbed by the nephron to stay in balance. The majority of Na^+ recovery is fixed, and is said to be constitutive with only a small percentage under variable control by the distal tubule, colon and sweat glands. The proportion of Na^+ recovered by the segments of the nephron is shown in Figure 14.17. Na^+ must first cross from the tubular fluid into the cell across the luminal or apical side of the cell. Since Na^+ ions are polar, they cannot cross a lipid bilayer by simple diffusion and this passage must be carrier mediated.

Sodium recovery

The majority of ion and fluid movement is dependent on the Na^+ gradient generated across the cell by the Na^+/K^+-ATPase pumps located on the blood side of the tubule cells.

The PCT

As previously discussed, from the tubule side of the PCT, non-electrolytes are transported into the cells of the tubule using a sodium dependent co-transporter, which can move these molecules 'uphill' against their concentration gradient using the potential energy of the Na^+ gradient. Non-electrolytes then pass into the blood by facilitated carriers 'downhill', and the sodium which has entered with them is returned to the blood by the Na^+/K^+-ATPase.

The PCT recovers 50–55% of the filtered sodium and water and almost all the glucose, amino acids and nucleosides. A key element of these processes is the Na^+/H^+ antiporter on the apical side of the cell, which recovers Na^+ for H^+ using the Na^+ gradient. The Na^+ then passes to the basolateral side where it is transported back to the blood via the Na^+/K^+-ATPase (Fig. 14.9).

The loop of Henle

The descending thin loop of Henle is water permeable, and as the fluid descends into the medulla the tubule contents are concentrated as the loop is exposed to the increasing concentration gradient in the ECF (see Fig. 14.15). On turning the loop, the wall of the thin ascending loop becomes less permeable to water, but permeable to Na^+ and urea. In all, some 25% of the remaining Na^+ passes from the loop into the ECF and is recovered by the counter-current flow of the vasa recta. The structure of the loop changes again to become the thick ascending loop of Henle, where the powerful $Na^+/K^+/2Cl^-$ carrier (BSC, bumetanide sensitive carrier), removes a further 15% of Na^+ into the cell. This process, which is sensitive to furosemide (see Ch. 4), dilutes the tubule fluid further and this Na^+ is removed from the cell by the usual Na^+/K^+-ATPase. The K^+ is recycled via K^+ channels back into the tubule and the Cl^- exits via Cl^- channels into the blood.

The DCT

In the DCT, which is the connecting segment, the dilute fluid emerging from the loop loses another 5–8% more Na^+ via a thiazide sensitive Na^+/Cl^- co-transport (TSC, see Ch. 4).

The collecting ducts

The fluid in the DCT becomes isotonic as salts and water are recovered into the peritubular vessels, aided by the high colloid osmotic pressure of these capillaries, and finally leaves the DCT to enter the collecting ducts. In this region there are two specific cell types with very different transport properties:

1. Principal (P) cells – more Na^+ is recovered by its passage via epithelial Na^+ channels (eNaC) on the apical side into the cells and K^+ exits back into the tubule via K^+ channels in exchange. This K^+ loss into the tubule can cause hypokalaemia (see Ch. 4). Sodium entry into the cells of the collecting ducts occurs through these selective eNaC which are opened in response to aldosterone and closed by atrial natriuretic peptides (ANP) (see Information box 14.2). With a low level of Na^+ there will be high levels of aldosterone, which will conserve Na^+ so Na^+ loss in urine can be reduced to as low as 1 mM.
2. Intercalated (IC) cells – these have a H^+-ATPase on the luminal side and can lower the pH of the tubular fluid to pH 4.5, generating in turn new HCO_3^-, which passes back across the basolateral face with Na^+ (Fig. 14.18). H^+/K^+-ATPase located on basolateral side of IC cells secretes H^+ and recycles K^+ via apical K^+ channels during K^+ repletion and reabsorbs K^+ via basolateral K^+ channels during K^+ depletion.

Control of GFR by the renal capillaries

Since the amount of sodium entering the renal tubules depends on the GFR it is critical that this filtration process is controlled by a number of mechanisms.

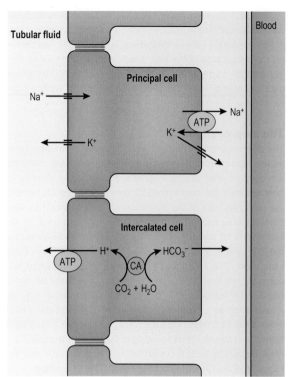

Fig. 14.18 Autoregulation. Transport pathways in principal cells and intercalated cells of the distal tubule and collecting duct. ATP, adenosine triphosphate; CA, carbonic anydrase.

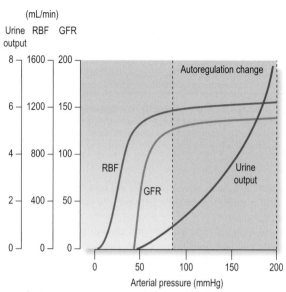

Fig. 14.19 The independence or autoregulation of renal blood flow (RBF) and glomerular filtration rate (GFR) to changes in blood pressure (BP) above 70 mmHg. Note that the lower part of the figure shows that urine flow does increase but only to a small degree as the BP rises. A further key point is that with a BP of <70 mmHg, the RBF and GFR fall with a decrease in BP which can lead to renal failure.

Autoregulation

The first step in sodium balance is to control the hydrostatic pressure driving fluid across the capillary walls; renal glomerular capillaries are unusual in having arterioles at both ends (see Fig. 14.18). These arterioles have sympathetic receptors with different sensitivity to norepinephrine (noradrenaline), the efferent arteriole being more sensitive than the afferent, so maintaining the net filtration force when the blood pressure (BP) falls. However, under high levels of sympathetic drive, the renal blood flow can fall and filtration is reduced. Normally, for values of arterial pressures between 70 mmHg and about 180 mmHg the renal blood flow (RBF) and GFR are constant, so that variation in blood pressure does not result in changes in renal haemodynamics and GFR (Fig. 14.19). The rate of urine formation increases with increasing blood pressure, but these changes are small in relation to the large change in blood pressure. Below 70 mmHg the GFR and RBF both fall and such low pressures can cause ischaemia and renal failure.

Glomerular–tubular balance

There is also an intrinsic mechanism in the PCT which increases the reabsorption of fluid and salts in proportion to any changes in the GFR. This may be related to the filtration fraction which would alter the peritubular colloid osmotic pressure, so increasing reabsorption. There may also be a flow dependent factor which increases GFR. In the event of volume contraction, glomerular-tubular balance is set upwards (increasing fractional reabsorption of sodium) and with volume expansion balance is set downwards (decreasing fractional reabsorption of sodium). These mechanisms ensure that although a single nephron may have a different GFR, the GFRs will match and contribute to the overall balance across the renal bed.

Receptors involved with sodium balance

The Na+ level in the blood is mainly controlled by the kidney. The 'level' of Na+ is 'detected' at multiple sites and with a multiple layer sensor system. As has been stated the level of Na+ reflects the volume of extracellular fluid so there is a need for 'volume' receptors. Since 'volume' cannot be measured directly it can be assessed indirectly by the degree of stretch in the walls of vascular structures containing various low and high pressure baroreceptors.

Baroreceptors

High pressure baroreceptors are located in the walls of carotid arteries and the aorta. These respond to dynamic changes in arterial pressure, being low pressure receptors that can measure an index of 'volume' by the distension of blood vessel walls. These are found in the great veins, atria and ventricles. There are also receptors in the vessels of the liver, the kidneys and the thorax.

The juxtaglomerular apparatus

The juxtaglomerular apparatus (JGA) shown in Figure 14.20 is a special modified part of the tubule that has three components.

- The first segment of the afferent arteriole, close to the glomerulus, is lined with granular cells which secrete the proteolytic enzyme renin into the blood in response to a fall in Na+ in the afferent blood supply.
- Second, these cells are also supplied with sympathetic nerves which respond to a fall in arterial pressure.
- Finally, around the afferent and efferent capillaries is a specialised group of mesangial cells through which runs the distal tubule with the specialised macula densa (MD) cells at the interface. The MD cells are especially sensitive to the delivery of chloride ions by the distal tubule. If this delivery is decreased, afferent arteriolar

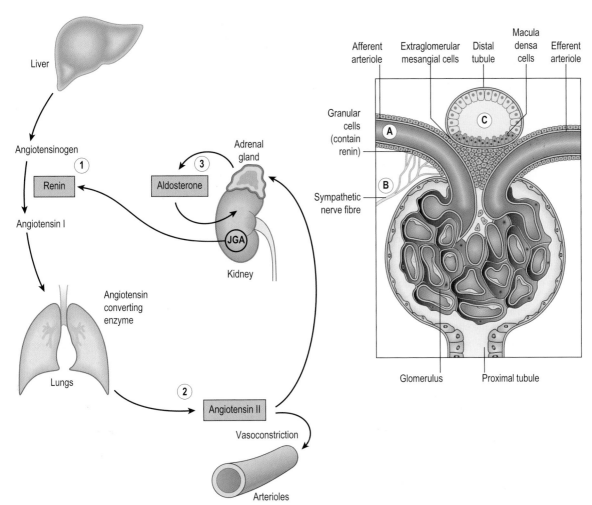

Fig. 14.20 The renin–angiotensin–aldosterone system. The numbers 1–3 show the sequence of steps in the activation of the system. The inset shows the juxtaglomerular apparatus (JGA) with major stimuli acting as triggers for renin release. A: fall in pressure in afferent arteriole; B: release of norepinephrine by sympathetic nerve endings on granular cells; C: fall in NaCl concentration in distal tubule. Note that angiotensin II has a number of additional actions not shown on this figure.

dilation occurs, which may be via prostaglandins and which restores the MD flow; this is termed tubulo-glomerular feedback.

This complex structure, the JGA, responds to:

- The perfusion pressure in the afferent arteriole
- The sympathetic nerve supply to the arterioles
- The 'sodium' concentration in distal tubule as reflected by the chloride delivery.

Renin–angiotension–aldosterone system

The JGA structures are the principal detectors of the renin–angiotensin–aldosterone system. If the ECF volume falls, the pressure distending the afferent arteriole falls, which will cause a sympathetic system discharge onto the afferent arteriolar granular cells. At the same time the supply of sodium '(Cl⁻)' ions to the distal tubule falls and these stimuli lead to the release of renin into the blood. Renin is an enzyme which acts on the peptide angiotensinogen, an α_2 globulin in the blood manufactured by the liver. Renin removes a four amino acid fragment to generate angiotensin I (10 amino acids). In various vascular beds, ACE, which is bound to the walls of the blood vessels, mostly in the lung, removes a further two amino acids to form the powerful vasoconstrictor peptide angiotensin II.

Role of angiotensin II and Na⁺ control

Angiotensin II has the following actions:

- It is a potent vasoconstrictor of blood vessels, so increases tubular perfusion rate and blood pressure
- It causes the release of aldosterone from the adrenal cortex
- It causes the release of vasopressin and stimulates the area postrema, causing thirst
- It increases the reabsorption of salt by the PCT and activates the sympathetic nervous system centrally.

All these actions cause Na⁺ retention, which eventually, by negative feedback, switches off the response.

Aldosterone

Angiotensin II is closely coupled to the release of aldosterone.

- Aldosterone acts on the late part of the DCT and on collecting ducts. It also acts on salivary and sweat glands, and on the colon.
- Aldosterone being lipid soluble crosses the cell wall and binds to a cytoplasmic receptor, and causes the synthesis of Na⁺ channel proteins, which increases the uptake of Na⁺ by the lumen side of the DCT cells. It also increases the Na⁺ transport on the blood side, via the Na⁺ pump,

which raises the cell potential difference (i.e. makes it more negative) and this increases the uptake of Cl⁻.

- Aldosterone potentiates Na⁺/K⁺/2Cl⁻ transport in the thick ascending loop of Henle.
- It causes the excretion of H⁺ ions by the DCT, therefore if in excess it can cause alkalosis.

Potassium

If the level of K⁺ in the plasma is elevated this acts directly on the adrenal cortex to cause the secretion of K⁺ into the lumen by the DCT, which is independent of the renin–angiotensin system.

Autoregulation and the DCT

The distal convoluted tubule is limited in its ability to handle large quantities of salt and water, so the flow of fluid and ions is also controlled by autoregulation, which is dependent on the local release of angiotensin II via the MD. Angiotensin antagonists cause a loss in the ability to autoregulate, so that as the blood pressure falls, the threshold of the ability to autoregulate occurs at a 'higher' pressure. Normally, angiotensin II release will increase the efferent arteriolar resistance as the blood pressure falls, so maintaining GFR.

Tubulo-glomerular feedback

The MD cells not only control the release of renin in response to a fall in the 'sodium' level but also function in tubuloglomerular feedback. A fall in chloride delivery to the distal nephron will cause afferent arteriolar dilation possibly mediated via prostaglandins. The release of renin via the angiotensin system will cause efferent vasoconstriction. Both of the above will increase GFR and raise the flow through the distal tubule towards normal.

Na⁺ balance summary

Sodium balance within the kidney depends on both physical factors, such as the cardiac output and blood pressure which are usually balanced by autoregulation, and on neuroendocrine factors. Autoregulation can be controlled by the 'myo-genic mechanism' of the smooth muscles of arterioles which contract in response to stretch, as is seen in most vascular beds, but in the kidney, the sympathetic system, acting through norepinephrine release, can act differentially on the efferent arterioles to maintain GFR when the blood pressure falls. The renin–angiotensin–aldosterone system acts to control not only the GFR, but also the release of renin and aldosterone, which can upregulate the expression of transporters such as the Na⁺/K⁺/2Cl⁻ carrier in the thick ascending loop of Henle, Na⁺/Cl⁻ co-transport in the DCT and recycling of urea in the inner medulla. Other neurohormones such as nitric oxide, ANP, kinin, adenosine, vasopressin and endothelin also play a complex role. This mixture of physical factors and neuroendocrine influences leads to the mechanism by which Na⁺ balance is achieved (Clinical box 14.9).

DIURETICS

When fluid balance is disturbed, if the kidneys are beginning to function less efficiently or in diabetes, the circulation becomes overfilled, leading to hypertension. In these states it is necessary to increase the urine flow with **diuretics** to reduce the fluid overload in the circulation. These are more accurately called natriuretics as they promote fluid excretion by

---

Clinical box 14.9 **Essential hypertension**

The elevation of blood pressure occurs with age, obesity and genetic factors. However, the role of the kidney and salt is still controversial. While there is no doubt that a high salt intake from processed foods can lead to hypertension, the exact mechanism has not been resolved. In youth, any excess salt is easily excreted, but with ageing this ability is lost. There is, however, no doubt that there is a strong link with the renal handling of salt. Experiments demonstrated that obstructing the renal artery caused hypertension in experimental animals. This response is related to the sodium detection systems within the kidney and the false error signal leads to the release of renin/angiotensin/aldosterone, thus causing an increase in total peripheral resistance, retention of sodium and expansion of the vascular volume, all of which lead to hypertension. Although a tremendous volume of research has investigated human hypertension, no uniform hypothesis has emerged. Some patients do not have elevated renin or blood volume and do not respond to diuretics so at present this condition is still an enigma. Drugs used in the medical treatment of hypertension are discussed in Chapter 4.

---

preventing salt reabsorption. These drugs have several sites of action along the nephron, with different mechanisms of action depending on the processes of water and salt recovery in the given segment of the nephron.

Most of the 180 L of water filtered into the nephron in 24 hours must be recovered to preserve homeostasis. The bulk of this fluid (some 70%) is reabsorbed by the PCT, the loops of Henle recover about 10–20%, leaving the thick ascending loop, the distal convoluted tubule and the collecting ducts to recover the final 10%, so only about 1 mL/min passes into the bladder as urine. The potential sites at which diuretics can act is shown in Figure 14.21 (see also Ch. 4).

Osmotic diuresis

Glucose is freely filtered by the capillaries of the nephron, and some 99% is normally recovered by the PCT. If there is an excess of plasma glucose, the recovery process becomes saturated and glucose remains in the tubular lumen; here, since glucose is a small molecule and osmotically active, it retains water in the urine which leads to a brisk osmotic diuresis, salt loss and 'raging thirst', seen in untreated diabetes mellitus. This defect was known from the times of the Ancient Greeks as flies were attracted to the sweet urine (mellitus is Greek for honey). The first test of urine involved tasting a tiny drop of the fluid, which revealed the glucose content of the urine of these patients. The concentration of glucose in both plasma and urine is now measured using 'dipsticks'.

Osmotic diuresis can be used clinically to increase urine flow by using an intravenous infusion of the sugar alcohol **mannitol** (Clinical box 14.10). Mannitol is a small, osmotically active molecule, but is not recovered by the glucose carriers or metabolised, and, being polar, remains trapped in the nephron.

Carbonic anhydrase inhibitors

The recovery of Na⁺ by the PCT depends on the low intracellular sodium concentration produced by the basolateral sodium pump (see above and Fig. 14.9). On the luminal side of the tubular cell, the exchange of H⁺ ions from the cell cytoplasm for Na⁺ ions leads to H⁺ ions in the tubular fluid. These H⁺ ions react with the filtered HCO_3^- ions, which generates CO_2. The CO_2 being lipid soluble passes into the cytoplasm of the PCT

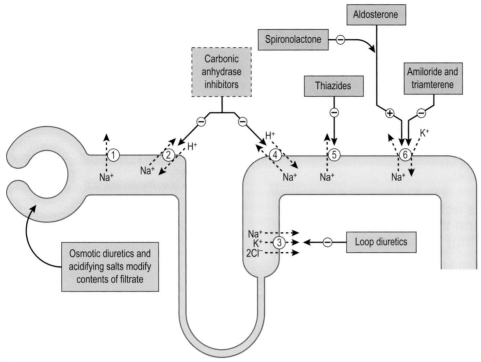

Fig. 14.21 **Main sites of action of diuretics and sodium absorption in the nephron.** 1: Na (passive Cl absorption); 2: Na$^+$/H$^+$ exchange; 3: Na$^+$/K$^+$/2Cl$^-$ co-transport; 4: Na$^+$/H$^+$ exchange; 5: Na$^+$/Cl$^-$ co-transport; 6: Na$^+$/K$^+$ exchange. Currently used diuretics are shown in solid boxes, agents not used for their diuretic action are in boxes with dashed lines.

Clinical box 14.10   **Use of mannitol during surgery**

Osmotic diuresis with mannitol is used during surgery when the urine flow has been reduced through blood loss or by the fall in blood pressure used to reduce bleeding during the surgical process. During surgery, most patients are given intravenous saline to maintain fluid volume, but if renal function is impaired, this added fluid can lead to overfilling of the circulation and eventually to pulmonary oedema. This is the reason the majority of surgical patients have a bladder catheter inserted during surgery so the flow of urine can be monitored directly and mannitol can be infused by the anaesthetist should the urine flow become too low. Other small molecules can be used as osmotic diuretics, such as urea, glycerine and isosorbide. It is important to note that urea and mannitol must be administered intravenously.

cells and is reconverted to H$^+$ and HCO$_3^-$ ions under the influence of the enzyme **carbonic anhydrase** which is bound to the wall of the PCT cells. The enzyme can be inhibited by a group of **carbonic anhydrase inhibitors** developed from sulphonamides (e.g. acetozolamide), which were found to cause a mild diuresis (Clinical box 14.11). The diuretic effect of carbonic anhydrase inhibition is weak because, although it has a major effect on the PCT, the retention of salt and water into the tubule is compensated by the recovery processes further along the nephron.

Clinical box 14.11   **Carbonic anhydrase inhibitor as a diuretic – acetazolamide**

Acetazolamide was the first synthetic carbonic anhydrase inhibitor, and is still in use to reduce intra-ocular pressure in **glaucoma** by inhibiting fluid secretion in the eye (see Ch. 4). It also reduces cerebrospinal fluid (CSF) secretion. Acetazolamide is also used to reduce the effect of high altitude by causing a cellular acidosis which opposes the alkalosis induced by the CO$_2$ loss in response to the hypoxic drive (see Ch. 13).

The thiazide diuretics

Thiazide diuretics block the Na$^+$/Cl$^-$ co-transport (TSC) in the distal convoluted tubule (DCT). Examples are chlorothiazide, hydrochlorothiazide and bendrofluazide (see Ch. 4). In this section of the nephron, the co-transport process helps the recovery of Na$^+$ and Cl$^-$ by the DCT, but although they are well tolerated, the diuresis is relatively mild, since the majority of the salt and water has been removed by the PCT and the thick ascending loop of Henle. They are, however, useful for reducing circulatory volume, especially in the treatment of age-related hypertension. Side effects include potassium loss, increased calcium retention and metabolic alkalosis (see Ch. 4). They also cause vasodilation so are ideal for the treatment of hypertension. They should be avoided in patients with gout as they can cause hyperuricaemia. Thiazide-like diuretics (metolazone and indapamide) act on TSC and are used more often in clinical practice.

Loop diuretics

This relatively newer group of diuretics act on the thick ascending loop of Henle and inhibit the key bumetanide sensitive, Na$^+$/K$^+$/2Cl$^-$ co-transport process (see Fig. 14.15). This carrier complex recovers large amounts of Na$^+$ from the lumen of the thick ascending loop so that the fluid entering the DCT has a low osmolarity. Blocking of this process by inhibitors leads to an added load of Na$^+$ passing into the DCT, which prevents recovery of water by the collecting ducts and cause a brisk dose-related diuresis. Examples include furosemide, bumetanide and ethacrynic acid (see Ch. 4). Loop diuretics act rapidly with a steep dose-response curve inducing a profound diuresis (Clinical box 14.12). These drugs are rapidly absorbed from the gastrointestinal tract and, being bound to plasma proteins, are not filtered into the nephron but are secreted by the PCT.

Diuretics acting on the late distal tubule and the collecting ducts (K^+ sparing)

Amiloride and triamterene

Amiloride and triamterene are sodium (Na^+) blockers. The principal cells in the late DCT and collecting ducts (see Fig. 14.21) have epithelial Na^+ channels (eNaC) in the luminal membrane which leads to the uptake of Na^+ from the tubules; this Na^+ is then returned to the blood via the basolateral sodium pumps. To balance the charge there are K^+ channels which transfer K^+ into the tubular lumen. Amiloride and triamterene block eNaC, so reduce the recovery of Na^+ in the late DCT. Although the recovery of Na^+ by these regions is important it is relatively small so the diuretic effect is limited, but they do prevent excessive K^+ loss.

Spironolactone

Spironolactone competes with aldosterone, and is a K^+-sparing diuretic (Clinical box 14.13). Aldosterone is the adrenal cortical mineralocorticoid which is responsible for the control of sodium in the kidney, sweat glands and colon. Aldosterone crosses the basolateral membrane of the late distal tubule and binds to cytosolic membrane receptors which are then translocated to the nucleus. This passage causes the production of multiple gene products which are thought to activate 'silent' Na^+ channels and Na^+ pumps and also increase the permeability of the tight junctions. The net effect of these actions is to enhance the NaCl transport back into the blood when Na^+ is low and cause the excretion of K^+ and H^+ ions into the lumen. Spironolactone competitively inhibits the binding of aldosterone to its receptors, leading to a loss of Na^+ into the urine. The efficiency of this drug depends on the endogenous level of aldosterone.

RENAL CONTROL OF ACID–BASE BALANCE

The kidney plays a vital role in the control of acid–base balance. The pH of the plasma is held close to 7.4 under normal

conditions. This value, which reflects a plasma H^+ concentration of 40 nM/L, depends on the balance between the concentration of HCO_3^- ions in the plasma, which is mainly controlled by the kidneys, and the arterial pCO_2 which is controlled by the respiratory system (see Chs 3 and 13).

Hydrogen ions

The CO_2 in the circulation is mostly derived from oxidation of glucose and, as the rate of metabolism changes, say in exercise, the increased production of CO_2 is detected by the central and peripheral chemoreceptors, which increase the rate of ventilation so the excess CO_2 is excreted via the lungs and the arterial pCO_2 is kept remarkably constant (see Ch. 13). Since these H^+ ions can easily be excreted via the lungs, they are termed **volatile.**

The arterial pH therefore depends on the balance between the HCO_3^- concentration and the pCO_2, i.e. kidney/lung. The $[HCO_3^-]$ is the prime buffer in the blood and is therefore affected by the production of **fixed** acids by the biochemical process of the body. These H^+ ions are defined as 'fixed' since they can only be excreted via the kidneys. They used to be defined as metabolic H^+ ions, which can be confusing, so now it is better to use the term non-respiratory H^+ ions (see below).

Sources of H^+ ions

Although all H^+ ions are protons, in biology it is convenient to categorise the H^+ ions in relation to their sources.

Cell metabolism produces 'volatile' H^+ ions

The aerobic metabolism of glucose to produce ATP and energy generates some 14000 mM of H^+ from bicarbonate (H_2CO_3) which is linked to ventilation and is rapidly adjusted to keep the pH constant. These are primarily 'volatile' H^+ ions and so can be rapidly 'blown off' or retained by the lungs.

'Fixed' H^+ ions

'Fixed' H^+ ions are generated from metabolic processes and the concentration depends largely on the diet. The total amount is relatively small (80–100 mM per 24 h) when compared to the 14000 mM of 'volatile acid', but the rate of excretion is slow in relation to the acidification process of the renal tubules, which can produce a minimum urinary pH of 4.5. The pH limit of 4.5 is set by the ability of the collecting duct intercalated cell H^+-ATPase to secrete H^+ into the tubule, which it can do to about 800 times of the value in the plasma. This value of 4.5 represents a minute concentration of free H^+ ions equivalent to 0.003 M of H^+ in the 1–2 L of urine which is produced per day at the rate of about 1 mL/min; it does, however, cause considerable discomfort when passed. The pH of plasma represents 40 nmol/L of H^+ so 100 mM is still a relatively large concentration.

There are, however, buffers in the urine which allow more H^+ ions to be secreted into the tubule yet keep the pH above the critical limit of 4.5. The kidneys must excrete H^+ ions at a rate equal to the rate of extra renal net acid production (0.3–1.0 mM/kg per 24 h).

Sources of non-respiratory H^+ ions

■ Dietary sulphates: amino acids such as methionine and cysteine, which contain 'S' groups, yield the equivalent of an intake of H_2SO_4 when they are metabolised to urea. In a normal mixed diet this represents an intake of 50–100 mM of 'fixed' H⁺ ions per day. This figure will be much higher for individuals who have a high dietary intake of meat, whereas for a vegetarian diet, the value will be much less.

- Phosphates: a further source of 'fixed' acid is the turnover and breakdown of phospholipids in neurons and DNA which produces the equivalent of some 50 mM of phosphoric acid (H_3PO_4) per day.
- Lactic acid: in health, the arterial pCO_2 only changes in extreme exercise when there is insufficient oxygen to supply the muscles (anaerobiosis) and lactic acidosis occurs (see Chs 3 and 13). The lactic acid, with a pK of 3, dissociates to release ions which act via the peripheral chemoreceptors to drive the ventilation at a rate greater than needed to keep the pCO_2 constant and so disturbs the normal relationship between CO_2 and the rate of ventilation for a given pCO_2. This causes a paradoxical fall in pCO_2 to a small degree. This excess ventilation caused by the raised H⁺ is termed hyperventilation and not the hyperpnoea of normal exercise when the pH is kept constant. Lactic acid is also produced during surgery when tissues are under-perfused and during heart failure when the blood pressure is reduced (see Ch. 3 for lactic acidosis).

Disease states

In disease states excess amounts of fixed acid can be produced, such as the keto acids α-ketoglutaric and α-hydroxybutyric acids in diabetes mellitus when the supply of glucose is insufficient and fat is metabolised instead (see Ch. 3).

Acid–base balance is vital for life

In comparison to the vast acid load of H_2CO_3, the above figure of 100–150 mM of fixed H⁺ ions appears to be small, but it must be remembered that these are strong acids which are not volatile, so can only be eliminated by the kidneys. In renal failure these fixed acids rapidly accumulate leading to acidosis, and if blood pH falls below 6.9, death will result (see Ch. 13).

The proteins in the body are used for construction of tissue and for the thousands of enzymes which control all our body functions. These enzymes are complex chains of amino acids folded in a three-dimensional form which brings their active sites to the surface of the molecule in a critical fashion. This folding of a molecule depends on various charged processes (e.g. hydrogen bonds) which are very sensitive to the acidity of their environment. If the body becomes acid, the activities of many of the enzymes change, e.g. conversion of lactate to glucose is decreased by 64% if the pH falls from 7.4 to 7.0.

Renal mechanisms of HCO_3^- control

The kidney can act in three prime ways to maintain the concentration of HCO_3^- ions constant in the plasma (see also Ch. 13).

1. Recovery of filtered HCO_3^-: the rate of filtration of HCO_3^- is directly proportional to the plasma HCO_3^- concentration and the GFR. But since no HCO_3^- is usually found in the urine, the majority of this must be reabsorbed by the nephron. The bulk of HCO_3^- recovery occurs in the PCT (80%), and by the end of the PCT the tubular fluid is acidified to a pH of 6.7 as the concentration of HCO_3^- decreases from 24 mM to 8 mM. There are two processes by which this is achieved.

2. Na⁺/H⁺ antiporter (see also Fig. 14.9): Na⁺ enters the cell down its concentration gradient in exchange for H⁺. This antiporter carrier called NHE3 is a one-to-one coupled process of Na⁺ for H⁺ so is electrically neutral and accounts for 65% of the H⁺ secretion. It can be inhibited with amiloride and by lithium which is used in psychiatry and competes with Na⁺. In addition, glucocorticoids and thyroid hormones also increase the activity of this antiporter.

3. H⁺-ATPase: there is also an H⁺-ATPase present which can also transfer H⁺ into the tubule lumen of the PCT using ATP which carries the remaining 35% of H⁺ secretion (see Fig. 14.9). The H⁺ movement into the tubule leads to a reaction with the filtered HCO_3^- to form carbonic acid, which immediately splits into CO_2 and H_2O (see also Fig. 14.9). The CO_2, being lipid soluble, passes into the tubule cells where under the influence of carbonic anhydrase (CA), both bound to the cell walls and free in the cytoplasm, it rapidly forms carbonic acid, which then splits non-enzymically into H⁺ ions and HCO_3^-. The H⁺ ions are then used by the antiport carrier again to recover more Na⁺ ions. The HCO_3^- ions pass to the basal lateral side of the cell where they are carried across the cell wall to the peritubular capillaries by an electrogenic Na⁺/3Na⁺/3HCO_3^- carrier. The H⁺ formed by the CA-catalysed reaction in the cell is used to recover more filtered HCO_3^- from the PCT (Fig. 14.9).

The Na⁺/H⁺ antiport can apparently use K⁺ instead of H⁺, so in alkaline states when the H⁺ level falls more K⁺ is lost into the tubule, resulting in the condition of hypokalaemic alkalosis (Table 14.5). Conversely, in acidosis, less K⁺ is lost and hyper-kalaemic acidosis can occur as K⁺ is retained in the blood. These conditions are observed in vivo, but this explanation may be a little simplistic.

HCO_3^- ions and pCO_2

The recovery of HCO_3^- ions is related to the pCO_2 so if the pCO_2 rises, more HCO_3^- is recovered. Hypercapnia (excess CO_2 in the blood) leads to an increased renal recovery of HCO_3^- and an increase in the HCO_3^-/pCO_2 ratio. This process is relatively slow and takes 2–3 days (see Ch. 13). After haemoglobin, HCO_3^- is the first line key buffer in the plasma. The production of fixed acids such as lactic acid in hard exercise and ketoacidosis in untreated diabetes mellitus leads to a rapid fall in the plasma HCO_3^- concentration by this 'buffering' process. To overcome this acidosis and to return the pH to normal, new HCO_3^- has to be generated and the excess fixed H⁺ ion excreted.

Loop of Henle and HCO_3^- ions

The loop of Henle is a key segment for the counter-current hypothesis and the differential permeability of the loops leads to a concentration of tubular fluid at the 'hairpin' turn. The loss of water over electrolytes leads to a rise in the tubular HCO_3^- concentration so the fluid becomes alkaline. This raised HCO_3^- is, however, removed by the thick ascending loop so fluid entering the DCT and the collecting ducts has returned to a low HCO_3^- concentration.

Table 14.5	Causes of hypokalemic alkalosis			
		Defective channel	**Clinical features**	**Management**
Bartter syndrome	Like 'loop diuretics'	Type 1 (BSC – Bumetanide sensitive channel)	Neonatal, polyuria, polydipsia, sensorineural deafness, sal carving, normal BP. Nephrocalcinosis. Chloride resistant hypokalaemic metabolic alkalosis, hypercalciuric	Electrolyte supplementation
		Type 2 (ROMK channel-Renal outer medullary potassium)		Potassium-sparing diuretic
		Type 3 (CLCKb)		NSAIDs
		Type 4 and Type 5 (Barttin, CLCNKA or CLCNKB*)		
Gitelman syndrome	Like 'thiazide diuretics'	TSC (Thiazide sensitive channels)	Adolescent and young adults, muscle cramps, tetany, normal BP, hypokalaemic metabolic alkalosis, hypocalciuria	As for Bartter syndrome
Liddle syndrome	Like 'aldosterone excess'	eNaC defect – increased sodium reabsorption	Hypertension, hypokalaemic metabolic alkalosis	Amiloride and triamterene (spironolactone is ineffective)

*$BSND$ encodes barttin, an essential β subunit that is required for the trafficking of the chloride channel ClC-K (ClC-Ka and ClC-Kb) to the plasma membrane in the TALH and the marginal cells in the scala media of the inner ear that secrete potassium ion-rich endolymph.

The distal nephron

In the tubular segment from the DCT to the end of the collecting ducts, there are two types of specialised epithelial cell. The principal cells have Na^+ and K^+ channels on their apical side, which lead to K^+ loss when the Na^+ load in the tubule is increased in diuresis. A second cell type, the intercalated cell, has a H^+-ATPase on the apical side and can secrete H^+ ions and can reduce the acidity of the tubule to the minimum pH 4.5, a gradient of ×800. This process leads to the production of more HCO_3^- in the cell, which is then exchanged for Cl^- ions on the basolateral side of the cell. In this case, these are newly generated HCO_3^- ions which can replace the lost HCO_3^- ions in the plasma. The Cl^- is recycled via a Cl^- channel as shown in Figure 14.9. This H^+-ATPase is induced by mineralocorticoids, such as aldosterone, which accounts for the observed alkalosis seen with excess of this steroid.

Renal buffers

To achieve the excretion of the fixed H^+ ions produced daily yet keep the pH above 4.5, urinary buffers are needed. These buffers depend on the urine being acid so although the direct loss of free H^+ is minute, the low pH plays a key role in the excretion of H^+ (see also Ch. 1).

Phosphate buffering

In the plasma at pH 7.4 'phosphate' ions depend on the equation:

$$HPO_4^{2-} + H^+ \rightleftharpoons H_2PO_4^-$$

and the equilibrium will lie to the left, since the pK of this reaction is 6.8. In acidic urine at a pH of 4.5, the ratio of HPO_4^{2-} to $H_2PO_4^-$ will switch from 4:1 at pH 7.4 to 1:200 at pH 4.5. This has the advantage of keeping the pH at 4.5 as the added H^+ is 'locked' into the $H_2PO_4^-$. This also saves a cation as there is one less negative charge to balance, usually by a Na^+. Although the concentration of HPO_4^{2-} in plasma is low, the molecule is retained in the nephron and with the recovery of water and salts so reaches a concentration of 30–50 mM per 24 h. This can therefore buffer the same amount of H^+ ions, which is about half the daily acid load.

The low urinary pH also has two further effects. First, some molecules with a pK close to 4.5 will become partial buffers so reduce their need for buffering. This is seen with the keto acids, so their effect on the pH is reduced. Secondly, the synthesis of NH_4^+ from glutamine depends on a low pH.

Ammonium synthesis

Ammonia (NH_3) can exist as ammonium ions (NH_3^+) in the reaction:

$$NH_3 + H^+ \rightleftharpoons NH_4^+$$

which has a pK of 9 and therefore the equilibrium will be far to the right (see also Ch. 3). The proximal tubule is the major site for the synthesis of ammonia mostly from the conversion of glutamine by glutaminase to glutamate. This enzyme is upregulated in acidosis. The reaction yields one ammonia molecule and when the glutamate is further converted to α-ketoglutarate, a further ammonia molecule is produced. The ammonia molecules react with H^+ ions and yield NH_4^+ ions. Since NH_3 is moderately lipid soluble it can cross the apical cell membranes whereas NH_4^+ has a low permeability and becomes trapped in the lumen once this has occurred. NH_4^+ can also travel on the Na^+/H^+ antiporter, which is sensitive to **amiloride**. NH_4^+ ions accumulate in the tubular fluid where the luminal pH is less than in the cell. The PCT H^+ ions are derived from CO_2 and as these are used to produce NH_4^+ this yields an HCO_3^- ion which crosses the basal side of the cell with Na and in this case effectively generates 'new' HCO_3^- ions (Fig. 14.22).

In the loop of Henle, both ionic and non-ionic diffusion occur as the concentration of HCO_3^- is raised by water abstraction. This alkalisation will cause NH_3 to leave the tubule in both the ascending thin loop and the thick ascending loop by non-ionic diffusion and enter the collecting duct with its low pH to again form NH_4^+ ions, which are then trapped in the collecting duct fluid.

The formation of ammonium ions 'absorbs' H^+ ions, so keeping the pH above the critical value of 4.5, and generates new HCO_3^- which replace the base loss by metabolic acidosis. A further advantage is that again the generation of a positive charge as NH_4^+ saves a cation, usually Na^+. In chronic acidosis, the production of NH_3 can be increased six times. Prostaglandins can, however, inhibit ammonia genesis.

In summary, the role of the kidney in excreting fixed H^+ ions is related to the plasma pH, which will induce more ammonia genesis, increase Na/H$^+$ activity in the PCT and more

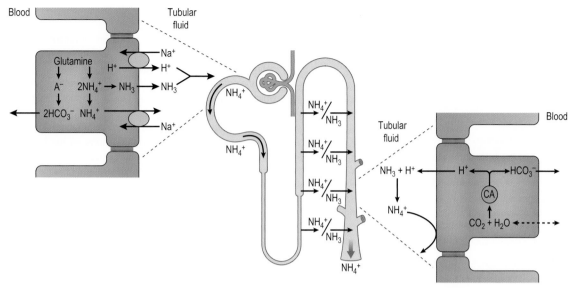

Fig. 14.22 Production, transport and excretion of ammonia by the nephron. Glutamine is metabolised to NH_4^+ and HCO_3^- in the proximal tubule. The NH_4^+ is secreted into the lumen and the HCO_3^- enters the blood. The secreted NH_4^+ is reabsorbed in the loop of Henle primarily by the thick ascending loop and accumulates in the medullary interstitium, where it exists as both NH_4^+ and NH_3. NH_3 diffuses into the tubular fluid of the collecting duct, and H^+ secretion by the collecting duct leads to accumulation of NH_4^+ in the lumen by the processes of non-ionic diffusion and diffusion trapping. CA, carbonic anhydrase.

H^+-ATPase in the collecting ducts. All these factors will help to replace the HCO_3^- lost by non-respiratory acidosis.

Abnormalities of acid–base balance
(also see Clinical box 14.14)

Metabolic acidosis (see Information box 14.3) is diagnosed by a low arterial pH and reduced serum bicarbonate. Compensation is by respiratory means with decrease in P_aCO_2. First step in investigation of cause of metabolic acidosis should involve calculation of serum anion gap (AG), which is the difference in plasma concentrations of major cation (Na^+) and major measured anions (chloride + bicarbonate). $AG = [Na^+] - [Cl] + [HCO_3]$ and normal is 12 ± 2 mmol/L.

The primary mechanism by which kidneys buffer acid load in the body is through urinary ammonia excretion. Urinary ammonia measurement is not measured by most laboratories and hence an indirect measurement involves calculation of the urinary anion gap (UAG) = [UNa + Uk+] – UCl⁻. UAG is normally positive (30–50 mmol/L). If negative suggests increased renal excretion of an unmeasured cation (NH_4^+).

Renal tubular acidosis (RTA) is a result of failure to excrete net acid load. AG is normal and different types are as follows:

- **Type I RTA** (distal) – characterised by inability to acidify urine, is due to reduction in net H^+ secretion (secretory defect) or abnormal permeability (gradient defect) in

---

Clinical box 14.14 Disturbances of acid–base balance

Disturbance of acid–base balance occurs when the blood pH deviates from around 7.4, disrupts normal cellular function, and is potentially life-threatening. The types of acid–base disorder are discussed in Chapters 3 and 13. Acid–base disturbance owing to defective renal regulation, otherwise known as metabolic acidosis or alkalosis, is the result of abnormalities in the regulation of 'fixed' H^+ excretion by the kidneys or defective renal buffer systems: bicarbonate, phosphate and ammonium.

Metabolic acidosis
Metabolic acidosis (blood pH <7.4) occurs when there is an increase in acids other than carbonic acid in the blood, with a decrease in plasma bicarbonate concentration, and may arise from:
- Excessive intake of acid
- Excessive fixed H^+ production, as in lactic acidosis and diabetic ketoacidosis (see Ch. 3)
- Decreased renal H^+ excretion, when the distal convoluted tubules fail to excrete H^+ ions, which also features ammonium deficiency and hypokalaemia, and occurs in renal failure
- Increased renal bicarbonate loss, which may be due to administration of carbonic anhydrase inhibitors (see above), damage to the renal tubules by drugs or heavy metals, or very rarely a condition known as proximal renal tubular acidosis, associated with low plasma renin and low plasma aldosterone concentrations
- Excessive loss of bicarbonate through the gastrointestinal tract, as in severe diarrhoea, and ileostomy.

Metabolic alkalosis
Metabolic alkalosis (blood pH >7.4) is primary excess of serum bicarbonate. It is relatively common, especially in hospital patients, often due to excessive loss of acid gastric contents (vomiting, gastric aspiration) and diuretic use causing chloride or potassium depletion. Severe metabolic alkalosis is life-threatening. Metabolic alkalosis may be due to chloride or potassium depletion, or a mixture of both. The mechanisms for excessive H^+ loss include:
- Loss of sodium, chloride and water in the distal nephron, which promotes potassium and H^+ secretion
- Potassium depletion, which increases bicarbonate reabsorption in the proximal tubules and stimulates ammonium synthesis
- Loss of ECF due the action of diuretics, which stimulates renin and aldosterone secretion (autoregulation), but also increases potassium and H^+ excretion.

Metabolic acidosis is divided into:
1. Chloride responsive alkalosis – principal causes of chloride-responsive are the loss of gastric secretions, ingestion of large doses of non-absorbable antacids, use of thiazide or loop diuretics
2. Chloride resistant alkalosis
   - Normal blood pressure – Bartter syndrome, Gitelman syndrome
   - Hypertension – primary hyperaldosteronism.

the distal nephron. Some patients have H^+/K^+-ATPase resulting in hypokalemic acidosis. Nephrolithiasis and nephrocalcinosis is very common. Patients may experience symptoms of hypokalaemia (musculoskeletal weakness, nephrogenic diabetes insipidus). Urine PH is usually above 5.5 and UAG is greater than zero.

Causes include idiopathic, autoimmune disorders (Sjögren syndrome, systemic lupus erythematosus (SLE)), genetic, drugs (amphotericin B, toluene (glue sniffing)), hyperparathyroidism, tubulointerstitial diseases.

Treatment involves correction of acidosis and hypokalemia. Sodium bicarbonate or potassium citrate can be used for long term management.

- **Type II RTA** (proximal) – usually 80–90% HCO_3 is reabsorbed in PCT. Type II RTA is due to decreased ability to reabsorb filtered HCO_3. Hypokalaemia is almost always seen and is due to activation of renin–angiotensin–aldosterone axis by intravascular volume depletion due to failure to loss of HCO_3. Proximal RTA often occurs due to widespread proximal tubule dysfunction (Fanconi syndrome) which is associated with glycosuria, aminoaciduria, phosphaturia and uricosuria. Urine pH is less than 5.5 reflecting distal compensatory mechanism.
  Management is similar to distal RTA.
- **Type III RTA** is a poorly decribed entity and refers to a combination of type I and type II RTA.
- **Type IV RTA** (hyperkalaemic, hyporeninaemic, hypoaldosteronism) is due to deficiency of aldosterone or resistance of its effects on distal tubule. It is differentiated from type I RTA by presence of hyperkalaemia, urine pH of less than 5.5 and less severe acidosis. Type IV RTA is often seen in patients with longstanding diabetes and lower level of renal function. Drugs associated with this condition include NSAIDs, ACE inhibitors, angiotensin receptor blockers, calcineurin inhibitors.

THE URINARY TRACT

Urine from the collecting tubules drains into the renal pelvis after leaving the pyramids. The urine is then carried by the ureters to the bladder, driven by active peristalsis since the pressure in the bladder is greater than in the renal pelvis. Urine stored in the bladder is voided through the urethra. These components constitute the urinary tract (Fig. 14.2).

URETERS

The ureters are composed of two layers of smooth muscle, a circular layer and a longitudinal layer, but the layers are poorly defined and autonomic ganglia are sparse. Autonomic drugs and their derivatives have little effect on ureteral peristalsis, which is initiated by pacemaker cells in the pelvis. As pressure in the renal pelvis rises to 14 cmH$_2$O, waves of peristalsis are initiated and the urine is forced towards the bladder at 2–3 cm/s.

The ureteral muscles maintain a tone so the ureters are normally empty unless there is an obstruction, usually a stone lodged in the lumen. The ureters and bladder are lined with urothelium, which is a compound epithelium with a specialised structure that is impermeable to CO_2, so can retain high levels of CO_2 in the urine.

The ureters enter the base of the bladder obliquely so are compressed when the bladder muscle contracts at the base of the bladder (Fig. 14.2). In addition, the lower section of the ureter is composed of more circular muscle than the initial section and both these properties limit the reflux of urine into the ureters during normal micturition (passing urine) as the bladder pressure rises when the bladder empties. There is also a reflex which increases ureteric tone as the bladder pressure rises, which also helps to prevent reflux. The kidney can easily be damaged by back pressure and by infection which can enter via this route (Clinical box 14.15).

Urinary tract obstruction

The urinary tract can be obstructed by three types of problem:

- Extrinsic – various factors in the abdominal cavity can externally compress the ureters, such as tumours, inflammation, fibrosis, infection, haemorrhage and trauma, which will lead to a decrease in flow of urine into the bladder
- Intramural – transitional cell cancer, infection, fibrosis and inflammation can all expand the wall and reduce the diameter of the lumen
- Intraluminal – calculi, bleeding and blood clot formation can also obstruct the ureters.

Congenital problems

A number of congenital problems can interfere with the transfer of urine from the renal pelvis to the bladder, such as pelvic/ureteral and ureteral/bladder discontinuity which can cause reflux and the ingress of infection (see Clinical boxes 14.16 and 14.17).

GROSS STRUCTURE OF THE BLADDER

Urine is formed continuously by the kidneys at a rate of at least 1 mL/min so must be stored within the bladder. The bladder consists of three layers of smooth muscle lined with **urothelium**. The outer layer is longitudinal muscle, the middle is a circular layer and there is an incomplete inner layer; together these form the detrusor urinae. There is also the trigone lying on the floor of the bladder at the back, which is a triangle of muscle between the ureter and the exit from the bladder, the urethra (Fig. 14.2). The ureters enter the bladder through this muscle layer and exit onto the surface of the trigone.

Maintenance of continence

Acting via the pelvic floor, continence is maintained by the sphincters of the bladder and the abdominal pressure compressing the bladder neck (see Fig. 14.2). The internal sphincter is an oblique muscle and not well defined. It leads to the urethral sphincter, which is mixed smooth and skeletal muscle, limited by the external sphincter, composed of only striated muscle and under voluntary control.

The cystometrogram records the pressure in the bladder as it fills and shows that the pressure rises in three phases. In the initial phase, the pressure rises rapidly to a small degree (Fig. 14.23). The pressure then rises more slowly over phase II. This is receptive relaxation when most of the bladder filling occurs. No contractions occur during this phase until the bladder has filled to 400 mL or so, when the pressure again rises steeply, phase III. This will only occur if the subject has been unable to empty their bladder and will cause a most unpleasant feeling of pain and 'urge to go'. Normal micturition is a complex active process involving both the parasympathetic and sympathetic systems. If the parasympathetic nerves are cut, the tone falls whereas when the sympathetic nerves are cut the tone rises. This process involves the intramural plexuses and is modified by a higher external input. When the bladder is filled externally, a 'blip' is seen as the pressure rises, then it decreases to a mean value. The tone of the bladder is indicated by the slope of phase II; if it is hypotonic it is flat indicating a flaccid bladder and if it is steep, this is a hypertonic over-reactive bladder. Insertion of the catheter into the bladder, and filling it, leads to a guard reflex increasing the tone in the urethra and the bulbocavernosi. These muscles exert a continuous tone which can be measured by a balloon catheter as it is passed into the bladder.

Nerve supply

The motor nerve supply to the bladder is complex, with a parasympathetic supply from the pelvic S2–S4 nerves, which has a mixed motor and sensory supply derived from the hypogastric and vesicle plexi. There is a sympathetic supply via the inferior mesenteric ganglia which passes via the hypogastric to the vesical plexus. Finally there is somatic control via S3–S4, the pudic motor control to the external sphincter.

The sensory supply is composed of pain and stretch fibres which receive inputs from a large variety of receptor types within the muscle wall with ascending sensory fibres as well as motor supply. The pelvic sensory fibres carry the desire to void urine.

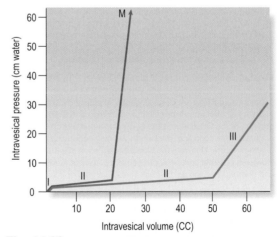

Fig. 14.23 **Schematic cystometrogram.** M indicates peak pressure during micturition contraction. Segment I, or the initial rise, is segment from zero to first point of inflection. Segment II, or the initial limb, begins at first inflection point and either ends at micturition contraction (*red line*) or, in the absence of micturition reflex, continues into segment III (*green line*). Segment III, or the ascending limb, is a sharply rising terminal limb.

The sympathetic supply is not vital to micturition, but in males it prevents sperm reflux during ejaculation. The main role of parasympathetic sensory fibres is in relation to the sensation of bladder fullness. Pain is mostly sympathetic.

Bladder filling and tone

Urinary bladder filling and tone can be studied using a double lumen catheter, filling the bladder via one tube and recording the pressure with a transducer connected to the other. Alternatively, a direct recording can be made via a suprapubic needle.

CONTROL OF MICTURITION

The ability of micturition to be controlled is a learned reflex. Both the abdominal pressure and the pelvic floor act to exert a force on the narrow neck of the bladder, so keeping it closed (Fig. 14.2). The outer sphincter in humans is made of somatic muscle. Coughing automatically increases this pressure so aids continence. In females, especially after repeated childbirth, these muscles become flaccid and stress incontinence can be a problem (Clinical box 14.18).

Clinical box 14.18   **Urinary incontinence**

Failure to control micturition results in **urinary incontinence**, also known as **enuresis**, the involuntary voiding of urine. Until young children learn to control micturition, urine is passed when the bladder is 'full'. **Primary nocturnal enuresis** is the condition in which the child has never been 'dry' at night.

Causes of urinary incontinence
Urinary incontinence may be associated with:
- Bladder defects
- Infection – cystitis, due to incomplete bladder emptying, VUR
- Weakness in bladder musculature – flaccid bladder, detrusor failure.
  Bladder outlet defects:
- Weakness in pelvic floor muscles leading to incompetence of the urethral sphincter – common in women – usually consequence of parturition, atrophic vaginitis, age
- Bladder outlet obstruction: prostatic enlargement, bladder calculi.
  Neurological bladder defects:
- Detrusor overactivity due to defect in central nervous system (CNS) inhibition – conditions include multiple sclerosis, cauda equina lesions, pressure from prolapsed intervertebral disc (S2–S4), stroke
- Intellectual impairment – e.g. **Alzheimer disease**.

Prostatic enlargement produces problems with micturition
Surgery in the lower abdomen can cause problems with micturition as a high pressure is needed to empty the bladder. In the male, obstruction can occur with benign and malignant growths of the prostate and this hyperplasia presses on the urethra. In this condition, micturition will only occur with a raised pressure. Normally the bladder empties at 30–40 cm H_2O. However, prostate problems can cause incomplete emptying and chronic retention as the neck cannot be held open. This leads to increased frequency and a small volume is voided on each occasion. Eventually this leads to a flaccid bladder as the urethra is damaged. Removal of the prostate can lead to stress incontinence as the urethra is now too short.

Problems with bladder emptying
Problems in emptying can occur with pain. An infection in the bladder called cystitis causes painful micturition. Spinal shock leads initially to difficulty in filling but with time this ability will return as lower spinal reflexes are still intact. The bladder in these cases can be induced to empty by squeezing the bladder and exceeding the pressure at which the reflex is initiated. Stroking the inner thigh, the Credé manoeuvre, has the same effect.

The micturition reflex

To enable the bladder to empty, it must first be filled to some 80% of its volume. Once in phase III, the pressure begins to rapidly rise and rhythmic contractions occur giving a sensation of fullness and a desire to void. This can be over-ridden in humans but once the pressure rises to a threshold the bladder will empty automatically. Under normal conditions the initiation of micturition depends on a graded series of autonomic reflexes, which once started go to completion; however, a normal person can inhibit the process at this stage and interrupt the flow. The micturition reflex depends on ascending signals to the pons and medulla which inhibit the normal descending inhibition and the guard reflex via a spinal route. The detrusor muscle contracts, which mechanically opens the internal sphincter and reflexly inhibits the external sphincter. This process flattens the floor of the bladder so the urethra is now open and fluid flows rapidly out as the detrusor contracts. Fluid flow through the urethra reinforces contraction of the bladder via pelvic plexuses and spinal reflexes. Once the smooth muscle in the bladder wall has maximally shortened, the tension falls and the guard reflex is initiated as the bladder starts to refill.

Renal tumours

Can be divided into benign or malignant.

Benign

- Cortical adenoma
- Oncocytoma
- Angiomyolipoma (80% associated with tuberous sclerosis)
- Medullary fibroma.

Malignant

Malignant renal tumours constitute 3% of adult cancers, common in the 6th to 7th decades; presentation is with loin pain, haematuria and mass (rare) but can be an incidental finding. Sporadic and familial (usually associated with von Hippel–Lindau disease):

- Primary – renal cell carcinoma (RCC), which has several subtypes:
  - Clear cell – commonest (80–90%)
  - Papillary – (10–15%)
  - Chromophobe – (4–5%)
- Metastatic tumour, e.g. ovarian carcinoma.

  Note: the commonest tumour of the ureter and bladder is transitional cell carcinoma.

RENAL DISEASES

The kidney has a large reserve in function so more than 75% can be destroyed before symptoms occur. While this is an advantage in one way in that homeostasis is protected, the onset of renal disease can be insidious and by the time symptoms appear it can be too late to treat the damage. The kidneys protect the organism against acidosis (fixed H^+) and hyperkalaemia (K^+) so, if renal function is lost, it is the consequence of the rise in these factors which could lead to the symptoms of disease and eventual death. Since the large reserve in function 'hides' incipient renal failure, the clinician must always be aware of clues which indicate the onset of renal dysfunction.

Routine blood tests can give early warning in the form of a rise in plasma creatinine and a rise in urea. However, if a patient is elderly with low muscle mass, the plasma creatinine may appear close to normal because of the low level of general metabolism and reduced creatinine production from a limited muscle mass. The same can occur with urea, especially if the intake for protein is reduced for economic reasons, poor dentition with difficulty chewing meat and due to isolation in the elderly.

Falls in the elderly are a major cause of hospital admissions and if bone fractures have occurred, loss of renal function must be considered as an underlying factor leading to calcium deficiency, such as disordered vitamin D production and osteoporosis with loss of calcium. The kidney plays a key role in the production of vitamin D (25-hydroxycholecalciferol), which is formed in the liver by a first hydroxylation, then undergoes a second hydroxylation in the kidney where it is converted into 1,25-dihydroxycholecalciferol, the active form of vitamin D (see Ch. 9).

GENERAL CLASSIFICATION OF RENAL DISEASE

There are two ways of classifying renal diseases: one is based on aetiology (e.g. pre-renal, renal or post-renal) and the other is by onset (acute or chronic). Pre-renal failure usually is due to problems with blood flow before it reaches the kidney and is the most common cause of renal failure seen in hospitalised patients. It is usually reversible, if identified early (see Clinical box 14.1).

Volume depletion triggers feedback systems used by the kidney to control sodium balance. The renin–angiotensin–aldosterone system is activated which promotes sodium retention and volume expansion. Compensatory sympathetic effects releases excess norepinephrine (noradrenaline) from the renal nerves facilitating vasoconstriction.

Drugs which inhibit prostaglandin release (e.g. NSAIDs) will have no adverse effects if the kidneys are intact, but may precipitate renal failure in susceptible individuals, because (in renal disease) maintenance of the GFR depends upon the vasodilator effect of prostaglandins. Obstruction of the drainage pathway by blockage of the ureters by stones can lead to back pressure on the nephron which will cause renal damage and, secondary to this, the dilated ureter can be a source of infection which will reflux into the kidneys and lead to septicaemia (see Clinical box 14.16).

Some of the common causes and presentations of intrinsic renal diseases are listed in Clinical boxes 14.19 and 14.20.

ONSET OF RENAL DISEASE

Renal failure can be acute (AKI, see below) with a sudden onset following an upper respiratory tract infection, or chronic (CKD) with a slow rise in plasma creatinine, which has an insidious progression with few symptoms at first but eventually increasing problems. A further classification of renal disease can be related to the site of damage, e.g. glomerulonephritis (inflammation of the glomeruli). Tubular disease involves damage to the tubular system that can be either focal and limited in its extent or global and widespread. The site of

---

Clinical box 14.19 Nephrotic syndrome and protein loss

The **nephrotic syndrome** is a group of disorders in which the permeability of the glomerular capillaries to protein macromolecules is increased. It is characterised by heavy proteinuria (>3.5 g of protein per day), hypoalbuminaemia, oedema, hyperlipidaemia. Peripheral oedema, which was thought to be due to loss of albumin and fall in colloid osmotic pressure (COP) but now has been identified as the consequence of increased Na^+ reabsorption by the collecting ducts leading to overfilling of the vascular space. In nephrotic syndrome the urine sediment is relatively inactive with few cells.

It is of interest that the rise in Na^+ excretion occurs before any changes in the level of albumin so the excess fluid was produced by the inappropriate activation of the renin–angiotensin–aldosterone system.

Common causes of nephrotic syndrome can be divided into:
- Primary (renal) – minimal change disease, focal segmental glomerular sclerosis and membranous nephropathy
- Systemic – amyloidosis, SLE and diabetes mellitus.

Clinical box 14.20 Nephritic syndrome and rapidly progressive glomerulonephritis

Nephritic syndrome is abrupt in onset of oliguria, haematuria, proteinuria of less than 3 g/day, oedema and hypertension. The urine sediment is active, often containing red cells and white cells with both cellular and granular casts. This syndrome reflects the influx of circulating inflammatory cells such as neutrophils, monocytes, macrophages and lymphocytes into the glomerulus. The severity of the glomerular injury reflects the degree of inflammation. Symptoms range from slight haematuria with no changes in glomerular filtration rate (GFR) to blockage of blood vessels, a rise in plasma creatinine and a fall in GFR. In this condition there are circulating antibodies against the glomerular basement membrane, immune complex and complement activation and circulating antibodies against neutrophil cytoplasmic antigens. It is usually self-limiting.

Common causes include post-streptococcal glomerulonephritis (GN), mild form of IgA nephropathy, membranoproliferative GN (MPGN).

Rapidly progressive glomerulonephritis (RPGN) is characterised by sub-acute onset of renal failure, haematuria, proteinuria (<3 g/day). Blood pressure is usually normal but patients may have other features of vasculitis. If renal biopsy shows >50%, it is described as crescentic GN.

RPGN is divided into:
- Anti-glomerular basement membrane (Anti-GBM) disease
- Pauci-immune GN – anti-neutrophil cytoplasmic antibody (ANCA) associated vasculitis (Wegener's granulomatosis, microscopic polyangiitis, Churg–Strauss syndrome)
- Immune complex GN – MPGN, post-streptococcal GN, infective endocarditis, IgA nephropathy, systemic lupus erythematosus.

---

such changes can be identified by a renal biopsy and careful histological examination, and also by blood chemistry where defects in the immune system can be identified.

ACUTE KIDNEY INJURY

Acute kidney injury (AKI) is defined as a sudden fall in renal function. This is accompanied by a fall in GFR and inability of the kidney to excrete toxic waste, so the plasma creatinine and urea values rise, which usually takes a week (see Fig. 14.1). The urine output falls, and oliguria (less than 400 mL per 24 h) occurs.

Acute kidney injury (AKI) has now replaced the term acute renal failure. This new terminology enables healthcare

Table 14.6 Classification of AKI

Stage	Serum creatinine criteria	Urine output criteria
1	Increase ≥26 μmol/L within 48h or increase ≥1.5 to 1.9 times reference SCr	<0.5mL/kg/h for >6 consecutive hours
2	Increase ≥2 to 2.9 times reference SCr	<0.5mL/kg/h for >12 hours
3	Increase ≥3 times reference SCr **or** increase 354 μmol/L **or** commenced on renal replacement therapy (RRT) irrespective of stage	<0.3mL/kg/h for >24 hours or anuria for 12 hours

professionals to consider the disease as a spectrum of injury. This spectrum extends from less severe forms of injury to more advanced injury when acute kidney failure may require renal replacement therapy. The most recent definitions proposed by the Acute Dialysis Quality Initiative (ADQI), RIFLE (Risk, Injury, Failure, Loss of function and End stage disease) and the Acute Kidney Injury Network (AKIN) have been based on rises in serum creatinine or reductions in urine output. For their classification of AKI see Table 14.6.

The commonest cause of AKI is pre-renal and treatment involves restoration of fluid balance and perfusion and treatment of the underlying cause. Urine analysis is normal with a low Na⁺. Fractional excretion of sodium is usually <1. A universal definition and staging system has been proposed to allow earlier detection and management of AKI by KDIGO (Kidney Disease: Improving Global Outcomes), which is a modification from the RIFLE and AKIN classification. Staging is performed by using serum creatinine or urine output criteria. It has been shown in many studies that as the stages increase, so does the risk of mortality.

Acute tubular necrosis

Ischaemia, endogenous and exogenous toxins produce tubular damage which can be very patchy and is a form of acute renal failure. It is the proximal straight tubule which is most sensitive to this damage and leads to loss of tubular epithelial cell structure, function and intratubular obstruction, resulting in decline of GFR.

Renal ischaemia is the most common cause of acute tubular necrosis (ATN). The effect of the duration of ischaemia is, however, very variable; some severe damage can occur with a reduction in RBF of only a few minutes whereas little damage is sometimes seen with much larger periods of interrupted flow. Abdominal and cardiac surgery have the highest incidence of ATN, which may relate to damage or stimulation to the neural inputs to the kidney. In the septic patient ATN may be related to the hypotensive effects of endotoxins.

Nephrotoxic agents

The mechanism by which the kidney is able to secrete a variety of toxins and drugs into the urine can malfunction and lead to nephrotoxicity. Antibiotics such as aminoglycosides and amphotericin B, used in the treatment of hospital-acquired infections, result in 10% of the cases of ATN. Occupational exposure to heavy metals also causes ATN and, in the clinical situation, platinum in the form of cisplatin used in cancer chemotherapy can cause renal toxicity. A further problem

has been introduced with the increased use of radiocontrast agents in urography and CT scans.

Endogenous toxins such as myoglobin in traumatic muscle crush injury can cause ATN, as do some forms of multiple myeloma associated with a high concentration of immunoglobulin light chains.

Drugs and the elderly

With the elderly and those who have pre-existing renal dysfunction, great care must be taken if drugs with known nephrotoxicity are used. The poor renal function results in the patient being exposed to a higher potentially toxic level as the drug is not cleared from the tubule cells for a longer period of time than in those with normal renal function. Digoxin is a case in point and the failing heart impairs the renal excretion so leading to digoxin toxicity.

Although the values of plasma creatinine and creatinine clearance give early warning of renal impairment in most patients, this can be misleading in the elderly with a low muscle mass, as the creatinine values may be only slightly elevated while renal function is depressed. In addition, if the subject is volume depleted, the conservation of sodium and water can over-ride the normal expected response and may lead to a poor clearance of drugs by tubular secretion. Even if the treatment is terminated, the retention of the drugs in the tubular cells can lead to continued damage. Treatment consists initially of maintenance of fluid and electrolyte balance. The use of diuretics such as **furosemide** and **metolazone** can help but great care must be taken with monitoring of renal function.

CHRONIC KIDNEY DISEASE

Chronic kidney disease (CKD) is a clinical syndrome caused by irreversible and progressive renal injury which is persistent for at least 3 months. This condition leads to a rise in plasma creatinine and in blood urea nitrogen (BUN), which is caused by a fall in GFR. In addition, other functions of the kidney are also impaired, such as the failure to secrete hormones such as erythropoietin and calcitriol, which can lead to anaemia and hypocalcaemia. The elevation of plasma urea is referred to as uraemia or azotaemia, and is seen in both chronic and acute renal failure. New classification of CKD (Table 14.7) is clinically used and the stages of CKD are mainly based on measured or estimated GFR calculated by MDRD (modification of diet in renal disease) equation. This staging is an important tool in early identification and management of CKD.

Table 14.7 Classification of CKD

	eGFR	
1	90+	Normal kidney function but urine findings or structural abnormalities or genetic trait point to kidney disease
2	60–89	Mildly reduced kidney function, and other findings (as for stage 1) point to kidney disease
3A	45–59	Moderately reduced kidney function
3B	30–44	
4	15–29	Severely reduced kidney function
5	<15	Very severe, or **end-stage** kidney failure (sometimes called **established renal failure**)

Additional suffixes: P=with proteinuria, e.g. stage 3P; T=post-renal transplant, e.g. stage 3T; D=on dialysis (always stage 5D).

Causes of chronic kidney disease

CKD can be caused by a wide variety of conditions:

- Diabetes mellitus is the commonest, which accounts for some 30–40% of the cases needing dialysis. Type 1 diabetes leads to chronic renal failure after about 10 years, the first signs being microalbuminuria accompanied by diabetic neuropathy and retinopathy. It can also occur in type 2 diabetes, which is also dependent on the duration of the condition and on good glucose control. The mechanisms underlying diabetic nephropathy are discussed in detail in Chapter 3.
- Hypertension is also a major cause of chronic renal failure, which causes thickening of the arterioles and nephrosclerosis, and is limited by reducing the blood pressure.
- The third most common cause of CKD is glomerulonephritis, which includes conditions such as membranous nephropathy, focal glomerular sclerosis, systemic lupus erythematosus and Goodpasture syndrome, which reflects immune damage to the glomerular basement membrane.

There are many other causes, such as long-term exposure to lead and other environmental toxins, misuse of analgesics, and various genetic problems such as polycystic kidney disease.

Progression of chronic kidney disease

CKD (Chronic Kidney Disease) is often a progressive disease but with the appropriate treatment the damage can be slowed although rarely completely halted. It is thought that the progressive nature of the condition is caused by the remaining healthy nephrons being subject to hyperfiltration and an increased plasma flow with a raised hydrostatic pressure. ACE inhibitors are most useful in the treatment of this progression by reduction of blood pressure and proteinuria. The accumulation of uraemic toxins can lead to neurological conditions with seizures and depressed sensory function.

Chronic kidney disease and hypertension

The failure in chronic renal failure of the kidneys to excrete adequate water and salt leads to hypertension, which in turn can lead to myocardial infarction and stroke. The disturbance in calcium homeostasis and acidosis leads to bone calcium depletion and osteomalacia. This condition is made worse by the use of aluminium-based antacids taken to bind phosphate.

The progress of chronic renal failure is monitored by plotting the reciprocal of the plasma creatinine against time, and changes in the slope of the line give an indication of whether the rate of renal failure is progressing or slowing.

Erythropoietin

The kidneys secrete the hormone **erythropoietin** (**EPO**), which maintains bone marrow production of red cells. A major complication of renal failure has been the loss of red cells owing to the lack of EPO production. Repeated blood transfusions may be necessary to maintain red cell volume. EPO is secreted by the fibroblast-like renal interstitial cells in response to changes in the pO_2 of blood. At high altitude, the pO_2 falls and the EPO is released, which increases red cell mass. This is also seen in chronic obstructive pulmonary disease, where the lung disease results in a low arterial pO_2, leading to polycythaemia (see Ch. 13).

Pharmacological renal damage and chronic renal failure

Table 14.8 lists some of the drugs which can cause acute interstitial nephritis, and renal function must be monitored during their use. The sites of damage vary, with the least common being the glomerulus. However, glomerular damage can be affected by gold and penicillamine used in the treatment of rheumatoid arthritis and to a small extent with NSAIDs. Aminoglycoside antibiotics need particular care as they are secreted by the tubule and can alter glomerular haemodynamics. The nephrotoxicity is related to peak dose rather than the steady state value so a smaller dose given at more frequent intervals is less toxic than a single large dose. Agents such as digoxin and cephalosporin, in contrast, depend on their steady state value and in CRF the dose must be

Table 14.8	The nephrotoxicity of some drugs, toxins and endogenous compounds
Drugs	
Aminoglycoside antibiotics	These accumulate in the lysosomes of the PCT cells and can generate reactive species, depending on the number of NH_3^+ groups. Very persistent accumulation for up to 4–6 weeks
Amphotericin	Predominantly produces tubular damage, but acute vasoconstriction may be responsible for rapid reductions in glomerular filtration rate which can return quickly to normal once the drug has been discontinued
Cephalosporins	Acute tubular damage – less frequent with the new generation of compounds
Polymyxin	Tubular damage and also neurotoxic
Rifampicin	Tubular damage and interstitial nephritis
Sulphonamides	Intratubular crystal aggregation may cause obstruction which can be cleared by alkali and fluid administration. Vasculitic damage has also been reported
Tetracyclines	Anti-anabolic and in some cases directly nephrotoxic
Cisplatin	A cytotoxic drug which is also nephrotoxic
Phenacetin	Nephritis

Continued

Table 14.8   **The nephrotoxicity of some drugs, toxins and endogenous compounds—cont'd**

Phenindione	Allergic glomerulonephritis
General anaesthetic agents	Mainly methoxyflurane – produces tubular damage and, as it is metabolised to oxalic acid, crystal deposition within the kidney may cause acute renal failure. This, however, is rare
Radiographic contrast	Strictly not a drug, but mentioned here as reports of nephrotoxicity following intra-arterial injection have been made. Dehydration should be avoided in patients with impaired renal function, and the use of isotonic contrast media may limit renal damage

Endogenous compounds	**Toxins**
Myoglobin	Heavy metals
Haemoglobin	Aluminium
Myeloma light chains	Environmental toxins
Crush injury	PO_4^{2-} = binders and antacids
Haemolysis, hypertension	
Leukaemia	

reduced to avoid toxicity. Cephalosporins induce a marked vasoconstriction and a fall in GFR with ischaemic damage in the long term. Note: absorption of 99% of the water by the nephron can lead to toxic concentration of drugs in the tubule cells.

Analgesic nephropathy is now less common with the withdrawal of combination tablets such as aspirin, phenacetin and caffeine. Chinese herbs such as *Aristolochia frangulin* have been identified as causing interstitial fibrosis and uroepithelial cancer. As with all drugs, patients differ in their sensitivity so care must be taken to monitor their effect on renal function.

RENAL REPLACEMENT THERAPY

Renal replacement therapy (RRT) involves life-supporting treatment for patients with end-stage renal failure (eGFR <15 mL/min). In acute kidney injury, support is usually required temporarily (dialysis), whereas in end-stage renal failure secondary to CKD, it is lifelong and in the form of dialysis or transplantation (see Clinical boxes 14.21 and 14.22). Best outcomes are with pre-emptive transplantation (before the patient ends up on dialysis). RRT is a very intensive treatment and not all patients can tolerate it (e.g. old age with multiple comorbidities). In such cases supportive and palliative care is a better option.

Clinical box 14.21   **Transplantation**

Best available treatment for end-stage renal disease is kidney transplantation. Patient survival is much better than on dialysis. Broadly this can be divided into:

Living donor transplants
Directed:
- Genetically related – father, mother, siblings etc.
- Emotionally related – partner, close friend etc.
- Paired/pooled kidney donation
- Incompatible – ABO or HLA.

Non-directed:
- Altruistic

Cadaveric (dead) transplants
- Donation after circulatory death (non-heart beating)
- Donation after brain death (heart beating).

Clinical box 14.22   **Dialysis**

Once a patient is oliguric and fails to respond to diuretic treatment, it is better to initiate dialysis at an early stage than wait until hyperkalaemia and uraemia develop. Once GFR falls below 10 mL/min renal replacement therapy should be initiated. Although dialysis can maintain most aspects of renal function, phosphate does not exchange easily, so it builds up. Phosphates binders can be given to help correct this problem although, being aluminium based, they can cause toxicity.

Peritoneal dialysis
The patient's peritoneum can act as a dialysis or semi-permeable membrane. Dialysate at body temperature is introduced via a soft catheter into the peritoneal cavity; 1–2 L of fluid can be introduced and left for 1–2 h (Fig. 14.24A). By the use of fluid with an appropriate composition, i.e. lower Na^+ and osmolarity made up with lactate, it is possible to withdraw water, potassium and urea from the patient. The fluid is then drained from the peritoneal cavity and replaced. Using this method it is possible for the patient to carry on a normal life while being dialysed. Much care in the technique is necessary to avoid infection but continuous ambulatory peritoneal dialysis can be continued for many weeks. The total removal of creatinine and urea by this method may be inadequate but hyperkalaemia and fluid balance can be achieved.

Haemodialysis
A more efficient way of replacing kidney function is to use haemodialysis, with a flat plate or hollow fibre dialyser (Fig. 14.24B). In these the blood flows through the system one way and the dialysate flows in the opposite direction. The membrane is made of various plastics, and permits the rapid removal of waste products in the blood and virtual complete replacement of renal function. A shunt must be constructed between, usually, a peripheral artery and vein so blood can be withdrawn with a roller pump and passed through the dialyser, cleansed and returned to the patient. This process takes 4–6 h and is performed three times per week. With a compliant patient, this can be done at home. This process is also used in haemofiltration which uses a more permeable membrane and can depend on the patient's own blood pressure to drive the blood through the filter. This process is more gentle and can run continuously for several days. Fluid is removed from the patient and a slightly smaller volume returned to balance the electrolytes and fluid volume.

Indication for dialysis
- Persistent hyperkalaemia (K > 6.5) with oligo-anuria
- Pulmonary oedema (diuretic resistant or with oligo-anuria)
- Severe metabolic acidosis
- Uraemic pericarditis (pericardial rub)

Haemofiltration
A continuous (usually 24–48 hours) and gentle form of dialysis, which is performed in haemodynamically unstable patients, exclusively in intensive care setting.

Clinical box 14.22 Dialysis—cont'd

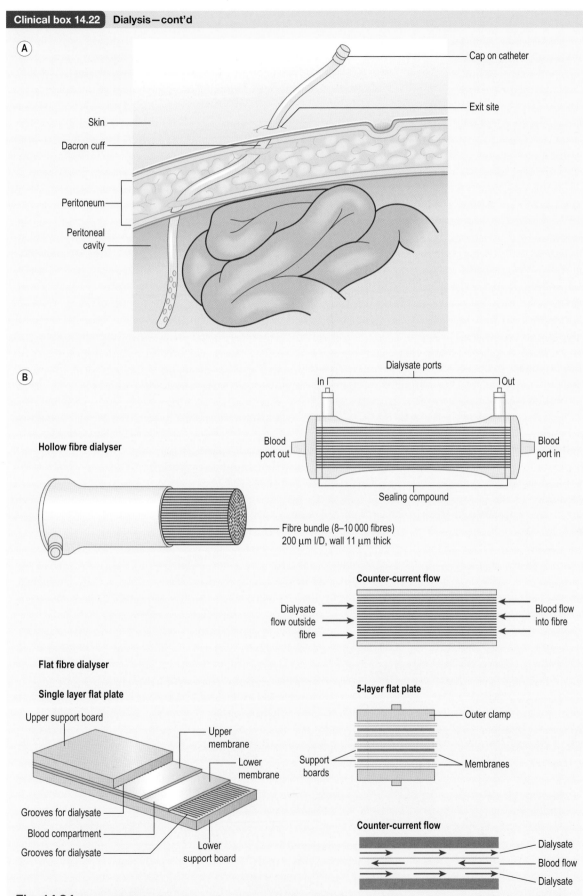

Fig. 14.24 **Haemodialysis.** Diagrams of flat plate and hollow fibre dialysers. Note the arrangements for increasing the surface area of the dialyser membrane.

15

The alimentary system

John Wilkinson

Introduction	**699**
Basic functions and structure of the alimentary system	699
Blood supply to the gastrointestinal tract	700
Overview of digestion and absorption	**701**
Physical digestion	701
Chemical digestion	701
Absorption	702
Surface anatomy of the abdomen	**709**
Abdominal regions	710
Quadrants	711
Microanatomy of the gastrointestinal tract	**711**
Innervation of the alimentary canal	713
Mouth	**714**
Teeth	714
Tongue	714
Mastication	714
Salivary glands	**714**
Functions of saliva	715
Composition of saliva	715
Secretory mechanisms	716
Control of salivary secretion	717
Pharynx and oesophagus	**718**
Swallowing	718
Stomach and duodenum	**719**
Anatomy of the stomach	719
Control of gastric secretions	**722**
Stimulation of gastric acid secretion	722

Inhibition of gastric acid secretion	723
Stimulation of pepsinogen secretion	724
Cellular mechanisms of gastric acid secretion	724
Gastric mucosal protection	726
Gastric motility	**727**
Gastric musculature	727
Electrical and contractile activity of gastric smooth muscle	727
Gastric motility during the interdigestive period	728
Gastric motility during a meal	728
Nausea, retching and vomiting	730
Exocrine pancreas	**730**
Pancreatic enzymes	730
Control of pancreatic juice secretion	734
The liver and biliary system	**734**
Anatomy of the liver	735
Functions of the liver	737
Some diseases of the liver	740
Gall bladder	742
Small intestine	**743**
Structure of the small intestine	744
Small intestinal fluid secretion	744
Small intestinal motility	745
Large intestine	**746**
Large intestinal fluid secretion	746
Musculature of the large intestine	746
Large intestinal motility	746
Motility of the rectum and anal canal	747
Defecation	747

INTRODUCTION

The chemical composition of food is complex and little of it is water soluble, therefore it cannot enter the body fluids unaltered. A series of digestive processes enables food to be broken down and absorbed. These processes take place in the alimentary canal, which consists of the mouth, oesophagus and gastrointestinal tract, and associated exocrine glands producing secretions that act on food.

BASIC FUNCTIONS AND STRUCTURE OF THE ALIMENTARY SYSTEM

The functions of the alimentary canal are concerned with storage, digestion and absorption of food together with the excretion of undigested food and waste products. Digestion is the process of breaking down complex food molecules, by mechanical and chemical methods, into simple ones that can be absorbed. The digestion products

together with salts and water are absorbed into the blood and lymphatic systems. In addition, the alimentary canal serves to protect the body from swallowed noxious agents and bacterial toxins.

Four activities of the alimentary canal can be identified. These are:

- Motility
- Secretion
- Digestion
- Absorption.

Motility is the term used to describe movements of the alimentary canal that are responsible for propelling partly digested food along the canal, and for mixing the food with the digestive secretions in order that digestion and absorption can take place in a regulated manner. These activities are inter-related. In health there is a balance, and we pay little attention to alimentary function. Disruption of one activity in disease leads to an imbalance and we become conscious of gastrointestinal function, e.g. pain and peptic ulceration, diarrhoea, constipation. Coordination of alimentary function depends on the combined action of the nervous, endocrine (circulating hormones) and paracrine (local hormones) systems. The anatomy of the alimentary system and associated glands is shown in Figure 15.1.

- The **mouth** or oral cavity consists of the lips, tongue, gums, teeth, hard and soft palate and the pharynx together with the salivary glands. Food is ingested, mixed with saliva, chewed and swallowed.
- The **oesophagus** is a muscular tube lying in the thorax and abdomen that connects the pharynx to the stomach. It is separated from the pharynx by the upper oesophageal sphincter. Food and drink are propelled to the stomach by the action of the oesophageal muscles.
- The **stomach** lies in the abdomen below the diaphragm. It is separated from the oesophagus and small intestine by the lower oesophageal (cardiac) and pyloric sphincters, respectively.
- The **duodenum** forms the first part of the small intestine. It receives the pancreatic and biliary ducts from the pancreas and liver, respectively.
- The **jejunum** and **ileum** are a continuation of the small intestine. The ileum terminates at the **ileo-caecal junction**.
- The large intestine consists of the **caecum** with the **appendix**, the **colon** (divided into three sections: ascending, transverse and descending) and the **rectum**.
- The **anus** is the opening at the end of the large intestine. An internal and an external anal sphincter control the opening.

BLOOD SUPPLY TO THE GASTROINTESTINAL TRACT

The gastrointestinal tract, liver, gall bladder, pancreas and spleen are supplied with blood from the splanchnic circulation in a number of parallel circuits (Fig. 15.2). Blood is delivered via three major arteries:

- **Coeliac artery** to the liver, gall bladder, pancreas, stomach and spleen
- **Superior mesenteric artery** to the pancreas, small intestine and most of large intestine
- **Inferior mesenteric artery** to the terminal portions of the large intestine and rectum.

The arterial supply divides into a capillary network within the digestive organs that subsequently drains into the hepatic portal vein, which enters the liver. The blood from the hepatic portal vein flows through liver sinusoids before being returned to the heart by the inferior vena cava. The liver also receives about 20–25% of its blood supply from the hepatic branch of the coeliac artery. Blood flow through the splanchnic circulation is enhanced during feeding.

The control of blood flow to the different mucosal and muscle layers (see Fig. 15.7) of the gastrointestinal tract is regulated independently. The neural, endocrine and paracrine mechanisms controlling gastrointestinal blood flow are shown in Table 15.1.

Mucosal blood flow is required to:

- Maintain viability of the mucosa
- Provide the precursors for secretory products
- Deliver hormones to their target cells
- Remove absorbed digestion products, toxins and drugs from the mucosa.

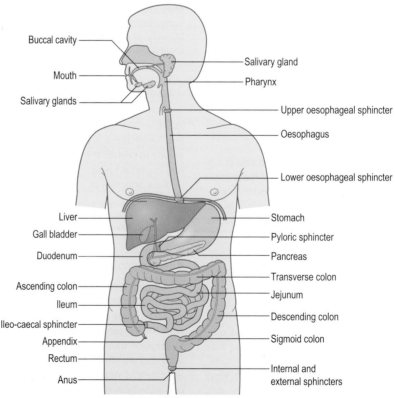

Fig. 15.1 **The alimentary canal and its associated glands.**

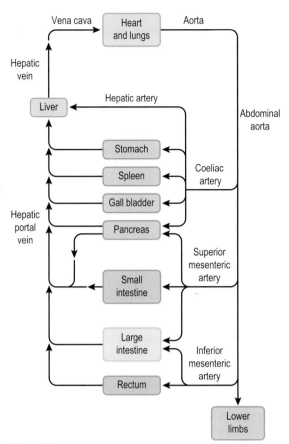

Fig. 15.2 **The splanchnic circulation.**

Table 15.1	Control of gastrointestinal blood flow	
Neural mechanisms	**Vasoconstrictor action (neurotransmitters)**	**Vasodilator action (neurotransmitters)**
Parasympathetic nerves		ACh, VIP
Sympathetic nerves	NE via α adrenoceptors	NE via β_2 adrenoceptors
Sensory nerves		CGRP, SP, NKA
Enteric nerves		ACh, VIP, NO
Hormonal mechanisms	Catecholamines (mainly epinephrine (adrenaline))	Gastrin
	Angiotensin II	Cholecystokinin
	Vasopressin	Secretin
Local mechanisms	Somatostatin	Adenosine
	Endothelin 1	Low pO_2
		Histamine
		Prostacyclin (PGI$_2$)
		Prostaglandin E$_2$

ACh, acetylcholine; CGRP, calcitonin gene-related peptide; NE, norepinephrine (noradrenaline); NKA, neurokinin A; NO, nitric oxide; SP, substance P; VIP, vasoactive intestinal polypeptide.

OVERVIEW OF DIGESTION AND ABSORPTION

Before nutrients can be absorbed, ingested carbohydrates, protein and fat have to be digested. Disruption of the normal mechanisms for either digestion or absorption

Clinical box 15.1 **Clinical conditions associated with impaired physical digestion**

Beginning in the mouth, pain from diseased mucous membranes or dental problems interferes with chewing (mastication), the first step in the process of breaking down large food particles. A number of systemic diseases are associated with oral manifestations. Common conditions include:

- Oral candidiasis (thrush) associated with diabetes mellitus, debilitating illness such as human immunodeficiency virus (HIV)/acquired immune deficiency syndrome (AIDS), cancer and blood dyscrasias, and chemotherapy.
- Mouth ulcers may be due to: infections, e.g. herpes simplex, erythema multiforme (Steven–Johnson syndrome); other ulcerations of the gastrointestinal tract, e.g. coeliac disease, regional ileitis (Crohn's disease), ulcerative colitis, disseminated (or systemic) lupus erythematosus, Behçet's disease; squamous cell carcinoma and other, less common tumours; and trauma including ill-fitting dentures.
- Absence of teeth or neuromuscular defects in old age (e.g. after a stroke) can interfere with mastication.
- Physical digestion in the stomach, i.e. storage of ingested food, mixing the contents to promote fat emulsification, enzyme and acid action, may be impaired through infiltration of gastric musculature by tumour ('leather bottle stomach') affecting motility. Pyloric stenosis from peptic ulceration or tumour delays gastric emptying. Surgical resection (partial gastrectomy) increases the rate of gastric emptying (see Clinical box 15.10).
- Conditions that affect small intestine motility are usually manifested by increased motility, and may lead to diarrhoea, abdominal pain and discomfort. Irritable bowel syndrome (IBS) is an example. Other causes include infection, food sensitivities, endocrine disease and radiation enteritis.

(malabsorption), or both, leads to disease. Two mechanisms for the digestion of ingested food can be identified. These are:

- Physical digestion
- Chemical digestion.

PHYSICAL DIGESTION

Physical digestion is produced by mechanical activity of the alimentary canal breaking down pieces of food into smaller particles. The food retains its complex chemical structure, but its surface area is increased to expose more sites to enzymic action. Physical digestion takes place in the:

- Mouth
- Antrum and pylorus of the stomach
- Small intestine.

It is dependent upon muscular contractions squeezing and grinding the food, and mixing it with secretions. In addition, bile salts and lecithin act as detergents to emulsify fat globules. These actions are produced by the physical properties of bile salts and lecithin, having fat- and water-soluble components in the molecules (see Clinical box 15.1).

CHEMICAL DIGESTION

Enzymes are responsible for chemical digestion. This involves the hydrolysis of the complex food molecules, i.e. being broken down into their simpler constituents, which are capable of being absorbed. Chemical digestion may occur by means of enzyme activity present in the lumen of the alimentary canal or on the luminal-facing membrane of the epithelial cells (enterocytes) in the small intestine.

Carbohydrate digestion

The predominant carbohydrates in the diet are:

- Starch and glycogen (polysaccharides)
- Sucrose and lactose (disaccharides)
- Fructose (monosaccharide).

Starch and glycogen are polymers comprising chains of glucose molecules joined together by α-1,4 glycosidic bonds and at branch points by α-1,6 glycosidic bonds. Salivary and pancreatic amylases catalyse the hydrolysis of the interior α-1,4 bonds but do not split either the terminal α-1,4 glycosidic bonds or the α-1,6 glycosidic bonds at the branches of starch and glycogen. The products of amylase action are maltose (a disaccharide), maltotriose (a trisaccharide) and α-limit dextrins (branched oligosaccharides) (Fig. 15.3). However, there are no transport systems for the absorption of these carbohydrates in the intestine. The oligosaccharides derived from starch together with maltose, sucrose and lactose are further digested by enzymes present on the brush border of enterocytes to their monosaccharides – glucose, galactose and fructose (Table 15.2 and Clinical box 15.2).

Protein digestion

The various sources of protein for digestion are from food and also desquamated gastrointestinal cells and digestive secretions. Proteins and polypeptides consist of amino acids linked together by a peptide bond formed between the amino terminal of one amino acid and the carboxy terminal of another (see Ch. 2). Protein digestion is accomplished by enzymes (protease or peptidase) hydrolysing peptide bonds either within a polypeptide chain or protein (endopeptidase) or at the free ends (exopeptidase). Thus a protein may be broken down to a mixture of small polypeptides and amino acids.

Protein digestion in the stomach

Peptic cells in the stomach secrete pepsinogens, the precursor of a family of enzymes known as pepsins. The acid contents of the stomach activate pepsinogens to pepsins and denature the structure of proteins. Pepsin is an endopeptidase and specifically hydrolyses peptide bonds containing an aromatic L-amino acid such as phenylalanine or tyrosine. Pepsin is inactivated by the alkaline pH found in the duodenum (Clinical box 15.3).

Protein digestion in the small intestine

Protein digestion in the small intestine occurs due to the presence of pancreatic proteases (Table 15.3). The most important are trypsin, chymotrypsin and carboxypeptidase. These are secreted as precursors into the duodenum and activated by enteropeptidase (enterokinase) secreted by the duodenal and jejunal mucosa. Enteropeptidase activates trypsinogen to trypsin. Once some trypsin is formed it acts autocatalytically to convert more trypsinogen to trypsin and also activates chymotrypsinogen to chymotrypsin. Trypsin, chymotrypsin and elastase are endopeptidases and convert protein into polypeptides. Carboxypeptidases release single amino acids from the carboxyl end of polypeptides. The pancreatic proteases active in the lumen of the intestine produce small peptides and some amino acids before being inactivated by autodigestion. The next stage of protein digestion occurs at the brush border of the enterocytes by the action of peptidases present in the luminal membranes to produce small peptides (di-, tri- and tetrapeptides) and single amino acids. Finally, small peptides (usually di- and tri-) are hydrolysed to single amino acids after they have been absorbed into the enterocyte (Fig. 15.3).

Fat digestion

The majority of the fats in the diet are triacylglycerols (triglycerides), consisting of glycerol to which three fatty acids are attached (see Ch. 2). Fats separate from the water phase of the partly digested food in the stomach and empty slowly. The contractile action of the stomach breaks the fat into small droplets and mixes them with the water phase. The nature of fats and their insolubility in the water create difficulties for their digestion by water-soluble lipases. There are three lipases:

- Lingual
- Gastric
- Pancreatic.

The lingual and gastric lipases have acidic pH optima and function in the stomach producing fatty acids and diacylglycerols (diglycerides) by attacking the outer ester linkages between glycerol and the fatty acids.

The major site of fat digestion is in the small intestine (see Information box 15.1). Fat enters the duodenum relatively slowly in order that there is time for the process of emulsification and fat hydrolysis. Fat is emulsified into droplets about 500–1000 nm in diameter by the action of bile salts with their hydrophobic side (fat soluble) dissolving in the fat and their hydrophilic side (water soluble) facing outwards in the water of the intestinal fluid. This process is aided by lecithin and cholesterol, which are also found in bile. The emulsifying agents reduce the surface tension of the fat droplets and keep them apart. These actions increase the surface area of the ingested fat. This allows an interaction between the water-soluble pancreatic lipase and the ingested fat. Pancreatic lipase (optimum pH 8.0) preferentially hydrolyses the bonds between glycerol and the fatty acid residues at positions 1 and 3 to produce 2-monoacylglycerols (monoglycerides) and free fatty acids. A small quantity of the 2-monoacylglycerols are hydrolysed to glycerol and a free fatty acid. The presence of fat digestion products, bile salts, cholesterol and phospholipids leads the emulsion to break up into smaller particles, known as mixed micelles, with diameters of up to 5 nm. The bile salts form an outer coat with the fatty digestion products in the centre. The micelles are small enough to diffuse between the microvilli of the enterocytes.

ABSORPTION

Absorption is the term used to describe the transfer of nutrients or their digestion products from the lumen of the alimentary canal to either the blood or lymph. The small intestine possesses efficient mechanisms for the absorption of nutrients and prevents their passage to the large intestine. The presence of nutrients in the large intestine produces diarrhoea resulting from water being drawn into the lumen by osmosis or by bacterial overgrowth. The absorbed molecules have to overcome a barrier (Fig. 15.4) made up of the:

- Unstirred layer of fluid covering the microvilli
- Glycocalyx covering the microvilli

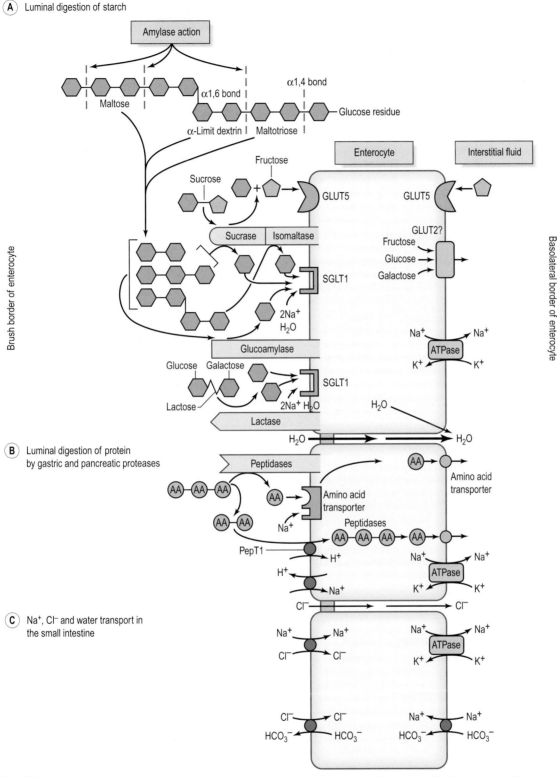

A Luminal digestion of starch

B Luminal digestion of protein by gastric and pancreatic proteases

C Na⁺, Cl⁻ and water transport in the small intestine

Fig. 15.3 **Digestion and absorption of carbohydrates and protein from the small intestine.** (A) Carbohydrate; (B) protein; (C) electrolytes and water. GLUT2, GLUT5, membrane glucose transporters; SGLT1, sodium/glucose-linked transporter; PepT1, peptide membrane transporter.

- Luminal plasma membrane
- Cytoplasm
- Basal or lateral border of the cell
- Intercellular space
- Basement membrane (basal and reticular lamina)
- Plasma membrane of the capillary or lymph vessel.

General principles of absorption

Most carbohydrate, protein and lipid absorption occurs in the small intestine, in the duodenum, jejunum and the early sections of the ileum. These sites, together with the stomach, are also where orally administered drugs are absorbed.

Table 15.2   The action of disaccharidases in the brush border of enterocytes

Enzyme	Substrate	Products
Glucoamylase (maltase)	Maltose	Glucose
	Maltotriose	Glucose
	α-Limit dextrins	Glucose
Isomaltase (α-Dextrinase)	α-Limit dextrins	Glucose
Sucrase	Sucrose	Glucose and fructose
	Maltose	Glucose
	Maltotriose	Glucose
Lactase	Lactose	Glucose and galactose

Clinical box 15.2   Enzyme deficiency

Deficiencies in enzymes concerned with carbohydrate digestion prevent the breakdown of oligo- and di-saccharides to monosaccharides that can be absorbed, so, instead, these are excreted undigested. This gives rise to diarrhoea after ingesting foods rich in these particular carbohydrates. A common example is milk intolerance due to lactase deficiency, a condition more common in some Asian and Mediterranean countries. It is not a major clinical problem, as most people with lactase deficiency simply avoid milk. A lactose tolerance test is available, but rarely used for adults.

Clinical box 15.3   Enzyme defects in protein digestion

Deficiency in pancreatic enzyme secretion, notably of trypsinogen and chymotrypsinogen, prevents the conversion of dietary protein into polypeptides for absorption. This can occur in chronic pancreatitis, mainly related to sustained alcohol overuse. Cystic fibrosis sufferers have the same enzyme deficiency. The inability of children with cystic fibrosis to digest protein and fat because of the lack of pancreatic enzymes, trypsin and lipase, leads to nutritional deficiencies in essential amino acids, fatty acids and fat soluble vitamins. High-dose pancreatic enzyme supplements to treat the resulting steatorrhoea, as well as nutritional supplementation, will be necessary.

Table 15.3   Gastric and pancreatic proteases

Precursor	Activator	Protease
Pepsinogens	Acid	Pepsins
Trypsinogen	Enteropeptidase	Trypsin
Chymotrypsinogen	Trypsin	Chymotrypsin
Procarboxypeptidase	Trypsin	Carboxypeptidase
Proelastase	Trypsin	Elastase

Disease of the membranes through which absorption takes place, and defects in the normal mechanisms for absorption, lead to nutritional deficiencies and also adverse or toxic drug effects. Absorption of solutes may occur by either passive or active processes. See Clinical box 15.4.

There are two types of passive diffusion. These are simple diffusion, where small molecules, such as O_2 and CO_2, and fat-soluble molecules diffuse through the lipid bilayer of the cell membrane, and facilitated diffusion, where the transported molecule moves through the membrane by means

Information box 15.1   Defects in chemical fat digestion

Failure of secretion of pancreatic lipase and deficiency in bile salts affects fat digestion in the small intestine. Pancreatic lipase deficiency occurs in many conditions, including chronic pancreatitis, carcinoma of the pancreas and cystic fibrosis. Deficiency in bile salts is usually due to obstruction, which may be intra-hepatic, as in cirrhosis of the liver, or extra-hepatic due to gall bladder disease, stones in the biliary tree or tumours. The resulting failure to digest fat leads to the excretion of undigested fat globules in the form of pale, bulky, offensive and sometimes frothy stools that float (steatorrhoea). Steatorrhoea may be confirmed by measuring the fat content of stools. The absorption of fat-soluble vitamins may also be impaired (see below).

of a protein carrier. In a passive process, the absorbed solute will move from a high to a low concentration. Passive processes do not require the use of energy from cellular metabolism.

Water and some solutes pass through membranes at a faster rate than would be expected from a knowledge of the lipid solubility. This suggests that there are routes through the membrane for water and small hydrophilic solutes. These may be in the spaces between the membrane phospholipids and through specific membrane proteins called aquaporins. Ions can diffuse through specific protein ion channels that span the membrane.

In contrast, an active process involves cellular energy to drive an absorbed solute against either a concentration gradient or an electrical gradient, i.e. an 'uphill' movement from a low to a high concentration or for a charged solute moving to a region of the same charge, e.g. Na^+ ions being transported out of cells. The two types of active transport either use ATP directly, as in the Na^+/K^+-ATPase pump, or as a source of energy to power secondary active transport.

For the absorption of many solutes in the alimentary canal there are carrier-mediated mechanisms that use the concentration gradient built up as a result of the primary active transport of Na^+. This process is known as secondary active transport. The carriers have binding sites for the organic molecules and for Na^+. The movement of Na^+ down its concentration gradient can lead to the simultaneous transfer of the organic molecule into the cell against its concentration gradient. Metabolic inhibitors which block the primary active transport system will lead to inhibition of the secondary active transport system once the potential energy stored in the Na^+ concentration gradient across the cell membrane has run down.

Carbohydrate absorption

The carbohydrate digestion products are glucose, galactose and fructose. A small quantity of these sugars is absorbed by passive diffusion through aqueous channels between enterocytes and in the cell membranes. The main transport mechanisms involve carrier proteins in the brush and basolateral borders of enterocytes. All the sugars enter the hepatic portal vein for delivery to the liver.

Glucose and galactose absorption

Glucose and galactose are absorbed by secondary active transport involving a sodium-dependent glucose and galactose transporter (sodium/glucose-linked transporter, SGLT1) in the brush border membrane of the enterocyte (see Fig. 15.3).

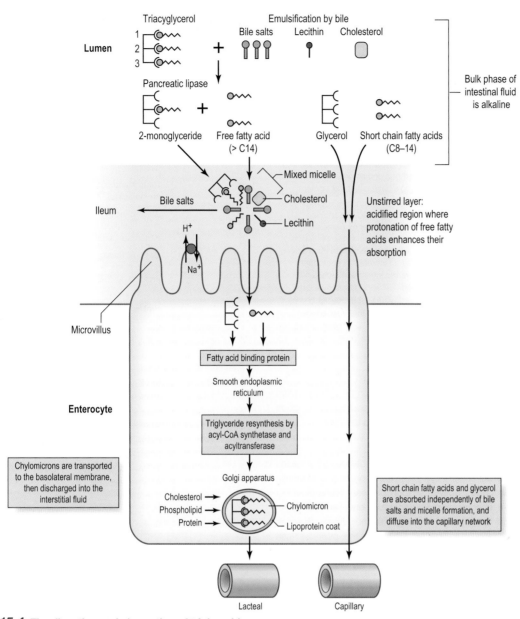

Fig. 15.4 **The digestion and absorption of triglycerides.**

The glucose and galactose compete for the sugar site on the transporter which also binds two Na⁺ ions at a different site. Once loaded, the transporter moves the Na⁺ down its electro-chemical gradient into the cell together with either the glucose or galactose. The Na⁺ diffuses into the intracellular fluid and is transported out of the cell by the Na⁺/K⁺-ATPase (sodium pump) on the basolateral membrane. The glucose and galac-tose accumulate in the cell until they are removed by simple diffusion and facilitated diffusion involving GLUT2, a trans-porter found in the basolateral borders of the enterocyte. The importance of GLUT2 has been questioned because patients with the rare Fanconi–Bickel syndrome in which GLUT2 trans-porters are defective absorb glucose from the intestine but not from the kidney tubules which also have GLUT2 transporters located on the basolateral borders of the tubular cells.

Fructose absorption

Fructose enters the enterocyte by facilitated diffusion us-ing the specific fructose transporter GLUT5, which does not require the co-transport of Na⁺ to function (Fig. 15.3). Young

children may have difficulty in absorbing fructose in fruit juices due to a less developed transport system compared with adults leading to the production of gas and diarrhoea. As with glucose and galactose, GLUT2 is believed to transport fructose across the basolateral border of the enterocyte to the tissue fluid; however, patients with Fanconi–Bickel syn-drome are able to absorb fructose. GLUT5 has been identi-fied in the basolateral border of human enterocytes and will provide a route for fructose transport to the tissue fluid.

Protein absorption

The proteases in the gastrointestinal tract produce a variety of peptides and free amino acids for absorption. The enterocytes have a relatively high cytosolic concentration of free amino acids for protein synthesis that, in turn, can make amino acid absorption more difficult. This difficulty is overcome by the absorption of di- and tripeptides that are subsequently hy-drolysed by peptidases to release free amino acids within the cell. This hydrolysis maintains a concentration gradient

Clinical box 15.4   **Diarrhoea**

Disease of the gastrointestinal tract prevents efficient absorption by compromising the transfer of nutrients across the intestinal epithelium. This can be caused by inflammatory processes through infection (gastroenteritis, dysentery and parasitic infestations), immune responses (Crohn's disease, ulcerative colitis, coeliac disease), hereditary digestive enzyme deficiency, presence of defective Na^+/glucose transporter (SGLT1) or through a reduction in surface area after surgical resection.

Clinically, diarrhoea occurs when there is an increase in daily stool weight to more than 300 g, increased fluid content and stool volume, and there is usually an associated increase in frequency of bowel action. Steatorrhoea occurs when there is impaired fat absorption and the stools have a high fat content. Diarrhoea may be:

- Osmotic – when the presence of undigested hypertonic substances draws fluid into the large bowel by osmosis
- Secretory – usually after intestinal resection, in the presence of toxins or laxative use, when fluid and electrolyte absorption is decreased at the same time as an increase in secretion
- Inflammatory – due to damage of the intestinal mucosa through infection or inflammation.

There is increased fluid and electrolyte loss as well as reduced absorption. The fluid and electrolyte loss can lead to severe dehydration and metabolic imbalance. Diarrhoea is one of the leading causes of death among children in developing countries.

Table 15.4   Amino acid transport systems in enterocytes

Site and system	Amino acid transporter	Co-transported ion
Apical membrane		
B	Neutral amino acids, e.g. alanine	Na^+
B°	Neutral and cationic (basic) amino acids, e.g. lysine and also cystine	Na^+
b^{o+}	Neutral and cationic amino acids	None
X_{AG}^-	Anionic (acidic) amino acids, e.g. glutamate, aspartate	$2 Na^+$, $1 H^+$, inward, $1 K^+$ outward
y^+	Cationic (basic) amino acids, e.g. arginine, lysine	None, but will also co-transport small neutral amino acids with Na^+
Imino	Proline and hydroxyproline	Na^+ and Cl^-
β	β amino acids: β-alanine and taurine	Na^+ and Cl^-
Basolateral membrane		
A	Most neutral and imino acids	Na^+
ASC	Neutral amino acids with 3–4 carbons	Na^+
b^{o+}	Neutral and cationic amino acids	None
L	Neutral amino acids with hydrophobic side chain	None
y^+	Cationic (basic) amino acids, e.g. arginine, lysine	None but will also co-transport small neutral amino acids with Na^+

for peptides across the luminal cell membrane. After passing across the basolateral membrane, the absorbed amino acids enter the hepatic portal vein for delivery to the liver.

Di- and tripeptide absorption

Di- and tripeptides are absorbed into the enterocyte by means of a brush border carrier PepT1. The transport of di- and tripeptides is a secondary active transport process. The movement of Na^+ down its concentration gradient, to enter an enterocyte in exchange for a proton moving into the lumen, provides the electrochemical energy for absorbing the peptides (see Fig. 15.3). The PepT1 transporter co-transports H^+ from the lumen and peptides into the cell down an electrochemical gradient for H^+. It is interesting to note that the absorption of β-lactam antibiotics (penicillins) and angiotensin-converting enzyme inhibitors (captopril) is by means of the PepT1 transporter.

Amino acid absorption

There are a number of transport systems (Table 15.4) for L-amino acids in the brush border of enterocytes which require the co-transport of Na^+ to allow the transfer of amino acids against a concentration gradient by means of secondary active transport. Facilitated diffusion of some amino acids also occurs. The presence of carrier systems working in parallel for single amino acids and small peptides in the intestine enhances the overall absorption of amino acids by allowing the uptake of the same amino acid, e.g. glycine in peptide form, as well as free amino acid. Five carrier mechanisms are present in the basolateral borders of enterocytes. Three amino acid carriers not requiring Na^+ to function transport the intracellular amino acids to the extracellular fluid for diffusion into the blood. The Na^+-requiring carriers provide amino acids from the circulation for protein synthesis in crypt cells.

Fat absorption

The process of fat absorption (Fig. 15.4) differs from that of carbohydrate and proteins. Short- and medium-chain-length fatty acids (C8–14) and glycerol are water soluble and diffuse

directly through the luminal and basolateral membranes of the enterocyte to enter the capillaries. The micelles, containing 2-monoacylglycerols and larger free fatty acids (chain length greater than 14 carbon atoms) in their cores, being water soluble, diffuse through the unstirred layer of water at the surface of the enterocyte at a faster rate than can be achieved by fat digestion products alone. The hydrophobic 2-monoglycerides and free fatty acids are delivered by this mechanism to the enterocytes of the jejunum where they are absorbed by diffusion through the lipid portions of the surface of the cell membrane.

The absorbed long-chain fatty acids and 2-monoglycerides bind to a fatty acid binding protein within the enterocyte, thus maintaining the concentration gradient across the cell membrane for these products. The fatty acid binding protein transfers the fatty acids and 2-monoglycerides to the smooth endoplasmic reticulum for the resynthesis of triglyceride by acyl-CoA synthetase and acyltransferase. The triglyceride is coated with lipoprotein, derived from cholesterol, phospholipid and apoprotein B in the rough endoplasmic reticulum to form a chylomicron which is transferred to the Golgi apparatus where the protein coat is glycosylated prior to exocytosis across the basolateral membrane. Chylomicrons (diameter 75–600 nm) are too large to enter capillaries but can diffuse through spaces in the walls of lacteals (lymphatic vessels) in the villi. The lacteals drain into larger lymphatic vessels leading to the thoracic lymphatic duct which, in turn, distributes the lymph to the venous system at the junction of the left subclavian vein and left jugular vein.

Bile salt absorption

The bile salts are ionised at intestinal pH and require a carrier mechanism for their absorption. The sodium-dependent carrier is present in the enterocytes of the terminal ileum. Absorption is by means of secondary active transport similar to that described for glucose or amino acid transport. The absorbed bile salts enter the venous system draining the ileum and are transported to the liver in the enterohepatic circulation. The liver extracts the bile salts and secretes them into the bile. The bile salt pool may recirculate two or three times during a large meal.

Vitamins

Vitamins (A, B, C, D, E and K) are organic compounds that the body is unable to synthesise; therefore, they must be absorbed from the small intestine (see Ch. 16).

Water-soluble vitamins

The water-soluble vitamins (B group and C) are absorbed by passive diffusion and in some cases secondary active transport. Specialised sodium-dependent transport systems exist for thiamine (B_1), niacin, folate and vitamin C in the apical membrane of enterocytes. A facilitated transport system is responsible for the exit of niacin, folate and thiamine across the basolateral border.

Vitamin B_{12}

The absorption of vitamin B_{12} (cobalamin) involves a complex series of events. Vitamin B_{12} in food is bound to proteins. The action of acid and pepsins in the stomach releases the vitamin B_{12}. The free vitamin B_{12} binds to glycoproteins, known as R proteins, that are present in the stomach contents derived from saliva and gastric juice. Another glycoprotein capable of binding vitamin B_{12} is intrinsic factor secreted by parietal cells. The affinity of intrinsic factor for ingested B_{12} is less than that of R proteins; therefore, most of the vitamin B_{12} in the chyme leaving the stomach and entering the intestine is bound to R protein. Once in the intestine the pancreatic proteases digest the R protein and vitamin B_{12} is free once again. It binds to intrinsic factor, which is resistant to digestion by pancreatic proteases. The vitamin B_{12} intrinsic factor complex passes along the small intestine to the terminal ileum where there are receptors in the brush borders of the enterocytes for the vitamin B_{12} intrinsic factor complex. Binding of the vitamin B_{12} intrinsic factor complex to the membrane receptor triggers endocytosis (receptor-mediated endocytosis) of the complex into the cell. Vitamin B_{12} is released from the complex within the cell and exported across the basolateral border and diffuses into the blood where it binds to transcobalamin II, a transport protein. See Information box 15.2.

Fat-soluble vitamins

The fat-soluble vitamins A, D, E and K entering the small intestine are solubilised by diffusion into micelles containing bile salts and fat digestion products (see Ch. 16). Absorption of these vitamins occurs by diffusion across the brush border of the enterocyte together with fatty acids and monoglycerides.

> **Information box 15.2**   **Vitamin B_{12} malabsorption**
>
> Vitamin B_{12} deficiency is caused by the malabsorption of vitamin B_{12}. The commonest cause is **pernicious anaemia**. There is atrophic gastritis leading to a failure in the production of **intrinsic factor**. This is an autoimmune condition, and is associated with other autoimmune diseases, such as thyroid disease and vitiligo. It is sometimes also associated with gastric carcinoma. Intrinsic factor antibodies are present, inhibiting the binding of intrinsic factor to B_{12} in the stomach, and also blocking the vitamin B_{12} intrinsic factor complex to receptors in the terminal ileum, where B_{12} would normally be absorbed. A 3–6-year store of vitamin B_{12} is present in the liver, so that patients with pernicious anaemia may take years to develop symptoms of anaemia. Treatment is by intramuscular injections of vitamin B_{12}. Other causes of vitamin B_{12} malabsorption include coeliac disease, surgical resection of stomach or ileum, and the long term use of drugs such as proton pump inhibitors.

> **Information box 15.3**   **Vitamin D deficiency**
>
> Chronic steatorrhoea could lead to malabsorption of fat-soluble vitamins. Although this could be the cause of vitamin D deficiency (**rickets**, **osteomalacia**), other factors are anticonvulsant therapy and renal failure, which interfere with vitamin D metabolism.

The fat-soluble vitamins are exported to the lymphatic system in chylomicrons. See Information box 15.3.

Absorption of electrolytes and water

Each day about 9 L of fluid enters the alimentary canal. This is derived from the diet (2 L) and the digestive secretions (7 L) (Fig. 15.5). In health about 99% of the water and electrolytes are absorbed into the blood as the fluid passes along the small and large intestine. The major site of fluid absorption is the jejunum and ileum (8.5 L), with a relatively small quantity being absorbed from the colon (0.4 L). The faeces contain about 0.1 L of water. The absorption of water is secondary to the uptake of electrolytes, in particular Na^+ and Cl^-, sugars and amino acids.

Pathways for electrolyte and water absorption

The electrolytes and water may be absorbed by passing between the enterocytes (paracellular route) via aqueous channels, through the tight junctions linking the cells together. The alternative route is by passing through the cells (transcellular route). This may involve both carrier-mediated mechanisms and passage through water-permeable channels (Table 15.5).

Water movement from the lumen of the intestine may occur via membrane proteins including the SGLT1, sodium/glucose co-transporter and channels named aquaporins that allow the passage of water. The unstimulated SGLT1 acts as a water permeable protein channel. When stimulated by the presence of Na^+ and glucose in the intestinal lumen it co-transports water together with Na^+ and glucose into the intestinal mucosal cell. In addition, the absorption of water is secondary to organic and ionic solute movement. The transfer of solutes across the intestinal epithelium creates an osmotic gradient between the lumen and the interstitial fluid and blood. Water is absorbed by osmosis via paracellular and transcellular routes (see Fig. 15.3). The principle of oral rehydration therapy, used to treat diarrhoea, is based on promoting water absorption, either by means of co-transport or by osmosis, following an isotonic drink containing glucose and electrolytes, including sodium chloride.

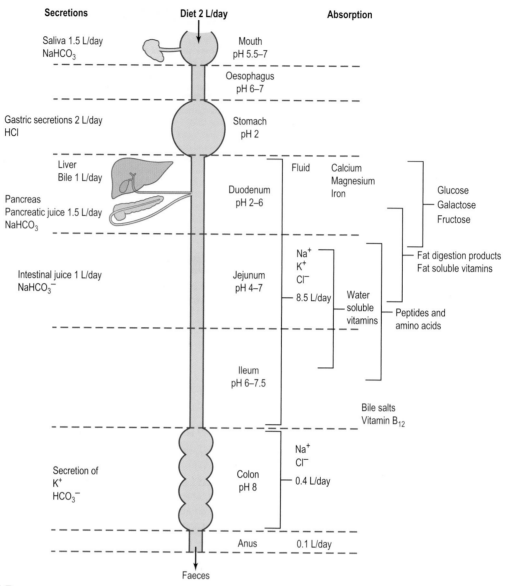

Fig. 15.5 Fluid and electrolyte input into the alimentary canal.

Calcium absorption

Dietary calcium is found in a variety of foods including dairy products. Calcium may exist bound to oxalates, phosphates and phytates or in the ionised form (Ca^{2+}) in the intestine. Ionised calcium is available for absorption by enterocytes in the upper small intestine. The free Ca^{2+} concentration in the cell is low, giving rise to a steep concentration gradient between the lumen and the cytoplasm. Ca^{2+} ions bind to a protein in the brush border and are transported down their concentration gradient into the cell. The free Ca^{2+} concentration in the cytoplasm is kept low by Ca^{2+} binding to calcium-binding proteins that are sequestered in intracellular organelles such as the endoplasmic reticulum. Ca^{2+} ions are exported across the basolateral border of the cell against an electrochemical gradient by active transport. There are two mechanisms:

- Ca^{2+}-ATPase – which uses energy derived from the hydrolysis of ATP to transfer Ca^{2+} out of the cell
- Na^+/Ca^{2+} exchanger – in which Na^+ moving down its electrochemical gradient into the cell drives Ca^{2+} extrusion.

The Ca^{2+}-ATPase mechanism is the more important one.

Calcium absorption is regulated by 1,25-dihydroxychole-calciferol, the active form of vitamin D which stimulates the synthesis of both calcium-binding proteins and Ca^{2+}-ATPase (see Ch. 10). Note: a high dietary phytate content, as in cha-patti flour, may inhibit calcium absorption.

Iron absorption

Dietary iron is present in two forms:

- The haem portion of haemoglobin, myoglobin and cytochromes
- An insoluble, non-absorbable state complexed with phytate, tannins and plant fibres. Insoluble iron salts may also form with hydroxide, phosphate and bicarbonate found in digestive secretions.

The acidic conditions of the stomach mobilise the iron compounds by converting the ions from the ferric (Fe^{3+}) to the ferrous (Fe^{2+}) state. Similarly, vitamin C reduces iron to the ferrous state and also forms soluble complexes with it that enhance absorption. Ferric ions are reduced to ferrous

Table 15.5 Electrolyte transport in the small and large intestine

Intestinal region	Na$^+$	K$^+$	Cl$^-$	HCO$_3^-$
Duodenum and jejunum	Actively absorbed • Co-transport with glucose, galactose, amino acids • Co-transport with Cl$^-$ • Counter transport exchange for H$^+$ • Diffusion through aqueous channels	Passively absorbed by diffusion through paracellular pathways as the luminal concentration rises after water absorption	Passively absorbed • Co-transport with Na$^+$ • Counter transport exchange for HCO$_3^-$ • Diffusion through paracellular channels	Absorbed as CO$_2$ following neutralisation of secreted H$^+$
Ileum	Actively absorbed as above but reduced importance of co-transport with organic solutes	Passively absorbed as above	Passively absorbed • Counter transport exchange for HCO$_3^-$ • Diffusion through paracellular channels	Passively absorbed • Counter transport in exchange for Cl$^-$ • Diffusion
Colon	Actively absorbed • Via Na$^+$ channels • Co-transport with Cl$^-$ Stimulated by aldosterone	Secretion Passive leakage from enterocytes through K$^+$ channels in their apical membranes when luminal concentration <25 mM Stimulated by aldosterone	Passively absorbed • Co-transport with Na$^+$ • Counter transport with HCO$_3^-$ • Diffusion through paracellular channels	Secretion Counter transport exchange with Cl$^-$

ions by duodenal cytochrome b ferric reductase in the brush border of the duodenal enterocyte.

The enterocytes of the duodenum absorb haem and ferrous ions by two separate mechanisms:

1. Haem is absorbed by endocytosis and digested in the enterocyte by haem oxidase to release ferric ions, carbon monoxide and biliverdin. The ferric ions are reduced to ferrous ions that bind to ferroportin 1 in the basolateral membrane for export from the cell.
2. Ferrous ions and a proton bind to a divalent metal transporter to cross the brush border. The movement of a proton down its concentration gradient into the enterocyte is the driving force for ferrous ion absorption. In the cytosol ferrous ions bind either to a storage protein, apoferritin, to form ferritin, or are transferred to ferroportin 1 in the basolateral borders of the cell for export to the tissue fluid.

An additional protein, hephaestin, is considered to have a role in the export of iron from the enterocytes to the plasma. It may be involved in the release of iron from its storage sites and transfer to ferroportin 1 for export to the tissue fluid. Ferrous ions diffuse into the blood and are transported around the body in association with transferrin, a plasma protein.

The absorption of iron needs to be regulated because:

■ There are no active excretory mechanisms
■ This metal plays an essential biological role in oxygen transport and redox reactions in cellular respiration.

In addition, iron is involved in the formation of reactive oxygen species that may be useful in killing bacteria. However, reactive oxygen species are also toxic to cells when large quantities are produced following excessive iron accumulation (see Ch. 16 and Information box 15.4).

Regulation of iron absorption

Iron transport is stimulated either through erythropoiesis following haemorrhage or moving to high altitude and decreased when iron stores are high. The development of the iron absorptive mechanisms in the immature enterocytes of the crypts is controlled by the uptake of transferrin-bound iron from the plasma. In states of iron deficiency the immature enterocyte becomes programmed to increase iron absorption by the upregulation of the divalent metal ion transporter and ferroportin 1 synthesis. An increase in iron accumulation in the body leads to a decrease in the synthesis of the transport systems involved in iron uptake and to the lysosomal degradation of ferroportin 1 initiated by the action of peptide hepcidin following its increased secretion from the liver. The accumulation of iron in the enterocyte stimulates apoferritin synthesis and ferritin formation to protect the body from iron overload. The ferritin is released into the intestinal lumen when the enterocytes are shed from the villus tip.

SURFACE ANATOMY OF THE ABDOMEN

The upper abdomen is bound by the lower rib (costal) margins formed by the seventh to tenth costal cartilages, and joined in the middle at the xiphisternum (Fig. 15.6). The lower abdomen extends to the inguinal ligaments and the pubis. The inguinal ligaments appear convex in thin people. To locate the surface positions of abdominal organs, the anterior surface of the abdomen could roughly be divided into nine regions, or four quadrants. The nine regions are demarcated by two vertical and two horizontal imaginary planes that transect the abdominal cavity.

Information box 15.4 Absorption of oral iron

The ferrous state is more readily absorbed than ferric iron, and oral iron supplement formulations are usually in the ferrous state. Iron absorption increases during pregnancy and iron deficiency anaemia. High dietary content of phosphates and phytate (in chapatti flour) can inhibit iron absorption by forming insoluble complexes.

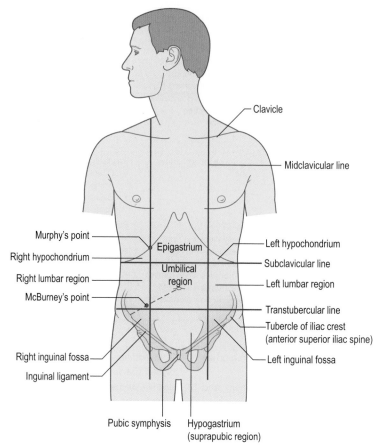

Fig. 15.6 **Surface anatomy of the abdomen.**

ABDOMINAL REGIONS

Abdominal regions are demarcated by four imaginary planes into nine regions. The two vertical planes pass through the midclavicular lines. The upper horizontal plane is marked by the lowest edge of the rib cage, the subcostal line, and the lower horizontal plane passes through the line drawn between the tubercles of the iliac crest: the transtubercular line. In practice, the anterior superior iliac spines (ASIS) are easier to feel than the tubercles, which are palpable a little way behind the ASIS. The plane passing through the ASIS is sometimes substituted for the transtubercular plane. From top to bottom in the midline, the regions are epigastric, umbilical and hypogastric (also known as suprapubic). The lateral regions are left and right hypochondrial, lumbar and inguinal (or iliac fossa).

Two important landmarks are McBurney's point, about one-third of the way on a line drawn from the right ASIS to the umbilicus, marking the base of the appendix where the point of maximal tenderness is felt in classical acute appendicitis. Murphy's point is roughly below the plane where the midclavicular line crosses the lower margin of the rib cage (costal margin) at about the level of the ninth costal cartilage, and is classically where the fundus of the gall bladder may be found. It is also the point of maximum tenderness in acute cholecystitis.

Epigastric region

Typically, pain and tenderness in the epigastrium are referred from the upper abdominal organs, such as the stomach and duodenum. Palpable masses usually arise from the stomach, and the pulsations of the abdominal aorta can also just be felt in thin people.

Umbilical region

Pain from intestinal obstruction, e.g. in acute appendicitis, could be referred to the area around the umbilicus. Pain and tenderness from disease of the transverse colon are also located in the umbilical region. The transverse colon is extremely variable in position, sometimes reaching down to the suprapubic region. Tumours of underlying structures and pulsations from the abdominal aorta are palpable here.

Suprapubic (hypogastric) region

Pain and tenderness from the lower bowel, e.g. descending colon and anal canal, bladder and uterus, and sometimes the fallopian tubes, are referred to this region. Enlargement or tumours of the pelvic organs, e.g. bladder and uterus, are palpable here.

Left and right hypochondrium

The spleen is situated behind the left lower ribs. Splenic tenderness and enlargement are felt in the left hypochondrium, although the spleen has to be enlarged to more than three times its normal size to be palpable. The liver and gall bladder are behind the rib cage on the right. An enlarged or tender liver and gall bladder may be palpated in the right hypochondrium.

Left and right lumbar region

The lumbar regions refer to the 'flanks'. Normally, the kidneys lie deep against the posterior abdominal wall and are not palpable. The lower poles of enlarged kidneys may be felt in the lumbar regions. The right kidney is usually lower than the left. Posteriorly, the angles formed by the ribs and the spine are the renal angles where maximal renal tenderness may be felt when the kidneys are dilated or inflamed. The ascending colon may be palpable in the right lumbar region and the descending colon in the left.

Left and right iliac fossa (inguinal region)

Pain and tenderness in the left iliac fossa could be related to problems with the descending or sigmoid colon, whereas signs in the right iliac fossa signify disease of the appendix, caecum or ascending colon. Deep iliac fossa pain may relate to fallopian tube disease. Masses in either iliac fossa are suspicious of underlying tumours, but sometimes a loaded colon or impacted faeces may be palpable.

The pulsations of the femoral artery are easily felt at the midpoint between the anterior superior iliac spine and the pubic symphysis along the inguinal ligament. A weakness in the inguinal canal can cause some abdominal contents to be forced through this potential weakness in the inguinal region (hernia) when the intra-abdominal pressure is significantly raised, as in coughing and lifting heavy weights.

This manifests as palpable 'bulges' medial to the femoral artery when a patient is asked to cough, particularly when standing.

QUADRANTS

For the purposes of description, the surface of the abdomen is also commonly divided into quadrants – the right and left upper and lower quadrants (the gall bladder and liver being palpable in the right upper quadrant, enlarged spleen in the left upper quadrant). The right lower quadrant is where the signs of disease in the appendix and caecum become evident, and the left lower quadrant is where signs of disease of the sigmoid colon become evident.

MICROANATOMY OF THE GASTROINTESTINAL TRACT

The gastrointestinal tract can be considered as a muscular tube 7–10 m in length, consisting of four major layers (Fig. 15.7). From the lumen these are:

- Mucosa
- Submucosa
- Muscle
- Serosa.

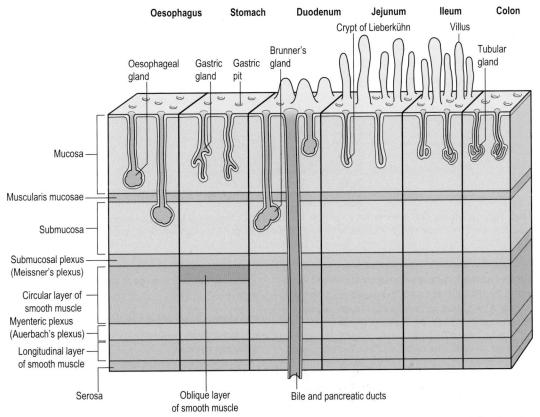

Fig. 15.7 General organisation of the layers of the alimentary canal together with features of specialised regions.

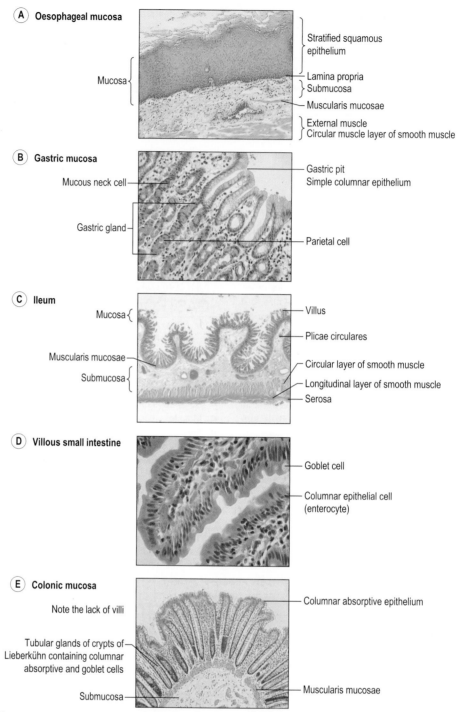

Fig. 15.8 Microanatomy of the alimentary system. Courtesy of Dr Gregory J Michael, Institute of Cell and Molecular Science, Barts and The London School of Medicine and Dentistry, Queen Mary University of London.

There are variations in the general structure related to the functions of the different regions of the gastrointestinal tract. The histological structure of the mucosal layers shows the greatest variation (Fig. 15.8). The **mucosa** consists of:

- A lining layer of **epithelial cells** that have secretory and absorptive functions
- The **lamina propria**, a connective tissue support for the mucosa, together with blood vessels and the glandular ducts in some regions
- The **muscularis mucosae**, a thin layer of smooth muscle cells which moves the epithelium, producing

mixing activity, and leads to folding of the mucosal layer.

The **submucosa** contains connective tissues, blood vessels and lymphatics together with nerves innervating structures within the mucosa.

In most regions of the alimentary canal the external **muscle** consists of two layers of smooth muscle: the inner layer in which the long axis of the muscle fibres is arranged in a circular manner around the canal (**circular muscle**) and an outer layer with the muscle fibres lying along the length of the canal (**longitudinal layer**). Contraction of the circular and longitudinal muscle layers narrows the lumen and shortens the canal, respectively. These muscles are responsible for mixing the food with the digestive secretions and for propelling the contents along the digestive tract. The first third of the oesophagus and the anal sphincter contain skeletal muscle.

The **serosa** is the outermost layer of the alimentary canal and is continuous with the parietal peritoneum lining the inner surface of the body wall. It consists of connective tissues covered with a squamous epithelium.

INNERVATION OF THE ALIMENTARY CANAL

Sensory and motor neurons are found within the wall of the alimentary canal. Major aggregations of neurons are found in:

- The **submucosal plexus** or **Meissner's plexus** on the outer edge of the submucosa adjacent to the circular muscle layer
- The **myenteric plexus** or **Auerbach's plexus** lying between the circular and longitudinal muscle layers.

The plexi are innervated by sensory neurons from the mucosa and muscle layers, and by preganglionic parasympathetic nerves and postganglionic sympathetic nerves from the central nervous system. The nerves, with their cell bodies within the alimentary canal, form the enteric nervous system.

The function of nerves within the alimentary canal is to co-ordinate muscular, secretory and absorptive activity in order that the digestive tract functions as a coordinated unit. Many functions of the alimentary canal continue to be coordinated following the cutting of the parasympathetic and sympathetic nerves innervating the canal. For this reason it may be said that the nerves within the alimentary canal constitute 'a little brain'. The central nervous system (or 'large brain') modifies the action of the enteric nervous system via the parasympathetic and sympathetic branches of the autonomic nervous system.

Table 15.6 shows the hormones and neuropeptides secreted by the alimentary system. Some gastrointestinal hormones and neuropeptides also act centrally on the hypothalamus to control appetite, hunger and satiety (see also Chs 8 and 16).

Table 15.6	**Gastrointestinal hormones and neuropeptides, their source, target organ and action**		
Hormone/neuropeptide	**Source**	**Target organ**	**Action**
Cholecystokinin	I cells in duodenum and jejunum and neurons in ileum and colon	Pancreas Gall bladder	↑ Enzyme secretion ↑ Contraction
Calcitonin gene-related peptide	Enteric neurons Splanchnic afferent nerves	Blood vessels Neurons	↑ Vasodilatation Sensory neurotransmitter
Enkephalins	Enteric neurons	Gastrointestinal smooth muscle Intestinal mucosa	↑ Contraction ↓ Fluid secretion
Enteroglucagon Glucagon-like peptide 1	L cells in the ileum, colon and rectum	Pancreas Stomach	↑ Insulin release ↓ Acid secretion ↓ Gastric emptying
Epidermal growth factors	Salivary and Brunner's glands	Gastrointestinal mucosa	↑ Growth and mucosal protection
Gastric-inhibitory peptide or glucose-dependent insulinotropic peptide	K cells in duodenum and jejunum	Pancreas Stomach	↑ Insulin release ↓ Acid secretion
Gastrin	G cells, antrum of stomach	Parietal cells in body of stomach Enterochromaffin-like cells Gastrointestinal mucosa	↑ Acid secretion ↑ Histamine secretion ↑ Growth
Gastrin-releasing peptide	Enteric neurons	G cells in antrum of stomach	Gastrin release
Ghrelin	Gr or X/A cells in the stomach adjacent to parietal cells	Anterior pituitary Hypothalamus Stomach	↑ Growth hormone release ↑ Feeding ↑ Acid secretion ↑ Motility and gastric emptying
Guanylin	Endocrine cells in ileum and colon	Small and large intestine	↑ Fluid secretion
Motilin	Endocrine cells in upper gastrointestinal tract	Oesophageal sphincter Stomach Duodenum	↑ Smooth muscle contraction migrating myoelectric complex
Neurotensin	N cells, throughout gastrointestinal tract	Gastrointestinal smooth muscle Gastrointestinal mucosa Stomach	Relaxation of LOS ↓ Antral motility ↑ Growth ↓ Acid secretion
Pancreatic polypeptide	Endocrine cells in ileum	Pancreas	↓ Enzyme and fluid secretion
Peptide YY	Endocrine cells in ileum and colon	Stomach Pancreas	↓ Vagally mediated acid secretion ↓ Enzyme and fluid secretion
Pituitary adenylate cyclase-activating peptide (PACAP)	Enteric neurons	Intestinal smooth muscle	Relaxation

Continued

Table 15.6 Gastrointestinal hormones and neuropeptides, their source, target organ and action—cont'd

Hormone/neuropeptide	Source	Target organ	Action
Secretin	S cells in small intestine	Pancreas	↑ HCO$_3^-$ and fluid secretion by pancreatic ducts
		Stomach	↓ Gastric acid secretion
Somatostatin	D cells of stomach and duodenum, δ cells of pancreatic islets	Stomach Intestine	↓ Gastrin release ↑ Fluid absorption ↓ Secretion ↑ Smooth muscle contraction
		Pancreas Liver	↓ Endocrine/exocrine secretions ↓ Bile flow
Tachykinins: substance P; neurokinin A	Sensorimotor neurons; enteric neurons	Longitudinal and circular layer smooth muscle	↑ Contraction
		Enteric nervous system	Stimulation of inhibitory and excitatory pathways
		Blood vessels	↑ Vasodilatation
		Small and large intestinal mucosa	↑ Fluid secretion
Vasoactive intestinal peptide	Enteric neurons	Gastrointestinal smooth muscle	↑ Relaxation
		Small intestinal mucosa	↑ Fluid secretion
	Pancreatic neurons	Pancreas	↑ HCO$_3^-$ and fluid secretion by pancreatic ducts

↑ increase; ↓ decrease; LOS, lower oesophageal sphincter.

MOUTH

The mouth or oral cavity consists of the lips, tongue, teeth, gums and hard and soft palate. Stratified squamous epithelial cells, kept moist by saliva, cover the surface of the oral cavity and tongue. Sensory nerves sensitive to pain, touch and temperature are present in the lining of the mouth together with taste buds in the dorsal surface of the tongue (see Ch. 8). The temperature and taste of ingested food and drink is sampled by the sensory receptors before chewing or drinking begins.

TEETH

In adults there are 32 permanent teeth that have different functions.

- Incisors – chisel shaped teeth for cutting and biting
- Canines – puncture and hold food
- Molars – grind and crush food.

The adult teeth are preceded by 20 deciduous or milk teeth. The deciduous teeth begin to appear at 6 months, the set is complete at 6–8 years and is replaced by permanent teeth at 10–12 years.

TONGUE

The anterior two-thirds of the tongue are composed of skeletal muscle fibres, covered by a layer containing seromucous glands and stratified epithelium. The secretions of these glands together with saliva ensure the tongue is moist to facilitate movement during chewing and swallowing food.

MASTICATION

The mastication, or chewing, process physically breaks food into smaller pieces. This voluntary and reflex behaviour serves to:

- Dissolve chemicals in saliva so that they can stimulate the taste buds
- Lubricate the food to ease swallowing
- Mix starch-containing food with salivary α-amylase
- Increase the surface area of food to facilitate digestion in the stomach and duodenum.

The absence of teeth and neuromuscular defects in the elderly after strokes can severely interfere with mastication.

SALIVARY GLANDS

Saliva is an exocrine secretion which enters the mouth from salivary glands by a duct system. There are two types of salivary secretion produced by different cells:

- Serous cells produce a watery secretion
- Mucous cells produce a thick mucus-rich secretion.

In human beings there are three pairs of salivary glands: parotid, submandibular and sublingual (Fig. 15.9). The glands vary in the type of saliva they produce.

The **parotid glands** lie in the cheeks anterior to the ear with their excretory ducts opening into the mouth opposite the second upper molar teeth. They are serous glands producing a watery secretion rich in amylase. These are the largest glands but they produce only 25% of the daily saliva.

The **submandibular glands** lie under the mandible with their excretory ducts entering the mouth under the tip of the tongue behind the central incisor teeth. They secrete 70% of the daily saliva production. These are mixed glands that contain serous and mucous cells, producing a more viscous secretion than the parotid glands.

The **sublingual glands** lie in the floor of the mouth just posterior to the mandible and have many small

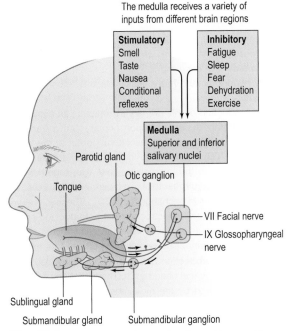

The medulla receives a variety of inputs from different brain regions

Stimulatory
Smell
Taste
Nausea
Conditional reflexes

Inhibitory
Fatigue
Sleep
Fear
Dehydration
Exercise

Medulla
Superior and inferior salivary nuclei

Parotid gland
Otic ganglion
Tongue
VII Facial nerve
IX Glossopharyngeal nerve
Sublingual gland
Submandibular gland
Submandibular ganglion

Fig. 15.9 Position of salivary glands and innervation.

Clinical box 15.5 Some clinical conditions of the salivary glands

Disease of the salivary glands may lead to impaired secretion of saliva, giving rise to **xerostomia** (dry mouth). This interferes with both chemical and physical digestion of food, and also increases the risk of oral infections and ulceration.

- Mumps is a common childhood infection of the salivary glands, characterised by pain and swelling, which temporarily affects salivation.
- Salivary duct calculi (stones) obstruct the flow of saliva and may cause pain and swelling of the gland.
- Salivary gland tumours are usually benign but may be malignant.
- Drugs with anticholinergic action inhibit saliva secretion.
- Sjögren's syndrome is an autoimmune condition in which saliva-secreting cells are destroyed. There may be associated parotid gland enlargement, with ensuing dry mouth. Dry eyes, skin and vagina are also clinical features. This condition can occur in association with other systemic autoimmune diseases (e.g. rheumatoid arthritis, thyroid disease). Difficulty with swallowing because of the lack of lubrication and mouth ulcers and oral infections may be a manifestation of systemic disease (see above).
- 'Water brash' is a symptom in which there is a sudden inflow of saliva into the mouth, but without the stimulation of food. This is sometimes associated with peptic ulceration and inflammatory bowel disease.

ducts opening into the mouth, some of them entering the submandibular duct. The cells of the sublingual glands are predominantly mucous cells; therefore, the secretion is thick and viscous due to the presence of mucus. These glands produce 5% of the total daily output. In addition, there are smaller salivary glands scattered over the tongue, buccal cavity and on the inner side of the lips. See Clinical box 15.5.

FUNCTIONS OF SALIVA

Saliva has three functions. These are:

- Lubrication
- Protection
- Digestion.

Lubrication

The water and mucus in saliva act as lubricants that aid the movement of the tongue to facilitate speech and swallowing of food. You may have noticed that it is difficult to talk when your mouth is dry. Swallowing a number of dry biscuits is also difficult unless they are accompanied by a drink.

Protection

The presence of food debris in the warm and wet environment of the mouth provides ideal conditions for bacterial growth and division. The mouth is protected from metabolic acids produced by bacteria by the buffering action of bicarbonate, phosphate and mucus in saliva. The saliva is saturated with calcium salts at neutral pH, so that the calcium in the teeth does not dissolve. However, calcium from the teeth will dissolve and the formation of dental caries will occur if the pH falls to 5.5, once saliva flow has been reduced after a meal. The presence of protein in saliva forms a protective coat on the teeth surface to reduce the adherence of bacteria

and to act as a barrier to acid. In addition, bacterial growth is limited by:

- Lysozyme, an enzyme responsible for breaking down bacterial cell walls
- Lactoferrin, an iron-chelating agent that binds iron to prevent its use by some bacteria requiring iron for growth
- Secretory immunoglobulin A, derived from plasma cells, which provides immunity against bacteria and viruses.

Large volumes of alkaline saliva are produced before vomiting. The alkali neutralises the gastric acid and inactivates the enzyme pepsin when it enters the oesophagus and mouth during vomiting.

Digestion

The digestive function of saliva is to dissolve food so that the chemical constituents can stimulate the taste buds, and to begin chemical digestion of carbohydrate and fat. Saliva contains an α-amylase or ptyalin which starts the digestion of starch by hydrolysing α-1,4 glycosidic bonds to produce maltose, maltotriose and oligosaccharides known as α-limit dextrans (see Fig. 15.3). Salivary amylase is active over the pH range 4–11 and has an optimum pH 7. Chewing mixes the saliva with food. The amylase present inside a bolus of swallowed food continues its activity in the stomach until the acid in the gastric secretions penetrates the bolus. Up to 75% of starch digestion may occur in the stomach before amylase is destroyed by gastric acid.

Salivary glands present on the tongue secrete a lingual lipase that digests fat. This enzyme is also active in the stomach and intestine.

COMPOSITION OF SALIVA

Saliva consists of water (99%) and dissolved chemicals (1%). In humans, it is less concentrated (hypotonic) than the plasma. The solid materials include organic and inorganic constituents.

Organic constituents

These consist of:

- Amylase (ptyalin)
- Lipase
- Kallikrein
- Lysozyme
- Mucus
- Immunoglobulin A
- Lactoferrin
- Blood group antigens, e.g. A and B.

Inorganic constituents

These are electrolytes, mainly Na^+, K^+, Ca^{2+}, Cl^-, I^-, PO_4^{2-} and HCO_3^-. The majority of electrolytes are found in lower concentrations than in the plasma. The exceptions are K^+ and HCO_3^-, which are found in higher contractions. The electrolyte composition and pH of saliva varies with flow rate. The increase in HCO_3^- concentration as flow rate increases accounts for the pH changing from being slightly acidic (pH 5.5–6.1) at resting flow rates to alkaline (pH 7.8) at high flow rates. The K^+ concentration is highest at the lowest flow rate.

SECRETORY MECHANISMS

The total production of saliva per day is 0.75 L to 1 L. The salivary glands produce large quantities of secretion per day relative to their size. The secretion of saliva is an active process requiring energy derived from cellular metabolism that in turn depends on a good blood supply.

The salivon

The functional unit of a salivary gland is termed a **salivon** (Fig. 15.10A). It consists of an acinus, an intercalated duct and a striated duct. The acinus is composed of pyramidal shaped acinar cells containing secretory granules. The acini are surrounded by contractile myoepithelial cells. The intercalated duct consists of cuboidal epithelial cells that may also be attached to myoepithelial cells. Columnar cells containing many mitochondria line the striated ducts. All the above components lie within a lobule surrounded by connective tissue. Striated ducts from adjacent lobules join together to form interlobular ducts and excretory ducts.

Mechanisms of secretion of saliva

Animal studies have demonstrated that saliva production can take place when the pressure in the duct system is greater than the arterial blood pressure in the arteries supplying the salivary gland. This observation indicates that the process of salivation is not due to the hydrostatic pressure of the blood producing an ultrafiltrate of plasma into the salivary glands and so is different from the production of urine (see Ch. 14). Furthermore, the composition of saliva varies with salivary flow rate. The secretion of saliva is believed to be a two-stage process.

Stage one – the primary secretion

The acinar and intercalated duct cells produce a primary fluid secretion containing amylase and electrolytes. Water moves by osmosis into the lumen of the acini and striated ducts. Experimental evidence indicates that it is either isotonic or slightly hypertonic and has a similar electrolyte composition to plasma.

The production of this primary secretion is an active one that is ultimately dependent upon primary active transport by the Na^+/K^+-ATPase in the basolateral border of the acinar cells (Fig. 15.10B) creating a Na^+ concentration gradient from the extracellular to the intracellular fluid. Na^+, together with Cl^- to maintain electroneutrality, diffuses into the cells. Cl^- also enters the cell in exchange for HCO_3^-. These ion movements increase the Cl^- electrochemical potential and create a diffusion gradient for Cl^- to leave the cell via channels in the apical membrane. The secretion of Cl^- by this mechanism drives the production of saliva. HCO_3^- may also leave the cell via the channel used by Cl^-. The secretion of Cl^- and HCO_3^- is facilitated by the movement of K^+ out of the cell through Ca^{2+}-activated K^+ channels, thus making the interior more electronegative.

K^+ and Na^+ diffuse into the duct system to maintain electroneutrality. K^+ enters the secretion via a channel in the luminal membrane. Na^+ moves through the junctions between the cells to enter the saliva. Water follows the ions and organic constituents of saliva by osmosis via aquaporin 5 water channels in the apical membrane and the paracellular route between cells.

Stage two – modification of the primary secretion

The striated, intercalated and excretory ducts modify the primary secretion by removing Na^+ and Cl^- and adding K^+ and HCO_3^-. This process is dependent upon the action of Na^+/K^+-ATPase in the basolateral border of the duct cells. As in the acinar cells, this primary active transport mechanism creates the conditions for the secondary transport systems to function. The Na^+/K^+-ATPase lowers the cellular concentration of Na^+ so that an electrochemical gradient exists between the lumen of the duct and the intracellular fluid for the diffusion of Na^+ into the cells through epithelial sodium channels, ENaC, in the apical membrane. Additionally, Na^+ may be exchanged for H^+ at this membrane. Cl^- is exchanged for HCO_3^- at the apical membrane. The action of this exchanger is controlled by the chloride channel known as cystic fibrosis transmembrane conductance regulator. The result of these ion movements is that NaCl is absorbed. The Na^+ is pumped out of the cell across the basolateral border by the Na^+/K^+-ATPase and the Cl^- leaves via a chloride channel. The removal of H^+ by Na^+/H^+ exchange in the basolateral membrane increases the intracellular pH and enhances the exchange of HCO_3^- for Cl^-. Cellular K^+ is secreted into the lumen via a K channel. In summary, the overall result is that Na^+ and Cl^- are removed and K^+ and HCO_3^- are added to saliva.

The duct cells are relatively impermeable to water. As saliva flows along the duct system more ions are removed than are added and it becomes hypotonic. The final composition of saliva depends upon the flow rate and, as a consequence, on the time that exchanges may take place across the duct cells. At low flow rates there is more time for Na^+,

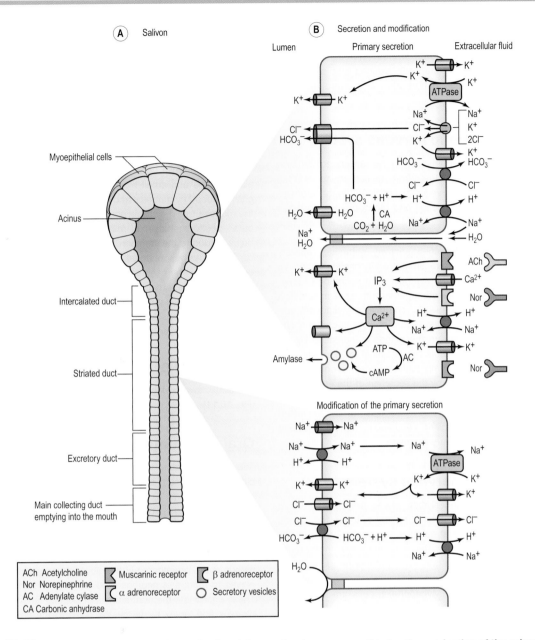

A Salivon

B Secretion and modification

Lumen Primary secretion Extracellular fluid

Myoepithelial cells

Acinus

Intercalated duct

Striated duct

Excretory duct

Main collecting duct
emptying into the mouth

Modification of the primary secretion

ACh Acetylcholine	Muscarinic receptor	β adrenoreceptor
Nor Norepinephrine	α adrenoreceptor	Secretory vesicles
AC Adenylate cylase		
CA Carbonic anhydrase		

Fig. 15.10 **General structure of a salivary gland and the mechanisms responsible for the production of the primary secretion and its modification.** (A) Salivon. (B) Secretion and modification.

Cl^- re-absorption and K^+ secretion. As the flow rate increases there is less time for ionic exchanges to take place, therefore the Na^+ and Cl^- content of saliva rises and the K^+ content falls. The HCO_3^- concentration of saliva increases with an increase in flow rate due to the action of stimulants of secretion on the acinar cells.

Secretion of organic constituents

Organic constituents of saliva such as amylase and mucus are secreted from zymogen and mucus-filled secretory granules found in the apical border of serous and mucous acini, respectively. Following stimulation of the cells, these granules fuse with the apical membrane, and their contents are secreted by exocytosis. Plasma proteins found in saliva, e.g. Immunoglobulin A, enter acinar cells across the basolateral

membrane by endocytosis and are transferred in a vesicle across the cell for export to the saliva by exocytosis.

CONTROL OF SALIVARY SECRETION

The salivary glands are primarily controlled by the autonomic nervous system (see Ch. 4). This is in contrast to the control of gastrointestinal, pancreatic and biliary secretions, which are controlled by gastrointestinal hormones and the autonomic nervous system. Both the parasympathetic and sympathetic divisions of the autonomic nervous system stimulate secretion, but the parasympathetic division is relatively more important.

The smell, taste and chewing of food, in addition to conditioned reflexes associated with the preparation and presentation of food, lead to increased salivary secretion via stimulation of the medullary salivary nuclei. The sight and thought of food might make you aware of the presence of saliva in the mouth without increasing its flow (as could reading this chapter!). Nausea also stimulates salivation. Sleep, fear, dehydration and exercise inhibit secretion.

Parasympathetic nervous system

The parasympathetic innervation of the salivary acinar cells, ducts and blood vessels arises from the salivary nuclei in the medulla via the facial nerve (cranial nerve VII) to the submandibular and sublingual glands and glossopharyngeal nerve (cranial nerve IX) to the parotid glands, respectively (see Fig. 15.9).

Increased parasympathetic activity stimulates salivary secretion, via the neurotransmitter acetylcholine acting on muscarinic receptors. The synthesis and secretion of amylase and mucus is increased, together with a rise in fluid flow and metabolism of the glands. The myoepithelial cells surrounding the acini and intercalated duct cells contract and expel saliva. Blood flow to the glands is increased by the vasodilator action of vasoactive intestinal polypeptide (VIP) released from the parasympathetic nerves in blood vessels. This action is reinforced by the secretion of the enzyme kallikrein from duct cells, which releases a vasodilator peptide (bradykinin) from α_2-globulins in the plasma. The increased blood supply meets the gland's demand for more oxygen and nutrients to sustain salivary secretion.

Sympathetic nervous system

Sympathetic nerve innervation arises from the thoracic segments 1–3 of the spinal cord and reaches the glands via the superior cervical ganglion. Sympathetic nerve action, via the neurotransmitter norepinephrine (noradrenaline) and the circulating hormone epinephrine (adrenaline), stimulates amylase, K^+ and HCO_3^- secretion via their action on adrenoceptors. Myoepithelial cells are stimulated to contract and expel preformed saliva. Blood vessels are constricted. The vasoconstriction restricts blood flow and salivary secretion.

Intracellular messengers producing salivary secretion

The neurotransmitters acetylcholine and norepinephrine act via their respective receptors to change the concentrations of intracellular second messengers (see Fig. 15.10B), which in turn influence the enzymes and channels involved in the secretory process. Acetylcholine acting via muscarinic receptors increases the free Ca^{2+} concentration within the cells via the production of inositol trisphosphate (IP_3), which releases Ca^{2+} from intracellular stores, and by the direct influx of Ca^{2+} from the extracellular fluid. Norepinephrine acts via α- and β-adrenoceptors. Stimulation of α-adrenoceptors increases the concentration of free Ca^{2+}. β-Adrenoceptor stimulation activates adenylate cyclase with the formation of cyclic adenosine monophosphate (cAMP). Rises in intracellular Ca^{2+} have a major effect in increasing the fluid secretion, while cAMP influences enzyme and mucus synthesis and secretion by exocytosis of secretory vesicles.

PHARYNX AND OESOPHAGUS

The oral cavity gives rise to the pharynx, which continues as the oesophagus and conveys food, drink and saliva to the stomach. The oesophageal mucosa is lined with stratified squamous epithelium. The mucosa and submucosa consists of longitudinal folds, in the absence of a swallowed food bolus. The muscularis mucosae is absent from the upper oesophagus but is developed near the stomach.

The submucosa consists of a network of collagen, and elastic fibres and small blood vessels. A thin layer of mucus produced by mucosal and submucosal glands lubricates the mucosa to aid swallowing. An inner circular layer and an outer longitudinal layer of muscle produce propulsion of a bolus of food to the stomach.

The upper oesophageal sphincter and upper third of the oesophagus in humans consists of skeletal muscle, with the lower third being smooth muscle. The middle third consists of a mixture of skeletal and smooth muscles. Both the skeletal and smooth muscles are arranged in an outer longitudinal and an inner circular layer.

SWALLOWING

The act of swallowing (deglutition) consists of three phases (Fig. 15.11).

Oral or voluntary phase

The process begins with a voluntary action initiated by the closing of the mouth and moving the tip of the tongue to the hard palate in order to separate the bolus of food to be swallowed (Fig. 15.11A). The back of the tongue moves up towards the hard palate and this action pushes the food into the pharynx where mechanoreceptors are stimulated to start the swallowing reflex. Sensory nerve impulses from the mechanoreceptors are propagated in the glossopharyngeal and vagal nerves to groups of neurons lying in the pons and medulla. These coordinate the contractions of skeletal muscles in the pharynx and larynx to deliver the bolus to the oesophagus without it entering the airways. The motor nerve pathways are present in cranial nerves VII, IX, X and XII (see Ch. 8).

Pharyngeal phase

The soft palate moves upwards and constriction of the posterior wall of the pharyngeal wall occurs to separate the oropharynx from the nasopharynx (Fig. 15.11B). In order to prevent food reflux into the nasal passages and lungs:

- Ventilation is inhibited
- Contraction of the laryngeal muscles closes the glottis and raises the larynx to create a funnel-like structure to direct the bolus into the oesophagus
- A sequence of peristaltic contractions starting in the upper pharynx propels the bolus of food through the pharynx towards the oesophagus and pushes the epiglottis over the glottis to prevent food entering the trachea
- The bolus passes into the oesophagus through the relaxed upper oesophageal sphincter (Fig. 15.11C).

The mechanisms described above protect against choking during swallowing. Either damage or depression of the

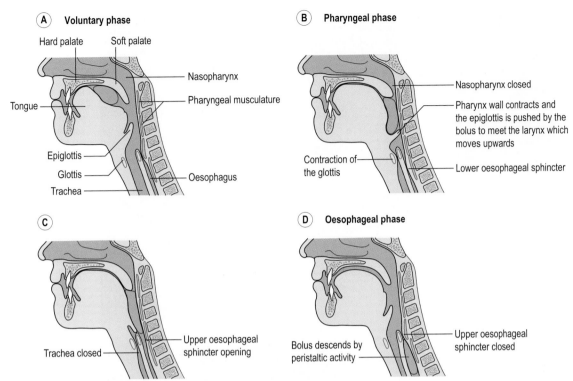

A Voluntary phase

Hard palate   Soft palate

Tongue

Nasopharynx

Pharyngeal musculature

Epiglottis
Glottis
Trachea

Oesophagus

B Pharyngeal phase

Nasopharynx closed

Pharynx wall contracts and
the epiglottis is pushed by the
bolus to meet the larynx which
moves upwards

Contraction of
the glottis

Lower oesophageal sphincter

C

Trachea closed

Upper oesophageal
sphincter opening

D Oesophageal phase

Bolus descends by
peristaltic activity

Upper oesophageal
sphincter closed

Fig. 15.11 **The major phases of the swallowing reflex.** (A) Voluntary phase. (B, C) Pharyngeal phase. (D) Oesophageal phase.

neural control mechanism after a stroke or by alcohol or general anaesthetics can lead to the entry of food or vomit into the airways.

Oesophageal phase

The upper oesophageal sphincter contracts once a bolus of food has passed. A peristaltic wave is initiated in the skeletal muscle just below the upper oesophageal sphincter (Fig. 15.11D). This is known as the primary peristaltic wave and its production is coordinated by the 'swallowing centre', a group of neurons distributed in the pons and medulla, via vagal nerve pathways. The circular muscle layer contracts and raises the pressure on the oral side of the bolus and pushes it into an area of low pressure. The longitudinal muscle contraction pulls the oesophagus over the bolus of food. The active muscles relax. This sequence of events is repeated in a distal direction and the wave of contraction travels in the direction of the stomach.

The terminal 1–2 cm of the circular smooth muscle of the oesophagus has a high degree of tension and acts as the lower oesophageal sphincter to prevent gastro-oesophageal reflux. As the bolus of food approaches the lower oesophageal sphincter it relaxes due to action along the vagal nerve pathway, which contains postganglionic neurons utilising vasoactive intestinal polypeptide and/or nitric oxide as a neurotransmitter(s). The peristaltic wave moves down the oesophagus at 2–5 cm/second and takes about 10 seconds to reach the lower oesophageal sphincter. If some of the bolus of food remains in the oesophagus it stimulates sensory nerves that in turn induce another peristaltic wave at the point of distension (see Fig. 15.12). A secondary peristaltic wave need not be preceded by the oral or pharyngeal phases of swallowing. It may also be induced by the reflux of the gastric contents into the oesophagus. Secondary peristalsis involves neural pathways within the wall of the oesophagus (see Clinical box 15.6).

STOMACH AND DUODENUM

The stomach is a hollow organ consisting of smooth muscle lined with a secretory mucosa that produces exocrine, endocrine and paracrine secretions (Table 15.7). It receives and stores food temporarily and contributes to digestion by mixing food with gastric secretions to form a semi-liquid material called **chyme**. Chyme is emptied into the duodenum at a controlled rate, in order to allow time for further digestion and absorption of digestion products in the small intestine. In addition, the stomach reduces the entry of bacteria and noxious chemicals into the small intestine.

ANATOMY OF THE STOMACH

Anatomically, the stomach (Fig. 15.13) is divided into five regions:

- Cardia
- Fundus
- Corpus (body)
- Pyloric antrum or antrum
- Pylorus.

The cardia lies adjacent to the lower oesophageal sphincter, which guards the entrance to the stomach. The fundus is the upper portion of the stomach, which together with the corpus or body, acts as a reservoir for food and swallowed air. The corpus is the site of secretion of hydrochloric acid, intrinsic factor and pepsinogen by specialised cells in the mucosal lining. The pyloric antrum is the region of the

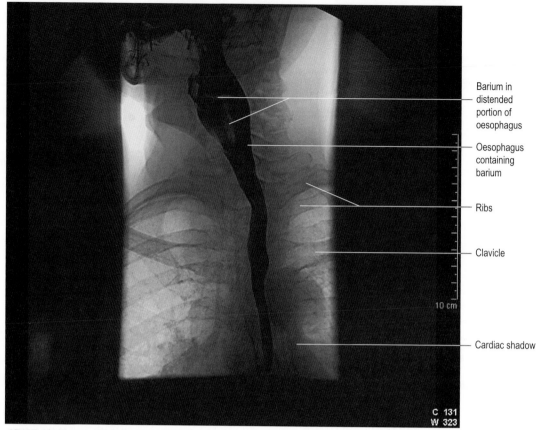

Barium in distended portion of oesophagus

Oesophagus containing barium

Ribs

Clavicle

10 cm

Cardiac shadow

C 131
W 323

Fig. 15.12 **Barium swallow.** The radio-opaque barium outlines a peristaltic wave in the oesophagus. Courtesy of the Radiology Department, Guy's and St Thomas' NHS Foundation Trust.

Clinical box 15.6 | **Clinical conditions associated with oesophageal disorders**

Oesophageal disorders manifest as symptoms experienced by the patient. These are commonly:

- Dysphagia: discomfort experienced as obstruction when swallowing solids or fluids
- Odynophagia: pain when swallowing
- Heartburn: retrosternal pain experienced as a burning sensation that may spread to the neck and across the chest, often worse in the supine position or bending over
- Reflux: when food or liquid regurgitates into the mouth without any rise in intra-abdominal pressure (as in vomiting).

Examples of oesophageal disorders causing symptoms include:

- Mucosal disorders, which may be:
  - Infective, such as candidiasis (thrush) of the mouth and tongue or the oesophagus, or tonsillitis
  - Inflammatory, as in GORD (see Clinical box 15.7) which may lead to ulceration and strictures.
- Motility disorders, which may be:
  - Neuromuscular, as in bulbar palsy, following strokes, myasthenia gravis
  - Achalasia of the cardia, where there is disturbance of the innervation of the smooth muscle and lower sphincter of the oesophagus due to inflammation of the myenteric plexus. Achalasia has an uncertain aetiology, but may be auto-immune, neurodegenerative or infective. The condition is characterised by dysphagia, regurgitation of food and drink and retrosternal pain. Food and liquids are retained in the oesophagus and may overflow into the lungs, leading to pneumonia.
- Oesophageal lesions such as strictures, pharyngeal pouch, malignant tumours, foreign bodies
- Pressure from thoracic structures such as mediastinal glands, cardiomegaly.

Table 15.7 | **Stomach secretions**

Type of secretion	Constituents
Exocrine	Hydrochloric acid
	Electrolytes including Na^+ and K^+
	Intrinsic factor
	Pepsinogen
Endocrine	Gastrin
	Ghrelin
Paracrine	Histamine
	Somatostatin

stomach adjacent to the duodenum and is involved in grinding solid food and mixing it with the gastric secretions. Small quantities of liquefied chyme are propelled into the duodenum through the pyloric sphincter.

Gastric and duodenal musculature

The gastric musculature consists of smooth muscle arranged in distinctive layers. As in other parts of the alimentary canal (see Figs 15.7 and 15.13B) there is an outer longitudinal layer and an inner circular layer which increases in thickness in the antrum and pylorus. Additionally, the fundus and corpus contain a specialised obliquely arranged layer of smooth muscle below the circular layer. The mucosal lining contains a thin layer of muscle, the muscularis mucosae.

The duodenal musculature consists of an outer longitudinal layer, continuous with that of the stomach, and an inner circular layer. A bundle of connective tissue separates the circular muscle layer of the pylorus from that of the duodenum.

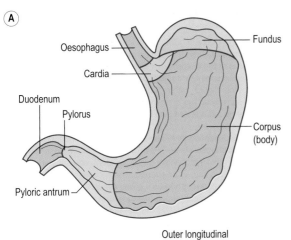

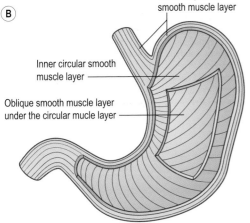

Fig. 15.13 **Anatomy of the stomach.** (A) Anatomical regions of the stomach. (B) Gastric musculature.

The gastric mucosa

The gastric mucosa is a relatively thick mucous membrane, which is smooth when the stomach is distended but thrown into folds or **rugae** when the stomach is empty. The luminal surface of the mucosa contains gastric pits from which branch tubular shaped glands reaching deeper into the mucosa towards the muscularis mucosae. There are three types of gastric gland:

- Cardiac
- Parietal (or oxyntic)
- Pyloric.

The glandular types, their sites, cell types, their secretion and functions are shown in Table 15.8. The surface layer of all regions of the mucosa contains columnar epithelial cells with nuclei in the basal region. These cells secrete mucus, sodium, potassium and bicarbonate ions. These secretions provide lubrication and act to protect the mucosa from digestion by acid and pepsin. The mucosa of the fundus and body regions contains the oxyntic glands (Fig. 15.14), which are divided into three regions:

- Base
- Neck
- Isthmus.

The base region contains predominantly peptic (or chief) cells. These cuboidal-shaped cells have well-developed rough endoplasmic reticulum and a Golgi complex typical of cells synthesising protein. These cells are the source of pepsinogen, the precursor of the protease pepsin. This region contains few parietal cells.

The neck region contains parietal (or oxyntic) cells and mucous neck cells. The parietal cells are large rounded cells with a large nucleus and cytoplasm containing many mitochondria and tubulo-vesicles. The presence of many mitochondria are typical of cells needing to provide energy for transport processes, in this case the secretion of hydrochloric acid. The cytoplasm also contains intracellular canaliculi (channels) which open into the lumen of the gland. These canaliculi swell in conditions producing acid secretion. This suggests they are the conduits for the secreted acid to reach the lumen of the gland. The parietal cells also synthesise and secrete a glycoprotein named intrinsic factor, which binds to vitamin B_{12} in the diet to form a vitamin B_{12}–intrinsic factor complex that is absorbed in the terminal ileum.

Table 15.8	Gastric glands, their cell types, exocrine, endocrine and paracrine secretions and functions			
Gland	**Site**	**Cell type**	**Secretion**	**Function**
Cardiac	Adjacent to the lower oesophageal sphincter	Mucous	Mucus	Lubrication
				Protection
Oxyntic	Fundus and corpus	Parietal (or oxyntic)	HCl	Digestion
				Antibacterial
				Activate pepsinogen to pepsin
			Intrinsic factor	Promotes vitamin B_{12} absorption in the ileum
		Peptic (or chief) cell	Pepsinogen	Pepsin – protein digestion
		D cell	Somatostatin	Inhibition of histamine release and acid secretion
		Gr or X/A	Ghrelin	Stimulation of feeding, gastric motility, acid secretion and growth hormone release
Pyloric	Pylorus and antrum	Peptic (or chief) cell	Pepsinogen	Pepsin – protein digestion
		Mucous	Mucus	Lubrication
				Protection
		G cell	Gastrin	Stimulation of gastric acid secretion
		D cell	Somatostatin	Inhibition of gastrin secretion

Region   Cell type

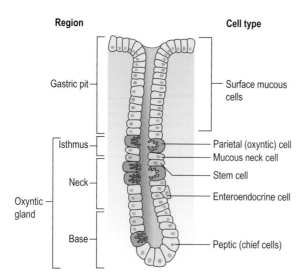

Fig. 15.14 **Structure of an oxyntic gland.**

The mucous neck cells have an irregular shape, with cytoplasm filled with mucous granules along the border adjacent to the lumen of the gland. The isthmus is the region connecting the neck to the gastric pit. It contains a mixture of parietal cells and surface mucous cells. The pyloric gland mucosa consists of chief cells and mucous cells producing pepsinogen and mucus. In addition to exocrine cells, the oxyntic glands and pyloric glands contain endocrine cells.

These hormone-producing cells contain granules near their basal border. The hormones are secreted into the tissue fluid and either act on adjacent cells (a local hormone or paracrine function) or enter capillaries and the hepatic portal circulation before reaching the systemic circulation and being delivered to their target organ via the arterial system (an endocrine function). Some cells such as the G cells of the pyloric antrum possess microvilli that project into the gastric lumen. It is believed that these microvilli contain receptors that are sensitive to the luminal contents and in turn control the secretion of their hormone in response to stimuli. In the case of the G cell, amino acids from the gastric lumen stimulate the release of gastrin. Other hormone-containing cells lie adjacent to either the exocrine or endocrine cells and control their function.

For example, enterochromaffin-like cells (ECL cells) containing histamine lie close to parietal cells and stimulate acid secretion. D cells containing somatostatin are also observed to have processes that terminate on parietal cells. Somatostatin is an inhibitor of acid secretion. The position of these cells suggests that they are stimulated by circulating hormones or neurotransmitters to release their products, in order to control adjacent cells in a paracrine manner.

CONTROL OF GASTRIC SECRETIONS

The rate of gastric secretion is determined by stimulatory and inhibitory mechanisms. For convenience, these mechanisms may be considered to occur in three overlapping phases (Fig. 15.15):

1. Cephalic phase
2. Gastric phase
3. Intestinal phase.

STIMULATION OF GASTRIC ACID SECRETION

The basal gastric acid secretion during the inter-digestive period increases when food is anticipated or consumed. The increase in acid secretion occurs by means of mechanisms having their origin in the head (cephalic phase), stomach (gastric phase) and intestine (intestinal phase) (Fig. 15.15).

Cephalic phase

Stimuli such as the thought, sight, smell, taste and chewing of food induce a reflex stimulation of acid secretion via the central nervous system and the vagal nerves. The vagus directly stimulates the parietal cells via the neurotransmitter acetylcholine.

There are two indirect vagal mechanisms of parietal cell stimulation:

- The release of the antral hormone, gastrin, from G cells following vagal stimulation by means of gastrin releasing peptide. The gastrin diffuses into the venous system and is delivered via the heart and arterial system to stimulate the parietal cells of the stomach (an endocrine mechanism).
- The release of histamine from enterochromaffin-like cells as a result of the action of acetylcholine released from postganglionic vagal nerves, and by the action of gastrin. Histamine diffuses from the enterochromaffin-like cells through the tissue fluid to stimulate the parietal cells (a paracrine mechanism).

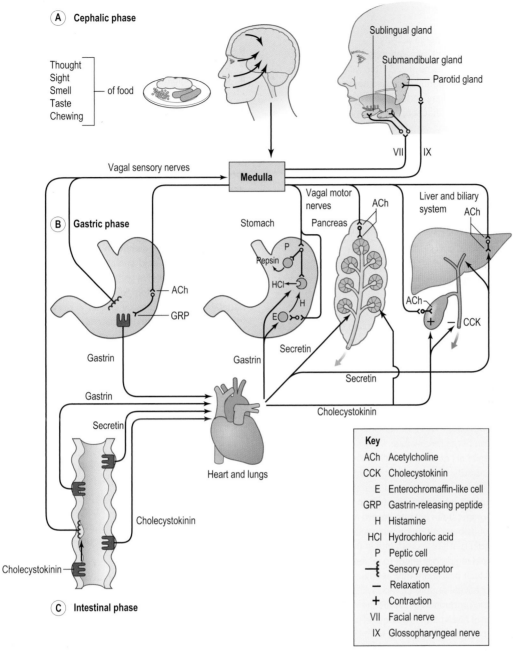

Fig. 15.15 Neurohumoral mechanisms stimulating gastric, pancreatic and biliary secretions.

Gastric phase

This phase is initiated by the presence of food in the stomach and involves physical and chemical mechanisms. Distension of the stomach stimulates stretch receptors that induce vago-vagal and intramural reflexes to induce acid secretion. The chemical composition of food buffers acid secretion and so causes a withdrawal of inhibitory mechanisms preventing gastrin release in addition to releasing gastrin directly. Protein digestion products, particularly the amino acids tryptophan and phenylalanine, are potent stimulants of gastrin secretion. Amino acids are detected by microvilli projecting into the lumen of the pyloric glands from the G cells. Gastrin secreted by the antral G cells consists of 17 amino acids (G17). Other stimulants of acid secretion are Ca^{2+}, caffeine and alcohol.

Intestinal phase

Chyme entering the intestine from the stomach produces a weak stimulation of gastric acid secretion via neural and humoral mechanisms. The upper small intestine contains intestinal gastrin, a peptide consisting of 34 amino acids (G34) that is released by the presence of food. The presence of another stimulant in the intestine, entero-oxyntin, has also been suggested. Entero-oxyntin activity may be due to the action of absorbed amino acids stimulating gastric acid secretion.

INHIBITION OF GASTRIC ACID SECRETION

Cephalic, gastric and intestinal inhibitory phases of acid secretion have been recognised (see Fig. 15.15).

Cephalic phase

1. **Withdrawal of vagal nerve activity**
   The cephalic phase of stimulation is over once eating is finished and food is removed. This will reduce vagal activity and consequently decrease acid secretion. Emotions, such as fear, sadness and depression, in addition to pain and nausea, act through central nervous mechanisms to inhibit vagal nerve activity from the medulla.
2. **Increased splanchnic nerve activity**
   Pain and fear lead to increases in splanchnic nerve activity with the release of norepinephrine, which produces vasoconstriction in the gastric arteries with a reduction in gastric blood flow. The delivery of oxygen, nutrients and gastrin to the stomach is decreased, and gastric acid secretion is inhibited.

Gastric phase

1. **Inhibition of gastrin release**
   Gastrin release from G cells is controlled by the pH of the antral contents through a negative feedback mechanism. Acid secretion leading to falls in antral pH below 3 inhibits gastrin release, and inhibition is complete when the pH falls to 1.5. This situation will occur towards the end of a meal when the buffering capacity of the gastric contents has been reduced and/or gastric emptying is nearing completion. Two mechanisms may contribute to the inhibition of gastrin release:
   - Changes in pH at the microvilli of the G cells reduce their sensitivity to the stimulatory action of amino acids
   - Acid stimulates the release of somatostatin from D cell terminals which are directed on to the adjacent G cells. Somatostatin inhibits gastrin release.
2. **Inhibition of acid secretion by prostaglandin E_2**
   Prostaglandin E_2 (PGE_2), produced in the gastric mucosa, exerts a local regulatory effect to inhibit histamine-stimulated acid secretion. PGE_2 stimulates EP_2 receptors that are negatively coupled to adenylate cyclase, and so inhibit the production of cAMP, the intracellular messenger of histamine. Prostaglandins also reduce the release of histamine and gastrin from ECL and G cells, respectively.

Intestinal phase

The entry of chyme into the small intestine from the stomach induces inhibition of gastric acid secretion. Experimental evidence suggests that a number of neural, hormonal and paracrine mechanisms are involved. These mechanisms, which are responsible for inhibition of acid secretion, need to be clarified.

Acidification of the small intestine inhibits gastric acid secretion. The neural mechanisms include withdrawal of vagal motor nerve activity as a consequence of vagal or splanchnic sensory nerves detecting low intestinal pH, and an enterogastric reflex in the splanchnic nerves.

Inhibitory hormonal mechanisms are stimulated by the presence of acid, hypertonic saline, glucose solutions, fats or monoglycerides in the intestine. The hormones involved are described as enterogastrones; that is, chemicals released from the small intestine that inhibit gastric function. There are several candidate enterogastrones:

- Cholecystokinin
- Secretin
- Vasoactive intestinal peptide
- Enteroglucagon/glucagon-like peptide
- Oxyntomodulin
- Gastric inhibitory peptide also known as glucose dependent-insulinotropic polypeptide
- Neurotensin
- Neuropeptide YY
- Somatostatin.

Intravenous infusion of each of the above candidate hormones produces inhibition of acid secretion, but that by itself does not establish a physiological role as an enterogastrone. To do so would require knowledge of the relationship between the delivery of acid, hypertonic and fatty solutions to the small intestine, with the release of the candidate hormones and their delivery to the gastric mucosa during the course of a meal. Inhibition of acid secretion during the intestinal phase may be due to additive or potentiating effects between candidate hormones. Enterogastrones inhibit acid secretion from parietal cells either directly or via the release of somatostatin from D cells adjacent to the parietal cells. An additional mechanism is by the inhibition of gastrin release from the antrum.

The intestinal phase of gastric acid secretion is predominantly inhibitory because removal of part of the small intestine leads to increased acid secretion.

STIMULATION OF PEPSINOGEN SECRETION

Pepsinogen secretion from the zymogen granules in the peptic (chief) cells is controlled in a similar manner to gastric acid secretion. The major mediator stimulating pepsinogen secretion is acetylcholine released from vagal nerves during the cephalic and gastric phases. Acetylcholine acts on muscarinic M_3 receptors on the peptic cell. In addition, acid secretion stimulated by the vagus induces pepsinogen secretion by two mechanisms:

- A local reflex in the intramural cholinergic nerves
- The release of the hormone secretin from the duodenum, which in turn acts on the peptic cells.

Gastrin and cholecystokinin (CCK) are also weak stimulants of pepsin secretion acting via CCK_A receptors. The importance of their role in controlling pepsinogen remains to be determined.

The intracellular messenger for acetylcholine, gastrin and cholecystokinin is Ca^{2+}. Receptor stimulation by these secretagogues leads to the production of inositol trisphosphate to release Ca^{2+} from intracellular stores. Secretin stimulates adenylate cyclase to produce cAMP from ATP. Rises in intracellular Ca^{2+} and cAMP initiate cytoskeletal activity that leads to the movement of zymogen granules containing pepsinogen to the apical surface of the cell, where they fuse with the membrane and discharge their contents by exocytosis.

CELLULAR MECHANISMS OF GASTRIC ACID SECRETION

Morphological changes in parietal cells (Fig. 15.16)

The apical cytoplasm of the parietal cell in the resting state is packed with tubulo-vesicles that contain K^+/H^+-ATPase

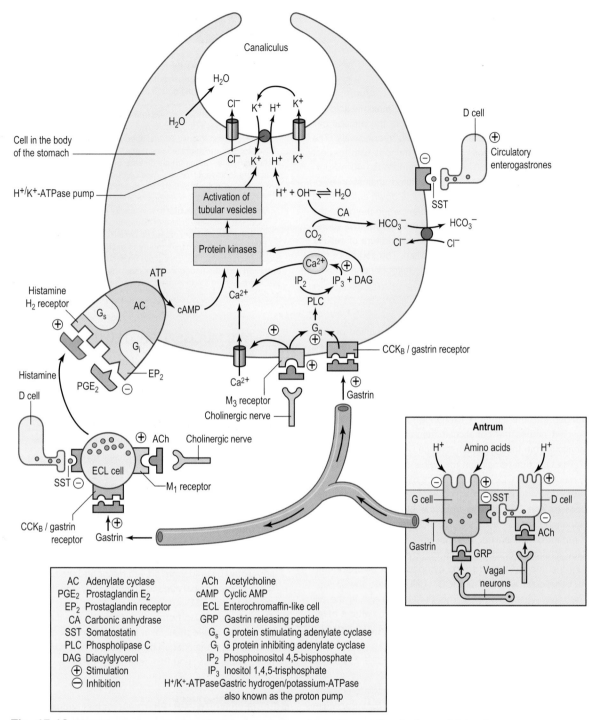

Fig. 15.16 **Physiological mechanisms in the control of gastric acid secretion by the parietal cell.**

(proton pump), which secrete H^+ in exchange for K^+. Stimulation of the cell with gastrin, acetylcholine or histamine is accompanied by cytoskeletal movements, causing the migration and incorporation of the tubulo-vesicles into the canalicular membranes. This action produces microvilli on the surface of the canalicular membranes which greatly increases the surface area and the number of proton pumps at the cell surface. Secretion occurs with the opening of K^+ and Cl^- channels in the canalicular membranes. The canaliculi swell when acid secretion begins. The tubulo-vesicles reform at the end of secretion and the microvilli disappear. Parietal cells are rich in mitochondria in order to provide sufficient ATP to power H^+ secretion.

Intracellular messenger for the action of acetylcholine, gastrin and histamine

Acetylcholine and gastrin acting via muscarinic M_3 and CCK_B gastrin receptors, respectively, stimulate phospholipase C which converts phosphoinositol 4,5-bisphosphate (IP_2) to inositol 1,4,5-trisphosphate (IP_3) and diacylglycerol (DAG). IP_3 stimulates Ca^{2+} release from intracellular stores to activate calmodulin-dependent protein kinase. DAG activates protein kinase C. Histamine acting on histamine H_2 receptors, activates adenylate cyclase to increase the formation of cAMP from ATP. cAMP-stimulated protein kinase A, Ca^{2+} and protein kinase C are involved in the changes in parietal cell function leading to the onset of acid secretion.

Ion movements during acid secretion

In human beings, it is estimated that during maximal acid secretion, the concentration of H^+ and Cl^- in the parietal cell secretion is 150 mmol/L and 170 mmol/L, respectively. The potential difference across the gastric mucosa with respect to the blood is about -60 mV at rest and falls to -40 mV during stimulation of secretion. Cl^- is secreted against an electrochemical gradient. Protons are moving down an electrical gradient and up a concentration gradient when the pH of the gastric juice is compared with that of the plasma. The secretion of hydrochloric acid requires the expenditure of cellular energy derived from aerobic metabolism. The source of this energy is ATP, produced by the many mitochondria packed into the cell.

Proton pump

The transport processes involved in the production of acid secretion are shown in Figure 15.16. The protons required for acid secretion are derived from water. With the opening of K^+ channels in the canalicular membrane, K^+ diffuses into the canaliculi and stimulates the proton pump from the luminal side to hydrolyse ATP. Protons derived from water are pumped into the lumen in exchange for K^+ ions, which are recycled across the canalicular membrane. Cl^- enters the canaliculi from the cytoplasm through Cl^- channels.

The OH^- that remains in the cell is converted to HCO_3^- by reacting with CO_2 in the presence of carbonic anhydrase. Carbon dioxide for this reaction is provided by cellular metabolism and by diffusion from the blood. The HCO_3^- is exchanged for Cl^- across the basal membrane by means of a carrier mechanism. The movement of HCO_3^- down its electrochemical gradient drives the inward transport of Cl^- from the interstitial fluid to the cytoplasm for secretion into the canalicular lumen. The HCO_3^- diffuses into the venous blood leaving the stomach. This produces a rise in the pH of arterial blood and a fall in the acidity of urine after a meal. The phenomenon is referred to as 'the alkaline tide of gastric secretion'.

Sodium pump

The sodium pump (Na^+/K^+-ATPase) in the basolateral membrane transports K^+ into the cell in exchange for intracellular Na^+. The accumulated K^+ moves down its electrochemical gradient through channels in the basolateral and canalicular membranes, producing a negative intracellular potential.

A Na^+/H^+ exchanger in the basolateral membrane transfers Na^+ into the cell down its electrochemical gradient in exchange for H^+ to provide Na^+ for the sodium pump and subsequent exchange for K^+ to maintain the K^+ content of the cell. Transfer of H^+ out of the cell increases the availability of OH^- to interact with CO_2 to produce HCO_3^-, thereby increasing the drive on Cl^- accumulation in the cell via the Cl^-/HCO_3^- exchanger. The energy for the accumulation of Cl^- within the cell and its diffusion into the canaliculus comes from the action of the sodium and proton pumps. The transfer of HCl into the canaliculus creates an osmotic flow of water to produce the gastric secretion. See Clinical box 15.8.

Clinical box 15.8 **Clinical conditions associated with disorders of gastric secretions**

Atrophic gastritis is a condition in which the glandular cells of the stomach are destroyed due to chronic inflammation caused by autoimmune disease or persistent *Helicobacter pylori* infection. Gastric acid, intrinsic factor and pepsin secretion is impaired or absent. The resulting clinical conditions include:

- Pernicious anaemia – an autoimmune disorder leading to loss of parietal cells in the gastric mucosa and the absence of intrinsic factor. Vitamin B_{12} malabsorption ensues leading to a macrocytic, megaloblastic anaemia.
- Achlorhydria – autoimmune disease of the parietal cells leading to absence or very much reduced gastric acid production in the stomach. The resulting raised pH inhibits activation of pepsin and leads to impaired protein digestion. Bacterial overgrowth due to low acidity may also occur, with associated malabsorption of nutrients and vitamins. There is also an increased risk of gastric cancer.

Over-secretion (hypersecretion) of gastrin leads to excess gastric acid production. This could be secondary to gastrin secretion from the endocrine pancreas, the Zollinger–Ellison syndrome, where the increased acidity of the stomach contents leads to duodenal ulceration.

GASTRIC MUCOSAL PROTECTION

The ability of the gastroduodenal mucosa to withstand the digestive action of hydrochloric acid, pepsin and bile (see Information box 15.5) depends on a number of factors:

- The mucous bicarbonate barrier, where protons are neutralised by bicarbonate ions to produce a neutral pH at the cell surface when the luminal pH is 2
- Phospholipids, covering the epithelial layer producing a protective coat
- Mucus secreted by the epithelial cells to trap the bicarbonate ions
- The action of prostaglandin E_2, stimulating phospholipid and mucus secretion
- The renewal of epithelial cells every 2 to 4 days from stem cells in the neck region of the gastric gland stimulated by epidermal growth factor and their migration to cover the luminal surface stimulated by transforming growth factor, TGF-α
- The delivery of bicarbonate ions from the basal border of the parietal cell to the lamina propria by mucosal blood flow, which is maintained by vasodilator neuropeptides, nitric oxide, PGE_2 and PGI_2 (see Table 15.1).

Information box 15.5 **Pharmacological inhibition of gastric acid secretion**

Drugs that inhibit gastric acid secretion are used to promote healing in peptic ulcers and reflux oesophagitis. Commonly used are the histamine H_2 receptor antagonists and proton pump inhibitors.

- H_2 receptor antagonists inhibit histamine action at all H_2 receptors competitively. The main clinical use is to inhibit gastric acid secretion by inhibiting histamine-, acetylcholine- and gastrin-mediated acid secretion by parietal cells; pepsin secretion is also reduced, with a decrease in gastric juice volume. Familiar preparations include cimetidine and ranitidine.
- Proton pump inhibitors act by the irreversible inhibition of H^+/K^+-ATPase, markedly reducing gastric acid secretion. Drugs such as omeprazole, a substituted benzimidazole, diffuse from the blood through the parietal cell cytoplasm into the canaliculi, where they are activated by acid. Following activation they bind irreversibly to sulphydryl groups in cysteine residues in the proton pump and inactivate it.

Peptic ulceration

Peptic ulceration occurs when the mucosal protective factors (Fig. 15.17) are reduced or overwhelmed by the action of aggressive factors (**acid**, **proteolytic enzymes** (e.g. pepsin) or **bile**) that digest the mucosal layer. See Clinical box 15.9.

Clinical box 15.9   **Peptic ulcers**

Infection with *Helicobacter pylori,* a Gram-negative organism with spiral morphology, causes ulceration. The bacterium secretes urease that converts blood urea to ammonia, which weakens the mucosal barrier, secretes toxins that destroy epithelial cells and produces platelet-activating factor, a potent ulcerogen and inflammatory mediator. *H. pylori* has also been identified as a cause of gastric cancer. *H. pylori* infection is associated with low socio-economic status, with a high prevalence of up to 90% of the population in developing countries. A higher prevalence is found in the older population in high-income countries.

Non-steroidal anti-inflammatory drugs (e.g. aspirin or indometacin) inhibit the enzyme cyclo-oxygenase and reduce the synthesis of protective prostaglandins (PGE_2 and PGI_2) from arachidonic acid, as well as causing irritation and death of epithelial cells thus weakening the gastric mucosal barrier. The arachidonic acid is converted by lipoxygenase to leukotriene LTB4, which causes neutrophil adhesion to the endothelium of small mucosal blood vessels and reduced blood flow. This leads to ischaemia, hypoxia and the release of proteases and reactive oxygen species from neutrophils, all of which damage the mucosa, causing ulceration and mucosal erosions that can bleed.

Ulceration also occurs with vasoconstrictor-mediated reductions in mucosal blood flow (see Table 15.1), caused by trauma and disease. Cigarette smoking, which causes vasoconstriction and mucosal ischaemia, is associated with increased risk of peptic ulceration.

Severe, recurrent duodenal ulcers occur with Zollinger–Ellison syndrome, where ectopic gastrin is secreted from an ectopic gastrinoma in the endocrine pancreas.

GASTRIC MOTILITY

For the purposes of describing gastric motility, the stomach is divided into two parts (see Fig. 15.13A):

- An upper orad portion containing the fundus and upper two-thirds of the corpus
- A caudad portion containing the lower third of the corpus and the antrum.

GASTRIC MUSCULATURE

The gastric musculature regulates the storage, mixing and emptying of the gastric contents. The smooth muscle cells in the stomach are arranged in four layers (Fig. 15.13B):

1. A longitudinal layer under the serosa and continuous with that of the oesophagus and duodenum
2. A circular layer continuous with that of the circular layers of the oesophagus and duodenum
3. An oblique layer inside the circular layer and found only in the orad region
4. A thin layer, the muscularis mucosae, at the base of the mucosa.

The muscle layers are innervated by intrinsic nerves of the myenteric plexus which receive branches from the submucosal plexus and parasympathetic vagal nerves from the medulla. Postganglionic nerves from the coeliac plexus also innervate the plexus regions.

ELECTRICAL AND CONTRACTILE ACTIVITY OF GASTRIC SMOOTH MUSCLE

The gastric musculature shows rhythmical contractile activity driven by the gastric pacemaker region in the greater curvature of the body of the stomach. This is driven by fluctuations

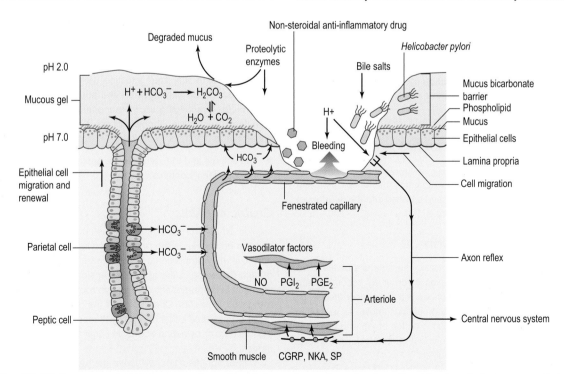

Fig. 15.17 **Factors contributing to gastric-mucosal protection and peptic ulceration.** Ulcerogenic factors: proteolytic enzymes, bile salts, *Helicobacter pylori*, non-steroidal anti-inflammatory drugs, vasoconstriction. CGRP, calcitonin gene-regulated peptide; NKA, neurokinin A; NO, nitric oxide.

in the membrane potential of the smooth muscles known as the **basic electrical rhythm** (**BER**), **pacesetter potentials** or **slow waves**. The frequency of these slow waves is about 3 per minute. The slow waves arise from **interstitial cells of Cajal** (**ICCs**). These smooth muscle-like cells occur as a single layer in plexus regions, with overlapping processes extending from the cell bodies of adjacent cells, to form a network providing communication with the smooth muscle layers via gap junctions. Slow wave activity spreads throughout the muscle layers. Some ICCs are found between the enteric nerve terminals and smooth muscles. The smooth muscle membrane potential may reach threshold at the peak of a slow wave potential. At threshold, L-type calcium channels open and an action potential will be generated with an influx of Ca^{2+} into the smooth muscle. The Ca^{2+} initiates contraction of the muscle. The strength of contraction is proportional to the frequency of the action potentials. The electrical activity spreads in a circular direction producing a band of contraction that propagates from the corpus of the stomach towards the antrum. This occurs because the electrical coupling between smooth muscle cells is faster in the circular than the longitudinal direction.

GASTRIC MOTILITY DURING THE INTERDIGESTIVE PERIOD

Contractile activity of the gastric musculature occurs in bursts at 90-minute intervals during the interdigestive period. These contractions begin in the orad portion of the stomach and sweep towards the antrum, pushing any residues (undigested food, e.g. bones, and other objects that may have been swallowed, desquamated cells, mucus, secretions) into the relaxing duodenum for onward propulsion along the small intestine. These bursts of activity are known as **migrating motor complexes** (**MMCs**). They act to prevent bacterial overgrowth and keep the stomach and intestine clean. MMCs depend on the enteric nervous system and are stimulated by the small intestinal hormone **motilin**. The antibiotic **erythromycin** also stimulates MMC production by acting on motilin receptors. Feeding inhibits the MMCs. Vagal nerve activity during the cephalic phase of feeding and gastrointestinal hormones **gastrin** and **cholecystokinin** released during digestion change the pattern of motility to that seen in the fed state.

GASTRIC MOTILITY DURING A MEAL

The pattern of gastric motility during feeding ensures that food is accommodated in the stomach, mechanically broken down, mixed with secretions and emptied into the duodenum at a regulated rate (Fig. 15.18).

Receptive relaxation

Following swallowing, the gastric musculature of the orad portion of the stomach relaxes in order to accommodate food, drink and gastric secretions without an increase in intragastric pressure. This phenomenon is known as receptive relaxation and is produced by the action of VIP and nitric oxide released from enteric nerves (Fig. 15.18A). The enteric nerves respond to such stimuli as:

- Sight, smell, taste of food – cephalic phase
- Oesophageal distension – oesophageal phase
- Gastric distension – gastric phase.

All phases of receptive relaxation include a vagal reflex. Sensory receptors in the oesophagus and stomach, via afferent vagal nerves, activate motor nerve pathways from the medulla to produce receptive relaxation. The reflex is known as a vagovagal reflex. The densest food tends to sink towards the caudad portion of the stomach, leaving the less dense foods such as oils and fat floating on the surface in the fundus. Gradually, the tension in the smooth muscles in the wall of the stomach increases as the gastric contents empty into the duodenum.

Mixing of gastric contents

The presence of food in the stomach stimulates powerful gastric peristaltic activity which begins in the body of the stomach and sweeps towards the antrum at the rate of 3 contractions per minute (Fig. 15.18A). The lumen of the antrum is narrowed by the contractile activity. Small particles and liquids are pushed towards the pylorus and large particles are forcibly propelled to the corpus of the stomach. This retropulsion of the antral contents into the corpus of the stomach helps to break down the food and mix it with the gastric secretions to form chyme.

Gastric emptying

A wave of contraction spreading over the antrum can sweep chyme into the duodenum, where the muscular wall is relaxed. The powerful peristalsis of the alimentary canal can propel a bolus of food from the oral to the anal end (Fig. 15.15C). Chyme flows from a region of high pressure to one of low. The pyloric sphincter between the antrum and the duodenum acts as a sieve to allow fluid and small particles to enter the duodenum but to retain larger particles in the stomach for further digestion. The motility of the gastroduodenal junction regulates gastric emptying and minimises retropulsion of the duodenal contents into the antrum.

Gastric emptying is regulated in order to match the supply of chyme to the small intestine with the rate at which the chyme can be can digested and absorbed (see Clinical box 15.10). Overloading the intestine leads to diarrhoea by stimulating peristalsis. The rate of gastric emptying is influenced by:

- The volume and the nature of the gastric contents
- The duodenal contents.

Gastric contents

Liquids empty from the stomach faster than solids, which need to be liquefied. The rate of emptying of liquid meals is approximately proportional to the square root of the volume of fluid remaining in the stomach. Tension in the wall of the stomach is proportional to the square root of the volumes of the gastric contents. Contraction of the gastric musculature may be stimulated either directly by the tension in the smooth muscle cells or by neural activity in either the enteric or vagal nerves.

Oils or liquefied fats will leave the stomach after aqueous solutions, in subjects who are either sitting upright or standing, because they float on the surface of the gastric contents.

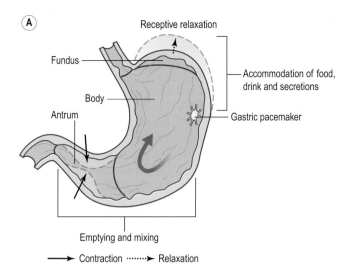

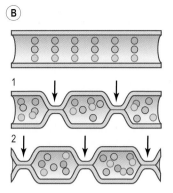

Segmentation of the intestine. Contraction of the intestinal wall in the sequence 1, 2 produces mixing

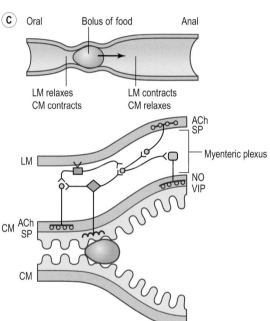

Peristalis propels a bolus of food from the oral to the anal end of the alimentary canal. Stimulation of a mechano- or chemosensitive neuron ◇ in the mucosa or stretch receptor ▢ initiates an ascending excitatory reflex and a descending inhibitory reflex.

LM   Longitudinal muscle
CM   Circular muscle
ACh Acetylcholine
NO   Nitric oxide
SP   Substance P
VIP Vasoactive intestinal peptide

Fig. 15.18 **Gastrointestinal motility.**

Duodenal contents

The composition of the chyme entering the duodenum from the stomach influences the rate of gastric emptying via a number of feedback mechanisms (see Ch. 16). The duodenum is sensitive to the following qualities of the chyme:

- pH
- Osmotic concentration
- Fat
- Amino acids and peptides.

Inhibition of gastric emptying occurs when the duodenal mucosa is exposed to:

- pH <3.5
- Hypertonic solutions
- Fatty acids with a chain length of 12–18 carbon atoms
- Tryptophan.

The neural and hormonal feedback mechanisms initiated by the stimulation of intestinal receptors are not completely understood. Reflex pathways involving both the central nervous system and the coeliac ganglia are present in the vagal and splanchnic nerves. The intestinal hormones, secretin, cholecystokinin and gastric inhibitory polypeptide, probably acting together during a meal, contribute to the inhibition of gastric emptying. The changes in neural and hormonal activity lead to alterations in gastric and duodenal motility.

Clinical box 15.10   **'Dumping' syndrome**

Dumping describes the symptoms of nausea, vomiting, bloating, sweating, palpitations and feeling faint after a meal in patients after partial gastrectomy or gastro-enterostomy. Decreased gastric emptying time results in the rapid 'dumping' of undigested stomach contents into the jejunum, leading to a rapid fluid influx into the jejunum in order to dilute the hypertonic contents. The pancreas may be stimulated to release excessive insulin, giving rise to hypoglycaemia. The symptoms may also occur in Zollinger–Ellison syndrome, where excessive gastrin secretion leads to over-production of acid, causing peptic ulcer disease. Dumping is also seen sometimes as a complication of cholecystectomy.

Acidification of the duodenum, for example, reduces gastric contractions and enhances the frequency and size of duodenal contractions. The presence of fats and fatty acids in the duodenum inhibits gastric and duodenal contractions but stimulates pyloric contractile activity.

These changes in gastrointestinal motility reduce the rate of gastric emptying. The inhibitory effects on gastrointestinal motility are known as enterogastrone actions. This name is derived from the hormone postulated to be produced in the intestine (*enteron*, Greek) that inhibits (*chalone*, Greek) the stomach (*gaster*, Greek). A single agent with the properties of enterogastrone has not been identified.

Other factors

Gastric emptying time can be increased by fear, pain and exercise, and reduced by excitement.

NAUSEA, RETCHING AND VOMITING

Vomiting or emesis is a complex series of responses in the gastrointestinal tract, respiratory tract and abdominal musculature leading to the forced expulsion of the gastric and sometimes the duodenal contents. There are three phases:

1. Nausea – a psychological event encompassing the feeling of wanting to vomit and often accompanied by gastric dilatation and upper intestinal contractions propelling the intestinal contents by reverse peristalsis into the stomach. Excessive salivation and pallor of the face may occur.
2. Retching – forceful, involuntary contractions of the diaphragm and abdominal muscles leading to the cardiac portion of the stomach being forced into the thorax.
3. Vomiting – rapid inspiration followed by reflex closure of the glottis and elevation of the soft palate to prevent vomitus entering the lungs and nasal cavity; contractions of the diaphragm and the abdominal muscles compress the stomach and expel the gastric contents into the oesophagus and mouth through the relaxed lower and upper oesophageal sphincters, respectively.

A variety of stimuli (Table 15.9) induce the complex responses involved in vomiting. The stimuli may be peripheral or central in origin. The hindbrain contains a group of chemoreceptors, known as the **chemoreceptor trigger zone** (CTZ) in the area postrema in the floor of the fourth ventricle that lies outside the blood–brain barrier. Circulating toxic agents stimulate these receptors. Vomiting may result from the summation of signals arising from several sources. Postoperative vomiting in the 24 hours following abdominal surgery may occur as a result of the combined influence of inhalation anaesthetic, the use of opioid analgesics for pain relief and reflexes from irritation to the gastrointestinal tract.

The neural pathways from higher regions of the brain (cortex and limbic system) and from peripheral sensory pathways (gustatory, motion, visual, gastrointestinal, liver) converge in the lateral reticular formation of the medulla oblongata of the hindbrain to control autonomic and somatic motor nerves involved in the visceral and somatic systems contributing to the vomiting response (Fig. 15.19). The neurons controlling the vomiting response are scattered throughout the medulla oblongata and do not lie in a discrete vomiting centre. The control of vomiting may be better described as being coordinated by a central pattern generator, representing the neuronal circuits involved in regulating the sequence of events in emesis. See Information box 15.6.

Table 15.9	Causes of vomiting
Central nervous system	Psychogenic factors – certain sights, smells, feelings, nervous dyspepsia, anorexia nervosa and bulimia
	Pain reflexes from injuries and disease, e.g. myocardial infarction
	Motion sickness
	Raised intracranial pressure
	Migraine
Alimentary canal	Pharyngeal irritation
	Distension or obstruction of organs
	Bacterial toxins
	Alcohol
	Therapeutic agents, e.g. non-steroidal anti-inflammatory drugs, antibiotics
	Salts of heavy metals, e.g. copper, mercury, zinc
Metabolic disorders	Diabetes, e.g. ketoacidosis, gastroparesis (delayed gastric emptying)
	Renal failure, e.g. uraemia
Therapeutic agents	Cancer chemotherapy, e.g. cisplatin, doxorubicin
	Radiotherapy
	Dopamine agonists, e.g. levodopa, bromocriptine
	Cardiac glycosides, e.g. digitalis
	Morphine and opioid analgesics
	Selective serotonin reuptake inhibitors, e.g. fluoxetine, paroxetine
Pregnancy	Causes unknown but may involve: • Altered function of the alimentary canal – delayed gastric emptying • Variation in intra-abdominal pressure • Metabolic and hormonal changes • Psychogenic factors

EXOCRINE PANCREAS

The exocrine pancreas is responsible for the secretion of enzymes for digesting carbohydrates, proteins and fats. It is composed of a system of ducts and acinar cells grouped into lobules which make up 98% of the pancreatic tissue. The pancreatic structure resembles that of salivary glands. The remaining 2% of the pancreas is composed of endocrine tissue which produces the hormones insulin and glucagon (see Ch. 10). The exocrine secretion, pancreatic juice, is composed of:

- Enzymes synthesised by acinar cells grouped into lobules
- An alkaline fluid secreted by the ductular epithelial cells.

The pancreatic juice flows along the main pancreatic duct which empties into the duodenum along with the bile duct (Fig. 15.20).

PANCREATIC ENZYMES

The pancreatic enzymes are synthesised in the rough endoplasmic reticulum of the acinar cells. They are transferred to the Golgi apparatus where they are directed to the condensing vacuoles for packaging into zymogen granules. These granules are found in abundance at the apical pole of the cell. Each zymogen granule contains several pancreatic enzymes (Table 15.10) whose relative concentration depends on the composition of the diet, e.g. a high

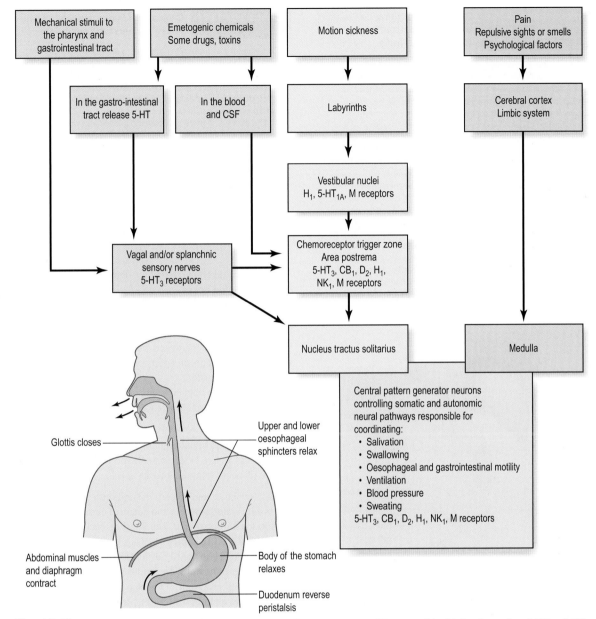

Fig. 15.19 **Stimuli and neural pathways controlling vomiting.** Receptors: CB_1, cannabinoid; D_2, dopamine; 5-HT$_{1A}$, 5-HT$_3$, 5-hydroxytryptamine; H_1, histamine; M, muscarinic; NK_1, neurokinin.

carbohydrate diet produces a high amylase component and a reduction in protease. See Clinical box 15.11.

Mechanisms of enzyme secretion

A rise in the intracellular Ca^{2+} concentration produced by neurohormonal agents (acetylcholine, gastrin and cholecystokinin) acts as a signal to induce exocytosis, in which the zymogen granules fuse with the apical membrane of the acinar cell and the contents are released into the acinar lumen (Fig. 15.21A). In addition to enzyme secretion, the acinar cells secrete a small quantity of isotonic fluid to wash the enzymes into the ducts. The increased intracellular Ca^{2+} concentration, produced by stimulants of enzyme secretion, activates protein kinases which produce an opening of Cl^- channels in the apical membrane. Cl^- diffuses from the cytoplasm to the acinar lumen. The gradient for Cl^- diffusion is maintained by the influx of Cl^- from the interstitial fluid across the basolateral membrane by means

of the $Na^+/K^+/2Cl^-$ transporter. This transfer is driven by the Na^+ gradient created by the Na^+/K^+ pump. The electronegative lumen attracts Na^+ to move from the interstitial fluid through cationic channels in the tight junctions between adjacent acinar cells. Water moves from the cells and interstitial spaces to the lumen of the duct system to produce an isotonic secretion. See Information box 15.7.

Alkaline secretion

The pancreas secretes 1–2 L of fluid per day. The pancreatic juice is alkaline (pH ~8) and isotonic to the blood. The major site for the production of the bicarbonate-rich juice is the duct system (Fig. 15.21B). The composition of the secretion varies with flow rate. At low flow rates the major ionic constituents are Na^+ and Cl^-. This contrasts with high flow rates where the predominant ions are Na^+ and HCO_3^-. The concentrations of K^+ and Na^+ at all flow rates are similar to

Gastric juice is composed of non-parietal and parietal cell secretions with different electrolyte compositions. Non-parietal cell secretions are produced at a constant flow rate and contain Na^+, K^+, Cl^- and HCO_3^-, while parietal cell secretions are produced at varying flow rates and contain H^+ and Cl^-. The electrolyte composition of gastric juice therefore varies with flow rate. At a low flow rate, the major components are Na^+ and Cl^- with lower concentrations of K^+ and H^+. However, at high flow rates, the major components are H^+ and Cl^- with lower concentrations of Na^+ and K^+.

The HCO_3^- secretion from non-parietal cells is neutralised by H^+ in the parietal cell secretion and can be measured in the absence of H^+ secretion. At all secretory rates the H^+, K^+ and Cl^- concentrations of the gastric juice exceed those in plasma, and the Na^+ concentration is less than that in plasma.

Prolonged vomiting or aspiration of gastric juice can lead to hypochloremic, hypokalaemic, metabolic alkalosis. Excessive loss of alkaline intestinal fluid leads to metabolic acidosis. Death may result unless intravenous infusions of NaCl, dextrose and K^+ are given. This is particularly in important in hyperemesis gravidarum – pronged vomiting in pregnancy.

The failure of the endocrine pancreas to secrete insulin, from the islets of Langerhans, is the primary cause of type 1 diabetes, and is also partially responsible for type 2 diabetes (see Ch. 3). Type 1 diabetes is caused by autoimmune destruction of Islet cells. Type 2 diabetes is associated with impaired insulin secretion, but also obesity and insulin resistance.

The exocrine pancreas secretes digestive enzymes concerned with all ingested macronutrients: carbohydrate, protein and fats. Failure of pancreatic cells to secrete these enzymes would lead to malabsorption and malnutrition. Absorption of some, particularly fat soluble, vitamins will also be impaired. Some clinical conditions leading to failure of the exocrine pancreas include:

- Chronic pancreatitis
- Cystic fibrosis
- Pancreatic cancer.

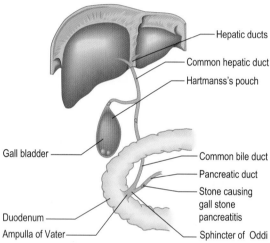

Fig. 15.20 Anatomical relationship between the liver, biliary system, pancreas and the small intestine. Adapted with permission from Kumar P, Clark M 2005 Clinical medicine, 6th edn. Elsevier Mosby, Edinburgh.

Labels:
- Hepatic ducts
- Common hepatic duct
- Hartmanss's pouch
- Common bile duct
- Pancreatic duct
- Stone causing gall stone pancreatitis
- Sphincter of Oddi
- Gall bladder
- Duodenum
- Ampulla of Vater

those in plasma. The concentration of Cl^- falls and that of HCO_3^- rises as flow rate increases.

The reciprocal changes in Cl^- and HCO_3^- concentrations with increases in flow rate may be accounted for by the mixing of two different secretions, one being a NaCl solution produced by the acinar cell, and the second solution being $NaHCO_3$ produced by the duct cells. The NaCl solution predominates at low flow rates. The secretion of $NaHCO_3$ increases with stimulation and dilutes the NaCl solution. At high flow rates, the increased secretion of $NaHCO_3$ leads to a high concentration of HCO_3^- and a low concentration of Cl^- in pancreatic juice.

The pancreatic duct cells can produce HCO_3^- concentrations of 140–150 mM. The HCO_3^- in the duct cells comes from two sources:

- HCO_3^- can be transferred from the interstitial fluid by means of a Na^+- HCO_3^- co-transporter
- CO_2 diffusion from the interstitial fluid.

CO_2, which is lipid soluble, diffuses into the cells where it reacts with water, aided by the action of carbonic anhydrase, to produce carbonic acid. The latter dissociates to produce H^+ and HCO_3^-. The supply of CO_2 is maintained by the duct cells exporting H^+ to the tissue fluid in exchange for Na^+ moving down its concentration gradient into the cells. The H^+ combines with HCO_3^- from the blood to form CO_2 and water.

The basal secretion of HCO_3^- from the duct cell is accounted for by the action of an anion exchanger in the luminal membrane. This mechanism transports HCO_3^- out of the cell into the lumen in exchange for Cl^- uptake. Cl^- is moving down its concentration gradient into the cell. The luminal Cl^- comes from the acinar cells' fluid secretion, and as a result of recycling through channels in the apical membrane of the duct cell.

Table 15.10 Pancreatic enzymes

Enzyme	Secreted as	Activation	Function
Amylase	Active enzyme		Starch digestion
Trypsinogen	Proenzyme	Activated by enteropeptidase to trypsin which act autocatalytically	Protein digestion
Chymotrypsinogen	Proenzymes	Activated by trypsin	
Procarboxypeptidase			
Proelastase			
Lipase	Active enzymes		Fat digestion
Cholesterol esterase			Cholesterol esters
Phospholipase			Phospholipids
Deoxyribonuclease	Active enzymes		Nucleic acid digestion
Ribonuclease			

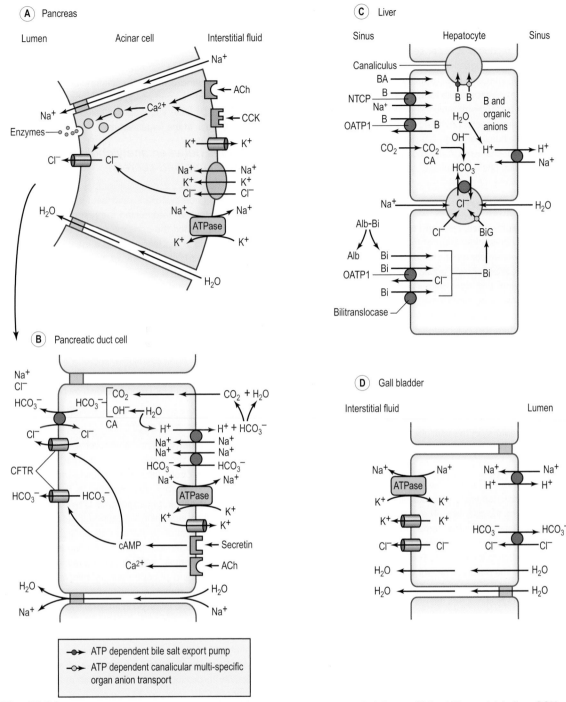

Fig. 15.21 Transport mechanisms involved in the formation of pancreatic juice and bile. ACh, acetylcholine; CCK, cholecystokinin; CA, carbonic anhydrase; CFTR, cystic fibrosis transmembrane regulator; B, bile salts; BA, bile acid; Bi, bilirubin; BiG, bilirubin glucuronide; Alb, albumin; NTCP, sodium taurochlorate co-transporting polypeptide; OATP1, organic anion transporting protein.

Information box 15.7   Pancreatitis

Pancreatic acinar cells are destroyed by acute or chronic inflammation and hereditary factors (e.g. cystic fibrosis), leading to failure to secrete pancreatic enzymes for the digestion of starches, proteins and fats. Nutritional deficiencies then ensue. Causes of pancreatitis include infection, alcohol, gall stones, tumours, heredity, trauma and surgery.

Stimulation of the duct cells with the hormone secretin leads to enhanced HCO_3^- secretion. The supply of Cl^- is insufficient to account for the concentrations of HCO_3^- achieved. Furthermore, high luminal HCO_3^- concentrations inhibit the Cl^-/HCO_3^- exchange at the apical membrane. The secretion of HCO_3^- under these circumstances is due to a Cl^--independent pathway. The cystic fibrosis transmembrane conductance regulator (CFTR) may serve as the pathway for HCO_3^- secretion to the duct lumen.

The lumen of the duct is electronegative with respect to the interstitial fluid. Na^+ enters the luminal fluid from the interstitial spaces by diffusion down this gradient. The resulting osmotic change draws water into the duct system to produce an isotonic secretion.

CONTROL OF PANCREATIC JUICE SECRETION

The pancreas produces a basal secretion of enzymes and fluid during the interdigestive period. This flow increases in parallel with the intestinal MMC activity. The parasympathetic nervous system is responsible for coordinating this secretory activity, aided by the hormone cholecystokinin.

Pancreatic juice secretion during a meal increases up to 20 times that of the basal secretion. It is determined by stimulatory and inhibitory mechanisms. As with gastric juice this occurs in three overlapping phases: cephalic, gastric and intestinal.

Cephalic phase

The thought, sight, smell, taste and chewing of food produce a reflex vagal nerve stimulation of the pancreatic acinar and duct cells to secrete pancreatic juice. The action of the vagus is mediated by acetylcholine acting on muscarinic M_3 receptors on the acinar and duct cells. Gastrin, released into the circulation by vagal activity to the gastric antrum, also contributes to pancreatic enzyme secretion. Gastrin, which has a similar structure to cholecystokinin (CCK), acts on CCK_A receptors on the acinar cells. Vagal nerve activity produces a pancreatic juice that is rich in enzymes.

Fear acting to increase sympathetic splanchnic nerve activity reduces pancreatic juice secretion. This action is produced by vasoconstriction due to the release of norepinephrine (noradrenaline) from the splanchnic nerves. Norepinephrine acts via α-adrenoceptors on the vascular smooth muscle, reducing blood flow to the pancreas, which inhibits secretion.

Gastric phase

The gastric phase consists of neural and hormonal components stimulating the pancreas. The gastro-pancreatic reflex is produced by distension of the stomach, leading to the stimulation of stretch receptors with afferent nerves in the vagus conveying information to the medulla. These nerves excite efferent vagal nerves to the pancreas (a vagovagal reflex) by means of the neurotransmitter acetylcholine. Gastrin released by protein digestion products stimulates the pancreatic acinar cells.

Intestinal phase

The intestinal contents play a major role in controlling pancreatic juice secretion. This is achieved by means of the hormones cholecystokinin and secretin, and the enteropancreatic vagovagal reflex.

Cholecystokinin is synthesised by I cells in the duodenal and jejunal mucosa. It is secreted in response to the presence of lipids such as monoglycerides and free fatty acids, amino acids and peptides, but not to carbohydrates or hydrochloric acid in the chyme. In animals, cholecystokinin enters the venous circulation and is delivered to the pancreas to stimulate enzyme secretion via CCK_A receptors situated on the acinar and duct cells. In humans, CCK_A receptors are absent from pancreatic acinar cells. It is suggested that cholecystokinin stimulates CCK_A receptors on vagal sensory nerves to produce a vagovagal reflex secretion of enzymes. The primary role of cholecystokinin is to stimulate enzyme secretion. Cholecystokinin alone has weak effects on fluid secretion but it potentiates the action of secretin.

Secretin is synthesised by S cells in the duodenal mucosa. It is released by hydrochloric acid in the chyme entering the small intestine from the stomach. Bile salts and lipids are much weaker stimulants of secretin secretion than hydrochloric acid. Secretin enters the circulation and is delivered to the pancreatic duct cells where it stimulates bicarbonate and, consequently, fluid secretion.

The **entero-pancreatic reflex** is stimulated by the presence of lipid, peptides and amino acids in the small intestine. The nutrients stimulate vagovagal reflexes with afferent and efferent pathways in the vagal nerves.

Interactions between acetylcholine, cholecystokinin and secretin

Interactions between the neurotransmitter acetylcholine and the hormones cholecystokinin and secretin at the cellular level are important in determining the response of the pancreas to a meal. When the concentration of either cholecystokinin or secretin in the blood during a meal is reproduced, by intravenous infusions of one of the hormones, the response of the pancreas is lower than that observed to a meal. The administration of the drug atropine, to block the action of acetylcholine released from the vagal nerves, or cutting the vagal nerves, reduces the effectiveness of both cholecystokinin and secretin in producing enzyme and bicarbonate secretion, respectively. The results of these observations suggest that when cholecystokinin, secretin and acetylcholine act together, they increase the sensitivity of the pancreas to stimulation. This phenomenon is known as potentiation.

Intracellular messengers for acetylcholine, cholecystokinin and secretin

The actions of acetylcholine, cholecystokinin and secretin depend on the production of intracellular messengers. Acetylcholine and cholecystokinin stimulate muscarinic and cholecystokinin receptors, respectively, in the acinar and duct cells. This results in phospholipase C hydrolysing phosphatidyl inositol to inositol 1,4,5-trisphosphate and diacylglycerol (DAG). Inositol trisphosphate releases Ca^{2+} from stores in the endoplasmic reticulum. The rise in intracellular Ca^{2+} activates calmodulin, which in turn increases the activity of protein kinases and phosphorylation involved in the processes of zymogen granule secretion. DAG activates protein kinase C, which is also involved in enzyme secretion from zymogen granules. The rise in intracellular Ca^{2+} also stimulates fluid secretion by acinar cells, probably by inducing phosphorylation of ion channels involved in the production of the secretion. Secretin stimulates an increase in adenylate cyclase activity to produce cyclic AMP, which in turn activates protein kinase C to promote enzyme and fluid secretion.

Inhibition of pancreatic secretion

Pancreatic function at the end of a meal is returned to the interdigestive state by the lack of stimulatory factors in the alimentary canal. There is an additional inhibitory mechanism that operates from the terminal ileum. The presence of fat in the terminal ileum and colon releases **peptide YY** (**PYY**) from intestinal L cells, an inhibitor of pancreatic enzyme secretion.

THE LIVER AND BILIARY SYSTEM

The liver is situated in the right hypochondrium, under the diaphragm, and behind and protected by, the lower ribs. Although embryologically developed from the foregut, the

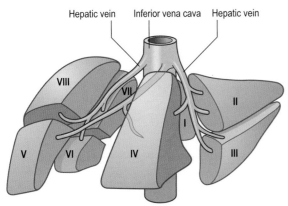

Fig. 15.22 **Segmental anatomy of the liver.** I, caudate lobe; II–IV, left hemi-liver; V–VIII, right hemi-liver. Adapted with permission from Kumar P, Clark M 2005 Clinical Medicine, 6th edn. Elsevier Mosby, Edinburgh.

liver performs much more than digestive functions. In health, the liver is not palpable on examination of the abdomen. The lower edge of the liver becomes palpable below the rib cage when the organ is enlarged through disease. The liver participates in a wide variety of processes that are discussed in many chapters in this book. This section is a summary of what the liver does, and what can happen in liver disease.

ANATOMY OF THE LIVER

The liver is a solid, pyramid-shaped organ enclosed by peritoneum. It is the largest internal human organ, weighing between 1.4 kg and 1.6 kg in the healthy adult.

Gross anatomy of the liver

The hepatic portal vein, hepatic artery and common bile duct (see below) enter the liver at the hilum (porta hepatis). The vessels and duct divide into right and left branches. Functionally, the parts of the liver supplied by these branches constitute a larger right and a smaller left lobe. Depending on the blood supply, the liver can be further subdivided into eight segments (Fig. 15.22). This has important clinical implications during surgery, when it is possible to resect individual segments.

Blood supply to the liver

The liver is a highly vascular organ, receiving 25% of the resting cardiac output, and is unique in that it has a dual blood supply of both arterial and venous blood, necessary for the performance of complex liver functions. The hepatic portal vein and hepatic artery enter the liver through a central area on the ventral surface of the liver, through which the common bile duct also enters. This area is known as the **hilum (porta hepatis)**.

- The portal vein carries blood from the gut, pancreas and spleen. Absorbed nutrients and products of digestion enter the liver directly from the gastrointestinal tract. Senescent (used, spent) red blood cells are delivered from the spleen (see Ch. 12). As much as 75% of the blood supply to the liver is via the portal vein.
- The hepatic artery, arising from the coeliac axis which originates from the abdominal aorta, ensures that the liver cells are well perfused and supplied with oxygen for metabolism.
- The hepatic vein drains into the inferior vena cava.

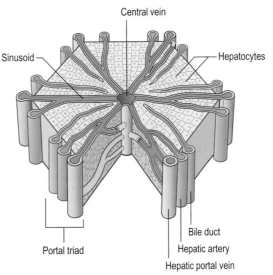

Fig. 15.23 **Microanatomy of a hepatic lobule.** The portal tract consists of a triad of an hepatic arteriole (a branch of the hepatic artery), a terminal portal venule (a branch of the portal vein) and a bile duct, which receives bile from bile ductules. Blood from the portal tract flows through the sinusoids into the central vein.

Microanatomy of the liver

Microscopically, liver cells (hepatocytes) make up the liver parenchyma (substance), forming hepatic plates that are one to two cells thick. The plates are separated from each other by large capillary spaces known as sinusoids. Bile canaliculi run in a network between the hepatocytes, receiving bile secretions, and join to form the intra-hepatic small bile ductules.

The hepatic plates are arranged into a large number of polyhedral liver lobules, which are hexagonal in cross-section (Fig. 15.23). There is a central lobular vein (also known as the terminal hepatic venule) in the middle of each lobule. At the periphery of each polygonal lobule are the portal tracts, which consist of a triad of vessels, also known as the portal triad, consisting of:

- An hepatic arteriole (a branch of the hepatic artery), which supplies oxygenated blood straight from the lungs and heart
- A terminal portal venule, which is a branch of the hepatic portal vein, draining blood from the stomach, intestine, pancreas and spleen
- A bile ductule, which drains into the bile duct, delivering bile (see below).

Arterial blood and portal venous blood mix as the blood flows through the sinusoids from the periphery of the lobule to the central vein. The central lobular veins converge to form the hepatic vein, which carries the blood to the inferior vena cava. The sinusoids do not have a basement membrane, and are lined by two cell types:

- Specialised, fenestrated vascular endothelial cells forming a lining with numerous gaps that facilitates transfer of metabolites between the plasma and hepatocytes.
- Mononuclear, phagocytic Kupffer cells that are part of the reticular endothelial system (see also Ch. 12). Kupffer cells, usually situated near the gaps between the endothelial cells, have a role in recycling senescent, non-functioning red blood cells; one of the products is bile.

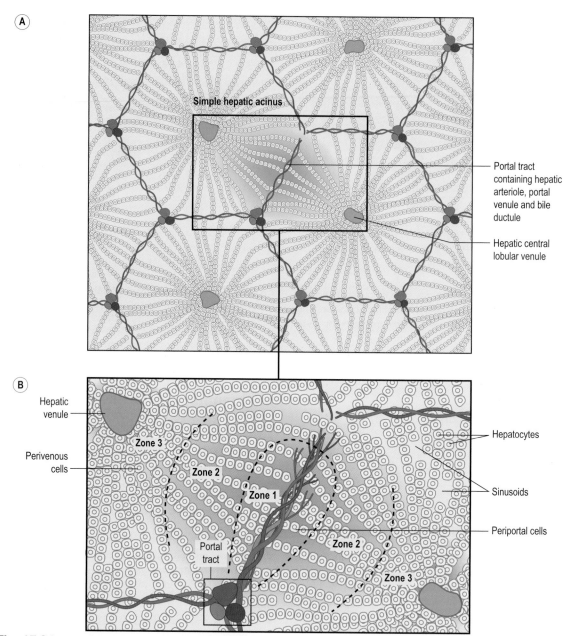

Ⓐ

Simple hepatic acinus

Portal tract
containing hepatic
arteriole, portal
venule and bile
ductule

Hepatic central
lobular venule

Ⓑ

Hepatic
venule

Perivenous
cells

Zone 3

Zone 2

Zone 1

Portal
tract

Zone 2

Zone 3

Hepatocytes

Sinusoids

Periportal cells

Fig. 15.24 **Hepatic acinus and metabolic zonation.** Hepatocytes in zone 1, nearest to the portal triad (tract), receive the most oxygen from the hepatic arteriole and nutrients from the portal venule; hepatocytes in the more peripheral zone 3, being more distant, receive less. The difference results in differential oxygenation of the cells, leading to different gene expression and metabolism. Adapted from from Young B, Woodford P, O'Dowd G, et al. 2013 Wheater's functional histology: a text and colour atlas, 6th edn. Churchill Livingstone, Philadelphia, with permission.

The hepatocytes are separated from the sinusoids by the space of Disse. The basolateral membranes of the hepatocytes face the space of Disse and are covered with microvilli to create a large surface area to facilitate absorption. The membranes also contain stellate cells that store vitamin A during their quiescent state and produce collagen when activated. The smallest functional unit of the liver is the acinus:

- The liver acinus consists of hepatocytes and sinusoids from two adjacent lobules supplied by one portal tract. Blood flowing through the hepatic sinusoids drains into the central lobular vein, so that there are two to each acinus (Fig. 15.24A).
- The hepatocytes nearest the portal tract, the periportal cells, are well supplied with oxygenated blood from the hepatic arteriole and nutrients from the terminal portal

venule (Fig. 15.24B). A difference in oxygen and nutrient concentration arises as the blood flows towards the central lobular vein. Hepatocytes nearest the vein, perivenous cells, are less well oxygenated. This phenomenon is known as metabolic zonation of the liver where the difference in oxygenation results in differential gene expression and metabolism. For example, periportal cells receive more oxygen than the perivenous cells and have a more oxidative metabolism, whereas the expression of glucokinase is mainly restricted to the perivenous cells (see Ch. 3).

The liver acinus is not to be confused with the basic hepatic lobule. In the acinus, the portal tract is central, with the central lobular veins at the periphery, whereas in the hepatic lobule, the central lobular vein is central with a portal tract at each corner of the hexagon.

FUNCTIONS OF THE LIVER

The liver participates in a wide range of biochemical processes, its functions including metabolism, catabolism, synthesis, elimination of toxic substances and storage. In addition, the liver has an immunological function. Among these functions, the liver has a pivotal role in metabolism, discussed in detail in Chapter 3. The interrelationship of carbohydrate, protein and lipid metabolism to maintain optimum blood glucose concentration is orchestrated in the liver.

The liver and carbohydrate metabolism

The liver has a major role in glucose metabolism to maintain the optimum level of circulating glucose essential to energy metabolism: glucose homeostasis (see Ch. 3).

- Glycogen synthesis and storage: after a carbohydrate-rich meal, glucose is mainly taken up by the perivenous cells, initially to synthesise glycogen. When blood glucose levels are high, e.g. after a meal, the liver stores glycogen.
- Owing to the presence of the enzyme glucose-6-phosphatase (G6Pase), unlike muscle, hepatic glycogenolysis releases glucose directly into the blood stream, thus acting as a reservoir for glucose.
- Gluconeogenesis: the liver is able to synthesise glucose from non-carbohydrate sources (e.g. amino acids and glycerol from fat metabolism), which is an essential source of glucose during starvation when glycogen stores are depleted.

The liver and protein metabolism

As a first step in protein metabolism, the nitrogen component of amino acids delivered to the liver via the portal vein is removed through transamination (catalysed by aminotransferases, also known as transaminases) and deamination in the liver (see Ch. 3). This function is disrupted in liver disease, and transaminase enzymes are clinical markers of hepatocyte damage (see Clinical box 15.9). One of the products of deamination is ammonia (NH_3), which is toxic and normally removed rapidly via the urea cycle in the liver. The liver thus fulfils its function in protein metabolism by catabolism and detoxification of waste products of metabolism. Protein synthesis is another important liver function (see Clinical box 15.12).

- Most plasma proteins are synthesised in the liver. Albumin is exclusively produced by the liver, and low plasma concentration, called hypoalbuminaemia, is common in liver disease. The implications for nutritional status, immunity and drug metabolism are discussed in Chapters 4 and 16. See also Clinical box 15.9.
- The liver also participates in the production of all the coagulation factors: prothrombin, fibrinogen and factors V, VII, IX, X and XIII. Defective production of one or all of these factors results in coagulation defects, with spontaneous bruising and prolonged bleeding after minor injuries. Laboratory measurement of prothrombin time (PT) assesses the functional concentration of these factors (see Ch. 12).
- Plasma α- and β-globulins are mostly synthesised by hepatocytes. This function is compromised in liver disease, affecting immunity. (See Clinical box 15.13.)

Clinical box 15.12 **Some clinical conditions associated with defects in hepatic protein synthesis**

- α_1-Antitrypsin deficiency is a rare genetic disorder associated with about 1% of chronic obstructive pulmonary disease (COPD). Onset of COPD at a young age and a family history are suggestive of α_1-antitrypsin deficiency, and may warrant genotype investigation. When arising in infancy, the condition presents with liver disease.
- Wilson's disease is an autosomal recessive condition in which hepatic caeruloplasmin synthesis is defective. Normally, dietary copper is absorbed from the upper gastrointestinal tract, transported to the liver bound to albumin, and thence incorporated into the copper-containing glycoprotein caeruloplasmin, concerned with plasma copper transport. Caeruloplasmin deficiency leaves the copper free, which is then deposited in the hepatocytes, causing chronic hepatitis, cirrhosis and ultimately liver failure, although the precise mechanism is unclear (see below). Biliary excretion of copper is also compromised. Copper deposits in the central nervous system, kidneys and bone cause further damage. Deposits of copper in the cornea give the characteristic Kayser–Fleischer rings.
- Ferritin, the protein concerned with iron storage, and transferrin, responsible for iron transport, are also synthesised by the liver (see Ch. 12). Although the mechanism of damage is unclear, defective hepatic synthesis of these proteins results in prolonged iron overload in the liver. Hereditary haemochromatosis is a condition in which iron is deposited in the liver (and other tissues), eventually leading to fibrosis (cirrhosis, see below) and liver failure.
- α-Fetoprotein is synthesised by the liver, predominantly in the foetal liver. Elevated maternal plasma α-fetoprotein concentration is used as a screening test for foetal open neural tube defects and as part of the triple test for Down syndrome. Regenerating hepatocytes synthesise α-fetoprotein, so high concentrations may be associated with carcinoma of the liver.

Clinical box 15.13 **Acute phase proteins**

The acute phase response refers to the body's defence mechanism against infections and inflammation, when the liver synthesises 'acute phase proteins', stimulated by pro-inflammatory cytokines (see Ch. 6). Plasma concentrations rise by 25% or more following the initial challenge, and the magnitude of the response reflects the severity of the infection or inflammatory process. Amino acids are needed as substrate for the increased hepatic protein synthesis. In severe, prolonged inflammatory (including carcinomas) or infective conditions, the amino acids are derived from muscle breakdown, resulting in the muscle wasting of chronic disease (cachexia). Of the acute phase proteins, changes in plasma concentration of C-reactive protein (CRP) are most marked, and values derived from laboratory measurement are used clinically as a marker of infection or inflammation.

The liver and lipid metabolism

Insoluble dietary lipids are transported to the liver, via the portal vein, as lipoproteins (Ch. 3); the liver has a central role in lipoprotein metabolism. The functions may be summarised to include:

- Synthesis of triacylglycerol (TAG) and removal of TAG from TAG-rich lipoprotein particles (hepatic triacylglycerol lipase HTGL)
- Synthesis of very-low-density lipoproteins (VLDL) and high-density lipoproteins (HDL)
- Synthesis of apolipoproteins that control lipoprotein metabolism

- Cholesterol: the liver has a major role in both synthesis and catabolism of cholesterol:
  - Cholesterol synthesis
  - Esterification of free cholesterol to cholesterol ester, catalysed by lecithin-cholesterol acyltransferase (LCAT)
  - Removal of cholesterol into hepatocytes for excretion as bile salts and sterols.
- Steroid and hormone synthesis from cholesterol by the cytochrome P450 system of hepatic microsomal enzymes
- Cytochrome P450 enzymes also participate in the biosynthesis of endogenous substances such as arachidonic acid, a precursor of prostaglandins and thromboxane. Thromboxane induces platelet aggregation and vasoconstriction, which initiates the normal coagulation mechanisms following injuries (see Coagulation cascade, Ch. 12).
- When there is excessive carbohydrate intake, the liver synthesises fatty acids using intermediates from the breakdown of sugars, some amino acids and other fatty acids.

The liver and red blood cells

The red cell membrane, like all cell membranes, is a lipid bilayer containing cholesterol. In severe liver disease, LCAT is decreased so that esterification of free cholesterol to cholesterol ester is reduced, increasing the ratio of circulating cholesterol to cholesterol ester. This changes cell membrane structure. In chronic obstructive liver disease, abnormal liver enzyme activity results in thinning of the red cell membrane, with an increase in membrane surface area, leading to macrocytosis. Microscopically, the abnormal red cells have a central dark area surrounded by a pale ring, giving the appearance of the 'bulls eye' in an archery target; these cells are known as target cells (codocytes).

The respiratory pigments responsible for the transport of oxygen, haemoglobin in red blood cells and myoglobin in muscle, contain haem, a porphyrin with a central iron core (see Ch. 12). Although haem is synthesised in most cells, the liver is the main non-red cell source of haem. The liver is also responsible for the catabolism of haem. Haemoglobin from senescent red blood cells is transported via the portal vein to the liver from the spleen (the graveyard of red blood cells). The spent red cells are phagocytosed by the Kupffer cells, where iron and globin are removed from haem. The iron is released and recycled via transferrin; the globin is also reused. Haem is then recovered by the Kupffer cells, and the porphyrin ring is broken down to bilirubin for excretion.

Metabolism of bilirubin

Bilirubin, a yellow pigment, is a product of haem catabolism, following the destruction of haem molecules by macrophages. The vast majority of bilirubin (75%) comes from the haemoglobin of senescent red blood cells. Macrophages are part of the reticulo-endothelial system, found in the spleen, bone marrow and the Kupffer cells lining liver sinusoids. After haemoglobin is degraded into haem and globin, the porphyrin ring of haem is cleaved by haem oxygenase, a cytochrome P450 enzyme (see Chs 3 and 4), to biliverdin with the release of iron. Biliverdin, which is water soluble, is enzymically reduced to bilirubin by biliverdin reductase. Bilirubin has low water solubility, therefore it is transported in the blood bound

to plasma albumin. On reaching the liver, the bilirubin–albumin complex dissociates and free bilirubin crosses the hepatocyte basolateral membrane by one of three mechanisms: either diffusion or transport by OATP1 or bilitranslocase (see below).

Following uptake by hepatocytes, free bilirubin is transported to the endoplasmic reticulum where it is conjugated with glucuronic acid to form bilirubin glucuronide. The conjugated bilirubin is more soluble and can be excreted by the hepatocyte into the biliary canaliculi via the transporter canalicular multi-specific organic anion transporter (cMOAT), then transported to the gastrointestinal tract via the biliary tree (see below). In the gastrointestinal tract, bacterial flora catabolise conjugated bilirubin to the colourless stercobilinogen (also called faecal urobilinogen), which is oxidised to the coloured stercobilin (also called faecal urobilin) for excretion in faeces.

Bilirubin, being yellow, gives the yellow coloration of bruises and the brown colour of faeces. Excess plasma bilirubin causes jaundice, a yellow discoloration of the skin and sclera (see Clinical box 15.11).

The liver and bile production

Among its many functions, the liver contributes to digestion by secreting bile (Table 15.11). Approximately 0.6–1.2 L is secreted per day in an adult. This exocrine secretion serves not only to aid digestion but also as a route for the excretion of metabolites produced by the liver.

Bile secretion

The components of bile diffuse from the sinusoids through spaces between the endothelium to the space of Disse, from where they are absorbed by the hepatocytes and formed into bile. The apical membranes of adjacent hepatocytes form the walls of the biliary canaliculi into which bile is secreted. The bile then flows through the biliary tree into the duodenum (see Fig. 15.20 and Clinical box 15.14):

- The biliary canaliculi join together to form bile ductules
- Bile ductules convey the bile to the bile ducts in the portal tracts at the periphery of the lobule
- Portal tracts drain into the intra-hepatic bile ducts that join to form hepatic ducts leaving each liver lobe
- The left and right hepatic ducts join to form the common hepatic duct just outside the liver
- The common hepatic duct joins the cystic duct from the gall bladder to form the common bile duct.

Table 15.11	Composition of human hepatic and gall bladder bile	
Component	**Hepatic bile (mmol/L)**	**Gall bladder bile (mmol/L)**
Na^+	150–160	230–240
K^+	4–5	6–14
Ca^{2+}	1.0–2.5	2.5–16
Cl^-	62–112	1–10
HCO_3^-	20–50	8–10
Bile salts	20–40	200–300
Bilirubin	1–3	5–30
Cholesterol	2–4	10–25
Phospholipids	3–7	18–40

Clinical box 15.14   Jaundice

Jaundice (icterus) is characterised by elevated concentrations of bilirubin in the plasma producing a yellow discoloration of the sclera of the eyes, skin and mucous membranes. Jaundice may be characterised as unconjugated hyperbilirubinaemia and obstructive or cholestatic jaundice.

Unconjugated hyperbilirubinaemia
Haemolytic jaundice occurs following excessive haemolysis of erythrocytes in newborn infants, and hereditary, autoimmune and non-immune disorders of erythrocytes. The hepatocytes cannot dispose of the increased amounts of unconjugated bilirubin, which accumulates in the blood (see Ch. 12).

Transient defects in the conjugation of bilirubin may occur in the newborn due to immaturity of the liver in which the glucuronidation pathway is not fully developed, leading to unconjugated bilirubin accumulating in the blood: physiological jaundice. Haemolytic disease of the newborn, due to rhesus incompatibility with maternal blood, results in massive intravascular haemolysis and severe unconjugated hyperbilirubinaemia, which may be complicated by bilirubin deposition in the central nervous system (CNS) – kernicterus – leading to brain damage. Congenital unconjugated hyperbilirubinaemia (e.g. Gilbert's syndrome) may be due to abnormalities in glucuronide conjugation or transport into the biliary canaliculi by cMOAT (see below).

Obstructive or cholestatic jaundice
- Intra-hepatic jaundice: caused by damage to liver cells produced by viruses, drugs, alcohol cirrhosis, or blockage of the intra-hepatic bile ducts leading to a failure of bile secretion.
- Extra-hepatic jaundice: produced by blockage of the extra-hepatic bile ducts. The obstruction may be due to gall stones in the biliary tree, or due to enlargement of an adjacent organ, such as carcinoma of the head of the pancreas.

Obstructive jaundice, however caused, leads to conjugated bilirubin accumulating in the blood. Some of this water-soluble form of bilirubin is excreted by the kidneys and gives the urine a dark yellow colour. Bile-containing conjugated bilirubin does not enter the intestine, and therefore cannot be transformed by intestinal flora to stercobilin, so that faeces in obstructive jaundice are pale coloured.

- Just before its termination in the duodenum, the common bile duct is joined by the pancreatic duct at the ampulla of Vater (hepatopancreatic ampulla)
- The termination of the common bile duct is in the duodenum, marked by an accentuation of its circular smooth muscle layer (sphincter of Oddi).

Cellular mechanisms of bile secretion
Bile is composed of water, electrolytes, bile salts, cholesterol, phospholipids and bilirubin (Table 15.11). Hepatocytes synthesise the primary bile acids, cholic acid and chenodeoxycholic acid, from cholesterol. These bile acids are metabolised by intestinal bacteria to the secondary bile acids, deoxycholic acid and lithocholic acid. They are absorbed from the intestine and circulate to the liver where they are eventually absorbed by hepatocytes to form bile. The bile acids are conjugated with glycine and taurine to form negatively charged bile salts, which have a greater water solubility than the bile acids at the near neutral pH of the intestinal contents. The enhanced water solubility is important in enabling the bile salts to aid the digestion of fats.

The secretion of bile depends on two separate, active secretory processes:

- Bile-salt-dependent secretion produced by the hepatocytes
- Bile-salt-independent secretion produced by the hepatocytes and duct cells.

Bile-salt-dependent secretion Bile formation begins with the absorption of bile salts and other organic and inorganic ions across the basolateral border of the hepatocyte by a variety of transporters. Bile salt uptake is dependent on two transporters and non-ionic diffusion (Fig. 15.21C).

The Na+ coupled transporter known as the sodium taurocholate co-transporting polypeptide (**NTCP**) can transfer both conjugated and unconjugated bile salts. The organic anion transport protein (**OATP1**) also transfers bile acids into hepatocytes in exchange for Cl−. In addition, unconjugated bile salts may enter the cell by non-ionic diffusion in their undissociated acid form.

The hepatocytes secrete bile acids and organic anions (e.g. bilirubin, glucuronide, glucuronidated bile acids) across their apical membrane into the canaliculi via two ATP-dependent pumps:

- ATP-dependent bile salt export pump (**BSEP**)
- ATP-dependent canalicular multi-specific organic anion transporter (**cMOAT**).

Na+ ions accompany the negatively charged bile salts and together they create an osmotic force for water movement into the bile canaliculi. The flow of water from the hepatocytes through the tight junctions between the hepatocytes brings other solutes by solvent drag, producing canalicular bile, which is isosmotic with plasma (~300 mosmol/kg). The bile acids form micelles with cholesterol and phospholipids entering the canaliculi from the hepatocytes. This effectively lowers their concentration and more cholesterol and phospholipid enter the bile.

Bile-salt-independent flow The hepatocytes produce a small bile-salt-independent secretion. The intra-hepatic bile duct cells, called **cholangiocytes**, have a similar function to pancreatic duct cells and produce an isotonic, bicarbonate rich secretion by the same mechanism as described for pancreatic juice secretion. In summary, the opening of Cl− channels in the apical membranes of the cholangiocytes leads to the diffusion of Cl− into the bile duct, with water movement by osmosis via aquaporin 1 channels. Cl− is exchanged for HCO_3^- produced by cholangiocytes. The bile has a higher concentration of HCO_3^- than the plasma and a lower Cl− concentration. The cholangiocytes have secretin receptors on their basolateral membranes and are stimulated to secrete bicarbonate by the intestinal hormone secretin. This leads to a watery alkaline secretion. Another intestinal hormone, cholecystokinin, potentiates the action of secretin.

The bile ducts also have the ability to reabsorb NaCl and water. This function is observed following removal of the gall bladder.

The liver and drug metabolism

The metabolism of drugs is discussed in detail in Chapter 4. The role of the liver is summarised here as a reminder to the reader. The liver metabolises most drugs, including alcohol. Orally administered drugs are absorbed by the small intestine and transported to the liver via the portal vein, then distributed to the relevant compartments in the body. Outcomes of hepatic drug metabolism include the production of less pharmacologically active metabolites, production of active metabolites that are more potent than the parent drug, conversion of inactive pro-drug to the active drug, production of toxic metabolites and elimination of inactive metabolites. When in the liver, the drug undergoes:

- First pass metabolism: some drugs, such as glyceryl trinitrate, are completely metabolised and inactivated by the liver so that this class of drugs cannot be administered orally. When a drug is partially inactivated by the liver, producing metabolites with reduced biological activity, a larger dose may be needed. In the elderly or patients with impaired liver function, a drug may not be sufficiently metabolised during first pass metabolism, potentially leading to toxic side effects. In such patients, the usual dose of the drug will need to be reduced.
- Phase I metabolic reactions: these involve microsomal enzymes in the hepatocytes (the mixed function oxidases), of which the cytochrome P450 system is the most important. This mechanism is also known as preconjugation, when the drug undergoes oxidation, reduction and hydrolysis. Oxidation is the most important reaction. Hepatic synthesis of cytochrome P450 enzymes is increased by some classes of drug, a phenomenon known as **enzyme induction**. Enzyme induction increases the rate of phase I reactions. Some drugs cause enzyme inhibition by reducing hepatic enzyme synthesis. These actions lead to reduction or enhancement of the therapeutic effects of drugs, and, particularly when several drugs are administered together, may lead to unwanted side effects. Not all phase I reactions are performed by cytochrome P450 enzymes, some are non-microsomal, located in the hepatic cytoplasm, notably alcohol dehydrogenase and xanthine oxidase (see Ch. 4).
- Phase II metabolic reactions are conjugation reactions where hepatic cytoplasmic enzymes conjugate a phase I metabolite (and sometimes an endogenous substance), most commonly by glucuronidation. The conjugate is nearly always pharmacologically inactive, more water soluble and easily excreted in the urine and/or bile. Conjugation with glutathione is the major pathway for drug detoxification. Unfortunately, some conjugates are more toxic than the parent drug, resulting in hepatotoxicity and potential liver failure. One example is acetaminophen (paracetamol), which taken in overdose is highly toxic (see Information box 4.6, Ch. 4). Some halogenated inhaled general anaesthetics are also hepatotoxic (Ch. 4). Alcohol is toxic to the liver and a major cause of liver disease.

The pharmacokinetics and pharmacodynamics of drugs determine hepatic response. The genes coding for the enzymes, transporters and receptors concerned with drug metabolism vary between individuals, so that each person's response to a drug is variable. Pharmacogenomics, a study of this individual variability, has clinical significance for the future development of medicines.

Immunological functions of the liver

As well as synthesising acute phase proteins necessary for the body's immune mechanisms (see above), immunologically active cells are present in the hepatic reticulo-endothelial system. The body's immune system can be severely impaired when these cells are destroyed in liver disease.

- **Kupffer cells** phagocytose and catalyse bacterial and other antigens absorbed from the gastrointestinal tract, acting as a protective barrier. These antigens are catalysed without the production of antibodies, thus preventing them from reaching and overwhelming other antibody-producing sites.
- The liver also participates in tissue repair. Following challenge from endotoxins, Kupffer cells release cytokines that, in turn, stimulate hepatocytes to release pro-inflammatory cytokines (see Ch. 6).

The liver and hormones

As mentioned previously, steroid hormones are synthesised in the liver. The liver converts inactive hormone to its active form, e.g. cholecalciferol to 25-hydroxycalciferol essential for vitamin D metabolism (see Chs 10 and 16). The liver is also the target for insulin, central for glucose homeostasis (see Ch. 3). The liver inactivates hormones, including insulin, glucagon, glucocorticoids, parathormone, thyroxine, growth and sex hormones. The rate of clearance is variable; for example, insulin is cleared in minutes, steroid hormones take days and thyroxine takes months (see Ch. 10).

Storage function of the liver

The liver is the main storage site for vitamins A, B_{12}, D and K. Iron is stored bound to ferritin in hepatocytes. The liver also functions as a storage site for glycogen.

SOME DISEASES OF THE LIVER

Some clinical conditions resulting from disorders of liver function have already been discussed. In general, liver disease may be the consequence of:

- Hepatocellular damage, when hepatocytes and Kupffer cells are destroyed, and the sinusoids and space of Disse are obliterated. Depending on the cause and severity of the damage, most, if not all, liver functions will be impaired to varying degrees.
- Biliary obstruction, also known as cholestasis, which can occur in small bile ducts intra-hepatically, or in the larger extra-hepatic bile ducts. Jaundice is a clinical manifestation of biliary obstruction and intra-hepatic disease (see Clinical box 15.11).

Hepatocellular disease

Hepatocellular inflammation, known as hepatitis, may be acute or chronic. In acute hepatitis, the portal tracts and lobules are infiltrated by lymphocytes, and the hepatocytes degenerate, become necrotic and are phagocytosed. This is followed by fibrosis when the stellate cells are activated to produce collagen (see above). Depending on cause and severity, single or small groups of cells may be affected (focal or spotty necrosis).

More severe damage leads to limited confluent necrosis with collapse of the acinar and lobular architecture (see Fig. 15.25). Bridges form between central veins and portal tracts, obstructing portal blood flow, which results in portal hypertension (see below). In the worst case, massive liver necrosis occurs involving numerous hepatic lobules with damage to a substantial part of the hepatic parenchyma. Massive liver necrosis results in fulminant hepatic failure,

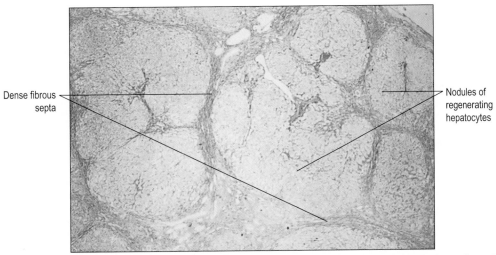

Dense fibrous septa

Nodules of regenerating hepatocytes

Fig. 15.25 **Cirrhosis of the liver.** The specimen is stained with Van Gieson stain so collagen is blue. Note disruption of normal lobular architecture (see Figs 15.23 and 15.24). Courtesy of Dr Gregory J Michael, Institute of Cell and Molecular Science, Barts and The London School of Medicine and Dentistry, Queen Mary University of London.

when encephalopathy develops (see below). Other changes include cholestasis in the acinar metabolic zone 3 and fatty change (steatosis). Steatosis (fatty deposits in hepatocytes) is commonly due to alcoholic hepatitis and drug toxicity.

In chronic hepatitis, lymphoid follicles are present in the portal tracts, which are infiltrated with lymphocytes and plasma cells. Mild to severe inflammation may be present, with further loss of definition in the acinus, changes in the hepatic lobule, confluent necrosis and fibrosis linking (bridging) the portal tracts. See Clinical box 15.15.

Some causes of hepatitis

Table 15.12 summarises the main causes of hepatitis.

Cirrhosis of the liver

The liver is unusual in having the ability to regenerate. Prometheus, the Titan in Greek mythology, was chained to a rock where an eagle ate his liver every day, but he grew a whole new one every night. Some of the pathological features in liver disease are related to cellular regeneration.

Cirrhosis of the liver is a separate entity from hepatitis, although it may be a consequence of hepatocellular damage caused by hepatitis. Hepatic cirrhosis results from hepatocellular necrosis followed by fibrosis, and nodular regeneration. The pathology is characterised by dense fibrous septa surrounding variable-sized nodules of regenerating hepatocytes (Fig.15.25). The normal lobular architecture is disrupted, leading to impaired liver function and obstruction to liver blood flow.

Worldwide, the commonest cause of cirrhosis is viral hepatitis, and the commonest cause of cirrhosis in developed nations is excessive alcohol ingestion. There is no known cure for cirrhosis. Management is aimed at prevention of disease progression and treatment of complications. Occasionally, liver transplantation is the treatment option. See Clinical box 15.16.

Portal hypertension

Portal hypertension is a serious complication of cirrhosis. The portal vein receives blood from the superior mesenteric and splenic veins, with a normal venous pressure of 5–8 mmHg within it. As a consequence of scarring through fibrosis and distortion of lobular architecture, venous blood flow is

> **Clinical box 15.15   Clinical features of hepatocellular failure**
>
> The clinical features of hepatic failure are related to the inability of hepatocytes to perform normal physiological functions for enzyme synthesis, protein and coagulation factor synthesis, metabolism and bile production. Measurement of biochemical markers for dysfunction in liver function tests is done when hepatic failure is suspected (see Clinical box 15.16).
>
> Jaundice (see Clinical box 15.14) is not strictly a consequence of hepatocellular failure, but of biliary obstruction from whatever cause. Intra-hepatic biliary obstruction, however, may be a consequence of cirrhosis and hepatitis, when there is distortion of normal hepatic architecture.
>
> Hepatocellular failure may be classified as chronic or acute. Chronic hepatic failure is most commonly seen in cirrhosis, which potentially has many causes, including hepatitis and alcohol misuse. Some patients with chronic hepatitis or in the early stages of cirrhosis may be asymptomatic, but biochemical tests may be abnormal. For example, macrocytosis (abnormal lipid synthesis) and an elevated γ-glutamyltransferase (cholestasis) may be the only clues to alcohol overuse. Other biochemical markers of liver function may be abnormal. Histology ranges from mild to moderate inflammation to cirrhosis, when features of portal hypertension, ascites and porto-systemic encephalopathy may develop progressively.
>
> Primary biliary cirrhosis is a condition in which there is progressive destruction of the bile canaliculi, resulting in cholestasis and eventually hepatocellular necrosis. Over time, this leads to fibrosis, cirrhosis and hepatic failure. The condition predominantly affects women, with onset at over 40 years of age. The aetiology is unknown, but autoimmune mechanisms have been implicated.
>
> Acute hepatic failure occurs when encephalopathy develops over a short period in patients with apparently normal livers. Acute hepatic failure is further classified as subacute when the encephalopathy develops from 2 to 12 weeks of the onset of symptoms (e.g. jaundice), and fulminant when encephalopathy develops in less than 2 weeks. Fulminant hepatic failure occasionally develops in patients with previous liver disease.
>
> Encephalopathy may be indicated by symptoms of altered mental state, such as confusion, disorientation and drowsiness, but may progress to hepatic coma, cerebral oedema and death. A peculiar smell, fetor hepaticus (an offensive odour due to liver disease), may be present on the patient's breath, caused by the presence of volatile, aromatic products of metabolism that accumulate in the blood and are excreted in expired breath.

Table 15.12	Causes of hepatitis	
Cause	**Acute hepatitis**	**Chronic hepatitis**
Viral	Hepatitis A–E: commonest cause of acute hepatitis is hepatitis A virus	Hepatitis B (sometimes plus hepatitis D), hepatitis C
	Epstein–Barr virus (infectious mononucleosis)	
	Cytomegalovirus	
	Yellow fever	
	Herpes simplex	
	Mumps	
	Rubella	
Non-viral, parasitic	Toxoplasmosis	Schistosomiasis
Drugs	Analgesics, e.g. paracetamol	Anti-tuberculosis, e.g. isoniazid
	Halogenated anaesthetics	Antibiotics, e.g. nitrofurantoin, ketoconazole
		Anti-epileptics, e.g. sodium valproate
		Antihypertensives, e.g. methyldopa, amiodarone
		Alcohol (rare)
Autoimmune		Associated with pernicious anaemia, Coombs' +ve haemolytic anaemia, thyroiditis
Genetic		Wilson's disease
		Gilbert's syndrome
		Hereditary haemochromatosis
		Non-alcoholic fatty liver
Other		Chronic hepatitis of unknown cause
		Inflammatory bowel disease (e.g. ulcerative colitis) gives rise to sclerosing cholangitis with subsequent hepatocellular damage, thus it is strictly a biliary tract disease, and not hepatitis

and sodium retention as the consequence of peripheral arterial vasodilatation. Some factors contributing to the formation of ascites include:

- Portal hypertension: this causes a rise in local hydrostatic pressure, which results in increased venous pressure in the capillary beds servicing the intestines and spleen, leading to increased hepatic and splanchnic lymph production and fluid transudation into the peritoneal cavity.
- Increased venous pressure in the splanchnic capillary bed: this reduces water absorption leading to the accumulation of extracellular fluid in the peritoneum. Hypoalbuminaemia due to failure of hepatic albumin synthesis also reduces plasma oncotic pressure, which further reduces water absorption.

Porto-systemic encephalopathy

- Porto-systemic encephalopathy is a neuropsychiatric condition seen in fulminant hepatic failure and advanced cirrhosis, which is potentially reversible, but may lead to coma and death.
- Failure of the liver to metabolise toxic endogenous (e.g. ammonia) and exogenous (e.g. drugs) substances results in an accumulation of these substances in the blood, which circulate to the central nervous system with consequent encephalopathy.
- In portal hypertension, portal blood bypasses the liver through the collaterals, to deliver toxic metabolites directly to the brain, leading to encephalopathy.

GALL BLADDER

The functions of the gall bladder are the storage, concentration and discharge of bile into the intestine. Bile leaving the liver in the hepatic duct between meals is diverted into the gall bladder as a consequence of the closure of the sphincter of Oddi. The gall bladder musculature relaxes to receive

obstructed, elevating portal pressure. When the portal venous pressure rises above 10–12 mmHg, porto-systemic anastomoses occur in the systemic venous system at sites where the venous system is pliant and collaterals are formed. Dilated collaterals are known as varices. The main sites for porto-systemic anastomoses include the gastro-oesophageal junction (oesophageal varices), the rectum (haemorrhoids), and the anterior abdominal wall via the umbilical vein (caput medusae – visible on inspection of the abdomen as snake-like varices radiating from the umbilicus). Oesophageal varices are thin-walled and superficial, thus likely to rupture, causing life-threatening haemorrhage, which may be compounded by coagulation defects.

Ascites

The presence of extracellular fluid in the peritoneal cavity is known as ascites. The mechanisms through which ascites accumulates are uncertain, but possibly include renal water the bile. The human gall bladder can accommodate to hold 20–50 mL of bile. Hepatic biliary secretion between meals is about 450 mL.

Bile is concentrated in the gall bladder

In the gall bladder the volume of bile is reduced and concentrated (Fig. 15.21D). The gall bladder concentrates the bile by reabsorbing Na^+, Cl^- and water. Na^+ and Cl^- ions, in the gall bladder lumen, are exchanged for protons and bicarbonate ions, respectively, from the cytoplasm of the epithelial cells. The Na^+ ions are removed from the epithelial cell along the basolateral border by the Na^+ pump. Chloride ions exit the cell via Cl^- channels in these membranes. The observation that the intercellular spaces dilate when fluid is being absorbed suggests that this is the route of fluid absorption. The accumulation of salt in the intercellular space will create an osmotic gradient for the transfer of water from the lumen of the gall bladder. Water passes from the lumen through channels in the membranes and between the cells along this gradient. The resulting solution becomes diluted as it flows towards and through the basement membrane of the epithelium and into capillaries.

The overall result is that the many components of gall bladder bile are more concentrated compared with hepatic bile (see Table 15.11). The bile remains isotonic to plasma because the micelle concentration increases. The aggregates of salts, phospholipids and cholesterol in the micelles have only a small osmotic activity.

The protons secreted by the gall bladder epithelium decrease bile pH and increase the solubility of calcium salts. In turn, this action reduces the possibility of gall stone formation caused by the precipitation of calcium salts. Epithelial cells also secrete mucus to protect their apical membranes from the damaging effects of bile salts. Excessive mucus secretion may contribute to gall stone formation. See Information box 15.8.

Emptying of the gall bladder

Neural and hormonal mechanisms control the emptying of the gall bladder and the expulsion of bile into the intestine during a meal. Vagal nerves release acetylcholine to cause gall bladder contraction during the cephalic phase of digestion. Fats in the small intestine stimulate the secretion of **cholecystokinin** which in turn causes smooth muscle contraction in the gall bladder and relaxation of the sphincter of Oddi to allow bile flow along the common bile duct into the intestine. Bile empties into the duodenum during periods in which the musculature is relaxed.

Enterohepatic circulation of bile salts

The liver does not have the capacity to synthesise de novo the quantity of bile salts needed to aid the digestion of fat in each day's meals, so the bile salts have to be recycled from the intestine to meet this need. The enterocytes along the length of most of the intestine are impermeable to conjugated bile salts. This effect maintains a high concentration of bile salts to promote fat digestion and absorption, which is usually complete before the terminal ileum is reached by the chyme.

The enterocytes of the terminal ileum possess transport mechanisms for conjugated and non-conjugated bile salts. A Na^+-dependent bile salt transporter is present in the brush border of the enterocytes that preferentially absorbs the negatively charged conjugated bile salts. The absorbed bile salts probably leave the epithelial cells by an anion exchanger.

Non-conjugated bile salts may be passively absorbed if they become protonated, which removes their negative charges, increasing their lipid solubility. Passive absorption accounts for about 10% of the recycling of the bile salts that can occur along the length of the small intestine and colon. The bile salts are transported in the hepatic portal vein to the liver where they are again extracted and secreted into the bile.

Bile salts that escape absorption from the small intestine are metabolised by colonic bacteria. This can involve deconjugation, which increases their lipid solubility and reabsorption. In addition, bacteria are responsible for the conversion of primary bile acids to secondary bile acids, which may be absorbed. Approximately 5% of the bile salts entering the duodenum are excreted each day. The liver synthesises this quantity each day to make up for the loss. Increases in bile salt excretion are matched by increases in the synthesis in order to maintain the bile salt pool.

Information box 15.8 Gall stones

Raised concentrations of bile salts, bile pigment (bilirubin from the breakdown of haem) and/or cholesterol may lead to precipitation of these substances in the biliary tree or gall bladder, causing irritation and the formation of gall stones.

- Irritation of the gall bladder wall gives rise to chemical cholecystitis and inflammation
- Gall stones cause obstruction in the biliary tree with an increased risk of infection – ascending cholangitis and cholecystitis, with further formation of gall stones
- Obstruction to the common bile duct prevents the secretion of bile into the small intestine so that fat digestion and absorption would be impaired
- Common bile duct obstruction also prevents the excretion of bilirubin, resulting in clinical jaundice
- The retention of some drugs and poisons normally excreted in bile could lead to toxicity and other adverse effects.

SMALL INTESTINE

The small intestine is the major site for the digestion and absorption of food, salts, water and orally administered drugs. The small intestine consists of the:

- Duodenum
- Jejunum
- Ileum.

It serves to:

- Mix digestive secretions with food and propel chyme along the intestine
- Digest and absorb nutrients
- Absorb the constituents of digestive secretions
- Regulate gastric function
- Synthesise and secrete hormones influencing feeding and gastric function
- Defend the body against invasion by microorganisms.

	Brunner's glands	Circular folds	Crypt of Lieberkühn	Villus shape	Paneth cells	Peyer's patches
Table 15.13						

Table 15.13 Structural features of the duodenum, jejunum and ileum

	Brunner's glands	Circular folds	Crypt of Lieberkühn	Villus shape	Paneth cells	Peyer's patches
Duodenum	++	+	+	Broad and short	+	+
Jejunum	–		+	Long finger-like	+	+
Ileum	–	+	+	Short finger-like	+	+

+, present; ++, present and distinguishing feature; –, absent.

STRUCTURE OF THE SMALL INTESTINE

The generalised structure of the alimentary canal was outlined above. The small intestine is 4–7 m in length. The duodenum is 25–30 cm in length and is recognised externally by an absence of mesentery. There are histological differences between the duodenum, jejunum and ileum (Table 15.13). The surface area of the mucosa is increased by the presence of outgrowths of the submucosa to form circular folds, the plicae circularis or valves of Kerkring, on which are found finger-like projections known as villi. The surface area of the luminal border of the enterocytes is enlarged by the presence of microvilli that create a large surface area for the final stages of digestion and absorption. The total increase in surface area of the intestine produced by the folding of the submucosa, mucosa and enterocyte surface is 600 times that of a cylinder with the same internal dimensions as the small intestine.

The villi contain smooth muscle fibres arranged along the length of their core which are attached to the central lacteal, a blind-ended lymph vessel. Contraction and relaxation of the muscle changes the length of the villi and in the process propel lymph along the lacteal vessels. Lymph flows into the lymphatic vessels in the submucosa and onwards through the abdomen to the thoracic lymph duct, which empties its contents into the junction of the left subclavian and internal jugular veins.

The intestinal glands or crypts of Lieberkühn are simple tubular glands lying between the bases of the villi. The crypts contain **stem**, **entero-endocrine** and **Paneth cells**. The stem cells become differentiated into enterocytes and goblet cells as they migrate from the crypts to the tip of the villus. The cells take 3–6 days to reach the tip of the villus where they are extruded and become part of the intestinal juice (succus entericus). The crypts are the source of the intestinal juice, an alkaline fluid similar in composition to extracellular fluid, containing the enzyme enteropeptidase which is responsible for activating trypsinogen. The intestinal juice also contains digestive enzymes derived from extruded enterocytes. The enterocytes begin to synthesise digestive enzymes, develop microvilli and become absorptive cells as they migrate along the villus.

Entero-endocrine cells play a role controlling digestion and local defence mechanisms. They synthesise and secrete intestinal hormones, e.g. cholecystokinin and secretin, and local hormones, e.g. 5-hydroxytryptamine (serotonin). Mechanical stimulation of enterochromaffin cells by the passage of the intestinal contents (chyme, parasites, bacteria) releases 5-hydroxytryptamine and leads to activation of the enteric reflexes, leading to, for example, intestinal fluid secretion and peristalsis. Chemical stimulation of enterochromaffin cells and release of 5-hydroxytryptamine by some anti-cancer drugs produces vomiting via stimulation of vagal nerve sensory pathways.

The Paneth cells are part of the intestinal defence system against bacteria and parasites. These cells secrete tumour necrosis factor-α (TNF-α), lysozyme and defensins. TNF-α produces inflammation in response to bacteria and parasites. Lysozyme destroys the peptidoglycan bonds in bacterial membranes leading to an influx of water and rupture of the bacteria. Defensins are proteins that produce ion channels in the cell membranes of invading organisms to increase their permeability.

The ileum contains **Peyer's patches** in the submucosa, and they extend into the mucosa where they are covered by an epithelial layer, containing enterocytes, M cells and **dendritic cells**. The M and dendritic cells are capable of taking up antigens and transferring them by exocytosis to the interstitial fluid for processing by macrophages, T and B lymphocytes. Processed antigens produce an immune reaction. The centre of the Peyer's patch contains a germinal centre for proliferating B cells. The Peyer's patches form part of the gut-associated lymphoid tissue (GALT), which includes lymphocytes found between epithelial cells in the intestinal mucosa and in the lamina propria of the mucosa, together with mast cells. The plasma cells secrete IgA antibodies which are transferred by enterocytes to the intestinal lumen, where they react with bacteria and toxins to prevent them becoming attached to epithelial cells. These immunological mechanisms and the non-immunological mechanisms, such as gastric acid secretion, intestinal fluid and mucus secretion, and peristalsis, assist in the defence of the body from luminal pathogens (see Ch. 6).

SMALL INTESTINAL FLUID SECRETION

The enterocytes in the crypts of Lieberkühn are responsible for intestinal fluid secretion. The volume of fluid produced is 1–2 L/day. The production of intestinal fluid secretion is driven by Cl^- secretion from enterocytes. The $Na^+/K^+/Cl^-$ transporter in the basolateral border transfers Cl^- into the cell from the interstitial fluid. The inward movement of the transporter occurs secondary to the action of the Na^+/K^+-ATPase which maintains a low Na^+ concentration in the cell. Cl^- enters the lumen of the intestine by diffusion through Cl^- channels in the apical membrane. These Cl^- channels are a protein known as the cystic fibrosis transmembrane regulator (CFTR). K^+ leaves the cell through K^+ channels in the basolateral border. The intestinal lumen become electronegative and that leads to the flow of Na^+ from the interstitial fluid through paracellular pathways (tight junctions). The movement of NaCl results in an osmotic gradient and the movement of water into the intestine.

In the absence of stimulation there is little fluid secretion. Intestinal fluid secretion is regulated by:

- The enteric nervous system
- Hormones
- Enterotoxins.

Chloride secretion is primarily controlled by the submucosal plexus of the enteric nervous system. Mechanical stimulation of enterochromaffin cells leads to the release of

5-hydroxytryptamine which stimulates sensory neurons to activate secretomotor neurons terminating on enterocytes. The neurotransmitters stimulating the enterocytes are acetylcholine and VIP, via muscarinic M_3 and VIP receptors, respectively. Axon reflexes within the mucosa may also stimulate secretion via substance P acting on neurokinin 1 (NK_1) receptors on the enterocytes. Mechanical stimulation of the mucosa also releases prostaglandins, which stimulate the secretomotor neurons. The intracellular messengers for acetylcholine and VIP are Ca^{2+} and cAMP, respectively. The elevation of the intracellular concentration of Ca^{2+} and cAMP leads to stimulation of the enterocytes and fluid secretion.

The intestinal hormone, guanylin, stimulates the guanylin receptor on the apical border of the enterocyte to increase the activity on guanylate cyclase and increase the intracellular concentration of cyclic guanosine monophosphate. This also leads to the opening of the Cl^- channels in the apical membrane. Antigen–antibody reactions at mast cells in the lamina propria and stimulation of these cells by substance P released during axon reflexes lead to histamine release. Histamine stimulates secretion by a direct effect on histamine receptors on the enterocytes and indirectly via cholinergic nerves.

Finally, bacterial toxins (enterotoxins) stimulate enterocytes both directly and by means of enteric reflexes.

SMALL INTESTINAL MOTILITY

In between meals the small intestine undergoes periodic contractile activity at intervals lasting 80–90 minutes. The propulsive waves (known as the migrating motor complexes, MMC) begin in the stomach (see above) and sweep along the small intestine, clearing it of debris and bacteria. Each MMC consists of four phases:

- **Phase I** – a prolonged quiescent period (45–60 minutes) with slow waves.
- **Phase II** – a period (30–35 minutes) of action potentials, apparently randomly superimposed on the slow waves, and sporadic contractions. This phase is associated with gastric acid, bile and pancreatic juice secretion.
- **Phase III** – a period (2–12 minutes) of activity with action potentials superimposed on each slow wave and regular contractions at the rate of 3 per minute in the stomach and 10–12 per minute in the small intestine.
- **Phase IV** – a period in which action potential production and contractile activity reduces and merges into phase I.

The MMC also prevents reflux of bacteria from the large intestine to the terminal ileum. The MMC has been described as the 'housekeeper of the small intestine'. However, within a few minutes of feeding this type of motility ceases.

The small intestine receives chyme from the stomach and digestive secretions from the pancreas, biliary tract and intestinal mucosa. The function of small intestinal motility after eating is to:

- Mix the nutrients in the chyme with the digestive secretions
- Bring the chyme into contact with the epithelial cells to promote the final stages of digestion
- Regulate the rate at which chyme is propelled along the small intestine to the caecum.

Two types of small intestinal motility are needed to fulfil these objectives. Mixing of the chyme with the secretions and bringing the mixture into contact with the mucosa is achieved by the process of **segmentation** (Fig. 15.18B). This is achieved by contractions of the circular muscle layer at short intervals along the intestine. The intestine in between the contracted regions is relaxed. The chyme is propelled a short distance orally and aborally from a point of contraction. The contracted circular muscles relax and are replaced by contractions in the formerly relaxed region. This type of motility will not be very effective in propelling chyme along the intestine to the caecum. It is, however, effective in mixing the chyme with secretions and in breaking up the unstirred layer of fluid adjacent to the epithelial cells to aid nutrient absorption.

Peristalsis propels chyme along the small intestine. This is achieved by contraction of the circular muscle layer on the oral side of the bolus of chyme and relaxation on the aboral side (Fig. 15.18C). The contractile action of the musculature pushes the bolus into the adjacent area of the intestine which is ready to receive it. Peristalsis consists of a repeated pattern of contraction and relaxation of the circular muscle layer of the small intestine. The peristaltic response is controlled by nerves in the enteric nervous system. Distension of the wall of the intestine stimulates mechanoreceptors in the mucosa and muscle layers that synapse with excitatory and inhibitory neural pathways, producing contraction of the circular muscle and relaxation of the longitudinal muscle layers at the point of stimulation. The reflex spreads into the adjoining region ahead of the bolus with the longitudinal muscles being stimulated to contract and the circular muscles to relax to create a dilated region to receive the bolus of chyme. Entry of the bolus stimulates the sensory receptors and the reflex is repeated to propel the bolus along the intestine.

As has been described for the stomach, smooth muscle cells in the small intestine are associated with slow waves of depolarisation to a plateau, followed by repolarisation. Action potentials superimposed on the plateau lead to a contraction. Slow waves are detected in adjacent parts of the intestine and are related in time but do not always give rise to action potentials. A region showing slow waves with action potentials may be separated from another one by a region with slow wave activity alone. This pattern of electrical activity is consistent with segmentation. Interstitial cells of Cajal generate slow wave activity. The frequency of slow waves in the duodenum is about 12 per minute, slowing to 10 per minute in the jejunum and 9 per minute in the ileum. This decline in frequency of pacemaker activity along the intestine is known as the **intestinal gradient**.

Intestino-intestinal inhibitory reflex

If a region of the intestine becomes distended or obstructed, contractile muscle activity in adjacent regions are inhibited. This is a response known as the intestino-intestinal reflex and depends upon the activation of sympathetic nerves via the coeliac ganglion and spinal cord.

Gastro-ileal reflex

An increase in gastric activity during a meal leads to the gastro-ileal reflex in which propulsive activity of the terminal ileum is increased and its contents are emptied into the caecum via the relaxed ileo-caecal sphincter. This reflex response may be mediated by the extrinsic innervation of the ileum. The gastric antral hormone gastrin

As the small intestine is the major site for digestion and absorption, disease would lead to malabsorption. The intestinal villi become flattened, greatly decreasing the surface area for water and nutrient absorption. The increased amount of partially digested nutrients and electrolytes in the intestinal contents make it hypertonic, thus drawing more water into the intestine, and further increasing the volume. Diarrhoea ensues, and if fats are not absorbed, steatorrhoea. Severe weight loss and vitamin deficiency may occur from malnutrition. Causes include:

- Infection – which may be acute or chronic, from gastrointestinal infections and infestations (e.g. *Giardia*), dysentery, cholera, human immunodeficiency virus (HIV) enteropathy, tuberculosis. The diarrhoea may be produced by enterotoxins. For example, the profuse diarrhoea and electrolyte imbalance in cholera is cause by the stimulation of Cl⁻ secretion by the irreversible activation of G proteins by cholera toxin. This leads to fluid loss via increased cAMP in enterocytes.
- Inflammation – which may be autoimmune, associated with connective tissue disorders (e.g. rheumatoid arthritis), ulcerative colitis, regional ileitis (Crohn's disease), gluten sensitive enteropathy (coeliac disease) leads to enterocyte destruction and loss of function.
  - Gluten sensitive enteropathy (coeliac disease) is an autoimmune, inflammatory disease of the upper small intestine. The immune response is triggered by exposure to the protein gliadin, contained in the gluten of cereals.
  - Crohn's disease, or regional ileitis, which affects the whole bowel, and ulcerative colitis, which affects the large bowel. The aetiology is not known, but may be associated with genetic predisposition, immunity and nutritional or infective factors. The inflammation may extend through all the layers of the intestine, and ulceration may occur (mainly in ulcerative colitis) leading to bloody diarrhoea.
- Ischaemic – occlusion of arterial or venous blood flow, which occurs more often in the elderly.
- Tumours – either tumours of the small intestine (e.g. adenocarcinoma, carcinoid tumour, polyps – Peutz–Jeghers syndrome), or more distal tumours causing abnormalities in enzyme or other secretions (e.g. Zollinger–Ellison syndrome).
- Radiation – radiation enteritis occurs after pelvic radiation with symptoms of diarrhoea and abdominal pain. This usually resolves after completion of treatment.
- Surgery/trauma – intestinal resection, especially after massive resection.
- Drugs – particularly antibiotics (e.g. amoxicillin), and rarely antibiotic-associated colitis due to damage by toxins produced by *Clostridium difficile*, bacteria and drugs that bind to bile salts (e.g. cholestyramine).

and duodenal hormone cholecystokinin have also been implicated in the response. These hormones increase contractile activity in the ileum and relax the ileo-caecal sphincter.

Interruption of the extrinsic innervation of the ileum, as in surgical vagotomy for peptic ulceration, may give rise to chronic diarrhoea. See Clinical box 15.17.

LARGE INTESTINE

The main function of the large intestine is to absorb water and electrolytes, and to evacuate faeces. The large intestine consists of the:

- Caecum
- Ascending, transverse, descending and sigmoid colon
- Rectum
- Anal canal.

The large intestine serves to:

- Absorb salt and water to produce semi-solid or solid faeces
- Absorb short chain fatty acids produced by colonic bacteria from unabsorbed carbohydrate entering the colon
- Act as a store for faeces
- Expel the faeces.

The mucosa of the colon does not have folds or villi like the small intestine but has numerous tubular glands (crypts of Lieberkühn). These are deeper than in the small intestine (0.4–0.6 mm) and are lined with many goblet cells, enterocytes, stem cells and entero-endocrine cells. The surface enterocytes have microvilli and an absorptive role.

LARGE INTESTINAL FLUID SECRETION

The secretions of the large intestine are similar to those found in the small intestine. However, the volume produced is less and the K^+ and HCO_3^- content is increased together with more mucus. K^+ enters the colonic secretion by both passive and active mechanisms. In the lumen a negative, transepithelial potential difference of up to 25 mV is enough to produce a diffusion of K^+ from the interstitial spaces through the tight junctions to the lumen. Active K^+ secretion occurs as a result of K^+ channels opening in the apical membrane and K^+ diffusion to the intestine. Uptake of K^+ at the basolateral membrane is due to the action of the $Na^+/K^+/Cl^-$ transporter and the Na^+/K^+-ATPase. Aldosterone increases the opening of the K^+ channels in the apical membrane. In addition, aldosterone enhances the absorption of Na^+ from the intestinal lumen leading to a rise in luminal negativity and an increase in passive secretion. It also stimulates the Na^+/K^+-ATPase, subsequently producing a greater active secretion of K^+. VIP and cholera enterotoxin, via an increase in intracellular cAMP, stimulate K^+ secretion. 5-Hydroxytryptamine stimulates a rise in intracellular Ca^{2+}, which also opens apical K^+ channels and promotes secretion. Faecal losses of K^+ by these mechanisms may be significant in secretory diarrhoea.

MUSCULATURE OF THE LARGE INTESTINE

The smooth muscle is arranged in an outer longitudinal and inner circular layers. The longitudinal muscle layer from the caecum to the rectum does not completely cover the large intestine but is arranged in three bands known as the **taeniae coli**. The layer fans out to cover the rectum. The circular muscle layer is continuous from the caecum to the anal canal. The layer becomes thicker to form the internal anal sphincter, which lies adjacent to the external anal sphincter composed of striated muscle.

LARGE INTESTINAL MOTILITY

The large intestine functions as two organs. The proximal part, consisting of the ascending and transverse colon, is the site for the bacterial production of fatty acids and their absorption together with electrolytes and water. Approximately 1.5 L of chyme per day enters the colon from the ileum. The water content of the faeces is 50–150 mL per day. The absorbed water contributes to the maintenance of water balance by the body. Absorption of fluid is aided by the segmental-like activity of the musculature. The colon is divided into segments known as **haustra**. Sequential circular muscle contraction and relaxation cause the position of the haustral folds to change after many minutes. This rate of change of position of the haustra contrasts with the more rapid changes in the position of small intestinal segments, which only last for seconds. This type of motility promotes fluid absorption.

The distal part of the colon (descending and recto-sigmoid region) is responsible for the final drying of the faeces and storage before defecation. The contractile movements of sigmoid colon cause retention of the colonic contents in the descending colon. This activity promotes drying of the faeces and a reduction in their volume. The faeces may be retained in the colon for 36 hours or longer in healthy people. In some cases of constipation the contractile activity of the sigmoid colon is enhanced and is absent in diarrhoea. These observations support the view that the contractile activity of the sigmoid colon promotes water absorption from the faeces.

One to three times a day, a propulsive motility described as **a mass movement** drives the faeces in an anal direction. The haustra and segmental activity are abolished for the duration of a mass movement. Mass movements are responsible for propelling faeces into the rectum. Filling of the rectum stimulates sensory receptors that give rise to the desire to defecate. The pattern of colonic motility is similar in both the fed and interdigestive states.

The regulation of colonic motility depends on the interstitial cells of Cajal giving rise to slow wave activity leading to contraction and their modification by the action of the intrinsic and extrinsic nerves. As in other parts of the alimentary canal there are intrinsic nerves with inhibitory and excitatory action on the smooth muscle. These nerves promote mixing and propulsive activity. The excitatory extrinsic innervation is via the vagus and pelvic nerves, with acetylcholine being the major neurotransmitter. The inhibitory extrinsic innervation is provided by the lumbar and sacral branches of the sympathetic nervous system terminating in the intramural plexuses. These nerves tonically inhibit colonic motility via the neurotransmitter norepinephrine. Feeding and distension of the upper regions of the gastrointestinal tract lead to **gastrocolonic reflexes**, in which mass movements are induced via the extrinsic nerve pathways. The afferent pathway is not well defined. The efferent pathway involves the vagus and pelvic nerves to the proximal and distal parts of the colon, respectively. In addition, the hormones gastrin and cholecystokinin are capable of stimulating colonic smooth muscle and may contribute to the response. Distension of the upper colon produces a **colono-colonic reflex** in which activity via the intrinsic nerves and extrinsic sympathetic nerves from the superior and inferior mesenteric ganglia leads to relaxation of the colon. See Clinical box 15.18.

MOTILITY OF THE RECTUM AND ANAL CANAL

During most of the day the upper portion of the rectum generates segmental activity, which tends to prevent emptying of the colonic contents into the rectum. These movements ensure that the rectum is usually empty. The levator ani muscles making up the pelvic floor are contracted and hold the rectum at

Clinical box 15.18 **Some clinical conditions associated with large intestine disorders**

Many conditions of the large bowel are associated with anatomical abnormalities. Diverticular disease is a common condition in the colon (up to 50% of the population over age 50). Although the precise aetiology is unknown, it appears that the high intraluminal pressure causes colonic mucosa to extrude through weak areas of musculature (usually near blood vessels) to form pouches, or diverticula. The diverticula could be obstructed by faecal material leading to infection and inflammation: diverticulitis. One serious complication is perforation leading to peritonitis.

Ulcerative colitis is an autoimmune inflammatory bowel disease affecting the colonic mucosa. Ischemia may occur in the colon, as in the small intestine. Other conditions are associated with neuromuscular incoordination. Hirschprung's disease in young children under age 1 is due to an aganglionic segment of the rectum leading to constipation and subacute obstruction with megacolon.

an angle of about 90° to the anal canal. This angle helps to maintain continence. The anal canal is tightly closed by the anal sphincters. The rectum fills following a mass movement from the descending and sigmoid colon. Distension of the rectum leads to the urge to defecate. The rectum acts as a storage organ.

DEFECATION

The presence of gas or faeces in the rectum stimulates stretch receptors in its wall and, via the myenteric plexus, stimulates a mass movement in the sigmoid colon and rectum, initiating the **rectosphincteric reflex**. This involves a reflex relaxation of the smooth muscle of the internal anal sphincter and contraction of the striated muscle of the external anal sphincter in order to maintain continence for up to a minute. The rectal contents enter the upper anal canal, producing sensory information that distinguishes between gas, liquid or solid, probably on the basis of the amount of distension produced. Defecation will occur if the circumstances are appropriate and the external anal sphincter relaxes.

Defecation is a reflex activity and is subject to conscious control (Fig. 15.26). The sacral region of the spinal cord (segments S2–S4) acts to integrate signals from the brain with those from stretch receptors in the rectal wall via afferent fibres in the pelvic nerves. Descending pathways from the cerebral cortex inhibit the somatic motor nerve activity in the pudendal nerves that innervate the external anal sphincter. The tonic flow of nerve impulses to the sphincter producing contraction is interrupted. The external anal sphincter relaxes and peristaltic activity of the rectum expels the faeces. Adopting a squatting position and lowering of the pelvic floor levator ani muscles allows the rectum to come into line with the anal canal. Expulsion of the faeces is aided by the development of high intrathoracic pressure produced by an inspiration followed by expiration against a closed glottis (Valsalva's manoeuvre) with contraction of the abdominal muscles. The intra-abdominal pressure can rise to 200 cm H_2O with the effect of squeezing the wall of the rectum and anal canal to aid expulsion of the faeces. In addition, this high intra-abdominal pressure reduces venous return to the heart with possible temporary adverse consequences on blood pressure and the circulation.

If the circumstances are inappropriate the act of defecation is postponed. The internal sphincter contracts and the

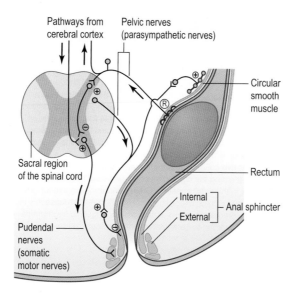

Pathways from cerebral cortex

Pelvic nerves (parasympathetic nerves)

Circular smooth muscle

Sacral region of the spinal cord

Rectum

Internal
External
Anal sphincter

Pudendal nerves (somatic motor nerves)

⊕ Stimulation   ⊖ Inhibition   ® Mechanoreceptor

Stimulation of distention sensitive mechanoreceptors produces a reflex contraction on the colonic side of the faeces and a relaxation of the internal and external anal sphincters via the pelvic and pudendal nerves. Pathways from the cerebral cortex can oppose this reflex.

Fig. 15.26 **Postulated neural mechanism for defecation.**

Clinical box 15.19 | **Constipation**

Constipation is a complex phenomenon, and is very common. A low dietary fibre intake is a common cause, as are drugs such as diuretics, analgesics and anticholinergic drugs. It occurs more often in the elderly. Increasing dietary fibre and fluid intake often relieves constipation. However, it is sometimes associated with serious bowel disease (e.g. intestinal obstruction, colonic cancer, ulcerative colitis), when a change in bowel habit or alternating diarrhoea and constipation are the more significant symptoms. Rarely, a dilated 'megacolon' occurs with chronic constipation. In young patients and children, constipation and megacolon may be due to the presence of an aganglionic rectal segment giving rise to chronic constipation (**Hirschsprung's disease**) caused by a failure in development of neural crest cells to migrate to parts of the intestine.

Training small children into a regular bowel habit of defecating at particular times of the day relies on the gastro-colonic reflex, when a natural, large peristalsis is most likely to occur in the colon, inducing defecation.

---

rectal contents are returned to the colon by retroperistalsis. The sensation to defecate disappears. The faeces are subject to further desiccation and reduction in volume in the colon. Repetition of these events may lead to constipation as the volume of the faeces is reduced and they are less effective at stimulating the stretch receptors in the rectal wall. See Clinical box 15.19.

16

Diet and nutrition

Amrutha Ramu, Penny Neild and Jeannette Naish

Introduction	749
DIET	**750**
Worldwide dietary patterns and food guides	**750**
Food guides	750
Food labelling	750
Dietary reference values	751
Nutritional requirements	**751**
Variations in nutritional requirements	752
NUTRITIONAL STATUS	**754**
Clinical assessment of nutritional status	**754**
Food intake	754
'Usual weight' and weight loss/gain	754
Body mass index	755
Children	**755**
Measures of body composition: adults	**755**
Estimating body fat	755
Other measurements of nutritional status	**756**
Plasma proteins	756
Vitamin status	756
Muscle strength	756
Immunological skin testing	756
Malnutrition screening tools	756
Energy and nitrogen balance	**756**
Conversion of macronutrients to energy	756
Energy balance	757
Nitrogen balance and protein requirements	759

MICRONUTRIENTS AND WATER	**765**
Vitamins	**765**
Water-soluble vitamins	765
Fat-soluble vitamins	766
Trace elements: minerals	**767**
Iron	767
Copper	767
Zinc	768
Selenium	768
Magnesium	768
Calcium	768
Phosphate	768
Iodine	768
Fluoride	769
Water and electrolytes	**769**
Water	769
Electrolytes	769
Water and electrolyte depletion	769
Water overload	770
THE CONTROL OF FOOD INTAKE	**771**
Appetite and satiety	**771**
The physiological control of eating	**771**
Peripheral satiety signals	771
Peripheral hunger signals	772
Long-term satiety signals	772
Diet and disease	**773**
Association between diet and disease	773
Diet and carcinogenesis	774
Nutrition and cancer treatment	775
Diet and cardiovascular disease	775
Malnutrition	779
Obesity	780

INTRODUCTION

In 2003, the Director General of the World Health Organization (WHO) unequivocally stated that 'proper nutrition and health are fundamental human rights'. Good nutrition underpins human health in the sense that it influences growth, physical and intellectual development and the ability to combat disease processes. 'Bad nutrition' or malnutrition, whether overnutrition (obesity) or undernutrition, is a major determinant of morbidity and mortality. Knowledge of the principles of nutrition is vital to the understanding of the prevention, diagnosis and treatment of clinical conditions.

DIET

WORLDWIDE DIETARY PATTERNS AND FOOD GUIDES

Eating habits and dietary patterns vary greatly according to demographic and cultural factors. Historically, most people in the developing world have consumed bulky low-energy diets where half or more of the total energy is supplied by cereals, starchy roots or fruits. Since industrialisation, most people in the developed world have increasingly consumed energy-dense diets, in which less than 25% of the total energy comes from cereals, and consumption of fats, alcohol, meat and dairy products is increased.

Although there is still great disparity between the developed and the developing world's dietary patterns, this distinction has been blurring since the 1970s and 1980s, as the developing world has also become increasingly industrialised. The Food and Agriculture Organization (FAO) of the United Nations was founded in 1945 to collect, analyse, interpret and disseminate information relating to nutrition, food, agriculture, forestry and fisheries. The FAO publishes the world food survey every 10 years. Figure 16.1 shows past and predicted changes in dietary patterns in developing countries. Diets in developing areas have become more energy-dense at the same time as the populations have become less physically active. In contrast, despite the huge and still increasing problems with obesity in the developed world, a significant minority of health-conscious people are choosing to consume relatively bulky, low energy-dense diets and may also engage in physically active recreation.

FOOD GUIDES

Many countries have developed their own dietary guides. These are often pictorial representations of nutrition recommendations and are usually regularly revised and updated. The food guides are a simple way of summarising the recommended balance of foods in the diet and provide a consistent message regarding dietary advice for the public. Examples can be found on the websites of the various national institutions for nutrition policy.

FOOD LABELLING

In most developed countries, there is public awareness of the healthy eating messages: the connections between diet, health and disease. However, to act on this knowledge, the general population needs nutritional information on specific foods, particularly on processed foods. Therefore, food labelling, quantifying the main nutrients, is important. In the UK (Fig. 16.2), such labelling is compulsory if a nutritional advantage is claimed for the product.

In recent years, manufacturers have started to include more nutritional labels with their products. In the European Union (EU), all food labelling is controlled principally by the Food Labelling Regulation 1996. All packaged food must have a label that states:

- The name of the food
- A list of ingredients in descending order of content, i.e. the first item listed is the largest ingredient
- Storage conditions and durability (best before or use-by date)
- The name and address of the manufacturer, packer or seller established within the EU.

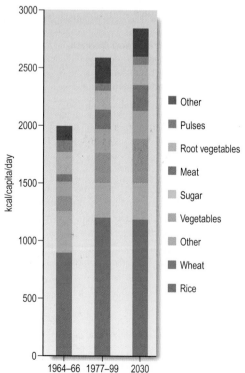

Fig. 16.1 **Dietary changes in developing countries 1964–66 to 2030.** From the Food and Agriculture Organization of the United Nations 2003 World Agriculture: towards 2015/2030, with permission.

Legend (top to bottom): Other, Pulses, Root vegetables, Meat, Sugar, Vegetables, Other, Wheat, Rice. Y-axis: kcal/capita/day. X-axis: 1964–66, 1977–99, 2030.

Nutritional Information		
Typical values	Per serving (1 pie)	Per 100g
Energy	914 kJ / 218 kcal	1423 kJ / 339 kcal
Protein	2.3 g	3.6 g
Carbohydrate	31.0 g	48.3 g
of which Sugars	16.6 g	25.8 g
Fat	9.4 g	14.6 g
of which Saturates	1.9 g	3.0 g
Fibre	0.7 g	1.1 g
Sodium	0.1 g	0.1 g
Per serving (1 pie)		
218 Calories 9.4 g Fat		
Guideline daily amounts		
Each Day	Women	Men
Calories	2,000	2,500
Fat	70 g	95 g
Official government figures for average adults		

More detailed information regarding carbohydrates and fats is sometimes given

Salt – sometimes given as sodium

Fig. 16.2 A UK food label.

Legislation was updated in the European parliament in 2011, aiming to promote healthier food choice to EU citizens, including such stipulations as:

- The actual food label must be visible, clear (a minimum print size) and accurate
- That energy, fat, saturated fat and carbohydrates with specific reference to salt and sugar content per 100 mL or per 100 g should be displayed. The recommended daily amount (RDA) should also be displayed
- Substances known as allergens should be displayed on the food label.

Nutrition claims (e.g. the food is a source of a particular nutrient), health claims (e.g. the food is in some way beneficial to health), and other claims for particular uses, may be made in relation to certain products.

Food labels are compulsory when nutritional advantages are claimed. Information contained on the labels should include:

- Nutrients – energy (kJ/kcal per kg), protein, fat and carbohydrates are expressed per 100 mL/100 g or per serving.
- More detailed information regarding carbohydrates and fats, as appropriate.
- Vitamins and minerals can only be declared if providing a significant amount (approximately one-sixth of the recommended daily amount).
- Fibre content – there are two methods available, the Englyst method (which measures non-starch polysaccharide) and the Association of Analytical Communities (AOAC) method, giving two different results. The UK has since adopted the AOAC method which provides a higher estimate of fibre content because it measures a much wider range of dietary fibre constituents. In 2007 the European Union regulations stated that in order to be able to able to label food a 'source of fibre' the product has to contain at least 3 g per 100 g or at least 1.5 g fibre per 100 kcal.
- Salt – this is sometimes expressed as sodium content.

DIETARY REFERENCE VALUES

Dietary reference values (DRVs) provide information on the amount of different nutrients that are needed for maintaining health in different groups of people in the UK. They are estimated requirements for a population rather than exact recommendation for individuals, whose energy expenditure and levels of physical activity will vary (Fig. 16.3). Worldwide, there is broad agreement on DRVs based on data from the WHO, FAO and other expert committees of the United Nations. Many countries have produced their own dietary reference standards. From the 1960s, the UK had used a single figure for each nutrient: recommended daily intake (RDI) or recommended daily amount (RDA). However, it was found that there was a large potential for misuse and misinterpretation of these single reference points. In response to this, in 1991 the dietary reference values (DRVs) guidelines were produced. These were re-calculated in 2011 by the Scientific Advisory Committee on Nutrition (SACN) partly due to the advancement in techniques used to calculate energy expenditure and partly the fact there is a growing obesity epidemic in the UK. RDAs were replaced in the UK by three DRVs: reference nutrient intake (RNI), estimated average requirement (EAR) and lower reference nutrient intake (LRNI). The RNI (Fig. 16.3) values are similar to the RDAs, and meet the nutrient needs of the vast majority (97%) of any healthy population. The RNI for different nutrients is set two standard deviations above the EAR, the amount of a nutrient which is needed daily on average in a large population of normal people. The LRNI is set two standard deviations below the EAR and represents a level of usual nutrient intake which is not likely to be sufficient in more than 97% of people. Thus an intake below the RNI does not suggest deficiency, but an intake below LRNI does.

NUTRITIONAL REQUIREMENTS

In 2004, the WHO released a global strategy on diet, physical activity and health with an aim to reduce death and disease burden worldwide as the number of deaths from

EAR Estimated average requirement:
half the population usually needs more than the EAR and half less.

LRNI Lower reference nutient intake:
sufficient for the few people who have low needs, but not meeting the needs of 97.5% of the population (2 standard deviations below the EAR).

RNI reference nutrient intake:
sufficient for about 97.5% of people (2 standard deviations above the EAR). If the average intake of a population is at RNI, the risk of deficiency is very small.

Safe intake:
range for which there is not enough information to estimate RNI, EAR or LRNI. Sufficient for almost everyone but not so large as to cause undesirable effects.

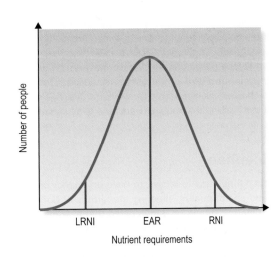

Fig. 16.3 **Dietary reference values for a population.** From Department of Health 1991 Dietary reference values for food energy and nutrients for the United Kingdom. HMSO, London (Report on Health and Social Subjects, No. 41), with permission.

Table 16.1 WHO guidelines for a healthy diet

Dietary factor	Goal*	Important sources
Fat	15–30	
Saturated fat	10	Meat fat, lard, dripping, butter, cheese and cream
Monounsaturated fat	By difference†	Olive and rape seed oil
Polyunsaturated fat	6–10	Vegetable oils, nuts, eggs, fish and liver
Trans fatty acids	<1	Margarine and other fat spreads
Carbohydrate	50–75‡	
Starches	33	Bread, cereal, rice, potatoes, pasta
Free sugars§	10	Sugar, fruit and cereals
Protein	10–15	Meat and meat products, milk and milk products, eggs, pulses, nuts and seeds
Fibre (non-starch polysaccharide)	18 g/day	Cereals, vegetables, fruit and nuts
Sodium chloride** (sodium)	<5 g/day; 2 g/day	Foods canned in brine, smoked or salted; yeast extract and stock cubes; 'discretionary' (added during cooking or at the table)

*Per cent of daily energy intake unless otherwise stated.
†This is calculated as: total fat − (saturated fatty acids + polyunsaturated acids + *trans* fatty acids).
‡Percentage of total energy including energy from ingested protein and fat, hence the wide range.
§The term 'free sugars' refers to all monosaccharides and disaccharides added to foods by the manufacturer, cook or consumer, plus sugars naturally present in honey, syrups and fruit juices. The suggested range should be seen in the light of the joint World Health Organization/Food and Agricultural Organization/United Nations University Expert Consultation on Protein and Amino Acid Requirements in Human Nutrition, Geneva, 9–16 April 2002.
**Salt should be iodised appropriately. The need to adjust salt iodination, depending on observed sodium intake and surveillance of iodine status of the population, should be recognised.

non-communicable diseases, such as cardiovascular disease, diabetes and cancer, continues to increase. Several of the risk factors associated with disease are related to diet and physical activity. The present WHO guidelines for a healthy diet for the prevention of chronic diseases were formulated in 2003 (Table 16.1). The recommendations are based on epidemiological and interventional studies that examined the relationship of lifestyle variables, including exercise, smoking, obesity and diet, with:

- Life expectancy
- Incidence of specific diseases, particularly cancer, coronary heart disease and stroke (see later).

VARIATIONS IN NUTRITIONAL REQUIREMENTS

Requirements for most nutrients vary with age and sex, and at times of physiological adaptation, e.g. during pregnancy, lactation and growth. Appropriate DRVs have thus been produced for these subgroups. In disease states such as infection, trauma, disorders of the gastrointestinal tract or metabolic abnormalities, requirements will vary. The DRVs for one nutrient assume that requirements for energy and all other nutrients are met.

Preconception

Preconceptional nutrition is known to have an impact on ovulation and sperm quality, affecting the fertility of both women and men. It should be remembered that a woman of childbearing age may not be aware of her pregnancy until near the end of the first trimester. Therefore, preconceptual nutritional advice is important and should emphasise a varied and balanced diet and a body weight within a desirable range.

Severe weight loss has an impact on ovulation. Body fat must make up at least 22% of body weight to maintain ovulation. Prolonged undernutrition, as in anorexia nervosa, can result in amenorrhoea. Conversely, obesity can also inhibit ovulation. Weight loss can induce spontaneous ovulation in previously anovulatory obese women. For example, weight reduction in overweight women with polycystic ovarian syndrome (PCOS) leads to ovulation and improves fertility.

Pregnancy

The energy demands of a pregnancy are usually estimated at approximately 323 MJ (77 000 kcal), although variations in activity levels account for major differences in the energy needs of individual women. Over the course of a full-term pregnancy, there should be an approximate weight gain of 12.5 kg, consisting of:

- 2.5 kg body weight
- 3.5 kg infant weight
- 6.5 kg placental weight.

During pregnancy, there are increased requirements for some, but not all, nutrients (Clinical box 16.1). The diet must provide sufficient energy and nutrients to:

- provide extra growth of the breasts, uterus and placenta, and to meet the mother's needs
- meet the requirements of the growing foetus
- allow the mother to lay down stores of nutrients for lactation.

Pregnancy is often an ideal opportunity for clinicians to promote healthier eating for the benefit of the baby, immediate family and the wider community, although there has been little research into the effects of this form of intervention.

Clinical box 16.1   Nutrition during pregnancy

Nutritional requirements increase during pregnancy due to the requirements of the growing foetus, and the mother's body being prepared for parturition and lactation.

- Energy: there are wide variations between individuals. Minimum threshold for maternal weight gain is 6.8 kg. Additional 838 KJ (200 kcal)/day required in the third trimester. Eat according to appetite.
- Protein: an additional 6 g/day to 51 g RNI.
- Vitamins:
  - Folate: poor **folic acid** status is associated with an increased risk of neural tube defects. In most developed countries, all women who are planning a pregnancy are recommended to consider folic acid dietary supplements and to try to include folate-rich foods and foods fortified with folic acid in their diet. Women who become pregnant should supplement their diet immediately (0.4 mg folic acid) until the twelfth week of pregnancy.
  - Vitamin A: an increment of 100 mg/day to 800 mg/day throughout pregnancy. High doses (>1500 mg) are known to be teratogenic.
  - Vitamin D: supplemented to achieve an intake of 10 mg/day.
  - Vitamin C: increase by 10 mg/day to 50 mg/day in the third trimester.
  - Iron: 14.8 g/day, with no recommended increase in pregnancy unless iron stores are inappropriately low at the beginning of pregnancy.

  Conditions that affect nutrition during pregnancy are:
- Nausea and vomiting
- Hyperemesis gravidarum
- Cravings, aversions and pica
- Heartburn
- Constipation.

Lactation

Lactation imposes a heavy nutritional demand on the mother. Requirements for energy, calcium and many other vitamins and minerals are increased. If the nutritional needs of lactation are not met, it is generally the mother who is affected and not the infant. Milk quantity and quality will be maintained at the expense of the maternal stores. Any significant fall in nutritional status, especially calcium, may have long-term consequences for the mother's health, particularly bone health. Lactating women should ingest at least 1200 mg calcium/day. Dehydration can occur if fluids are not replaced – requirement is about 2 L/day.

Aspects of the maternal diet can affect breast milk. High intakes of alcohol and caffeine should be avoided. Strong tasting or highly spiced foods can alter the taste of breast milk, which may cause distress to the infant. Infants who are highly sensitive to allergens such as cow's milk protein can react to, or may be sensitised to, the presence of these antigens in breast milk, although cow's milk exclusion for the mother is rarely justified.

Infancy

Infancy is a period of rapid growth and development. Compared with adults, infants have increased requirements per kilogram of body weight for energy, protein, iron and calcium. Mothers should be encouraged to breastfeed for at least 4 months, because breast milk provides the best form of nourishment. When breastfeeding is not possible, infant formulae, which are based on cow's milk and modified to mimic breast milk, may be used.

NUTRITIONAL STATUS

Assessment of nutritional status identifies individuals who are at risk of under- or over-nutrition. In the hospital setting, undernutrition (often used synonymously with **malnutrition**) is the major concern as it tends to be under-diagnosed. However, in the general population in the developed world, and increasingly elsewhere too, *obesity* is a significant issue, at least in part because of its associated metabolic syndromes (see below).

CLINICAL ASSESSMENT OF NUTRITIONAL STATUS

There is no single parameter that accurately measures nutritional status. Assessment of dietary intake, body composition, functional testing, clinical presentation and laboratory measures all reflect aspects of nutritional status and should be considered together. In children, nutritional status needs to be considered in relation to age, and growth is of major importance.

FOOD INTAKE

Detailed assessment of dietary intake is the province of the fully trained dietitian. However, a simple dietary history is often useful to doctors and other clinicians. For example, the number of meals and the quantity, content and variety of snacks consumed can give clues to whether intake is a factor for weight change. Basic enquiries into diet and the timing of meals and snacks can be usefully incorporated into routine questions about lifestyle. The relation of gastrointestinal symptoms with food intake can be of great clinical importance.

Detailed dietary assessment

A full quantitative dietary assessment is time consuming and, depending on the method used, often subjective. Table 16.2 summarises the most commonly used methods of recording intake. Misreporting is common as people can feel guilty or embarrassed about aspects of their diet. In addition, food choices may be influenced when intake is recorded by the patient. All food intake varies by day of the week and season.

Once completed, a dietary record can be analysed into its constituent nutrients by using food composition tables or computer packages based on them. Information on dietary balance, deficiencies and surpluses, specific nutrients and compliance with previously given advice can be obtained from such programs. For example, comparisons can be made with age- and gender-specific dietary reference values (DRV).

'USUAL WEIGHT' AND WEIGHT LOSS/GAIN

'Usual weight' may be constant or variable. If variable, the weight at which the patient feels best should be identified, as well as the weight immediately before illness or when weight loss commenced. Previous records of body weight are helpful. Usual weight allows estimation of **percentage weight loss** once current weight has been measured:

$$\text{Percentage weight loss} = \frac{\text{Previous weight} - \text{current weight}}{\text{Previous weight}} \times 100$$

Percentage weight gain is calculated by reversing previous and current weights. The timing of the weight change should be noted; whether the weight loss is intentional or unintentional is important:

- In **intentional weight loss** produced by well-designed dieting, the lean body mass component may represent only 25% of the decrease in weight
- In disease-related **unintentional weight loss**, 60% or more of the loss may be lean.

Weight measurements are distorted by fluid retention or loss. However, day-to-day weight comparisons may provide useful clinical information in assessing changes in hydration.

Table 16.2	Methods for recording food intake		
Type	**Definition**	**Uses**	**Disadvantages**
Weighed food record	Record with weights of portions served, and plate waste	When a quantified measure of nutrient intake is required, e.g. in specialised research studies	Not all foods fully weighed, as logistically this can be difficult and can lead to poor compliance
Unweighed food record	Estimated record using portions described in household measures (spoon, cups, etc.)	Semiquantitative measure used to identify meal patterns, food choices, e.g. associations between food and symptoms	Can be hard to quantify specific nutrient intakes
24-hour recall	The respondent is asked to recall all food eaten within the past 24 hours	As a quick assessment of food choices/meal patterns	Past 24 hours may not be representative of usual intake
Food frequency questionnaire	A questionnaire consisting of a list of foods. The respondent has to say how often each food is eaten – per day/week/month	For identifying foods eaten less often, which may be of special interest and not included in short-term food records, e.g. when trying to identify certain nutrients consumed over a larger period of time	May not be a good assessment of total diet
Diet history	Respondent is asked detailed questions about usual intake. The aim is to get a comprehensive 7-day estimate of intake	Method used by the majority of dietitians in clinical practice for fast assessment and immediate advice	Information can be difficult to obtain, and often misreported

BODY MASS INDEX

To be clinically informative, body weight needs to be expressed as a function of height. The most widely used stature-adjusted weight index is the body mass index (BMI) otherwise known as the Quetelet index (QI).

$$\text{BMI or QI} = \frac{\text{weight (kg)}}{\text{height (m}^2)}$$

BMI (QI) is useful for identifying underweight and overweight individuals (Table 16.3). BMI, like body weight itself, does not differentiate between fat or lean body mass. Oedema and ascites may result in a higher BMI and an overestimate of muscle mass while heavily muscled individuals, such as body builders, may have a BMI that suggests that they are 'overweight'.

One should also take into account racial diversity, reflected in a variety of 'healthy' BMI ranges suggested for different countries or ethnic groups. It is important to be aware that, although a range of values is given for a healthy BMI, the risk of disease can be increased at the upper limit of that range. For example, the risk of type 2 diabetes increases progressively over a BMI of $23\,\text{kg/m}^2$, which is within the 'normal' range (18.5 to $24.99\,\text{kg/m}^2$).

CHILDREN

The weight and height of children are assessed against standard growth charts to identify whether the weight and height are appropriate for the age of the child. Both are expressed in centiles, which tells us whether a child is above or below the average height or weight for their age, and whether they are growing at the expected rate; that is, whether they are following the same centile over time. Children who become malnourished first lose weight compared with their age and height (**wasting**); with more prolonged undernutrition, their growth becomes affected and height centile diminishes relative to normal or their previous situation (stunting). Height centile increase can occur with effective refeeding of malnourished children (catch up growth). An example of a growth chart used in the UK is shown in Figure 10.13. They are adapted for age and gender.

MEASURES OF BODY COMPOSITION: ADULTS

Measures of body composition are important in a clinical setting. They allow not only initial assessment but also monitoring of any change in body composition that may be due to disease.

For measurement of body composition, the body is usually divided into compartments consisting of fat mass (lipids) and fat free mass. There are a number of methods used to estimate body composition, depending on which measurements need to be obtained. They differ in their advantages, cost, complexity and availability, some being used only in the research environment.

ESTIMATING BODY FAT

There are several methods of estimating body fat, which range from simple to more complex.

One commonly employed is anthropometry, where, by using simple tools, the percentage of body fat can be estimated by measurements taken at selected anatomical sites where fat is deposited:

- Skinfold thickness
- Arm circumference
- Waist circumference and waist/hip ratio.

Skinfold thickness

Skinfold measurement, also called the 'pinch test', assesses the thickness of a fold of skin at selected body sites where adipose tissue is normally deposited, such as over the biceps, triceps, subscapular and suprailiac regions, and thigh and calf muscles. More accurate estimates of adiposity are obtained by measuring skinfold thickness at several sites. In clinical practice, triceps skinfold thickness is most often used as an estimate of body fat reserves.

Arm circumference

The mid upper arm circumference (MUAC) is a useful measure of both fat and muscle protein stores. The measurement is taken with a tape measure, midway between the tip of the acromion and olecranon process in the non-dominant arm to the nearest centimetre, with the dominant arm hanging relaxed. MUAC correlates fairly well with BMI, and has been used as a quick and convenient method of estimating nutritional status of children in field studies and is increasingly being used in adults.

Table 16.3	The international classification of underweight, overweight and obese adults according to BMI	
Classification	**BMI (kg/m²)**	
	Principal cut-off points	**Additional cut-off points**
Underweight	<18.50	<18.50
Severe thinness	<16.00	<16.00
Moderate thinness	16.00–16.99	16.00–16.99
Mild thinness	17.00–18.49	17.00–18.49
Normal range	18.50–24.99	18.50–22.99
		23.00–24.99
Overweight	≥25.00	≥25.00
Pre-obese	25.00–29.99	25.00–27.49
		27.50–29.99
Obese	≥30.00	≥30.00
Obese class I	30.00–34.99	30.00–32.49
		32.50–34.99
Obese class II	35.00–39.99	35.00–37.49
		37.50–39.99
Obese class III	≥40.00	>40.00

Adapted from WHO (1995, 2000, 2004).
BMI values, being ratios, are the same for males and females, and vary with age. Overweight and obesity may impair health, but the degrees of excessive fat accumulation vary between populations. Therefore, the health risk associated with increasing BMI differs for different populations.

Waist circumference and waist/hip ratio

Strong correlations have been found between subcutaneous and intra-abdominal fat (on computed tomography (CT)), with waist and hip circumferences and waist/hip ratios. Measurement of waist alone may have greater sensitivity for predicting complications of obesity, such as coronary heart disease, than the waist/hip ratio. In Caucasians, a waist measurement of >94 cm in men and >80 cm in women is associated with increased risk. The risk is substantially increased in men with a waist >102 cm and in women >88 cm.

OTHER MEASUREMENTS OF NUTRITIONAL STATUS

PLASMA PROTEINS

Serum albumin is often incorrectly used as an indicator of nutritional status, with levels often remaining normal in undernutrition, which is uncomplicated by disease. The decrease in serum albumin concentration during infection, cancer, burns and after trauma or surgery is related primarily to increased vascular permeability. While undernutrition may exacerbate disease-related hypoalbuminaemia, albumin concentration primarily reflects a disease process, and it is better considered as an 'index of disease severity' rather than a nutritional indicator. Serum albumin can also be depressed by dilution during refeeding or excessive rehydration. It should be interpreted in combination with some other estimate of the acute-phase response, such as C-reactive protein or the erythrocyte sedimentation rate (ESR).

The same problems apply to other plasma proteins which are used as nutritional indicators, such as pre-albumin, transferrin and retinol-binding protein. However, these may be more sensitive as nutritional indicators because they have a shorter half-life in the circulation and can respond to dietary change more quickly.

VITAMIN STATUS

Vitamin deficiencies can be detected either by biochemical assays or by physical symptoms (see below). The detailed assessment of vitamin status is beyond the scope of this chapter. The relatively common presentation of macrocytic anaemias necessitates vitamin B_{12} and folate assays, but other vitamin deficiencies are unmeasured and often overlooked. Specific deficiency syndromes are outlined below.

MUSCLE STRENGTH

Studies have shown that malnutrition leads to impaired muscle strength, and nutritional support may rectify this before improvements in weight are seen.

IMMUNOLOGICAL SKIN TESTING

Adequate nutrition is essential for the maintenance of a normal immune system. A reduced blood total **lymphocyte count** may be indicative of protein calorie malnutrition. Delayed hypersensitivity is particularly affected by undernutrition, and, in the past, skin tests for mumps, tuberculin and *Candida* have been used clinically to monitor nutrition.

MALNUTRITION SCREENING TOOLS

Research has shown that, not only are a significant number of patients already malnourished on entry to hospital, but that hospital admissions are also often associated with a deterioration in nutritional state. The causes of this are invariably multifactorial, but the associated effects on morbidity and mortality are reflected in the high rates of readmission, lengthier hospital stays, susceptibility to infection and impaired wound healing in such patients. This has prompted some countries to develop national guidelines that recommend mandatory assessment of the nutritional status of all patients in hospital as well as those who are at risk in the community, in order to identify those who may require nutritional support. In the UK, these have been developed by the National Institute of Clinical Health and Excellence (NICE). Many hospitals and other healthcare settings will have their own screening tools that combine features from the history and clinical examination, which are then ranked and combined to produce a score indicating malnutrition risk. In UK, the Malnutrition Universal Screening Tool (MUST) is a five-step process based on BMI and weight loss designed to identify patients who are at risk of malnutrition or obesity, and includes management guidelines. In other parts of Europe, the nutritional risk screening (NRS-2002) is often employed, whereas the Mini Nutritional Assessment (MNA) and more complex Subjective Global Assessment (SGA) are used more commonly in the USA and Canada.

ENERGY AND NITROGEN BALANCE

Energy is required for metabolic processes such as active transport of molecules and ions, synthesis of tissue, thermoregulation, and voluntary and involuntary muscle movement. Dietary intake of food provides the body with the macronutrients – carbohydrates, fats and proteins – that are converted to energy. Each one of these has a slightly different energy content, the approximations of which are shown in Table 16.4.

CONVERSION OF MACRONUTRIENTS TO ENERGY

After absorption, macronutrients may pass through a number of different pathways of metabolism, shown in Figure 16.4, but ultimately the energy comes from the tricarboxylic acid (TCA) cycle and the mitochondrial process of oxidative phosphorylation (see in detail in Ch. 3).

Table 16.4	Energy values for macronutrients and alcohol as measured by indirect calorimetry	
Nutrient	**kJ/g**	**kcal/g**
Carbohydrates	17.2	4.1
Protein	23.8	5.7
Fats	39.7	9.5
Alcohol	29.7	7.1

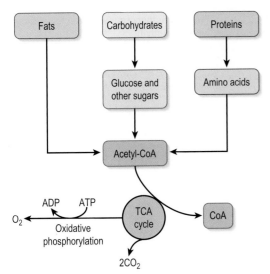

Fig. 16.4 Metabolic pathways for converting macronutrients to energy.

ENERGY BALANCE

Positive energy balance results in weight gain and the deposition of fat and glycogen, whereas a negative energy balance leads to weight loss and the depletion of glycogen and fat stores and ultimately muscle loss. The chemical energy content of food (measured in calories or joules) is the amount of energy that would be released from food if it was burned in oxygen in a fixed volume. This can be undertaken experimentally using a bomb calorimeter, which measures the heat produced per unit of food.

In healthy people, most of the energy in food is absorbed – around 97% of the energy in carbohydrate, 95% in fat and 92% in protein. Less energy is absorbed from protein because nitrogen is metabolised to urea and not fully oxidised, so that some of the energy from protein is not available to the body (see Ch. 3).

Basal metabolic rate (BMR) and resting energy expenditure

BMR is the energy that is used by the body to maintain basic physiological functions, including metabolic processes, cell membrane pumps and intracellular pumps.

Resting energy expenditure (REE) is the energy used by a normal, post-absorptive (about 12 hours fasting) individual at rest, but not asleep, under thermoneutral conditions. Measurements of REE are used as surrogates for BMR, though are, in reality, about 10% greater than BMR. Although BMR varies among people of equal height and weight, owing to ethnic and geographical differences, individual BMRs remain relatively constant over a number of years.

There are a number of factors that can affect BMR, including age, sex, obesity, climate, medications and disease. In the acutely unwell patient, even in the absence of fever, metabolic demands may increase significantly. The measurement of these stress factors can be difficult, but accurate clinical assessment is required in order to ensure the individual obtains sufficient calories.

Total energy expenditure

Total energy expenditure (TEE) is composed of:

- Resting energy expenditure (around 60–70% of TEE)
- Exercise/ physical activity (10–30%)

- Food induced thermogenesis (up to 10%)
- Growth in children
- Disease processes.

Measuring energy expenditure

BMR can be measured at rest by direct calorimetry (direct measurement of heat exchange in a chamber), or indirect calorimetry, which uses a canopy over the head to measure oxygen consumption and carbon dioxide generation from which energy consumption can be calculated. In practice, BMR is estimated from the Schofield (1985) predictive equations, which are based on the analysis of a large number of measurements of BMR and can predict individual BMR reasonably accurately.

Oxygen consumption and carbon dioxide production can also be measured during exercise either by collecting exhaled gases in portable Douglas bags (an airtight bag which collects expired gases via a one-way valve) or by studying the subject in a chamber calorimeter. Energy expenditure can alternatively be measured by administering a drink of doubly labelled radioactive water and monitoring the relative decay of ^2H and ^{18}O from the body. The difference between the decay of ^2H and ^{18}O allows estimation of CO_2 production and total energy consumption. This method has the advantage that the subject is free to move about.

Total energy expenditure and the effect of physical activity

The total amount of energy used up in a day will depend on the individual's BMR, the nature of their occupation (whether sedentary or labour intensive), and the amount of physical activity undertaken in leisure and the pursuit of sports. The heat derived from food is not measured separately, but is included in measurements or estimations of energy expenditure.

Energy expenditure during daily living

Daily energy output for the activities of daily living can be estimated from the BMR and the individual's physical activity level (PAL), an index derived from experimental studies of energy expenditure for physical activity over 24 hours. Energy expenditure during activities of daily living is best measured by the doubly labelled water method, which allows measurements to be made over periods of days or weeks. PAL is expressed as a ratio of total energy expenditure and the resting energy expenditure (BMR). Total daily energy requirement can be calculated from a table of PAL, calibrated for the subject's leisure and work occupation, which provides a multiple by which the estimated BMR can be multiplied. For any one individual, these values are obtained from reference tables (Table 16.5). The most commonly used units are kcal/24 h or kJ/24 h.

An estimated average requirement (EAR) for energy can be calculated by multiplying the BMR by the appropriate PAL (see Table 16.5). The PAL index takes into consideration occupational as well as non-occupational activities because an individual with a sedentary occupation may undertake a lot of non-occupational activity, and vice versa. Physical activity makes a variable contribution to the total energy expenditure, which, over average 24-hour periods, is nearly always less than the BMR.

An individual at rest would be using energy for maintaining BMR only, i.e. a PAL of 1. Many people in the developed world have sedentary occupations (light activity) and are

Table 16.5	Physical activity levels (PALs)					
Non-occupational activity	**Occupational activity**					
	Light		**Moderate**		**Moderate/ heavy**	
	M	**F**	**M**	**F**	**M**	**F**
Non-active	1.4	1.4	1.6	1.5	1.7	1.5
Moderately active	1.5	1.5	1.7	1.6	1.8	1.6
Very active	1.6	1.6	1.8	1.7	1.9	1.7

Department of Health 1991 Dietary reference values for food energy and nutrients for the United Kingdom. HMSO, London (Report on Health and Social Subjects, No. 41).

non-active, or only moderately active, outside work. From the corresponding PAL of 1.4 and 1.5 (Table 16.5), it can be seen that their energy consumption is mainly due to BMR: only about a third of it (0.4–0.5) is due to physical activity. For example, for a woman who has a BMR of 6000 kJ, has a sedentary occupation and is moderately active outside of work, the total daily energy output is:

$$6000 \text{ kJ} \times 1.5 = 9000 \text{ kJ}$$
(4.2 kJ is equivalent to 1 kcal)

Estimates of energy consumption for different types of activity

More accurate estimates of energy consumption during a 24-hour period can be made by keeping a diary of each activity, then calculating the total by adding all the different components. The energy used during each activity is calculated by reference to **physical activity ratios (PAR)** for different activities. PAR is an index of the energy expenditure for the duration of a particular activity compared with a reference activity, such as BMR, expressed as the estimated energy cost **per minute** for the specific activity relative to the measured energy cost **per minute** for the reference activity. This index is used to compare the energy consumption of various activities by different people (Table 16.6).

Energy expenditure during exercise

Energy needs during exercise vary depending on whether it is intense, over a short period (e.g. 100 m sprint), or sustained endurance exercise, such as running a marathon (see Clinical box 16.2).

Anaerobic carbohydrate metabolism

During short bursts of intense activity (e.g. sprinting, weight lifting), close to maximum oxygen consumption (VO_{2max}) takes place when the exercising muscles depend on their own individual stores of adenosine triphosphate (ATP), supported by glucose from the muscle's own store of glycogen. This allows for brief periods when energy consumption is substantially greater than can be supplied by circulating substrates and oxygen. This is called 'anaerobic' metabolism. It builds up lactate and an oxygen debt, which have to be compensated for later. Lactate is recycled to the liver for gluconeogenesis (Cori cycle) (see Ch. 3).

Aerobic carbohydrate metabolism

During more prolonged exercise, 'aerobic' metabolism takes place, in which muscle stores of ATP run out very quickly if

Table 16.6	Physical activity ratios (PARs) for different types of activity	
	PAR	**Example activity**
PAR 1.2 (range 1.0–1.4)	Lying at rest	Reading
	Sitting at rest	Watching television, reading, eating
	Standing at rest	
PAR 1.6 (range 1.5–1.8)	Sitting	Sewing, playing piano, driving
	Standing	Light kitchen work, ironing, office or laboratory work
PAR 2.1 (range 1.9–2.4)	Standing	Household chores, cooking
PAR 2.8 (range 2.5–3.3)	Standing	Vacuuming, making beds, showering
	Walking	3–4 km/h, cricket
	Industrial	Painting and decorating, machine tool, tailoring
PAR 3.7 (range 3.4–4.4)	Standing	Gardening, sailing
	Walking	4–6 km/h, golf
	Industrial	Motor vehicle repairs, bricklaying
PAR 4.8 (range 4.4–5.9)	Standing	Chopping wood, heavy gardening, volleyball
	Walking	6–7 km/h
	Exercise	Moderate swimming, gentle cycling, slow jogging
	Occupational	Labouring, digging/ shovelling, felling trees
PAR 6.9 (range 6.0–7.9)	Walking	Uphill with load, cross-country, climbing stairs
	Exercise	Average jogging, cycling
	Sports	Football, tennis, more energetic swimming, skiing

Clinical box 16.2   **Energy needs for sport: advice for sportsmen and sportswomen for optimising performance**

The advice on energy intake is aimed at enabling individuals to:
- Compensate for the high energy consumption produced by training and competition to maintain an optimal body weight (water, protein and fat)
- Ensure that the muscles and the liver contain plenty of stored glycogen prior to the event
- Replace glycogen quickly and optimally after sport or between events
- Maintain hydration during the sporting activity and salt replacement during prolonged endurance exercise.

they cannot be replenished. Energy during prolonged exercise can be provided by:

- The exercising muscle's glycogen stores
- Circulating energy substrate – glucose derived from hepatic glycogenolysis and gluconeogenesis
- Fatty acids derived from adipose tissue.

Training increases the capacity of the muscle mitochondria to oxidise circulating substrate, especially fatty acids, to produce ATP (see below, TCA cycle). This delays the time at which the relevant muscle's glycogen runs out and the athlete becomes especially fatigued ('hits the wall').

NITROGEN BALANCE AND PROTEIN REQUIREMENTS

Nitrogen balance is the difference between the amount of nitrogen that is ingested and the amount lost from the body. It indicates whether the body is **anabolic** or **catabolic** in terms of net protein metabolism; whether the lean tissue is increasing (positive nitrogen balance) or decreasing (negative nitrogen balance). Nitrogen is ingested in the form of dietary proteins, which are metabolised in the liver and excreted, mainly as urea, in the urine.

Dietary nitrogen

Nitrogen makes up about 16% of the weight of most proteins, i.e. 6.25 g protein contains 1 g nitrogen. Table 16.7 shows how a (numerically convenient) intake of 62.5 g protein, which equates with 10 g nitrogen, is balanced quantitatively by nitrogen excretion. Healthy adults have a net zero nitrogen balance, with ingestion of food by day balancing losses of nitrogen by day and night. Nitrogen balance is positive during growth, weight regain and, pregnancy, and negative during starvation, protein deprivation, nutrient imbalance, trauma and sepsis.

In clinical practice, true nitrogen balance is seldom assessed. However, it should be remembered that, whereas in the normal individual a high nitrogen intake is balanced by a higher resulting output, it may not be possible, or indeed desirable, to achieve such balance in a patient in a catabolic state, who is losing excessive amounts of protein due to sepsis or trauma, even with significantly increased nitrogen intake.

Protein requirements

A positive nitrogen balance is seen during growth (nitrogen intake exceeds excretion), and sufficient nitrogen intake is required for cell renewal and to replace nitrogen excretion in adults. Adults in the developed world tend to eat more protein than they need; often more than the RNI of approximately 45 g/day for a non-pregnant woman and 55 g/day for a man.

Essential and non-essential amino acids

Twenty amino acids are needed for the manufacture of proteins in humans. These are traditionally categorised into essential/indispensible and non-essential/dispensible, although it should be noted that in metabolic terms there is an essential need for all the amino acids, as all are required within metabolic pathways The essential amino acids cannot be synthesised endogenously and thus must be taken from the diet. Some amino acids are 'conditionally' essential; their rate of synthesis may not be sufficient to meet demand under all conditions and so may need to be taken by the diet. Non-essential amino acids are those that can be synthesised from other amino acids or precursors. These are listed in Table 16.8.

Table 16.7	Adult nitrogen balance	
Nitrogen intake (diet)	**Nitrogen output (excretion)**	
62.5 g protein	Urine	8.50 g (7 g as urea)
	Faeces	0.75 g
	Other	0.75 g
	Total	10.0 g

Table 16.8	Classification of amino acids	
Essential	**Non-essential**	**Conditionally essential**
Isoleucine	Alanine	Arginine
Leucine	Aspartic acid	Glutamine
Valine	Asparagine	Histidine
Lysine	Cysteine	
Methionine	Glutamic acid	
Threonine	Glycine	
Phenylalanine	Proline	
Tryptophan	Serine	
	Tyrosine	

Obligatory nitrogen loss

Obligatory nitrogen loss is the amount of nitrogen excreted when protein is excluded from a diet otherwise adequate in energy, electrolytes, minerals, vitamins and trace elements. In this highly artificial situation, the daily excretion of nitrogen in the urine and faeces declines over a few days to a minimum (Fig. 16.5).

Minimum nitrogen requirement

In the absence of growth, nitrogen requirement is estimated by summing the obligatory loss in urine to faecal and other (e.g. skin, sweat) excretions on a protein-free diet (the so-called factorial method). However, an otherwise adequate diet providing only this amount of nitrogen (even as high-quality or first class protein) does not achieve zero balance; the balance remains slightly negative because ureagenesis increases. A better way of finding minimum requirements in adults is by balance studies in which high-quality protein is gradually added to an otherwise complete diet until zero balance is obtained. In children, growth rates must be taken into account. Adults can maintain nitrogen balance on 96 mg N/kg per day.

Nitrogen excretion

Unlike glucose and fatty acids, amino acids do not have storage depots, so amino acids are stored in structural and functional protein. Most nitrogen is excreted in the urine as

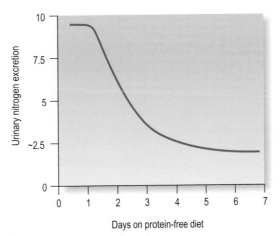

Fig. 16.5 Obligatory nitrogen loss: minimum urinary nitrogen excretion – protein-free diet. Urine nitrogen loss on a protein-free, otherwise adequate diet reaches equilibrium of about 2.5 g by about day 5–7. However, if only 2.5 g of nitrogen are supplied in the otherwise protein-free diet, nitrogen losses will increase marginally because of increased ureagenesis, and nitrogen balance is not quite achieved. Slightly more is required for balance.

urea, with smaller amounts as creatinine and uric acid, for example. The nitrogen containing amino group is removed from the amino acid, and the remaining carbon skeleton is then metabolised for gluconeogenesis and protein synthesis (see Ch. 3). The waste product is ammonia, NH_3, which is highly toxic and rapidly converted to **urea.** Urea is excreted principally through the kidneys. The breakdown of amino acids for use in gluconeogenesis is the main source of urea, and plays a major part in nitrogen balance. When fasting, more amino acids are mobilised for gluconeogenesis, and the metabolic pathways reverse during feeding towards protein synthesis. During feeding, as more protein is eaten, more amino acids are metabolised and more urea nitrogen is excreted so that nitrogen balance is maintained. Losses of nitrogen in the faeces approximate 1 g/day and are relatively constant.

Energy and protein metabolism during fasting and feeding

In healthy people, intracellular metabolism to produce energy is regulated by hormones (Ch. 3). During the fed state, energy stores are laid down for use during periods of fasting (Table 16.9). It is normal to fast overnight or for short periods during the day, but the body adapts if longer periods of fasting occur. The hormones insulin, glucagon, epinephrine (adrenaline), cortisol and growth hormone are involved in the regulation of energy metabolism, exerting short-term effects on the direction of metabolic pathways (Information box 16.1, Fig. 16.6; see also Ch. 3).

The anabolic, fed, high-insulin state results in net storage of protein and glycogen. The catabolic, fasted, low insulin state results in mobilisation of, firstly, glycogen for maintenance of blood glucose, and, subsequently, amino acids (especially 3C alanine) as substrate to make 6C glucose (gluconeogenesis–alanine cycle). 5C glutamine is an amino acid which is a major energy substrate for rapidly turning over cells such as enterocytes and lymphocytes. It is partially metabolised there to 3C alanine before this is returned to the liver. During brisk exercise, when a low insulin state prevails, the exercising muscles take up glucose, which may not be fully oxidised. Lactate is produced and recycled after anaerobic glycolysis back to the liver for gluconeogenesis (Cori cycle) (Ch. 3.)

Table 16.9	Fuel stores in an average person	
Fuel source	**In weight (g)**	**In energy (kJ)**
Fat		
Plasma free fatty acids	0.4	16
Plasma triacylglycerols	4.0	156
Intramyocellular triacylglycerol	300	11 700
Adipose tissue	12 000	468 000
Carbohydrate		
Plasma glucose	20	360
Liver glycogen	100	1800
Muscle glycogen	350	6300
Whole body protein	10 000	168 000

Adapted from Geissler C, Powers HJ (eds) 2005 Human nutrition, 11th edn. Elsevier, Edinburgh.
Note: The principal component of body weight (water) provides no energy. Protein is structural and is therefore not all available for energy production. Glycogen and protein in the body are in the hydrated state and so weigh much more, kilojoule for kilojoule, than fat, which is stored in adipose tissue. Adipose tissue contains relatively little water.

Information box 16.1	Effect of insulin in the fed and fasted states

During the fed state, the active metabolic pathways are for fuel breakdown, storage of excess fuel through glycogen and lipid synthesis, and protein synthesis (anabolism) (see also Ch. 3). These processes are induced by insulin, an anabolic hormone, to:
- Increase glycogen synthesis in the liver and muscle
- Increase hepatic glycolysis
- Increase glucose uptake into muscle
- Increase lipogenesis and decrease lipolysis
- Increase cellular uptake of amino acids and net protein synthesis.

In fasting, which can begin a few hours after the last meal, the direction of the metabolic pathways is reversed to break down stored fuels to produce energy. Protein synthesis also slows down. The level of circulating insulin falls. (In the stress of disease or trauma the action of insulin is opposed by increased levels of glucagon, epinephrine, cortisol and growth hormone.) Glycogenolysis, lipolysis, ketogenesis and gluconeogenesis are promoted.

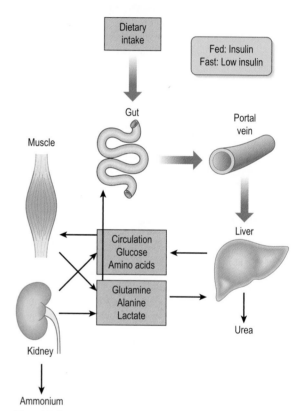

Fig. 16.6 Carbohydrate and amino acid metabolism during fasting and feeding.

Fed state

When nutrients are abundant, metabolic processes are geared to the catabolism of macronutrients and anabolism of the excess products for storage against lean times.

Absorbed carbohydrate in the fed state

After a meal, blood glucose rises, as shown in the **blood glucose response curves** in Figure 16.7. Some foods produce a blood glucose response very similar to that of glucose, the reference food; others produce a much flatter curve. Glucose is made available for:

- Metabolism
- Storage as glycogen (principally in muscle and liver)
- In more extreme excess, lipogenesis.

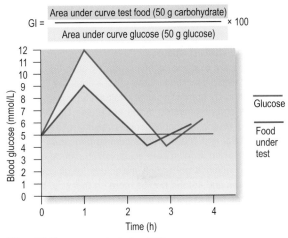

$$GI = \frac{\text{Area under curve test food (50 g carbohydrate)}}{\text{Area under curve glucose (50 g glucose)}} \times 100$$

Fig. 16.7 **Glycaemic index (GI).**

Table 16.10	Classification of foods by glycaemic index
Glycaemic index	**Foods**
High (70–100)	Bread (white or wholemeal), glucose, fruit juices, honey, mashed potatoes
Intermediate (56–69)	Granary bread, rice
Low (<55)	Pulses, beans, peas, legumes, oat and oat-based cereals, pasta, raw fruit

Many physical and chemical characteristics of carbohydrates affect how quickly they are absorbed: reflected in how quickly blood sugar rises and falls after they are eaten. The **glycaemic index** (GI) describes this response in relation to glucose (see Fig. 16.7), and foods can be classified as having low, intermediate or high GI (Table 16.10). This is used in the management of diabetes: low GI foods are recommended as an aid to restricting glucose intake. In the UK, low GI foods are recommended to the general population as part of a balanced diet. However, estimating the total GI of a meal is not practical in clinical situations because there are many factors which affect the GI, including:

- Pectin to amylopectin ratio in the food (mainly fruit)
- Degree of ripeness (fruit) and method of preparation (e.g. mashing increases the GI of potatoes)
- Size of the meal
- Addition of fat.

Absorbed fat in the fed state

Dietary fat is about 95% triacylglycerol (TAG) (also known as triglyceride), with cholesterol and phospholipids making up the other main components. Dietary fats in the form of TAG are digested by pancreatic enzymes in the intestine to form free fatty acids and 2-monoacylglycerol (MAG), which are absorbed by the enterocytes (Ch. 15). The enterocytes re-esterify some of the free fatty acids and MAG to synthesise TAGs. Chylomicrons are then assembled from TAGs, cholesterol, apoproteins and phospholipids. Most TAGs enter the systemic circulation as chylomicrons, via the thoracic duct. Medium- and short-chain fatty acids pass directly into the liver via the portal vein. Cholesterol (like bile acids) is absorbed in the last 100 cm or so of the terminal ileum.

In the fed state, the excess of circulating TAG is stored in adipose tissue whose lipid content reflects dietary fatty acid composition. When there is excess carbohydrate intake, it is principally stored as glycogen. Biochemically, dietary carbohydrate can be, but is not usually, converted to fatty acids in the liver and stored as TAG in adipose tissue.

Protein in the fed state

During the fed state, rates of body protein synthesis exceed rates of protein breakdown back to free amino acids, and net protein accumulation (positive nitrogen balance) occurs. The digestion of protein takes place firstly in the stomach by denaturation by stomach acid, then secondly in the small intestine by the action of pancreatic proteases to form a mixture of free amino acids and small peptides, following which a series of carrier systems transport them into the gut cells where they enter the portal blood for transport to the liver. Some amino acids, e.g. glutamine, are metabolised in preference to glucose in the gut, mainly to alanine (see Ch. 3). Alanine can enter gluconeogenesis, or, together with other amino acids, be used for the synthesis of liver structural or export proteins. Final degradation of amino acids results in the formation of glucose or glycogen from the carbon skeleton, and urea from the amino groups. A relatively small proportion of ingested amino acids, particularly the branched chain amino acids valine, leucine and isoleucine, say 25%, leave the liver to circulate generally to be available for protein synthesis. The liver therefore acts to protect the rest of the body from sudden potentially toxic surges in free amino acids.

In healthy individuals who have adequate protein consumption, 24-hour dietary intake and excretion of nitrogen should be equal (nitrogen balance). This will include periods of positive nitrogen balance (during feeding), where the rate of protein synthesis is higher than protein catabolism, and periods of negative nitrogen balance (overnight usually), where the rate of synthesis is lower than protein catabolism.

Fasted state

When fasting, metabolic processes tend towards mobilisation of stored energy substrates to meet the energy requirements for maintaining essential biological functions. Metabolic pathways are not independent and in times of substrate deficit the body has the ability to metabolise its stored energy substrates for energy (Fig. 16.8; Information box 16.2) (Ch. 3).

The need for glucose in the fasted state

During fasting, and after all the glucose from a meal has been metabolised, blood glucose is maintained at a relatively constant 'post-absorptive' level by:

- Drawing on reserves of glycogen in the liver, i.e. glucose is produced via **glycogenolysis** (Ch. 3)

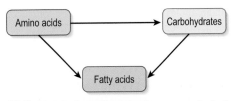

Fig. 16.8 **Metabolic pathways of energy substrates in the fasted state.** Fatty acids cannot be converted to either carbohydrates or amino acids, but are oxidised via acetyl-CoA (if there is plentiful oxaloacetate as a result of glycolysis).

pyruvate) substrates are cycled back to the liver for gluco-neogenesis (see Ch. 3).

Information box 16.2 **Metabolism of stored energy substrates in the fasted state**

During fasting:
- The carbon chains of some (glucogenic) amino acids, particularly alanine, can be converted to glucose.
- Fatty acids cannot be converted to glucose or amino acids (only the glycerol component can be a small contributor to glucose).
- Fatty acids can only be oxidised via acetyl-CoA entering the TCA cycle if there is plentiful oxaloacetate from glucose or glycogen metabolism.
- Deficiency of oxaloacetate results in acetyl groups forming keto acids which can be, and are, metabolised during prolonged fasting or starvation. In starvation, as the brain switches from metabolising glucose (derived at first from glycogen and subsequently from protein/amino acids) to keto acids (derived from fat), it reduces the need for gluconeogenesis from amino acids and therefore 'spares protein'.

- **Gluconeogenesis,** when glucose is synthesised from lactate or non-carbohydrate (mainly protein) sources in the body (Ch. 3).

The main stores for glycogen are in the liver and muscle. Hepatic glycogenolysis provides an almost immediate source of glucose during short-term fasting (e.g. overnight) for maintaining normal blood glucose concentration. The hormone glucagon activates hepatic glycogenolysis. Skeletal muscle glycogen cannot leave the muscle, so muscle glycogenolysis (activated by epinephrine) does not increase blood glucose and can only meet the energy requirements for muscle contraction during exercise (Ch. 3).

Glucose from hepatic glycogenolysis is sufficient only for between 12 and 24 hours and cannot replace all the glucose needed for essential functions. To meet all the requirements, as hepatic glycogen depletes, gluconeogenesis in the liver and kidneys becomes important. Non-carbohydrate substrates for gluconeogenesis include (Ch. 3):

- Lactate – from anaerobic glycolysis in red blood cells and from active skeletal muscle. Starting with lactate, gluconeogenesis is conceptually the reverse of anaerobic glycolysis, though there are slight differences in the pathway.
- Glycerol from fat metabolism – TAGs in adipose tissue are broken down to glycerol and free fatty acids by lipolysis (see Ch. 3). These fatty acids cannot be made into glucose. The glycerol component diffuses into the bloodstream to be reconverted to glucose in the liver and kidneys – a minor supply quantitatively.
- Amino acids from protein muscle breakdown – the main amino acids used in gluconeogenesis are alanine and glutamine, from muscle protein hydrolysis.

With prolonged fasting, the body minimises the drain on structural proteins by reducing the need for glucose and therefore gluconeogenesis from protein. This is achieved by muscles using fat for fuel, especially ketones (see below), and the brain adapting to using more ketone bodies.

Decreased insulin – fasting state

The post-absorptive and fasting states are signalled by a low level of circulating insulin associated with raised plasma glucagon concentration (Information box 16.1). This results in glycogenolysis, lipolysis, ketogenesis and net protein breakdown. 5-Carbon (glutamine) and 3-carbon (alanine, lactate,

Fat in the fasted state

Fatty acids are oxidised, acetyl group by acetyl group, in a process called β-oxidation. Acetyl groups enter the TCA cycle for oxidation by combining with oxaloacetate, derived from glycolysis and regenerated in the cycle (see Ch. 3). During prolonged fasting, gluconeogenesis results in depletion of oxaloacetate, and acetyl groups derived principally from fat are diverted into forming keto acids, which can be oxidised. The brain, which is normally a major user of glucose, uses glucose less and ketone bodies more. In this way, the body uses ketone bodies derived from fat rather than glucose derived from protein. Water-soluble ketone bodies consist of:

- Acetoacetate
- β-Hydroxybutyrate
- Acetone.

Free fatty acid is mobilised from adipose tissue, and the liver also increases the rate of fatty acid production. Hepatic β-oxidation of fatty acids forms acetyl-CoA, which can have one of two metabolic fates:

- React with oxaloacetate to form citrate (and continue to complete oxidation)
- React with acetyl-CoA to form acetoacetate and subsequently other ketone bodies.

This is determined by the rate of β-oxidation and the availability of oxaloacetate. If β-oxidation is high and oxaloacetate low, ketone bodies form. Water-soluble ketone bodies from hepatic ketogenesis can be readily transported in aqueous solution in the blood to various tissues (mainly the heart, muscle and the brain). The ketone bodies can cross the blood–brain barrier to become the dominant energy source there.

Prolonged fasting/starvation

During short-term starvation (overnight fast, up to 3 days), glucose from glycogen and, later, ketone bodies, provide fuel for muscle, kidneys and intestine. With prolonged fasting (more than 3 days), the brain also converts to the use of ketone bodies for more than 50% of its energy metabolism (Table 16.11). This metabolic switch allows glucose to be conserved, reducing the demand to degrade muscle protein for gluconeogenesis (Ch. 3). The concentration of ketone

Table 16.11 **Fuel used by the brain on days 3 and 40 of a prolonged fast**

Starvation	Day 3	Day 40
Fuel used (g)		
Glucose	100	40
Ketones	50	200
Other glucose	50	40
Endogenous source of fuel used (g)		
Lipolysis	180	180
Muscle protein breakdown	75	20
Hepatic glucose	150	80
Ketones	150	150

Note the increased use of ketones by the brain and the reduced hepatic glucose production by day 40 and the reduction in net muscle protein breakdown.

The clinical effects of starvation reflect the biochemistry. For example, as a result of muscle protein breakdown for gluconeogenesis, there is type 2 fibre atrophy in skeletal muscle (including respiratory muscle), leaving only the fat burning and posture maintaining (type 1) fibres. This results in:

- Wasting and other demonstrable changes in muscle physiology
- Muscle fatigue and decreased ability to do physical work
- Diminished respiratory function (e.g. forced expiratory volume in 1 second (FEV_1)).

The pulse rate slows and circulating volume and cardiac output decreases.

The ability to produce heat is compromised so that there is increased risk of hypothermia in a cold environment. Respiratory muscle weakness reduces ventilation, increasing the likelihood of respiratory disease (e.g. pneumonia). The patient becomes weak and apathetic.

bodies may increase dramatically as starvation continues from days into weeks. The low insulin state of starvation thus has qualitative metabolic parallels with diabetic ketoacidosis.

With prolonged starvation, nitrogen excretion in the form of urea diminishes, reflecting reduction of the drain on protein, but does not go as low as the obligatory minimum loss (the amount of nitrogen lost when dietary protein is excluded, see Fig. 16.5) seen in protein deprivation. Clinical box 16.3 sets out some clinical effects of starvation.

Metabolic response to stress: sepsis and trauma

Nutritional support of sick patients requires understanding of the metabolic changes that occur in illness, summarised in Information box 16.3. These occur in response to the secretion of cytokines and classical hormones, and perhaps other unknown factors, considered here separately from the changes that occur simultaneously in the inflammatory response, which are dealt with elsewhere in this book (see Ch. 6).

The metabolic rate rises depending on the severity of the stress and the body temperature of the patient. Burns are notorious for increasing BMR, which may rise to nearly double the normal rate. It should, however, be remembered that it is

Cytokines are proteins that are produced by a variety of cells in response to exogenous challenge (Ch. 6):

- Pro-inflammatory:
  - Tumour necrosis factor-α (TNF-α)
  - Interleukin 1
  - Interleukin 6.
- Classical hormones are secreted by specialised glands mainly in response to stress (Ch. 10):
  - Cortisol
  - Catecholamines
  - Glucagon.

The metabolic responses can be summarised under the following headings:

- Energy metabolism
  - Changes in metabolic rate
  - Increased glucose turnover and insulin resistance
  - Lipid metabolism
- Protein metabolism
  - Changes in whole body protein turnover and nitrogen balance
  - The acute phase response.

the *total* energy expenditure of the patient that determines how much energy is needed for energy balance. In trauma and sepsis, physical activity almost always reduces dramatically and this reduction in energy need offsets any increase in basal metabolism so the energy requirements of most ill patients are seldom much more than those of active people.

Energy metabolism during illness

Although there is a low level of physical activity during illness, which reduces energy expenditure, other changes use energy and so increase expenditure, for example:

- The inflammatory response (Ch. 6)
- Pyrexia
- Infection
- Sepsis
- Physical trauma (especially burns).

Information box 16.4 summarises the energy needs of very sick patients.

Insulin and the inflammatory response

Blood glucose is raised despite an elevated plasma insulin concentration during stress – 'insulin resistance' (see Chs 3 and 10). This is accompanied by an increase in the levels of pro-inflammatory cytokines and the hormones; cortisol, catecholamines and glucagon. The metabolic turnover of glucose is increased:

- There is increased uptake of glucose by immune cells, mediated by non-insulin-dependent systems
- Glucose metabolism, by both glycolysis and oxidation, is increased, with an increase in blood lactate levels so that gluconeogenesis (from lactate) also increases
- Glycogen synthesis and storage is reduced.

The increase in circulating glucose enables the body to meet the increased energy need during illness.

Protein metabolism in illness

Owing to increased energy needs during trauma and sepsis (see above), amino acids are released from muscle to be made available for gluconeogenesis. Blood glucose level is therefore relatively high and produces a secondary rise in plasma insulin. An elevated blood glucose level in the face of raised plasma insulin is termed **insulin resistance** (see above).

The result of increased amino acid breakdown for gluconeogenesis is an increase in nitrogen excretion, so that unless dietary sources of amino acids increase, there will be a negative nitrogen balance. This effect is enhanced in big and heavily muscled, well-nourished men. It is diminished in a warm environment and in people with a smaller muscle mass. Intake of exogenous amino acids helps to limit protein loss from the body, but urinary nitrogen losses remain high because of sustained protein catabolism. If feeding fails, depletion of tissues becomes a threat to survival.

Protein metabolism and acute phase response in illness

In acute illness, although the rate of protein synthesis increases (in the liver and immune cells), the rate of protein degradation is comparatively higher, resulting in the net loss of body protein from the less essential organs (e.g. muscle). The provision of amino acids in the diet reduces nitrogen losses substantially; however, patients generally do not regain muscle mass until the underlying pathology is resolved.

Protein synthesis provides substrate for the repair of tissue and for host defence mechanisms including the acute phase response. There is a diversion in synthesis away from somatic and circulating proteins, such as albumin, towards acute phase proteins, of which there are over 30. These include:

- Haptoglobin
- Caeruloplasmin
- α_2-Macroglobulin
- β_1-Antitrypsin
- Fibrinogen
- C-reactive protein
- α_1 Acid glycoprotein
- Ferritin.

A prolonged increase in acute phase protein synthesis is accompanied by a reduction in albumin synthesis, one of several causes of clinically observed hypoalbuminaemia, which will not respond to dietary intake until the underlying pathology is successfully treated.

Tracer studies, used more for research, use stable isotopes to determine the rates of amino acid metabolism. These can give a more precise indication of the determinants of nitrogen balance, telling us whether changes in protein synthesis or breakdown to constituent amino acids is dominant. In inflammatory and infective states turnover/breakdown tends to increase if food intake is maintained.

MICRONUTRIENTS AND WATER

Some essential components of the human diet, such as vitamins, electrolytes and trace elements (iodine, zinc, magnesium), are only needed in tiny amounts. Water is another essential part of the diet. Although dietary deficiency of vitamins and minerals is uncommon with a balanced diet in developed countries, supplementation of electrolytes, vitamins and trace metals become important for people on artificial diets or parenteral feeding. The absorption and transport of vitamins and minerals are discussed in Chapter 15.

VITAMINS

Vitamins are organic molecules that are needed in small (microgram to milligram) amounts in the diets of higher animals and man. They are present and serve similar purposes in most forms of life, but humans cannot synthesise them so they have to be ingested in the diet. Although grouped together under 'vitamin', they are not chemically related to each other. They are classified according to their solubility in fat or water. Although only required in small amounts, without them deficiency diseases occur (see below).

Most vitamins function as coenzymes or as antioxidants (see later sections). Except in illness, dietary vitamin deficiencies are relatively rare in developed nations, but seen more often in developing countries, in association with macronutrient malnutrition. Vitamin supplements should not be necessary with otherwise well-balanced diets in people who are not ill or pregnant.

Dietary vitamin supplementation (e.g. ascorbic acid, β-carotene, α-tocopherol) as a means of reducing cardiovascular disease or cancer risk has not been demonstrated to be effective in randomised controlled trials. However, epidemiological studies have shown that a high intake of fruit and vegetables) is associated with reduced cardiovascular morbidity and mortality. The recommendation for an adequate daily intake of fruit and vegetables as sources of micronutrients is uncontroversial.

Vitamins as coenzymes

Some enzymes require the presence of coenzymes or cofactors in order to function (see Ch. 2), of which many are derived from B vitamins. Coenzymes are often involved in oxidation–reduction (redox) reactions, where they act as either electron donors or acceptors. They enable chemical reactions to move in a direction otherwise prevented by an energy gradient.

Vitamins as antioxidants

Protection from damage caused by free radicals may be prevented by the action of a number of antioxidants such as vitamin E, vitamin C and vitamin A (β-carotene), which form non-reactive, stable radicals.

WATER-SOLUBLE VITAMINS

Water-soluble vitamins are derived from the diet. Their absorption requires the use of transport proteins, actively and passively from the gut lumen into the enterocytes. Some of these vitamins then use a further transport protein to be actively moved from the cells into the bloodstream. Apart from vitamin B_{12}, storage is minimal in humans, so that water-soluble vitamin excess or toxicity is unknown. Deficiencies occur either because of poor diet or malabsorption and can lead to disease conditions. It is not generally appreciated how common deficiencies of water-soluble vitamins are among non-alcoholic patients admitted to hospital. For example, subclinical B_1 deficiency can all too easily be converted to clinical deficiency with lactic acidosis if glucose infusions or parenteral nutrition feeds are provided without inclusion of this vitamin.

The B vitamins

The B complex vitamins are coenzymes. In the activated form, they carry electrons and chemical groups in numerous metabolic processes. They are widely distributed in meat, liver, poultry, eggs, dairy products, fish, wholegrain cereals, legumes and grains. Deficiency states often present with multiple B vitamin deficiencies (see Clinical box 16.4).

Vitamin B_1 (thiamine)

Vitamin B_1 is a coenzyme in carbohydrate metabolism (pentose phosphate, hexose monophosphate pathway) and in pyruvate metabolism. The body stores very little vitamin B_1 so a regular intake is necessary. It is present in the husk of rice, in wheatgerm and in seeds. Thiamine is actively transported out of enterocytes into the bloodstream, which is a process that is inhibited by alcohol. This can explain why patients with alcohol dependence, who are also often undernourished, are prone to thiamine deficiency.

Clinical box 16.4   **Some vitamin B deficiencies**

Vitamin B_1 deficiency impairs glucose metabolism
The commonest form of thiamine deficiency, beriberi, occurs in populations dependent on rice diets of highly polished rice, which removes the thiamine. Large caloric requirements, as in the catabolic state, can give rise to beriberi. Alcohol inhibits thiamine absorption in the intestines, leading to deficiency. Wernicke–Korsakoff syndrome is the result of thiamine deficiency associated with the combination of chronic alcohol misuse and malnutrition. In thiamine deficiency there are raised levels of pyruvate, which inhibits glycolysis and leads to the accumulation of lactate. The accumulation of both pyruvic acid and lactic acid causes acidosis which, in severe cases, can lead to coma and death.

Vitamin B_3 deficiency
Niacin deficiency leads to pellagra, which is rare and is related to some drugs, e.g. isoniazid. Superficial glossitis leads to dermatitis, giving sunburn-like lesions on exposed skin. Pressure sores, diarrhoea, dementia and death ensue. Excessively high doses of niacin are hepatotoxic.

Vitamin B_6 deficiency
Pyridoxine is needed for neurotransmitter synthesis (e.g. serotonin, norepinephrine), so deficiency can lead to symptoms of irritability and depression and peripheral neuropathy. Dietary deficiency is rare but peripheral neuropathy associated with administration of the anti-tuberculous drug isoniazid is well known. The use of the contraceptive pill can also increase pyridoxine requirement and can theoretically lead to a deficiency state.

Vitamin B₂ (riboflavin)

The coenzymes flavine mononucleotide (FMN) and flavine adenosine dinucleotide (FAD) are derived from vitamin B_2. They are required for carbohydrate and fat metabolism and a wide variety of oxidation and reduction reactions central to all metabolic processes (Ch. 3). Deficiencies lead to angular stomatitis, glossitis, dermatitis, cheilosis and cataracts. Sources include liver, milk, meat, fish and some leafy vegetables.

Vitamin B₃ (niacin)

Nicotinic acid and nicotinamide are also known as niacin (vitamin B_3), an essential part of the human diet as it forms the active part of nicotinamide adenine dinucleotide (NAD^+) and nicotinamide adenine dinucleotide phosphate ($NADP^+$). Energy for ATP synthesis is derived from oxidation of these nucleotides (see Ch. 3). Both vitamins B_2 and B_3 have a central role in the transduction of energy in the electron transport chain of mitochondria. Niacin can be synthesised from tryptophan in the presence of other B vitamins such as riboflavin, pyridoxine and/or thiamine.

Vitamin B₆ (pyridoxine)

Vitamin B_6 is a cofactor in glycogen and amino acid metabolism. A high dietary protein intake increases pyridoxine requirement.

Biotin

Biotin functions as a coenzyme in lipogenesis, gluconeogenesis and the breakdown of branch chained amino acids (see Ch. 3). A growth factor for cells, it is synthesised by intestinal flora. Some dietary constituents, such as the raw egg white protein avidin, bind with biotin to prevent its absorption, leading to deficiency. Clinical consequences include dermatitis, depression and muscular pains, but deficiency is very rare outside the context of artificial nutrition.

Pantothenic acid

Pantothenic acid is part of coenzyme A and is widely available in all plant and animal foods. Deficiency in humans is very rare.

Folic acid

The physiologically active, reduced form of folic acid, dihydrofolic acid, acts as a coenzyme in single carbon transfer during nucleic acid (DNA) and amino acid synthesis. Folic acid is therefore most needed by rapidly dividing cells (see Clinical box 16.5).

Vitamin B₁₂ (cobalamin)

Vitamin B_{12}, together with folic acid, is involved as a coenzyme in the conversion of homocysteine to methionine (see above). It also acts as a coenzyme for methylmalonyl-CoA

Clinical box 16.5 **Folic acid deficiency**

Deficiency of folic acid is one of the most common vitamin deficiencies. Increased demand, such as during pregnancy and the demand of rapid foetal growth, could precipitate folate deficiency. This feature is also exploited, as antifolate drugs are used against rapidly dividing bacterial cells (antibiotic trimethoprim) and cancer cells (cytotoxic methotrexate).

Folate deficiency causes a macrocytic, megaloblastic anaemia (see Ch. 12). The features are similar to vitamin B_{12} deficiency. High intake of folate reduces plasma concentrations of homocysteine.

Clinical box 16.6 **Vitamin B₁₂ deficiency**

Vitamin B_{12} is well stored and deficiency takes months or years to develop. Eventually, deficiency leads to a methionine deficiency in the spinal cord, giving rise to a neurological disorder, subacute combined degeneration of the cord, which can occur without megaloblastic anaemia. The megaloblastic anaemia in vitamin B_{12} deficiency is probably associated with a deficiency of reduced folate (see Ch. 12). For this reason, until the cause is finally established, a macrocytic, megaloblastic anaemia should not be treated with folic acid alone because of the risk of precipitating subacute combined degeneration of the cord.

Vitamin B_{12} is the only water-soluble vitamin stored mainly in the liver. Pernicious anaemia, an autoimmune gastritis which results in lack of gastric intrinsic factor required for the absorption of vitamin B_{12}, is one cause of deficiency; gastric resection is a cause of intrinsic factor deficiency. Malabsorption due to chronic pancreatitis can occur as a result of failure to secrete a pancreas-derived activating component of intrinsic factor. Small-intestinal bacterial overgrowth causes deficiency, commonly in the elderly. Extensive (100 cm or more) ileal resection, for example because of Crohn disease, prevents absorption of vitamin B_{12}. Vegans, who eat no animal products, are at risk of dietary vitamin B_{12} deficiency.

---

mutase. Vitamin B_{12} is synthesised by bacteria and only available in foods of animal origin (see Clinical box 16.6).

Vitamin C (ascorbic acid)

Vitamin C is essential in the human diet, and abundant in citrus fruits and green vegetables. Ascorbic acid, the physiologically active form, is a reducing agent in hydroxylation reactions. Its role as an antioxidant in preventing cancer and atherosclerosis has attracted much attention but as yet there is no evidence of its effectiveness. It also takes part in the synthesis of epinephrine (adrenaline) and steroids.

Vitamin C is a cofactor in several collagen synthesis reactions; severe deficiency leads to scurvy, a condition in which there is capillary fragility, giving rise to bruising and subcutaneous haemorrhages, bleeding and swollen gums, muscle weakness, anaemia and poor wound healing. Although common in the days of long sea voyages when fresh fruit and vegetables were not available, scurvy is now rare except among the very elderly with poor diets. Vitamin C deficiency is associated with impaired immunity and, in epidemiological studies, is associated with a faster rate of loss of bone mineral density.

FAT-SOLUBLE VITAMINS

Fat-soluble vitamins are stored in the liver and adipose tissue. They have to be absorbed with fat and are less easily absorbed from food than water-soluble vitamins. Enthusiastic supplementation, however, can lead to toxicity and overdose. Vitamins A and D function like hormones and are toxic in overdose.

Vitamin A

Vitamin A is a generic term used to describe a collection of related compounds. The main physiologically active forms of vitamin A are retinaldehyde and retinoic acid, which are derived from retinol. These are collectively known as retinoids.

A number of carotenoid pigments in plants can also form retinol, the most important being β-carotene. Retinaldehyde is involved in the visual system and retinoic acid modulates gene expression and tissue differentiation.

Clinical box 16.7   **Vitamin A deficiency**

Retinol is an intracellular pigment that is bound to rhodopsin in the cells of the retina and acts like a hormone. When exposed to light, it dissociates and initiates a signal to the brain which is perceived as light. Vitamin A deficiency thus leads to 'night blindness', or visual impairment in poor light. Retinoic acid acts as a typical steroid hormone. It increases the synthesis of proteins controlling epithelial cell differentiation. Deficiency can lead to corneal softening (defective epithelial growth and keratinisation leading to **xerophthalmia**) causing partial and, if severe, permanent blindness. Under famine and starvation conditions, vitamin A deficiency is the commonest cause of blindness. Vitamin A deficiency also occurs in liver failure and in malabsorption as a result of steatorrhoea.

The main dietary source of vitamin A in developed countries is from retinol palmitate which is an ester of retinol (free retinol being chemically unstable so found in small amounts) found in animal sources, such as liver, milk, cod liver oil, butter, cheese and margarine. The provitamin is β-carotene, widely distributed in green vegetables. Enough is stored in the liver as retinol palmate to last about a year. Two specialised proteins, serum retinol binding protein (SRBP) and cytosolic binding proteins, are needed to distribute vitamin A from the liver to its active site. High concentrations of the retinoids (not carotenoids) are toxic, particularly in pregnancy.

β-Carotene has been shown to have antioxidant activity and is found in lower levels in patients with cancer compared with controls. However, so far, trials have not shown a beneficial effect of supplementation. As mentioned above, a diet high in β-carotene would be one that is high in fruit and vegetables and generally lower in saturated fat, therefore could be considered more 'healthy' (Clinical box 16.7 describes vitamin A deficiency).

Vitamin D (calciferol)

Vitamin D is really a hormone synthesised from cholesterol (produced in the liver) in the skin following exposure to ultraviolet rays in sunlight. Dietary intake is only necessary when exposure to sunlight is inadequate; dietary sources include cod liver oil, eggs, dairy products, fortified milk and margarine (see Clinical box 16.8 for vitamin D deficiency). The effect of sunlight leads to the synthesis of ergocalciferol (D_2) and cholecalciferol (D_3), which are further metabolised to hydroxylated derivatives – first in the liver (25 position) and then in the renal tubules (1 position) to 1,25-hydroxyvitamin D_3, the active form of vitamin D (Ch. 10).

Vitamin E (tocopherols)

Vitamin E is incorporated in the lipid cell membrane structure, lipoproteins and adipose tissues, and is an antioxidant. There are eight vitamers of vitamin E, known as

Clinical box 16.8   **Vitamin D deficiency**

Vitamin D affects Ca^{2+} metabolism and bones (see Ch. 11 for details). Deficiency leads to rickets in children and osteomalacia in adults. This can occur when a lack of sunshine combines with dietary deficiency due to inadequate intake of milk and oily fish, or malabsorption from foodstuffs that bind with dietary vitamin D to prevent absorption.

the tocopherols. Although it is associated with fertility in some animals, with a role in spermatogenesis and ovum implantation, there is no proven association in human beings. Widely available in vegetable oils, dietary vitamin E deficiency is rare as there are relatively large tissue reserves. The exceptions are in fat malabsorption, rare genetic disorders, cholestatic hepatobiliary disease and in very-low-weight premature infants, where deficiency causes haemolytic anaemia and thrombocytosis. Dietary sources include seeds, margarines and vegetable oils, especially wheatgerm and sunflower seed oils.

Vitamin K

Vitamin K acts as a coenzyme in activating precursors (clotting factors) produced by the liver in the coagulation cascade (see Ch. 12). Dietary deficiency causes haemorrhagic disease. Although dietary deficiency is uncommon, it occurs with fat malabsorption. Coagulation disorders, owing to vitamin K deficiency, can also occur in liver disease (e.g. alcoholic cirrhosis) and in newborn infants. In newborn infants with very immature livers and sterile guts, vitamin K deficiency occurs because it is mostly made by the normal bacterial flora of the jejunum and ileum not present in newborns. Anticoagulants of the dicoumarin group (warfarin or rat poison) act by inhibiting the action of vitamin K. Vitamin K may be used to reverse haemorrhagic conditions from dicoumarin overdose. Dietary sources include green leafy vegetables, vegetable oils and fermented dairy products.

TRACE ELEMENTS: MINERALS

Trace amounts of some minerals are necessary for metabolic processes and are therefore essential in the human diet. All are toxic in high concentrations, and a number of deficiency syndromes have been recognised. Unbound metal ions carry a charge and can lead to the formation of free radicals.

IRON

Iron is essential for many metabolic processes, especially for the oxygen-carrying capacity of haemoglobin (see Ch. 12). The average body content of iron is 3–5 mg, two-thirds of which is in haemoglobin.

Iron is absorbed in the ferrous Fe^{2+} form. It is transported in the oxidised ferric Fe^{3+} form, bound to transferrin and is stored mainly in the liver, spleen or bone marrow as ferritin. Iron in the diet is present in the haem form (found in haemoglobin) from animal sources and the non-haem form from vegetables and pulses. The haem form is much easier to absorb, hence vegan diets may be predisposed to deficiency. Iron absorption is enhanced by vitamin C. Iron deficiency is the most common vitamin deficiency worldwide affecting more than 2 billion people. Clinical box 16.9 discusses iron deficiency and overload.

COPPER

Dietary sources of copper include legumes, nuts, animal sources and water (from copper pipes) Copper is incorporated into the oxygenase enzymes, particularly superoxide dismutase, which is a scavenger of superoxide and other

Clinical box 16.9   Iron deficiency and overload

Iron deficiency anaemia can occur with dietary deficiency, increased demand or excessive blood loss and results in microcytic hypochromic anaemia:

- Deficiency is seldom due to dietary inadequacy but can be associated with extreme, unbalanced diets such as the vegan diet.
- Increased demand from excessive blood loss in women of childbearing age or from overt or occult gastrointestinal bleeding. Iron deficiency anaemia in men or post-menopausal women should trigger a search for gastrointestinal pathology, particularly colon cancer.
- Malabsorption of iron is rarely a problem but occurs in coeliac disease.
- There is increased demand during both pregnancy and rapid growth in childhood.
  Iron overload leads to hepatomegaly and cirrhosis.

Excessive iron stores in the liver may be caused by:

- Repeated blood transfusions causing haemosiderosis, e.g. in β-thalassaemia
- Unusually excessive dietary intake, as in some South African tribes that use iron cooking pots
- Hereditary haemochromatosis.

Clinical box 16.10   Copper deficiency and overload

Copper deficiency due to malabsorption occurs in **Menke syndrome**, a rare, sex linked, recessive genetic disorder. In children with this condition, there is failure to thrive, mental retardation and bone defects, with characteristic kinky, brittle hair.

    Wilson disease is an inborn error of metabolism and an autosomal recessive disorder. Biliary excretion of copper is severely impaired leading to copper deposits in:

- Liver – resulting in cirrhosis
- Kidneys – with tubular degeneration
- Basal ganglia – causing tremor, involuntary movements and dementia
- Cornea – as Kayser–Fleischer rings.

reactive oxygen species (see below). It is also necessary for collagen synthesis. Copper deficiency is quite rare and occurs with excessive loss, as in chronic renal dialysis and in malabsorption. The latter occurs in Menke disease. It has been seen in patients receiving long-term parenteral nutrition with copper-free feeds and in premature infants fed cow's milk (see Clinical box 16.10).

ZINC

Zinc is involved in many metabolic processes as coenzymes and metalloproteins. Zinc is widely available in all foods. Although of low toxicity, excessive zinc intake interferes with copper absorption and can lead to copper deficiency. Clinical box 16.11 discusses zinc deficiency.

Clinical box 16.11   Zinc deficiency

A very rare hereditary disorder, acrodermatitis enteropathica, is characterised by zinc malabsorption, leading to growth retardation, diarrhoea, hair loss, skin lesions and *Candida* infections. Zinc supplementation reverses all the symptoms. Zinc deficiency can also be caused by increased loss, as in renal disease and major burns. Patients on total parenteral nutrition also need regular assessment of zinc status and supplementation. Zinc depletion prevents wound healing and compromises the immune system so that the patient is more susceptible to infections. Sexual development and spermatogenesis may also be impaired.

SELENIUM

Selenium is part of the antioxidant glutathione peroxidase and is also found in most cells. Dietary sources include shellfish, offal, brazil nuts and cereals. Low selenium is thought to impair immune and thyroid function, decrease antioxidant status and increase susceptibility to viral infections. Selenium intake varies worldwide as a result of varying soil composition and therefore the variable selenium content in staple foods such as wheat. Deficiency is rare except for Keshan disease, which is endemic in some areas in China where the soil selenium content is extremely low or absent. Muscle pains and cardiomyopathy may result. Total parenteral nutrition can also lead to selenium deficiency.

MAGNESIUM

Magnesium is an intracellular ion involved in maintaining electropotentials in nerves and skeletal muscle. The amount of magnesium consumed is the main determinant of the amount absorbed, although parathyroid hormone (PTH) and vitamin D probably increase absorption. Its main dietary source is from green vegetables, legumes, nuts, seeds and unrefined grains and as well as animal products – although dairy products contain low amounts. The main control of plasma magnesium levels is by the kidneys.

CALCIUM

Nearly all (99%) the body's calcium in adults is found in the skeleton (about 1 kg). Plasma concentration is about 2.25–2.60 mmol/L. The recommended daily intake of calcium in adults in the UK is:

- Adult (19–50 years) RNI = 700 mg
- Lactation = 700 mg + 550 mg.

    Calcium absorption and metabolism are discussed in Chapters 10 and 15. Lack of oestrogen and corticosteroid therapy in particular are implicated in loss of calcium from the skeleton and osteoporosis in later life. Calcium is mainly found in milk and dairy products; vegetables contain a small amount. In some countries (e.g. the UK) flour is fortified with calcium. Calcium requirements increase during pregnancy and lactation. Deficiency is associated with vitamin D deficiency. Adolescent girls frequently do not consume enough calcium. It is estimated that a third of women and a sixth of men will have an osteoporotic fracture at some time in their life.

PHOSPHATE

Phosphate is needed for phosphorylation, an essential process in most metabolic pathways. Daily oral intake for adults is similar to that of calcium. Phosphate is widely available and well absorbed from food, so that dietary deficiency is unknown. Plasma phosphate levels are regulated by PTH (see Ch. 10). Low levels are associated with hyperparathyroidism. High phosphate concentrations are seen in hypoparathyroidism and renal failure.

IODINE

Iodine is a constituent of thyroid hormones. Seafoods and seaweed are rich in iodine. Iodine is also available in milk, which is now the major source of iodine in Western countries.

Deficiency causes goitre and brain damage. Endemic goitre occurs in mountainous regions where iodine is absent in the soil. Salt is also iodised to help eradicate iodine deficiency.

FLUORIDE

Epidemiological evidence suggests that dental caries is more prevalent in areas with lower levels of fluoride in drinking water. There are few dietary sources of fluoride apart from shellfish. Fluoridation of drinking water and toothpaste may help. Fluorosis, resulting from fluoride overdose, causes damage to dental enamel with pitting and discoloration.

WATER AND ELECTROLYTES

Water and electrolytes are essential constituents of the human body and are found in three compartments within the body:

- Intracellular fluid (ICF)
- Interstitial fluids
- Plasma.

The typical volumes of fluid distributed in the various compartments are described in Chapters 2 and 4. The intracellular compartment is separated from the extracellular compartment by the lipid cell membrane. In the extracellular compartment, plasma is separated from the interstitial fluids by the capillary membranes. The biochemical composition and volume of body fluids in health are kept constant through homeostatic mechanisms (see Ch. 2). In disease, the control mechanisms are altered, so that there could be disturbance in fluid volume and altered biochemical composition.

WATER

Most of the water in the body is in the lean body mass. The fat-free mass of adults is about 72% water. The amount of water in an adult is therefore dependent on the amount of adipose tissue in their body. Men tend to have a higher percentage of water content than women because women store more fat per unit weight.

Daily water requirements

The water requirement for an average adult varies between 1.5 L and 3 L per day (30–35 mL/kg body weight), of which 0.5 to 1 L is to replace insensible loss, i.e. from skin and respiration. The daily output of water is the sum of losses in the urine, faeces and sweat, and will vary according to the environmental temperature, body temperature, amount of physical activity and weight. The amount of water lost in the urine is determined by urine concentration or dilution by the kidneys, which in turn is regulated by vasopressin (also called anti-diuretic hormone (ADH)). The mechanism is discussed in detail in Chapter 14.

The daily water requirement increases substantially during vigorous exercise because of loss through sweating. Children also need more water. To estimate daily fluid balance and fluid requirement in clinical practice, the urine, faecal and other intestinal (e.g. diarrhoea, vomit or gastric aspirate) losses are summed, and then a nominal 500–1000 mL for insensible (sweat) loss is added.

The amount that a person drinks can be in excess of requirement, based on thirst and to some extent habit (Ch. 8).

Water is obtained from foods and drinks and from water formed during metabolism. The water formed during metabolism is relatively small at roughly 275 mL/day. For patients who are unable to drink (e.g. postoperatively) or have suffered severe losses, as with burns or haemorrhage, hydration must be maintained by intravenous infusion. Fluid balance can be monitored either by careful input and output charting or by monitoring the changes in body weight from day to day.

ELECTROLYTES

The plasma electrolytes that are clinically important include the sodium and potassium cations (Na^+ and K^+), and the chloride and bicarbonate anions (Cl^- and HCO_3^-). Clinical laboratory measurements of plasma concentration are used for the diagnosis of metabolic disturbances, such as diabetic ketoacidosis, renal failure and so on. Electrolytes are dissolved in water and, as with water, divided into intracellular and extracellular compartments. The molecules dissolved in water contribute to the **osmotic pressure** in their separate compartments (see also Chs 2 and 14). The osmotic gradient created by the different electrolyte concentrations in each compartment enables water to move between the compartments.

Although water is freely diffusible across the barriers between compartments, the movement of water-soluble electrolytes and molecules is restricted by the lipid cell membrane. Water-soluble molecules have to be transported across these membranes via ion pumps, of which the Na^+/K^+-ATPase pump is the most active. The energy-consuming process in which Na^+ is driven out of cells and K^+ is driven into cells is reduced during fasting, so that Na^+ moves into cells and K^+ moves out. The opposite occurs with refeeding (see Refeeding syndrome, below). One of the ion pump's functions is nerve transmission (see Ch. 8). Other ion pumps transport glucose, amino acids and calcium.

WATER AND ELECTROLYTE DEPLETION

Fluid depletion could be due to:

- Severe water deprivation, as in postoperative patients unable to drink, unconscious patients or abnormalities with thirst mechanisms
- Loss of electrolytes and water, as in severe, prolonged vomiting and diarrhoea
- Excess water loss due to pituitary (failure of ADH secretion) or renal (failure to respond to ADH) problems or **diabetes insipidus**
- Excess water loss through osmotic diuresis, e.g. drug induced, hyperglycaemia
- Loss of plasma, as in severe burns
- Haemorrhage, when blood as well as water and electrolytes are lost.

Oral rehydration with water and electrolytes is the method of choice, whenever possible. Intravenous fluid replacement is needed when the fluid loss is severe, the patient is unconscious, or when the patient cannot drink.

Intravenous fluid replacement

A variety of intravenous fluids are available for severely dehydrated patients in whom oral rehydration is contraindicated. Table 16.12 shows the electrolyte content of the principal

Table 16.12	Constitution of solutions for intravenous infusion			
	Na$^+$ (mmol/L)	K$^+$ (mmol/L)	HCO$_3^-$ (mmol/L)	Energy (kJ (kcal)/L)
5% Dextrose	–	–	–	838 (200)
Dextrose saline solution	30	–	–	670 (160)
Normal saline	150	–	–	–
Hartmann's solution	131	5	29 (lactate) +2 mmol Ca	–

intravenous fluids used in clinical practice. Note that dextrose saline is a maintenance solution for use when there is no excessive fluid loss or Na$^+$ depletion, whereas 0.9% ('normal') saline is a replacement solution with a Na$^+$ content approximating that of plasma. However, compared with plasma values, there is excess Cl$^-$ relative to Na$^+$, which can result in hyperchloraemic acidosis (i.e. sodium and chloride are equimolar in normal saline whereas there is less chloride than sodium in plasma), so a more physiologically balanced solution such as Hartmann's may be preferable and better tolerated. Both Hartmann's solution and normal saline contain more than a day's requirement of Na$^+$ per litre. They are therefore fluid replacement and not fluid maintenance solutions and carry the risk of salt and water overload and oedema.

WATER OVERLOAD

Water overload occurs if the intake exceeds renal excretion and is uncommon with normal renal function, except with very excessive drinking. It does, however, occur if 5% dextrose or a hypo-osmolar solution is infused over-enthusiastically. The effect is to dilute sodium content: hyponatraemia (Na$^+$ <135 mmol/L). If uncorrected, hyponatraemic encephalopathy can occur. Hyponatraemia has been reported with excessive intake of sports drinks and water after strenuous exercise, e.g. after running a marathon. It can also occur after excessive dextrose infusions postoperatively, particularly if there is a degree of impaired glomerular filtration. This can be avoided by giving isotonic normal saline.

THE CONTROL OF FOOD INTAKE

The interactions between energy balance and food intake for humans is complex. The increasing prevalence of obesity and its associated disease states has focused attention on the physiological mechanisms that control nutritional intake and energy expenditure. These mechanisms are potential targets for intervention, whether through use of anti-obesity drugs or the use of psychological therapies, in the quest for effective treatment of obesity.

APPETITE AND SATIETY

Appetite refers to a desire to eat, which may be influenced by the sight, taste and smell of food, social and cultural patterns of eating behaviour and psychological factors (e.g. depression). Hunger is the feeling of a pressing need to eat, and satiety is the feeling during, or soon after, a meal that enough has been eaten. Eating as a goal-directed behaviour and motivation for eating (or not) is discussed in Chapter 8. Eating is a basic function to sustain life, which also gives enjoyment. For human beings, satiety does not necessarily terminate eating, and nor is it hunger that always initiates eating. The central neuroendocrine regulation of eating is discussed in Chapter 8.

THE PHYSIOLOGICAL CONTROL OF EATING

A complex system of signals indicating satiety (satiety signals) balances the drive to eat. These include:

- Peripheral signals arising from the gut
- Hormones signalling energy balance and fat stores.

These signals are integrated through a network of feedback mechanisms in which the hypothalamus plays the leading role. The brainstem and higher cortical networks also play their part (Fig. 16.9).

PERIPHERAL SATIETY SIGNALS

Satiety signals originating in the gut are carried via afferents in the vagus to the nucleus of the solitary tract (nTS) in the brainstem (Fig. 16.9). These signals are initiated by:

- Gastric fullness, gastric distension, when the stretch receptors in the stomach walls are stimulated by overfilling the stomach, and gastric emptying
- The balance of chemical content in the lumen of the gut
- Peptides and hormones secreted by the stomach and small intestine in response to the presence of food.

Gastric distension and emptying

Filling the stomach leads to distension, which reduces the desire to eat. For example, pyloric ligation (in animal experiments, to prevent gastric contents from entering the duodenum) results in stomach distension that appears to induce satiety. Balloons inflated in the stomach induce satiety in

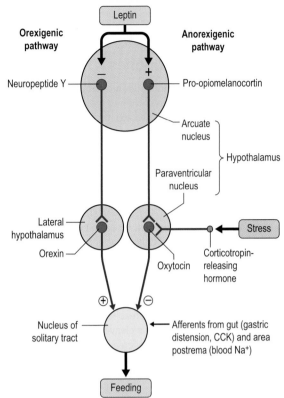

Fig. 16.9 Postulated pathways for the regulation of appetite and energy balance. Increased leptin secretion is a long-term satiety signal, increased CCK (cholecystokinin) in the short term reduces appetite. Decreased leptin levels increase appetite (hunger). Hunger (during starvation and weight loss) increases appetite and reduces energy expenditure. Satiety should reduce eating and increase energy expenditure.

rats. This appears to be true in humans as well: endoscopically placed gastric balloons help obese patients lose weight. Cancer of the stomach is a common pathological cause of early satiety when infiltration of the stomach wall with cancer cells leads to rigidity and limited distension so that smaller than normal feeds make the patient 'feel full'. However, a full stomach does not always stop someone from eating more.

The *rate* of gastric emptying is an important component in determining gastric fullness. It depends upon the physical form of the meal eaten, its volume, energy density, fat content and many other variables, including stress, smoking and whether the food is eaten in an habitual form. In man, for any particular fixed proportions of constituents, the higher the *volume* of a feed, the *slower* the gastric emptying. Animal studies indicate that slower gastric emptying gives rise to a greater sense of satiety.

Balance of chemical contents in the gut

The presence of food in the duodenum, jejunum and ileum delays gastric emptying, probably mediated by intestinal receptors for acidity, osmolality, fat, glucose and amino acids. A jejunal infusion of a mixture of casein hydrolysate, oleic acid and maltose, designed to simulate the composition of normal chyme in the jejunum, inhibits gastric acid secretion and delays gastric emptying. The results of altering the proportions of the constituents in the infusion suggest that carbohydrate and fat have the principal inhibiting effect on acid secretion, whereas carbohydrate, fat and protein delay stomach emptying.

Peptides and hormones

A variety of peptides and hormones are secreted by the stomach and small intestine in response to the presence of food, stimulating the pancreas to secrete digestive enzymes and hormones, the gall bladder to contract and empty bile into the duodenum, promote or inhibit stomach and gut motility, and act as short-term chemical signals to inhibit excessive eating (see also Ch. 15). Among these, the best characterised include:

- **Cholecystokinin** (CCK) – a hormone secreted in the duodenum, jejunum and terminal ileum in response to the presence of food. CCK reduces appetite and inhibits eating. It also acts as a neurotransmitter in the hypothalamus to inhibit eating (see Information box 16.5).
- **Glucagon-like peptide-1 (GLP-1)** – the ileal brake is a signal which reduces gastric emptying and inhibits upper intestinal motility when food reaches the ileum. It is mediated by GLP-1, which is cleaved from proglucagon and expressed in the gut, pancreas and brain.
- **Oxyntomodulin** – also proglucagon-derived and secreted by ileal cells in proportion to ingested calories, this peptide lessens hunger and food intake.
- **Peptide YY (PYY)** – secreted in the ileum and colon and also part of the 'ileal brake'. It is related to neuropeptide Y (NPY), inhibits pancreatic exocrine secretion and slows down gastric and small bowel transit of food. Intestinal PYY reduces appetite (whereas hypothalamic NPY increases food intake) but the effect may be independent of central pathways.

PERIPHERAL HUNGER SIGNALS

Peripheral hunger signals arise from the intestine, mediated by the hormone ghrelin. Hunger is not usually experienced until after near-complete gastric emptying (about 1.5–3 hours after eating) and peaks about 2–4 hours after onset. Hunger ratings in experimental subjects continue to increase after complete gastric emptying, indicating that while an empty stomach may give rise to hunger, it cannot be the whole cause.

Ghrelin

Ghrelin is a 28 amino acid peptide hormone that has orexigenic effects, increasing appetite, weight and blood sugar. The main source of ghrelin is from the gastric parietal cells (and small amount from the small intestine and hypothalamus). This acts on ghrelin receptors in the hypothalamus to stimulate GHrF (growth hormone releasing factor) which acts on pituitary GH receptors causing release of growth hormone (see Information box 16.5). Ghrelin levels are increased during fasting and decrease on eating. With bariatric surgery (see below), the use of sleeve gastrectomy removes the majority of ghrelin producing cells, hence results in reduced ghrelin levels which may also contribute to the weight loss achieved with these procedures. It is also possible that

---

| **Information box 16.5** | **Action of cholecystokinin and ghrelin** |

Upper gastrointestinal tract peptides and neurotransmitters released in response to the presence of food (see above) are carried via vagal afferents to the nTS.

- **CCK**: there is early evidence from animal experiments that brainstem POMC (pro-opiomelanocortin) neurons may transmit CCK satiety signals to the hypothalamus. Further clues may come from the link between the intraventricular injection of leptin and insulin with the enhanced effect of peripherally administered CCK.
- **Ghrelin**: most of the evidence for the mechanisms of the action of ghrelin has been derived from animal experiments. It appears that vagal afferents carry ghrelin signals to inhibit POMC neurons in the nTS. The inhibited nTS neurons then send further signals to the arcuate nucleus to synapse with the NPY neuron. Ghrelin signalling on the brain is thereby mediated by NPY/ agouti-related peptide neurons (AgRP) in the arcuate nucleus to increase appetite and feeding. There is also evidence indicating that there may be anatomical links between ghrelin and NPY, and that ghrelin may activate NPY directly.

| **Clinical box 16.12** | **Ghrelin in disease** |

Plasma concentrations of ghrelin in patients with anorexia nervosa are higher than normal. As body weight rises to near normal levels, ghrelin concentration falls. Conversely, ghrelin levels are lower in obese people compared with lean controls. The relationships between the conditions and ghrelin concentration are not yet clear. Ghrelin levels are extremely high in the plasma of patients with Prader–Willi syndrome, characterised by extreme obesity and an almost insatiable appetite.

---

it has longer term effects on the regulation of body weight. In rodent studies, administration of ghrelin resulted in increased appetite and weight gain. However, in obese subjects, levels are found to be decreased. Ongoing research may elucidate its role in energy homeostasis and obesity (see below) (see Clinical box 16.12).

LONG-TERM SATIETY SIGNALS

The peripheral signals to eat or not to eat are short-term responses to food. Longer-term signals are in response to the overall energy requirements and expenditure of the body–energy homeostasis (see Fig. 16.9). Discovery of the hormone **leptin** in 1994 led to the understanding of how endocrine and metabolic signals might orchestrate the integration of food intake, energy expenditure and fat storage.

Leptin

Leptin was originally discovered in mice that were found to be naturally obese. This was due to a homozygous mutation in the Ob gene that encodes leptin, causing deficiency. Intravenous injection of leptin into these mice resulted in reduced feeding and weight loss and improved hyperinsulinaemia, hyperglycaemia and diabetes. Leptin deficiency has since been found in humans, but it is rare.

Leptin is a hormone synthesised and secreted by white adipose tissues (see Fig. 16.9). The leptin receptors, of which there are several isoforms, are found in the hypothalamus (as well as a number of other tissues, including stomach and placenta). During starvation, plasma leptin concentration falls and it is thought that in humans this is a very powerful signal to increase appetite and eating (orexigenic) and to decrease

BMR in order to conserve energy. It has been shown that, in animals, low circulating leptin also inhibits growth and reproduction so it likely to have a role in reproductive signalling.

Plasma leptin levels reflect the size of adipose tissue in fat stores, where a higher concentration is found in obesity. As the plasma leptin concentration increases, it has the effect on the hypothalamus of increasing satiety and suppressing appetite (anorexigenic), It also increases BMR and energy expenditure when the hypothalamus activates the peripheral nervous system to increase fat breakdown for gluconeogenesis.

In obesity, however, despite elevated leptin levels, satiety is not achieved. There have been findings of leptin receptor mutations as well as gene mutations causing production of non-functional leptin, but it is possible that at high levels the signalling is weak or the brain becomes insensitive to its actions, suggesting possible leptin resistance. Research is ongoing.

Insulin

Before leptin was discovered, research was focused on the role of insulin in human energy homeostasis. Evidence from animal experiments suggests that insulin has a role in the central (brain) physiological regulation of energy homeostasis (see Fig. 16.9). Experimental mice lacking insulin receptors in the brain became obese. It has also been reported that intraventricular administration of insulin and leptin into the brain potentiates the action of peripherally given CCK to stop feeding, leading to sustained weight loss.

Oestrogen

Although there is as yet no direct evidence for the cellular mechanisms of the anorexigenic action of oestrogens, evidence from animal experiments is emerging. Oestrogen receptor expression has been localised in parts of the hypothalamus, namely the arcuate nucleus. Oestrogen appears to target the anorexic pro-opiomelanocortin (POMC) neuron.

DIET AND DISEASE

Diet is strongly implicated in the aetiology of some of the most prevalent diseases: obesity and its complications including coronary heart disease, hypertension and therefore heart failure and stroke, and many cancers. Nonetheless it has proven difficult to demonstrate causality between diet and disease because of the huge size and economic cost of the clinical trials needed to do so.

Much depends on epidemiological association of disease with diet and then animal studies to test hypothetical mechanisms. Other approaches are case–control and cohort studies, which have validity only if they follow a large enough sample of the general population over a sufficiently long period (see Ch. 7). Most studies create a highly artificial situation in which changes are made in the amount of a single nutrient. This is confounded by diet being made up of a large number of foods, each containing many macro- and micronutrients, and that a change in one type of food with the intention of changing one nutrient in the diet will also change other nutrients. These difficulties are compounded by the fact that there is a variable latent effect between (repeated) exposure to nutrient intake and pathological response.

ASSOCIATION BETWEEN DIET AND DISEASE

Given the difficulties involved in research, it is remarkable how much progress has in fact been made in defining the effects of diet and dietary change. Diet is estimated to explain around 30% of cancers in the Western world, and perhaps 20% in the developing countries. Theories regarding ageing, formation of atheroma and cancer are based on the effects of cellular damage by free radicals.

Reactive oxygen species or free radicals

Oxygen atoms bind together by sharing electrons (paired) in their outer shells to form O_2 molecules (see Ch. 2 and Information box 16.6). When the outer shells are full, the molecule is stable and inert (or unreactive). During chemical reactions, the bond between electrons sometimes splits to give a free, unpaired electron. The molecule is known as a 'free radical'. Reactive oxygen species are oxygen molecules that have gained an extra, unpaired electron, and are known as **superoxide** when a single electron is added.

The molecule containing the oxygen radical becomes highly unstable and reactive, because it tries to 'steal' an electron from another molecule to stabilise itself. Within cells, the free oxygen radical captures an electron from the nearest molecule, which loses an electron and becomes a free radical. This sets off a chain reaction that ends by disrupting the cell. Thus reactive oxygen species are toxic, causing tissue damage. However, they have a positive role in immunological defence systems where they enter cancer or bacterial molecules and disrupt them.

At human body temperatures, O_2 is stable. The vast majority of O_2 in the body is used in producing energy (90%) and in redox reactions (9%). Less than 1% is converted to free radicals (reactive oxygen species). Free radicals are alleged to play a role in more than 60 different health conditions, including ageing, cancer and atherosclerosis.

Formation of reactive oxygen species

Free radicals are highly reactive compounds that are formed in the body during normal metabolic processes or introduced from the environment. Oxygen, although essential to life, is the source of the potentially damaging free radicals. Environmental sources of free radicals include exposure to ionising radiation (from industry, sun exposure, cosmic rays, and medical X-rays), ozone and nitrous oxide (primarily from automobile exhaust), heavy metals (such as mercury, cadmium and lead), cigarette smoke (both active and passive), alcohol, unsaturated fat and other chemicals and compounds from food, water and air.

Metal ions are normally bound to transport or storage proteins (e.g. iron in haemoglobin, myoglobin or methaemoglobin). In cells, metal ions that are not bound to protein donate electrons to O_2 to form reactive oxygen species.

Information box 16.6	**Redox reactions**

- **Oxidation** occurs when a molecule loses an electron – an oxidising agent therefore is a molecule that gains an electron. Oxygen is a common oxidising agent.
- **Reduction** occurs when a molecule gains an electron – a reducing agent therefore is a molecule that loses an electron.

Body defence against cancer or invading bacteria

Phagocytic action of white blood cells involves enzymic action that adds an electron to the O_2 molecules around the bacteria to form **superoxide**, which reacts with itself to give another reactive oxygen species, hydrogen peroxide. Hydrogen peroxide destroys the bacteria by generating free radicals that eventually disrupt the cells.

Oxidative stress

Oxidative stress occurs when the production of reactive oxygen species exceeds the body's defences against them (see Information box 16.7).

Defence against reactive oxygen species – antioxidants

The antioxidant defences are both endogenously produced and dietary and can be summarised to be:

- Enzymatic – superoxide to hydrogen peroxide, hydrogen peroxide to water (catalase and glutathione peroxidase)
- Non-enzymatic – glutathione, urate, ubiquinones, albumin, bilirubin, vitamins A, E and C, β-carotene.

There are normal metabolic processes that 'mop up' the tiny amount of free radicals produced:

- Proteins that bind metals such as iron and copper (transport and carrier protein) trap metal ions that activate redox reactions.
- Detoxifying enzymes that mop up metal ions – **superoxide dismutase, catalase, glutathione peroxidase**.
- Anti-oxidant vitamins A, C and E are reducing agents that donate H atoms to free radicals caused by action of

reactive oxygen species in proteins, lipids and DNA (see later); for example, vitamin A protects against damage by sunlight.

DIET AND CARCINOGENESIS

Diet can influence carcinogenesis through general mechanisms, which apply to most or all cancers, or through specific toxicities which increase the risk of a particular cancer (Clinical box 16.13). Epidemiological studies suggest that certain dietary components increase the risk of cancer, whereas others appear to be protective (Table 16.13). The evidence that cancer is preventable by consuming a balanced diet comes from:

- Differences in incidence between communities
- Changes in incidence in migrant people
- Changes in incidence over time
- Identification of causes in animal research
- Intervention trials (randomised controlled trials).

Dietary constituents themselves can have effects on aspects of DNA expression and cell signalling, which in turn may increase the risk of cancer development (mutagens), usually by forming mutagen-DNA adducts (Table 16.14). Mutagens can be diluted; it may that by drawing water into the colon, dietary non-starch polysaccharides, such as fibre and resistant starch, help protect against colon cancer.

Antioxidants

One general protective component that emerges repeatedly in population studies is a high intake of fruit and vegetables. One mechanism postulated is that the presence of antioxidants, such as vitamin C, carotenoids (e.g. lycopene from tomatoes), fat-soluble vitamin E and the trace element

---

Information box 16.7 **Factors associated with oxidative stress**

- Cells of the immune system produce excessive amounts of reactive oxygen species in response to overwhelming infections and cancers, and to 'challenges' that may be local, as in arthritis and atherosclerosis, or systemic, as in systemic lupus erythematosus
- Deficiencies in antioxidant enzymes and/or vitamins
- Excessive products of certain types of enzyme reactions, e.g. fatty acid oxidation (see Ch. 3)
- Metal overload, as the result of repeated blood transfusions in thalassaemia major
- Drugs, such as antibiotics and cytotoxic agents, and alcohol and nicotine from tobacco smoking
- Environmental factors (including diet)
- Hyperbaric oxygen.

Clinical box 16.13 **Dietary recommendations for reducing cancer risk**

The Committee on Medical Aspects of Food Policy (COMA) working party has produced guidelines on dietary practices intended to reduce the risk of the most common types of cancer:
- Maintain a healthy body weight
- Consume a variety of fruits and vegetables (at least five portions/day)
- Eat plenty of cereal food – whole wheat or wholemeal
- Limit consumption of red meat to no more than 90 g/day (or 8–10 portions/week)
- Moderate alcohol consumption (3–4 or 2–3 units per day for men and women, respectively)
- Avoid high dose supplements as a means of cancer protection.

Table 16.13 **Dietary components associated with increased cancer risk**

Dietary factor	Proposed reason for increased risk	Type of cancer
Excessive food intake – obesity	A result of its effects on oestrogen production	Breast, colorectal, endometrial
High intake of meat and meat products	Increased exposure to carcinogens such as heterocyclic amines or *N*-nitroso compounds	Colorectal, breast, prostatic, pancreatic
Lack of fruit and vegetables	Fruit and vegetables have a protective effect due to a wide range of antioxidants, vitamins and anticarcinogens	Colorectal, lung, prostatic, cervical, breast, pancreatic, gastric, oesophageal
Lack of dietary fibre	Low-fibre diets pass along the gastrointestinal tract more slowly, thus the mucosa is exposed to potential carcinogens for longer	Colorectal, pancreatic

Source: COMA 1998 (this report discusses the evidence of associations as being not, moderately, or strongly consistent).

Table 16.14 Mutagenic dietary constituents

Food	Mutagen	Cancer produced
Red/processed meat, especially char-grilled	Polycyclic hydrocarbons, heterocyclic amines, N-nitroso compounds	Colon
Fatty foods	Saturated fat	Breast, colon,
Salt fish	Salt and nitrosamines	Oral cavity, nasopharynx, oesophagus and stomach
Alcohol	Alcohol + smoking combined especially	Oropharynx and oesophagus; breast
Mouldy/rancid foods	Aflatoxin	Hepatocellular

selenium, inhibit oxidation and therefore DNA damage and tumour initiation. Lycopene, a carotenoid pigment found in red fruits, which concentrates in prostate tissue, has been particularly implicated as protective in prostate cancer. Evidence from clinical trials, however, has not convincingly demonstrated the effectiveness of supplementation with these substances in prevention of cancer. Folic acid is alleged to be protective through its effect on increasing DNA methylation. Hypermethylation can lead to the inactivation of genes that suppress tumour formation.

Obesity

Obesity is another main general nutritional risk factor for cancer. This is particularly true for those cancers that may be influenced by hormones (e.g. post-menopausal breast, prostate, endometrium, testis), because excess adipose tissue results in the increased production of oestradiol. Obesity also increases the risk for cancers of the pancreas, oesophagus, kidney and colon. Bile salt excretion and oesophageal reflux are also increased in obese individuals.

NUTRITION AND CANCER TREATMENT

There are many aspects of cancer that can affect nutritional status:

- Reduced appetite (depression and anxiety)
- Physical symptoms such as dysphagia, early satiety and food-induced abdominal pain as well as malabsorption and increased losses
- Abdominal symptoms, taste changes, nausea, vomiting, pain, diarrhoea due to anti-cancer treatment
- Dry mouth (xerostomia), sore mouth or oesophagitis due to mucositis
- Increased metabolic rate (due to tumour load and cytokine production).

Treatment for cancer, whether curative or palliative, can involve surgery, radiotherapy, chemotherapy, or a combination of all three. However, nutrition is also important. The main aims of nutritional therapy are to:

- Restore or maintain good nutritional status, to enable patients to better metabolically handle the stress of treatment(s) and to recover, especially from surgery
- Overcome complications of treatment by providing nutritional support, e.g. advising on a soft diet or enteral nutrition in those who have problems swallowing, and providing artificial nutrition to those who cannot eat enough
- Improve outcome – the prevention of weight loss and protein energy malnutrition can enhance immune responses and improve quality of life. Bone marrow suppression, for example, is prolonged in the presence of poor nutrition.

At all stages of the disease, the dietitian has an important role. Early referral is likely to result in better nutritional outcomes.

DIET AND CARDIOVASCULAR DISEASE

Epidemiological studies have shown an association between diet, coronary heart disease (CHD), peripheral vascular disease (PVD) and stroke. The main disease process underlying cardiovascular disease is atherosclerosis (see Chs 3 and 11). Age, sex and family history are unmodifiable risk factors for cardiovascular disease, but there are many modifiable risk factors that are diet related. A poor diet can indirectly influence the development of cardiovascular disease by increasing obesity and associated risk factors such as hypertension, hypertriglyceridaemia and type 2 diabetes.

Dietary prevention of atherosclerosis

Dietary prevention of atherosclerosis focuses on (see Clinical box 16.14, Information boxes 16.8 and 16.9):

- Preventing the accumulation of lipid and its composition
- Changing the composition of circulating and stored lipid
- Reduction of the process of oxidation or glycation
- Prevention of hypertension, which increases the risk of infarction.

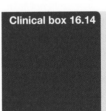

Clinical box 16.14 **Cardioprotective diet (adapted from NICE guidance on lipid modification 2010 (primary care): Cardiovascular risk assessment and the modification of blood lipids for the primary and secondary prevention of cardiovascular disease)**

- People at high risk of, or with, cardiovascular disease (CVD) should be advised to eat a diet in which total fat intake is 30% or less of total energy intake, saturated fats are 10% or less of total energy intake, intake of dietary cholesterol is less than 300 mg/day and, where possible, saturated fats are replaced by monounsaturated and polyunsaturated fats. It may be helpful to suggest they look at NHS Choices for further practical advice.
- People at high risk of or with CVD should be advised to eat at least five portions of fruit and vegetables per day, in line with national guidance for the general population. Examples of what constitutes a portion can be found at NHS Choices.
- People at high risk of or with CVD should be advised to consume at least two portions of fish per week, including a portion of oily fish. Further information and advice on healthy cooking methods can be found at NHS Choices.
- Pregnant women should be advised to limit their oily fish to no more than two portions per week. Further information and advice on oily fish consumption can be found at NHS Choices.
- People should not routinely be recommended to take omega-3 fatty acid supplements for the primary prevention of CVD.

Correction of hyperlipidaemia (see also Ch. 3) has a major impact: a 1% reduction in population blood cholesterol is associated with a 3% reduction in the risk of coronary heart disease.

- **If no lipid profile is available**: the dietary approach is to advise low total fat (especially saturated fatty acids), high soluble fibre and reduced alcohol, with replacement of refined carbohydrates by complex carbohydrates
- **If a lipid profile is available**: the dietary approach depends on the specific picture of dyslipidaemia, advice being matched to the desired effects (Information box 16.9).
  The emphasis of advice differs slightly according to the specific picture of dyslipidaemia.

Atherogenesis

Excess low-density lipoprotein (LDL) (due to smoking, hypercholesterolaemia, hypertension or diabetes) leaks from plasma into the extracellular space, where it becomes oxidised. Oxidised LDL is cytotoxic to endothelial cells, promotes inflammation, and is immunogenic. Its products are mitogenic and attract macrophages. The abnormality in the arterial wall that starts as oxidised LDL is taken up there by macrophages. Lesions progress from fatty streaks to atherosclerotic plaques as a result of lipid deposition, connective tissue proliferation and fibrin and thrombus accumulation. Atherogenesis is similar to a process of chronic inflammation within the arteries. The artery becomes narrowed. A tear in the plaque is often the precipitating cause for the formation of a large thrombus, which may occlude the artery and cause infarction, whether myocardial, cerebral or peripheral.

Prevention focuses on the accumulation of the lipid and its composition, on the reduction of the process of oxidation or glycation, and the prevention of hypertension, which increases the risk of infarction. As LDL per se is not toxic, the oxidation process is important in the accumulation of modified lipid in the vessel wall. Oxidised LDL also inhibits the production of nitric oxide (a vasodilator) in the endothelium. Oxidation is inhibited by vitamin E. Oxidation processes *may* be modified by dietary and endogenous antioxidants.

Vitamin C and carotenoids are present in vegetables and fruits, while vitamin E comes especially from seed and vegetable oils. Dietary intake of these nutrients is inversely proportional to the incidence of coronary heart disease.

Homocysteine

Hyperhomocysteinaemia is associated with an increased risk of coronary heart disease, colon cancer and stroke. Homocysteine is a sulphur-containing amino acid, which uses B vitamins for conversion to other amino acids. Folic acid (B_9) and B_{12} are needed for conversion to methionine (this is reversible) and B_6 is needed for conversion to cysteine. Folic acid and vitamin B_{12} and B_6 supplements, particularly combined, reduce plasma homocysteine.

It is unclear at present whether raised plasma levels themselves cause disease or whether it is a marker of disease, as reduction in plasma levels has not been shown to improve mortality and morbidity in cardiovascular disease.

Diet and hypertension

In patients with hypertension, diet is an important element in the prevention of cardiovascular disease. This is particularly important for patients with metabolic syndrome (or syndrome X), consisting of:

- Hypertriglyceridaemia with low HDL cholesterol
- Insulin resistance (fasting glucose 6.1 mmol/L or more)
- Central obesity (waist circumference >102 cm men and >88 cm women)
- Hypertension (blood pressure 130/85 mmHg or more).

This syndrome arises from interplay between genetic propensity (e.g. defective insulin receptor genes), sedentary lifestyle and poor diet. Patients are at risk of diabetes, coronary artery disease, left ventricular failure and stroke. Treatment involves preventive diet, weight loss, exercise and medication.

Dietary approach to hypertension

Excessive alcohol is associated with hypertriglyceridaemia, hypertension and stroke. High vegetable intake is preventive. An appropriate diet includes fruits, vegetables, low-fat dairy foods, grains, poultry, fish and nuts and with a reduction in fats, red meat, sweets and sugar-containing drinks.

| **Information box 16.9** | **Lipid profile and dietary approach for hyperlipidaemia** |

Lipid profile	Dietary advice
Raised total and LDL cholesterol; normal HDL cholesterol and TAGs	Reduce SFA intake, partially substitute with MUFA Encourage sources of soluble fibre Moderate sources of dietary cholesterol if excessive
Raised TAG; normal total LDL and HDL cholesterol	If obese, encourage weight loss by reduction of SFA Replace high intakes of refined CHO with more complex sources Reduce or avoid alcohol intake
Raised total and LDL cholesterol and TAG	If obese, encourage weight loss by reduction of total and SFA Partial substitution with MUFA Replace high intakes of refined CHO with more complex sources Reduce or avoid alcohol intake Moderate sources of dietary cholesterol if excessive
Low HDL cholesterol	Encourage regular exercise Modest alcohol intake (1–2 units per day) can be encouraged Moderate sources of dietary cholesterol if excessive

CHO, carbohydrates; MUFA, monounsaturated fatty acid; SFA, saturated fatty acid; LDL, low-density lipoprotein; HDL, high-density lipoprotein; TAG, triacylglycerol.

Large-scale population studies, such as the Intersalt Study, have established the relationship of sodium intake with raised blood pressure. Sodium restriction is well recognised as being effective in hypertension; the Mediterranean diet (see below) enhances the effect of sodium restriction in reducing blood pressure.

Cardioprotective diets

Epidemiological evidence has highlighted the lower risk of cardiovascular disease in the Mediterranean population. Randomised controlled trials support a Mediterranean diet as cardioprotective in high-risk populations (Information box 16.10). Nevertheless, these guidelines should be viewed in the context of a general healthy diet, and lifestyle factors should also be considered, including smoking cessation, increased physical activity and stress management.

Some therapeutic diets

In some diseases, a specific therapeutic diet is an integral part of treatment, and the importance of adherence to such diets should not be under-estimated. The following sections aim to describe briefly the general dietary principles and the significance of dietary therapy in some relatively common disease states.

Dietary treatment of coeliac disease

Coeliac disease is an inflammatory disorder of the gut with a strong genetic susceptibility. It is caused by an immune reaction to gluten, resulting in an inflammatory infiltrate in the lamina propria of the proximal small intestine with flattening of the villi, an increased proportion of intra-epithelial lymphocytes to enterocytes and increased crypt cell proliferation (see Ch. 15). This leads to malabsorption of all macro- and micronutrients, particularly fat-soluble vitamins and calcium. The condition is commonest in Caucasians, with an estimated prevalence of at least 1:300 in Europe and North America.

Diet is the single most important factor in the treatment of coeliac disease. Symptoms usually improve within a few weeks of following a gluten-free, well-balanced diet, and the intestinal mucosa recovers within a few months. Gluten-containing foods, however, are a source of other essential nutrients, such as trace minerals and vitamins. A totally gluten-free diet may rarely lead to deficiency states, e.g. thiamine and niacin, which are used to fortify gluten-containing wheat flour. It is important to recognize gluten-free sources of such micro-nutrients and dietetic input is often helpful in this regard.

Dietary restrictions in renal disease

The main aims of dietary management in renal disease are to limit the consequences of deteriorating renal function by maintaining nutritional status and minimising complications. Diet is modified only in severe or end-stage disease, when appetite is often severely suppressed and weight loss common. Dietary management of the renal patient has to be closely linked to clinical management and renal replacement therapy. Blood biochemistry should be regularly monitored and treatment adjusted accordingly.

Protein

Protein intake has to be adequate to avoid malnutrition. Low-protein diets cause problems with compliance and may negatively impact on nutritional status, putting the patient at a higher risk of morbidity at the onset of haemodialysis. Current daily recommendations suggest a protein intake of 0.8–1.0 g/kg body weight for conservative management of chronic renal failure. This is increased slightly to 1.2 g/kg ideal body weight in haemodialysis and continuous ambulatory peritoneal dialysis (see Ch. 14).

Energy

There must be sufficient energy provided to prevent weight loss. In haemodialysis and continuous ambulatory peritoneal dialysis, energy requirements are often taken to be greater than or equal to 147 kJ/kg of ideal body weight (IBW). Malnutrition, which is linked to a poor outcome, is prevalent in 40–50% of patients on haemodialysis and continuous ambulatory peritoneal dialysis.

Potassium

Potassium restriction is often necessary because the ability to excrete potassium is impaired in chronic renal failure. This can lead to hyperkalaemia, causing cardiac arrhythmias or cardiac arrest. Blood biochemistry monitoring will indicate whether a low potassium diet is required. Potassium is abundant in a normal diet, and rich sources are found in pure fruit juices, bananas and any fruit or vegetable which has not been boiled in water. The intake of these foods should be restricted. The intake of meat, cheese, milk and fish should also be reduced if necessary.

Phosphate

Hyperphosphataemia is common in chronic renal impairment. High-protein foods tend to be high in phosphate, so limiting phosphate without limiting protein can be difficult. Phosphate binders are commonly prescribed, such as calcium carbonate or calcium acetate, which have the added advantage of providing extra calcium.

Sodium and fluid

In renal failure, sodium and fluid retention lead to oedema and hypertension. A no-added salt (<100 mmol/day) diet is advised if the patient has oedema or hypertension. Fluid restriction is usually required only during end-stage renal failure when urine output has diminished: fluid intake is often restricted to 500 mL plus the previous day's urine output.

Dietary control in diabetes mellitus

Dietary principles for type 1 and type 2 diabetes are very similar (see Information box 16.11), the main emphasis being on improving glycaemic control, thus:

- Alleviating acute and chronic symptoms of hyperglycaemia
- Reducing the risk of cardiovascular disease and other diabetic complications
- Achieving, or maintaining, ideal body weight.

Information box 16.10	**Recommendations for a cardioprotective diet**

- Maintain an ideal weight
- Increase consumption of fish – especially oily fish
- Increase consumption of fruit and vegetables (at least five servings a day)
- Replace saturated fats with monounsaturated fats
- Divide fat intake between at least three regular meals per day
- Reduce total fat intake and replace with foods containing complex starches
- Avoid excessive alcohol intake
- Limit salt intake.

Many patients presenting with type 2 diabetes are initially treated with diet alone. The doctor, dietitian and diabetes nurse specialist should work closely to ensure the delivery of nutritional advice tailored to the patient's needs and medication, with monitoring and evaluation of progress.

Exercise in diabetes

Being overweight is a risk factor for type 2 diabetes, and weight reduction to a desirable range improves glucose tolerance. Daily exercise benefits the diabetic patient by lowering blood glucose and free fatty acids and reducing insulin resistance. Exercise also helps weight control, and reduces the risks of cardiovascular disease.

Lipid lowering

A lipid-lowering diet is incorporated into the diabetic diet because most people with diabetes have hyperlipidaemia (see Clinical box 16.18). Disturbance of lipid metabolism in relation to poor glycaemic control means that those with diabetes have a greater risk of cardiovascular disease. Cigarette smoking must be discouraged. Lipid-lowering drugs are also highly effective.

Artificial nutrition

The term nutritional support is used to describe the provision of artificial feeds to maintain or improve nutritional status during illness. Nutrition should be supplied by the simplest, safest, most cost-effective approach. Supplementation of the patient's diet using ordinary nutrient-dense foods is the first step. If this is unsuccessful, liquid sip feeds may be introduced to provide some or all of the food needed. If this line of approach fails then artificial nutrition may be required:

- Enteral nutrition – consists of feeding liquid, artificial food via a tube directly into the stomach or small intestine
- Parenteral nutrition – this is intravenous feeding.

Nutritional assessment, discussed earlier in this chapter, should be performed to estimate nutritional requirements before starting artificial feeding. Calculation of fluid and electrolyte needs is part of this process.

Enteral nutrition

Enteral feeding is preferred to parenteral nutrition because it helps maintain gut mucosal integrity, as well as being more physiological and with less potential complications. It also costs less. The route of delivery will depend largely on the accessibility and condition of the gastrointestinal tract. Clinical box 16.15 sets out the indications and methods for enteral feeding.

Complications of enteral feeding

The most common complications of enteral feeding are:

- Tube blockage
- Tube mis/displacement, leading to oesophageal reflux or aspiration into the lungs
- Refeeding syndrome is a risk in malnourished and fasted patients (see below).

Gut infections, constipation, nausea, distension, dumping syndrome and diarrhoea may also occur. Gastrostomy and jejunostomy insertion may be complicated by peritonitis or abdominal wall sepsis.

Parenteral nutrition

Parenteral feeding is a method of delivering nutrition intravenously when the gastrointestinal tract is not functioning or is inaccessible. The term **total parenteral nutrition** implies that no other food is being taken intestinally, although it is often loosely used as a synonym for parenteral nutrition. Based on the patient's calculated requirements, parenteral feeds have to be nutritionally complete and contain a full complement of vitamins, trace elements and minerals, and prepared under sterile conditions. Excess feeding could be lethal (see Clinical box 16.16 for complications).

Parenteral feeding is indicated only when enteral intake is impossible, insufficient or undesirable. It may be used, e.g. in the context of intestinal perforation or ileus in critical illness, or in the longer term at home for patients with chronic intestinal failure due to short bowel or to intestinal pseudo-obstruction. Parenteral nutrition is delivered through peripheral or central veins. The choice is influenced by the condition and accessibility of veins in the arms and neck, the osmolarity of the feed, and the proposed duration of such feeding.

MALNUTRITION

Here, malnutrition is taken to mean under-nutrition, as in common usage. This could be from insufficient daily intake of protein and energy, inadequate micronutrient intake or an unbalanced intake of macronutrients (see later).

- Macronutrient malnutrition: related to severe, prolonged deficiency in protein and energy intake, known as **protein–energy malnutrition** (**PEM**). This will usually also be associated with deficiencies in micronutrient intake. Sustained PEM leads to loss of muscle mass and fat. Starvation, an extreme form of PEM, could be fatal if continuous for 2–3 months, depending upon initial body stores of fat and protein, and micronutrient status (Clinical box 16.17).
- Micronutrient deficiency: inadequate intake of vitamins and trace minerals in the diet (see later). This may also occur in the context of obesity.

In developing countries, whole populations may suffer from sustained, long-term malnutrition due to failure of crops, war, economic policies etc. In developed nations, although poverty can be a factor in malnutrition, it is more often due to an unbalanced intake of macronutrients, obesity being a common outcome.

Malnutrition and disease states

Malnutrition is commonly caused by or associated with disease

- Anorexia: psychological – depression; eating disorder, e.g. anorexia nervosa; reduced central control of appetite in cancer
- Inability to eat or swallow, persistent vomiting
- Increased energy expenditure and net protein breakdown (catabolic state): cancer, burns, wounds, sepsis, postoperative state (see below).
- Side effect of drugs
- Immobility, e.g. old age.

Diagnosis of malnutrition

Malnutrition may not be easily recognised, particularly in hospital, and is associated with many medical conditions. Formal screening or assessment processes should be followed to document weight loss and weight for height quantitatively (see above).

Refeeding syndrome

This is a potentially lethal condition and can occur when refeeding malnourished patients via any route. It causes metabolic disturbance leading to severe fluid and electrolyte shifts. Figure 16.10 shows the pathogenesis and features of the refeeding syndrome.

In prolonged starvation the body undergoes adaptive changes. Due to low glycogen stores, the body attempts to preserve protein (i.e. prevent muscle loss) by using fat stores for gluconeogenesis. Despite this, there is a gradual depletion of visceral muscle (e.g. cardiac and respiratory muscle) and reduction in energy stores (ATP). There is also a reduction in production of triiodothyronine (T3) levels which in turn causes a reduction in metabolic rate. This leads to downregulation of various intracellular pumps which usually maintain electrolyte gradients and concentrations between the intracellular and extracellular space. As a result there is leakage of phosphate, magnesium and potassium out of cells, whilst sodium and water move into cells.

In the fed state, i.e. when refeeding these patients, they will once again utilise glucose. This causes an increase in insulin secretion which causes intracellular movement of phosphate, potassium and magnesium, with resulting depletion intravascularly. Thiamine (a cofactor) utilisation also increases. The increase in metabolic rate associated with refeeding leads to an increase in demand for the depleted energy stores and increased stress on the weakened heart and lungs, thus leading to risk of cardiac and respiratory failure.

Groups at particular risk should be intensively monitored with supplementation of phosphate, potassium, magnesium and B vitamins, as required. These are shown in Table 16.15.

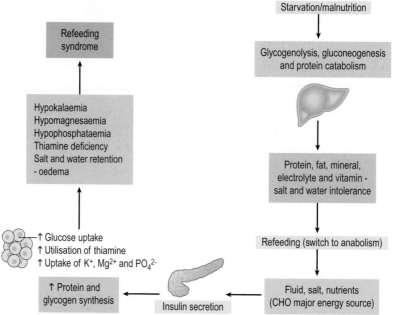

Fig. 16.10 Pathogenesis and features of the refeeding syndrome. (After Stanga Z, et al. 2008 Nutrition in clinical practice – the refeeding syndrome: illustrative guidelines for prevention and treatment. Eur J Clin Nutr 62(6): 687–94, with permission).

Table 16.15	Indications for refeeding

- Patients with anorexia nervosa
- Patients with chronic alcoholism
- Oncology patients
- Postoperative patients
- Elderly patients (comorbidities, decreased physiological reserve)
- Patients with uncontrolled diabetes mellitus (electrolyte depletion, diuresis)
- Patients with chronic malnutrition:
  - Marasmus
  - Prolonged fasting or low energy diet
  - Morbid obesity with profound weight loss
  - High stress patient unfed for >7 days
  - Malabsorptive syndrome (such as inflammatory bowel disease, chronic pancreatitis, cystic fibrosis, short bowel syndrome)
- Long term users of antacids (magnesium and salts bind phosphate)
- Long term users of diuretics (loss of electrolytes)

Clinical box 16.18	Increased risk of disease associated with obesity

Obesity, defined as BMI >30, carries an increased risk for:
- Diabetes (especially type 2)
- Coronary heart disease
- Hyperlipidaemia
- Hypertension
- Stroke
- Gall stones
- Some cancers (breast and colon for example)
- Infertility
- Sleep apnoea/respiratory problems
- Arthritis
- Joint and back pain
- Poor self-esteem.

Avoidance of refeeding syndrome

The key is to be cautious but to ensure that patients are not underfed. Feeding rates should be initiated at no more than 50% of patients usual energy requirements and gradually increased. Serum electrolytes (PO_4, Mg, K) should be monitored and replaced as necessary from the beginning and thiamine given promptly to prevent development of Wernicke-Korsakoff syndrome (a triad of confusion, nystagmus and ataxia) due to thiamine deficiency.

OBESITY

Obesity is the result of excess fat deposition in adipose tissue. In clinical practice, obesity is defined as Quetelet Index or BMI of 30+ (see above). It is only in relatively recent times that the impact diet obesity on general health has been recognised (Clinical box 16.18). Risks to health rise with increasing BMI, especially as it increases above 30, and also depends on body fat distribution (Fig. 16.11).

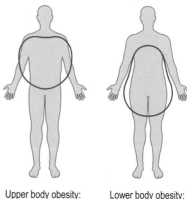

Upper body obesity: Apple shaped

Lower body obesity: Pear shaped

Fig. 16.11 Obesity classified according to body fat distribution. Health risks are higher with upper body obesity.

Obesity can be seen epidemiologically as a condition of affluence; its prevalence is increasing in developed countries, but it is also becoming common in the developing world. Over two-thirds of adults in the developed world have a BMI over 30 (Fig. 16.12). WHO figures for over 20s have shown

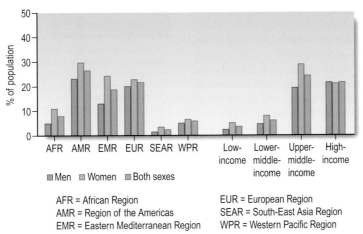

Fig. 16.12 **Age standardised prevalence of obesity (i.e. BMI ≥ 30 kg/m²) in adults aged ≥ 20 years, by WHO region and World Bank Income Group, comparable estimates, 2008.**

that the worldwide prevalence of obesity has nearly doubled between 1980 and 2008, being highest in those countries with high, upper-middle incomes. This is the equivalent of over half a billion adults worldwide.

Of even more concern is the rise in childhood obesity, also increasing in prevalence predisposing the next generation to the associated health risks (see Fig. 16.13). Obesity is now considered as one of the most important public health concerns of our time.

Aetiology of obesity

The cause of obesity is the prolonged excess of energy input over output (energy imbalance), causing the body to store the unused energy as fat deposits in adipose tissue. Each kilogram of adipose tissue represents the storage of about 29 330 kJ (7000 kcal). Just 838 kJ (200 kcal) per day excess might therefore be expected to result in an increase in weight of about 11 kg in a year if there was no compensatory increase in energy expenditure. Basal metabolic rate is closely related to lean body mass, which rises only a little as people become obese (adipose tissue is about 75% fat, 25% lean). It is thus remarkable how well the body balances energy intake to expenditure day by day.

It might be imagined that there would be teleological advantage in storing some energy at least in times of plenty, to guard against times of food shortage; it is precisely this safety mechanism which promotes obesity during prolonged periods in which shortage is never experienced. Once a person has become obese and the fat stores have been established, s/he will remain obese if energy input and output remain equal. An increase in energy intake above expenditure depends on the following:

- Appetite and the mechanisms involved in control (see above)
- Psychogenic and social aspects of eating (see later)
- Exercise and environmental factors
- Genetic factors.

Obesity tends to run in families but this is not necessarily entirely genetic; nonetheless genetic factors may play a part through appetite regulation. BMR correlates with lean body mass, and obese people do not have a lower BMR than non-obese people, because their lean body mass is modestly elevated compared with non-obese people.

Psychogenic factors

Food consumption patterns are often learned. A common assumption is that we need to eat three filling meals per day. Many young children are trained into this habit, and continue it into adult life. The calories ingested may be greater than those utilised, especially if the person has a sedentary lifestyle, in which case the patterns learned as a growing child are no longer appropriate. Eating is sometimes associated with comfort or tension release – weight gain is often seen during or after psychologically stressful situations.

Environmental factors and exercise

Because of their impact on exercise, environmental factors influence the prevalence of obesity. For example, in the UK, obesity has been increasing rapidly despite reductions in food and energy intake. As reliance on labour-saving devices, cars and a reduction of manual occupations increases, energy needs have decreased. Children in particular have fewer opportunities to run around, and intensive UK school curricula are crowding out sporting and leisure activities. Coinciding with this is the increased consumption of high-energy convenience meals and snacks.

As a race, humans have evolved to guard against energy deficit more efficiently than energy excess (see above), hence the resulting prevalence of obesity in times of plenty. This becomes particularly important when previously rural/agrarian populations change to a more Westernised and urban

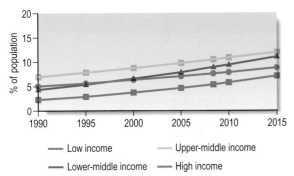

Fig. 16.13 **WHO Infant and young children overweight trends from 1990 to 2015, by World bank Income Group.**

mode of living; a classic example of this is the Pima Indians in southern USA. The traditional diet of the Sierra Madre (Mexico) Pima Indians is a low-fat diet (15% of energy as fat). They are physically active as farmers and sawmill workers. But in the past 50 years lifestyle changes in the Pimas of Arizona, who now consume a high-fat diet (50% of energy as fat) and lead a more sedentary lifestyle, have resulted in an epidemic of obesity and diabetes. The Pimas of Mexico have a much lower incidence of obesity and diabetes than their genetic kindred in Arizona.

Treatment of obesity

There are three categories of treatment for obesity:

- Dietary
- Pharmacological
- Surgical.

The latter two categories should not be viewed as an alternative to diet, but complementary.

Dietary management

The long-term goal of any dietary management programme is to change eating habits, behaviours and attitudes for life. Ideally, a multidisciplinary team approach is taken with attention given to any psychological factors influencing behavioural patterns. Weight-reducing diets should be attainable and flexible. It is important that they encourage a general healthy eating pattern that can be continued after the desirable amount of weight has been lost (see Information box 16.12, for example).

A slow but steady rate of weight loss is likely to be more effective than extremely restrictive diets that not only can reduce metabolic rate, but also are impractical and can result in difficulties with compliance. Diets that reduce overall intake will inevitably mean a reduction not only of energy but also of other nutrients; thus some patients may benefit from vitamin or mineral supplements.

Information box 16.12	Example of a weight-reducing diet

The diet must provide a deficit in energy balance, reducing intake to below energy requirements. The easiest way of doing this is to reduce total fat intake because fat is the highest energy-containing food (38 kJ/g). For example, a reduction of 2100–4200 kJ per day should result in a weight loss of 0.5–1 kg per week, allowing for an energy value of about 29 330 kJ per kg adipose tissue which is made up of about 75% fat and 25% lean tissue. This is considered a healthy rate of weight loss that minimises loss of lean body mass, and maximises energy liberated from adipose stores.

A psychological model for dietary modification

Advice for weight reduction from changing eating behaviour may be complied with better if it fits in with the psychological model for dietary modification. When dietary modification is needed to achieve a healthier state, the objective is to modify aberrant eating behaviour to achieve appropriate change. This is, however, a one-dimensional view of the patient–practitioner relationship. It is necessary to consider how the patient feels about changing habits – they may not want, or feel they need, to make any changes.

Since it was first developed in the early 1980s, the cycle of change model (Fig. 16.14) has been influential in our understanding of behaviour, especially of addictive behaviours (see also Ch. 8 for details of addiction). Change can be understood as a six-step repeating process with central features of resistance and resilience. Knowledge of where a patient is in the cycle of change makes it easier to begin the process of achieving change. A person can enter or leave the cycle at any point. It is usual for people to travel through the cycle a few times before reaching a stable change. For example, if an obese patient is in the pre-contemplative stage, i.e. they are unaware, unwilling or too discouraged to change, then giving weight-reducing advice at this time will be a waste of time. In this situation, discussion of the risks

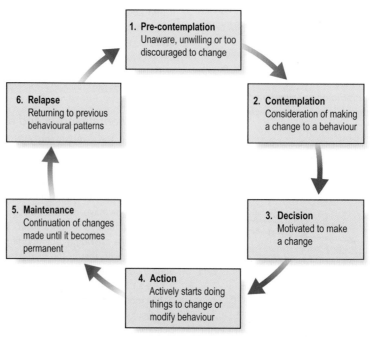

Fig. 16.14 **Six stages in the cycle of change.**

associated with obesity and the advantages of losing weight will be of greater benefit, with the idea of moving the patient into the contemplative or decision stage.

Pharmacological management

This is limited, due to the poor safety profile that has been associated with anti-obesity drugs. At present in the UK the only drug licensed for use is orlistat.

Appetite suppression

Sibutramine is a centrally acting appetite suppressant which blocks the re-uptake of serotonin (known to suppress appetite) and norepinephrine (noradrenaline) (which can affect metabolic rate). The increase in serotonin concentration in the synaptic cleft thus decreases food intake. Adverse reactions include an increase in heart rate and a smaller reduction in blood pressure. The effectiveness of appetite suppressants is limited because people do not eat purely in response to hunger.

Inhibition of fat absorption

Orlistat is a pancreatic lipase inhibitor, which binds to dietary fat and so blocks its digestion and absorption. To minimise the risk of adverse gastrointestinal effects caused by the unabsorbed fat in the bowel, patients have to reduce their habitual fat intake to less than 30% of total energy. Consequences of failure to comply with fat restriction include fatty loose stools and faecal incontinence. A meta-analysis comparing orlistat with a placebo supports a weight loss of about 2.9 kg.

Surgical management

Surgical procedures have been recommended as a treatment option for patients with morbid obesity that meet certain criteria (Information box 16.13). Morbid obesity here is defined as those with a BMI of 40 kg/m^2 or $\geq$35 with other significant disease (e.g. hypertension, diabetes).

The role of surgery in treatment of obesity has increased significantly as it has been shown to be an effective method for not only weight loss but also shown to improve metabolic profile, for example type 2 diabetes and cardiovascular risk with some procedures. These procedures, with the exception of gastric band, have been shown to reduce ghrelin levels and increase PYY and GLP1 which likely contribute to the weight loss seen post procedure, although it is not clear why all these changes occur (see Fig. 16.15).

Information box 16.13	Recommendations for consideration of bariatric surgery

Candidate criteria:
- They are aged 18 years or over
- They have been receiving treatment in a specialist obesity clinic at a hospital
- They have tried all other appropriate non-surgical treatments to lose weight but have not been able to maintain weight loss
- There are no specific medical or psychological reasons why they should not have this type of surgery
- They are generally fit enough to have an anaesthetic and surgery
- They should understand that they will need to be followed-up by a doctor and other healthcare professionals such as dietitians or psychologists over the long term

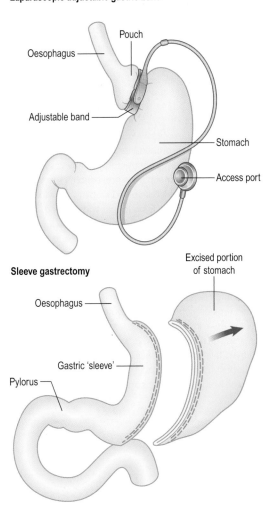

Laparoscopic adjustable gastric band

Sleeve gastrectomy

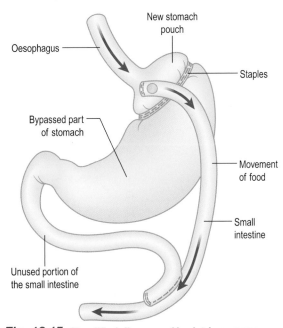

Roux-en-Y gastric bypass procedure

Fig. 16.15 Simplified diagram of bariatric surgery.

Bariatric surgery can be divided into two broad categories:

- Restrictive. This is must commonly done by placement of a gastric band fitted around the body of the stomach to make a small pouch for food to enter, thus restricting the capacity of the stomach. This restriction of the size of the stomach makes the patient feel full after eating a small amount of solid food. As there is no surgical resection involved it is a potentially reversible procedure. However, the percentage of excess weight lost tends to be less than seen with other procedures and there is no change in gut hormones. Sleeve gastrectomy involves removal of the fundus of the stomach so is irreversible. The vertical band gastroplasty, which involved stapling the stomach, carries a higher risk and is no longer widely used.
- Malabsorptive/restrictive. The two main procedures in this category are roux-en-Y gastric bypass and bilio-pancreatic diversion (BPD). These procedures achieve greater weight loss than the purely restrictive procedures but also carry a higher operative mortality and risk of macro- and micronutrient deficiencies, hence will require lifelong replacement post procedure.
  - Roux-en-Y involves division of the stomach to form a small gastric pouch which causes restriction. Food leaves this pouch, bypassing the rest of the stomach, duodenum and proximal jejenum via a shorter limb, thereby reducing the absorption of food.
  - BPD achieves even greater weight loss and resolution of comorbidites but is a more complex anastomosis with the diverted food joining pancreatic and biliary juices at the position of the terminal ileum. As well as the short-term operative risk, long-term complications include nausea, vomiting, diarrhoea, heartburn, macronutrient and micronutrient deficiency.

Increasing physical activity

Unfortunately, as obesity develops, there is a tendency for physical activity to decline. Physical exercise improves glucose tolerance and diminishes insulin resistance. Regular exercise can increase energy expenditure and metabolic rate – its most important role in maintenance of weight loss. Any increase in physical activity will be of some benefit, including walking up stairs instead of taking the lift, or walking instead of using a car. This is important for severely obese people who are limited in the kind of activity they can undertake.

Prevention of obesity

The best treatment for obesity is prevention:

- Prevention of weight gain in lean subjects
- Prevention of any further weight gain in already obese adults
- Adequate nutritional education about a balanced diet for school children. Fatness at the age of 13 is a strong predictor of adult obesity, and the earlier in life obesity develops, the greater the risk of mortality.

Index

Note: Page numbers followed by *f* indicate figures, *b* indicate boxes and *t* indicate tables.

A

Abdomen
  quadrants, 711
  regions, 710–711
  surface anatomy of, 709–711, 710f
Abdominal aorta, 501–502, 501f
Abducens (VI) nerve, 346, 346t
Abduction
  condyloid or ellipsoidal joint, 424–425
  definition of, 425b
ABO blood group system, 23
  antibodies, 606–607, 607t
  antigens, 604–606
  changes, 606
  transfusion medicine, 604–608, 605f, 605t
Abortion Act (1967), 282
Abscess
  formation of, 251b
  repair complications, 256
Absolute risk reduction (ARR), 300
Absorption, 702–709
Accessory ligaments, 422
Accessory muscles, of respiration, 628b
Accessory (XI) nerve, 346t, 348
Acetoacetate, 95
Acetyl-CoA carboxylase (ACC)
  lipogenesis, 96–98, 97f
  regulation of, 98
Acetyl coenzyme A (acetyl-CoA), 71
  oxidation of
    in ketogenic pathway, 95–96, 95f
    in TCA cycle, 94–95
  production of, for lipogenesis, 98–99
Acetylation, 38, 112
Acetylcholine, 514
  breakdown of, 434
  inactivation of, 142
  inhibition of, 142b
  interactions with cholecystokinin and secretin, 734
  intracellular messenger for, 725–726, 734
  neurotransmission, 362
  release of, 142
  storage of, 142
  synthesis of, 141
Acetylcholine receptors (AChRs)
  muscle innervation, 433–434
  myasthenia gravis, 435b
Acetylcholinesterase (AChE)
  inhibitors, 123b
Achondroplasia, 170b, 414b
Acid-base balance, 10–14
  abnormalities of, 689–690
  control of, 12–14
  disturbances, 14b, 14f, 14t, 639–640, 689b
  glutamine in, 85–86
  renal control of, 686–690
    hydrogen ions, 686–687
    renal buffers, 688–690

Acid-base balance (Continued)
  renal mechanism of bicarbonate control, 687–688
Acid hydrolases, 45–46
Acid secretion, ion movements during, 726
Acidosis
  definition, 11
  due to prolonged vomiting, 732b
  effects on drug absorption and distribution, 104
  metabolic. see Metabolic acidosis
Acids, 16–19
  dissociation constant (K), 12
  sources of, 11
  strength of, 16b
  see also specific acid
Acne, 447b
Acquired autoimmune haemolytic anaemia (AIHA), 583–585, 585f, 585t
Acquired haemophilia, 602
Acquired tolerance, 249
Acromegaly, 463b, 463f, 564
Actin filaments, 44
Action potentials, 356–358, 357f
  conduction of, 358
  depolarisation, 357
  generation of, 357–358
  hyperpolarisation, 357
  propagation of, 358f
Activated partial thromboplastin time (APTT), 600f, 601
Activation energy, 19
Activators, 167
Active membrane transport, 543
Active transport, 49
Acupuncture, 380b
Acute coronary syndromes (ACS), 534–539
Acute hepatic failure, 741b
Acute kidney injury (AKI), 657b, 693–694, 694t
Acute lung diseases, 615b
Acute lymphoblastic leukaemia (ALL), 592, 594f
Acute myeloid leukaemia (AML), 592, 594f
Acute myocardial infarction, complications of, 538t
Acute neurological disorders, respiratory failure, 650b
Acute phase proteins, 250, 737b
Acute renal failure
  acute tubular necrosis, 694
  nephrotoxic agents, 694
Acute tubular necrosis (ATN), 694
Acyl-carrier protein (ACP), 98
Acyl-CoA synthetase, 93
Adaptive immune system, 235–240, 236f
  B lymphocytes, 238–240
  null lymphocytes, 240
  T lymphocytes, 235–238
Addison disease, 456b
Adduction, condyloid or ellipsoidal joint, 424

Adenoma-carcinoma sequence, 274f
Adenomas, 263, 456
Adenosine, neurotransmission, 363–364
Adenosine diphosphate (ADP)
  glycolysis, 67
  in rigor mortis, 440b
Adenosine monophosphate (AMP), 67
Adenosine triphosphate (ATP), 28b
  energy storage, 57
  muscle metabolism, 440–441
  reactions yielding, 69
  regulator of, 67
  rigor mortis, 440b
  structure of, 28f, 58f
Adhering junctions, 46
Adhesins, 215
Adiponectin, 54
Adipose tissue, pathway of triacylglycerol uptake and storage by, 90f
Adipose triglyceride lipase (ATGL), 91
Adoption studies, 186
Adrenal cortex, 468
Adrenal gland
  innervation of, 139
  structure of, 468, 468f
Adrenal medulla
  nerve supply to the heart, 515
  stress and, 468–469
Epinephrine (adrenaline)
  anaphylactic shock, 148–149
  conversion from norepinephrine (noradrenaline), 146
  neurotransmission, 363
  regulation of vasoconstriction tone, 550
  shock treatment, 561
Adrenergic neuron blocking drugs (ANBs), 147
Adrenergic receptors (adrenoceptors), 148–151
  agonists, 148–149
  antagonists, 149–150
Adrenocortical insufficiency, 456b
Adult regression equations, 631b
Adult respiratory distress syndrome (ARDS), 560, 615b
Aerobic carbohydrate metabolism, 758
Aerobic glycolysis, 71–72
Afferent lymph vessels, 257
A fibres, 554
Afterload, 526
Agents of destruction, 234
Agnosias, 401
Agonist drugs, 135–136
Airflow, measuring rates of, 630–631
Airways
  collapse, flow-related, 635–636
  resistance, 631–634, 633f
Alanine, glucose-alanine cycle, 81
Alanine transaminase (ALT), 85b
Alar plate, 339f
Albinism, 83b
Albumin, 26f, 39, 40
  drugs that bind to plasma, 108t
  fatty acids, 90
Aldoses, 21, 21f
Aldosterone, 556, 683–684
  and spironolactone, 686

Adenoma-carcinoma sequence, 274f
Alimentary canal, 700f
  fluid/electrolyte input into the, 708f
  innervation of, 713
  layers of, 711f
Alimentary system
  blood supply to, 700, 701f, 701t
  effects of muscarinic receptor agonists on, 144
  functions/structure of, 699–700
  metabolism of drugs in, 117
  microanatomy of, 711–713, 711f, 712f
  pathogen entry via, 226
Alkali, sources of, 11
Alkaline phosphatase, 41
Alkaline secretion, pancreas, 731–733
Alkalosis
  definition, 11
  effects on drug absorption and distribution, 104
  metabolic. see Metabolic alkalosis
  respiratory. see Respiratory alkalosis
Alkaptonuria, 83b
Alleles, 278t
Allocation concealment, 278t, 306–307, 306b
Allopurinol, metabolism, 111
Allosteric effectors, binding of, 61
Allosteric modulation of drug-receptor interaction, 136
Alopecia, 447b
α-Adrenoceptors, 148
  antagonists, 150
α₁-Antitrypsin deficiency, 737b
α-Fetoprotein (AFP), 271t, 737b
α-Helix, 34, 35f
α Thalassaemia, 588
Alternative hypothesis (H₁), 278t, 294
Alternative splicing, 36–37
Altitude
  acclimatisation to, 646–647
  challenges to normal respiration, 646–647
  physiological responses to high, 646
Aluminium, nephrotoxicity of, 695t
Alveolar cells
  type I, 621
  type II, 621
Alveolar tension, 637
Alveoli, 619–621, 620f
  partial pressures of gases in, 637
Alzheimer disease, 38b, 400b
Amelanosis, 83b
Amelia, 281b
Amiloride, 686
Amino acid derivative, 452t
Amino acid metabolism, 83–88
  absorption, 83–84
  errors in, 33b
  essential amino acids, 87–88
  gluconeogenesis, 87, 87f
  inborn errors, 83b
  metabolic classes of, 83, 84f
  nitrogen in, 84–87
  signalling molecules, 88

Amino acids, 20, 32–33
  absorption, 706
  branched-chain, 84
  classification, of, 32–33, 759t
  dissociation of, 32
  essential, 87–88
  excitatory, 360–362
  fate of, in liver, 87b
  found in human proteins, 32t
  inhibitory, 362
  neurotransmitters, 88, 360–362
  proximal convoluted tubule, 668
  side chains of, 33f
  stereoisomers of, 32f
  structure of, 32–33
  transport systems, 706t
Aminoglycoside antibiotics
  nephrotoxicity, 695t
  side effects of, 142b
Aminotransferases
      (transaminases), 84
Ammonia, 86
  -induced encephalopathy, 88b
  amino acid metabolism, 85f
  pH value, 11t
Ammonium ions
  in ammonium synthesis, 688
  in metabolic acidosis, 85b
Ammonium synthesis, 688–689
AMP-activated protein kinase
      (AMPK), 68
Amphetamine, overdose, 105b
Amphiarthroses, 418
Amphipathic molecules, 26
Amphotericin, nephrotoxicity, 695t
Amygdala, functions, 397t
Amyloid, formation of, 254
Amyloidosis, 254b
Amylopectin, 21–22
Amylose, 21–22
Anabolic pathways, 19
Anabolism, 57–58
Anaemia of chronic disease (ACD),
      582–583
Anaemia(s), 576–589
  acquired
      due to blood loss, 582
      due to chronic disease,
          582–583
      due to deficiencies, 578–581
  causes of, 578t
  classification, 578
  clinical indication, 577t
  disordered erythropoiesis, 572b
  due to haemolysis, 583–586
  general features of, 576–577
  inherited, 585–589
  physiological adaptations to, 577
  renal failure, 656b
  symptoms and signs of, 577t
Anaemic hypoxia, 638b
Anaerobic carbohydrate
      metabolism, 758
Anagen phase, hair growth, 447
Anal canal, motility of, 747
Analgesic neuropathy, 696
Analgesics, opioid, 380b
Anaphylactic shock, 559
Anaphylactoid reactions, 559
Anaphylaxis, 559
Anastomoses, arteriovenous
      (AVAs), 505
Anatomical axes, 340f
Anatomical dead space, 629–630
Androgen insensitivity
      syndrome, 480b
Androgen receptor
      insensitivity, 490t
Androgens, 25t, 479, 480f, 480t
Anergy, 249
Aneuploidy, 163
Aneurysm, 539
Angelman syndrome, 181, 181b
Angina, 531, 535f
  nitric oxide and, 55b
  stable, 534
  treatment of, 534
Angioneurotic oedema, 242

Angiotensin converting enzyme
      (ACE), 556
Angiotensin-converting enzyme
      (ACE) inhibitors, 123b
Angiotensin I, 556
Angiotensin II, 550–551, 556
  role of, 683
Angle of Louis, 626
Anhydramnios, 662–663
Animal models, polygenic diseases,
      186
Anion gap (AG), 20
Anions, proximal convoluted
      tubule, 669t
Ankle
  fractures, 424b
  joint, 424f
Annulus fibrosus, 409b
Annulus fibrosus cordis, 494
Anorexia nervosa, 394b
Anorexigenic pathway, 394
Anosmia, 392b
Anoxia, 65, 638b
Antabuse effect, 123b
Antagonists, 133
  see also specific antagonist
Anterior cerebral arteries, 353
Anterior cruciate ligament, 430b,
      431b
Anterior longitudinal ligament, 409b
Anterior spinal artery, 354
Anterior tibial compartment
      syndrome, 408b
Anterograde transport, 45
Anti-arrhythmic drugs, 520
Anti-cancer drugs, 28b
  targeting nuclear and intracellular
      receptors, 132, 132b
  see also specific drugs
Anti-platelet therapy, 533
Antibacterial drugs, 133t
  targeting nuclear and intracellular
      receptors, 132
Antibiotics
  aminoglycoside. see
      Aminoglycoside antibiotics
  and pharmacogenomics, 207
Antibodies, 240–241
  classes, functions of different,
      242t
  complexes, 241, 241f
  functions of, 241
  heavy chains of, 240
  light chains of, 240
  production, 606–607
  screening, 609–610
Anti-cardiolipin antibody, 604
Anticholinesterase drugs, 142–143
  irreversible, 143, 143b
  medium-acting, reversible, 142
  short-acting, reversible, 142
Anticoagulants, natural, 599
Anti-D prophylaxis, 607f
Antidiuretic hormone (ADH), 556
Antigen-presenting cells (APCs),
      237, 237f, 569
Antigen receptors, 233–234
Antigens, 234
  blood group, 604
  endogenous, 237
  exogenous, 237
  recognition of, 238
  T-dependent, 239
  T independent, 239
Antiglobulin test, 610, 611f
Antioxidants, 774–775
Anti-phospholipid syndrome (APS),
      604
Antiport transport mechanism, 94
Antiporters, 106
Antiports, 50
Antisense oligonucleotides, 209
Anxiety
  disorders, 397b
  serotonin, GABA and, 363b
Aortic arch, 500–501, 501f
Aortic regurgitation, 496b, 498b
Aortic stenosis, 496b, 498b

Aortic valves, 494, 497f
Apex beat, 494
  character of, 495b, 496f
Apical ectoderm ridge (AER), 172
Aplasia (agenesis), 262
Apneusis, 643b
Apneustic centre, breathing, 642
Apnoea, 643b
Apocrine glands, 447
Apolipoprotein(s), 92
Aponeuroses, 429–430
Apoptosis, 48, 259
  transforming growth factor-β, 250
Apparent volume of distribution,
      109
Appetite, 771
  suppression, 783
Apraxias, 401
APUD (amine precursor uptake and
      decarboxylation) cells, 618
Aquaporin membrane proteins
      (AQPs), 80
Aquaporins
  diffusion, 543
  proximal convoluted tubule, 668
Aqueous pores, diffusion through,
      106
Arachidonic acid, 23, 25f
Arachnoid mater, 350
Archaea, 213
  as model organisms, 204
Arcuate popliteal ligaments, 430b
Arginine, urea cycle, 86
Arithmetic mean, 278t
Arm circumference, 755
Arrector pili, 448
Arterial blood pressure
  regulation of, 554–556
  systemic, 554–566
Arterial system, 500–502
Arterial thromboembolism, 539b
Arteries, 529
  elastic, 529, 529f
  muscular, 529, 529f
  in respiratory system, 623
Arteriosclerosis, non-
      atherosclerotic, 533
Articular capsule, 420
Articular cartilage, 406, 420
Articular discs, 422
Ascending aorta, 500–501
Ascending sensory pathways, 379,
      379b
Ascites, 742
Ascorbic acid. see Vitamin C
Aspartate aminotransferase (AST),
      85b
Aspirin, 25, 67b
  angina, 536b
  overdose, 105b
  potentiates action of warfarin,
      108b
Association cortex, 341
Association of analytical
      communities (AOAC)
      method, 751
Asthma, 248b, 615b
  airway resistance, 633–634
  respiratory failure, 649
Astrocyte-neuron lactate shuttle,
      356
Atelectasis, 615b, 634b
Atherogenesis, 776
Atheromatous plaque, 530, 530f
Atherosclerosis, 23b, 530–533
  dietary prevention of, 775–776,
      775b
  prevention and treatment of, 533
  risk factors for, 532–533
Atherosclerotic plaque, evolution
      of, 530–532
Atomic mass, 16, 16t
Atomic number, 16
Atoms, 16
Atresia, 262
Atria, 494, 507
Atrial fibrillation (AF), 518, 519f
Atrial flutter, 518

Atrial natriuretic peptide (ANP), 556
Atrial septal defects (ASDs), 507
Atrial systole, 524
Atrioventricular (AV) node, 513
Atrioventricular (AV) valves, 494,
      497f
Atrioventricular canal, 506–507,
      506f
Atrioventricular cushions, 506–507
Atrioventricular nodal re-entrant
      tachycardia (AVNRT), 518
Atrioventricular re-entrant
      tachycardia (AVRT), 520
Atrophy, 260
  pathological, 260b
  physiological, 260b, 260f
Attention, cognitive process and,
      401
Auditory system, 388–392
Auerbach's plexus, 713
Autocrine effects, 452
Autocrine signalling, 238
Autolysis, 45–46
Autonomic motor reflex, 139, 140f
Autonomic nervous system (ANS),
      138–153, 513, 515f
  anatomical and pharmacological
      subdivisions of, 138f
  anatomy of, 140, 141f
  drug targets in, 141b
  functions of, 138–139
  neurotransmitters, 138
  overview of, 139–140
  parasympathetic system. see
      Parasympathetic nervous
      system
  receptors of, 140–153
  sympathetic system. see
      Sympathetic nervous system
Autoreactivity, 249
Autoreceptor, 360
Autoregulation, sodium balance,
      682, 682f, 684
Autosomal dominant form of
      polycystic kidney disease
      (ADPKD), 663
Autosomal dominant inheritance,
      177–178, 177f
Autosomal recessive inheritance,
      178–179, 178f
Axon hillock, 358
Axonal transport, 45
Azathioprine, 113b
Azidothymidine (AZT), 31, 31b

B

B cell
  activation of, 239–240
  response of, 240, 240f
  self-tolerance breakdown, 249
  switching off, 240
B lymphocytes, 238–240
Bacille-Calmette-Guérin (BCG)
      vaccine, 215b
Bacteria, 213–216, 213b
  adhesion of, 227
  attacking the host, 229
  body defence against, 774
  classification of, 215
  disordered immunological
      response to, 248b
  food poisoning, 226b
  host organ dissemination of, 227
  invasion of, 227
  as model organisms, 204
  replication of, 215–216
  structure of, 214, 214f
  surface features of, 215
  unusual types of, 215
Bactericidal drugs, 132
Bacteriostatic drugs, 132
Bainbridge reflex, 555
Balanced mutation, 173
Ball and socket joints, 425, 427b,
      429b
Baltimore classification, 217

Bankart lesion, 428b
Bariatric surgery, 783b, 783f
Barium swallow, 720f
Barlow's test, 429b
Baroreceptor reflex, 554–555, 554f
    regulation of, 555
Baroreceptors, 554, 554f, 645, 682
    dynamic response, 554, 554f
    static response, 554, 554f
Barr bodies, 179
Bartter syndrome, 688t
Basal cell carcinoma, 446b
Basal ganglia, 339, 341, 343f,
    372–373, 373f
    control of eye movements, 374
    functional derangements of, 374f
Basal metabolic rate (BMR),
    645–646, 757
Basal plate, 338, 339f
Base excision repair (BER), 168
Base pairing, 29f
Basement membrane, glomerular,
    664
Bases, 16–19
Basic electrical rhythm (BER),
    727–728
Basic Local Alignment Search Tool
    (BLAST), 202
Basilar artery, 354
Basket cells, 371
Basophils, 235, 244–245, 569
Beau's lines, 448
Bell's palsy, 347b
Benign neoplasms
    characteristics of, 265–268, 267t
    macroscopic features and
        growth pattern of, 266, 266f
Benzothiazepines, 512b
Beriberi, 71b
β-Adrenoceptors, 148
    antagonists, 150
    metabolism, 149
β₂-Adrenoceptors, respiratory
    system, 149
β-blockers, 515, 515b
β-Bungarotoxin, 142b
β-oxidation, 94–95
β-Sheet, 34, 35f
β Thalassaemia, 588–589
Bias, 278t, 298b
Bicarbonate
    formation of, 639b
    loop of Henle, 687
    and pCO₂, 687–688
    renal mechanism of, 687–688
    renal reabsorption, 13f
Bicarbonate/carbon dioxide buffer
    system, 11–12
Bicipital muscle, 443
Bile
    concentrated in the gall bladder,
        743
    production, liver and, 738–739,
        738t
    secretion, 738–739
Bile acids, 25
Bile salt absorption, 707
Bile-salt-dependent secretion,
    739
Bile-salt-independent flow, 739
Bile salts, enterohepatic circulation
    of, 743
Bilharzia, 223b
Biliary obstruction, 740
Biliary secretions, 723f
Biliary system, 734–743
Biliopancreatic diversion (BPD),
    784
Bilirubin
    metabolism of, 738–739
    urine, 670, 671t
Binary data, 278t
Bioavailability, 117
Biochemistry, 1, 15–56
Bioequivalence, 117
Bioinformatic tools, 198–199
Biological agents, 213
Biological barriers, 233

Biological weapons, 143b
Biology, energy cycle in, 18–19
Biotin, 766
Biot's respiration, 643b
Bipolar neurons, 353
Birth defects, an epidemic of,
    281b
Black urine disease, 83b
Bladder
    cystometrogram, 691f
    filling and tone, 692
    gross structure of, 691–692
    maintenance of continence, 691
    major components of, 658f
    nerve supply, 691–692
Bleeding time, 600, 600f
Blending theory, 155
Blisters, 446b
Blood, 54
    carbon dioxide carriage, 12f,
        639–640
    carriage of oxygen by, 637–639
    cells. see Blood cells; Red cells;
        White blood cells
    deoxygenated, 623
    film, 600
    group. see Blood groups
    and its constituents, 567–570
    key features, 567b
    loss. see Blood loss
    low albumin levels in, 40b
    measuring hormones in, 458
    oxygenated, 623
    partial pressures of gases in,
        637
    pH value, 11t
    plasma. see Plasma
    production, 590
    red cells. see Red cells
    tests for renal function, 670–671
    transfusion. see Blood
        transfusion
    transport of substances in, 51
    in urine testing, 671t
    white blood cells. see White
        blood cells
Blood-brain barrier, 355–356, 356f,
    643
    circumventricular organs,
        355–356
Blood cells, 567–568, 569f
    production, 570–571
    production disorders, 589–596
    red. see Red cells
    white. see White blood cells
Blood-CSF barrier, 351
Blood flow
    autoregulation of, 552–553,
        553f
    control of, 547–549
    drug distribution and, 106
    mechanics of, 546–553
    types of, 547, 547f
    velocity of, 546–547, 547t
Blood glucose, 473b
    concentration, 62b
    maintenance of, 64, 64f
    regulation of, 63
    sources of, 63–64
    utilisation of, 64, 64f
Blood glucose response curves,
    760, 761f
Blood groups
    antibody production, 604
    antigens, 604
    definition of, 604
    systems, 604–608
    tests, 609, 610f
Blood islands, 506
Blood loss
    acute, 582
    anaemia due to, 582
    chronic, 582
Blood pressure
    classification of, 562t
    different ranges of, 554f
    long-term control of, 556
Blood-testis barrier, 478

Blood transfusion, 608–610
    avoiding transmission of variant
        Creutzfeldt-Jakob disease
        (vCJD), 608b
    guidelines for safe, 608–609
    non-red cell, 610–611
    reactions, 609
    tests, 609–610
Blood vessels, 528–553, 528f
    adrenergic effects on, 149b
    pulmonary, 624–625
Body, system of, 2–3
Body fat, estimating, 755–756
Body fluids
    distribution of, 7f, 109f
    effect of solutes on, 8–9
    homeostatic control of, 7–9
    variation in pH of, 104t
Body mass index (BMI), 755, 755t
Body temperature, 5
    control of, 5f
    heat gain mechanisms, 5–6
    heat loss mechanisms, 5
Body weight
    loss/gain, 754
    'usual,' 754
Bohr effect, 574, 638
Bolus flow, 547, 547f
Bone marrow
    failure, 585
    infiltration, 585
    microenvironment, 570–571
    regeneration of, 255
Bone marrow stroma, 570
'Bone seekers,' 108b
Bone(s), 54, 403–449
    appendicular skeleton, 406
    appositional growth, 411
    axial skeleton, 406
    blood and nerve supply of, 411
    cell types, 405f
    cellular content of, 405–406
    compact, 410
    flat, 406
    formation, 406
    growth, 412–415
        factors affecting, 414
        interstitial, 411
        in length, 412–414, 413f
        in thickness, 414
    healing of, 255, 417–418
    irregular, 406
    long, 406, 410f
    matrix, 405
    microanatomy, 405–406
    ossification, 406
    parathyroid hormone (PTH), 415
    regeneration of, 255
    remodelling, 414–415, 415f
    scans, 404
    short, 406
    spongy, 410f, 411
    structure of, 406–411
    tumour, 408b
    types of, 408b
Bony callus, 255, 418
Bottleneck effect, 174, 175f
Botulinum toxin, neuromuscular
    blockade, 434b
Botulism, 142b
Bovine spongiform encephalopathy
    (BSE), 223b
Bowel Cancer Screening
    Programme, 272
Bowman's capsule, 659
Box and whisker plot, 292–293, 295f
Brachial arteries, 432
Brachial plexus, 348
Brachial pulse, 502
Brady-arrhythmia, 538t
Bradycardia, adrenoceptor
    antagonists, 151
Brain
    blood supply, 353–356
    anterior cerebral circulation,
        353–354
    arterial, 353–355, 353f
    loss of, 353b

Brain (Continued)
    posterior cerebral circulation,
        354
    venous drainage, 355
    cortical areas, 402f
    death, 402
    development, 338–339, 338f
    glycogenolysis in, 77
    imaging techniques, 356b
    magnetic resonance (MR) image
        of, 344f
    metabolic requirements of, 356
    metabolism, 353–356
    reward system, 398–399
    ventricular system, 351f
    vesicles, 340f
Brain natriuretic peptide (BNP), 556
Brainstem, 339, 341–344, 344f,
    365–367
    vestibular testing of, function
        of, 389b
Breast development, 488–489, 491f
Breast Screening Programme, 272
Breastfeeding, vertical transmission
    of pathogens, 230
Breath-hold diving, 647
Breath-holding, 643b, 647
    prolonging, 647
Breath sounds, 618
    abnormal, 618b
Breathing
    bronchial, 618b
    control of, 642–645, 642f
    diaphragm and other muscles
        used in, 627–628
    higher centre control of, 645
    mechanics of, 627–636
    patterns, 643b
    pulmonary pressure changes
        during ventilation, 628–629
    respiratory centre, 642
    respiratory receptors, 642–645
    work of, 631–636
British Isles Network of Congenital
    Anomaly Registers
    (BINOCAR), 283
Brittle bone disease. see
    Osteogenesis imperfecta
Broad street pump, 277–280, 281f
Brodmann's areas, 341, 343f
Bronchial arteries, 623
Bronchial smooth muscle, 618
Bronchial veins, 623
Bronchiectasis, 615b, 634b
Bronchitis, acute, 615b
Bronchoconstriction, 633–634
Brown fat, 60–61
Brown-Séquard syndrome, 369b,
    369f
Buccal drug administration, 118
Buffer capacity, 11
    of the main buffer systems in the
        blood, 11t
Buffer systems, 11–12
Bulbus cordis, 506
Bundle branch block
    left, 522, 522f
    right, 522, 522f
Burns, 446b
Bursae, 431
    inflammation of, 431b
    local injections into, 118
Butyrylcholinesterase, 142
Bystander lysis, 244

C

C3, central role of, 244
C1 complex, 243f
C-peptide, 471
C5a, 244
CA125, 271t
Cachexia, 250
Cadherins, 46
Caenorhabditis elegans (round worm),
    as model organisms, 204
Calciferol. see Vitamin D

Calcified cartilage, 413
Calcitonin, 271t
    calcium homeostasis, 416
Calcitonin gene-related peptide,
        source, target organ, and
        action of, 713t
Calcium, 768
    absorption, 708
    homeostasis, 475
    second messenger system,
        129–130
Calcium channel antagonists,
        124–125
Calcium-channel blockers
    angina, 536b
    therapeutic uses of, 512b
Calcium chelators, 108b
Calcium hydroxyapatite, 54
Calcium-induced calcium release
        (CICR), 510
Calmodulin, 548
Calsequestrin, 440
Canaliculi, 410
Cancellous bone, 406
Cancer
    body defence against, 774
    genes, 188–190
    genetics, 187–190
    inheritance of, 187
    mortality and incidence of, 287b
    registration, 283
    risk
        dietary components associated
            with increased, 774t
        dietary recommendations for
            reducing, 774b
    treatment, and nutrition, 775
Candidate genes, 192
Capillaries, 541–542, 542f
Capillary bed, 542
Capillary endothelial cells, 621
Capillary exchange, 542–543
    influence of blood flow on, 543
Capillary hydrostatic pressure,
        545f
    increased, 545, 545f
Capillary permeability, increased,
        545, 545f
Capillary structure, 541–542
Capsid, 216
Capsule, bacteria, 215
Carbamino haemoglobin, 12
Carbamoyl phosphate synthetase
        (CPS-1) deficiency, 86b
Carbohydrate
    absorbed, in fed state, 760–761
    absorption, 704–705
    digestion, 702, 703f
        enzyme deficiency in, 704b
    metabolism during fasting and
        feeding, 760f
Carbohydrate metabolism, 63–82
    blood glucose
        key pathways maintain and
            utilise, 64
        regulation of, 63
        sources of, 63–64
    glucose
        transport, 64
Carbon atom, 16b
Carbon dioxide
    in blood, carriage of, 12f
    carriage by blood, 639–640
    dissociation curve, 639, 640f
    and oxygen therapy, 643b
    transport, 574–575, 574f
Carbon isotopes, atomic mass
        of, 16t
Carbon monoxide
    poisoning, 648
Carbon monoxide diffusing capacity
        (D_LCO), measuring, 636b
Carbonic anhydrase (CA), 639, 667
Carbonic anhydrase inhibitors,
        684–685
    as diuretic, 685b
Carcinoembryonic antigen
        (CEA), 271t

Carcinogenesis, 273–275
    chemical carcinogens, 273
    and diet, 774–775
    effect of hormones on, 274
    effect of radiation on, 274
    genes and inherited cancer
        syndromes, 274
    genes associated with cancer
        and oncogenesis, 273
    host factors, 274
    infective carcinogens, 273–274
    multistep theory of, 275
    neoplastic cells, 273
Carcinoma in situ, 261–262, 261f,
        263
Cardiac arrhythmias, 518–520
Cardiac axis deviation, 518b
Cardiac conduction system, 513
Cardiac cycle, 522–525, 523f
    phases of, 524t
Cardiac dysrhythmias, adrenoceptor
        antagonists, 150
Cardiac failure, adrenoceptor
        antagonists, 151
Cardiac muscle, 20b, 55
    contraction, 510–511, 511f
    metabolism, 512
    relaxation, 511–512
Cardiac nerves, 514–515
Cardiac output (CO), 525–528
Cardiac prevention, components
        of, 334t
Cardiac resynchronisation therapy,
        for heart failure, 528b
Cardiac tamponade, 494
Cardiogenic shock, 537–539,
        558–559
Cardiomyocytes, 510, 511f
Cardioprotective diets, 777, 777b
Cardiopulmonary reflexes, 555
Cardiovascular disease
    adrenoceptor agonists in,
        148–149
    β-adrenoceptor antagonists,
        150
    phenotype series associated
        with, 177t
    renal failure, 656b
Cardiovascular reflexes, central
        regulation of, 555
Cardiovascular system, 493–566
    adaptations to anaemia, 577
    arteries. see Arteries
    blood flow, 546–553
    blood pressure, 554–566
    blood vessels. see Blood vessels
    cardiac cycle. see Cardiac cycle
    clinical anatomy of, 493–505
    effects of muscarinic receptor
        agonists on, 144
    functions of, 493
    heart, 493–496
    microcirculation. see
        Microcirculation
    shock. see Shock
Carnitine, 183b
Carnitine deficiency, 94
Carnitine shuttle, 94, 94b, 94f
Carpal tunnel, 425
Carpal tunnel syndrome, 427b
Carrier-mediated transport, 48–50,
        104–106
Carrier proteins, 105–106,
        124, 667
Cartilage, 53
Cartilaginous joints, 419
Case-control studies, 186, 278t,
        296b, 297–302, 299b, 299t
    analysing and interpreting data
        from, 299–302
        biological gradient, 301, 301f
        biological plausibility, 302
        coherence of the evidence, 302
        consistency of findings, 300
        demonstration of reversibility,
            301, 302f, 303f
        relationship in time, 301,
            301f

Case-control studies (Continued)
        specificity of the association,
            300–301
        strength of the association,
            299–300
    comparing risk, 300b
    selecting the sample for,
        298–299
Catabolic pathways, 19
Catabolism, 57–58
Catagen phase, hair growth, 447
Catalase, 46
Catalytic proteins, 39
    enzymes, 40–42
Cataract, 382b
Catechol-O-methyltransferase
        (COMT), 148
Catecholamines, 144, 454f
    adrenal, 454–455
    metabolism of, 147–148
    receptor-mediated differential
        effects of, 551–552, 551t
    vasoconstriction by, 551,
        552f
    vasodilatation by, 552
Categorical data, 314, 314f
Catenins, 46
Cations
    proximal convoluted tubule, 669t
Cauda equina, 345
Caveolae, 547
Cavernous sinus, 355
C5b, 244
CD nomenclature, 235
CD14 receptor, 235
CD4 T lymphocytes, 237
    cytokines released by, 239t
CD8 T lymphocytes, 236–237
    cytokines released by, 239t
cDNA selection, 193
Cell, 1, 43–56
    biology, 1
    death, 259
    differentiation, 259
    growth, 259
        decreased, 260
        increased, 259
    membrane, 1
    proliferation of, 259
Cell adhesion, and recognition, 46
Cell biology, 15–56
Cell cycle, 159–163, 159f
    in neoplasia, 259
Cell junctions, 46
Cell membranes, 43–48
    of bacteria, 214
    of fungi, 218
    passive diffusion across, 104
    proteins in, 44
Cell signalling, types of, 47f
Cell surface (membrane) receptors,
        47
Cell surface molecules, 234
Cell wall
    of bacteria, 214
    of fungi, 219
Cells, of the nervous system,
        352–353
    see also Glial cells; Neurons
Cellular glucose metabolism, 10
Cellular protein targeting, 38
Cellulose, 22
Cellulose acetate electrophoresis,
        589, 589f
Cementum, 54
Central auditory pathways,
        390–392, 391f
Central autonomic networks,
        392–395, 393f
Central chemoreceptors, 643
Central control, failure in, 9
Central nervous system (CNS), 55,
        339–345
    drug distribution to, 107
    effects of muscarinic receptor
        antagonists on, 144
Central nervous system ischaemic
        response, 560

Centrioles, 44–45
Centromere, 157
Centrosomes, 44–45
Cephalosporins, nephrotoxicity, 695t
Ceramide, 26
Cerebellar disorders, motor signs
        in, 372b
Cerebellar hypotonia, 371b
Cerebellum, 344, 369–372
    anatomy, 369–370, 370f
    cognitive deficits, 372b
    cortex and circuitry, 371–372, 371f
    folia, 369
    functional subdivisions, 370
    input-output relations, 370t
Cerebral arteries, 354f
Cerebral circulation, 504
Cerebral cortex, 340–341, 343f
Cerebral hemispheres, 339, 341f
Cerebral oedema, 356b
Cerebral venous thrombosis, 355b
Cerebrocerebellum, 370, 371b
Cerebroside, 26
Cerebrospinal fluid (CSF), 20, 350
    absorption, 352
    composition, 351t
    functions, 352
    intrathecal injections, 118
    lumbar puncture, 351b
    secretion and circulation,
        351–352
Cerebrovascular accidents. see
        Stroke(s)
Cerebrum (telencephalon), 338, 339
Cervical Screening Programme, 272
Cervical spondylosis, 407b
C fibres, 554f, 555
Chain elongation, lipogenesis, 98
Charcot-Marie-Tooth disease, 173
Chemical antagonism, 136b, 137
Chemical barriers, 233
Chemical bonds, 16–17
    different types of, 17f
    potential energy of, 18–19, 19t
Chemical carcinogens, 273
Chemical composition of human
        body, 20–42
Chemical digestion, 701–702
Chemical elements, that form the
        human body, 20
Chemical reactions, 18
Chemical synapses, 358
Chemical weapons, 143b
Chemokines, in inflammatory
        response, 252
Chemoreceptor reflexes, 555
Chemoreceptor trigger zone (CTZ),
        730
Chemotactic factors, 235
Chemotherapy, polycythaemia
        rubra vera, 592
Chest
    anterior surface of, 626, 626f
    lateral surface of, 626
    posterior surface of, 626, 626f
Chest leads, 515–516, 515f, 515t
Cheyne-Stokes respiration, 643b
Childbirth, pathogen entry via, 227
Children, nutritional status of, 755
Chinese restaurant syndrome, 88b
Chiral centre, 18
χ^2 distribution, 316, 317f
χ^2 test, 316–317, 318b, 318t
Chlamydia, 215
Chloride
    proximal convoluted tubule, 668
    transport in, loop of Henle, 680
Chloride shift, 639b
Chloroplast, 45
Cholangiocytes, 739
Cholecalciferol, 25
Cholecystokinin (CCK), 734, 772,
        772b
    interactions with acetylcholine
        and secretin, 734
    intracellular messenger for, 734
    source, target organ, and action
        of, 713t

Cholera, 277, 280t, 281f
Cholestasis. see Biliary obstruction
Cholesterol, 24–25
  reverse transport, 93
  structure of, 25f
Cholinergic pathways, major, 362t
Cholinergic receptors, 143–144
  drugs acting at, 143t
  see also Muscarinic receptors
  see also Nicotinic receptors
Cholinesterase, drug hydrolysis, 112b
Chondroblasts, 53, 404
Chondrocytes, 53, 404, 411
Chorionic gonadotropin, 487–488
Chorionic somatomammotropin, 487–488
Choristoma, 262
Choroid epithelial cells, 55
Christmas disease, 601
Chromatids, 157, 158f
Chromatin, 30
Chromatin loops, 158f
Chromosomal abnormalities, sex, 490b
Chromosomal comparative genomic hybridization (CGH) arrays, 194
Chromosomal disorders, 156
Chromosomal mosaicism, 182
Chromosome translocations, 590
  in non-Hodgkin lymphoma (NHL), 595
Chromosomes
  abnormalities, 163–165
  deletions, 163
  DNA and, 157–165
  duplications, 165
  fungi, 218
  karyotypes, 157
  structure, 161f
  translocations, 163
  walking, 192f
Chronic kidney disease (CKD), 657b, 694–696
  causes of, 695
  classification of, 694t
  erythropoietin, 695
  and hypertension, 695
  progression of, 695
Chronic lymphocytic leukaemia (CLL), 593–595
Chronic muscle disease, respiratory failure, 650b
Chronic myeloid leukaemia (CML), 593
Chronic obstructive pulmonary disease (COPD), 614b, 615b
  GOLD (Global Initiative for Obstructive Lung Disease) guidelines on, 649
  measuring airflow limitation in, 632b
  respiratory failure, 649
Chronic progressive external ophthalmoplegia (CPEO), 182b
Chronic renal failure, pharmacological renal damage and, 695–696
Chronotropic effects, 513, 513b
Chylomicrons, 531t
  lipoprotein metabolism, 92
  disorders of, 89b
Chyme, 719
Cilia, 45, 51
  action, as lung defence against infection, 650
  and macrophages, 619
Circadian rhythm, 5
Circle of Willis, 353, 353f
Circular muscle, 443
Circumventricular organs, 355–356
Cirrhosis, of liver, 741–742, 741f
Cis-trans isomerism, 18
Cisplatin, nephrotoxicity, 695t
Cisterns, 350

Citrate, 68–69
  lipogenesis, 96
  phosphofructokinase-1, 68
Citrate agar, 589
Citrate synthase, 59
Clara cells, 619
Claudication, 531
Clavicles, 626
Clinical disagreement, strategies for preventing or minimising, 332b
Clinical significance, 311
Clinical trials, 278t, 305
  analysing and interpreting the results, 310–311
  blinding to avoid bias, 307–308
  calculating sample size, 307
  ethical considerations during, 306
  ethical principles, 308–310
  evaluation of clinical effectiveness, 305–313
  interpreting the results, 312–313
  measures of treatment effect, 311, 311t
  outcomes measurement, 307, 309b, 310
  outcomes of interest: end-point definition, 308
  randomisation to minimise bias, 306–307, 307b
  selecting the sample, 305–306, 306b
Clonal deletion (central tolerance), 249
Cloning, 192–194
Cloning vectors, 192
Clot-busting drugs, 599b
Clusters of Orthologous Groups (COGs), 202
Co-enzymes, 58
  involved in metabolism, 58t
Co-transmission, 359
Coagulation cascade, 598–599, 598f
  common pathway, 598–599
  extrinsic pathway, 598
  intrinsic pathway, 598
Coagulation system, 251
Coagulation tests, 600–601
Coarctation of the aorta, 564
Cobalamin. see Vitamin B_{12}
Cobalamin-folate metabolism, 582f
Cocaine, 147b
  addiction, 399b
Cochlea, 388f, 389–390, 390f
Cochlear implants, 391b
Codons, 36
Coefficient of relationship (COR), 178–179, 179t
Coeliac disease, dietary treatment of, 777
Coenzyme A (CoA), 27, 58, 58t
Coenzymes, 19, 42
  involved in metabolism, 42t
Cognition, 399
Cohort studies, 278t, 296b, 302–304, 304t
  analysing and interpreting data from, 303–304, 304b
  association between genotype and risk factor, 304–305
  interaction with environmental factors, 305, 305f
  selecting the sample for, 302, 304b
  Whitehall studies, 302–303
Cold receptors, 378
Collagen, 40, 448
Collagen diseases, 449b
Collateral ventilation, 621
Collected data, common problems with, 282b
Collecting ducts (CD), 659
  diuretics acting on the late distal tubule and, 686
Collectins, 235
Colles' fractures, 427b
Collinearity, 278t

Colloid osmotic pressure (COP), 9, 544
  filtration forces, 665
Colloid solutions, 561b
Colloids, 544
Colon cancer, 187
Colono-colonic reflex, 747
Colony-stimulating factors, 252
Colorectal cancer, adenoma-carcinoma sequence for, 274f
Commensalism, 224
Commissures, 339
Common iliac arteries, 502
Communicable disease surveillance, 283, 283b
Comparative mortality index (CMI), 290
Comparing proportions, 318b
Compartments, body fluid in, 7f
Competitive inhibition, 42
  of alcohol dehydrogenase, 42b
Competitive protein binding, 108
Complement, 241–244
  alternative pathways, 243–244, 243f
    factors that encourage positive feedback of, 244
    factors that inhibit, 243
  bronchial fluid, 650–651
  central role of C3, 244
  classical pathways, 242, 243f
  lectin pathways, 242, 243f
  lytic sequence, 243f, 244
Complement pathway, 235
Complement system, in inflammatory response, 251
Complementarity determining regions (CDRs), 235
Complex carbohydrates, 23
Complex joint, 428
  knee, 430b
Complex lipids, 26
Compliance
  clinical trials, 309b
  lungs, 634, 635f
Compounds, functional groups and classes of, 18t
Computed axial tomography (CAT), 404
Computed tomography (CT), 404
Concentric contractions, 435
Concordance, 185
Conditional logistic regression analysis, 318
Confidence interval, 278t, 295–296, 295b
Confidential enquiries, 282
Confounding, 278t, 289b
Congenital abnormalities of the kidneys and urinary tract (CAKUT), 662b
Congenital adrenal hyperplasia (CAH), 469b, 469f, 490t
Congenital anomalies notification, 283
Congenital disease, 205, 205t
Congenital disorders, renal agenesis, 662–663
Congenital heart defects, complications of, 507b
Congenital rubella syndrome, immunisation, 324t
Conjugation
  bacteria, 216
  by glucuronidation, 112
Connective tissue, 53–54, 448–449
Connective tissue metaplasia, 260–261
Connexins, 46, 358
Connexon, 46
Consanguinity
  rare disorders and, 179
  and recessive disorders, 178–179
Consciousness, 395
  disorders of, 395b

Conserved Domain Database (CDD), 202
Conserved sequences, 193
Constipation, 748b
Contamination, clinical trials, 309b
Contiguous gene syndrome, 163
Continence, maintenance of, 691
Contingency table, 278t, 295t
  of survey data, 315t
Continuous capillaries, 542
Continuous effects models, 184
Contractile process, 510–512
Control centre, 3
Conus medullaris, 345
Coombs test, 610
Copper, 767–768
  deficiency and overload, 768b
Copy number arrays, 198
Cor pulmonale, 500b, 625b
Coracohumeral ligament, 427b
Cori cycle, 81, 760
Corneal (blink) reflex, 369
Coronary angiography, 536f
Coronary artery bypass graft surgery (CABG), 536b
Coronary artery disease (CAD), 185, 534
  diagnostic tests for, 535t
Coronary blood flow, 504, 504f
Coronary circulation, 503–504
Coronary heart disease
  high risk strategy for, 325, 326t
  primary prevention of, 325
Coronary sinus, 503
Corpus callosum, 339
Corpus haemorrhagicum, 483
Correlation, 317
Correlation coefficient (r), 278t, 317
Cortex
  cerebral. see Cerebral cortex
  of lymph node, 257
Cortical collecting duct, 680
Corticospinal tract, 365
Corticospinal tract fibres, 366b
Corticosteroid Randomisation after Significant Head injury (CRASH) trial, 306
Cortisol, 76
  actions of, 469–470
  Cushing syndrome, 100b
  deficiency, 470b
Cortisol-binding globulin (CBG), 25, 26t
Cortisone, 113b
Cough, 644
  different types of, 644b
Counter-current hypothesis, 678–680
Counter-current mechanism, 680
Covalent bonds, 17
  non-polar, 17f
  polar, 17f
Covalent modification
  regulation of phosphorylase kinase, 77
  reversible activation and deactivation by, 62
CpG islands, 182
Crackles, 618b
Cranial nerves, 346–348, 346t, 347f
  reflexes, 369
  see also specific nerve
Craniosynostosis syndromes, 418b
C-reactive protein (CRP), 234
Creatine kinase (CK), 41
Creatine phosphate, muscle metabolism, 441
Creatine supplementation, 441
Creatinine clearance, renal failure, 672–673
Creutzfeldt-Jakob disease (CJD), 38, 223b
Cri-du-chat syndrome, 163
Crohn disease (CD), 249b, 253, 746b
Cross-match (compatibility test), 610

Cross-over, clinical trials, 309b
Cross-sectional studies, 296b, 297, 298t
  interpreting the data from, 297
  sampling for, 297
Cross tolerance, 137
Crossed extensor reflex, 368
Crossover analysis, in metabolic pathway, 68b
Crude rate, 278t
Crude touch sensations, 379
Cryoprecipitate, 611
Cryptorchidism, 478
Crystalloid solutions, 561b
Cubital fossa, 432b
Cumulative meta-analysis, 319–320, 320f
Curare, 153, 434b
Cushing syndrome, 457b, 470b, 470f
Cushing's reflex, 350b
Cushing syndrome, 564
  cortisol, 100b
Cut-point, 328
Cutaneous circulation, 505, 505f
Cutaneous reflexes, 368
Cyanosis, 639b
Cyclic adenosine monophosphate (cAMP), 27, 48, 514
  stimulation/inhibition of, 129f
Cyclic guanosine monophosphate (cGMP), 27
  activation of, by nitric oxide, 129b
  second messenger system, 129f
Cyclic nucleotide system, 128–130
Cyclin-dependent kinases (CDKs), 159, 259
Cyclo-oxygenase (COX), 25
Cyclophosphamide, 113b
Cyproterone, 132b
Cystic fibrosis, 173b, 179, 619b
  protein augmentation, 208
Cystometrogram, schematic, 691f
Cytochrome P-450
  drug metabolism, 110, 111t
  metabolites of, 113
Cytokines, 47, 245
  in illness, 763b
  released by CD4 and CD8 activated T lymphocytes, 239t
Cytokinesis, 161
Cytoplasm, 1, 44
Cytoskeletal elements, structure of, 44f
Cytoskeletal proteins, 40, 40t
Cytoskeleton, 44–45
Cytosol, 1
  proteins synthesized in, 38
Cytosolic HMG-CoA synthase, 95b

D

Danio rerio (zebrafish), as model organisms, 204
Darwin, Charles, 2
Data
  categorical, 314, 314f
  distribution of, 291–293, 291f
  examining from different sources, 283
  independent data, 313
  interpretation of, 286–289
    clustering, 288
    environmental factors, 288–289, 288f
    health-related behaviours, 288
    healthcare facilities, 288
    inadequacies, 286
    migration, 289
    socio-economic factors, 288
  measures of centre, 292
  measures of spread, 292
  ordered, 292–293
  paired (dependent), 313
  patterns in, 314, 314f

Data (Continued)
  qualitative, 313
  quantitative, 313, 314f
  statistical assessment of, 313–319
    χ^2 test, 316–317
    degrees of freedom, 314, 315b
    multivariate analysis, 318–319
    t-test, 315–316
DAXX (death domain-associated protein), 250
Deafness, 390b
Deamination, amino acid metabolism, 85–86
Declarative memory, 399–401
Decompensated shock, 560
Deep brachial artery, 432b
Deep diving, effects of pressure in, 647
Deep fascia, 441
Deep vein thrombosis (DVT), 540, 540b
Defecation, 747–748, 748f
Defensins, 651
Deformation, definition of, 205
Degrees of freedom, 278t
Dehydration, clinical manifestations of fluid imbalance, 10b
Denaturation, 34
Dendritic cells, 238
  antigen presentation, 238
  in asthma, 248b
  epidermal, 445
Dense bodies, 547
Dentine, 54
Deoxyribonucleic acid. see DNA (deoxyribonucleic acid)
Deoxyribose, 21
Dependent variable, 278t
Depolarisation, action potentials, 357
Depression, 398b, 400–401
Depth, perception of, 386
Dermatome, 348, 349b, 349f
Dermis, 446–447
Desaturation, lipogenesis, 98
Descriptive studies, 280–291
Desferrioxamine, 207
Desmosomes (macula adherens), 445, 510
Development
  genes and, 169
  mediators of, 169–170
Developmental dislocation of the hip (DDH), 429b
Developmental disorders, of nervous system, 339, 340b
Dexamphetamine, 146b
dHAND, 171
DHEA (dehydroepiandrosterone), 470b
Diabetes insipidus, renal fluid balance, 677b
Diabetes mellitus, 63b, 472–474
  clinical features of, 82b
  diagnosis of, 473b, 473f
  dietary control in, 777–778, 778b
  exercise in, 778
  heritability of, 185b
  ketone bodies accumulate, 96b
  maturity-onset diabetes of the young, 66b
  metabolic defects in, 82b
  type 1, 63b, 82b, 473
  type 2, 63b, 82b, 473, 473t
    insulin resistance in, 74b
Diabetic ketoacidosis, 96b, 474, 474f
Diacylglycerol (DAG), 26, 130
Diagnostic test
  calculations, 328t, 329–331
  characteristics, 327–331, 327t
  evaluating, 331–333
  and non-dichotomous values, 328
  result with clinical information, 331f
  true and false, 328b
Diakinesis, 162

Dialysis, 696b
Diapedesis (transmigration), 251
Diaphragm, 627
Diaphysis, 406
Diarrhoea, 706b
Diastole, 522
Diazepam, 119b
Dicrotic notch, 524
Diencephalon, 338, 341
Diet, 3, 750–753
  affecting bone mass, 417
  and carcinogenesis, 774–775
  cardioprotective, 777
  and cardiovascular disease, 775–779
  dietary patterns, 750–751, 750f
  dietary reference values, 751, 751f
  and disease, 773–784
  food guides, 750–751
  food labeling, 750–751, 750f
  and hypertension, 776–777
  therapeutic, 777–778
  WHO guidelines for healthy, 752t
Dietary fats, 24
Dietary fibre, 22
Dietary reference values, 751, 751f
Diffusion, 543
  channel-based, 543
  free, 543
  gas exchange, 636–637
Diffusion force, 356–357
Diffusion-limited diffusion, 543
Digestion, 701–709
  carbohydrate, 702
  chemical, 701–702
  fat, 702
  physical, 701
  protein, 702
Digoxin, 49, 49b, 102
  acting on protein transporters, 105b
  pharmacodynamics of, 102
  pharmacokinetics of, 102
  unwanted effects of, 102
Dihydropyridine derivatives, 512b
Dihydropyridine (DHP) receptors, 440
Dihydroxyacetone-P (DHAP), 91
1,25-Dihydroxyvitamin D (dihydroxycholecalciferol), 416
Diluting segment, and DCT, 680
2,4 dinitrophenol (DNP), 60–61
Dipeptide absorption, 706
Diphtheria, immunisation, 324t
Diploid cell, human, 157
Diploid chromosomes, 162f
Dipole, 17
Direct calorimetry, 645
Disaccharidases, action of, 704t
Disaccharides, 21, 23t
Discontinuous capillaries, 542
Disease
  effect of tonicity in, 8b
  incidence, 280
  occurrence, 280–281
  outcome, 281–282
  prevalence, 281
  surveillance, 282–283
D-isomers, 21
Disordered protein structure, clinical conditions associated with, 38b
Disruption, definition of, 205
Disseminated intravascular coagulation (DIC), 560
  fibrin degradation products, 599
  thrombocytopenia, 602
Dissemination, clinical trials, 313
Distal convoluted tubule, 659, 681
  autoregulation and, 684
Disulfiram, 123b
Disulphide bond(s), 35b
Disynaptic reflexes, 367
Diuretic drugs, 115–116, 684–686
  acting on collecting ducts, 686
  acting on the distal tubule, 115
  acting on the loop of Henle, 115
  acting on the proximal tubule, 116

Diuretic drugs (Continued)
  carbonic anhydrase inhibitors, 684–685
  loop, 685
  main sites of action of, 685f
  osmotic, 116
  osmotic diuresis, 684
  potassium sparing, 115–116, 686b
  sites for actions of, 114f
  thiazide, 115, 685
Diver's reflex, 648
Diverticular disease, 747b
Diving
  ascent from depth, effects of pressure during, 647
  challenges to normal respiration, 647
Dizygotic twins, 185
DNA binding domain, 131
DNA (deoxyribonucleic acid), 28–31, 157
  and chromosomes, 157–165
  cloning, 193f
  complementary, 37t
  damage, 31, 168–169
    from environmental factors, 168
    repair mechanisms, 168–169
    spontaneous, 168
  databanks, 187b
  deletion, 29b, 172–173, 173b
  double helix, 29, 30f
  and genes, 166–168
  insertions, 172–173, 173b
  methylation, 182
  non-coding, 166
  organisation of, 158f
  repair genes, 190
  replication, 159
  secondary structure of, 29
  strands, complementarity of, 30
  structure of, 30f
  tertiary structure of, 30, 30f
  transcription factors. see Transcription factors
DNA-dependent DNA polymerase, 217
DNA-dependent RNA polymerase, 217
DNA glycosylases, 31
DNA helicase, 31
DNA ligase, 31
DNA polymerase III, 31
DNA proofing and repair, 31
DNA replication, 31, 31f
Dobutamine, 149, 562
Dopamine, 461, 561–562
  neurotransmission, 363, 363t
Dorsal column lesions, 376b
Dorsal column-medial lemniscal pathways, 377f
Dorsal horns, 345
Dorsal motor nucleus, 555
Dorsal root ganglia, 348
Dorsal striatum, 341
Dosage mapping, 191
Dose-response curves
  for comparing potency, 134f
  graded, 132–133, 134f
  quantal, 135, 135f
Down syndrome, 156–157
Drosophila (fruit fly), as model organisms, 204
Drowning, 648
Drug absorption, 103–106, 103f
  carrier-mediated transport, 104–106
  diffusion through aqueous and intercellular pores, 106
  endocytosis. see Endocytosis
  exocytosis. see Exocytosis
  fate of drugs in the stomach, 117
  ion trapping, 104
  lipid solubility, 103, 103b
  passive diffusion through lipid membranes, 103–104
  physico-chemical properties of drugs, 116–117
  surface area for, 116–117

Drug antagonism, 136–137, 136*b*
Drug clearance, 120
Drug detoxification, 112
Drug distribution, 103*f*, 106–109
  accumulation in fat and
    redistribution in other
    tissues, 107
  apparent volume of distribution,
    109
  into aqueous compartments, 109
  binding of drugs to proteins,
    107–108
  blood flow, 106
  in the body, 108–109, 109*f*
  capillary permeability, 106–107
  gap junctions, 106–107
  plasma concentration curves,
    120*f*, 122*f*
  to special organs, 107
Drug excretion, 103*f*, 113–116
  glomerular filtration, 114
  hepatobiliary excretion and
    enterohepatic circulation, 116
  renal system, 113–116, 114*f*
  tubular reabsorption, 114
  tubular secretion, 114
Drug metabolism, 103*f*, 109–113
  associated with gene traits, 207*b*
  conversion of inactive pro-drug
    to active metabolite, 113
  detoxification, 112
  factors affecting, 112–113
  first pass, 117–118
  in the gastrointestinal tract, 117
  hydrolysis, 111–112
  phase I metabolic reactions
    (pre-conjugation reactions),
    110–112
  phase II metabolic reactions
    (conjugation reactions), 112
  reduction, 111
Drug-receptor binding, strength
  of, 136
Drug targets, 123–132
  carrier proteins, 124
  enzymes, 123–124
  ion channels, 124–125
  receptors, 125–126
Drug(s)
  absorption. *see* Drug absorption
  classification of, according to
    performance, 133–135
  degree of ionisation of, 104
  distribution. *see* Drug distribution
  dosage, and para-amino hippuric
    acid, 669
  efficacy, 134–135
  and efflux transporters, 669–670
  and elderly, 694
  environmental contaminants and,
    112–113
  excretion. *see* Drug excretion
  factors that affect performance
    of, 135–137
  half-life, 119–120
  ionised and non-ionised forms
    of, 104
  metabolism. *see* Drug
    metabolism
  multiple dosing, 122
  potency, 133–134, 134*f*
  routes of administration, 116–119
  safety and effectiveness of,
    132–137
  safety margins of, 121–122
  selectivity, 133, 134*b*
  sequestration in tissues, 108, 137
  solubility, 116
  specificity, 133
  steady state concentration of,
    121–122, 121*f*, 122*f*
  in the stomach, 117
  targets. *see* Drug targets
  tolerance, 137
  toxic doses, 121–122
Dry chemistry, urine testing, 670
Dual-energy X-ray absorptiometry
  (DXA scanning), 404

Duchenne muscular dystrophy,
  442*b*
Ductus arteriosus, 508–509, 509*f*
Ductus venosus, 508, 509*f*
Duffy antigen receptor for
  chemokines (DARC), 176
Duffy blood group systems, 608
Dukes' staging system, neoplasms,
  271
'Dumping' syndrome, 729*b*
Duodenal musculature, 720
Duodenum, 700, 719–722
  structural features of, 744*t*
Dura mater, 349–351
Dwarfism, 463*b*
Dyneins, 45
Dysgenesis, 262
Dyslipidaemias, 89*b*
Dysplasia, 260, 261–262, 261*f*
Dyspnoea, 643*b*
Dystrophin gene, 200

E

Eadie-Hofstee plot, 41*f*
Early diastolic murmur, 498*b*
Early Pregnancy Factor (EPF), 488
Eating. *see* Food intake
Eccentric contractions, 435
Eccrine glands, 447
Ectoderm, 51
Ectopic beats, 518
Ectopic pregnancy, 487*b*
Edinger Westphal nucleus, 346
Effector, 3
Efferent lymph vessels, 257
Efferent neurons, 353
Efflux transporters, 669–670
eHAND, 171
Ehlers-Danlos syndrome, 38
Eicosanoids, 24
  second messenger system, 130
Eicosapentaenoic acid, 23
Einthoven's triangle, 516, 516*f*
Eisenmenger syndrome, 508*b*
Ejection click, 498*b*
Ejection systolic murmur, 498*b*
Elastic cartilage, 53
Elastic (yellow) cartilage, 404
Elastin, 40, 448
Elbow joint, 423*b*, 423*f*
  dislocation, 423*b*
  tennis elbow, 423*b*
Electrical force, 356–357
Electrical synapses, 358
Electrocardiogram (ECG), 515–516
  12-lead, 516*t*
  deflections, determinants of,
    516*t*
  normal, 516–517, 517*f*, 517*t*
Electrocardiography, 515–517
Electrochemical gradient, 106
Electroencephalography, 395*b*
Electrolytes, 769
  absorption of, 707
  depletion, 769–770
  transport of, 709*t*
Electron sharing, 17
Electron transfer chain (ETC), 18
Electron transport chain, 59–60, 60*f*
  coupling of, 60–61
  inhibition of, 61
  uncoupling, 60–61
Electrophiles, 18
Electrophoresis, haemoglobin,
  589*b*
Embryonal neoplasms,
  nomenclature of, 265*t*
Embryonic stem cell
  transplantation, 208
Emesis. *see* Vomiting
Emotion, 396–398, 397*f*
  expression, 397, 398*b*
  recognition, 397
Emphysema, 615*b*
  respiratory failure, 649
Empyema, 251*b*, 621

Enalapril, 113*b*
Enamel, 54
Encephalopathy, 741*b*
  NH_3-induced, 88*b*
  porto-systemic, 742
End-diastolic volume (EDV), 524
End-systolic volume (ESV), 524
Endergonic reactions, 19
Endfeet, 438
Endocardial cushions, 506–507
Endochondral ossification,
  411–412, 412*f*
Endocrine activity, 234
Endocrine axes, 456*b*
Endocrine disease, 455–457
Endocrine effect, 452
Endocrine glands, 451, 452*f*
Endocrine hypertension, 563
Endocrine system, 451–455
  comparison of nervous systems
    and, 451*b*
Endocrine testing, 456–457
Endocrinology, 451–491
  ageing, 491–492
  concepts in, 455–457
  control of blood calcium,
    475–476
    calcium homeostasis, 475
    and phosphate concentrations,
      475–476
  control of glucose metabolism,
    471–474
    endocrine pancreas, 471–474
    plasma glucose concentration,
      471
  endocrine homeostasis, 464–476
  endocrine regulation, 459–461
  endocrine system, 451–455
  growth hormone, 461–463
  neuroendocrinology. *see*
    Neuroendocrinology
  pregnancy, 464–466
  reproductive physiology,
    478–491
Endocytosis, 50, 50*f*, 106
Endomysium, 441
Endoneurium, 348–349
Endoplasmic reticulum (ER), 45
  in the liver cells, 45*b*
Endospores, bacteria, 215
Endosteum, 410
Endothelial cells
  haemostasis, 597
  in inflammatory response, 252
Endothelial damage, 530
Endothelium, role in haemostasis,
  597–598, 597*f*
Endotoxins, 229
Energy
  balance, 756–764, 756*t*
  consumption
    estimates of, for different types
      of activity, 758
    methods for estimating,
      645–646
  conversion of macronutrients to,
    756, 757*f*
  expenditure
    during daily living, 757–758
    measuring, 757
    total, 757
  for gluconeogenesis, 80–81
  intake in renal disease, 777
  metabolism, 1, 57–100
    during fasting and feeding,
      760–761, 760*t*
    during illness, 763
    in muscles, 75*b*
  needs
    for sport, 758*b*
    of very sick patients, 763*b*
    in pregnancy, 752
  output, 61, 61*t*
  substrates, in fasted state,
    metabolism of, 761*f*, 762*b*
Englyst method, 751

Enhancers, 167
Enkephalins, source, target organ,
  and action of, 713*t*
Enteral nutrition, 778
Entero-pancreatic reflex, 734
Enterocytes, 43
  transport of sugars across, 50*f*
Enteroglucagon, source, target
  organ, and action of, 713*t*
Enterohepatic circulation, 116
  of bile acids, 25
Enthesis, 430–431
Environmental contaminants and
  drugs, 112–113
Enzyme activity, regulation of, 42
Enzyme cofactors, 42
Enzyme deficiency, 704*b*
Enzyme histochemistry, 43
Enzyme induction, 740
Enzyme inhibition, 42
Enzyme kinetics, 40
Enzyme-linked immunosorbent
  assay (ELISA), 459*b*
Enzyme-linked receptors, 127, 131
Enzymes
  binding of allosteric effectors, 61
  as biomarkers, 41*b*
  classes of, 41*t*
  drug targets, 123–124
  induction, 110*b*, 113, 113*b*
  inhibition, 110*b*, 113
  inhibitors, 123
Eosinophils, 246, 569
  in asthma, 248*b*
  in chronic inflammation, 253
  role in inflammation, 246
Ependymal cells, 55
Ephedrine, 146*b*
Epidemics, 231, 277
Epidemiology, 2, 277–335
  basic concepts in, 291–296
  as the detective, 277–280
  epidemiological approach,
    277–291
  epidemiological enquiry, 291–319
    accuracy of the distribution
      summary, 293
    contingency tables, 293
    distribution of data, 291–293,
      291*f*
    health education and
      promotion. *see* Health
      education and promotion
    investigation by experiment,
      305–313
    investigation by observation,
      296–305, 297*b*
    investigation by review,
      319–321
    observational studies. *see*
      Observational studies
    statistical assessment of data,
      313–319
    statistical concepts used in,
      293–296
  terminology, 278*t*
Epidermal dendritic cells, 445
Epidermal growth factors, source,
  target organ, and action
  of, 713*t*
Epidermis, 445
Epidural anaesthesia, 351*b*
Epidural (extradural or peridural)
  space, 350
Epidural injection, 118
Epigastric region, 710
Epilepsies, 400*b*
Epimers, 21
Epimysium, 441
Epinephrine. *see* Adrenaline
Epineurium, 348–349
Epiphyseal arteries, 411
Epiphyseal growth plate, 412
Epiphyses, 406
Epithalamus, 341
Epithelial cells, 43*f*
  types of, 52*f*
Epithelial metaplasia, 260

Epithelial neoplasms, 263
  nomenclature of, 265t
Epithelial tissues, 51–53
Epitopes, 235
Equilibrium potentials, 356–358
Erlanger/Gasser classification of
  nerve fibres, 350t
Erythrocyte sedimentation rate
  (ESR), 597b, 597f
Erythrocytes. see Red cells
Erythropoiesis
  disordered, 572b
  growth factors in, 571–572
  stromal molecules in, 572–573
  transcription factors in, 571
Erythropoietin (Epo), 408–410, 570t
  chronic kidney disease, 695
  control of red cell mass, 571–572
  negative feedback loop, 572, 572f
Escherichia coli, 228b
Essential amino acids, 32, 87–88, 759
Essential fatty acids, 24
Essential hypertension, 684b
Essential thrombocythaemia, 592
Esterification, 88
Estimated average requirement
  (EAR), 751, 757
Eu-FEDS (eutherian fetoembryonic
  defence system), 249
Eubacteria, 213
Eukaryotes, 213
Eukaryotic cell, 43f
Eupnoea, 627, 643b
Evidence-based medicine,
  334–335
Evidence-based treatment, 207
Exchange reactions, 18
Excitation-contraction coupling,
  438–440
  of smooth muscle, 548–549, 549f
Excitation-secretion coupling, 359
Excitatory postsynaptic potential
  (EPSP), 360
Excitotoxicity, 362b
Exercise
  affecting bone mass, 416–417
  challenges to normal respiration,
    646, 646t
  in diabetes, 778
  energy expenditure during, 758
  obesity management, 784
Exergonic reactions, 19
Exocrine glands, 52–53
  effects of muscarinic receptor
    agonists on, 144
Exocytosis, 50f, 51, 106
Exons, 36–37, 166
Exotoxins, 229
Expiration, 628
  variations in pulmonary blood
    flow, 625
Expiratory reserve volume (ERV),
  629
Expiratory wheezes, 618b
Expressed sequence tags (ESTs),
  193
Expression arrays, 197
Expression cassette, 209
Expression profiles, 187
External ear, 389, 390f
Extracapsular ligaments, 422
Extracellular compartment, 7
Extracellular compartment,
  interstitial fluid, 8
Extracellular fluid (ECF), 20
  composition of, 20t
  drug distribution, 109f
Extracellular ligand-binding
  domain, 131
Extracellular matrix (ECM), 21, 53
  collagens and proteins present
    in, 39–40
Extracellular matrix proteins, 170
Extracellular pathogens, 227
Extradural haemorrhage, 350b
Extrafusal fibres, 367
Extramedullary haemopoiesis, 570
Extraocular muscles, 373, 374f, 375t

Extravascular haemolysis, 584f
Exudate, 251
Eye(s)
  anatomy, 381–382, 382f
  effects of muscarinic receptor
    agonists on, 144
  effects of muscarinic receptor
    antagonists on, 144
  movements, 346, 373–374
  optics of the, 381
  pathogen entry via, 226

F

F 1,6-BPase deficiency, 81b
F-actin, 437
Facial (VII) nerve, 346t, 347
Facilitated carriers, 668
Facilitated diffusion, 48–49
Facilitated transport, 49f
Fainting, mechanisms involved
  in, 557b
False substrates, 124, 124b
Falx cerebri, 350
Familial adenomatous polyposis,
  187
Familial combined hyperlipidaemia,
  89b
Familial dysbetalipidaemia, 89b
Familial hypercholesterolaemia, 47,
  178, 207, 532b
Familial Mediterranean fever, 179
Fanconi's anaemia, 585–586
Fascia, 429–430
Fascicles, 348–349
Fasted state, pyruvate, 70
Fasting, prolonged, 762–763, 762t
Fasting lipid profile, 92b
Fat
  absorbed, in fed state, 761
  absorption, 706–707
  absorption, inhibition of, 783
  accumulation of drug in, 107
  digestion, 702
    defects in chemical, 704b
  in fasted state, 762
Fat (adipose) tissue, 54
Fat metabolism, regulation of, 100
  in fasting (post-absorptive) state,
    100
  in fed (absorptive) state, 100
Fat-soluble vitamins, 707, 766–767
Fatty acid binding proteins
  (FABPs), 90
Fatty acid elongase, 98
Fatty acid synthase (FAS)
  lipogenesis, 96, 98
Fatty acid transport proteins
  (FATP), 90
Fatty acids, 23–24, 24b, 90
  carnitine shuttle, 94, 94f
  dietary, 89
  endogenously synthesized, 89, 89f
  essential, 88
  fine-tuning of, 99–100
  free, 88
  oxidation, 93–96
    activation and transport into
      mitochondria, 93–94
    β-oxidation, 94–95
    carnitine shuttle, 94
    ketogenesis in liver, 95–96
  polyunsaturated, 88
  protein-bound, 90
  sources of, 88–89
  synthesis, 96–99
Fatty liver, 54
Fatty streaks, 530
Fava (broad) beans, 67b
Fear, pathways of, 397
Fed state, pyruvate, 70, 70f
Feed forward activation, 42
Feedback error correction,
  371–372
Feedback loops, 42
Feedforward, 6
  control, examples of, 6b

Feeding, regulation of, 394, 394f
Feet, normal flora, 224f
Female reproductive endocrinology,
  481
Female reproductive tract, 481 f,
  181–184
Ferritin, 737b
  iron deficiency and, 579
Fertilisation, 486–488
Fetoplacental circulation, 508
Fever, 6b
  in response to infection, 231b
  as systemic effect of acute
    inflammation, 252
Fibre content, in food labelling, 751
Fibrillin, 35
Fibrinogen, 54
Fibrinolysis, 598
  inhibitors, 600
Fibroblast growth factor, 169
Fibroblast growth factor receptor
  (FGFR), 169
Fibroblasts, 53
  in granulation tissue, 254
Fibrocartilage, 54
Fibrocartilaginous callus, 255
Fibrocollagenous tissues, 53, 53f
Fibronectin, 40
Fibrous cap formation, 531
Fibrous joints, 418–419
Fick equation, 624, 624b, 636
Fick's law, 104
Filtration pressure, 544, 544f
Fimbriae, 215
  bacteria, 215
First-order kinetics, 119–120, 120f
Fisher's exact test, 278t
Fixed hydrogen ions, 686
Flagella, 45
  bacteria, 215
Flavin adenine dinucleotide (FAD),
  27, 58t
Flexion withdrawal reflex, 368
Flippases, 43–44
Flow-limited diffusion, 543
Flow-volume loop, 631, 633f
Fluid balance, 3
  behavioural control of, 9
  behavioural effects leading to
    disturbance of, 9b
  causes for homeostatic failure
    in, 9b
  homeostatic control of, 9
  hormonal control of, 9
  renal control of, urine
    concentration and dilution,
    678–680
Fluid chart, 20
Fluid compartments, 7–9
  homeostatic failure in, 7b
  of human body, 20
Fluid imbalance, clinical
  manifestations of, 10b
Fluid mosaic model, 43, 44f
Fluid replacement, 561, 561b
Fluids
  excess loss of, 10
  movement of, 8
Flukes, replication of, 223
Fluorescence in situ hybridization
  (FISH), 164b, 165t, 191, 191f
  normal/abnormal human
    karyotype, 164f
Fluorescence Resonance Energy
  Transfer (FRET), 197
Fluoride, 769
Fluorouracil, 124b
Foam cells, 531
Foetal abnormalities, screening
  for, 489b
Foetal alcohol syndrome, 205b
Foetal circulation, 508–509, 509f
Foetal development, 488, 489f
Foetal haemoglobin, elevated, 587
Foetus, drug distribution to, 107
Folate, 581
  deficiency, 581, 582t
    laboratory findings in, 581, 583t
  importance of, 580–581

Folic acid, 766
  deficiency, 766b
Follicle stimulating hormone (FSH),
  460, 479
Follicular dendritic cells, 257
Follow-up, clinical trials, 309b
Fontanelles, 418
Food and Agriculture Organization
  (FAO), 750, 750f
Food intake, 754
  control of, 771–784
  methods for recording, 754t
  peripheral hunger signals, 772
Foramen ovale, 507
Foramen primum, 507
Foramen secundum, 507
Forced expiratory volume (FEV),
  630–631, 632f
  measurement of, 631b
Forced respiration, 627, 628f
Forced vital capacity (FVC), 629,
  632f
Ford, E.B., 172
Foreign body granulomas, 253
Founder effects, 173–174, 174f
Fragile X syndrome, 173b
Fragment crystallisable (Fc) region,
  241
Frameshift mutation, 29b
Free diving, effects of pressure
  in, 647
Free radicals, 773–774
Free water clearance, 677t
Frequency distribution plot, 135,
  135f
Fresh frozen plasma (FFP), 611
Frozen shoulder, 428b
Fructose, 21
  gluconeogenesis from, 81
  glycolysis, 65
  intolerance, 81b
  metabolism defects of, 81b
Fructose-1,6-bisphosphate
  (F-1,6-BP), 67
Fructose-2,6-bisphosphate
  (F-2,6-BP), 68
Fructose 6-phosphate (F6P), 67
Fructose absorption, 705
Fructose kinase deficiency,
  81b
Fuel metabolism
  diabetes mellitus and, 63b
  layout of, 58f
  regulation of, 61–62
  stored and transported between
    tissues, 63
Fuel stores, 760t
Full blood count, 600
Functional barriers, 233
Functional residual capacity (FRC),
  629, 630
  measurement of, 630b
  pulmonary diseases that affect,
    630b
Funduscopy, 384b, 384f
Fungi
  classification of, 219, 219t
  general features of, 218b
  invasion of, 227
  structure of, 218–219
Furosemide, 670b
Fused tetanus, 435
Fusiform muscle, 443

G

G-actin, 437
G-protein coupled receptors
  (GPCRs), 127–131
  molecular structure of, 128f
  neurotransmission, 360
  and signal transduction
    mechanism, 128
  speed of transmembrane
    signalling, 131
  termination of transmembrane
    signals, 131

G proteins, 48, 76
  ion channel modulation by, 131
  and signal transduction, 128
  types of, 128
GABA transaminase, 362
GABA$_A$ receptor, 127, 362b
Gag reflex, 369
Gait
  analysis, 444
  defects, 444b
Galactokinase deficiency, 81b
Galactosaemia, 81, 207
Galactosamine, 21
Galactose, 21
  absorption, 704–705
  glycolysis, 65
Galactose-1-phosphate (Gal-1-P),
  81b
Galactose-1-phosphate uridyl
  transferase, deficiency, 81b
Gall bladder, 742–743
  emptying of, 743
Gall stones, 743b
Gametocytes, protozoa, 220
γ-Aminobutyric acid (GABA), 88
Ganglion cysts, 431b
Gap junctions, 46, 106, 510
  electrical synapses, 358
Gas-blood barrier, 620–621, 620f
Gas exchange, principles of,
  636–637
Gaseous exchange, 613
Gasping, 616b
Gasser classification of nerve
  fibres, 350t
Gastric distention, 771
Gastric emptying, 728–730, 771
  duodenal contents, 729–730
  gastric contents, 728
Gastric glands, 721t
Gastric-inhibitory peptide, source,
  target organ, and action
  of, 713t
Gastric juice, pH value, 11t
Gastric motility, 727–730
  during the interdigestive period,
  728
  during a meal, 728–730, 729f
  mixing of gastric contents, 728
Gastric mucosa, 721–722
Gastric musculature, 720, 727
Gastric proteases, 704t
Gastric secretions, 722–727, 723f
  cellular mechanisms of, 724–726,
  725f
  disorders of, 726b
  gastric mucosal protection,
  726–727, 727f
  inhibition of, 723–724
    cephalic phase, 724
    gastric phase, 724
    intestinal phase, 724
  pharmacological inhibition of, 726b
  stimulation of, 722–723
    cephalic phase, 722
    gastric phase, 723
    intestinal phase, 723
Gastric smooth muscle, electrical/
  contractile activity of,
  727–728
Gastrin
  intracellular messenger for the
  action of, 725–726
  source, target organ, and action
  of, 713t
Gastrin-releasing peptide, source,
  target organ, and action
  of, 713t
Gastro-ileal reflex, 745–746
Gastro-oesophageal diseases,
  722b
Gastrocolonic reflexes, 747
Gastroenteritis, 226b
GATA-1, 571
GATA-2, 571
Gate control theory, 379, 380f
Gaussian distribution curve, 291f,
  292

Gaze
  shift, 374
  stabilization, 374
GC islands, 193
GenBank, 200
Gene expression
  blood production and, 590
  regulation of, and transcription,
  62
General anaesthetics (GAs),
  151–153
  inhaled, 151
  intravenous, 151
  muscle relaxants, 153
  nephrotoxicity, 695t
  pharmacodynamics of,
  151–153
  unwanted effects of, 153
Gene(s)
  deletion, 181b
  and development, 169
  duplications, 173
  expression, 156
  families, 200–202
  identifying disease, 190–204
  testing, 204–205
  transfer, 208–209
Genetic code, 36t, 156
  mutation, 38b
Genetic counselling, 204–205
Genetic linkage, 195
  and monogenic disease, 194
  and polygenic disease,
  196–199
Genetic medicine, 207–210
Genetic penetrance, 176, 176b
Genetics, 2, 155
  ethics, 204
  factors affecting drug
  metabolism, 112
  genetic disease, diagnosis and
  therapy, 204–210
  human genetic variation,
  172–176
  modern, basis of, 156–157
  modes of inheritance,
  177–183
Genome, 156
  bacteria, 214
  mapping, 190–199
  microarrays, 197–198
Genomic imprinting, 181–182
Genomic instability, 190
Genomic library, 192
Genomic sequencing, 207b
Genomics, 156
Genotypes, 176
Germ cell neoplasm, 265
Germline, 156
Gerota's fascia, 657
Gestational hypertension, 564
Ghrelin, 772
  action of, 772b
  in disease, 772b
  source, target organ, and action
  of, 713t
Gigantism, 463b
Gitelman syndrome, 688t
Glandular epithelial cells, 52–53
Glandular metaplasia, 261b, 261f
Glaucoma, 382b
Glenohumeral ligaments, 427b
Glial cells, 56, 352
Gliding synovial joint, 422–423
Global Alert and Response (GAR),
  284
Global infectious disease
  surveillance, 284
Global Registry of Acute Coronary
  Events (GRACE) score,
  537b
Glomerular basement membrane
  (GBM), 661
Glomerular capillaries, 661, 661f
Glomerular filtration, 114, 114f
  barrier, 661
  and production of primary urine,
  664–665

Glomerular filtration rate (GFR),
  656, 657f, 682f
  control of, by the renal
  capillaries, 681–682
  inulin, 672
  renal clearance, 672
  urea clearance, 673
Glomerular-tubular balance, 682
Glomerulonephritis, 657b
Glossopharyngeal (IX) nerve, 346t,
  347
Glucagon, 76, 472
  regulation of gluconeogenesis,
  81
  starvation, 68
Glucagon-like peptide 1 (GLP-1),
  772
  source, target organ, and action
  of, 713t
Glucocorticoid resistance
  syndrome, 178
Glucocorticoids, 25t
  effects of, 470t
  therapeutic use of, 470b
Glucokinase (GK), 66b, 67
  regulation of, 66f
Gluconeogenesis, 22, 78–82, 762
  amino acids in, 87f
  Cori and glucose-alanine cycles,
  81
  energy for, 80–81
  from glycerol, 80
  from lactate, 78–79
  pathway of, 79f
  precursors of, 78–80
  from protein, 79–80
  regulation of, 81–82
  from sugars, 81
Glucosamine, 21
Glucose, 4, 21, 63
  absorption, 50, 704–705
  anaerobic catabolism of, 65–71
  blood. see Blood glucose
  forms of, 22f
  need for, in fasted state, 761–762
  phosphorylation, 66–69
  red cell energy, 576
  tolerance curve in diabetes, 82b
  transport of, 64, 64t
  urine testing, 671t
Glucose-6-phosphate
  dehydrogenase (G6PD), 67
  deficiency, 67b, 586–587
  haemolytic anaemia and, 67b
Glucose-6-phosphate (G6P), 66
  glycolysis, 67
Glucose-alanine cycle, 81
Glucose-dependent insulinotropic
  peptide, source, target
  organ, and action of, 713t
Glucose homeostasis, scheme
  for, 4f
Glucose metabolism, homeostatic
  control of, 4
Glucose phosphate, 63
Glucose phosphorylation, 66–69
Glucose tolerance curve in
  diabetes, 82b
Glucose transport, 64, 64t
Glucose transporters (GLUTs), 64
  GLUT1, 64
  GLUT2, 64
  GLUT3, 64
  GLUT4, 64
Glucuronidation, conjugation by,
  112
Glutamate
  ammonium synthesis, 688
  metabolism, 361f
  neurotransmitters, 360
Glutamate receptors, 127
Glutamine
  in acid-base homeostasis, 85–86
  dietary, 84
Glutathione, conjugation, 112
Glutathione reductase, 198b
Gluten sensitive enteropathy, 746b
Glycaemia, 63

Glycaemic index (GI), 761, 761f
  classification of foods by, 761t
Glycated protein, clinical features
  resulting from, 82b
Glycation, 531
Glycerol
  gluconeogenesis from, 80
  glucose in fasted state, 762
Glycerol 3-phosphate (gl-3-P), 91
Glycerophospholipids, 26
Glyceryl trinitrate (GTN), drug
  administration, 119b
Glycine
  neurotransmitters, 362
Glycogen, 22, 72, 72b
  breakdown of, 75
  structure of, 73
  synthesis of, 72–75
Glycogen storage diseases, 78b
Glycogen synthase (GS), 72–73
Glycogen synthesis
  control of, 73–74
  non-invasive techniques for, 74b
  regulation of, 73f
Glycogenesis, 64
Glycogenin, 73
Glycogenolysis, 3, 64, 75
  genetic defects in, 78
  glucose in fasted state, 761f
  mechanism of glucagon
  regulation of, 76, 76f
  regulation of, 75–76
    muscle and brain, 77
Glycolipids, 88
Glycolysis, 61t, 64, 65–71, 68b
  advantages and disadvantages
  of, 63b
  and associated metabolic
  pathways, 65f
  energy-producing stage of,
  69–71, 69f
  energy-using reactions in, 66–69
  energy-utilising steps in, 66f
  importance of the anaerobic
  nature of, 65–66
Glycoproteins, 23
  chemical nature of hormones,
  452t
Glycosaminoglycans (GAGs), 23,
  23t
Glycosidic bonds, 21
Glycosuria, 472–473
  in thiazide diuretics, 115
Glycosylation, 38
Goal-directed behaviours, 398–399
Goblet cells, 52–53, 619
Goitre, 465b
Golgi apparatus (Golgi complex),
  45
Golgi cells, 371
Golgi tendon organ reflex, 368
Gomphosis, 419
Gonadal mosaicism, 182
Gonadotropin-releasing hormone
  analogues, 132b
Goodpasture syndrome, 247
Gorlin syndrome, 170
Goserelin, drugs targeting nuclear
  receptors, 132b
Granulation tissue
  in bone, 255
  granulomas and, 254
Granule cells, 371
Granules, bacteria, 214
Granulocyte colony-stimulating
  factor (G-CSF), 570t
Granulocyte macrophage colony-
  stimulating factor (GM-CSF),
  570t
Granulomas
  chronic inflammation and, 253
  and granulation tissue, 254
  stimulants of, 253–254
Grapefruit juice, enzyme inhibition,
  110b
Grave disease, 248, 457b
Great arteries, 508
Great cerebral vein, 355

Gregor Mendel's experiments, 155
Grey matter, 345
Groin, normal flora, 224f
Growth, 461
  charts, 462f
Growth factors, 47
  in erythropoiesis, 571–572
  functions, 570t
  haemopoiesis, 570–571
  therapeutic use, 571b
Growth hormone (GH), 461–463
  abuse of, 463b
  actions of, 462–463
  dynamic testing for excess, 458b, 458t
  metabolic effects of, 463t
  regulation of, 461, 462b, 462f
  replacement, 463b
Guanylin, source, target organ, and action of, 713t
Guillain-Barré syndrome, 358b, 650b
Gut, balance of chemical contents in, 771–772

H

Haematocrit, 7b, 567
Haematology, 567–611
  blood groups and transfusions, 604–611
  haemopoietic system. see Haemopoietic system
  haemostasis. see Haemostasis
  oncogenesis and disorders of blood cell production, 589–596
  red cells, 571–589
  terms used in, 568t
  thrombosis. see Thrombosis
Haematopoietic stem cells, 51
  transplantation, 208
Haemodialysis, 697f
Haemoglobin, 573, 573f, 575–576, 638
  buffer system, 12
  deoxygenated, 574f
  disorders, 587–589
    see also Specific disorder
  electrophoresis, 589b
  embryonic, 575t
  foetal. see Foetal haemoglobin
  oxygenated, 574f
  production throughout life, 575–576, 575f
Haemoglobin-oxygen dissociation curve, pyruvate kinase and, 70b
Haemoglobinuria, 577b
Haemolysis, anaemias due to, 583–586
Haemolytic anaemia
  G6PD deficiency, 67b
  pyruvate kinase deficiency and, 70b
Haemolytic disease of the newborn (HDN), 607b
Haemophilia, 181
Haemophilia A, 180–181, 601
Haemophilia B, 601
Haemophilus influenzae meningitis, immunisation, 324t
Haemopoiesis
  regulation of, 570–571
  role of stem cells in, 570, 570f
Haemopoietic neoplasms, 263–265
Haemopoietic receptors, 571
Haemopoietic stem cells, 506
Haemopoietic system, 567–571
  see also Blood
Haemoptysis, 644
Haemorrhage, 557
Haemosiderin, iron deficiency, 579

Haemostasis, 596–604
  coagulation cascade, 598–599, 598f
  coagulation factor disorders, 601–602
    acquired, 602
    inherited, 601
  coagulation system, 600–601
  endothelium, 597–598, 597f
  fibrinolytic system, 599–600
  natural anticoagulants, 599
  normal mechanisms, 596–601
  platelets, 597–598, 597f, 598f
  thrombocytopenias, 602–603
  thrombophilias, 603–604
Hair, 35b, 447–448
  structure of, 447
  types of, 448
Hair follicle, structure of, 447–448
Haldane's effect, 639
Halothane, 152
Hamartoma, 262
Haplo-insufficiency, 178
Haplotype, 173
Haustra, 746–747
Haversian system, 410
Health beliefs, 323
Health claims, 751
Health education and promotion, 321–335
  approaches to, 321
  essentials for effective, 322
  ethical considerations in, 322–323
    case scenario: a new diagnosis of diabetes, 322–323
  health education, 321–323
  high-risk strategy, 322
  population strategies, 321–322
  prevention, 323–335
  strategies for, 321–322
Health inequalities, 285–286, 285f
  in UK, 286, 286b
Health of populations, measures for, 284–285
Health outcomes, changes in, 286, 287f
Health surveys, 285
Hearing, 347
Heart, 493–496, 494t
  adrenergic effects on, 149b
  apex of, 494
  asymmetrical, 171
  cellular structure and function of, 510–528
  chambers, 494, 495f, 506–508
  conduction pathways in, 514f, 514t
  development of, 506–508, 506f
    congenital heart abnormalities, 507b
  effects of muscarinic receptor antagonists on, 144
  efficient functioning of, 514b
  electrical activation of, 512–522
  electrical axis of, 517, 517f
  embryology of, 505–510
  muscle, structure of, 510
  nerve supply to, 513–515
  sounds and murmurs, 495–496, 497f, 498f
  valves, 494–495
Heart block, 520–522, 521f
Heart failure, 525–528, 538t
  cardiac resynchronisation therapy for, 528b
  causes of, 526, 527t
  oedema in, 546b
  pathophysiological mechanisms activated by, 526–527, 527b
  treatment of, 527–528, 527b
Heart sounds, 498b
Heat gain mechanisms, 5–6
Heat loss mechanisms, 5
Heavy metals, nephrotoxicity, 695t
Helicobacter pylori, 228b

Helminths, 222–223
  adhesion of, 227
  classification of, 222–223
  general characteristics of, 222b
  replication of, 223
  transmission of, 222f
Hemidesmosomes, 445
Heparin, as an anticoagulant, 601
Heparin-induced thrombocytopenia (HIT), 603
Hepatic acinus, 736f
Hepatic circulation, 504–505
Hepatic failure, in paracetamol overdose, 112b
Hepatic glycogen phosphorylation, regulation of, 77–78, 77f
Hepatic glycogenolysis
  enzyme regulation of, 76–77
  hormone regulation of, 76
  pathways for, 75f
  regulation of, 76
Hepatic lobule, microanatomy of, 735f
Hepatic portal system, 504–505
Hepatitis, causes of, 742t
Hepatobiliary excretion, 116
Hepatocellular disease, 740–741
Hepatocellular failure, 741b
Hepatocytes, 45b
HER-2, 271t
Hereditary nonpolyposis colorectal cancer, 187
Hereditary spherocytosis, 586, 586b
Hering-Breuer lung inflation reflex, 644
Heritability, 185–186, 185t
Heterochromatin, 157
Heteroreceptor, 360
Heterotopia, 262
Heterozygous familial hypercholesterolaemia, 89b
Hexokinase (HK), 66
  regulation of, 66f
Hexose monophosphate shunt, 67
Hexoses, 21
Hiccups, 616b
High acuity vision, 384b
High-density lipoprotein (HDL), 531t
  lipoprotein metabolism, 92–93
  reverse cholesterol transport, 93
High-performance liquid chromatography (HPLC), 589
Higher cortical functions, 399–401
Hilum, 735
Hinge joint, 423–424, 424b
Hip fractures, 429b
Hippocampal cognitive maps, 400b
Hirschsprung disease, 748b
Hirsutism, 447b
Histamine, 244
  in inflammatory response, 252
  intracellular messenger for the action of, 725–726
  neurotransmission, 363
Histogram, 278t
Histology, 43b
Hodgkin disease, 595
Homeobox (HOX) genes, 166
Homeostasis
  definition, 3–14
  kidney, 655
Homeostatic control
  of fluid balance, 9
  of hydrogen ions, 10–14
Homeostatic failure, clinical effects of, 7b
Homeostatic regulation mechanisms, 3–6
Homeotic mutations, 166
Homocysteine, 776
Homogentisic acid oxidase, deficiency of, 83b
Homologous recombination, 169

Homologues, 161, 200
  types of, 202f
Homology modelling, 202
Homozygous familial hypercholesterolaemia, 89b
Homunculus, 365
Horizontal transmission, of pathogens, 230–231
Hormone replacement therapy (HRT), 491–492
Hormone secretion
  kidney, 655
  negative feedback regulation of, 455
  patterns of, 455, 455f
Hormone sensitive lipase (HSL), 91, 91f
Hormone signalling, 76, 76f
Hormones, 47, 452
  action of, 62
  chemical nature of, 452t
  eating, 772
  gastrointestinal, 713t
  in illness, 763b
  measuring
    in blood, 458
    techniques for, 459b
  and stress, 467–470
  that influence haemoglobin production, 572
  transport in blood, 455b
"Housemaid's knee," 431b
β-Human chorionic gonadotrophin (β-HCG), 271t
Human chromosome karyotype, 159f
Human genetics, 155–210
Human genome, 157–172
Human Genome Project (HGP), 199–204
  statistics of, 200
  using data from, 200, 201f
Human growth hormone (hGH), 413
Human immunodeficiency virus (HIV), 31, 218b
  replication of, 31b
Human leucocyte antigen (HLA), 236
Human transmissible spongiform encephalopathies, 223b
Huntington disease, 173b, 178
  basal ganglia and, 373b
  penetrance and phenotypic expression, 176b
  RNAi in, 209
Hyaline cartilage, 53, 404
Hydrocarbon chains, 18
Hydrocephalus, 352b
Hydrochloric acid, pH values, 11t
Hydrocortisone, 238
Hydrogen bonds, 17
  protein structure, 34
Hydrogen ion dissociation constant (pKa), 104, 104t
Hydrogen ions, 68
  acid-base balance, 686–687
  disease states, 687
  fixed, 686
  homeostatic control of, 10–14
  partial pressure of, 10
  renal excretion of, 13f
  sources of non-respiratory, 686–687
  volatile, 686
Hydrolases, 41t
Hydrolysis, 111–112
Hydronephrosis, 691b
Hydrophobic interactions, 17, 34
Hydrostatic pressure, 8
3-Hydroxy-3-methylglutaryl-CoA (HMG-CoA)
  cytosolic HMG-CoA synthase, 95b
  mitochondrial HMG-CoA synthase, 95b
Hydroxyapatite, 406
3-Hydroxybutyrate, 95
β-Hydroxybutyrate, 95

5-α Hydroxylase deficiency, 490t
Hydroxyurea, 207
Hyperbilirubinaemia, unconjugated, 739b
Hypercalcaemia, 476f, 477b, 512b
Hypercapnia, respiratory failure, 650
Hypercholesterolaemia, 89b
Hyperglycaemia, 4, 66b
Hyperkalaemia, 512b
Hyperlipidaemia, 92b
 dietary approach to the control of, 776b
 secondary, 89b
Hyperosmolar non-ketotic states (HONK), 474
Hyperparathyroidism, 477b
Hyperplasia, 259
 pathological, 260b
 physiological, 259b
Hyperpnoea, 643b
Hyperpolarisation, action potentials, 357
Hyperprolactinaemia, 457b, 461b
Hyperpyrexia, 440b
Hypersensitivity, 246–248
 type 1, 246t, 247, 247f
 type 2, 246t, 247
 type 3, 246t, 247
 type 4, 246t, 248
 type 5, 246t, 248
Hypertension, 562–566
 adrenoceptor antagonists, 150
 aetiology of, 562
 chronic kidney disease and, 695
 diagnosis of, 562
 diet and, 776–777
 drug-induced, 564
 due to chronic kidney disease, 563
 endocrine causes of, 563–564
 main cause of, 563t
 pathophysiology of, 562–563
 portal, 741–742
 pregnancy-induced, 564
 renal failure, 656b
 secondary, 563–564
 treatment of, 565–566, 565t
Hyperthermia, 4
Hyperthyroidism, 457b, 467b, 467f
Hypertriglyceridaemia, polygenic, 89b
Hypertrophic cartilage, 413
Hypertrophy, 259
 pathological, 260b, 260f
 physiological, 259b
Hyperventilation, 643b
Hypervolaemia, 7b
Hypo-osmotic, 8
Hypoalbuminaemia, 108
Hypocalcaemia, 476f, 512b
Hypochlorous acid (HOCl), 67b
Hypochondrium, left and right, 710
Hypoglossal (XII) nerve, 346t, 348
Hypoglycaemia, 4, 62b, 474, 474f
 adrenoceptor antagonists, 151
 excessive alcohol intake, 78b
 glucokinase, 66b
Hypokalaemia, 512b
 digoxin toxicity, 102
 loop diuretics, 115
Hypokalemic alkalosis, causes of, 688t
Hypoparathyroidism, 477b
Hypophosphataemic rickets, 180
Hypopituitary states, 460b
Hypoplasia, 262
Hypopnoea, 643b
Hypoproteinaemia, 108
 renal failure, 656b
Hypotension, 560
Hypothalamic-pituitary-testicular axis, 479–481, 479f
Hypothalamo-pituitary-adrenal axis, 469, 469f
Hypothalamo-pituitary-thyroid axis, 456b, 456f

Hypothalamus, 341
 functional anatomy of, 458, 459f
 neural and vascular connections between pituitary and, 460f
Hypothermia, 4
Hypothesis tests, 294
Hypothyroidism, 467b, 467f
Hypoventilation, 643b
Hypovolaemia, 7b
Hypovolaemic shock, 557, 558f
Hypoxia, 638b
 digoxin toxicity, 102
Hypoxia-inducible factor 1 (HIF1), 66
Hypoxia response elements (HREs), 66
Hysteresis, 634

I

I/i blood groups, 608
Idiopathic adhesive capsulitis, 428b
Ileum, 700
 structural features of, 744t
Iliac fossa, left and right (inguinal region), 711
Iliofemoral ligament, 429b
Illness
 cytokines and hormones in, 763b
 energy metabolism during, 763
 protein metabolism in, 763–764
 and acute phase response in, 764
Immune response, 233
Immune system
 adaptive, 235–240, 236f
 autoimmune disease, 249–250
 cellular defences of, 244–246
 hypersensitivity, 246–248, 246t
 innate, 234–235, 236f
 other substances important to, 250
 tolerance, 249
Immune thrombocytopenic purpura (ITP), 603
Immunisation, 324–325, 324t
 public perception and immunisation coverage, 324–325
Immunity, 233–258
 immunological defence system, 233–250
 invading immunogen, detection and destruction of, 233–234
 lymphoid organs, 257–258
 non-immunological defence system, 233
Immunoassay (IA), 459b, 459f
Immunogens, 233
 detection and destruction of invading, 233–234
Immunoglobulin A (IgA), functions of, 242t
Immunoglobulin D (IgD), functions of, 242t
Immunoglobulin E (IgE), functions of, 242t
Immunoglobulin G (IgG), functions of, 242t
Immunoglobulin M (IgM), functions of, 242t
Immunoglobulins, 40, 241f
Immunohistochemistry, 43
Immunological defence system, 233–250
Immunological skin testing, 756
Immunology, 2
Immunometric (sandwich) assays, 459b
Impulse transmission, 20
Inactivated vaccines, 232, 232t
Inadequate fluid intake, 10
Inborn errors of metabolism
 amino acid, 83b
 sugar, 81b
Incidence, 278t, 280

Incomplete penetrance, 196
Incontinentia pigmenti, 180
Independent variable, 278t
Indirect calorimetry, 645
Infant death, cause of, 169
Infantile autism, 184b
Infections, 213–232
 bacterial. see Bacteria
 biological agents of, 213
 burden of, 213, 213f
 disease manifestation, 231
 extrinsic causes of disease, 212t
 fungi. see Fungi
 helminths. see Helminths
 incubation period of, 231
 intrinsic causes of disease, 212t
 local versus general, 231
 pattern of disease, 231–232
 persistence, 231
 prions, 223
 symbiotic relationship between infectious agents and humans, 224–225
Infectious disease surveillance, and information sources, 283–284
Infective carcinogens, 273–274
Inferior mesenteric artery, 502
Inferior sagittal sinus, 355
Inferior vena cava, 503
Infertility, 491
Inflammation
 acute, 250–252
  cellular events, 251
  initiation of inflammatory response, 251–252
  outcome of, 252
  phagocytosis and killing microbes, 251
  systemic effects of, 252
  vascular events of, 250–251
 chronic, 252–255
  complications of, 254–255
  initiation of, 252–253
  manifestation of, 253–254
  outcomes of, 255
 mediators of, 251f
 repair and, 255–257
Inflammatory arthritis, 254b
Inflammatory bowel disease, 249b
Inflammatory response, insulin and, 763
Influenza, 231b
 antigenic variation of, 229
Informed consent, 306b
Inhalation drug administration, 119
 general anaesthetics, 152
Inhaled foreign bodies, lung diseases associated with, 252b
Inhibitory postsynaptic potential (IPSP), 360
Innate immune system, 234–235, 236f
 lung defences against infection, 650–651
Inner ear, 389–390
Inosine monophosphate (IMP), 27
Inositol phosphates, 130
Inositol triphosphate (IP₃) second messenger system, 130f
Inspiration, 627–628
 variations in pulmonary blood flow, 625
Inspiratory reserve volume (IRV), 629
Insulin, 62, 476b
 administration of, 119b
 control of secretion of, 471–472, 472f
 decreased, in fasting state, 762
 effects of, in fed and fasted states, 760b
 inflammatory response and, 763
 regulation of gluconeogenesis, 81
 resistance, 763
 satiety, 773
 synthesis, 471–472

Insulin-like growth factor 1 (IGF-1), 413, 462, 463t
Insulin resistance, 64
Insulin signalling, 48
Integral membrane proteins, 44
Integrated learning, systemic approach, 56
Integrins, 46
Integumentary system, definition, 403
Intention-to-treat analysis, 310–311
Intentional weight loss, 754
Intercalated discs, 510
Intercellular adhesion molecule (ICAM), 46
Intercellular pores, diffusion through, 106
Intercostal spaces, 626
Interdecile range, 278t
Interferons, 47, 250
Interim analyses, 310
Interleukin-2, 238
Interleukin 3 (IL-3), 570t
Intermediate-density lipoprotein (IDL), 531b
 lipoprotein metabolism, 92
Intermediate filaments, 45
Internal mammary artery, 501b
International Classification of Diseases (ICD), 282
Interneurons, network of, 353
Internodal tracts, 513
Interosseous membranes, 418
Interphase, 159–163
Interquartile range, 278t, 292–293
Interspinous ligaments, 409b
Interstitial cells of Cajal (ICCs), 727–728
Interstitial fluid (ISF), 7
Intervention bias, clinical trials, 309b
Interventricular septum, 507–508
Intervertebral foramen, 409b
Intestinal gradient, 745
Intestine, normal flora, 224f
Intestino-intestinal inhibitory reflex, 745
Intracapsular ligaments, 422
Intracellular compartment, 7, 8
Intracellular fluid (ICF), 1, 20
 composition of, 20t
 drug distribution, 109f
Intracellular messengers, producing salivary secretion, 718
Intracellular parasites, 219–220
Intracellular pathogens, 227
Intracellular receptors, 48, 127, 131–132
 drugs that target, 131–132
Intracellular signal cascade, 46
Intracerebral haemorrhage, 350b
Intracranial haemorrhage, 350b
Intraepithelial neoplasia, 261–262
Intrafusal fibres, 367
Intramembranous ossification, 412, 413f
Intramuscular drug administration, 118
Intranasal drug administration, 119
Intrapleural pressure, 628
Intrapulmonary pressure, 628
Intrathecal injection, 118
Intravascular fluid (IVF), 7
Intravascular volume, 7b
Intravenous drug administration, 118
 general anaesthetics, 151
Intravenous fluid, replacement, 769–770, 770t
Introns, 36–37, 166
Inulin clearance, 672, 672f
Inverse agonists, 136
Inversions, 165
Iodine, 464, 768–769
 deficiency, 464
Ion channels, 49, 49f
 as drug targets, 124–125
 modulation by G-proteins, 131
 proteins, 106

Ion channels (Continued)
    proximal convoluted tubule, 667
    use dependency and drug action
        on, 125b
Ion gradient, 20
Ion trapping, 104
    therapeutic application of, 105b
Ionic bonds, 16–17
    protein structure, 34
Ionotropic receptors, 126f, 127
    molecular structure of, 127f
    see also Ligand-gated ion
        channels
Ions, 16
Iris, 381
Iron, 767
    cellular uptake, 579f
    daily requirement, 579t
    deficiency, 578–580
        causes of, 580, 580t
        diagnosis, 579b
        laboratory findings in, 580,
            580f, 580t
    deficiency and overload, 768b
    homeostasis, 579
    loss, 579
    metabolism, 578–579
Iron absorption, 708–709, 709b
    regulation of, 709
Irreversible, competitive
    antagonism, 137
Ischaemia, 553
Ischaemic heart disease (IHD),
    534–539, 534f
    effects of adrenoceptor
        antagonists on, 151
Ischaemic hepatocellular damage,
    560
Ischiofemoral ligament, 429b
Islets of Langerhans, 471, 471f
    cell types in, 471t
Isochromosome, 165
Isocitrate dehydrogenase, 59, 95
Isoelectric focusing (IEF), 589
Isoenzymes, 41
    of cytochrome P-450, 111t
Isoleucine, 88
Isomerases, 41t
Isomerism, 21
Isotopes, 16
Isovolumetric contraction, 523f,
    524
Isovolumetric relaxation, 523f,
    524
Itch receptors, 378

J

J-receptors (juxtacapillary
    receptors), 644
Japanese pufferfish, 199
Jaundice, 739b, 741b
Jejunum, 700
    structural features of, 744t
Jenner, Edward, 231–232
Joint capsule, 420
Joint proprioceptors, 644–645
Joint(s), 403, 418–432
    anatomical movements, 425f
    ball and socket, 425
    blood and nerve supply of, 422
    bony, 418
    cartilaginous, 419
    fibrous, 418–419
    hip, 429f
    knee, 430b, 430f
    movement of, 425b
    saddle, 425, 426b
    shoulder, 428f
    synovial, 419–428
    vertebral column, 407b
Jugular venous pressure (JVP),
    503
Jugular venous pulse, 503
Juxtaglomerular apparatus (JGA),
    682–683
Juxtaglomerular cells, 556

K

Kallman syndrome, 490t
Kappa, 278t
Kappa statistic, 332b, 332t
Karyotyping, 191
Kearns-Sayre syndrome, 182b
Kell blood groups, 607
Keratin, 35
Keto acid decarboxylase, 83b
Ketogenesis
    fine-tuning, 99–100
    liver, 95–96
α-ketoglutarate dehydrogenase, 59
Ketone bodies, 62b
    accumulation, 96b
    prolonged fasting/starvation,
        762–763
    role of, in fuel homeostasis, 96
    utilisation, 96
Ketones, urine testing, 671t
Ketonuria, 82b
Ketose(s), 21, 21f
Khan, Genghis, 173–174
Kidney disease, failure due to, 9
Kidney(s)
    as an endocrine tissue, 476b
    anatomy of, 657–662
    control of acid-base balance,
        686–690
    development of, 662–663
    function tests. see Renal function
        tests
    functions of, 655
    gross structure, 657–659
    nephron, 659
    normal and abnormal ascent, 663f
    permanent, 662–663
    renal pyramids, 658–659
    vasculature, 659–661
Kinase-linked receptors, 131
Kinases, 38
Kinesins, 45
Kinin system, 251
Klinefelter syndrome, 490f, 490t
Koch's postulates, 233
Koilonychia, 448
Krebs' cycle, 58
Kulchitzky cells, 618
Kupffer cells, 740
Kuru, 223b
Kussmaul's respiration, 640, 643b
Kwok's Quease, 88b
Kyphosis, 407b

L

L-type calcium channels, 510
Labile cells, 255
Labour, 488–491
Lachman test, 431b
Lactate, 70
    gluconeogenesis from, 78–79
    glucose in fasted state, 762
    production of, 69–71
Lactate dehydrogenase (LDH),
    70–71
Lactation, 489–491, 491f
Lactic acidosis, 10b, 71b
    type A, 71b
    type B, 71b
Lactobacilli, 225
Lactoferrin, 650
Lactose, 21
Lacunae, cartilage, 410
Lamellae, 410
Lamina propria, 712
Laminar blood flow, 547, 547f
Laminar flow, 631
Laminin, 40
Langerhans cells, 238
Langerhans' cells, epidermis,
    445
Language, 401, 402b
Lanugo, 448
Laplace's equation, 635
Laplace's law, 526

Large intestine, 700
    clinical conditions associated
        with, 747b
    fluid secretion, 746
    motility, 746–747
    musculature of, 746
Laryngotomy, 616b
Larynx, 617, 617f, 626
Lateral (fibular) collateral ligament,
    430b
Lateral horns, 345
Lateral motor pathways, 365, 366f
Leber's hereditary optic neuropathy
    (LHON), 182b
Lecithin, 26
Lecithin-cholesterol acyl
    transferase (LCAT), 93
Left ventricular aneurysm, 538t
Legg-Calves-Perthe disease, 429b
Leishmaniasis, 220
Lemon juice, pH values, 11t
Leptin, 54
    satiety, 772–773
Lesch-Nyhan syndrome, 28
Leucine, 88
Leucine zipper, 167
Leucocytes. see White blood cells
Leukaemias, 592–595
    acute, 592–593, 593t, 594b, 594f
    chronic, 593–595, 593t, 595f,
        595t
Leukotrienes, 244
    in inflammatory response, 252
Levodopa, 145b
Liddle syndrome, 688t
Life and death, patterns of,
    280–291
    births and deaths, 282
    descriptive studies, 280–291
    disease surveillance, 282–283
    health inequalities, 285–286, 285f
    health of populations, measures
        for, 284–285
    interpretation of data, 286–289
    measuring disease occurrence,
        280–281
    measuring disease outcome,
        281–282
    monitoring adverse reaction to
        drugs, 284
    morbidity, 280
    mortality, 280
    standardisation of rates, 289–291
Life expectancy, 284–285
Ligaments, vertebral column, 409b
Ligand-binding domain, 125–126
Ligand-gated ion channels, 127
    drug targets, 124, 125
    neurotransmission, 359, 360f
Ligases, 41t
Likelihood ratio (LR), 278t, 330–331
Limb development, 171–172
Limbic system
    cerebral hemispheres, 339
    emotion, 396–398
    structures, 341, 343f
Lines of Zahn, 540, 540f
Lineweaver-Burk plot, 41f
Link reaction, 61t
Linkage disequilibrium, 194
Linkage mapping, 194f
Linkage studies, 186
Linoleic acid, 24
Linolenic acid, 24
Lipid, 21–23
    essential fatty acids, 88
    fasting lipid profile, 92b
    lowering, 778
    metabolism, 88–100
    storage of, 90
Lipid profile, 776t
Lipid solubility, of drugs, 103
Lipid theory, general anaesthetics,
    152
Lipogenesis, 96–99
    chain elongation, 98
    desaturation, 98
    fine-tuning, 99–100

Lipogenesis (Continued)
    malate shuttle, 98–99, 99f
    rate of, 98
    regulation of fatty acid synthase,
        98
    stage 1, 96–98
    stage 2, 98
Lipolysis, 91
Lipoprotein, 530–531
    different types of, 531t
Lipoprotein lipase (LPL), 90
    deficiency, 89b
Lipoprotein metabolism, disorders
    of, 89b
Lipoproteins, 24, 91–93
    classes and functions, 92–93
    fuel transport and overflow
        pathway, 93
    measurement of, 92b
    metabolism, 93
    receptors, 93
    structure, 91f
Lithium, drug targeting
    phosphatidylinositol
        pathway, 130b
Live attenuated vaccines, 232, 232t
Liver
    anatomy of, 735–736, 735f
    blood supply to, 735
    and carbohydrate metabolism,
        737–738
    diseases of, 740–742
    and drug metabolism, 109,
        739–740
    fate of amino acids in, 87b
    functions of, 737–740
    and hormones, 740
    immunological functions of, 740
    ketogenesis in, 95–96
    and lipid metabolism, 737–738
    metabolic zonation, 736f
    microanatomy of, 735–736, 735f
    phosphofructokinase-2, 68
    and protein metabolism, 737,
        737b
    and red blood cells, 738
    regeneration of, 255
    storage function of, 740
Liver cells, endoplasmic reticulum
    in, 45b
Liver disease, on first pass drug
    metabolism, 117–118
Liver function tests, 742b
Liver steatosis, 54
Local hormones, 452
Local vasoactive hormones, 553
Lock and key mechanism, 40
Locomotion, 368, 443–444
Locus heterogeneity, 195
Logarithm of the odds (LOD)
    scores, 194–196
Logistic regression, 318
London Medical Gazette, 277–279
Long-term potentiation, 400–401
Loop diuretics, 115, 685, 686b
Loop of Henle, 659, 681
    ammonium synthesis, 688
    and bicarbonate ions, 687
    diuretics acting on, 115
    transport properties of, 679–680
Lordosis, 407b
Loss-of-function mutations, in RB1
    gene, 188
Loss of heterozygosity (LOH),
    188–189, 189f
Low-density lipoprotein (LDL)
    receptors, defect in, 47b
Low-density lipoproteins (LDLs),
    51b, 531, 531t
    atherogenesis, 776
    in diabetes mellitus, 82b
    disorders of, 89b
    lipoprotein metabolism, 92
Lower motor neuron syndrome,
    367b
Lower reference nutrient intake
    (LRNI), 751
Lumbar region, left and right, 711

Lung bud, 651
Lung-irritant receptors, 644
Lung ventilation, acid-base balance related to
  disturbance of, 12b
Lung(s)
  blood volume in, 624
  closing capacity and posture, 636
  compliance, 634, 635f
  defences against infection, 650–651
  development of
    abnormalities of, 652b
    alveolar phase, 652
    canalicular phase, 651
    and changes in newborn, 651–653
    early, 651, 652f
    inadequate, 652b
    pseudoglandular phase, 651
    saccular phase, 651–652
  diffusion capacity of, 636–637
  gross anatomy of, 617–623, 617f
  inflation and deflation of, 634–635
  normal flora, 224f
  perfusion, 640–642
  and pleural cavity, 627
  pressure-volume relationship, 634, 634f
  receptors, 644
  respiratory distress syndrome of the newborn, 653
  surface marking of, 627f
  surface tension, 635
  surfactant, 635
  ventilation, 640–642
  volume and capacities, 629–630, 629f
Lunula, 448
Lupus anticoagulant, 604
Luteinising hormone (LH), 460
Lyases, 41t
Lymph, 20
Lymph nodes, 257–258, 591b
  structure of, 257–258, 258f
Lymphatic drainage, reduced, 545
Lymphocytes, 569
  in asthma, 248b
  count, 756
Lymphoid organs, 257–258
Lymphoid system, 590–591
Lymphoid tissues, 591b
  primary, 591
  secondary, 591
Lymphomas, 595
  Hodgkin disease, 595
  non-Hodgkin, 595
Lyon hypothesis. see Lyonisation
Lyonisation, 179
Lysis, 18
Lysosomal storage disease, 26
Lysosomes, 45–46, 234
Lytic sequence, 243f, 244

M

M1/motor strip, 365
Macromolecules, 21t, 665
Macrophage-activating factors (MAFs), 245
Macrophages, 237, 245–246, 569
  alveolar, 621
  cilia and, 619
  functioning, 246
  in granulation tissue, 254
  in granulomas, 253
  in inflammatory response, 252, 651
  pulmonary, 650
  role in inflammation, 245–246
  struggling, 246
Macrovascular disease, in diabetes mellitus, 82b
'Mad cow disease,' 223b
Magnesium, 768

Magnetic resonance imaging (MRI), 404
  brain, 344f
  spinal cord, 344f
Major histocompatibility complex (MHC), 236
Malaria, 221b
Malarial parasites, 220, 221f
Malate shuttle, 98–99, 99f
Male reproductive endocrinology, 468–469
Male reproductive tract, 478, 478f
Malformation, definition of, 205
Malignant hypertension, 564–565
Malignant hyperthermia, 440b
Malignant melanoma, 446b
Malignant neoplasms
  behaviour of, 268
  characteristics of, 265–268, 267t
  differentiation and grade of, 267–268, 267f
  local invasion, 268, 268b
  macroscopic features and growth pattern of, 266, 266f, 267f
  metastasis of, 268, 268f
  screening for, 272–273
Malnutrition, 779–780
  consequences of, 779b
  diagnosis of, 779–780
  and disease states, 779
  screening tools, 756
Malnutrition Universal Screening Tool (MUST), 756
Malonyl-CoA, 98
Maltose, 21
Mammals as model organisms, 202–203
Mannitol, 116
  use during surgery, 685b
Mannose, 21
Mannose-binding lectins (MBL), 234
Maple syrup urine disease, 83b
March haemoglobinuria, 585
Marfan syndrome, 170
Mass screening, 326, 326b
  reasons for, 326t
Mast cells, 235, 244–245
  activation of, 244
  in asthma, 248b, 634
  in inflammatory response, 251
  substances released by, 244–245
Mastication, 714
Matching, 278t, 298–299
Matrix, mitochondria, 45
Maturity-onset diabetes of the young (MODY), 66b
Maximal respiratory pressures, 628–629
Mean, 278t, 292
Mean cell volume (MCV), 578
Measles
  immunisation, 324t
  mumps and rubella (MMR) vaccine, 324, 325t
Mechanical nociceptors, 378
Mechanoreceptors, 555
  non-hairy skin, 376t
  skin, 376
Medial calcific sclerosis, 533
Medial motor pathways, 365–367, 366f, 366t
Medial (tibial) collateral ligament, 430b
Median, 278t, 291f, 292
Median effective dose (ED_{50}), 135
Median lethal dose (LD_{50}), 135
Median toxic dose (TD_{50}), 135
Mediastinum, 591b
Medical therapy, treatment of angina, 536b
Medulla, 344
  in lymph nodes, 257
  respiratory centre, 642
Medullary cavity, 408
Megaloblastic anaemia, 580–581

Meiosis, 158, 161–163
  anaphase I, 162
  anaphase II, 162
  interphase I, 161
  metaphase I, 162, 162f
  metaphase II, 162
  in neoplasia, 259
  prophase I, 161–162
    diplonema, 162
    leptonema, 161
    pachynema, 162
    zygonema, 161–162
  prophase II, 162
  telophase I, 162, 163f
  telophase II, 162
Meissner's plexus, 713
Melanocytes, 445, 446b
Membrane associated transporter protein (MATP), 174
Membrane attack complex (MAC), 241
Membrane-bound guanylate cyclase, 128
Membrane transport, 48–51
Memory, 399–401
Menarche, 486t
Mendel, Gregor, 2
Mendelian disorders, 177–183
Ménière disease, 387b
Meninges, 349–351, 350f
  arachnoid mater, 350
  dura mater, 349–351
  pia mater, 351
Meningitis, 228b
Menisci, 422
  knee joint, 430b
Menke syndrome, 768b
Menopause, 491
Menstrual cycles, 482–483
  first phase of, 482, 483f
  luteal phase/secretory phase of, 483
  ovulation, 483
  second phase of, 483, 484f
Merkel's cells, 445
Merozoites, 220
Mesenchymal neoplasms, 263
  nomenclature of, 265t
Mesoderm, 51
Mesolimbic system, drug act on, 398b
Mesonephros, 662
Mesosome, bacteria, 214
Messenger RNA (mRNA), 31
  production of, 167f
Meta-analysis, 319–321, 320f
Metabolic acidosis, 13b, 640, 689, 690b
  ammonium ion in, 85b
Metabolic alkalosis, 13b, 640
Metabolic defects, in diabetes mellitus, 82b
Metabolic energy generation, 19
Metabolic flux, 182–183
Metabolic fuels, 19b
Metabolic hyperaemia, 499–500
Metabolic ketoacidosis, 82b
Metabolic manipulation, 207
Metabolic pathways, 58b
Metabolism
  action of hormones, 62
  definition, 1
  inborn errors of, 182–183, 183f
  regulation of fuel, 61–62
  regulation of gene expression and transcription, 62
  reversible activation and deactivation by covalent modification, 62
Metabolites
  conversion of inactive pro-drug to active, 113
  enzyme inhibition by, 113
  excretion, 113–116
Metabolome, 184
Metabotropic receptors. see G protein-coupled receptors (GPCRs)
Metachromatic leucodystrophy, 209

Metanephros, 662
Metaphyseal arteries, 411
Metaphyses, 406
Metaplasia, 260–262
  connective tissue, 260–261
  epithelial, 260
  glandular, 261b, 261f
  myeloid, 260–261
  squamous, 261b
Metastasis, 268, 268f
  clonal evolution of, 268
  mechanism of invasion and, 268b
  patterns and sites of, 268
Metencephalon, 338
Methaemoglobin, 576b
Methanol poisoning, treatment of, 42
Methotrexate, 28
α-Methyldopa, as false substrates, 124b
Methylxanthines, 129
Michaelis-Menten curves, 41f
Micro RNAs (miRNA), 31
Microangiopathic haemolytic anaemia (MAHA), 585
Microbes, 200
Microcirculation, 541–545, 541f
  regulation of flow in, 552–553
Microfilaments, 44
Microhomology-mediated end joining (MMEJ), 169
Micronutrients, 765–770
Microsatellites, 186, 196
  instability, in cancer cells, 190f
Microsomal oxidation reactions, 110
Microtubule-associated proteins, 45
Microtubules, 44
Microvascular disease, in diabetes mellitus, 82b
Microvilli, 44, 51
Micturition, control of, 692
Micturition reflex, 692
Mid-diastolic murmur, 498b
Mid upper arm circumference (MUAC), 755
Midbrain, 343
Middle cerebral arteries, 353–354
Middle ear, 389, 390f
Migraine, 150
Migrating motor complexes (MMCs), 728
Migration inhibition factor (MIF), 245
Milk, pH values, 11t
Mineralocorticoids, 25t
Minerals, diet, 767–769
Minimisation, 278t
Minisatellites, 196
Minor Grove Binder (MGB), 197
Mismatch repair (MMR), 169
Mitochondria, 45
  fatty acid oxidation, 93–94
Mitochondrial disorders, 182
Mitochondrial DNA, 30–31, 157
  mutation, 182b
Mitochondrial HMG-CoA synthase, 95b
Mitochondrial ketogenic pathway, 95f
Mitochondrial monoamine oxidase (MAO), 111
Mitochondrial myopathy, encephalopathy, lactic acidosis with stroke-like episodes (MELAS), 182b
Mitochondrion, energy transfer in, 60f
Mitosis, 160–161, 160f
  anaphase, 160–161
  metaphase, 160
  in neoplasia, 259
  prophase, 160
Mitral regurgitation, 496b, 498b
Mitral stenosis, 496b, 498b
Mitral valve, 494, 497f
Mixed function oxidase (MFO) system, 110

Mode, 278t, 291f, 292
Model organisms, 202–204
Molecular chaperones, 34
Molecular clock hypothesis, 202
Molecular interactions, principles of, 16–19
Molecular mimicry, 254b
Molecular Modeling DataBase (MMBD), 202
Molecular phylogenetics, 201–202, 203f
Mönckeberg's sclerosis, 533
Monoamine oxidase inhibitors (MAOIs), 148b
Monoamine oxidase (MAO), catecholamines metabolism, 147–148
Monoamine oxidase (MAO) inhibitors, 564
Monoamines, 362–363
see also Specific monoamine
Monocarboxylate transport proteins (MCT1-4), 70–71
Monocyte colony-stimulating factor (M-CSF), 570t
Monocytes, 245–246, 569
Monogenic disease, genetic linkage and, 194
Monogenic disorders, 156
Monosaccharides, 21, 22f
Monosodium glutamate (MSG), 88b
Monosynaptic reflexes, 367
Monozygotic twins, 185
Morbidity, 280, 285
Mortality, 280
and life expectancy, 284–285
Mosaicism, 182
Motilin, source, target organ, and action of, 713t
Motility, 699–700
Motivation, 398–399
Motor control and pathways, 364–374
Motor cortex, 365
primary, 365
somatotopic mapping, 365f
Motor neurons, 353, 366–367
Motor reflexes, 367–368
Motor units, 434–435
Mountain sickness, 647
Mouth, 714
normal flora of, 224f
Movements, locomotion, 443–444
mRNA, 37t
bacterial, 214
Mucins, 650
Mucociliary escalator, 619, 619f
Mucopolysaccharides, 23
Müllerian-inhibitory factor, 170
Multi-hit carcinogenesis, 187, 188f
Multi-polar neuron, 55f
Multifactorial diseases
characteristics of, 184–186
genetic epidemiology of, 185
Multiphasic screening, 326
Multiple dosing, 122
Multiple myeloma, 596, 596t
Multiple sclerosis, 358b
Multipotent stem cells, 51
Multivariate analysis, 318–319
Murmurs, 495–496, 497f
Muscarinic receptors, 144
agonists, 144
antagonists, 144
Muscle contraction
excitation-contraction coupling, 438–440
calcium removal and muscle relaxation, 440
cross-bridge formation, 440
intracellular calcium release, 438–440
muscle length and tension, 440
isotonic versus isometric, 435
Muscle fibre, 435–438
contractile proteins, 436–438
sliding filament model of muscle contraction, 438, 438f

Muscle fibre (Continued)
thick filaments, 437–438
thin filaments, 437
types of, 441
Muscle stretch receptors, 644
Muscle(s), 40, 54–55, 403–449
fatigue, 441
glycogenolysis in, 77
growth and repair, 442
nomenclature, 442–443
phosphofructokinase-2, 68
spindles, 367–368
strength, 756
tone, 368, 435
types of, 54f, 55t
Muscularis mucosae, 712
Musculoskeletal system, 403
Mutagenic dietary constituents, 775t
Mutation, 155, 172
Mutualism, 224
Myasthenia gravis, 248
Mycelia, 219
Mycoplasma, 215
Myelencephalon, 338
Myelin membrane, 44
Myelodysplastic syndromes (MDS), 592
Myelofibrosis, 592
Myeloma, multiple, 596, 596t
Myeloproliferative disease, 591–592
Myenteric plexus, 713
Myocardial contractility, 525–526
Myocardial infarction, 534–537
complications of, 537–539
Myocardial revascularisation, 536b
Myoclonic epilepsy with ragged red fibres (MERRF), 182b
Myocytes, 54
Myofibrils, 55
Myofilaments, 55
Myoglobin, 573, 638–639
saturation curve, 573f
Myosin, 40
Myosin light-chain kinase (MLCK), 548
Myosin light chain phosphatase (MLCP), 548

N

N-acetylglutamate, 86
N-methyl-D-aspartate (NMDA) receptors, 362
Na⁺/ K⁺-ATPase, 49, 49b, 49f
Nail clubbing, 448
Nail matrix, 448
Nail-patella syndrome (NPS), 195, 195f
Nail pitting, 448
Nail plate, 448
Nails, 448
Nasal cavity, 616–617
Natriuretic peptides, 681b
Nausea, 730
Necrotic cell death, 259
Negative chronotropic effect, 102
Negative feedback, 4–6, 5f
loop, 4f
Negative feedback regulation, hormone secretion, 455
Negative predictive value (NPV), 329
Nematodes, replication of, 223
Neocortex, 340, 342f
layers, 342t
Neonatal alloimmune thrombocytopenic purpura (NAITP), 608b
Neonatal circulation, 509f, 510
Neonatal tolerance, 249
Neoplasia, 259–275
blood, 590
cell cycle, 259
defects of development, 262–263
epidemiology of, 263, 264f

Neoplasia (Continued)
growth, differentiation and development, 259–263
pathology of, 263–268
Neoplasms
benign, characteristics of, 265–268
diagnosis of, 270–271, 271f
effects on host, 269
immunological effects, 269
local effects, 269
metabolic effects, 269
embryonal, 265t
epithelial, 263
germ cell, 265
haemopoietic, 263–265
histologic features, 266–267
malignant, characteristics of, 265–268
mesenchymal, 263, 265t
nervous system, 265, 265t
nomenclature and classification of, 263–265
paraneoplastic syndromes, 269–270
prognosis of, 272
staging of, 271–272
variation in cell growth and differentiation, 259
Neoplastic cells, biology of, 273
Neostigmine, 123b
Nephric ducts, 662
Nephron, 659
development of, 663f
diagrammatic representation of major sites in, 664f
distal, 688
production, transport and excretion of ammonia by, 689f
renal tubule, 659
collecting ducts (CD), 659
distal convoluted tubule, 659
loop of Henle, 659
proximal convoluted tubule (PCT), 659
renal corpuscle, 659
structure of, 660f
Nephrotic syndrome, and protein loss, 693b
Nephrotoxic agents, 694
Nephrotoxicity, 670
Nerve fibre classification, 349
Nerve impulses, 20, 356
Nerves, peripheral. see Peripheral nerves; Peripheral nervous system
Nervous system, 337–402
arterial blood supply, 353–355
blood-brain barrier, 355–356
blood supply, and brain metabolism, 353–356
brain death, 402
cells of, 352–353
central. see Central nervous system (CNS)
central autonomic networks, 392–395
cognition. see Cognition
consciousness, 395
embryology, 337–339
emotion, 396–398
gross anatomy, 339–351
higher cortical functions, 399–401
motivation and goal-directed behaviours, 398–399
motor control and pathways, 364–374
neoplasms, 265, 265t
neural signals. see Neural signals
peripheral. see Peripheral nervous system
sensory systems. see Sensory systems
sleep and wakefulness, 395–396
special senses, 381–392
ventricular system, 351–352
Nervous tissue, 55–56

Neural arch, 409b
Neural crest cells, 171
Neural signals, 356–364
Neural stem cells, 51b
Neural tube defect (NTD), 205b
Neuraxis, 341–342
Neuroblasts, 55–56
Neuroendocrinology, 455–463
Neurofibromatosis type II, 177
Neurogenic inflammation, 378b
Neurogenic shock, 559
Neurokinin A, source, target organ, and action of, 713t
Neurolemma, 348–349
Neurological complications, renal failure, 656b
Neuromuscular blockade, 434
Neuromuscular junction, 434f
Neuronal ceroid lipofuscinosis (Batten disease), 208
Neuronal development, 171
Neurons, 55
chemistry, 353
connectivity, 353
morphology, 352–353
size, 352–353
types of, 352f
Neuropeptides, 359
gastrointestinal, 713t
Neurotensin, source, target organ, and action of, 713t
Neurotransmission, 359–364
Neurotransmitter receptors, 359–360
Neurotransmitters, 47, 359–364, 361t
amino acids as, 88
autonomic nervous system, 138
classical, 359
diffusion, 360
effect of general anaesthetics on release of, 152
enzymatic destruction, 360
inactivation, 360
parasympathetic system, 141–144
peptide (neuropeptides), 359
release, 359
reuptake, 360
sympathetic nervous system, 144–151
Neurulation, 338–339, 338f
Neutrons, 16
Neutrophils, 245, 568–569
inflammatory responses in, 651
role in inflammation, 245
Next generation sequencing (NGS), 198, 199t
NF-kB essential modulator (NEMO), 180
N-glycosylation, 23
Niacin. see Vitamin B₃
Nicotinamide adenine dinucleotide (NAD), 18, 58t
Nicotinamide adenine dinucleotide phosphate (NADP), 18, 58t
Nicotinamide adenine dinucleotide phosphate (NADPH), reduced, 67
Nicotine, nicotinic agonists, 143–144
Nicotinic receptors (nAChRs), 127
agonists, 143–144
antagonists, 144
Nitric oxide
in inflammatory response, 252
second messenger system, 129, 129f
Nitric oxide synthase (NOS), 553
Nitrite, urine testing, 671t
Nitrogen
in amino acid metabolism, 84–87
balance, 756–764, 759t
dietary, 759
excretion, 759–760
minimum requirement, 759
obligatory loss, 759, 759f
Nitrogen balance, 87
Nitrogen narcosis, 647

Nitrous oxide (N₂O), 152
Nociceptors, 378
Nodal bradycardia, 518, 519f
Non-adrenergic autonomic nervous system mediated vasodilatation, 551
Non-cardiogenic pulmonary oedema, 560
Non-coding DNA, 166
Non-competitive antagonism, 136b, 137
Non-competitive inhibition, in enzymes, 42
Non-dihydropyridine derivatives, 512b
Non-essential amino acids, 759
Non-haematopoietic stem cell transplantation, 208
Non-Hodgkin lymphoma (NHL), 595
Non-homologous end-joining (NHEJ), 169
Non-immune haemolytic anaemias, 585–586
Non-immunological defence system, 233
Non-microsomal oxidative reactions, 110–111
Non-parametric statistical tests, 313
Non-polar molecular interactions, 17
Non-ST elevation acute coronary syndromes (NSTEACS), treatment of, 537b
Non-ST elevation myocardial infarction, 535–537
Non-steroidal anti-inflammatory drugs (NSAIDs), 25
  administration of, 119b
Non-thrombotic emboli, 541
Norepinephrine (noradrenaline), 88
  conversion to epinephrine (adrenaline), 146
  drugs acting on the synthetic sequence of, 145b
  extraneuronal uptake, 147
  neuronal uptake, 147
  neurotransmission, 363
  release, 146–147, 146f
  storage, 146
  synthesis, 145–146, 145f
  termination of action of neuronally released, 147, 147f
Noradrenergic and adrenergic pathways, 363t
Norepinephrine. see Noradrenaline
Normal flora, 224–225, 224f
Northern blotting, 197
Nose, normal flora, 224f
Notification of infectious diseases, 283
NREM sleep (non-rapid eye movement), 396
Nuclear bag fibres, 367
Nuclear chain fibres, 367
Nuclear envelope, 45
Nuclear factor kB, 172b
Nuclear localisation sequences, 38
Nuclear magnetic resonance, 202
Nuclear receptors, 131–132
  drugs that target, 131–132
Nucleic acid(s), 28–31
  primary structure of, 29
  strand of nucleotides in, 29f
Nucleoid, bacteria, 214
Nucleoli, 45
Nucleophiles, 18
Nucleophilic attack, 18
Nucleoplasm, 45
Nucleoside phosphates, 27t
Nucleosides, 26–27
Nucleosomes, 30, 158f
Nucleotide excision repair (NER), 169
Nucleotides, 26–27
  recycling of, 28
  structure of, 27f
  synthesis and degradation of, 27–28

Nucleus, 45
Nucleus ambiguous, 555
Nucleus of the solitary tract (NST), 347
Nucleus tractus solitarius (nTS), 550, 550f
Null hypothesis (H₀), 278t, 294
Null lymphocytes, 240
Number needed to treat (NNT), 311
Nutrients, 62
  in food labelling, 751
  ingestion of, 19
Nutrition, 3
  artificial, 778–779
  and cancer treatment, 775
  claims, 751
  enteral, 778
    complications of, 778
  parenteral, 778–779, 778b, 779b
Nutritional requirements, 751–753
  in infancy, 753
  in lactation, 753
  preconception, 752
  during pregnancy, 752, 753b
  variations in, 752–753
Nutritional status, 754–764
  of children, 755
  clinical assessment of, 754–755
  dietary assessment, detailed, 754
  energy and nitrogen balance, 756–764
  measures of body composition: adults, 755–756
  other measurements of, 756

O

Obesity, 473, 780–784
  aetiology of, 781–782, 781f
  age standardized prevalence of, 781f
  cancer risk, 775
  classification according to body fat distribution, 780f
  dietary management of, 782
  environmental factors and exercise, 781–782
  increased risk of disease associated with, 780b
  increasing physical activity, 784
  pharmacological management of, 783
  prevention of, 784
  psychogenic factors of, 781
  psychological model for dietary modification, 782–783, 782f
  surgical management for, 783–784, 783f
  treatment of, 782–784
Observational studies, 296–297, 296b
  case-control studies, 296b, 297–302, 299b, 299t
  cohort studies, 296b, 302–304, 304f
  cross-sectional studies, 296b, 297, 298t
  role of genetics in, 304–305
Obstructive pulmonary disease, 615
Obstructive sleep apnoea, 643b
Occupation theory, 135–136
Occupational lung diseases, 615b
OCTN2 gene, 183b
Oculocutaneous albinism, 178
Oculomotor disorders, 375b
Oculomotor (III) nerve, 346, 346t
Oculomucocutaneous syndrome, 151
Odds ratio, 300b
Oedema, 10, 40b, 545
  clinical manifestations of fluid imbalance, 10b
  in heart failure, 546b
Oesophagus, 700, 718–719
  disorders of, 720b

Oestrogens, 25t
  affecting bone mass, 416
  satiety, 773
Off-centre cells, 376, 385
O-glycosylation, 23
Oil spots, 448
Okazaki fragments, 31
Olfactory (I) nerve, 346, 346t
Oligohydramnios, 662–663
Olsalazine, 113b
Omeprazole, acting on protein transporters, 105b
On-centre cells, 376, 385
On-centre ganglion cell, 385f
Oncholysis, 448
Oncogenes, 189–190
  blood disease, 590
  mutations, 590
  and tumour suppressor genes, 590
  viral activation, 590
Oncogenesis, blood cell, 589–596
Oncotic pressure, 544
One-tailed test, 278t, 294, 316
Open neural tube defects, 339b
Opening snap, 498b
Opioid receptors, 364, 364t
Opioids, neurotransmission, 364
Optic disc, 383
Optic (II) nerve, 346, 346t
Opticokinetic reflexes, 374
Oral drug administration, 116
Oral rehydration therapy, 50b
Oral tolerance, 249
Orexigenic pathway, 394
Organ development, anomalies of, 262
Organ formation, 171
Organ of Corti, 391f
Organic anion transport, 668–669
  representative compounds secreted by, 669t
Organic biomolecules, 20–21
Organic cation transport, 670
Organic compounds, 17–18
Organic molecules, spatial arrangement of, 18
Organogenesis, 171–172
Organophosphates, 143
Organs and tissues, 51–56
Orlistat, 783
Ornithine, urea cycle, 86
Orthologous genes, 173
Orthologues, 200
Orthopnea, 643b
Orthostasis, 556
Orthostatic hypotension, 556
Osmolality, 670
Osmolarity, 8, 656b
Osmoreceptors, 556
Osmotic diuresis, 684
Osmotic diuretics, 116
Osmotic fragility test, 586f
Osmotic movement, of water, 8f
Osmotic pressure, 8
Ossification, 406
  endochondral, 411–412
  intramembranous, 412, 413f
  primary, 412
  secondary, 412
Osteitis, lower leg pain, 408b
Osteitis deformans, 415b
Osteoarthritis, 420b
Osteoblasts, 54
Osteoclasts, 54
Osteocytes, 54, 405
Osteogenesis imperfecta, 38, 406b
  penetrance and phenotypic expression, 176b
Osteogenic progenitor cells, 405
Osteoid, 54
Osteomalacia, 416b, 767b
Osteomyelitis, chronic, 252
Osteoporosis, 54b, 416b
Outcome, 278t
  measuring, 281–282
Outliers, 292

Ovarian cycles, 482–483
Ovary, hormonal control of, 481–483, 482f
Oxaloacetate (OAA), 94
Oxidases, 46
Oxidation, 18, 773b
  activation and transport into mitochondria, 93–94
  β-oxidation, 94–95
  carnitine shuttle, 94
  drug metabolism, 110–111
  fine-tuning, 99–100
  ketogenesis in liver, 95–96
Oxidation-reduction (redox) reactions, 18
Oxidative decarboxylation, 71
Oxidative glucose metabolism, 71–72
Oxidative phosphorylation, 58, 60
  coupling of electron transport chain and, 60–61
Oxidative stress, 774, 774b
Oxidoreductases, 41t
Oxygen
  carriage by the blood, 637–639
  consumption, 645–646, 646t
  high levels (toxicity), 648
  release. see Oxygen release therapy, carbon dioxide and, 643b
Oxygen dissociation curve, 573–574, 574f, 638, 638f
Oxygen release
  role of acid in, 574
  role of 2,3-DPG (diphosphoglycerate), 574
Oxyntic gland, 722f
Oxyntomodulin, 772

P

Pacemaker cells, 512–513
Pacemaker potential, 512–513, 513f
Packed cell volume (PCV), 7, 567, 568b
Paediatric weight growth charts, 292, 294f
Paget disease, 415b
Pain
  lower leg, 408b
  modulation mechanisms, 380b
  neck, 407b
  pathways, 378–379, 378f
  phantom, 381
  referred, 381, 381f
  regulation, 379–381
  sensations, 378–381
Palmitate, 98
Palmitic acid, 23, 96
Palmitoyl-CoA, 98
Pancreas, 471–474
  control of pancreatic juice secretion, 734
  exocrine, 730–734, 732f
Pancreatic β cell, 66b
Pancreatic enzymes, 730–733, 732b, 732t
Pancreatic islets, 471
Pancreatic juice
  formation, 733f
  secretion, 734
    cephalic phase, 734
    gastric phase, 734
    inhibition of, 734
    intestinal phase, 734
Pancreatic polypeptide, source, target organ, and action of, 713t
Pancreatic proteases, 704t
Pancreatic secretions, 723f
Pancreatitis, 733b
Pandemics, 231
Pangenesis, theory of, 155
Pan-systolic murmur, 498b
Panting, 643b

Pantothenic acid, 766
Papillomas, 263
Para-amino hippuric acid (PAH), 669
Paracetamol, overdose, hepatic failure in, 112b
Paracrine effect, 452, 452f
Paracrine signalling molecules, 169
Paradoxical embolism, 539
Paralogous genes, 173
Paralogues, 201
Paralytic poliomyelitis, 650
Parametric statistical tests, 313
Paraneoplastic endocrinopathies, 270, 270t
Paraneoplastic syndromes, 269–270, 270t
Parasagittal meningioma, 365b
Parasitism, 224
Parasympathetic nervous system
  anatomy of, 140, 141f
  neurotransmitters and receptors, 141–144, 142f
  overview of, 139
  salivary secretion, 718
Parasympathetic supply, 513–514
Parathyroid hormone (PTH), 415, 455
  control of blood calcium and phosphate concentrations and, 475
Paravertebral ganglia, 140
Parenteral drug administration, 118
Parenteral nutrition, 778–779
Parietal cells, morphological changes in, 724–725, 725f
Parkinson disease, treatment, 374b
Parotid glands, 714
Paroxysmal nocturnal dyspnoea, 643b
Paroxysmal nocturnal haemoglobinuria (PNH), 585
Partial agonist drugs, occupation theory, 136
Partial pressure of gases
  in air, 637, 637t
  in alveoli and blood, 637
Parturition. see Labour
Passive diffusion, 48f, 103–104
Patched (PTC), 170
Patent ductus arteriosus (PDA), 510b
Patent foramen ovale (PFO), 507b
Pathogen associated molecular patterns (PAMPs), 233–234
Pathogen recognition receptor (PRR), 234
Pathogen-reduced plasma (PRP), 611
Pathogens, 225–231
  environmental exploitation, 227
  host entry, 225–227, 225f
  progress of infections, 227–231
    adhesion, 227
    attacking the host, 229
    exit, 229–230
    host organ dissemination, 227–228
    invasion, 227
    survival within the host, 228–229
    transmission, 230–231, 230f
Pathology, 2
Patterning, 170–171, 171f
  anterior/posterior axis formation, 170
  dorsal/ventral axis development, 170–171
  left/right axis formation, 170
Peak expiratory flow rate (PEFR), 631, 632f, 633b
Pelvic floor, maintenance of continence, 691
Penicillin, 123b
Penicillin G, administration of, 119b

Pennate muscle, 443
Pentose phosphate pathway, 67
Pentoses, 21
Pepsinogen, secretion, 724
Peptic ulceration, 727, 727b, 727f
Peptide bond, 34, 34f
Peptide deformylase, 207b
Peptide YY, 772
  source, target organ, and action of, 713t
Peptides, 33
  chemical nature of hormones, 452t
  eating, 772
  hormones, 452–455
  neurotransmission, 364
Percentage weight loss, 754
Percentile, 278t
Percutaneous coronary intervention (PCI), 536b
Perfusion
  adaptations to anaemia, 577
  uneven, 641, 641f
Periaqueductal grey (PAG) matter, 343
Pericarditis, 494b, 538t
Pericardium, 493–494
Perichondrium ossification, 411
Perimysium, 441
Perineum, normal flora, 224f
Perineurium, 348–349
Periodic breathing, 643b
Periodontal ligament, 419
Periosteal arteries, 411
Periosteal bone collar, 411–412
Periosteum, 408
Peripheral arterial pulses, 502–503, 502f
Peripheral chemoreceptors, 643–644
Peripheral membrane proteins, 44
Peripheral nerves, 348
  structure, 348–349, 350f
Peripheral nervous system (PNS), 55, 345–349
  somatic nervous system. see Somatic nervous system
Peristalsis, 745
Peritubular capillaries, 661, 668
Permanent cells, 255
Permeability and conductance, 357b
Permeases, 48–49
Peroxisome proliferator-activated receptors, 80, 80b
Peroxisomes, 46
Personal genomics, 198
Perthe disease, 419b, 429b
Petechial haemorrhages, skin with, 602f
Pethidine, drug hydrolysis, 112b
Peutz-Jeghers' polyp, 262f
P-glycoproteins (PGPs), 106
pH, 68–69
  effects on physiological processes, 11
  phosphofructokinase-1, 68
  physiological range of, 11
  renal control of, 13–14
  respiratory control of, 12
  urine testing, 671t
  values, for some fluids, 11t
Phaeochromocytoma, 145b, 563–564
Phagocytes, 235
Phagocytosis, 50, 245
  and killing of microbes, 251
Phagosomes, 50
Pharmacodynamics, 102, 123–137
  definition, 1
  drug targets, 123–132
  safety and effectiveness of drugs, 132–137
Pharmacodynamic tolerance, 137
Pharmacogenomics, 156, 205–207
Pharmacokinetic antagonism, 136b, 137

Pharmacokinetics, 103–122
  absorption, 103–106, 103f
  definition, 1
  mathematics of, 119–122
  routes of administration, 116–119
Pharmacology, 1–2, 101–153
Pharynx, 617, 718–719
Phenacetin, nephrotoxicity, 695t
Phenindione, nephrotoxicity, 695t
Phenobarbital, 103b
Phenocopies, 196
Phenotypes, 176
Phenotypic expression, 176b
Phenylalanine, 183
Phenylalanine hydroxylase, 83b
Phenylalkylamines, 512b
Phenylketonuria (PKU), 33, 83b
Philadelphia chromosome, 163, 590, 590f
Phosphatases, 38
Phosphate buffering, 688
Phosphate(s), 768
  buffer system, 12
  intake in renal disease, 777
Phosphatidic acid, 26
Phosphatidylserine, structure of, 26f
Phosphodiesterase inhibition, 129
Phosphoenolpyruvate carboxykinase (PEPCK), 78
Phosphofructokinase-1 (PFK-1), 67
  energy status of cell, 67
  regulation of, 68–69
Phosphoglucose isomerase, 67
Phospholipase A2, 128, 130
Phospholipase C, 128, 130
Phospholipids, 26, 88
5-Phosphoribosyl pyrophosphate (PRPP), 27
Phosphorylase-a, 77
Phosphorylase-b, 76
Phosphorylase kinase, regulation of, 77
Phosphorylation, 38, 57
Phosphorylation-dephosphorylation sequence, 42
Photoabsorption, in imaging, 404
Photoreceptors, 383–385
  absorption curves, 384f
  dysfunction, 384b
Phototransduction, 383–384
pH partitioning of drug molecules, 104, 105f
Physical activity, total energy expenditure and, 757–758
Physical activity level (PAL), 757, 758f
Physical activity ratio (PAR), 758, 758f
Physical barriers, 233
Physical digestion, 701, 701b
Physical maps, 191
Physiological antagonism, 136b, 137
Physiological dead space, 629–630
  measurement of, 630b
Pia mater, 351
Pili, bacteria, 215
'Pinch test,' 755
Pinocytosis, 50, 543
Pituitary adenylate cyclase-activating peptide (PACAP), source, target organ, and action of, 713t
Pituitary gland
  functional anatomy of, 458, 459f
  names for, 460b
  neural and vascular connections between hypothalamus and, 460f
Pivot joints, 424
Place coding, 392
Placebo effect, 309b, 380–381
Placenta, 486b
  hormone production by, 487
  pathogen entry via, 227
  steroid biosynthesis by, 488f
  structure of early, 487f

Planar joint, 422–423
Plaque rupture, 531–532
Plasma, 7, 567
  frozen, 611
  pathogen-reduced, 611
  selected transport proteins in, 26t
Plasma calcium, 475f
  levels, on cardiac excitation, 512b
Plasma cell
  disorders, 596
  features, 596f
Plasma cholesterol, high levels of, 47b
Plasma glucose, regulation of, 471, 471f
Plasma membrane, 1
  of bacteria, 214
Plasma oncotic pressure, decreased, 545, 545f
Plasma potassium levels, on cardiac excitation, 512b
Plasma proteins, 756
Plasma/serum, tests performed on, 54b
Plasmids, bacteria, 214
Plasmodium falciparum, 221–222
Plasmodium falciparum erythrocyte membrane protein 1, 222
Plasmodium falciparum malaria, 174f
Plasmodium malariae, 222
Plasmodium ovale, 222
Plasmodium vivax, 221
Platelet-activating factor (PAF), in inflammatory response, 252
Platelets, 246, 569–570
  antigens, 608
  impaired production, 602
  increased destruction, 602–603
  inherited disorders, 602
  role in haemostasis, 597–598, 597f, 598f
  tissue repair and, 255–256
  transfusion, 610
Pleura, 621
Pleural effusion, 621, 621b
  diagnosis of, 326b
Pleural rub, 618b
Pleurisy, 615b, 621
Pneumocytes
  type I, 621
  type II, 621
Pneumonia, 615b
Pneumotaxic centre, breathing, 642
Pneumothorax, 615b, 621, 622b
Poiseuille's equation, 632
Poisons, oxidative phosphorylation, 60
Polar covalent bonds, 17
Polycystic kidney disease, 663, 664b
Polycystic ovarian syndrome (PCOS), 491b
Polycythaemia
  in myeloproliferative disease, 591–592
  secondary, 573b, 573t
  types of, 591f
Polycythaemia rubra vera (PRV), 592
Polygenic diseases, 156, 183–187
  genetic linkage and, 196–199
  monogenic versus, 184f
  tools to investigate, 186–187
Polygenic hypercholesterolaemia, 89b
Polygenic hypertriglyceridaemia, 89b
Polymerase chain reaction (PCR), 197f
Polymodal nociceptors, 378
Polymorphisms, 172–176
  consequences of genetic mutation, 173
  mutational events leading to, 172–173
Polymyxin, nephrotoxicity, 695t

Polypeptide chain, elongation of, 37
Polypill, 533b
Polyploidy, 163
Polyribosomes, 37
Polysaccharides, 21–22
Polysomes, 37f
Polysynaptic, reflexes, 367
Polyunsaturated fatty acids (PUFA), 88
Polyuria, diabetes mellitus, 82b
Pons, 344
Popliteal fossa, 433b, 433f
Population census, 285
Population drift, 174–176, 175f
Pore size, 665
Porin, 45
Positional cloning, 192
Positive feedback, 6
    examples of, 6b
    loop, 6f
Positive inotropic effect, 102
Positive predictive value (PPV), 278t, 329
Positron emission tomography (PET), 404
Post-capillary venules, 542
Posterior cerebral arteries, 354
Posterior cruciate ligament, 430b
Posterior longitudinal ligament, 409b
Posterior parietal cortex, lesions, 377b
Posterior spinal arteries, 354
Post-streptococcal glomerulonephritis (PSGN), 248b
Post-transcriptional modifications, of mRNA, 36–37
Post-translational modifications, 36
    of proteins, 38
Postural hypotension, 556
Posture
    closing capacity and, 636
    and movements, 443–444
Potassium
    intake in renal disease, 777
    sodium balance, 684
Potassium ions (K⁺) concentration, changes in, 20b
Potassium sparing diuretics, 115–116
Potential energy, of chemical bonds, 18–19
Potter's sequence, 662–663
Potter syndrome, 662–663
Pott's fracture, 424b
Power calculations, 307, 308b
    nomogram for, 309f
PR interval, 517, 517t
Prader-Willi syndrome, 181, 181b
Prausnitz-Kustner (PK), 247
Pre-capillary sphincters, 542
Pre-capillary (terminal) arterioles, 542
Pre-prohormone, 452–453
Pre-test probability, 329, 332–333
Preconceptional nutrition, 752
Precordial leads, 515–516
Predictive values, effect of prevalence on, 330, 330t
Predictor, 278t
Prednisone, 113b
Prefrontal cortex, emotion, 398
Pregnancy, 486–491
    contraception and termination of, 487b
    establishment of, 486–487, 487f
    fertilisation, 486–488
    foetal development, 488
    infertility, 491
    nutritional requirements during, 752, 753b
    parturition. see Labour
    terminations of, 282
    tests, 488
Preload, 525

Premotor and supplementary motor cortices, 365
Preproinsulin, 472f
Pressure difference, 546, 546f
Pressure-volume loop, 524–525, 524f
Presynaptic autoreceptors, 146
Presynaptic heteroreceptors, 146
Presynaptic receptors, 360
Prevalence, 278t, 281
Prevention, 323–335
    primary, 324–325
    secondary, 325–333
    tertiary, 334–335
Prevertebral ganglia, 140
Primary biliary cirrhosis, 741b
Primary carnitine deficiency, 183b
Primary centre, breathing, 642
Primary hyperaldosteronism, 564
Primary motor cortex, 365
Primary ossification, 412
Primary proliferative polycythaemia (PPP), 591
Primase, 31
Primordial follicles, 481
    development, 481, 482f, 483f
Prinzmetal's angina, 534
Prions, 38, 213, 223
Pro-drugs, 124
    inactive, 113
Probability test, 294–296
Probenecid, acting on protein transporters, 105b
Procaine, drug hydrolysis, 112b
Prochlorperazine, 119b
Progestogens, 25t
Prokaryotes, 213
Prolactin, secretion, 461, 461f
Proliferating cartilage, 413
Proline, 33
Pronephric ducts, 662
Pronephros, 662
Propranolol, 150
Proprioception, touch and, 376–378
Propriospinal fibres, 345
Prospective cohort studies, 186
Prospective study, 278t
Prostacyclin, 25
Prostaglandins, 245
    ammonium synthesis, 688–689
    in inflammatory response, 252
    synthesis of, 25b
Prostanoids, 25b
Prostate Cancer Risk Management programme, 272
Proteasomes, 46
Protein augmentation, 208
Protein buffers, 12
Protein C
    activated resistance, 603
    deficiency, 603
Protein Data Bank (PDB), 202
Protein denaturation, 34
Protein-energy malnutrition (PEM), 779
Protein kinase A (PKA), 128
Protein kinases, in signal transduction, 130
Protein metabolism
    during fasting and feeding, 760–761
    in illness, 763–764
    acute phase response, 764
Protein modelling, 202
Protein-nucleic acid interactions, 39
Protein processing, 38f
    in endoplasmic reticulum, 38
    in Golgi apparatus, 39
Protein requirements, 759
Protein S, deficiency, 603
Protein subunits, cooperativity between, 34–36
Protein theory, general anaesthetics, 152

Protein(s), 33–42, 665
    absorption, 705–706
    binding of drugs to, 107–108
    chemical nature of hormones, 452t
    destined for secretion, 38
    digestion, 702, 704b
    in fed state, 761–764
    functions of, 39
    gluconeogenesis from, 79–80
    glycated, clinical features resulting from, 82b
    intake in renal disease, 777
    primary structure of, 34
    processing, 36–39
    quaternary structure of, 34
    secondary structure of, 34, 35f
    secretion, 39
    structure of, 34–36
    synthesis, 36–39
    tertiary structure of, 34
    urine testing, 671t
Proteinuria, 670–671
Proteoglycans, 23, 38
Proteolysis, 42
Proteolytic cleavage, 38
Proteome, 184
Proteomics, 156
Prothrombin time (PT), 600f, 601
Proton pump, 726
Protons, 16
Proto-oncogenes, 189
Protozoa, 219–222
    characteristics of, 219, 219b
    classification of, 219–220
    occurrence of, 220f
    reproduction of, 220–222, 221f
    structure of, 220
Provisional callus, 255
Proximal convoluted tubule (PCT), 681
    amino acids, 668
    anions and cations, 669t
    aquaporins, 668
    carrier proteins, 667
    chloride, 668
    facilitated carriers, 668
    functions of, 665–670, 666f
    ion channels, 667
    peritubular capillaries, 661, 668
    recovery of bicarbonate by, 667
    sodium, 668
    sodium pump, 667
    sodium recovery, 681
    sugars, 668
    tight junctions, 665–667
    water, 667–668
PrP^c, 223
PrP^{sc}, 223
Pseudocholinesterase, 142
Pseudounipolar neurons, 353
Puberty, 484–486
    age of, 484t
    events of, 486t
    failure of, 486b
    Tanner classification of, 485f
Pubofemoral ligament, 429b
Pulmonary arterial pressure, 624
Pulmonary artery, 623
Pulmonary blood flow, 624–625
    effect of gravity on, 625
    variations in, 625
Pulmonary capillaries, 623
Pulmonary circulation, 497, 499–500, 499f
    anatomy of, 623–625
    clinical conditions associated with defects in, 625b
Pulmonary diffusion capacity, 636–637
Pulmonary embolism, 540–541, 615b, 642b
    diagnosis of, 329–330, 329t
Pulmonary fibrosis, 615b
Pulmonary lymphatics, 622–623
Pulmonary oedema, 622–623, 622f, 625b
Pulmonary regurgitation, 496b
Pulmonary stenosis, 496b

Pulmonary stretch receptors, 644
Pulmonary valves, 494, 497f
Pulmonary vein, 623
Pulmonary venous pressure, 624
Pulmonary ventilation, 629–631
    lung volumes and capacities, 629–630
    measuring rates of airflow, 630–631
Pulp cavity, 54
Pulsus bigeminy, 102
Pupillary reflexes, 382, 383b, 383f
Pure water, 11t
Purines, 26–28
    excess, 28b
    neurotransmission, 363–364, 364t
    structure of, 27f
Purkinje cells, 371
Pus, 251
p value, 294–295, 316
P wave, 516, 517t
Pyridoxine. see Vitamin B₆
Pyrimidines, 26–28
    structure of, 27f
Pyruvate, 59
    amino acid metabolism, 84
    production of, 69–71
Pyruvate carboxylase (PC), 98–99
Pyruvate dehydrogenase complex (PDC), 70, 71–72
    deficiency, 71b
    regulation of, 70f, 71–72, 72f
Pyruvate kinase, 70
    deficiency, 70b
    haemolytic anaemia and, 70b

Q

Quiet respiration, 627

R

Radial pulse, 502
Radiographic contrast nephrotoxicity, 695t
Radioimmunoassay (RIA), 459b
Radioulnar interosseous joints, 418
Random, definition, 278t
Randomised controlled trial (RCT), 278t, 296b
    vs. reviews, 320–321
Rapid eye movement (REM) sleep, 396
Rapidly progressive glomerulonephritis (RPGN), 693b
Rathke's pouch, 458
Rbtn2/LMO2, 571
Reaction rate of enzymes, 40–41
Reactive hyperaemia, 553, 553f
Reactive oxygen species, 773–774
    antioxidant defense against, 774
    formation of, 773–774
Receiver operating characteristic (ROC) curves, 328, 328f
Receptive relaxation, 728
Receptor-mediated endocytosis, 51, 51b, 543
Receptor-operated non-selective channels (ROCs), 548
Receptors, 47–48, 125–126
    acetylcholine, 433–434
    activation and efficacy, 136
    antagonism, 136b, 137
    binding of ligand to, 126
    classification, 126–132
    cross-reaction in, 234
    desensitisation, 137
    drug targets, 125–126
    general structure of, 126f
    immune system, 233–234
    lipoproteins, 93
    non-specific, 234
    scavenger, 93
    specific, 234
Reciprocal translocation, 163

Recombinant vaccines, 232
Recombination frequency, 195
Rectal drug administration, 118
Rectosphincteric reflex, 747
Rectum, motility of, 747
Red cell membrane, 575
  disorders, 586
Red cells, 246, 567, 571–589
  anaemias. see Anaemia(s)
  breakdown of, 577f, 584f
  enzymes, 576, 586–587
  erythropoiesis. see
    Erythropoiesis
  fate of old, 576
  glycolysis and, 65
  haemoglobin. see Haemoglobin
  maintenance and recycling of,
    576
  mechanical fragmentation, 585
  production during life, 572–573
  red cell membrane. see Red cell
    membrane
  transport of oxygen by
    haemoglobin, 573–574
Red pulp, of spleen, 258
Redox reactions, 773b
Reduction, 18, 111, 773b
Reed-Sternberg cells, 595, 596f
Refeeding syndrome, 779–780,
  780f, 780t
Reference nutrient intake (RNI),
  751
Reflex arc, 139–140, 140f
Refractive errors, 382b
Refractometry, 670
Refractory period, 512
  action potentials, 358
  absolute, 358
  relative, 358
Regeneration, 255
Regional circulations, 503–505,
  503t
Regression, 317
Rehabilitation programme,
  components of, 334t
Relative polycythaemia, 592
Relative risk, 300, 300b
Renal agenesis, congenital,
  662–663
Renal blood flow (RBF), 682f
Renal buffers, 688–690
Renal clearance
  of drugs, 120
  methods of measuring, 673
  of molecules, 672, 673f
Renal collecting system,
  development of, 663f
Renal control of pH, 13–14
Renal corpuscle, 659
Renal diseases, 692–696
  acute kidney injury, 693–694
  chronic kidney disease, 694–696
  dietary restrictions in, 777
  general classification of, 693
  onset of, 693
Renal failure, 656, 657b
  clinical consequences of, 656b
Renal function, 663–690
  clearance methods to assess,
    674
  control of acid-base balance,
    686–690
  control of fluid balance,
    674–680
  glomerular filtration. see
    Glomerular filtration
  impairment, in digoxin toxicity,
    102
  production of primary urine,
    664–665
  proximal convoluted tubule, 659
  refractory, 670
  tests. see Renal function tests
Renal function tests, 670–674
  creatinine clearance, 672–673
  dry chemistry, 670
  osmolality, 670
  renal clearance, 672

Renal function tests (Continued)
  renal handling of molecules,
    671–674, 671f
  specific gravity, 670
  urea clearance, 673
Renal glomerulus, 659
Renal microvasculature, 659–661
Renal pyramids, 658–659
Renal replacement therapy, 696
Renal sympathetic denervation,
  566b
Renal system, 655–697
  balance of fluid intake and loss,
    656
  excretion of drugs and
    metabolites, 113–116
  kidneys. see Kidney(s)
  nerve supply to the renal tract,
    662
  overview of, 655–656
  renal failure. see Renal failure
  urinary tract, 658f, 690–692
  urine volume and composition,
    655
Renal tubular acidosis (RTA), 689
Renal tubule, 659
  collecting ducts (CD), 659
  distal convoluted tubule, 659
  loop of Henle, 659
  proximal convoluted tubule
    (PCT), 659
Renal tumours, 692
Renal vasculature, 659–661, 661f
Renal water excretion, calculation
  of, 677
Renin, 556
Renin-angiotensin-aldosterone
  system, 556, 559, 683–684,
  683f
Renovascular hypertension, 563
Reperfusion therapy, 538b
Repolarisation, 511–512
  action potentials, 357
Research and Surveillance Centre
  (RSC), 283
Reserpine, 146b
Residual volume (RV), 629
  measurement of, 630b
Resistant hypertension, 565–566
Resolution, 255
Respiratory acidosis, 12, 12b, 640
Respiratory airways, 616
Respiratory alkalosis, 640
Respiratory burst, 245
Respiratory chemoreceptors,
  642–644
Respiratory disease
  classification of common,
    614–615, 615b
  epidemiology and social impact
    of, 614, 614t
  smoke and, 614, 614f
Respiratory distress syndrome of
  the newborn, 653
Respiratory diverticulum, 651
Respiratory failure, 648–650
  causes of, 648–650, 650b
  clinical effects of, 649–650
  type I, 649
  type II, 649
Respiratory pigments, 638–639
Respiratory quotient (RQ), 645,
  645b
Respiratory reflexes, 616b
Respiratory system, 613–653
  abbreviations, 625t
  adrenoceptor agonists in, 149
  anatomy of, 615–627
    pulmonary circulation,
      623–625, 623f
    surface, 626–627
    upper airways, 616–617, 616b,
      616f
  changes at normal delivery, 653
  conducting airways, as defences
    against infection, 650
  energy production and oxygen
    consumption, 645–646

Respiratory system (Continued)
  inflammatory responses in, 651
  matching lung ventilation to lung
    perfusion, 640–642
  upper airways, as defences
    against infection, 650
Respiratory tissue, histological
  composition of, 620t
Respiratory tract, pathogen entry
  via, 226
Resting cartilage, 412
Resting energy expenditure (REE),
  757
Resting membrane potential, 20,
  356, 357f
Restitution, 255
Restriction fragment length
  polymorphism, 196
Restrictive pulmonary disease, 615
Retching, 730
Reticular formation, 341–342
Reticular network, in lymph nodes,
  258
Reticulospinal tracts, 365–366
Retina, 383–386, 383f
  processing, 385
Retinoblastoma
  penetrance and phenotypic
    expression, 176b
  two-hit theory of carcinogenesis,
    188
Retinoblastoma gene (RB1), 188,
  591b
Retinoids, 766
Retrograde transport, 45
Retrospective study, 278t
Retroviruses, 189, 203–204
Rett syndrome, 182
Reverse cholesterol transport,
  92–93
Reversible competitive antagonism,
  137
Rexed's laminae, 345
Rhesus system, 606
  antibodies, 607
  haplotypes and relative
    population frequencies,
    606t
Rheumatic fever, 248b
Rheumatoid arthritis, 253, 254b,
  421b, 448
Rhombencephalon, 338
Ribcage, 627
Riboflavin. see Vitamin B$_2$
Ribonucleic acids (RNAs), 28, 31
  secondary structure of, 31
Ribose, 21
Ribosomal RNA (rRNA), 31, 157
Ribosomal tRNA binding sites, 37f
Ribosomes, 36
  bacteria, 214
  fungi, 218
  structure of, 37f
Ribozymes, 209
Rickets, 767b
Rickettsia, 215
Rifampicin, nephrotoxicity, 695t
Right-to-left (arteriovenous) shunts,
  624
Rigor mortis, 440b
Ring chromosomes, 163
Risk, health education and
  promotion, 322
RNA-dependent DNA polymerase
  (reverse transcriptase), 217
RNA-dependent RNA polymerase,
  217
RNA modification, 209
RNAi, 209
Robertsonian translocation, 163
Rod cell phototransduction, 385f
Root canal, 54
Rostral ventrolateral medulla, 550
Rotenone, 61
Roux-en-Y gastric bypass, 784
Royal College of General
  Practitioners (RCGP), 283,
  284b

Rubrospinal tract, 365
Rule of nines, 446t
Ruptured plantaris tendon, 408b
Ryanodine-sensitive type 1 (RYR1)
  calcium channels, 440

S

Saccades, 374
Saccharomyces cerevisiae (baker's
  yeast), as model organisms,
  204
Saddle joint, 425, 426b
Saliva
  composition of, 715–716
  digestion, 715
  functions of, 715
  lubrication, 715
  pH values, 11t
  protection, 715
  secretion
    control of, 717–718
    mechanisms of, 716–717, 717f
    of organic constituents, 717
Salivary glands, 714–718
  clinical conditions of, 715b
  position/innervation of, 715f
  structure of, 717f
Salivon, 716
Salt, food labelling, 751
Saltatory conduction, 358
Salvage pathways, 28
Sample, 278t
Sampling frame, 278t
Sanger sequencing, 191
Sarcoidosis, 253, 253b
Sarcolemma, 438
Sarcomeres, 55, 437f
Sarcoplasmic reticulum (SR),
  skeletal muscle, 438
Satellite cells, 55, 442
Satiety, 771
  long-term signals of, 772–773
  peripheral signals of, 771–772,
    771f
  regulation of, 394, 394f
Saturated fatty acids, 23
Saturation kinetics, 120
Scalp, normal flora, 224f
Scandinavian Simvastatin Survival
  Study (4S), 305
  results from, 312t
  selecting the sample for,
    306–307
Scapula, 626, 626f
Scattergram, 278t, 317, 319f
Scavenger receptors, 93, 234
Schindylesis, 419
Schistosomiasis, 223b, 253
Sciatic nerve, 433b
Scleroderma, 448
Scoliosis, 407b
Screening, 325
  calculations, 328t, 329–331
  case scenario: breast screening,
    333, 333t
  clinical suspicion, 332–333
  consistency of findings, 333
  criteria for population screening
    strategies, 326–327
  ethical considerations, 327
  harming the patient, 333
  measuring clinical agreement,
    331–332
  strategies, 326
  test characteristics, 327–331,
    327t
  true and false, 328b
  vs. diagnosis, 326
Sea squirt, 199
Sea water, pH values, 11t
Sebaceous glands, 447
Sebum, acne, 447b
Second messenger systems,
  128–130
Secondary active transport, 49–50,
  50f

Secondary ossification centres, 412
Secretin, 734
　interactions with cholecystokinin
　　and acetylcholine, 734
　intracellular messenger for, 734
　source, target organ, and action
　　of, 713t
Secretomotor neurons, 353
Segmentation, small intestinal
　　motility, 745
Selectins, 46
Selection bias, 278t, 304
Selective screening, 326
Selective serotonin reuptake
　　inhibitors (SSRIs), serotonin
　　and, 363
Selenium, 768
Self-tolerance, 249
Semilunar valves, 494, 497f
Seminiferous tubules, 478, 478f
Sensation, 346
Sensitivity, 278t
　analysis, 311
　effect of prevalence on, 330,
　　330t
　screening test, 328
Sensor, 3, 5
Sensory systems, 375–381
　receptive field structure, 376
　receptor transduction, 375–381
　stimulus modalities, 375t
Septic shock, 229b, 559
Septum primum, 507
Septum secundum, 507
Sequence, definition of, 205
Sequence tagged sites, 191, 191t,
　　192f
Seronegative spondylarthritis, 254b
Seronegative
　　spondyloarthropathies, 431b
Serotonin, 88
　anxiety, 363b
　neurotransmission, 363, 363t
Serum sickness, 247
Sesamoid bones, 406
Sex chromosome
　monosomy, 163
　trisomy, 163
Sex-hormone-binding globulin, 26t
Sexual differentiation
　disorder of, 490b, 490t
　of internal genitalia, 489f
Sexual function, regulation, 395
Shear stress, 530, 531f
Sheath of Schwann, 348–349
Shock, 556–562
　cellular damage in, 560
　clinical signs of, 560
　homeostatic mechanisms
　　activated by, 559–560
　prognosis in, 562
　treatment of, 560–562
Short stature, causes of, 463t
Short tandem repeats (STRs), 196
Shoulder
　dislocations, 428b
　frozen, 428b
　joint, 428f
Sickle cell crisis, 588f
Sickle cell disease, 38, 172b, 587
　description, 3
　genetic mutation, 173
　laboratory findings, 587, 588t
　precipitants, 587
　screening, 587b
Sickle cell trait, 174f
Sign, definition of, 3, 278t
Signal recognition particle (SRP), 38
Signalling cascades, 39f
Signalling cassettes, 39
Signalling molecules, 88, 169–170
Signalling proteins, 39
Signal transduction
　cascades, 47–48
　in cells, 46–47
Silencers, 167
Single breath carbon monoxide
　　(CO) testing, 636–637

Single copy genes, 166
Single gene disorders, 156, 186
Single nucleotide polymorphisms,
　　172, 196–197
　arrays, 197–198
　DARC gene, 176f
　database, 199
　MATP gene, 175f
Sinoatrial (SA) node, 512–513
Sinus arrhythmia, 518
Sinus bradycardia, 518
Sinuses, lymph nodes, 258
Sinusoidal capillaries, 542
Sinus rhythm, 512–513, 518, 519f
Sinus tachycardia, 518, 519f
Sinus venosus, 506
Sjögren syndrome, 449
Skeletal muscle, 55, 432–443, 432f,
　　443b
　amino acid release by, 84–85
　circulation, 505
　connective tissue, 441
　contractile process, 438–440,
　　439f
　definition, 432
　fibre, 435–438
　glycogenolysis in, 77
　names, 443
　neuromuscular junction, 434f
　nomenclature, 442–443
　sensory innervation, 435
　shape, 442–443, 442f
　structure, 436f
　vertebral column, 407b
Skeletal muscle pump, 530f
Skeletal system, 404–418
　cartilage, 404–405
Skeleton, definition of, 403
Skin, 444–448
　dermis, 446–447
　hypodermis (subcutaneous
　　layer), 447
　normal flora, 224f
　pathogen entry via, 225–226
　structure, 444–447, 445f
Skinfold thickness, 755
Sleep, 395–396
　arousal system, 396, 396f
　NREM (non-rapid eye
　　movement), 396
　REM (rapid eye movement), 396
Slipped disc, 409b
Slipped upper femoral epiphysis
　　(SUFE), 419b
Slow acetylator status, 112
SMAD, 250
Small airway diseases, 615b
Small intestine, 743–746
　disease, 746b
　fluid secretion, 744–745
　motility, 745–746
　protein digestion in, 702, 703f,
　　704f
　structure of, 744
Small nuclear RNAs (snRNA), 31
Smell, 346, 392
Smith fractures, 427b
Smooth muscle, 55
　excitation-contraction coupling
　　of, 548–549, 549f
　muscarinic receptor agonists, 144
　proliferation, 531
Smooth pursuit, 374
SNARES, 359
Sneezing, 616b
Snow, John, 277
Sodium
　proximal convoluted tubule, 668
　transport, loop of Henle, 680
Sodium balance
　autoregulation and distal
　　convoluted tubule, 684
　control of, 680–684, 680t
　juxtaglomerular apparatus,
　　682–683
　receptors involved with, 682
　renal sodium handling, 681–684
　tubulo-glomerular feedback, 684

Sodium chloride, 17f
Sodium/Glucose Linked
　　Transport-1 (SGLT1), 50
Sodium pump, 726
Solenoid, 158f
Somatic cell mosaicism, 182
Somatic cells, 156
Somatic disorders, 156
Somatic motor reflex, 140, 140f
Somatic nervous system, 346–349
Somatosensory cortex, 377
　functions of, 377f
　primary, 377, 377f
　secondary, 377
Somatostatin, 461
　source, target organ, and action
　　of, 713t
Somatotropin, 460
Sonic hedgehog, 170
Sound, 388–389
　frequency coding, 392
　localisation of, 392
SOX family genes, 170
Spare receptors, 136
Spasticity, 367b
Special surveillance systems, 284
Specific gravity, urine testing, 670,
　　671t
Specificity, 234, 278t, 298–299
　screening test, 328
Spectrin, 575
Spermatogenesis, 479f, 480–481,
　　481f
Spherocytosis, hereditary, 586,
　　586b
Sphincter muscle, 443
Sphingolipids, 26
Sphingomyelin, 26
　structure of, 26f
Sphingosine, 26
Spinal cord, 344–345, 367–369
　arterial blood supply, 354
　cauda equina, 345
　central canal, 344
　development, 338–339, 340f
　diseases, 369b
　injury, 368–369
　localisation, 345b
　magnetic resonance (MR) image
　　of, 344f
　Rexed's laminae, 345
　transverse section through, 345f
Spinal nerves, 348, 348f
Spinal shock, 368
Spinocerebellum, 370, 371b
Spirochaetes, 214
Spironolactone, 115, 686
Splanchnic circulation, 701f
Spleen, 258, 258f
Splicing, 36–37
Spongy (cancellous) bone, 406
Sporozoites, 220
Squamous cell carcinoma, 446b
Squamous metaplasia, 261b
SRY (sex-determining region on the
　　Y chromosome) gene, 170
Stable angina, 534
　diagnosis of, 535b
Stable cells, 255
Stagnant anoxia, 638b
Standard deviation (SD), 278t, 292
　of normal platelet counts, 293b,
　　293f, 295f
Standard error, 278t
Standardisation
　choice of method for, 291
　direct method of, 289b, 289t, 290
　indirect method of, 290, 290b,
　　290t
Standardise, definition, 278t
Standardised mortality ratio (SMR),
　　278t, 290
Standing, 444
Staphylococcus aureus, virulence
　　of, 229b
Starches, 21–22
Starling forces, 543–544, 544f
Starling's law, 525, 525f

Starvation
　clinical effects of, 763b
　ketone bodies accumulate, 96b
　prolonged, 762–763
　pyruvate, 70f
Statin cholesterol lowering therapy,
　　533
Statistical significance, 311, 312f
Steady state distribution, 104
ST elevation myocardial infarction,
　　537, 538f
　treatment of, 538b
Stellate cells, 371
Stem cell factor (SCF), 570t
Stem cells
　differentiation of, 571f
　multipotent, 570
　role in haemopoiesis, 570, 570f
Stem cell therapies, 208–209
　ex vivo approach, 208
　in vivo approach, 209
Stereoisomers, 18
Sternal angle, 626
Sternum, 626
Steroid hormones, 25, 25t, 48,
　　453–454, 453f
　chemical nature of, 452t
Steroid synthesis, 453, 454f
Steroidogenesis
　hormonal control of, 482f
　rate limiting step of, 453, 454b
Sterol ring, 24
Stillbirths, 282
Stomach, 700, 719–722
　anatomy of, 719–722, 721f
　and drug administration, 117,
　　117b
　protein digestion in, 702
　secretions, 720t
Stop codon, 167–168
Straight sinus, 355
Stratification, 278t
Stratum basale, 445
Stratum corneum, 445
Stratum granulosum, 445
Stratum lucidum, 445
Stratum spinosum, 445
Stress
　adrenal cortex and, 469
　adrenal medulla and, 468–469
　hormones and, 467–470
　metabolic response to, 763
Stress fracture, 408b
Stretch reflex, 367, 368f
Stridor, 618b
Stroke(s), 354b, 538t
　excitotoxicity and, 362b
　haemorrhagic, 354b
　occlusive, 354b
Stroke volume, 524
Stromal molecules in
　　erythropoiesis, 572–573
Structural proteins, 39–40
ST segment, 517
Subarachnoid haemorrhage, 350b
Subarachnoid space, 350
Subcutaneous drug administration,
　　118
Subdural haemorrhage, 350b
Subfertility, 491
Sublingual drug administration,
　　118
Sublingual glands, 714–715
Submandibular glands, 714
Submucosa, 712
Submucosal plexus, 713
Substance P, source, target organ,
　　and action of, 713t
Subthalamus, 341
Subunit vaccines, 232, 232t
Succinylcholine, 434
Sucrose, 21
Sugar-derived acids, 21
Sugars
　gluconeogenesis from, 81
　inborn errors of metabolism, 81b
　proximal convoluted tubule
　　(PCT), 668

Sulphonamides, nephrotoxicity, 695t
Summation, 360, 361f
Superficial fascia, 441
Superficial muscle, 443f
Superior colliculi, 343
Superior mesenteric artery, 502, 700
Superior sagittal sinus, 355
Superior vena cava, 503
Superoxide, 773
Suprapubic (hypogastric) region, 710
Supraspinous ligaments, 409b
Suprasternal notch, 626
Sural nerve, 433b
Surround (lateral) inhibition, 376
Surveillance, 326
Suture, fibrous joint, 418
Suxamethonium, 153
  hydrolysis, 112b
  nicotinic agonists, 144
Svedberg units, 214
Swallowing, 718–719, 719f
  oesophageal phase, 719
  oral/voluntary phase, 718
  pharyngeal phase, 718–719
Sweat glands
  description, 447
  innervation of, 139
Sweat test, 173b
Symbiosis, 224
Sympathetic nervous system
  anatomy of, 140, 141f
  neurotransmitters and receptors of, 144–151
  overview of, 139
  salivary secretion, 718
  vasoconstriction, 550
Sympathetic stimulation, 76–77
Sympathetic supply, 514–515
Sympathomimetic agents, 561
Sympathomimetic amines, 144–145
Sympathomimetic drug treatment, 561–562
Sympathomimetics, clinical importance of indirectly acting, 146b
Symporters, 106
Symports, 50
Symptom, definition, 278t
Synaesthesia, 375b
Synapses, 358, 359f
  chemical. see Chemical synapses
  electrical. see Electrical synapses
Synapsin I, 359
Synaptic cleft, 358
Synarthroses, 418
Synchondroses, 419
Syndesmosis, 418
Syndrome, definition of, 205
Synovial fluid, 421–422
Synovial joints, 419–428, 419f
  accessory ligaments, 422
  articular capsule, 420
  articular cartilage, 420
  articular discs, 422
  structure, 419–422
  synovial fluid, 421–422
  synovium, 420–421, 420f
  tendons and ligaments, 428–431
  types of, 422–428, 422f
Synoviocytes, 420
Synovium, 420–421, 420f
Synthesis, 18
Systemic circulation, 497, 499f, 500–503, 500f
Systemic lupus erythematosus (SLE), 449
Systemic vascular resistance (SVR), 546
Systemic viral infection, 228
Systole, 522
Systolic click, 498b

T

Tachykinins
  peptides and, 364
  source, target organ, and action of, 713t
Tachyphylaxis, 137
Tachypnoea, 560, 643b
Taeniae coli, 746
Tal-1/SCL, 571
Tangier disease, 89b
Tanner classification, of pubertal development, 485f
Tapeworms, replication of, 223
Taq polymerase, 197
TaqMan assay, 198f
Targeted allele-specific mutation screening, 196–197
Taste, 392
  central pathways of, 392, 393f
TATA box sequence, 166
Tau, 45
Tay-Sachs disease, 173
  protein augmentation, 208
T cell receptor, 236f
T cells
  activation and killing, 238
  self-tolerance breakdown, 250
  switching off activated, 238
T-distribution, 278t, 315f, 316
Tectospinal tract, 365
Tectum, 343
Teeth, 54, 714
  normal flora, 224f
Tegmentum, 343
Telencephalon (cerebrum), 338, 339
Telogen phase, hair growth, 447
Telomeres, 157
Temperature
  body. see Body temperature
  sensations, 378–381
    pathways, 378–379, 378f
Tendon reflexes, 367, 367b
Tendon(s)
  insertion, 441
  local injections into, 118
  origin, 441
Tendon sheaths, 431
Tennis elbow, 423b
Tentorium cerebelli, 350
Teratogens, 205
  birth defects caused by, 205b
Terminal ganglia, 140
Terminal hairs, 448
Terry's nails, 448
Tertiary healthcare delivery, components for, 334
Testes, 478
Testosterone, 479, 479f
Tetanus, 440
  fused, 435
  immunisation, 324t
  unfused, 435
Tetracyclines, nephrotoxicity, 677b, 695t
Tetrad chromosome formation, 162f
Tetralogy of Fallot, 508b
Tetraploidy, 163
Th0 cells, 238
Thalamic nuclei, 344t
Thalamus, 341
Thalassaemias, 207, 587–589, 589b
  laboratory findings, 589
  α thalassaemia, 588
  β thalassaemia, 588–589
  major, 588
Thalidomide, 281b
  teratogenesis, 172b
Therapeutic index (TI), 121–122
Therapeutic ratio, 135
Therapeutic window, 122, 122f
Thermal nociceptors, 378
Thermogenin, 60–61
Thermoneutral zones (TNZ), 6
Thermoreceptors, 378
Thermoregulation, 4–6, 394

Thiamine. see Vitamin B$_1$
Thiazide diuretics
  description, 685
  pharmacodynamics of, 115
Thiazolidinediones (TZDs), 80b
Thiopental, 103b, 107b
Thiopurine-S-methyl-transferase (TPMT), 207b
Thirst, 9
  in diabetes mellitus, 82b
  and drinking, regulation of, 395
Thoracic aorta, 501
Thorax, surface markings of, 626–627
Threshold effects models, 184
Threshold stimulus, action potentials, 357
Throat, normal flora, 224f
Thrombin clotting time (TCT), 600f, 601
Thrombocythaemia, essential, 592
Thrombocytopenias, 602–603
  caused by impaired platelet production, 602
  caused by increased platelet destruction, 602–603
Thromboembolism, 539–541
Thrombolytic therapy, 538b
Thrombophilias, 603–604
  acquired, 603–604
  inherited, 603, 603t
Thrombophlebitis, 408b
Thrombopoietin (Tpo), function, 570t
Thrombosis, 596–604
Thromboxane A$_2$, 25
Thrombus formation, 539–540
Thymus, 591
Thyroglobulin, 454–455
Thyroid-binding globulin, 26t
Thyroid function
  control of, 466
  tests of, 466b
Thyroid gland, 464–466
  anatomy of, 464f
  histology of, 464f
  hormone synthesis in, 465, 465f
  regulation of metabolism and, 464–466
Thyroid hormone receptors, 466
Thyroid hormones, 454–455, 454f
  actions of, 466t
  in blood, 466
  synthesis of, 465f
Thyroid stimulating hormone (TSH), 460
Thyrotoxicosis, 457b, 467b
Thyroxine-binding globulin (TBG), 466
Thyroxine (T$_4$)
  functions of, 466
  peripheral metabolism of, 466
Tidal volume, 629
Tight junctions, 46, 106
  blood-brain barrier, 355
  drug distribution to special organs, 107
  proximal convoluted tubule, 665–667
Timolol, 119b
Tingible body macrophages, 257
Tiredness, adrenoceptor antagonists, 151
Tissue plasminogen activator (tPA), 599
Tissue repair
  complications of, 256
  factors that hamper, 256–257
  inflammation, 255–256
  proliferation, 256
  regeneration, 255
  remodelling, 256
Tissues
  adaptations to anaemia, 577
  repair. see Tissue repair
T lymphocytes, 235–238
  cytokines released by CD4 and CD8 activated, 239t

TNM (Tumour, node, metastasis) staging system, 271–272
  of breast adenocarcinoma, 272b
Tocopherols. see Vitamin E
Toll like receptors (TLRs), 235
Tomato juice, pH values, 11t
Tongue, 714
Tonicity, 8
Tonofilaments, 445
Tonsils, 591
Topical drug administration, 118–119
Total body clearance, 120
Total body water, 7, 108
Total energy expenditure, 757
Total lung capacity (TLC), 629
Total parenteral nutrition, 778
Toxic chemicals, 576b
Trabeculae, 411
Trace elements, 767–769
Trachea, 617, 626
Tracheobronchial tree, 617–619, 618f
Transaminases, transamination, 84
Transamination, 81
  in amino acid metabolism, 84, 85f
Transcellular fluid, drug distribution, 109f
Transcription, 36, 36f, 166–168
  of DNA to messenger RNA, 166f
  regulation of, 167
Transcription factors, 170
  in erythropoiesis, 571
Transcriptome, 184
Transcytosis, 51, 543, 543b
Transdermal drug administration, 118–119
Transducin, 383–384
Transduction, 189
  bacteria, 216
  mechanism, 125–126
Transfection, 189–190
Transferases, 41t
Transferrin, 26t, 51b
  iron deficiency, 579
Transfer RNA (tRNA), 31, 157
  structure of, 32f, 168f
Transformation, bacteria, 216
Transforming growth factor-β, 170, 238, 250
Translation, 36, 37, 37f, 166, 167–168
Translocations, chromosome, 590
Transmembrane receptor, 125
Transmembrane signals, amplification of, 130–131
Transplantation, 696b
Transport (binding) proteins, 40
Transporters, 105–106
  competition for, 114b
  coordinated action of, 50
  drug targets, 124
  drugs acting on, 105b
Transposition of the great arteries, 508b
Transposons, of bacteria, 216
Trans-splicing, RNA, 209
Transverse sinus, 355
Trapping exons, 193
Trendelenburg's sign, 444
Triacylglycerols (TAGs), 23, 72, 88, 91, 761
  components, 24f
  dietary, 88
  pathway of, and storage by adipose tissue, 90f
Triamterene, 686
Tricarboxylic acid cycle (TCA cycle), 58, 59, 59f, 61t
  control of, 59
  oxidation of acetyl-CoA, 94–95
Tricuspid regurgitation, 496b
Tricuspid stenosis, 496b
Tricuspid valve, 494, 497f
Tricyclic antidepressants, 147b
Trigeminal neuralgia, 379b
Trigeminal (V) nerve, 346, 346t
Triglycerides, 23, 761
  digestion/absorption of, 705f
Trioses, 21f

Tripeptide absorption, 706
Triploidy, 163
Trisomy, 163
Trisomy 21, 156*b*
Trochlear (IV) nerve, 346, 346*t*
Tropomyosin, 437
Troponin, 437
Troponin I, 534–535, 536*t*
Troponin T, 534–535, 536*t*
Truncus arteriosus, 506
Trypanosomes, 220
Tryptophan, 362
Tryptophan hydroxylase, 111
T-test, 315–316
   criteria for applying, 316
   evaluating probability for,
      315–316
   independent group, 315
   paired, 315
   t-distribution, 315*f*, 316
T-tubules, 438, 510, 511*f*
Tuberculosis, 215*b*, 253
   immunisation, 324*t*
Tubular permeability, 679*f*
Tubular reabsorption, 114, 114*f*
Tubular secretion, 114, 114*f*
Tubulo-glomerular feedback, 684
Tumour-like developmental lesions,
   262–263
Tumour markers, 270–271, 271*t*
Tumour necrosis factor, 250
Tumour suppressor genes,
   188–189
   human blood disease, 590
   retinoblastoma, 176*b*
Tunica adventitia, 529
Tunica externa, 529
Tunica intima, 528
Tunica media, 528–529
Turbulent blood flow, 547, 547*f*
Turner syndrome, 490*b*, 490*f*, 490*t*
T wave, 517
Twin studies, 185–186
   biases in, 186
Two-site non-competitive assay,
   459*b*
Two-tailed test, 278*t*, 294, 316
Tyramine, 146*b*
Tyrosinase, 83*b*
Tyrosine, 88
Tyrosine hydroxylase, 111
   regulation of, 145

U

Ubiquitin, 46
Ulcerative colitis (UC), 249*b*,
   747*b*
Ulcers, 257*b*
Ultrasound, 404
Umbilical region, 710
Uncouplers, 60–61
Unfused tetanus, 435
Unintentional weight loss, 754
Uniporters, 48–49, 105–106
Univariate analysis, 318–319
Unstable angina, 534
Upper motor neuron syndrome,
   367*b*
Urea
   nitrogen excretion, 759–760
   transport in loop of Henle, 680
Urea clearance, 673
Urea cycle, 86–87, 86*f*
   defects of, 86*b*
   regulation of, 86–87
Ureteric buds, 662
Ureteric colic, 690*b*
Ureters, 690–691
Urethra, normal flora, 224*f*
Urinary incontinence, 692*b*
Urinary plasminogen activator
   (uPA), 599
Urinary tract, 690–692
   major components of, 658*f*
   obstruction. see Urinary tract
      obstruction

Urinary tract infections, 226
Urinary tract obstruction, 690–691
   clinical consequences of, 691*b*
Urine
   analysis, 670, 671*t*
   composition, 655
   concentration of, 678*f*
   counter-current hypothesis,
      678–680
   osmolarity gradient, 678
   pH values, 11*t*
   refractory, 670
   relative density of, 670
   specific gravity, 670
   tests, 670–671, 671*t*
   vasa recta hypothesis, 678–680
   volume, 655
Urine protein to urine creatinine
   ratio, 671*b*
Urobilinogen, urine testing, 671*t*
Urogenital tract, pathogen entry
   via, 226
Urothelium, 691
'Usual weight,' of body, 754
U-turn, 34
U wave, 517

V

Vaccination
   aim of, 232
   prevention of infection by,
      231–232
Vagina, normal flora, 224*f*
Vagus (X) nerve, 346*t*, 347
Valine, 88
Valvular heart disease
   causes and clinical
      consequences of, 496*b*
   murmurs in, 498*t*
Van der Waals forces, 17
Vaptans, nephrotoxicity, 677*b*
Variable number of tandem repeats
   (VNTRs), 196
Variant angina, 534
Variant Creutzfeldt-Jakob disease
   (vCJD), 223*b*, 608*b*
Vasa recta, 678–680
   transport in loop of Henle, 680
Vasa vasorum, 529, 623
Vascular adhesion molecule
   (VCAM), 46
Vascular endothelium, muscarinic
   receptor agonists, 144
Vascular myocytes, 547, 548*f*
Vascular recruitment, 505
Vascular smooth muscle
   contraction, 548
   structure of, 547
Vascular stasis, 560
Vasculature, development of,
   508–510
Vasoactive intestinal peptide,
   source, target organ, and
   action of, 713*t*
Vasodilation, 550, 551*f*
   metabolic byproduct, 553
Vasodilatory shock, 559
Vasopressin, 556, 674–677
   action of, 676*f*
   release, 674
   renal control of fluid balance,
      674–680
   secretion, 675*f*
   urine volume, 9
Vasopressin receptors, 674–677,
   677*b*
Vasovagal syncope, 557*b*
Vaughan-Williams classification,
   520, 520*t*
Vector Alignment Search Tool
   (VAST), 202
Veins, 528–529
   in respiratory system, 623
Vellus hairs, 448
Venesection, polycythaemia rubra
   vera, 592

Venous sinuses, 355*f*
Venous system, 503
Venous thromboembolism, 538*t*,
   539
Venous thrombosis
   evolution of, 540*f*
   risk factors for, 539*t*
Ventilation, uneven, 641
Ventilation-perfusion mismatch,
   641–642
Ventilation-perfusion ratio,
   641–642
Ventricles, 338, 351, 494, 506*f*,
   507–508
Ventricular arrhythmia, 538*t*
Ventricular diastole, 524
Ventricular fibrillation (VF), 519*f*,
   520, 537
Ventricular hypertrophy, 526
Ventricular rupture, 538*t*
Ventricular septal defect (VSD),
   congenital, 508*b*
Ventricular system of the brain,
   351–352, 351*f*
Ventricular systole, 524
Ventricular tachycardia (VT), 519*f*,
   520
Vergence, 374
Vermis, lesions, 371*b*
Verotoxin-producing *E. coli* (VTEC),
   228*b*
Vertebra, typical, 409*b*, 409*f*
Vertebral arteries, 354
Vertebral body, 409*b*
Vertebral column, 407*b*, 407*f*
Vertebral notches, 409*b*
Vertical transmission, of pathogens,
   230
Very-low-density lipoproteins
   (VLDLs), 531*t*
   in diabetes mellitus, 82*b*
   disorders of, 89*b*
   lipoprotein metabolism, 92
Vesicoureteric reflux (VUR), 691*b*
Vessel wall, 528–529
Vestibular apparatus, 388*f*
Vestibular hair cell, 388*f*
Vestibular pathways, central, 388
Vestibular system, 386–388
Vestibulocerebellum, 370
Vestibulocochlear (VIII) nerve,
   346*t*, 347
Vestibulo-ocular reflexes, 374,
   389*f*
Vestibulospinal tracts, 365
Viraemia, primary, 228
Viral infection, non-Hodgkin
   lymphoma, and 595
Virchow's triad, 539
Virions, 216
Viruses, 213, 216–218
   adhesion of, 227
   attacking the host, 229
   and cancer, 218, 218*t*
   classification of, 217, 218*t*
   general features of, 216*b*
   host cell infection, 216–217
   host organ dissemination of, 227
   invasion of, 227
   nucleocapsid structure of, 216
   replication of, 217*f*
Visceral sensation, 381
Vision, 346, 381–386
   central visual pathways, 386
Visual cortex, 387*f*
Visual pathways, 386*f*
Visual perception, 386
Visual system, processing
   pathways in, 387*f*
Vital capacity (VC), 629
Vitalograph, 630–631
Vitamin A, 766–767
   deficiency, 767*b*
Vitamin B₁
   deficiency, 765*b*
   diet, 765
Vitamin B₂, 766
   deficiency, 765

Vitamin B₃
   deficiency, 765*b*
   diet, 766
Vitamin B₆
   deficiency, 85*b*, 765*b*
   diet, 766
Vitamin B₁₂, 581, 707, 766
   deficiency, 581, 583*t*, 766*b*
   importance of, 580–581
   malabsorption, 707*b*
Vitamin C, 766
Vitamin D, 25, 476*b*, 767
   calcium homeostasis, 416
   control of blood calcium and
      phosphate concentrations
      and, 475, 475*f*
   deficiency, 477, 656*b*, 707*b*, 767*b*
Vitamin E, 767
Vitamin K, 767
Vitamin(s), 765–767
   absorption of, 707
   as antioxidants, 765
   as coenzymes, 765
   fat-soluble, 766–767
   status, 756
   water-soluble, 765–766
Vocal resonance, 619
Volatile anaesthetics, 151, 152
Volatile hydrogen ions, 686
Volkmann's canals, 410
Voltage-gated ion channels
   drug targets, 124, 125*f*
   potassium, 357
   sodium, 357
Voltage-sensitive calcium channels
   (VSCCs), 548
Voluntary muscle, 54
Vomiting, 730
   causes of, 730*t*
   prolonged, 732*b*
   stimuli/neural pathways
      controlling, 731*f*
von Willebrand disease (vWD),
   601–602

W

WAGR syndrome, 163
Waist circumference, 756
Waist/hip ratio, 756
Wakefulness, 395–396
Walking, 444
   stabilisation, 444
   stance phase, 444
   swing phase, 444
Warfarin, aspirin potentiates action
   of, 108*b*
Warm receptors, 378
Wasting, 755
Water, 769
   absorption of, 707
   balance, 656*t*
   content, of human body, 20
   daily requirements, 769
   depletion, 769–770
   dissociation, 17*f*
   and electrolytes, 7–9, 20*b*
   exchange, 543–544
   micronutrients and, 765–770
   overload, 770
Water-soluble vitamins, 707,
   765–766
Wegener's granulomatosis, 449
Weight
   loss/gain, 754
   'usual,' 754
Weight-reducing diet, 782*b*
Wernicke-Korsakoff syndrome,
   765*b*
Western clawed frog, 200
Whiplash injury, 407*b*
White blood cells, 568
   transfusion, 611
White fibro-cartilage, 404
White matter, 345
White pulp, of spleen, 258
Whitehall II, 303

Whole-genome association studies (WGAS), 187
Whooping cough, 2, 277b, 298f
    epidemiology, 277
    immunisation, 324t
Wilson disease, 737b, 768b
Wingless (Wnt) genes, 170
Wolf-Hirschhorn syndrome, 163
Wolff-Parkinson-White syndrome (WPW), 520
Wolffian duct, 662
World Health Organization (WHO), 282, 283–284, 324
Woven bone, 418
Wrist fractures, 427b
Wrist joint, 426f

X

Xanthine oxidase, 110
Xeroderma pigmentosum (XP), 169b
X-inactivation, 157
Xiphisternum, 626
X-linked inheritance, 179–181
    dominant, 179–180, 180f
    recessive, 180–181, 180f, 181f
X-ray crystallography, 202
Xyphoid process, 626

Y

Years of life lost, 284–285
Yeasts, 219
Yellow nail syndrome, 448

Z

Zero-order kinetics, 120, 120f
Zinc, 768
    deficiency, 768b
Zinc finger motif, 167
Zoonoses, 230f
Zwitterions, 32
Zygapophyses, 409b